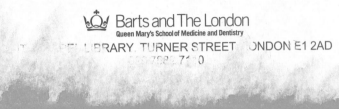

PHYSICAL THERAPIES IN SPORT AND EXERCISE

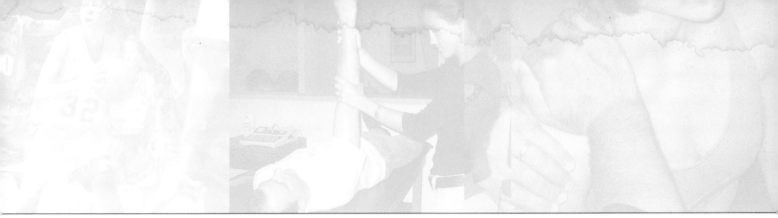

Senior Commissioning Editor: Sarena Wolfaard

Associate Editor: Claire Wilson

Project Manager: Anne Dickie

Design: Stewart Larking

Illustrator: Joanna Cameron

Illustration Manager: Merlyn Harvey

PHYSICAL THERAPIES IN SPORT AND EXERCISE

Second Edition

Edited by

Gregory S Kolt

BSc BAppSc(Phty) GradDipEd
GradDipBehavHlthCare PhD
Professor and Head of School, School of
Biomedical and Health Sciences, University of
Western Sydney, Sydney, Australia;
Adjunct Professor, Faculty of Health and
Environmental Sciences, Auckland University of
Technology, Auckland, New Zealand

Lynn Snyder-Mackler

BA CertPhysTher MS ScD
Alumni Distinguished Professor and Academic
Director, Graduate Program in Biomechanics and
Movement Sciences, Department of Physical
Therapy, University of Delaware, Newark,
Delaware, USA

Foreword by
James R Andrews MD

Founding member of the Alabama Sports Medicine and
Orthopaedic Center (ASMOC) and the American Sports
Medicine Center (ASMI) in Birmingham, Alabama; Chairman
and Medical Director of ASMI.

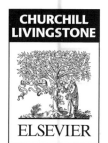

CHURCHILL
LIVINGSTONE

ELSEVIER

Edinburgh   London   New York   Oxford   Philadelphia   St Louis   Sydney   Toronto   2007

CHURCHILL LIVINGSTONE

An imprint of Elsevier Limited

First edition 2003

ISBN: 978-0-443-10351-3

British Library Cataloguing in Publication Data
A catalogue record for this book is available from the British Library

Library of Congress Cataloging in Publication Data
A catalog record for this book is available from the Library of Congress

Note
Neither the Publisher nor the Editors assume any responsibility for any loss or injury and/or damage to persons or property arising out of or related to any use of the material contained in this book. It is the responsibility of the treating practitioner, relying on independent expertise and knowledge of the patient, to determine the best treatment and method of application for the patient.
The Publisher

ELSEVIER your source for books, journals and multimedia in the health sciences

www.elsevierhealth.com

Working together to grow libraries in developing countries

www.elsevier.com | www.bookaid.org | www.sabre.org

ELSEVIER **BOOK AID International** **Sabre Foundation**

The Publisher's policy is to use paper manufactured from sustainable forests

Printed in China

Contents

Contributors vii

Preface. x

Acknowledgments xi

Foreword. xii

Foreword to the first edition. xiii

Abbreviations and acronyms xv

About the editors. xvii

1   The role of the physical therapies in sport, exercise and physical activity   1
Gregory S. Kolt and Lynn Snyder-Mackler

Section 1   Management principles for musculoskeletal and neural tissue in the physical therapies

2   Muscle   9
Peter J. McNair and Andrew G. Cresswell

3   Tendon   26
Jill Cook

4   Ligament   42
Gabriel Y. F. Ng

5   Bone   59
Pekka Kannus and Kim Bennell

6   Nerves   82
Robert J. Nee, David S. Butler and Michel W. Coppieters

7   Cartilage   100
Stefano Zaffagnini, Marc Safran and Elizaveta Kon

Section 2   Concepts in managing sport and exercise injuries

8   Motor control.   115
Paul W. Hodges

9   Pain.   133
Gregory S. Kolt

10   Exercise-based conditioning and rehabilitation   149
Rafael F. Escamilla and Robbin Wickham-Bruno

11   Psychology of injury and rehabilitation   171
Gregory S. Kolt and Britton W. Brewer

12   Screening for sport and exercise participation   190
Lisa Casson Barkley and Michael J. Axe

13   Clinical outcomes in sport and exercise physical therapies   206
James J. Irrgang and Robert G. Marx

14   Electrophysical agents in sport and exercise injury management   220
Lynn Snyder-Mackler, Laura A. Schmitt, Katherine Rudolph and Sara Farquhar

15 **Prevention of injury** 236
Timothy E. Hewett, Kristin Briem and Roald Bahr

Section 3 Regional sport and exercise injury management

16 **Spine** 255
Tara Jo Manal and Anthony Delitto

17 **Shoulder** 283
Brian J. Tovin and Jason P. Reiss

18 **Elbow** 308
Michael M. Reinold and Kevin E. Wilk

19 **Wrist and hand** 338
Paul LaStayo, Susan Michlovitz and Michael Lee

20 **Pelvis, hip and groin** 365
Michael T. Cibulka

21 **Knee** 382
Terese L. Chmielewski, Susan M. Tillman and Lynn Snyder-Mackler

22 **Patellofemoral joint** 402
Kay Crossley, Sallie Cowan, Kim Bennell and Jenny McConnell

23 **Foot, ankle and lower leg** 420
D. S. Blaise Williams III and Jack Taunton

24 **Rehabilitation of lower limb muscle and tendon injuries** 440
Thomas C. Windley, Suzanne Werner, Nicola Maffulli and Jack Taunton

Section 4 The role of sport and exercise physical therapies in active groups

25 **Children and adolescents** 459
*Heather Southwick, Christine Ploski, Lyle J. Micheli, Elly Trepman
and Lizanne Backe Barone*

26 **Older exercise participants** 484
Jennifer E. Stevens

27 **The active female** 499
Amanda Weiss-Kelly and Martin Kilbane

28 **Athletes with disability** 525
Zoë Hudson and Amy Brown

Section 5 Medical considerations for rehabilitation practitioners
in sport and exercise

29 **Pharmacological agents in sport and exercise** 541
Andrew Garnham

30 **Medical imaging of injury** 558
Douglas N. Mintz

31 **Medical issues in sport and exercise** 578
Bruce Hamilton and Mark Gillett

Index 599

Michael J Axe MD
First State Orthopaedics; Clinical Professor, Department of Physical Therapy, University of Delaware, Newark, DE, USA

Lizanne Backe Barone NP
Nurse Practitioner, Division of Sports Medicine, Children's Hospital, Boston, MA, USA

Roald Bahr MD PhD
Chair, Oslo Sports Trauma Research Center, Professor and Chair, Department of Sport Medicine, Norwegian School of Sport Sciences, Oslo, Norway

Lisa Casson Barkley MD FAAFP
Dean, College of Health and Public Policy, Head Team Physician, Delaware State University, Dover, DE, USA

Kim Bennell BAppSci(Physio) PhD
Professor and Foundation Director of the Centre for Health, Exercise and Sports Medicine, Faculty of Medicine, Dentistry and Health Sciences, University of Melbourne, Victoria, Australia

Britton W Brewer BA MA PhD
Professor, Department of Psychology, Springfield College, Springfield, MA, USA

Kristin Briem BSc MHSC
Doctoral Student, Department of Physical Therapy, University of Delaware, Newark, DE, USA

Amy Brown MPT SCS
Staff Physical Therapist, Christiana Care PT PLUS, Smyrna, DE, USA

David S Butler BPhys MAppSc GDAMT
Director, Neuro Orthopedic Institute, Adelaide City West, South Australia, Australia

Terese L Chmielewski PhD PT SCS
Assistant Professor, Department of Physical Therapy, University of Florida, Gainesville, FL, USA

Michael T Cibulka PT DPT MHS OCS
Assistant Professor, Physical Therapy Program, Maryville University, St. Louis, MO, USA

Jill Cook BAppSci PostGradDip PhD
Associate Professor, School of Exercise and Nutrition Sciences, Deakin University, Victoria, Australia

Michel W Coppieters PT PhD
Research Fellow, School of Health and Rehabilitation Sciences, University of Queensland, St Lucia, Brisbane, Australia

Sallie Cowan BAppSci PostGradDip PhD
Post Doctoral Research Fellow, Centre for Health, Exercise and Sports Medicine, University of Melbourne, Victoria, Australia

Andrew G Cresswell BEd MSc PhD
Associate Professor, School of Human Movement Studies, University of Queensland, Brisbane, Australia

Kay Crossley BAppSci PostGradDip PhD
Senior Lecturer, School of Physiotherapy, University of Melbourne, Victoria, Australia

Anthony Delitto PhD PT
Professor, Chair, Department of Physical Therapy, School of Health and Rehabilitation Sciences, University of Pittsburgh, Pittsburgh, PA, USA

Rafael F Escamilla BS MS PhD MPT CSCS
Professor, Department of Physical Therapy, California State University, Sacramento, CA, USA

Sara Farquhar BS MPT
Doctoral Candidate, Interdisciplinary Program in Biomechanics and Movement Science, Department of Physical Therapy, University of Delaware, Newark, DE, USA

Andrew Garnham MBBS DipRACOG FACSP
Senior Lecturer, School of Exercise and Nutrition Sciences, Deakin University, Burwood, Victoria, Australia

Mark Gillett BSc(Hons) MBBS FRCS(A&E) FFEM FFSEM(UK&I) DipIMC RCSEd
Lead Physician, EIS West Midlands, and Clinical Director, Emergency Department, Good Hope Hospital, Sutton Coldfield, West Midlands, UK

Bruce Hamilton BPhEd MBChB DTM&H FACSP FFSEM(UK)
Chief Medical Officer, UK Athletics, West Midlands, UK

Timothy E Hewett PhD
Director, Associate Professor, Cincinnati Children's Hospital, Sports Medicine Biodynamics Center, Human Performance Laboratory; University of Cincinnati College of Medicine, Department of Pediatrics and Orthopaedic Surgery, Biomedical Engineering and Rehabilitation Sciences, Cincinnati, OH, USA

Paul W Hodges BPhty(Hons) PhD MedDr(Neurosci)
Professor and NHMRC Principal Research Fellow, NHMRC Centre of Clinical Research Excellence in Spinal Pain, Injury and Health, School of Health and Rehabilitation Sciences, University of Queensland, Brisbane, Australia

Zoë Hudson GradAssocPhys MCSP SRP PhD
Associate Director and Senior Clinical Lecturer, Academic
Department of Sports and Exercise Medicine,
Barts and the London School of Medicine and Dentistry,
Queen Mary University of London, Mile End Hospital,
London, UK

James J Irrgang PhD PT ATC
Director of Clinical Research and Associate Professor, Department
of Orthopaedic Surgery, University of Pittsburg School of Medicine,
Pittsburgh, PA, USA

Pekka Kannus MD PhD
Professor, Injury and Osteoporosis Research Centre, UKK-Institute,
Tampere, and Section of Orthopaedics and Traumatology, University
and University Hospital of Tampere, Finland

Martin Kilbane
Clinical Site Coordinator, HealthSouth, Westlake, OH, USA

**Gregory S Kolt BSc BAppSc(Phty) GradDipEd
GradDipBehavHlthCare PhD**
Professor and Head of School, School of Biomedical and Health
Sciences, University of Western Sydney, Sydney, Australia; Adjunct
Professor, Faculty of Health and Environmental Sciences, Auckland
University of Technology, Auckland, New Zealand

Elizaveta Kon MD
Assistant Professor, Orthopaedic Department and Biomechanics
Laboratory, Istituti Ortopedici Rizzoli,
Bologna, Italy

Paul LaStayo PhD PT CHT
Associate Professor of Physical Therapy, Division of Physical
Therapy, University of Utah, Salt Lake City, UT, USA

Michael Lee PT DPT CHT
Clinical Director, Maximum Impact Physical Therapy,
Tucson, AZ, USA

**Jenny McConnell BAppSci(Phty) GradDipManTher
MBiomedEng**
McConnell Institute, Sammamish, WA, USA

Peter J McNair PhD MNZCP
Professor, School of Physiotherapy, Auckland
University of Technology, Auckland, New Zealand

Nicola Maffulli MD MS PhD FRCS(Orth)
Professor of Trauma and Orthopaedic Surgery, Keele
University School of Medicine, Stoke on Trent, UK

Tara Jo Manal PT DPT OCS SCS
Director of Clinical Services and Orthopedic Residency Program,
Department of Physical Therapy, University of Delaware,
Newark, DE, USA

Robert G Marx MD, MSc, FRCSC
Associate Professor of Orthopedic Surgery, Weill Medical College of
Cornell University, Hospital for Special Surgery, New York, NY, USA

Lyle J Micheli MD
Director, Division of Sports Medicine, Children's Hospital Boston,
Boston, MA, USA; Clinical Professor of Orthopaedic Surgery,
Harvard Medical School Boston, MA, USA

Susan Michlovitz PhD PT CHT
Adjunct Associate Professor, Program in Physical Therapy,
Columbia University, New York, NY; Hand Therapy Consultant,
Ithaca, NY, USA

Douglas N Mintz MD
Associate Professor of Clinical Radiology, Weill College of Medicine,
Cornell University; Associate Attending Physician, Hospital for
Special Surgery; Associate Attending Physician, New York-
Presbyterian Hospital, New York, NY, USA

Robert J Nee MAppSc PT ATC
Associate Professor, Co-ordinator – Transition DPT Program,
School of Physical Therapy, Pacific University, Hillsboro, OR, USA

Gabriel Y F Ng PhD MPhty ProfDipPhty
Professor and Associate Head, Department of Rehabilitation
Sciences, Hong Kong Polytechnic University,
Hong Kong, China

Christine Ploski PT MS PCS MAc LAc
Supervisor, Department of Physical and Occupational Therapy
Services, Children's Hospital, Boston, MA, USA

Michael M Reinold PT DPT ATC CSCS
Athletic Trainer, Boston Red Sox Baseball Club; Research Fellow,
Department of Orthopedics, Massachusetts General Hospital; Senior
Physical Therapist, Massachusetts General Hospital Sports Center,
Adjunct Faculty, Northeastern University, Boston, MA

Jason P Reiss MPT OCS
Clinical Director, Sports Rehabilitation Center, Atlanta, GA, USA

Katherine Rudolph PhD PT
Assistant Professor, Department of Physical Therapy,
University of Delaware, Newark, DE, USA

Marc Safran MD
Professor, Co-Director, Sports Medicine,
Department of Orthopaedic Surgery, Stanford University,
Stanford, CA, USA

Laura A Schmitt PT DPT OCS SCS ATC
Physical Therapist, Physical Therapy Clinic, University of Delaware,
Newark, DE, USA

Lynn Snyder-Mackler BA CertPhysTher MS ScD
Alumni Distinguished Professor and Academic Director, Graduate
Program in Biomechanics and Movement Sciences, Department of
Physical Therapy, University of Delaware,
Newark, DE, USA

Heather Southwick MSPT
Physical Therapist, Department of Physical Therapy and
Occupational Therapy Services, Children's Hospital Boston,
Boston, MA, USA

Jennifer E Stevens PhD MPT
Assistant Professor, Department of Physical Medicine and
Rehabilitation, University of Colorado at Denver and Health Sciences
Center, Denver, CO, USA

Jack Taunton MSc MD DiplSportMed(CASM)
Professor and Director, Allan McGavin Sports Medicine Center,
and Division of Sports Medicine, Department of Family Practice,
University of British Columbia, Vancouver, British Columbia, Canada

Susan M Tillman PT CSCS SCS
Clinical Coordinator, Shands Rehab, UF&Shands Orthopaedic and
Sports Medicine Institute, Gainesville, FL, USA

Brian J Tovin PT DPT MMSc SCS ATC FAAOMPT
Founder and Director, Sports Rehabilitation Center, Atlanta, GA, USA

Elly Trepman MD
Assistant Professor, Section of Orthopaedic Surgery,
University of Manitoba, Winnipeg, Manitoba, Canada

Amanda Weiss-Kelly BA MD
Director Paediatric Sports Medicine and Assistant Professor, Case
Western Reserve University, Rainbow Babies and Children's Hospital,
OH, USA

Suzanne Werner RPT, PhD, ATC
Associate Professor, Chairman, Stockholm Sports Trauma Research
Center, Karolinska Institutet, Stockholm, Sweden

Robbin Wickham-Bruno MS PT SCS ATC
Physical Therapist, The Therapy Connection, Indianapolis, IN, USA

Kevin E Wilk DPT
Clinical Director, Champion Sports Medicine, Birmingham,
AL, USA

DS Blaise Williams III PhD MPT
Director, Human Movement Research Laboratory, School of Allied
Health Sciences, Department of Physical Therapy, East Carolina
University, Greenville, NC, USA

Thomas C Windley PT MPT PhD
Co-founder and Partner, Premier Physical
Therapy and Sports Performance, Middletown, DE, USA

Stefano Zaffagnini MD
Associate Professor, Istituti Ortopedici Rizzoli, Bologna, Italy

In developing the concept and framework for *Physical Therapies in Sport and Exercise* we were conscious of two guiding principles: the need for a book that supports its content with evidence, and the need to go beyond standard sports medicine texts and provide a resource specifically for those who work in the physical and manual therapies. We also undertook to produce a resource that was valuable from an international perspective, and took into account the variety of approaches to the physical therapies across the world. The approach has been successful; the first edition was published not only in English, but also in Japanese, Spanish, Portuguese and Greek. In relation to an evidence-based text, one is reliant on the published literature that supports or refutes the wide variety of approaches that practitioners are now incorporating in their management of injury. Only relatively recently has this body of evidence built to a level that affords practitioners appropriate confidence in the effectiveness of the techniques they use.

The form of the book is unchanged in this second edition, but we have added chapters to three sections, one on cartilage to the first section where other tissues relevant to sports rehabilitation are discussed, a chapter on injury prevention to complement other chapters that deal with management concepts for injury and one on rehabilitation of lower limb injuries. Other chapters have been updated with the most recent literature and available evidence, and, in several instances, completely rewritten with new authors. We hope that with a resource such as this book, practitioners will explore new approaches to managing injury. The breadth of topics covered in this book is testament to the ever-increasing knowledge that competent practitioners are required to possess. Merely possessing this knowledge is insufficient; we must place it into an applied context with patients, athletes and the general population with which we work. The use of physical therapy in the sport and exercise environment is gaining rapid momentum in all regions of the world. Its place in mainstream medicine and health, however, is dependent on using approaches that have demonstrated acceptability and efficacy. Not only should this book be seen as a resource for practitioners, but as a platform from which researchers draw ideas for further investigation. Take the opportunity to draw upon the extensive reference lists provided in each chapter to further your reading and knowledge. But most of all use what is in the text to broaden the approaches you take with your patients.

Gregory S. Kolt, Sydney
Lynn Snyder-Mackler, Delaware

Acknowledgments

Many people have contributed in a variety of ways to bring this edition to fruition. Sarena Wolfaard, the Commissioning Editor, saw a place for a second edition and gave encouragement for the project to commence. Claire Wilson worked on this edition in its initial stages as the Development Editor until Claire Bonnett took over. They are both thanked for their efficiency, attention to detail, advice and prompt responses to the large number of emails that crossed the globe in making this edition happen. Rachel Holley was invaluable in the administration of the project – with 62 busy contributors from 10 countries, working on 31 chapters, this was no small task. Bonnie Brannigan undertook much of the time-consuming proof reading, while Neil Snowling provided invaluable support as an editorial assistant. Thanks also go to the many people who used the first edition of the book and provided valuable feedback on it, and to the publishers who translated the first edition into Spanish, Japanese, Portuguese and Greek. My professional life has been shaped by two very important people, both of whom are somewhat responsible for me completing this project: my academic mentor, the late Professor Rob Kirkby who provided an unparalleled enthusiasm for academia from which I have learnt; and David Zuker, one of the pioneers of sport physical therapy, who taught me so much. Last, but certainly not least, is my family. Emma, Daisy Chayne and Satchel provide a balance in my life, many great and fun reasons to have time away from the book and other work and the encouragement and support to complete the project. Throughout my life, my parents have taught me the importance of learning and education, and have given me unfaltering support for anything I have taken on.

Gregory S. Kolt

My doctoral students, sports PT residents and colleagues in the Department of Physical Therapy, and Biomechanics and Movement Sciences program, at the University of Delaware contributed in tangible (many were contributors, read early drafts) and intangible ways. My family (Scott, Alexander, Noah, Moms and Dad) and the army of people (especially Jill Heathcock and Dana Crumpler) who keep our home life healthy during Scott's valiant fight with ALS inspire all I do. Sara Farquhar continues to be academic publishing's loss and my gain, and provided invaluable editorial assistance.

Lynn Snyder-Mackler

The foreword, conveniently, is defined as a declaration expressed by a third party who is knowledgeable with the materials that the editor(s) wish to present. In the foreword to the first edition, Professor Per Renström expertly outlined the need for optimal injury management from team physicians and physical therapists. This is true in light of increased physical activity as a health benefit and the consequence of acute, noncontact and overuse injuries. He mentioned the obligation for expertise in rehabilitation of certain musculotendinous tissue injuries to be research based. Proper use of modalities and exercise techniques in order to promote patient well-being were essential elements, as he stated, in their text. On a personal note, Per Renström mentioned that a physical therapist accompanied him in his clinic. The author of this second edition foreword learned from his mentor the value of physical therapy after orthopedic surgery to enhance the benefits of successful surgery, such as shorter recovery time and to promote patient satisfaction. Also, rehabilitation techniques are tailored specifically for each surgical procedure in order to facilitate early return to prior activity levels.

The first edition of this text is recognized for its merits and its contents and by the fact that the text has been translated into four foreign languages. In order to enhance its proven worth, chapters were updated, research was refreshed and new authors' opinions adopted. Including the cartilage chapter along with emphasis on rehabilitation of the lower limb has added considerable substance. An international flavor continues. The new chapter on injury prevention is most copious in light of increased activity in all categories from children, adults, females, elderly and to the disabled with the inevitable injuries and with the need for physical therapy.

A 'walk through', to use the editors' verbiage, describes the activity of certain members of the Alabama Sports Medicine and Orthopaedic Center group in reviewing this text. The research and biomechanic elements of the group are most pleased with chapters on the components of the musculoskeletal system (Chapters 2 to 5). General sports medicine physicians applaud the contents of the medical chapters (28 to 31). Imaging was very helpful. Obviously, the chapters pertaining in general to the shoulder, elbow and knee received special interest for the orthopedic surgeons in the group.

Of particular note was the etiology of ACL injuries in the female athlete. The topic outlined the current theories as to the causes of noncontact ACL interruptions, as well as a proposed rehabilitation schedule to be implemented in preventative management. With the dramatic increase in pre-adolescent and adolescent shoulder and elbow injuries in throwing sports, the chapter on injury prevention was most significant. Incidentally, the information is in concert with the new pitching guidelines invoked by the Little Leagues for all teams in that program. Ancillary professionals in the group surveyed each new chapter for its content of sports physical therapy management techniques and found the results to be excellent. A physical therapist, not in our group, but whose expertise is valued, was asked to read the text and evaluate material from her perspective. She writes that 'I was very impressed by the text and I believe that many therapists in the field would benefit from reading this book. I look forward to referencing this text when I come across athletes with specific problems.' Of all the chapters she mentioned, her favorite from the point of view of helpfulness was motor control, Chapter 8.

After evaluation of this second edition by a cross section of members of an orthopedic sports medicine group, it would appear that the educational values of this new text have been enhanced by the editors' determination to produce current subject matter in sports physical therapy that when utilized will benefit the giver and the receiver. Their endeavors are to be lauded.

James R Andrews MD

Based on extensive scientific evidence, it is clear that inactivity is definitely the largest risk factor for poor health and disease. Physical activity is, on the other hand, beneficial for health and this also has some scientific support. This message has been spread during the last 20–30 years to a large part of the world. People have started to become more active although they are not as active as they should be. There is a renewed interest in different types of physical activity and exercise, particularly for the elderly and young children of school age. The benefits of physical activity are obvious for the elderly as it strengthens bone mass and prevents hip fractures. For the young, there is not as much scientific support to show the benefits; however, it is important to try to get into the habit of carrying out some physical activity regularly from an early age. It is, nonetheless, never too late to start being physically active.

Many people enjoy watching top level sport in sport arenas and on television, and there is huge mass media interest in many aspects of sport. This puts increasing pressure on top level athletes: they have to practice harder, for longer periods of time, with higher intensity and with less time to recover. Contact and collisions during games are getting rougher. All these factors increase the risk for injury. Athletes sustain injuries both of traumatic and overuse character, and overuse injuries, particularly, tend to increase both in frequency and in complexity. Unfortunately, there is not enough focus on prevention, which is a pity, as most overuse injuries can be prevented.

With the increasing awareness of the benefits of being physically active, the injury problem for the general population is also increasing among recreational athletes. Elderly people are tending to be more physically active today and this often generates some injury or pain problem. Active people often have a strong desire to recover as fast as possible after an injury.

There is increasing pressure to receive optimal injury management not only from physicians but also from physical therapists. The habit of including a physical therapist in the management team is gradually increasing and most people see much benefit from this. I have a physical therapist with me during all my clinics, which means that we can give every patient a rehabilitation program on the spot, and this is usually very much appreciated. This arrangement also makes sure that patients will see experts in the patients' specific injury, as the therapist can direct patients to where they need to go.

Physical therapy is a complex part of medicine and includes not only different aspects of exercises but also expertise on how different modalities can be used effectively. Rehabilitation exercises have been fairly extensively studied in the literature and they are well covered in this book in the first section, which describes management principles for musculoskeletal tissues in physical therapy. This section provides major coverage on the structural biomechanics of the tissues in relation to the response of tissue injury to healing. The competition between healing and exercise is perhaps the most intriguing problem that the physical therapist faces. The therapist must introduce an exercise program to the injured person, which is as effective and extensive as possible without compromising healing of the tissue. There are very few objective ways of dosing the level of physical therapy exercises and therefore the skill and knowledge of the therapist is essential.

Modalities such as ultrasound, electrical stimulation and other types of heat treatment have historically played major roles in physical therapy. They are still used widely all around the world, mostly because people undergoing rehabilitation like them as they give a feeling of wellbeing. The problem is, however, that scientific support for the efficacy of the most common modalities is limited and this means that there is a great need for more research in this area. This book, therefore, fills a gap, as it outlines the evidence to support or refute the role of modalities in sports medicine.

It is also important for the physical therapist to be updated on what is new in the field. During the last few years there has been major interest in exercises that improve motor control and balance. There is also huge interest in why eccentric exercise is so effective in dealing with painful chronic tendinopathy and why a major overload seems to make the exercise even more effective. How effective is stretching? This book discusses these aspects as well.

As mentioned above, one of the problems that physical therapists face today is a lack of scientific study supporting the efficacy of different treatment techniques. It is therefore important to have a book like this, which outlines the available science of today and presents the current concepts of injury management. The physical therapist needs to know what to do. This is especially important today as most management in medicine must be evidence-based.

In sections 3 and 4 of the book, management of different regions, and management of different groups are described. People with special risk factors are discussed and this allows physical therapists to plan programs for a special group in detail. Towards the end of the book, there is a discussion about drugs, doping and other medical issues, which can be of benefit to some physical therapists active in sport.

This book will be a great addition to the existing literature for physical therapists active in sport, physical exercise and activity. It is very well designed and well planned and covers the whole field. The editors have managed to recruit some of the leading experts in the world, covering most of the important fields in sports physical therapy. Current concepts of injury management and the increasingly important role the physical therapist plays in the field of sports, physical exercise and activity are described. The major advantage of this book is that the discussions are comprehensive and based on the scientific evidence available.

This is a high-quality book in an increasingly important field. It is my sincere opinion that this book will not only be very beneficial but also enjoyable to read for everyone active in the field of physical therapy, sports and physical activity.

Per Renström, Stockholm, 2003

AAS	anabolic androgenic steroids
AC	alternating current
ACI	autologous chondrocyte implantation
ACJ	acromioclavicular joint
ACL	anterior cruciate ligament
ADL	activities of daily living
ADP	adenosine diphosphate
ADR	autonomic dysreflexia
AIGS	abnormal impulse generating site
ALCL	accessory lateral collateral ligament
ALL	anterior longitudinal ligament
APL	abductor pollicis longus
ASIS	anterior superior iliac spine
ASL	airway surface liquid
ATFL	anterior talofibular ligament
ATP	adenosine triphosphate
ATPase	adenosine triphosphatase
BMD	bone mineral density
CAD	coronary artery disease
CAL	coracoacromial ligament
CBST	cognitive behavioral stress management
CBT	cognitive-behavioral technique
CGRP	calcitonin gene-related peptide
CHL	coracohumeral ligament
CIND	carpal instability non-dissociative
CMC	carpometacarpal
CNS	central nervous system
CO	cardiac output
CP	cerebral palsy
CPG	central pattern generators
CPM	continuous passive motion
CSF	cerebrospinal fluid
CT	computed tomography
CTS	carpal tunnel syndrome
DASH	Disabilities of the Arm, Shoulder and Hand Index
DC	direct current
DEXA	dual emission X-ray absorptiometry
DHEA	dehydroepiandrosterone
DHLNL	dihydroxylysinonorleucine
DHP	dihydropyridine
DIP	distal phalangeal
DISI	dorsiflexion intercalated segment instability
DJD	degenerative joint disease
DRG	dorsal root ganglion
DRUJ	distal radioulnar joint
DSST	digit symbol substitution test
DXA	dual energy X-ray absorptiometry
EAT	eating attitudes test
EBM	evidence-based medicine
EBP	evidence-based practice
ECG	electrocardiogram
ECRB	extensor carpi radialis brevis
ECRL	extensor carpi radialis longus
ECU	extensor carpi ulnaris
EDC	extensor digitorum communis
EDI	Eating Disorders Inventory
EDNOS	eating disorders not otherwise specified
EEG	electroencephalogram
EIA	exercise-induced asthma
EIB	exercise-induced bronchospasm
EMG	electromyography
EPB	extensor pollicis brevis
EPL	extensor pollicis longus
ERT	estrogen replacement therapy
ES	effect size
ESWT	extracorporeal shock-wave therapy
FCR	flexor carpi radialis
FDP	flexor digitorum profundus
FDS	flexor digitorum superficialis
FEV1	forced expiratory volume in 1s
FOOSH	fall on outstretched hand
FPL	flexor pollicis longus
FSH	follicle stimulating hormone
GABA	gamma-aminobutyric acid
GAG	glycosaminoglycans
GHJ	glenohumoral joint
GI	glycemic index
GnRH	gonadotrophin releasing hormone
GRF	ground reaction forces
GRIT	gripping rotatory impaction test
GTO	golgi tendon organ
HALE	healthy active life expectancy
HBO	hyperbaric oxygen
HBV	hepatitis B
HCV	hepatitis C
HHMD	histidinohydroxymerodesmosine
HIV	human immunodeficiency virus
HLA	human leukocyte antigen
HLBS	high-load brief stress
HLNL	hydroxylysinonorleucine
HO	hyperbaric oxygen
HOCM	hypertrophic obstructive cardiomyopathy
HP	hydroxypyridinoline
HR	heart rate
HSV	herpes simplex virus
HVPC	high-volt pulsed current
IBSA	International Blind Sports Association
IGF	insulin-like growth factor

IGHLC	inferior glenohumeral ligament complex
IOC	International Olympic Committee
IP	interphalangeal
IPC	International Paralympic Committee
IRRST	internal resistance strength test
ITBFS	iliotibial band friction syndrome
ITP	interval throwing program
IVF	intervertebral foramen
LCL	lateral collateral ligament
LH	luteinizing hormone
LHB	long head of biceps
LLLD	low load, long duration
LLPS	low-load prolonged stress
LOC	loss of consciousness
LT	lunotriquetal
LUCL	lateral ulnar collateral ligament
MCL	medial collateral ligament
MCP	metacarpophalangeal
MGHL	middle glenohumeral ligament
MMP	matrix metalloproteinase
MPQ	McGill Pain Questionnaire
MRI	magnetic resonance imaging
MTP	metatarsophalangeal
MVIC	maximum voluntary isometric contraction
NCSP	neutral calcaneal stance position
NCV	nerve conduction velocity
NMES	neuromuscular electrical stimulation
NRS	numerical rating scale
NSAID	non-steroidal anti-inflammatory drug
OA	osteoarthritis
OATS	osteochondral autograft transfer system
OCD	osteochondritis dissecans
OCP	oral contraceptive pill
ORIF	open reduction with internal fixation
PAR-Q	Physical Activity Readiness Questionnaire
PCL	posterior collateral ligament
PEFR	peak expiratory flow rate
PEMF	pulsed electromagnetic fields
PET	positron emission tomography
PFJ	patellofemoral joint
PFP	patellofemoral pain
PFPS	patellofemoral pain syndrome
PGHL	posterior glenohumeral ligament
PIP	proximal interphalangeal
POL	posterior oblique ligament
PPI	present pain intensity (scale)
PRE	progressive resistance exercise
PRI	pain rating index
PROM	passive range of motion
PSIS	posterior superior iliac spine
RCL	radial collateral ligament
RCSP	resting calcaneal stance position
RCT	randomized controlled trial
rER	rough endoplasmic reticulum
RICE	rest, ice, compression and elevation
RM	repetition maximum
ROM	range of motion
RSA	Roentgen stereophonogrammetric analysis
RSN	radial sensory nerve
RYR	ryanodine receptor
SAID	specific adaptations to imposed demands
SCD	sudden cardiac death
SCFE	slipped capital femoral epiphysis
SCI	spinal cord injury
SCJ	sternoclavicular joint
s.d.	standard deviation
SEM	standard error of measurement
SFMPQ	Short-Form McGill Pain Questionnaire
SGHL	superior glenohumeral ligament
SHB	short head of biceps
SIJ	sacroiliac joint
SIP	Sports Inventory for Pain
SIRAS	Sport Injury Rehabilitation Adherence Scale
SIS	second impact syndrome
SL	scapholunate
SLAC	scapholunate advanced collapse
SLAP	superior labral anterior posterior
SMOC	Sports Medicine Observation Code
SMT	spinal manipulative therapy
SPECT	single photon emission computer tomography
STJ	scapulothoracic joint
SUI	stress urinary incontinence
SV	stroke volume
TENS	transcutaneous electrical nerve stimulation
TERT	total end-range time
TFCC	triangular fibrocartilage complex
UCL	ulnar collateral ligament
UPS	unexplained underperformance syndrome
URTI	upper respiratory tract infection
US	ultrasound
USOC	United States Olympic Committee
VAS	visual analog scale
VEGF	vascular endothelial growth factor
VL	vastus longus
VML	vastus medialis longus
VMO	vastus medialis oblique
VRM	variable resistance machine
VRS	verbal rating scale
WADA	World Anti-Doping Agency

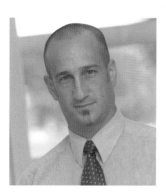

Gregory S. Kolt is Professor and Head of the School of Biomedical and Health Sciences at the University of Western Sydney, Australia, and an Adjunct Professor in the Faculty of Health and Environmental Sciences at Auckland University of Technology, New Zealand. A graduate of the University of Melbourne and La Trobe University, he is co-editor of the comprehensive book *Psychology in the Physical and Manual Therapies*, the journal *Physical Therapy in Sport* and sits on editorial boards of several other health care and sports medicine journals. In addition to being a highly experienced physical therapist, he has additional qualifications in psychology (particularly health psychology and sport and exercise psychology), exercise science and education. He has undertaken extensive research in physical therapy, health psychology and health-related physical activity and has held a variety of appointments with national sports teams in Australia and New Zealand as both a physical therapist and psychologist. Dr Kolt has published extensively and regularly presents his work at international conferences and courses.

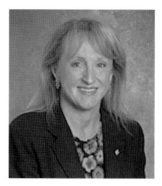

Lynn Snyder-Mackler is Alumni Distinguished Professor in the Department of Physical Therapy and the Academic Director of the Graduate Program in Biomechanics and Movement Sciences at the University of Delaware, USA. She is an internationally recognized clinician and clinical researcher in sports rehabilitation. Dr Snyder-Mackler is a graduate of the Johns Hopkins University, the University of Pennsylvania and Boston University. She is a Board Certified Sports Physical Therapist who maintains an active sports physical therapy practice at the University of Delaware and serves as a rehabilitation consultant to collegiate, amateur and professional teams. She served as the head trainer for the beach volleyball venue at the 1996 Olympic Games in Atlanta. She concentrates her clinical practice and research in areas of the knee and shoulder rehabilitation, and electrical stimulation of muscle. She has authored many research publications in the areas of knee and shoulder rehabilitation and neuromuscular electrical stimulation, and regularly speaks to international audiences on these topics. Her research has won several major awards for helping patients and practitioners and answering critical questions in sports rehabilitation.

The role of the physical therapies in sport, exercise and physical activity

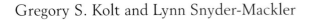

Gregory S. Kolt and Lynn Snyder-Mackler

CHAPTER CONTENTS

Introduction 1
Sports rehabilitation specialists and physical therapists 2
Injury in sport, exercise and physical activity 3
The need for an evidence base in the physical therapies 3
A walk through *Physical Therapies in Sport and Exercise*. 4
Summary 5

Introduction

Sport, exercise and physical activity pursuits are important in most societies. A result of participation in such activities, however, is the risk of injury. Not only does injury occur during competitive sport activities, but through preparation for such events, as well as during the general physical activities and exercise that an increasing number of people are becoming involved in for health benefits.

The field of sports medicine has developed as a result of increased participation rates in sport, exercise and physical activity, and the specific medical needs of participants (Matheson & Pipe 1996). Sports medicine is a multidisciplinary field that involves health professionals from a variety of professions. Whilst resources do not always allow for a large and multidisciplinary sports medicine team, the following personnel are often involved in the prevention and management of sport and exercise related injuries:

- Family physician (primary care physician)
- Sports physician
- Orthopedic surgeon
- Radiologist
- Physical therapist/physiotherapist
- Massage therapist
- Podiatrist
- Dietician/nutritionist
- Psychologist (often sport psychologist)
- Athletic trainer/sports trainer
- Chiropractor and osteopath
- Sport scientists including biomechanists and exercise physiologists
- Other health professionals including orthotists, nurses, dentists, occupational therapists and optometrists
- Coach
- Fitness coach or adviser.

Although this combination of professionals is ideal, in the majority of settings, sports medicine teams will be far smaller depending on the needs and demands of a particular sport and the availability of sports medicine practitioners.

People involved in sports medicine work towards several common goals. Two important goals are returning an individual to their preinjury level of functioning in the shortest possible time, and implementing strategies to avoid reinjury. Obviously there are several ways to rehabilitate each injury that an athlete presents with. Where possible, physical therapists should focus on techniques that have some level of proven efficacy. Despite the growing body of evidence of physical therapy methods, there are, however, still a plethora of physical management methods that are being implemented on the basis of anecdotal evidence alone.

Sports rehabilitation specialists and physical therapists

In the context of this book, the terms 'sports rehabilitation specialist' and 'physical therapist' are used to describe the set of professions that use physical techniques and skills in the prevention, management and rehabilitation of injury. For example, health professionals that would use these skills and techniques include physical therapists, physiotherapists, athletic trainers, athletic therapists, sports trainers, massage therapists, podiatrists, sports physicians, chiropractors and osteopaths. Many of these professionals do not rely exclusively on physical methods to carry out their role, but usually combine such methods with other skills (e.g. psychological or behavioral techniques, pharmacological therapy and electrophysical agents). The terms 'physical therapists' and 'sports rehabilitation specialists' will be used in a broad sense throughout this book.

Of the many professions listed above, several deal with issues that encompass more than sport and exercise alone. For example, physical therapy or physiotherapy is concerned with far reaching issues including cardiorespiratory problems, neurological conditions, physical developmental issues and treatment of terminally ill people. Therefore, the aspect of those professions that deal with injury in sport and exercise is a specialized field that requires an expert knowledge, usually obtained through a combination of formal study and clinical experience. In the USA, a specialist certification process in sports physical therapy is possible through the American Physical Therapy Association. In Australia, postregistration university graduate programs in sports physiotherapy, in combination with other relevant experience, contribute to becoming a sports physiotherapist. In several other countries, a mixture of graduate study and clinical experience provide the skills to work in the area of sport and exercise physical therapy. Given the lack of consistency of requirements across countries to work in the area of sports physical therapy, and that some countries lack any specific requirements in this area, the International Federation of Sports Physiotherapy recently developed and adopted a series of competencies relevant to sports physical therapy practitioners (refer to www.sportsphysiotherapyforall.org for further details).

The role of physical therapists has changed dramatically over the past 30 years. Whereas traditionally, those involved in the physical therapies were required to work under the guidance and referral of a medical practitioner, many physical therapists are now considered primary contact practitioners. The ability to consult with and manage patients directly is different in each country. For example, in Australia, physiotherapists were granted primary contact status in the 1970s with other countries more recently following this lead. In the USA, direct access to physical therapists is controlled by the laws in each state; currently, 42 of the 50 individual states allow direct access. Advanced practice options (specialization) have expanded practice opportunities to include ordering radiographic tests, providing injections, and in some cases prescribing medication. Physical therapists are becoming the musculoskeletal primary care providers of choice in much of the world. In many countries, however, the techniques that can be carried out by physical therapists are still somewhat restricted and guided by medical practitioners. In reading this book, therefore, physical therapists should be aware of their roles in the health and medical system of the country in which they work.

Not only are more physical therapists now working as primary contact practitioners, but the philosophy or approach to physical therapy has changed. Traditionally the main emphasis was on rehabilitation; however, more recently a major focus on preventive physical therapy has emerged for several reasons. In the case of elite athletes, time out from sport due to injury can result in decreased performance rankings (individual and team), and, in many cases, loss of earnings. In the cases of recreational or lower-level competitive athletes, time away from sport due to injury can result in a loss of enjoyment, reduced level of fitness, loss of social opportunities, and decreased health status. The older population is a new group that is increasingly involved in exercise and physical activity. The fitness, health and social rewards of their involvement can be affected when refraining from such activity due to injury or poor health.

The medical needs of people involved in sport, exercise, and physical activity are best addressed through the team approach of sports medicine professionals. The various professions involved in the ideal sports medicine team have been listed above. It is apparent that individuals in the sports medicine team have a level of overlap in terms of their skills. In many situations, practitioners are required to be multiskilled. For example, if the sole practitioner with a sports team traveling overseas to a competition is a sports physician, it would be useful for that individual to be familiar with basic soft tissue techniques. Furthermore, physical therapists should be familiar with methods of creating orthotics for use with athletes when an orthotist is not available.

Traditionally, medical models have been biased towards a medical practitioner as the primary contact practitioner (Brukner & Khan 2001). The sports medicine model is based on a number of people as the possible primary contact practitioner (e.g. medical practitioner, physical therapist, podiatrist). This means that each member of the team should have a high level of understanding of the role of other team members so that referral can be instigated where necessary, and so that collaborative treatment can be implemented.

An integral link in the modern day sports medicine team is the coach. Given that coaches are usually the individuals with the highest level of contact with the athlete, they form a vital link between the physical therapist and athlete. Coaches can be involved in the decision-making process regarding time away from sport and return to activity. Also, they can play an important role in deciding on alternative activities that athletes can perform when restricted from sport-specific skills.

Injury in sport, exercise and physical activity

Participation rates in sport and recreational activities have grown in recent times, giving rise to increased injury rates that have been described as a public health issue (Caine et al 1996). This increased participation is not surprising given the evidence of some of the physical and psychological benefits of exercise and physical activity (e.g. Taylor et al 2004, Warburton et al 2006); however, the costs involved in rehabilitation of people injured through such activities, the loss of sport and work participation time, the risk of long-term injury and the consequent reduced quality of life, are all major public health problems.

Several aspects of participation can contribute to the incidence and severity of injury in sport. These include the nature of the activity, and the gender, age and physical condition of the participant. Although most injuries in sport and exercise involve the musculoskeletal system, many other systems of the body can be involved (cardiorespiratory, neurological, etc.) In general, sport and exercise injury can be defined as any injury that is sports or physical activity related and results in keeping the individual out of practice, activity or competition, or requires the individual to seek medical attention (Noyes et al 1988).

One of the contributing factors to the increasing number of injuries in sport is the changing sport and exercise population. That sport and exercise have been promoted as healthy activities means that a larger number of older people are participating in increased amounts of physical activity. Also, children and adolescents are participating in greater amounts of sport at younger ages (see Adirim & Cheng 2003, Caine & Maffulli 2005, Maffulli & Bruns 2001, Maffulli & Caine 2005).

The need for an evidence base in the physical therapies

Optimal medical practice involves rational interpretation of research evidence and application of such evidence to clinical settings (Hart 2000). Physical therapy is an area that, until recently, was based on a small and often flawed body of research and evidence. We often rely on the journals that publish research to guide our clinical practice. We should be aware, however, that despite the best efforts, flawed research still sometimes appears in mainstream journals (Altman 1994, Chalmers & Altman 1999). Evidence-based medicine (EBM) has been described as the conscientious, explicit and judicious use of current best evidence in making decisions about the care of individual patients (Hart 2000). Several authors

have written extensively on EBM (e.g. Sackett 1992, Sackett et al 1996, Sackett et al 1997, Straus & Haynes 2002, Straus & Jones 2004, Straus et al 2004, Straus et al 2005). Furthermore, many journals now endorse the reporting standards for controlled trials published by the CONSORT group (Begg et al 1996, Moher et al 2001a). The CONSORT guidelines are designed to facilitate uniform reporting of clinical intervention results and to allow readers to determine efficiently whether sources of bias threaten internal or external validity of the findings (Moher et al 2001a). Notably, the CONSORT guidelines do not make a distinction between efficacy and effectiveness studies. Rather, the focus is on components of the reporting for all clinical interventions, regardless of their purpose. Preliminary data indicate that the use of CONSORT does indeed help improve the quality of reports of randomized controlled trials (Eggar et al 2001, Moher et al 2001b) by reducing unclearly reported allocation concealment by 22% after 4 years (Moher et al 2001b).

In sports medicine, the combination of clinical expertise and the best available evidence from systematic research can assist the practitioner in ensuring the most efficacious approach to patient management. The chapters of this book have, where possible, reported techniques and approaches to injury management that are supported by appropriate evidence. It is clear, however, that there are still several areas of the physical therapies in sport and exercise that lack sufficient evidence.

To address the dearth of evidence for clinical techniques in physical therapy, the American Physical Therapy Association developed a Clinical Research Agenda (Guccione et al 2000). The Clinical Research Agenda was developed to help guide the systematic progression of the scientific basis of the physical therapy profession. Many of the 72 research questions in the agenda can be related to the physical therapies as they apply to sport, exercise and physical activity. Examples of research questions identified as important in the Clinical Research Agenda include:

- What are the reliability and validity of assessment and pronation of the foot in patients with knee pain?
- How can patient characteristics and environmental factors be used to predict adherence to home programs?
- What are the factors that motivate patients to adhere to a plan of care?
- Does immediate postoperative physical therapy intervention affect the rate of recovery of function in patients following orthopedic surgery, and, if so, how?
- What is the relative effectiveness of immobilization versus mobilization in patients with musculoskeletal impairments on tissue healing and recovery of function?
- What is the effect of various intensities and durations of interventions on the rate and degree of functional recovery after anterior cruciate ligament injury?

It is efforts like the Clinical Research Agenda that can help prioritize and guide research that will benefit the sports physical therapy profession. Jette et al (2003) examined the beliefs, attitudes, knowledge and behaviors of physical therapists towards evidence-based practice and found a positive attitude towards the inclusion of evidence-based practice within the profession. Respondents also indicated an interest in learning or improving the skills necessary to implement such practices.

A walk through *Physical Therapies in Sport and Exercise*

Sports physical therapy does not have a unitary model, and thus we have assembled a group of researchers, practitioners and educators who represent the diversity of approaches in working with sport and exercise to contribute chapters to this book. The authors come from physical therapy, psychology, sports medicine, athletic training, orthopedic surgery, pediatrics, radiology, biomechanics and nursing, and represent countries as diverse as the USA, Australia, New Zealand, Hong Kong, the UK, Finland, Sweden, Italy, Norway and Canada. As previously mentioned, the chapters of this book have, where possible, reported techniques and approaches to injury management that are supported by appropriate evidence.

This book is divided into five sections:

Section 1: Management Principles for Musculoskeletal and Neural Tissue in the Physical Therapies. This section deals with five groups of body tissue: Muscle (Ch. 2), Tendon (Ch. 3), Ligament (Ch. 4), Bone (Ch. 5), Nerves (Ch. 6) and Cartilage (Ch. 7). These chapters provide coverage of the basic structure and biomechanics of the tissues, the principles relating to the adaptation of the tissue to mechanical load, and the response of the tissue to injury and healing.

Section 2: Concepts in Managing Sport and Exercise Injuries. The chapters in this section provide general information that is important in the management of injuries from the various regions of the body. Chapter 8, Motor Control, covers the theory and application of motor control and motor relearning in the management of sport and exercise related injury. Chapter 9, Pain, outlines the mechanisms and theories of pain perception, and presents strategies to assess and manage pain from both a physical and cognitive-behavioral perspective. Chapter 10, Exercise-based Conditioning and Rehabilitation, outlines the evidence for the use of various forms of exercise in injury prevention and management. Chapter 11, Psychology of Injury and Rehabilitation, works through the psychological factors that affect the onset and rehabilitation of injury. Also, issues related to rehabilitation adherence and the role of physical therapists in applying basic cognitive-behavioral techniques is covered. Chapter 12, Screening for Sport and Exercise Participation, focuses on the principles and practical application of screening procedures that are used for sport and exercise participation. Issues related to general health, and sport-specific health and fitness, are addressed. Chapter 13, Clinical Outcomes in Sport and Exercise Physical Therapies, covers a range of outcome measures that can be used in the sport and exercise physical therapies. This addresses both clinical measures and condition-specific functional measures.

Chapter 14, Electrophysical Agents in Sport and Exercise Injury Management, evaluates, from a scientific perspective, various electrophysical agents commonly used by sport physical therapists. The emphasis is on outlining the evidence to support or refute the role of such modalities in sports medicine. Chapter 15, Prevention of Injury, describes the general principles and models of injury prevention (and associated research) in sport and exercise.

Section 3: Regional Sport and Exercise Injury Management. The chapters in this section deal with the Spine (Ch. 16), Shoulder (Ch. 17), Elbow (Ch. 18), Wrist and Hand (Ch. 19), Pelvis, Hip and Groin (Ch. 20), Knee (Ch. 21), Patellofemoral Joint (Ch. 22), Foot, Ankle, and Lower Leg (Ch. 23) and Rehabilitation of Lower Limb Muscle and Tendon Injuries (Ch. 24). In each of these chapters the content focuses on sport-specific applied anatomy, examination and the management of common and less common sport- and exercise-related injuries to the region.

Section 4: The Role of Sport and Exercise Physical Therapies in Active Groups. Four groups of people are covered in this section: children and adolescents, older exercise participants, active females and athletes with disability. Chapter 25, Children and Adolescents, outlines the assessment and management of conditions specific to this age group. In particular, injuries and conditions specific to the immature musculoskeletal system are highlighted. Chapter 26, Older Exercise Participants, focuses on the assessment and management of conditions specific to older people involved in sport, exercise and physical activity. In particular, the impact of aging on the systems of the body is addressed, as well as the benefits that can be gained from participation in sport and exercise and guidelines for exercise participation. Chapter 27, The Active Female, focuses on conditions specific to women involved in sport and exercise. In particular, issues related to bone health are covered, as are the anatomical and physiological considerations for women. Other areas included are the menstrual cycle and performance, the female athlete triad and exercise during pregnancy. Chapter 28, Athletes with Disability, presents information on the benefits of exercise and sport for people with disability, classification of athletes with disability and injury management and assessment for a variety of disability groups in sport.

Section 5: Medical Considerations for Rehabilitation Practitioners in Sport and Exercise . Section 5 has three chapters dealing with a variety of medical considerations for physical therapists working in sport and exercise. Chapter 29, Pharmacological Agents in Sport and Exercise, deals with therapeutic pharmacological agents and the impact they have on injury repair, exercise participation and physical therapies management. The chapter also covers the effects of performance enhancing drugs on athlete health and wellbeing, and the International Olympic Committee Anti-Doping Code. Chapter 30, Medical Imaging of Injury, provides those working in the physical therapies with an understanding of the various imaging modalities used in diagnosing sport and exercise related injuries. Chapter 31, Medical Issues in Sport and Exercise, covers common medical emergencies in sport and exercise including head injuries, cardiovascular conditions and conditions related to environmental influences.

The specific aim of this chapter is to outline the role of physical therapists in recognizing and providing first-aid management to athletes with medical conditions.

Summary

Despite the many existing books that deal with sports physical therapy, the aim of this text is to provide a logical approach to the management of sport and exercise injuries that considers the available evidence for the efficacy and effectiveness of a variety of management approaches.

References

Adirim TA, Cheng TL 2003 Overview of injuries in the young athlete. Sports Medicine 33:75–81

Altman DG 1994 The scandal of poor medical research. British Medical Journal 308:283–284

Begg C, Cho M, Eastwood S et al 1996 Improving the quality of reporting of randomized controlled trials. The CONSORT statement. Journal of the American Medical Association 276:637–639

Brukner P, Khan K 2001 Clinical sports medicine, 2nd edn. McGraw Hill, Sydney

Caine DJ, Maffulli N 2005 Epidemiology of pediatric sports injuries. Individual sports. Medicine and Sport Science, vol 48. Karger, Basel

Caine DJ, Caine CG, Lindner KJ 1996 Epidemiology of sports injuries. Human Kinetics, Champaign, IL

Chalmers I, Altman DG 1999 How can medical journals help prevent poor medical research? Some opportunities presented by electronic publishing. Lancet 353:490–493

Eggar M, Juni P, Bartlett C 2001 Value of flow diagrams in reports of randomized controlled trials. Journal of the American Medical Association 285:1996–1999

Guccione AA, Va A, Goldstein M et al 2000 Clinical research agenda for physical therapy. Physical Therapy 80:499–513

Hart LE 2000 Evidence-based sports medicine. In: Kumbhare DA, Basmajian JV (eds) Decision making and outcomes in sports rehabilitation. Churchill Livingstone, Edinburgh

Jette DU, Bacon K, Batty C et al 2003 Evidence-based practice: beliefs, attitudes, knowledge, and behaviors of physical therapists. Physical Therapy 83:786–805

Maffulli N, Bruns W 2001 Training and injuries in young athletes. In: Maffulli N, Chan KM, Macdonald R, et al (eds) Sports medicine for specific ages and abilities. Churchill Livingstone, Edinburgh

Maffulli N, Caine DJ 2005 Epidemiology of pediatric sports injuries. Team sports. Medicine and Sport Science, vol 49. Karger, Basel

Matheson GO, Pipe AL 1996 Twenty-five years of sports medicine in Canada: thoughts on the road ahead. Clinical Journal of Sports Medicine 6:148–151

Moher D, Shulz KF, Altman D 2001a The CONSORT statement: revised recommendations for improving the quality of reports of parallel-group randomized trials. Journal of the American Medical Association 285:1987–1991

Moher D, Jones A, Lepage L 2001b Use of the CONSORT statement and quality of randomized controlled trials. A comparative before-and-after evaluation. Journal of the American Medical Association 285:1992–1995

Noyes FE, Lindenfeld TN, Marshall MT 1988 What determines an athletic injury (definition)? Who determines an injury (occurrence)? American Journal of Sports Medicine 16 (1, suppl):65–68

Sackett DL 1992 Evidence-based medicine: A new approach to teaching the practice of medicine. Journal of the American Medical Association 268:2420–2425

Sackett DL, Rosenberg WM, Gray JA et al 1996 Evidence based medicine: what it is and what it isn't. British Medical Journal 312:71–72

Sackett DL, Richardson WS, Rosenberg W et al 1997 Evidence-based medicine. Churchill Livingstone, New York

Strauss SE, Haynes RB 2002 Evidence-based medicine in practice. American College of Physicians Journal Club 136(3):A11–A12

Strauss SE, Jones G 2004 What has evidence based medicine done for us? British Medical Journal 329(7473):987–988

Strauss SE, Green ML, Bell DS et al 2004 Evaluating the teaching of evidence based medicine: conceptual framework. British Medical Journal 329(7473):1029–1032

Strauss SE, Ball C, Balcombe N et al 2005 Teaching evidence-based medicine skills can change practice in a community hospital. Journal of General Internal Medicine 20:340–343

Taylor AH, Cable NT, Faulkner G et al 2004 Physical activity and older adults: a review of health benefits and the effectiveness of interventions. Journal of Sports Sciences 22:703–725

Warburton ER, Nicol CW, Bredin SSD 2006 Health benefits of physical activity: the evidence. Canadian Medical Association Journal 174:801–809

Section One

Management principles for musculoskeletal and neural tissue in the physical therapies

2 Muscle 9
3 Tendon 26
4 Ligament 42
5 Bone 59
6 Nerves 82
7 Cartilage 100

Muscle

Peter J. McNair and Andrew G. Cresswell

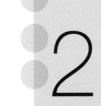

CHAPTER CONTENTS

Introduction 9

Gross structure of muscle 9

The contractile process 12

Factors influencing maximum force generation in a
muscle 13

Structures that influence the elasticity of muscle 16

Injury and disuse 17

Summary 22

Introduction

There are three types of muscle tissue within the body – skeletal muscle (striated voluntary), cardiac muscle (striated involuntary) and visceral (non-striated involuntary or smooth). This chapter will focus on skeletal muscle. Skeletal muscles develop force through contraction, which gives us the possibility of movement and interaction with our surroundings. In many pathological conditions muscle has been affected; either directly through injury or disease, or indirectly as a result of immobilization regimes. For the physical therapist to rehabilitate patients efficaciously, an understanding of muscle function is important. This chapter provides a foundation on which effective muscle training programs might be built. Its purpose is to examine the structure of muscle, its biomechanical characteristics and how those characteristics influence its function. This chapter will focus on the factors that influence the force generation capacity of muscle. It will also describe the changes that occur when muscle is in states of injury and disuse. Although the focus is predominantly on muscle structure, we recognize the importance of neural activation in generating force. This area, however, is beyond the scope of this chapter (see Chapter 6).

Gross structure of muscle

Fiber structure

To the naked eye, skeletal muscle is primarily made up of fibers. These fibers are grouped into bundles of approximately 10 to 20 fibers, each of which is called a fascicle. Each fascicle is surrounded by connective tissue (perimysium) that separates it from its neighboring fascicles. Muscle is built up from many such fascicles and is enclosed in a further thicker layer of connective tissue, the epimysium. Collagen fibers in all the layers of connective tissue are connected to the tendons at the end of the muscle. In this way, every individual muscle fiber is connected to the tendon and any force development from a muscle fiber will be exerted on the tendon.

At a microscopic level, each muscle fiber contains thousands of smaller units (myofibrils) which are responsible for contraction of the muscle (Fig. 2.1). A myofibril has a diameter of approximately 1 μm and is comprised of light and dark bands (striations) when viewed under a light microscope (Hess

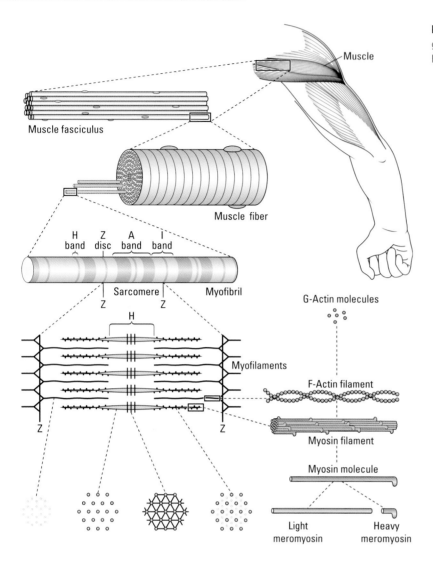

Figure 2.1 • The organization of skeletal muscle, from a gross to molecular level. (Reproduced from Guyton & Hall 2000 with the permission of WB Saunders.)

1967). The striations result from the myofibrils comprising two types of filaments (proteins): a thicker and darker, highly refractory A-band representing the myosin filament (containing 6 polypeptides, 2 heavy and 4 light chains, with a diameter of approximately 11 nm), and a thinner (7 nm) lighter and less refractory I-band representing the actin filament consisting of actin and two regulatory proteins troponin and tropomyosin (Huxley 1972). Both the myosin and actin filaments represent the smallest functional unit of the muscle. The myosin filaments are located centrally within a sarcomere and are held together at the M-region. The actin filaments make connections to the Z-disks, the boundary units between sarcomeres, where they receive partial structural support.

Close observation of the thicker myosin filament reveals that it has a head and tail configuration. The tail is comprised of two heavy molecular chains that are wound around each other. At one end of this chain are two globular heads. Attached to the myosin heads are two shorter and lighter amino acid chains.

The function of these light chains is to partially stabilize the myosin head and partly to modulate the interaction of actin and myosin (McComas 1996).

Actin is a globular protein comprised of approximately 300–400 actin molecules bound together in a chain approximately 1 μm long. Two such chains are twisted together to form a double-helical thin filament. Two strands of tropomyosin lie along the length of the actin filament, stiffening it. Troponin is a complex polypeptide and attaches to tropomyosin. One of the polypeptides, troponin T, attaches to tropomyosin, while troponin I binds to actin and indirectly prevents interaction with the myosin filament (Figs 2.2 and 2.3).

The sarcomere contains additional proteins other than actin and myosin to help organize the structure of the sarcomere. Proteins such as vimentin, desmin and synemin develop myofibril stability while integrin may help connect myofibrils to surrounding connective tissues. The protein nebulin appears to maintain the lattice array of actin (Labeit et al 1991), while titin,

A

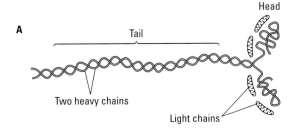

Head

Tail

Two heavy chains

Light chains

B

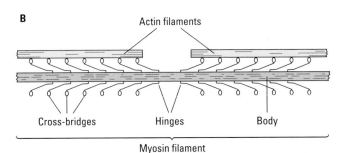

Actin filaments

Cross-bridges   Hinges   Body

Myosin filament

Figure 2.2 • A: Myosin molecule. **B:** Many myosin molecules and their relationship to the actin filaments. (Reproduced from Guyton & Hall 2000 with the permission of WB Saunders.)

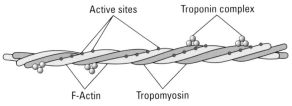

Active sites   Troponin complex

F-Actin   Tropomyosin

Figure 2.3 • Actin filament, composed of two helical strands, together with troponin and tropomyosin. Attached to one end of each tropomyosin molecule is a troponin complex that initiates contraction. (Reproduced from Guyton & Hall 2000 with the permission of WB Saunders.)

one of the largest proteins, are seen as thin strands connecting the myosin filament to the Z-disc (Trinick 1991). These strands are approximately 1 μm in length and are considered to be a longitudinal stabilizer for the myosin filament by keeping it centered within the sarcomere. It appears additionally to provide a degree of elasticity to the sarcomere when undergoing stretch, and also function as a template for the growth of the myosin filament.

Fiber types

Not all muscle fibers look alike; some fibers appear redder than others. A deep red color comes mostly from a denser network of capillaries leading to an increased amount of myoglobin, a red pigment with oxygen binding capability. Using histological methods such as enzyme histochemistry, it can be seen that the more red fibers contain higher amounts of oxidative enzymes and mitochondria. Such fibers are termed Type I fibers, and they

have greater aerobic capacity. There is a gradual change of color to paler whiter fibers that are larger in diameter, have fewer mitochondria and oxidative enzymes, but greater amounts of glycolitic enzymes. These paler fibers are known as Type II fibers and have a greater anaerobic capacity. Certain muscles have large percentages of Type I and II fibers (e.g. soleus or triceps brachii, respectively), while most are generally more mixed in their composition.

The so-called 'speed' or rate of shortening of each fiber type is also different. The rate of shortening is dependent on the characteristics of the myosin (i.e. how quickly ATP is broken down by the head of the myosin molecule, and how fast each cross-bridge cycle can be performed). In general, Type I fibers are constituted of slow myosin and are often referred to as slow-twitch fibers, while Type II fibers are made up of faster myosin and are called fast-twitch fibers. Fiber classification based on histochemical methods (i.e. typically staining for the enzymes myosin ATPase, phosphorylase, succinate dehydrogenase and malate) has determined that further classification of the Type II fibers is possible: Type IIA, Type IIAB and Type IIB (Gollnick et al 1972, Johnson et al 1973, Pette et al 1999, Thorstensson 1976) and Type IIC (Billeter et al 1980) are apparent. The difference between the Type IIA and B fibers is related to their relative aerobic ability, with Type IIA having greater aerobic potential. The IIC fibers are considered to have the foundation to form either Type IIA or IIB fibers. More recently, even more detailed ATPase staining techniques has revealed at least seven fiber types in human skeletal muscle with a Type IC and IIAC being added (Pette et al 1999). The technique of immunocytochemistry has been able to identify an additional fiber type based on the properties of myosin heavy chain isoforms (Larsson et al 1991). This newly identified Type IIX lies between IIA and IIB (Schiaffino & Reggiani 1994, Smerdu et al 1994), and it seems likely that in human skeletal muscle the earlier classified Type IIB fibers are actually of the Type IIX.

In general, the slow aerobic-oxidative Type I fibers are used continuously in the maintenance of posture while the faster anaerobic-glycolitic Type II fibers are used more intermittently for force development. When the force twitch of these fibers is recorded, and the interval between the onset of the twitch and the peak force is measured, the faster fiber types can have contraction times as low as 20 ms, while the slower fibers have times as protracted as 140 ms. In whole muscle, however, the muscle twitch depends on the fiber type proportions of the muscle. For example, the triceps surae has a high percentage of slow twitch fibers (approximately 80%, Gollnick et al 1974), and has a contraction time of approximately 120 ms (Sale et al 1982), while the biceps brachii has a higher percentage of fast twitch fibers (approximately 62%, Johnson et al 1973, Nygaard et al 1983) which results in a contraction time of only 65 ms (Bellemare et al 1983). Aging is generally associated with a reduction in muscle fiber size (sarcopenia) with Type II fibers being the most affected (Korhonen et al 2006, Larsson et al 1979). This, along with the fact that aging results in a greater expression of slow myosin heavy chain isoforms (Hameed et al 2003, Short et al 2005), results in a decrease in the ratio of the Type II to Type I fiber area. These changes are believed to result in an overall decrease in muscle force producing capacity and shortening velocity (Frontera et al 2000, Klitgaard et al 1990). In contrast, exercise, training and rehabilitation are known stimuli that can lead to fiber size increase (hypertrophy) and plastic changes in muscle fiber type. A change from Type IIB to IIA appears readily possible (Pette & Staron 1997) after specific training, and in some exceptional circumstances a change from Type I to II can occur. Whether significant changes in the direction of fast to slow occur is not presently known.

The contractile process

Force is generated in a muscle fiber when actin and myosin filaments interact. This event commences with action potentials spreading across the muscle fibers at approximately $3–5\,\mathrm{m\,s^{-1}}$. The potentials also spread deep within the fibers by way of the T-tubules (Peachey 1965a, 1965b), which have close contact with the terminal cisternae of the sarcoplasmic reticulum. The gap between these two structures is bridged by two proteins – a dihydropyridine receptor (DHP) and a ryanodin receptor (RYR). During rest, the ryanodin receptor channels are closed and Ca^{2+}

remains within the sarcoplasmic reticulum. Depolarization of the T-tubules results in activation of the dihydropyridine receptors which in turn causes the ryanodin receptor to open its Ca^{2+} channel and rapidly release Ca^{2+} along its concentration gradient out from the sarcoplasmic reticulum, thereby increasing cytostolic Ca^{2+} (Peachey 1965a, 1965b).

Figure 2.4 shows the transverse tubule–sarcoplasmic reticulum system. At rest, the binding sites for myosin on the actin filament are covered; however, with the release of Ca^{2+}, troponin undergoes a conformational change. This change lifts the tropomyosin molecule away from the actin filament and exposes sites on the actin filament for myosin head attachment, and allows the contraction to commence. Pumps in the sarcoplasmic reticulum continuously pump Ca^{2+} back into the sarcoplasmic reticulum. At rest, this event results in the concentration of Ca^{2+} in the sarcoplasmic reticulum being higher than that in the cytosol. When neural activation of a muscle ceases, Ca^{2+} is released from troponin and quickly pumped out of the cytosol. Tropomyosin then returns to its original position on actin and prevents any further binding of myosin to actin. Since the pump has to transport Ca^{2+} against its concentration gradient, adenosine triphosphate (ATP) is required to provide the necessary energy.

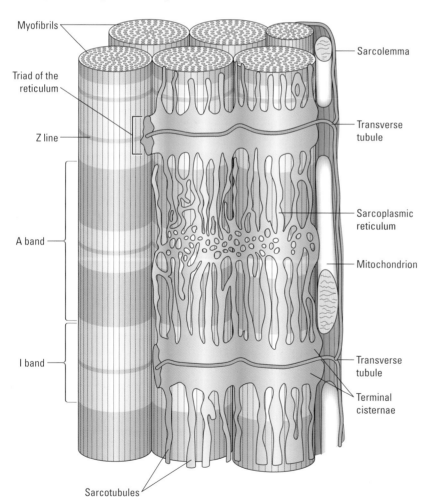

Myofibrils
Triad of the reticulum
Z line
A band
I band
Sarcotubules
Sarcolemma
Transverse tubule
Sarcoplasmic reticulum
Mitochondrion
Transverse tubule
Terminal cisternae

Figure 2.4 • The transverse (T) tubule-sarcoplasmic reticulum system. This illustration was drawn from frog muscle, which has one T-tubule per sarcomere, located at the z line. Mammalian skeletal muscle has two T-tubules per sarcomere, located at the A–I junction. (Reproduced from Guyton & Hall 2000 with the permission of WB Saunders.)

The force development is a result of the myosin heads, also called cross-bridges, bending while attached to the actin filament (Huxley & Simmons 1971, Narici 1999). After the cross-bridges have bent, they are released from actin, straighten, and then re-attach to a new actin site (Fig. 2.5). These events are termed cross-bridge cycling, and form the basis of the sliding filament theory (Huxley 1957, Huxley & Hanson 1954, Huxley & Simmons 1971). For their occurrence, energy is needed, and that is obtained by the splitting of ATP to adenosine diphosphate (ADP) and inorganic phosphate (P).

A single action potential that spreads over the fiber gives rise to a momentary increase in force that is called a muscle twitch (Huijing 1998). If rapidly repeated action potentials travel across the muscle fiber, Ca^{2+} cannot be pumped back into the sarcoplasmic reticulum before the next action potential arrives and the next release of Ca^{2+} takes place. This results in repeated cross-bridge cycling and a rapid summation of individual force twitches. If the action potentials arrive with a short inter-potential interval, individual twitches cannot be discerned from the force trace and the muscle is said to have reached tetanus. A muscle fiber generates its maximal force during tetanus (Fig. 2.6).

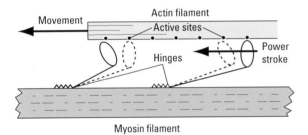

Figure 2.5 • Crossbridge formation and motion. (Reproduced from Guyton & Hall 2000 with the permission of WB Saunders.)

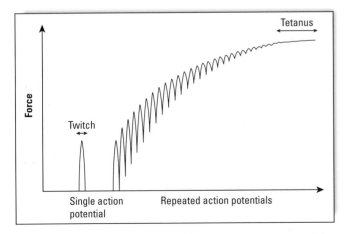

Figure 2.6 • Force change associated with a single action potential, and the effect of repeated action potentials.

Factors influencing maximum force generation in a muscle

In vitro and in vivo measurements of muscle force

In vitro recordings of maximal forces can readily be gathered from either single muscle fibers or single muscles activated by electrical stimulation. It is difficult to study force development of single muscles in humans, primarily due to tetanic stimulation of muscle being extremely painful to the subject, spread of current to nearby muscles is difficult to control, and if the subject is operating the intensity control, it is not certain whether complete activation of the muscle has taken place (Herbert & Gandevia 1999, Westing et al 1990). Furthermore, it is not currently possible in humans to directly measure the force developed by the muscle. Methods for measurement of muscle forces have been developed for animal preparations, with buckle-type force transducers being used by several research groups (Gregor et al 1988, Walmsley et al 1978, Whiting et al 1984). This type of transducer is placed around the tendon of a freely moving animal, and gives a signal that is proportional to the muscular force. A similar type of buckle transducer has also been implanted with some success around the Achilles tendon in humans (Fukashiro et al 1995, Gregor et al 1991, Walmsley et al 1978); however, the transducer output gives Achilles tendon force and not the forces of the individual muscles of the triceps surae. Moreover, the difficulty of transducer calibration and discomfort to the subject has limited their extended use. A more recent and somewhat less invasive technique has been the use of fiberoptics, where a thin fiberoptic cable is placed though the tendon and the light distortion as a result of increased tension can then be used to estimate tendon and muscle force (Erdemir et al 2004, Finni et al 1998).

Less invasive measurements of muscle force usually involve voluntary muscle activation and the use of a load cell or dynamometer. For their calculation, a knowledge of two lever arm distances is also needed. The first being that between the force transducer and the center of rotation of the joint, and the second is the lever arm between the center of rotation of the joint and line of action of the muscle force (Fig. 2.7). These distances are particularly difficult to ascertain when the center of rotation of a joint shifts as the joint rotates through its range of motion. Traditionally, such measures have been obtained from cadavers (Spoor et al 1990); however, the recent use of magnetic resonance imaging (MRI) and ultrasonography has allowed more accurate and straightforward estimation of in vivo joint-muscle lever arm lengths for the elbow (Fukunaga et al 2001), rotator cuff (Juul-Kristensen et al 2000a, 2000b), spine (Tveit et al 1994), knee (Narici et al 1988, Spoor & van Leeuwen 1992) and ankle (Fukunaga et al 1996) joints.

The calculations presented in Fig. 2.7 apply to muscle actions that are isometric. To measure muscle forces when a joint is in motion, knowledge of the moment of inertia of the moving limb and the angular acceleration of the joint is required.

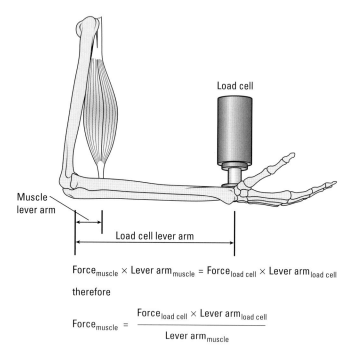

Force$_{muscle}$ × Lever arm$_{muscle}$ = Force$_{load\ cell}$ × Lever arm$_{load\ cell}$

therefore

$$Force_{muscle} = \frac{Force_{load\ cell} \times Lever\ arm_{load\ cell}}{Lever\ arm_{muscle}}$$

Figure 2.7 • The lever arms and forces associated with the calculation of torques.

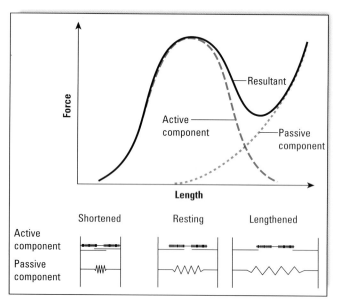

Figure 2.8 • The force–length relationship, and the interaction of the contractile and passive elements.

The moment of inertia is usually obtained from tables based on measurements taken on cadaveric specimens. Angular acceleration is usually acquired from recording the motion of interest with an electrogoniometer, optoelectronic movement analysis system or by video.

Force–length relationship

The amount of force a muscle fiber can develop during maximal activation is dependent on the number of established cross-bridges. This, in turn, means that the force that can be developed is dependent on the length of the muscle (Gordon et al 1966, Rack & Westbury 1969). During maximal activation, the greatest force development occurs with the muscle at its resting length (a sarcomere length of approximately 2.2 μm). At shorter lengths, the thin actin filaments begin to interfere with each other due to their overlap, cross-bridge formation is hindered and force development is reduced. As the sarcomere becomes even shorter (below approximately 1.7 μm), the decrease in force is thought to be related to the forces that are required to deform the thicker myofilament. Reduced Ca^{2+} release from the sarcoplasmic reticulum at shorter than optimal lengths (Rudel & Taylor 1971), however, may also be a contributing factor to the force reduction. At lengths above 2.2 μm, fewer binding sites are available for the myosin heads. This results in a reduction in active force production. To counter this loss of force, the stretch of passive tissues within the muscle (epimysium, perimysium, endomysium, titin, and nebulin) and tendon increases the passive force and hence total force is less affected (Fig. 2.8). The amount of force development by

the passive tissues varies between muscles in accordance with differences in architecture and the amount of connective tissue (Woittiez et al 1983).

Force–velocity relationship

A muscle can actively shorten if an external load generates less force than that being produced internally (often termed a concentric muscle action). The velocity of muscle shortening and its relationship to force development is well documented (Fenn & Marsh 1935, Hill 1938), with higher forces being generated at slower shortening velocities. As shortening velocity increases, the rate of cross-bridge cycling increases, the average force exerted by each cross-bridge decreases and there may even be fewer cross-bridges attached. If a muscle is not working against a load, then it can reach maximal shortening velocities in the order of 10 muscle lengths per second (Edman 1979). Most muscles, however, have distinctly slower maximum shortening velocities, but are surprisingly constant over a large range of sarcomere lengths (Edman 1979).

If the force generated by an external load is greater than the force being produced internally, the muscle undergoes active lengthening (often termed an eccentric muscle action). Depending on the experimental techniques used, the maximal force recorded for a lengthening muscle action can be similar to or greater than that recorded for an isometric muscle activation. For isolated muscle preparations (in vitro), the force developed during lengthening increases rapidly above its isometric value, and at fast lengthening velocities can reach 1.8 times that developed isometrically (Abbott & Aubert 1951, Katz 1939). This large increase is probably due to the rate of cross-bridge detachment being slower than during shortening actions at the same velocity (Rassier & Herzog 2005), and to a stiffening of titin within the parallel elastic elements of muscle fibers (Pinniger et al 2006). A reduction in detachment rate would result in the cross-bridges remaining attached and being forcibly stretched until detachment finally takes place. Stretching beyond the normal range of cross-bridge attachment thereby results in utilization of elasticity within the cross-bridge and thus increased force development (Abbott & Aubert 1951, Edman 1979).

The advent of the isokinetic dynamometer has enabled the experimenter to record the net joint torque while moving the limb through a prescribed range of motion at a specified angular velocity. The in vivo relationship between muscle force and linear velocity of muscle shortening or lengthening is then inferred from the measurement of angle specific or peak joint torques recorded at various angular velocities. Several studies on the force–velocity relationship have been made in humans for the knee extensors (Harris & Dudley 1994, Perrine & Edgerton 1978, Thorstensson et al 1976, Westing et al 1988), elbow flexors (Hortobagyi & Katch 1990, Komi 1973, Pousson et al 1999) and plantar flexor muscles (Fugl-Meyer et al 1980, Gerdle & Langstrom 1987, Pinniger et al 2000).

Most data for shortening muscle action appear similar to those for isolated muscle. However, compared to isolated muscle, in vivo force measurements appear to plateau and be slightly lower as the velocity approaches zero (Perrine & Edgerton 1978). Isometric torques are, however, most often greater than the torques recorded during shortening muscle actions. During in vivo lengthening muscle action, the maximum joint torque generally fails to increase above the isometric value, regardless of length-ening velocity (Aagaard et al 1995, Dudley et al 1990, Westing et al 1991). However, there does appear to be slight differences between muscle groups, and the level of training of the subjects under investigation (Aagaard et al 1996, Dudley et al 1990). For example, subjects who have been provided with practice sessions will often be able to generate higher forces. Thus, the inability to exceed forces produced isometrically, regardless of the angular velocity, may reflect a neural inhibitory process that limits voluntary torque production (Westing et al 1990, 1991). Some support for this idea comes from comparing levels of voluntary muscle activation across velocities during lengthening, shortening, and isometric actions (Aagaard et al 2000, Westing et al 1991), as well as from data collected during in vivo torque measurements produced via percutaneous electrical stimulation (Dudley et al 1990, Westing et al 1991).

The power that a muscle can generate (the rate at which it can produce work) can be deduced from the force–velocity relationship (Hill 1938). Power can be measured as the product of force and velocity, and can be viewed as the area under the force velocity curve (Fig. 2.9). It is zero when the muscle action is isometric, and when the muscle is not working against a load. Generally, it has been observed that maximum power is developed at velocities corresponding to 30–40% of the maximal shortening velocity of the muscle. This can read-ily be identified in cycling where changing gears results in load changes that allow the muscle to continuously work at its opti-mal shortening velocity (Sargeant et al 1981). Unfortunately

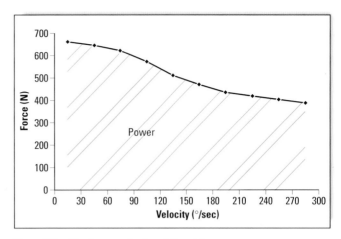

Figure 2.9 • The force–velocity relationship.

due to aging, there is a reduction in muscle mass and a reduc-tion in optimal velocity of shortening which contribute to an overall decrease in muscle power of approximately 10% per decade (Kostka 2005).

Muscle architecture

Muscle architecture cannot be overlooked when consider-ing the maximal force that a muscle might generate. The most commonly measured architectural features of muscle are related to volume, fiber length and pennation angle. Until recently, such measurements have been difficult or impossi-ble to gather for living human muscle, and cadaver material has provided much of the available information (Wickiewicz et al 1983). The advent of MRI, and in particular ultrasound equipment, has allowed in vivo measurements of muscle fiber architecture during not only rest, but also during active, iso-metric, shortening and lengthening muscle actions (Herbert & Gandevia 1995, Narici 1999, Rutherford & Jones 1992). Studies that have used such equipment have shown that pen-nation angle and fiber length, and thus physiological cross-sectional area, are dependent on joint position and the level of muscle activation (Herbert & Gandevia 1995). For example, for the medial gastrocnemius, pennation angle and fiber length decrease as the ankle joint angle increases, thereby resulting in an increase of the physiological cross-sectional area (Narici et al 1996). Increased voluntary activation of the medial gastrocnemius resulted in a 35% decrease in fiber length, and a 100% increase in pennation angle resulting in a 35% increase in physiological cross-sectional area (Narici et al 1996). Such findings cast some doubt on the calculations of cross-sectional area, and thus force potential that have previously been calcu-lated using data gained from cadavers.

The theoretical force potential of a muscle can be calcu-lated if the maximum force that can be generated per unit of cross-sectional area and the cross-sectional area of the muscle is known. The former variable appears to be at best $40\,\mathrm{N\,cm^{-2}}$. However, this value, depending on the study, varies between 15 and $40\,\mathrm{N\,cm^{-2}}$ (Edgerton et al 1990, Kanda & Hashizume

1992, Nygaard et al 1983). The wide range in these values may be attributed to differences in gender and muscle architecture (Ettema & Huijing 1994). It is also evident that the maximum force per unit area is not dependent on muscle fiber type (Bottinelli et al 1996, Herbert & Gandevia 1995). Thus, the amount of total force produced by a muscle is directly related to its cross-sectional area. Although there are differences in the diameters of fibers within a muscle, the largest contributor to the different forces produced by different muscles is the absolute number of muscle fibers. Such numbers can range from approximately 4.0×10^4 for the first dorsal interossei to 1.0×10^6 for the medial gastrocnemius (Feinstein et al 1955).

The physiological cross-sectional area of muscle can be calculated with a knowledge of the mass and density ($1.056\,\mathrm{g\,cm^{-3}}$) of the muscle together with information related to fiber length. Mass and density are determinants of the muscle's volume, which are reflected in the different shapes of muscles in the body. The diversity in shape of each muscle often results in the line of pull of individual fibers being quite different, and this can influence their force capability. Generally speaking, muscles are grouped according to the orientation of their fasciculi. These fasciculi are most often arranged either parallel or oblique to the final direction of pull at their insertion. Some muscles (e.g. sartorius) have fibers primarily parallel to the line of pull. Others (e.g. biceps brachii) can also have a similar arrangement in the belly of a fusiform muscle and the fibers converge to a tendon at either one or both ends of the muscle. Such muscles have longer muscle fibers and hence will have greater displacement potential, and are more effective at changing length quickly.

The length of a muscle fiber is determined by the number of sarcomeres in series. There are quite large differences in the number of sarcomeres per fiber, with long strap muscles like sartorius, which adducts and flexes the leg, having approximately 15.5×10^4 sarcomeres per fiber while the shorter plantar flexors, soleus and medial gastrocnemius have approximately 1.4×10^4 and 1.5×10^4 sarcomeres per fiber, respectively (Wickiewicz et al 1983). These numbers are often based on the premise that individual fibers run the full length of the muscle. In a number of instances, however, this is not the case. For instance, several of the longer strap muscles (e.g. rectus abdominis) have discrete compartments, defined by fibrous bands. These compartments result in significantly shorter muscle fiber lengths with sarcomere numbers in the region of 5.5×10^4 (Chleboun et al 2001, McComas 1996). Such compartmentalization is likely to make force transmission throughout the muscle more complicated than if fibers extend the entire length of the muscle.

A limitation of muscles with longer muscle fibers is that they are less effective at generating force. The potential to generate force will be proportional to the number of sarcomeres in parallel. Fasciculi that are oblique to the line of pull are often described as being pennate (feather-like). Pennate muscles (e.g. gastrocnemius) typically have a long tendon running through the muscle to which short muscle fibers are attached at angles that generally range from 5 to 20°. The fiber organization of a pennate muscle ensures a relatively large physiological cross-sectional area since there can be many more fibers packed within the muscle. A larger cross-sectional area results in an increase in force potential even though the force contribution of each fiber is reduced due to its angle of pull. Pennate muscle fibers have significantly fewer sarcomeres in series than parallel fibered muscle. Therefore, for the same decrease in fiber length, the relative shortening per sarcomere length will be greater for a short fiber (Narici 1999). The muscle is therefore less suited to situations that demand long length changes or high velocity length changes.

Structures that influence the elasticity of muscle

The connective tissues of muscle can be divided into three structures that are based on their position within muscle. Epimysium envelops the entire muscle, perimysium surrounds bundles of muscle fibers and endomysium provides a cover for the basement membrane of individual muscle fibers. Endomysium and perimysium are linked to one another, and these tissues are thought to provide a framework on which the muscle fibers attach and gain support. When muscle is stretched, it is thought that endomysium and perimysium are largely responsible for the passive tension generated in muscle at high sarcomere lengths. Purslow (1989) and Purslow & Trotter (1994) examined the morphology and mechanical properties of both endomysial and perimysial tissues. These authors noted that at resting muscle lengths the endomysial network was composed of wavy collagen fibrils arranged with a mean orientation to the muscle fibers of 60°. Perimysium was more organized with a cross-ply structural arrangement of crimped collagen fibers at a similar angle. A more complex arrangement has recently been described by Jarvinen et al (2002) who described endomysium and perimysium as having longitudinal and circularly organized collagen fibers. The complexity of this network varied across muscles, which probably reflected differences in requirements related to function. Purslow (1989) and Purslow & Trotter (1994) observed that tensile stiffness was minimal at the resting length in both endomysial and perimysial tissues. When the muscle fibers were stretched to high sarcomere lengths, the angle of the collagen fibers to the muscle fibers in both endomysium and perimysium decreased, and the respective wavy and crimped appearance of these tissues was lost. Thus at high sarcomere lengths, it has been suggested that both endomysium and perimysium may prevent overstretching of muscle (Purslow 1989, Purslow & Trotter 1994).

It is also apparent that the contractile elements have elastic properties. Short-range stiffness is a term used to describe the ratio of change in force to change in length of the muscle fibers when stretched. When muscle fibers are activated, short-range stiffness is noted until fibers are stretched past approximately 1% of muscle length (Malamud et al 1996). Thereafter, a yielding of the fibers is noted and resistance in the tissues decreases. It has been shown that the short-range stiffness increases with muscle activation levels, and hence has been related to the number of cross bridges formed between actin and myosin at the time of a rapid stretch (Ford et al 1981). It is has also been shown that Type I muscle fibers are stiffer than Type II fibers (Malamud et al 1996), and these findings have been related to the time course of the detachment and reattachment of cross-bridges.

Research involving x-ray techniques (Huxley et al 1994) has shown that elasticity lies within the myofilaments, and particularly within a protein named connectin (also termed titin) (Horowits et al 1986). Biochemical techniques have shown that individual filaments of connectin are attached from the z-line to the central region of the thick filament. Between the z-line and the myosin filament, the connectin is most elastic, whereas the section of connectin that is bound to the myosin filament is considerably less so (Higuchi 1996). Horowits (1992) has shown that much of the resting tension in sarcomeres is due to connectin, and that at long sarcomere lengths, connectin becomes considerably more resistant to stretch. Connectin's role is also to center the thick myosin filament within the sarcomere, that is, prevent myosin from moving toward either z-line (Horowits et al 1986). This is particularly important when actin and myosin are interacting to generate force. In doing so, connectin will also keep sarcomere length relatively constant across the length of the muscle fiber during muscle activation.

Injury and disuse

It is apparent that when muscle is injured, the damage results in a decrease in the force generation capacity of muscle. Similarly, when joints are immobilized, muscles near to that joint are affected, and their capacity to generate force decreases. This section describes the changes that occur to muscle structure with injury and disuse. Due to ethical constraints, most experiments in muscle healing have been undertaken using animals, primarily rodents. Borisov (1999) examined how well these animals represent the processes occurring in humans and stated that although there are similarities in the structure of the contractile mechanisms in skeletal muscles, there are distinct differences in the intensity and time course over which the restoration processes occur across species. He also suggested that the phylogenic age of the species is an important factor influencing the regenerative processes. Therefore, caution should be exercised when making inferences concerning the behavior of human tissues in response to injury and disuse.

The mechanism of injury

Two models are commonly used to induce an injury to muscle, and they supposedly simulate the contusion and strain injury paradigms. In the former, a mass (e.g. steel ball) is projected by a spring like device or by gravity to strike the tissue of interest. The shape of the mass and its momentum at impact will determine the magnitude of the injury. To simulate strain injuries, the animal's musculotendinous unit is exposed and one end is attached to an electromechanical device that lengthens the tissues at a particular rate. These rates range between 1 and $10\,cm\,min^{-1}$, which is relatively slow compared to the velocity

of lengthening that can occur during functional activities. The resistance of tissue to stretching (force) is also often measured. Despite the uniformity of each of the procedures to create the injury, some authors (Minamoto et al 1999) have noted considerable variation in the extent of damage inflicted on different animals.

To assess the extent of damage that has occurred as a result of these insults, researchers will kill some of the animals immediately after the injury, dissect out the muscle of interest, and provide a qualitative description of the injury site using light or electron microscopy. The healing process can also be monitored by regular histological and immunohistochemistry (Kasemkjwattana et al 1998). These techniques might be used to monitor the expression of molecules such as desmin and vimentin, and thus provide measures of fiber regeneration and fibrosis, respectively. Researchers may also electrically stimulate the muscle soon after injury, and describe the change in maximal force that the muscle can generate.

Regeneration of the contractile elements

Although the mechanisms of injury are different for contusion and strain injuries, the regeneration of the contractile elements follows a similar pattern, and begins with the activation of satellite cells. Normally these cells are non-active in adults, and lie between the basal lamina and the sarcolemma of the muscle fiber (Mauro 1961). There is evidence that the number of satellite cells varies according to fiber type, with greater numbers observed in Type I muscle fibers (Snow 1983). Recent evidence (Zammit et al 2004) suggests that satellite cells may be self proliferating and hence some are activated for the repair of damaged fibers while others replicate to maintain the satellite cell pool. Contact with the basement membrane, and the presence of various molecules is thought to inhibit their activity (Anderson 2000, Bischoff 1990). When the basal lamina of the muscle fiber is disrupted during injury, a number of events have been implicated in activating mitotic activity in the satellite cells. They include the shear forces as the injury occurs, hypercontraction of the myofibrils, retraction of the damaged fibers and the release of human growth factors and chemicals such as nitric oxide (Anderson 2000). Thereafter, the satellite cells become less adherent to the basement membrane, become more active and proliferate. The expression of genes and DNA synthesis important to regeneration then commences.

Hurme et al (1991a) reported that immediately after the trauma, muscle fibers that are ruptured retract and a gap is formed. At the ends of the retracted ruptured fibers, the intact sarcomeres have been observed to be hypercontracted immediately after the injury, and this activity is thought to block the inflow of inflammatory cells into the fiber and hence restrict their activity. Within hours, a membrane is formed that separates the intact sarcomeres of a fiber from the injury site (Carpenter & Karpati 1989).

At the time of trauma, numerous blood vessels are also torn, and the gap between the retracted fibers is initially filled with blood. The release of cytokines at the time of injury attract leucocytes and macrophages to the injury site (Robertson et al 1993). The relative contributions of different inflammatory cells to muscle regeneration are not known. There is evidence that satellite cells can regulate the degree to which inflammatory cells come to the damaged area (Chazaud et al 2003). Within the first 2 days after injury the macrophages become the dominant inflammatory cell at the injury site and their role is to remove necrotic tissue which includes cellular fragments and sarcoplasm from the damaged fibers (Grounds 1991). There is also some evidence to support their role in mediating satellite cell proliferation through chemotaxis (Kuschel et al 2000). Between 5 and 7 days after injury, the number of leucocytes and macrophages decreases considerably. Their numbers, however, can be influenced by physical activity in the first few days after injury. In this respect, Lehto et al (1985) noted that 5 days after injury, there were few inflammatory cells observed in animals that had been immobilized. In contrast, significant numbers of these cells were still present in animals mobilized with a treadmill running program 2 days after injury.

It is apparent that the fibers tear in a manner that leaves remnants of the tube like structure of the basal lamina intact but often with ragged ends (Hurme et al 1991a). The ragged edges of the basal lamina act as scaffolding for activated satellite cells, which are termed myoblasts. These fuse with one another to form a myotube within days of the injury (Fig. 2.10). Where

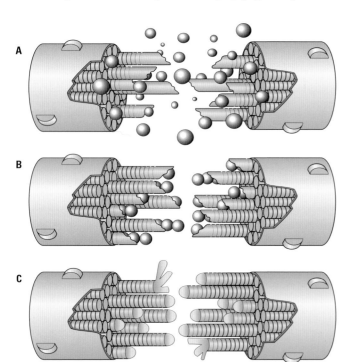

Figure 2.10 • A: The proliferation of satellite cells and subsequently myoblasts occurs in the first day after injury. **B:** Myoblasts are attracted to the ends of the surviving fibers. They subsequently fuse and growth begins. **C:** The new myotubes grow toward the central region from the periphery. Some myotubes split at their tips possibly to increase the chance of reuniting with the approaching myotubes from the other side of the injury site.

this process occurs in the old basal lamina, it is more likely that the new myotubes will fuse with the capped off surviving fibers. These myotubes then take on the characteristics (fast or slow fiber types) of the muscle fiber to which they have joined (Zhang & Dhoot 1998). Zhang & Dhoot (1998) commented that perhaps specific myoblasts might only fuse with specific types of fibers. In most instances, the growth of the myotube is across the gap between the retracted fibers. Some authors (e.g. Jarvinen & Lehto 1993) have described the new fiber as having a gradient of maturity, with areas closest to the original fiber displaying features more like undamaged muscle and the tip being the least developed.

Hurme et al (1991a) observed that at 7 days post injury, myotubes had grown within the damaged basal lamina and a new basal lamina was apparent. Once the myotube leaves the remnants of the old basal lamina and begins to traverse the central gap between fibers, it has been observed to split into multiple branches. It is thought that splitting may improve the chances of one branch being able to successfully pass through the collagen tissue of the central zone (Hurme et al 1991a). Lehto et al (1985) reported that the myotubes were more interlaced amongst the granulation tissue in rats that were immobilized immediately after injury compared to animals that had experienced early mobilization.

The stimulus for the myotubes to continue growing is not known; however, Hurme et al (1991a) suggested three factors that may be involved in the process. First, satellite cells may migrate along the new myotube to the tip. Second, the tip may grow from interactions with undifferentiated cells encountered in the central zone. Finally, there is also evidence of vesicular structures within the myotube that could supply essential materials to the tip. The maturation of myotubes into myofibers has been observed to occur after approximately 14 days (Kaariainen et al 1998). Whether the myofibers from each side of the injury site meet and subsequently fuse is questionable. Kaariainen et al (2000) suggested that the tip may adhere to the intervening scar tissues and form a 'mini musculotendinous junction'. While the scar tissue may decrease over months, and the tips become closer and interlaced, they may never actually fuse. Recent research by Aarimaa et al (2004) showed that maintaining close apposition of the muscle fibers after injury significantly reduced the presence of these new junctions, and that the regeneration of fibers was greatly enhanced with the overall strength of the tissue notably improved.

Regeneration of the connective tissue elements

Jarvinen & Lehto (1993) suggested that there are two competitive processes occurring during muscle regeneration after injury: regeneration of the myofibrils and the production of scar tissue. Like myofibril regeneration, there is a sequence of events that occur to lay down collagen in the injured area. These events are linked to and are important for the successful regeneration of the myofibrils.

Within hours of the injury, fibronectin is observed at the injury site. This substance, which is derived from plasma, adheres to strands of fibrin and forms scaffolding on which fibroblasts attach in the next few days (Lehto et al 1985). The fibroblasts produce Type I and III collagen, the latter being observed earlier. In rats, by 5 days it has been observed that connective tissue made up of Type III collagen together with granulation tissue is seen extensively in the gap between the retracted fibers, and it provides the initial strength of the injured area (Lehto et al 1985). As the repair process continues, Type I collagen becomes more predominant.

Lehto et al (1985) reported that a treadmill-running program instigated 2 days after injury for rats led to a sustained presence of fibronectin and a fibrin clot in the damaged area. Interestingly, in the following weeks, these rats developed a dense network of scar tissue in the endomysial and perimysial structures. Furthermore, increased deposits of fat at the injury site were also observed. In contrast, animals that had been immobilized for 5 days had much greater resorption of scar tissue 8 weeks after injury. A ramification of excessive scar tissue is that the extensibility of the tissues is reduced. In this respect, Kaariainen et al (1998) reported that strain values remained at approximately 50% of control values at a 56-day follow-up of rat muscles that had sustained a laceration injury.

In respect to the strength of the tissues, stretching the muscle to failure has been shown to primarily occur at the site of injury during the first week after injury (Jarvinen & Lehto 1993, Kaariainen et al 1998). Thereafter, the site of injury becomes increasingly more likely to be within the intact myofibers. Jarvinen & Lehto (1993) suggested that this finding is due to the increased amount of scar tissue at the injury site, and Kaariainen et al (1998) commented that it may indicate that the strength of the adhesions of the myotubes to the newly laid connective tissue is greater than that of the atrophied muscle fibers. These authors (Kaariainen et al 1998) reported that although force to failure was significantly decreased (50% of control values from day 10 to 56 following injury), when the cross-sectional area of the tissue was accounted for, the injured muscle had recovered its strength by day 21.

Thus, in summary, it seems that there is a need to provide a period of rest soon after injury. In doing so, the amount of scar tissue laid down is limited and less dense, and the regenerating myofibrils can penetrate this tissue more easily. In doing so, it is speculated that normal muscle performance might be achieved. Alternatively, mobilizing the muscle early after the injury will strengthen the tissue more quickly; however the density of connective tissue may act as a physical barrier that prevents the myofibrils from joining. Intuitively, this barrier might affect muscle activation patterns, and the additional junction caused by the scarring may predispose the area to recurring injury in the future. Furthermore, it is apparent that the scar tissue can affect the extensibility of the tissues. Muscle atrophy can be a source of structural weakness in the muscle, and so while the rehabilitation process may require a short period of immobilization, it should not be prolonged. The length of time of immobilization, however, is not known for the

human model. In the rat, it appears to be between 3 and 5 days.

When muscle is damaged by a contusion type injury, it is apparent that damage occurs not only to the muscle fibers but also to the nerves supplying those fibers. This damage can extend from minor disruption of myelin to complete rupture of the intramuscular nerves depending on the location of the injury and the forces involved. Hurme et al (1991b) noted that in the first 1–2 days following damage, phagocytic cells were present in the perineurial sheath. The depolarization of the nerves was affected with spontaneous action potentials being observed intermittently from 5 days after injury. These potentials were not present at 14 days and these authors suggested that this provided evidence that reinnervation was occurring at this time.

The effect of immobilization on muscle

After many injuries, a joint is placed in an immobilized state and muscle activity about the joint decreases. While the muscles may not be damaged, an inactive muscle undergoes rapid changes in structure, and consequently function. The most obvious change is muscle atrophy. Normally, a balance between protein synthesis and degradation maintains the mass of the contractile elements. Within hours of immobilization, protein synthesis decreases, and over a day protein degradation increases. Currently, there is much interest in identifying genes involved in the regulation of muscle contractile proteins. Changes in gene expression allow an appreciation of the pathways that might be operating as muscle becomes atrophied, and provide markers for the assessment of therapeutic interventions which might limit atrophy. Stevenson et al (2003) identified 309 genes that were activated during disuse atrophy. They noted that these genes could be clustered into groups that reflected the time at which particular atrophic processes occurred, and that some genes may activate for short periods, while others remain active throughout the entire immobilization period.

Three prominent and related chemical pathways are involved in the degradation of proteins: calpain, lysomal cathepsin and ubiquitin-proteasome (Kandarian & Stevenson 2002). While the last pathway has been shown to play the major role in protein degradation, to be most effective, it relies on others. For example, for protein breakdown to commence, the normal orientation and architecture of the actin and myosin within the sarcomere must be disrupted. Chemicals such as calpain have been shown to cleave/cut bonds (i.e. titin, nebulin) important to the structural integrity of the sarcomeric proteins leading to their disassembly and subsequent breakdown by the ubiquitin-proteasome pathway. Although calpain has a specific chemical inhibitor, its activation levels are also influenced by the amount of calcium within the sarcomere. Increased levels of Ca lead to increased amounts of calpain. The mechanism that stimulates increased calcium levels to be released is not known, although recent findings (see review by Powers et al 2005) suggest that oxidative stress may influence the removal of calcium within the muscle cell. Oxidative stress occurs when antioxidants are of insufficient numbers to buffer the increase in oxidants that occur with inactivity. Powers et al (2005) highlight the importance of oxidative stress, and suggest that both the calpain- and proteosomal-mediated pathways can be influenced by this mechanism. There is also evidence that the supplementation of antioxidants such as vitamin E (Appell et al 1997), and the application of heat (Selsby & Dodd 2005) can decrease oxidative stress and reduce the amount of muscle atrophy.

The magnitude and the rate of change in these processes differ across muscles and individual animals (Booth & Seider 1979, Goldspink 1977). Goldspink (1977) reported that over a 3-day period of immobilization with the muscle in a shortened state, the net weight of the animals' muscles decreased by 30%. Nicks et al (1989) examined whether such changes reflected modifications to either fiber size or fiber number. These researchers observed that following immobilization for 8 weeks, the fiber area of a rat's triceps brachii was decreased by 42%, whereas fiber numbers were unchanged. The position in which a muscle is immobilized influences the magnitude of atrophy considerably. Muscles that are immobilized in a shortened position are most affected. When muscles are immobilized in a lengthened state, they may increase in weight. For instance, Goldspink (1977) noted a 10% increase in muscle weight in the extensor digitorum muscle after three days of immobilization.

Related to these changes in muscle mass is a modification in the number of sarcomeres in series. In the early 1970s, Tabary et al (1972) reported that immobilization of a cat's soleus muscles in a plaster cast for four weeks in a shortened position led to a 40% decrease in sarcomeres in series. Tabary et al also noted that when these muscles were immobilized in a lengthened position, a 20% increase in sarcomeres in series occurred. Goldspink et al (1974) explored whether these changes were affected by denervation of the muscle. These researchers noted that sarcomere numbers did not appear to be under neural control, and they suggested that the mechanism was a local response to altered tension in the muscle.

The ultrastructural changes that occur following immobilization of muscles in a shortened position involve segmental necrosis, predominantly though not exclusively at the ends of the muscle fibers as compared to the mid region of the muscle. The work of Baker & Matsumoto (1988) provides an excellent description of this process. These authors immobilized the ankle joints of rats in maximal plantarflexion for up to 4 weeks. Within 2 days of immobilization, swelling of the mitochondria and sarcoplasmic reticulum had occurred, and by 5 days, the structure of the sarcomeres was breaking down and in many areas appeared kinked. By 7 days, fibers had lost their striated appearance with sarcomere structure being lost completely. These changes continued for approximately 2 weeks. By 4 weeks, although still immobilized, many fibers appeared to be regenerating. Normal sarcoplasmic structure was observed and although the regenerating myofibrils were thinner than normal, they exhibited defined I and Z bands, and hence a distinctive sarcomere structure. Thus, the segmental necrosis at the ends of the fibers allows the length of the fiber to be adjusted. This

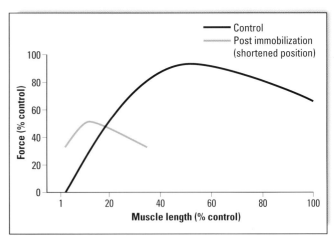

Figure 2.11 • The force–length relationship in normal muscle, and muscle that has been immobilized in a shortened position. Note the shift in the position of peak forces towards shorter muscle lengths and the decreases in force able to be generated.

in turn will affect the muscle mechanics (e.g. the length–tension relationship of the muscle). A muscle after immobilization in a shortened state, when stimulated electrically at different muscle lengths, will exhibit lesser peak force, and that force will be at a shorter muscle length compared to pre-immobilization (Williams & Goldspink 1978) (Fig. 2.11). After immobilization, most researchers allow their animals to exercise without restriction within their cages. It is apparent that even after a remobilization period similar to that of immobilization, the cross-sectional area of many muscle fibers remains significantly less than that of controls (Itai et al 2004). Where training (usually treadmill running) is instituted after immobilization, the size difference between control and previously immobilized muscle fibers is considerably less, though care in the exercise prescription is needed at the commencement of such programs as fibers are easily damaged immediately after immobilization.

It has been of interest whether a particular fiber type is more affected by immobilization in a shortened position. The findings generally indicate that Type I fibers undergo greater changes than Type II fibers. Lieber et al (1988), however, have challenged these findings. These authors have argued that many studies have compared slow and fast muscles without due consideration for the normal activity level of the muscles and the subsequent change in use that occurs with immobilization. As well, that these muscles are often immobilized at different lengths will influence the magnitude of atrophy. This will be most apparent when muscles with different fiber lengths and fiber length to muscle length ratios are compared. Finally, the number of joints that a muscle spans might also affect the magnitude of the atrophic response. In a study that controlled for these factors, Lieber et al (1988) concluded that the type of muscle to be affected most by the immobilization process was a single joint muscle containing a relatively large proportion of Type I fibers. It should be noted that structural changes are not confined to just the fibers per se, they have also been observed in other cellular structures. For instance, Leivo et al (1998) reported transient mitochondria swelling, with changes to their cristae and matrix following immobilization. Furthermore, the activity of enzymes such as nicotinamide adenine dinucleotide-tetrazolium reductase (NADH-TR), important for aerobic metabolism, was disrupted.

Together with structural changes, one might expect electromyographic activity in muscle immobilized in a shortened position to decrease. Fournier et al (1983) observed decreases in activation levels to approximately 50% of control values in animal muscles (soleus and medial gastrocnemius) immobilized in a shortened position for 4 weeks. These authors noted that there was a trend for a greater decrease in activity in the soleus compared to medial gastrocnemius muscle. Hnik et al (1985) also commented on large decreases in electromyography (EMG) activity after 10 days of immobilization, but only in the soleus muscle. The tibialis anterior, which is a more phasic type muscle, was not affected by immobilization in a shortened position. A consistent finding across these studies is that EMG activity was least affected when the muscle was immobilized in a lengthened position. The findings of these studies also indicated that EMG activity was not a major factor influencing the degree of atrophy observed in the muscles during the immobilization process. In a study involving humans whose arms were immobilized in plaster, Duchateau & Hainut (1990) examined motor unit activity, and observed that the motor unit firing rate at recruitment was similar in control and immobilized muscles; however, the maximal firing rate was lower in immobilized muscles, and this decrease was greater in low threshold motor units.

A common finding associated with immobilization is an increase in the connective tissue (endomysial, perimysial and epimysial) relative to the muscles' contractile tissues. Williams & Goldspink (1984) reported increases in perimysial tissue within 2 days of immobilization, whereas changes in endomysial tissues took approximately a week to become apparent. The magnitude of the changes can be substantial. For instance, Jozsa et al (1990) immobilized rat calf muscles in a shortened position for 3 weeks. Normal volume density of connective tissue of the soleus and gastrocnemius was 2–3%. After one week of immobilization, this had increased to 10 and 12%, respectively. After 3 weeks, the amount was 30% in both muscles (Fig. 2.12). Williams & Goldspink (1984) reported that the connective tissue laid down during immobilization was less aligned in respect to the muscle fibers. These changes in the size and structure of connective tissue are likely responsible for the increased stiffness of muscle immobilized in a shortened position (Tabary et al 1972), and to decreased range of motion Williams (1988). Jarvinen et al (1992) has also shown that after 7 and 21 days of immobilization, elongation at the point of failure was decreased by 21 and 36%, respectively.

Interestingly, Williams & Goldspink (1984) observed that increases in collagen content preceded any significant loss of sarcomeres in series. This finding would imply that early stiffness changes are associated with increased collagen within the muscle. Later work by Williams et al (1988) showed that

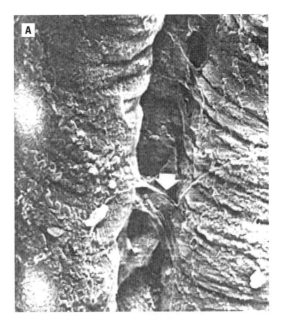

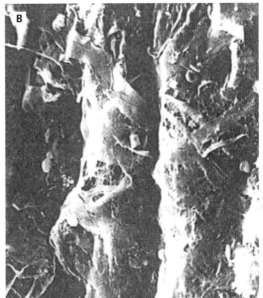

Figure 2.12 • A microscopic view of normal muscle fibers **(A)** and fibers that have been immobilized **(B)**. Note the increased amount of connective tissue adhesions. (Reproduced with permission and copyright of the British Editorial Society of Bone and Joint Surgery [Jozsa et al 1990].)

these connective tissue changes can be modified by muscle activation. In this study, Williams et al electrically stimulated muscles immobilized in a shortened position, and noted that they lost more sarcomeres in series than unstimulated muscles; however, increases in collagen content within the muscle were not observed. Thus, it seems that either maintaining the immobilized muscle in a lengthened state or applying electrical stimulation can regulate collagen content. An important question is whether intermittent lengthening can minimize the loss of sarcomeres in series when muscle is immobilized in a shortened position. Williams also addressed this question in two studies (Williams 1988, 1990). In the earlier study, Williams (1988) showed that 15 minutes of passive stretching every second day over 10 days was sufficient to prevent an increase in connective tissue within the muscle; however, fiber lengths and hence range of motion remained significantly decreased. In the second study (Williams 1990), where animals were immobilized for 2 weeks, sarcomeres decreased by 19% and range of motion was reduced by 41% in animals that were not stretched. However, she reported that 30 minutes of stretching per day was sufficient to prevent a loss of sarcomeres in series, and maintain range of motion at control levels.

Recently, there has been considerable interest in the effect of lengthening normal muscle tissue. This work has been stimulated by studies that showed that leg lengthening procedures were at times unsuccessful because patients were often encumbered with muscle contractures and subsequently a loss of joint range of motion (Simpson et al 1996). It was suspected that the rate of stretching might be a factor influencing the poor results, and to investigate this problem, rabbits underwent osteotomies and had their tibias lengthened at different rates until 20% increase in tibial length had occurred (Simpson et al 1996, Williams et al 1999). The main findings of these studies were that if rates were too high, then significant increases in connective tissue were observed, muscle fibers were damaged and sarcomeres were not added in series. At medium rates of lengthening, sarcomeres were added to the muscle fibers; however, moderate increases in connective tissue were observed. At low levels of lengthening, sarcomeres were added to the muscle fibers as would be expected, and increases in connective tissue were minimal. Thus, it would appear that low rates of stretch are needed to attain optimal adaptations in both the contractile and passive elements of the muscle when it is stretched.

Summary

Muscle is a complex structure, and we are continuing to discover new knowledge concerning its structure and function. For effective control of motion, it is important that our muscles function correctly. In many tasks, we are required to activate our muscles to high levels. Muscle force potential is governed by its structure, architecture and neural activation. Injury, disease and disuse can be particularly detrimental to this potential. An understanding of muscle function, and its reaction to pathology is important when designing and implementing effective training programs to limit and correct decreased muscle performance.

Acknowledgments

The authors would like to thank Jill Collier for her advice concerning the structure of the chapter, and Stephen Stanley for his advice and technical expertise in drawing the figures.

References

Aagaard P, Simonsen E B, Trolle M et al 1995 Isokinetic hamstring/quadriceps strength ratio: influence from joint angular velocity, gravity correction and contraction mode. Acta Physiologica Scandinavica 154:421–427

Aagaard P, Simonsen E B, Trolle M et al 1996 Specificity of training velocity and training load on gains in isokinetic knee joint strength. Acta Physiologica Scandinavica 156:123–129

Aagaard P, Simonsen E B, Andersen J L et al 2000 Neural inhibition during maximal eccentric and concentric quadriceps contraction: effects of resistance training. Journal of Applied Physiology 89:2249–2257

Aarimaa V, Kaariainen M, Vaittinen S et al 2004 Restoration of myofiber continuity after transection injury in the rat soleus. Neuromuscular Disorders 14:421–428

Abbott B C, Aubert X M 1951 Changes of energy in a muscle during very slow stretches. Proceedings of the Royal Society of London, Series B 139:104–117

Anderson J E 2000 A role for nitric oxide in muscle repair: nitric oxide-mediated activation of muscle satellite cells. Molecular Biology of the Cell 11:1859–1874

Appell H J, Duarte J A, Soares J M 1997 Supplementation of vitamin E may attenuate skeletal muscle immobilization atrophy. International Journal of Sports Medicine 18:157–160

Baker J, Matsumoto D 1988 Adaptation of skeletal muscle to immobilization in a shortened position. Muscle and Nerve 11:231–244

Bellemare F, Woods J J, Johansson R et al 1983 Motor-unit discharge rates in maximal voluntary contractions of three human muscles. Journal of Neurophysiology 50:1380–1392

Billeter R, Weber H, Lutz H et al 1980 Myosin types in human skeletal muscle fibers. Histochemistry 65:249–259

Bischoff R 1990 Interaction between satellite cells and skeletal muscle fibers. Development 109:943–952

Booth F, Seider M 1979 Early change in skeletal muscle protein synthesis after limb immobilisation of rats. Journal of Applied Physiology: Respiratory Environmental and Exercise Physiology 47:974–977

Borisov A 1999 Regeneration of skeletal and cardiac muscle in mammals: do nonprimate models resemble human pathology? Wound Repair and Regeneration 7:26–35

Bottinelli R, Canepari M, Pellegrino M A et al 1996 Force-velocity properties of human skeletal muscle fibres: myosin heavy chain isoform and temperature dependence. Journal of Physiology 495:573–586

Carpenter S, Karpati G 1989 Segmental necrosis and its demarcation in experimental micropuncture injury in skeletal muscle. Journal of Neuropathology and Experimental Neurology 48:154–170

Chazaud B, Sonnet C, Lafuste P et al 2003 Satellite cells attract monocytes and use macrophages as a support to escape apoptosis and enhance muscle growth. Journal of Cell Biology 163:1133–1143

Chleboun G, France A, Crill M et al 2001 In vivo measurement of fascicle length and pennation angle of the human biceps femoris muscle. Cells Tissues Organs 169:401–409

Duchateau J, Hainaut K 1990 Effects of immobilization on contractile properties, recruitment and firing rates of human motor units. Journal of Physiology 422:55–65

Dudley G A, Harris R T, Duvoisin M R et al 1990 Effect of voluntary vs. artificial activation on the relationship of muscle torque to speed. Journal of Applied Physiology 69:2215–2221

Edgerton V R, Apor P, Roy R R 1990 Specific tension of human elbow flexor muscles. Acta Physiologica Hungarica 75:205–216

Edman K A 1979 The velocity of unloaded shortening and its relation to sarcomere length and isometric force in vertebrate muscle fibres. Journal of Physiology 291:143–159

Erdemir A, Hamel A J, Fauth A R et al 2004 Dynamic loading of the plantar aponeurosis in walking. Journal of Bone and Joint Surgery (Am) 86A:546–552

Ettema G J, Huijing P A 1994 Effects of distribution of muscle fiber length on active length-force characteristics of rat gastrocnemius medialis. Anatomical Record 239:414–420

Feinstein N, Lindegard B, Nyman E et al 1955 Morphological studies of motor units in normal human muscles. Acta Anatomica 23:127–142

Fenn W O, Marsh B S 1935 Muscular force at different speeds of shortening. Journal of Physiology 85:277–297

Finni T, Komi P V, Lukkariniemi J 1998 Achilles tendon loading during walking: application of a novel optic fiber technique. European Journal of Applied Physiology and Occupational Physiology 77:289–291

Ford L, Huxley A, Simmons R 1981 The relation between stiffness and filament overlap in stimulated frog fibres. Journal of Physiology 311:219–249

Fournier M, Roy R R, Perham H et al 1983 Is limb immobilisation a model of muscle disuse? Experimental Neurology 80:147–156

Frontera W R, Suh D, Krivickas L S et al 2000 Skeletal muscle fiber quality in older men and women. American Journal of Physiology, Cell Physiology 279:C611–618

Fugl-Meyer A R, Gustafsson L, Burstedt Y 1980 Isokinetic and static plantar flexion characteristics. European Journal of Applied Physiology and Occupational Physiology 45:221–234

Fukashiro S, Komi P V, Jävinen M et al 1995 In vivo Achilles tendon loading during jumping in humans. European Journal of Applied Physiology 71:453–458

Fukunaga T, Roy R R, Shellock F G et al 1996 Specific tension of human plantar flexors and dorsiflexors. Journal of Applied Physiology 80:158–165

Fukunaga T, Miyatani M, Tachi M et al 2001 Muscle volume is a major determinant of joint torque in humans. Acta Physiologica Scandinavica 172:249–255

Gerdle B, Langstrom M 1987 Repeated isokinetic plantar flexions at different angular velocities. Acta Physiologica Scandinavica 130:495–500

Goldspink D 1977 The influence of immobilisation and stretch on protein turnover of rat skeletal muscle. Journal of Physiology 264:267–282

Goldspink D, Tabary J, Tabary C et al 1974 Effect of denervation on the adaptation of sarcomere number and muscle extensibility to the functional length of the muscle. Journal of Physiology 236:733–742

Gollnick P, Armstrong R, Saubert C et al 1972 Enzyme activity and fibre composition in skeletal muscle of untrained and trained men. Journal of Applied Physiology 33:312–319

Gollnick P D, Sjodin B, Karlsson J et al 1974 Human soleus muscle: a comparison of fiber composition and enzyme activities with other leg muscles. Pflugers Archiv – European Journal of Physiology 348:247–255

Gordon A M, Huxley A F, Julian F J 1966 The variation in isometric tension with sarcomere length in vertebrate muscle fibres. Journal of Physiology 184:170–192

Gregor R J, Roy R R, Whiting W C et al 1988 Mechanical output of the cat soleus during treadmill locomotion: in vivo vs in situ characteristics. Journal of Biomechanics 21:721–732

Gregor R J, Komi P V, Browning R C et al 1991 A comparison of the triceps surae and residual muscle moments at the ankle during cycling. Journal of Biomechanics 24:287–297

Grounds M 1991 Towards understanding skeletal muscle regeneration. Pathology Research and Practice 187:1–22

Hameed M, Orrell R W, Cobbold M et al 2003 Expression of IGF-I splice variants in young and old human skeletal muscle after high resistance exercise. Journal of Physiology 547:247–254

Harris R T, Dudley G A 1994 Factors limiting force during slow, shortening actions of the quadriceps femoris muscle group in vivo. Acta Physiologica Scandinavica 152:63–71

Herbert R D, Gandevia S C 1995 Changes in pennation with joint angle and muscle torque: in vivo measurements in human brachialis muscle. Journal of Physiology 484:523–532

Herbert R D, Gandevia S C 1999 Twitch interpolation in human muscles: mechanisms and implications for measurement of voluntary activation. Journal of Neurophysiology 82:2271–2283

Hess A 1967 The structure of vertebrate slow and twitch muscle fibers. Investigative Ophthalmology 6:217–228

Higuchi H 1996 Viscoelasticity and function of connectin/titin filaments in skinned muscle fibres. Advances in Biophysics 33:159–171

Hill A V 1938 The heat of shortening and the dynamic constants of muscle. Proceedings of the Royal Society Series B 126:136–195

Hnik P, Vejsada R, Goldspink D et al 1985 Quantitative evaluation of electromyogram activity in rat extensor and flexor muscles immobilised at different lengths. Experimental Neurology 88:515–528

Horowits R 1992 Passive force generation and titin isoforms in mammalian skeletal muscle. Biophysical Journal 61:392–398

Horowits R, Kempner E, Bisher M et al 1986 A physiological role for titin and nebulin in skeletal muscle. Nature 323:160–164

Hortobagyi T, Katch F I 1990 Eccentric and concentric torque-velocity relationships during arm flexion and extension. Influence of strength level. European Journal of Applied Physiology and Occupational Physiology 60:395–401

Huijing P A 1998 Muscle, the motor of movement: properties in function, experiment and modelling. Journal of Electromyography and Kinesiology 8:61–77

Hurme T, Kalimo H, Lehto M et al 1991a Healing of skeletal muscle injury: an ultrastructural and immunohistochemical study. Medicine and Science in Sports and Exercise 23:801–810

Hurme T, Lehto M, Falck B et al 1991b Electromyography and morphology during regeneration of muscle injury in rats. Acta Physiologica Scandinavica 142:443–456

Huxley A F 1957 Muscle structure and theories of contraction. Progress in Biophysics and Chemistry 7:255–318

Huxley A F, Simmons R M 1971 Proposed mechanism of force generation in striated muscle. Nature 233:533–538

Huxley A, Stewart A, Sosa H et al 1994 X-ray diffraction measurements of the extensibility of actin and mysosin filaments in contracting muscle. Biophysical Journal 67:2411–2421

Huxley H E 1972 Molecular basis of contraction in cross-striated muscle. In: Bourne G (ed) Molecular basis of contraction in cross-striated muscle. Academic Press, New York, p 302–387

Huxley H E, Hanson J 1954 Changes in the cross-striations of muscle during contraction and stretch and their structural interpretation. Nature 173:973

Itai Y, Kariya Y, Hoshino Y 2004 Morphological changes in rat hindlimb muscle fibres during recovery from disuse atrophy. Acta Physiologica Scandinavica 181:217–224

Jarvinen M, Lehto M 1993 The effects of early mobilisation and immobilisation on the healing process following muscle injuries. Sports Medicine 15:78–89

Jarvinen M, Einola S, Virtanen E 1992 Effect of the position of immobilization upon the tensile properties of the rat gastrocnemius muscle. Archives of Physical Medicine and Rehabilitation 73:253–257

Jarvinen T A, Jozsa L, Kannus P et al 2002 Organization and distribution of intramuscular connective tissue in normal and immobilized skeletal muscles. An immunohistochemical, polarization and scanning electron microscopic study. Journal of Muscle Research and Cell Motility 23:245–254

Johnson A, Polgar J, Weightman P et al 1973 Data on the distribution of fibre types in thirty six human muscles. Journal of the Neurological Sciences 18:111–129

Jozsa L, Kannus P, Thoring J et al 1990 The effect of tenotomy and immobilisation on intramuscular connective tissue. Journal of Bone and Joint Surgery (Br) 72B:293–297

Juul-Kristensen B, Bojsen-Moller F, Finsen L et al 2000a Muscle sizes and moment arms of rotator cuff muscles determined by magnetic resonance imaging. Cells Tissues Organs 167:214–222

Juul-Kristensen B, Bojsen-Moller F, Holst E et al 2000b Comparison of muscle sizes and moment arms of two rotator cuff muscles measured by ultrasonography and magnetic resonance imaging. European Journal of Ultrasound 11:161–173

Kaariainen M, Kaariainen J, Järvinen T et al 1998 Correlation between biomechanical and structural changes during the regeneration of skeletal muscle after laceration injury. Journal of Orthopedic Research 16:197–206

Kaariainen M, Järvinen T, Järvinen M et al 2000 Relation between myofibers and connective tissue during muscle injury repair. Scandinavian Journal of Medicine and Science in Sports 10:332–337

Kanda K, Hashizume K 1992 Factors causing difference in force output among motor units in the rat medial gastrocnemius muscle. Journal of Physiology 448:677–695

Kandarian S C, Stevenson E J 2002 Molecular events in skeletal muscle during disuse atrophy. Exercise and Sport Sciences Reviews 30:111–116

Kasemkjwattana C, Menetrey J, Somogyl G et al 1998 Development of approaches to improve the healing following muscle contusion. Cell Transplant 7:585–598

Katz B 1939 The relations between force and speed in muscular contraction. Journal of Physiology 96:45–64

Klitgaard H, Mantoni M, Schiaffino S et al 1990 Function, morphology and protein expression of ageing skeletal muscle: a cross-sectional study of elderly men with different training backgrounds. Acta Physiologica Scandinavica 140:41–54

Komi P V 1973 Measurement of the force-velocity relationship in human muscle under concentric and eccentric actions. Medicine and Sport 8:224–229

Korhonen M T, Cristea A, Alen M et al 2006 Aging, muscle fiber type and contractile function in sprint-trained athletes. Journal of Applied Physiology 101:906–917

Kostka T 2005 Quadriceps maximal power and optimal shortening velocity in 335 men aged 23–88 years. European Journal of Applied Physiology 95:140–145

Kuschel R, Deininger M, Meyermann R et al 2000 Allograft Inflammatory Factor-1 is expressed by macrophages in injured skeletal muscle and abrogates proliferation and differentiation of satellite cells. Journal of Neuropathology and Experimental Neurology 59:323–332

Labeit S, Gibson T, Lakey A et al 1991 Evidence that nebulin is a protein-ruler in muscle thin filaments. FEBS Letters 282:313–316

Larsson L, Grimby G, Karlsson J 1979 Muscle strength and speed of movement in relation to age and muscle morphology. Journal of Applied Physiology 46:451–456

Larsson L, Edstrom L, Lindegren B et al 1991 MHC composition and enzyme-histochemical and physiological properties of a novel fast-twitch motor unit type. American Journal of Physiology 261:C93–101

Lehto M, Duance V, Restall D 1985 Collagen and fibronectin in a healing skeletal muscle injury. Journal of Bone and Joint Surgery (Br) 67B:820–828

Leivo I, Kauhanen S, Michelsson J E 1998 Abnormal mitochondria and sarcoplasmic changes in rabbit skeletal muscle induced by immobilization. Acta Pathologica, Microbiologica, et Immunologica Scandinavica 106:1113–1123

Lieber R, Friden J, Hargens A et al 1988 Differential response of the dog quadriceps muscle to external skeletal fixation of the knee. Muscle and Nerve 11:193–201

McComas A J 1996 Skeletal muscle form and function. Human Kinetics, Champaign, IL

Malamud J, Godt R, Nichols R 1996 Relationship between short range stiffness and yielding in type-identified chemically skinned muscle fibers from the cat triceps surae muscles. Journal of Neurophysiology 76:2280–2289

Mauro A 1961 Satellite cells of skeletal muscle fibers. Journal of Biophysics Biochemistry and Cytology 87:225–251

Minamoto V, Grazziano C, De Fatima Salvino T 1999 Effect of single and periodic contusion on the rat soleus muscle at different stages of regeneration. Anatomical Record 254:281–287

Narici M 1999 Human skeletal muscle architecture studied in vivo by non-invasive imaging techniques: functional significance and applications. Journal of Electromyography and Kinesiology 9:97–103

Narici M V, Roi G S, Landoni L 1988 Force of knee extensor and flexor muscles and cross-sectional area determined by nuclear magnetic resonance imaging. European Journal of Applied Physiology and Occupational Physiology 57:39–44

Narici M V, Binzoni T, Hiltbrand E et al 1996 In vivo human gastrocnemius architecture with changing joint angle at rest and during graded isometric contraction. Journal of Physiology 496:287–297

Nicks D, Beneke W, Key R et al 1989 Muscle fibre size and number following immobilisation atrophy. Journal of Anatomy 163:1–5

Nygaard E, Houston M, Suzuki Y et al 1983 Morphology of the brachial biceps muscle and elbow flexion in man. Acta Physiologica Scandinavica 117:287–292

Peachey L D 1965a The sarcoplasmic reticulum and transverse tubules of the frog's sartorius. Journal of Cell Biology 25 (suppl):209–231

Peachey L D 1965b Transverse tubules in excitation-contraction coupling. Federation Proceedings 24:1124–1134

Perrine J J, Edgerton V R 1978 Muscle force velocity relationships under isokinetic loading. Medicine and Science in Sports and Exercise 10:159–166

Pette D, Staron R 1997 Mammalian skeletal muscle fiber type transitions. International Review of Cytology 170:143–223

Pette D, Peuker H, Staron R S 1999 The impact of biochemical methods for single muscle fibre analysis. Acta Physiologica Scandinavica 166:261–277

Pinniger G J, Steele J R, Thorstensson A et al 2000 Tension regulation during lengthening and shortening actions of the human soleus muscle. European Journal of Applied Physiology 81:375–383

Pinniger G J, Ranatunga K W, Offer G W 2006 Crossbridge and non-crossbridge contributions to tension in lengthening muscle: force-induced reversal of the power stroke. Journal of Physiology 573:627–643

Pousson M, Amiridis I G, Cometti G et al 1999 Velocity-specific training in elbow flexors. European Journal of Applied Physiology and Occupational Physiology 80:367–372

Powers S K, Kavazis A N, DeRuisseau K C 2005 Mechanisms of disuse muscle atrophy: role of oxidative stress. American Journal of Physiology, Regulatory, Integrative and Comparative Physiology 288: R337–344

Purslow P 1989 Strain induced reorientation of an intramuscular connective tissues network: implications for passive muscle elasticity. Journal of Biomechanics 22:21–31

Purslow P, Trotter J 1994 The morphology and mechanical properties of endomysium in series-fibred muscles: variations with muscle length. Journal of Muscle Research and Cellular Motility 15:299–308

Rack P M, Westbury D R 1969 The effects of length and stimulus rate on tension in the isometric cat soleus muscle. Journal of Physiology 204:443–460

Rassier D E, Herzog W 2005 Force enhancement and relaxation rates after stretch of activated muscle fibres. Proceedings Biological Sciences 272:475–480

Robertson T, Maley M, Grounds M et al 1993 The role of macrophages in skeletal muscle regeneration with particular reference to chemotaxis. Experimental Cell Research 207:321–331

Rudel R, Taylor S R 1971 Striated muscle fibers: facilitation of contraction at short lengths by caffeine. Science 172:387–389

Rutherford O M, Jones D A 1992 Measurement of fibre pennation using ultrasound in the human quadriceps in vivo. European Journal of Applied Physiology and Occupational Physiology 65:433–437

Sale D, Quinlan J, Marsh E et al 1982 Influence of joint position on ankle plantarflexion in humans. Journal of Applied Physiology: Respiratory, Environmental and Exercise Physiology 52:1636–1642

Sargeant A J, Hoinville E, Young A 1981 Maximum leg force and power output during short-term dynamic exercise. Journal of Applied Physiology: Respiratory, Environmental and Exercise Physiology 51:1175–1182

Schiaffino S, Reggiani C 1994 Myosin isoforms in mammalian skeletal muscle. Journal of Applied Physiology 77:493–501

Selsby J T, Dodd S L 2005 Heat treatment reduces oxidative stress and protects muscle mass during immobilization. American Journal of Physiology, Regulatory, Integrative and Comparative Physiology 289: R134–139

Short K R, Vittone J L, Bigelow M L et al 2005 Changes in myosin heavy chain mRNA and protein expression in human skeletal muscle with age and endurance exercise training. Journal of Applied Physiology 99:95–102

Simpson A, Williams P, Kyberd P et al 1996 The response of muscle to leg lengthening. Journal of Bone and Joint Surgery (Br) 77B:630–636

Smerdu V, Karsch-Mizrachi I, Campione M et al 1994 Type IIx myosin heavy chain transcripts are expressed in type IIb fibers of human skeletal muscle. American Journal of Physiology 267:C1723–1728

Snow M 1983 A quantitative ultrastructural analysis of satellite cells in denervated fast and slow muscles of the rat. Anatomical Record 207:593–604

Spoor C W, van Leeuwen J L 1992 Knee muscle moment arms from MRI and from tendon travel. Journal of Biomechanics 25:201–206

Spoor C W, van Leeuwen J L, Meskers C G et al 1990 Estimation of instantaneous moment arms of lower-leg muscles. Journal of Biomechanics 23:1247–1259

Stevenson E J, Giresi P G, Koncarevic A et al 2003 Global analysis of gene expression patterns during disuse atrophy in rat skeletal muscle. Journal of Physiology 551:33–48

Tabary J, Tabary C, Tardieu C et al 1972 Physiological and structural changes in the cat's soleus muscle due to immobilisation at different lengths by plaster casts. Journal of Physiology 224:231–244

Thorstensson 1976 Muscle strength, fibre types and enzyme activities in man. Acta Physiologica Scandinavica Supplementum 443:1–45

Thorstensson A, Grimby G, Karlsson J 1976 Force-velocity relations and fibre composition in human knee extensor muscles. Journal of Applied Physiology 40:12–16

Trinick J 1991 Elastic filaments and giant proteins in muscle. Current Opinion in Cell Biology 3:112–119

Tveit P, Daggfeldt K, Hetland S et al 1994 Erector spinae lever arm length variations with changes in spinal curvature. Spine 19:199–204

Walmsley B, Hodgson J A, Burke R E 1978 Forces produced by medial gastrocnemius and soleus muscles during locomotion in freely moving cats. Journal of Neurophysiology 41:1203–1216

Westing S H, Seger J Y, Karlson E et al 1988 Eccentric and concentric torque-velocity characteristics of the quadriceps femoris in man. European Journal of Applied Physiology and Occupational Physiology 58:100–104

Westing S H, Seger J Y, Thorstensson A 1990 Effects of electrical stimulation on eccentric and concentric torque-velocity relationships during knee extension in man. Acta Physiologica Scandinavica 140:17–22

Westing S H, Cresswell A G, Thorstensson A 1991 Muscle activation during maximal voluntary eccentric and concentric knee extension. European Journal of Applied Physiology and Occupational Physiology 62:104–108

Whiting W C, Gregor R J, Roy R R et al 1984 A technique for estimating mechanical work of individual muscles in the cat during treadmill locomotion. Journal of Biomechanics 17:685–694

Wickiewicz T, Roy R, Powell P et al 1983 Muscle architecture of the lower limb. Clinical Orthopaedics and Related Research 179:275–283

Williams P 1988 Effect of intermittent stretch on immobilised muscle. Annals of the Rheumatic Diseases 47:1014–1016

Williams P 1990 Use of intermittent stretch in the prevention of serial sarcomere loss in immobilised muscle. Annals of the Rheumatic Diseases 49:316–317

Williams P, Goldspink D 1978 Changes in sarcomere length and physiological properties in immobilised muscle. Journal of Anatomy 127:459–468

Williams P, Goldspink D 1984 Connective tissue changes in immobilised muscle. Journal of Anatomy 138:343–350

Williams P, Catanese T, Lucey E et al 1988 The importance of stretch and contractile activity in the prevention of connective tissue accumulation in muscle. Journal of Anatomy 158:109–114

Williams P, Simpson A, Kyberd P et al 1999 Effect of rate of distraction on loss of range of joint movement, muscle stiffness, and intramuscular connective tissue content during surgical limb-lengthening: a study in the rabbit. Anatomical Record 255:78–83

Woittiez R D, Huijing P A, Rozendal R H 1983 Influence of muscle architecture on the length-force diagram of mammalian muscle. Pflugers Archiv – European Journal of Physiology 399:275–279

Zammit P, Golding J, Nagata Y et al 2004 Muscle satellite cells adopt divergent fates: a mechanism of self renewal. Journal of Cell Biology 166:347–357

Zhang J, Dhoot G 1998 Localized and limited changes in the expression of myosin heavy chains in injured skeletal muscle fibers being repaired. Muscle and Nerve 21:469–481

Tendon

Jill Cook

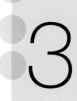

CHAPTER CONTENTS

Introduction 26

Tendons – anatomy and histology 27

Blood and nerve supply to tendon 29

Tendon structures 30

Biomechanical properties of tendons 30

Physiology of normal tendons 31

Tendon pathology 33

Tendon repair 36

Summary 37

Introduction

Tendon is a continuum of connective tissue that simply and effectively transfers force produced by contractile cells of muscles to their target, which is usually bone. They usually cross, and attach close to, a joint which permits rapid joint movement (Benjamin & Ralphs 1996).

Tendons have several functions other than directing muscle contraction. They act proprioceptively, and as both shock absorbers and energy storage sites (Benjamin & Ralphs 1995). In sport, these features are critical, as they enhance athletic function.

Tendons vary in length and size throughout the body. They can be long, broad, flat, round or aponeurotic; they may wind around bony pulleys, enclose sesamoids or fit into small areas (e.g. carpal tunnel). The peritendinous structures of tendons vary as much as the tendons themselves. Very organized and highly structured peritendon present in the long finger flexors and extensors is in contrast with negligible peritendon in the tendons of the hip adductors and knee extensors.

Tendon injury and pain affects individuals in the sporting and industrial population groups more than the general population, thought to be due to the loading profiles in these populations. The prevalence of tendon injury varies between studies depending on the tendon studied and the diagnostic criteria used. In the workplace, tendon injuries represent between 15 and 30% of medical cases, and in the sporting population the prevalence is reported up to 50% in such conditions as patellar tendinopathy in basketball players (Cook et al 1998).

A subpopulation of the general population have tendon pathology without pain; these individuals do not present for medical care or indeed have any idea that they have an abnormal tendon. Although many of these individuals will not develop symptoms, a proportion will experience an acute tendon rupture without warning (Kannus & Józsa 1991). This presentation of tendon injury (rupture without prior symptoms) can be devastating to the individual, as rehabilitation after rupture is prolonged.

Although tendon injury is a disabling and recurrent condition that is resistant to treatment, there are still many limitations on our understanding of the nature of tendon injury, repair and treatment. Although much of the pathology and etiology of tendinitis remains unclear (Almekinders 1998), new imaging and tissue sampling techniques have improved our understanding of overuse tendon disease in humans, and along with molecular and cellular investigations, understanding of tendon pathology and pain is improving rapidly.

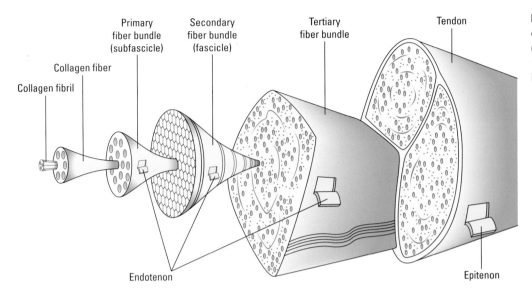

Collagen fibril
Collagen fiber
Primary fiber bundle (subfascicle)
Secondary fiber bundle (fascicle)
Tertiary fiber bundle
Tendon
Endotenon
Epitenon

Figure 3.1 • The hierarchical organization of tendon structure. (Reproduced from Khan et al 1999a with the permission of Adis Press.)

All tendons have similarities in microanatomy, histology, and pathology (Fig. 3.1). This chapter will outline the anatomical structure and physiological and biomechanical properties of tendon tissue in both the normal and pathological state. Cellular and molecular responses of tendon will not be discussed in detail and readers are directed to the biological literature for this detail.

Tendons – anatomy and histology

As tendons come under the umbrella term connective tissue, their structure is characteristic of this genre: a small cellular component that builds and maintains a much larger extracellular matrix. Macroscopically, healthy tendons are glistening and white, firm to touch but pliable (Józsa & Kannus 1997). Microscopically, the main components of tendon are the cells (tenocytes) and the extracellular matrix (collagen, ground substance, neurovascular and connective tissue structures, and assorted other important but low-volume proteins).

Tenocytes

Tenocytes are the cellular components of tendon tissue that manufacture all the extracellular components of tendon. Consequently, tenocytes are rich in the organelles responsible for protein synthesis and transport, such as rough endoplasmic reticulum (rER) and Golgi apparatus. Despite this critical function, tenocytes are reported as being sparse in tendon (Khan et al 1999a) with a low respiratory quotient that indicates a low metabolic rate (O'Brien 1997). Tendons cells are resilient to low oxygen levels (Rempel & Abrahamsson 2001) and respond positively to mechanical loads (Almekinders et al 1993).

Tenocytes are spindle shaped longitudinally and stellate in cross-section with numerous cell processes extending between the collagen fibers (Kraushaar & Nirschl 1999, O'Brien 1997). Both epitenon cells and tenocytes communicate via these cell processes (Banes et al 1995). Tenocytes move along the collagen fibers, tightening and structuring the matrix, and will remodel an expanded matrix.

Tenocytes are not primarily regulated from a central source but react to local stimuli (Leadbetter 1992). Tenocytes are deformed by, and respond to, mechanical load (Banes et al 1995), and change shape, function and composition in response to this load (Frank & Hart 1990, Sarasa-Renedo & Chiquet 2005). Tenocytes also communicate with each other in response to load (Shirakura et al 1995).

Extracellular matrix

The extracellular matrix comprises the majority of tendon volume, and provides the strength and flexibility inherent in tendon. The main components of the extracellular matrix are collagen, ground substance and neurovascular and connective tissue. Other protein components including elastin, COMP and tenascin-C will not be discussed in this chapter. The reader is referred to the literature for further discussion of the role and distribution of these proteins (Kjaer 2004).

Collagen

Collagen, which endows tendon with its impressive tensile strength, is present in tendons as tightly packed fibers. Normal tendons consist mainly of type I collagen and small amounts of type III collagen found only in the endotendon of normal tendon (Williams et al 1984). Type I collagen has a large diameter (40–60 nm) and links together to form tight fiber bundles. Type III collagen is smaller in diameter (10–20 nm) and forms looser, more reticular bundles.

Collagen comprises 30% of wet tendon weight and 80% of dry weight. Collagen gives a tendon stiffness, rigidity and strength when loaded, and flexibility when bent, compressed, twisted or sheared.

The majority of collagen fibers run in the direction of stress (Frost 1990) with a spiral component, but some fibrils run perpendicular to the line of stress (Józsa et al 1991). The ratio of axial to nonaxial fibers is between 10:1 to 26:1 (Józsa et al 1991). The larger diameter ($>1500\,\text{Å}$) fibers in longer tendons do not extend along the full length of the tendon (Benjamin & Ralphs 1995), but smaller diameter fibers may (Kirkendall & Garrett 1997).

Collagen fibers are formed in tendon cells and have a specific hierarchical order. In normal tendon, this structural order of collagen has five different levels (Robins 1988) and is described from microscopic to macroscopic structure (Fig. 3.1).

Level 1

Procollagen is formed in the rough endoplasmic reticulum of tenocytes as three polypeptide chains. Each procollagen chain consists of 1500 amino acid residues. Two of these chains are α-1 chains and the third is an α-2 chain with a different amino acid sequence. In the Golgi apparatus, procollagen forms a helix and is then transported to, and excreted from, the cell membrane in vacuoles via the cellular skeletal system of microtubules and microfilaments (O'Brien 1997). Procollagen is converted to insoluble tropocollagen in the extra-cellular matrix by cleaving the terminal extensions at both ends of the molecule.

Level 2

Five tropocollagen molecules aggregate spontaneously to form collagen fibrils. There is an ordered overlap of one quarter of each tropocollagen molecule in fibrils which is responsible for the striated appearance of collagen on electron microscopy (Gross 1992). This overlap reinforces the collagen and leaves no weak transverse point where stress could cause disruption (O'Brien 1997, Robins 1988, Scott 1995).

Level 3

Fibrils, which are visible on electron microscopy, aggregate into bundles, forming fibers that are visible on light microscopy.

Level 4

Fibers collect into fiber bundles hexagonal in shape and up to a third of a square mm in size.

Level 5

Fibers bundles group into fascicles surrounded by endotendon (O'Brien 1997). Fascicles are the longitudinal striations seen on ultrasonographic examination.

There is a regular sinusoidal pattern or 'crimp' in the extracellular matrix due to the tertiary structure of collagen that is maintained in part by elastic fibers. This crimp has a periodicity of $100–200\,\mu\text{m}$ (Robins 1988). Crimp facilitates shock absorption and allows tendon to stretch and recover fully. The so-called 'toe' area on the stress/strain curve represents crimp stretch.

Crosslinks bond collagen helices. They are essential for the tensile strength of tendon and assist in maintaining tendon shape. Crosslinks between three adjacent collagen molecules occur with hydroxylysylpyridinoline and lysylpyridinoline, glycation crosslinks with pentosidine occur increasingly in older tissue (Banks et al 1999). The tendon strength gained from crosslinks is reinforced by interaction between collagen and the proteoglycans in the ground substance.

Ground substance

Ground substance is found between collagen fibers and contributes to the viscoelastic properties of tendons. Although inconspicuous in normal tendon, ground substance still plays a very important role in the structure of the extracellular matrix of tendon. Ground substance organizes connective tissue by orientating and ordering collagen fibrils, and thus determines the ultimate tissue and organism shape (Scott 1995).

Ground substance also has other important roles in tendon physiology and metabolism. Ground substance attaches to, and surrounds, collagen fibrils (Vogel et al 1984), helping collagen fibrils adhere to and slide past each other (Selvanetti et al 1997). Water, which comprises 60–80% of the weight of ground substance, allows gas and nutrient diffusion (O'Brien 1997, Scott 1988).

Ground substance is formed by an association between a protein core and glycosaminoglycan (amino sugar) chains. Decorin constitutes most of the protein core in tendon associated with a single glycosaminoglycan chain. This hydrophilic proteoglycan forms a tadpole-like ground substance that constitutes up to 80% of adult tendon. The bulbous proteoglycan part binds to specific sites of the collagen fiber (the D band) and the glycosaminoglycan chain associates and holds the protein parts, and hence the collagen, a specified distance apart. Most proteoglycans are oriented at 90° to the collagen fiber, others are randomly arranged or lie parallel to the fiber (Scott 1988). Other small proteoglycans (biglycan, lumican and fibromodulin) are also found in tendon. Aggrecan and versican, large proteoglycans associated with cartilage, complete the other 20% of proteoglycan content of mature tendon (Fig. 3.2) (Vogel & Meyers 1999).

Tendons vary in composition throughout their length, dependent on the forces placed on specific parts of the tendon. These forces determine the levels and type of proteoglycans, dependent on their loading history. Tendons are subject to tensile loading and both collagen and proteoglycans resist and transmit these tensile forces (Cribb & Scott 1995). However, biological movement also causes compression and shearing of tissue, and tendons have weaker resistance to these forces (Selvanetti et al 1997). Tendons that consistently undergo compressive, bending or shearing forces have a higher amount of, and larger, proteoglycans (Giori et al 1993, Scott 1988). It appears that the compression of the tenocytes stimulates this proteoglycan response. Extra aggrecan protects the tendon by increasing resistance to compression, thus protecting neurovascular structures and allowing collagen fascicles to slide relative to one another (Vogel 2004).

Connective tissue

All bundles of collagen fibers and fascicles are surrounded by connective tissue called endotendon. The endotendon carries

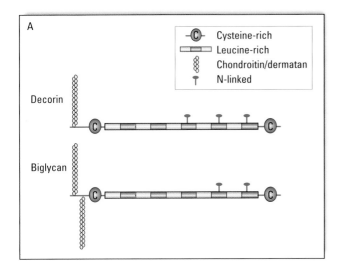

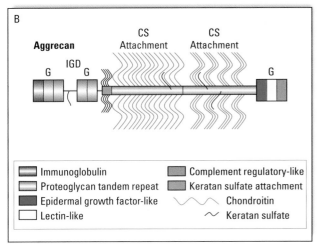

Figure 3.2 • A: Schematic diagrams of decorin and biglycan, two dermatan/chondroitin sulfate-containing small leucine-rich proteoglycans. **B:** Schematic diagram of the major large chondroitin sulfate-containing proteoglycans that form aggregates with hyaluronan (hyalectins). CS = chondroitin sulfate; IGD = interglobular domain; G = globular domain. (Diagrams provided by Professor Chris Handley with permission.)

the blood vessels, nerves and lymphatic vessels into and through the tendon. It appears to be the most important conduit of blood supply into the tendon (Ahmed et al 1998, Clancy 1990). The endotendon allows some movement between collagen bundles while still binding the collagen fibrils together (Józsa et al 1991).

Fascicle bundles aggregate to form a tendon and they are surrounded by peritendon. This contains two layers of connective tissue, the paratenon and the epitenon, which allow glide relative to surrounding tissue. The epitenon and paratenon consist of a dense network of meshed collagen fibrils (Józsa et al 1991). These layers of connective tissue are well vascularized and innervated.

The peritendinous structures vary in tendons depending on mechanical stress on the tendon and friction from surrounding structures. The paratenon can vary from a simple structure with loose, fatty areolar tissue to a complex double layered sheath lined with synovial cells (Clancy 1990). Paratenon with synovial cells is called tenosynovium; a double layer sheath without synovial cells is termed a tenovagium.

As all tendon connective tissue is continuous within the tendon, and in parts, continuous with muscle and bone connective tissue, it is the primary tissue to continue neurovascular structures across the muscle/tendon/bone unit. The importance of the peritendon and its cells is not fully understood, but the cells are more sensitive and reactive to stimuli than intratendinous cells (Rempel & Abrahamsson 2001) and they may have more influence on tendon structure and pathology than is currently known. Exercise has been shown to increase the prostaglandin in peritendon (Langberg et al 1999a); this in turn could influence the tendon proper (Khan et al 2005).

Blood and nerve supply to tendon

Blood supply

Tendon is a relatively avascular structure compared to tissue such as muscle and skin, but for the metabolic demands that it has, tendon is well vascularized tissue (Benjamin & Ralphs 1995, Hess et al 1989, Kirkendall & Garrett 1997). Tendon blood supply is variable, and affected by compression, torsion and friction. Intratendinous blood flow has been shown to be lower at tendon insertions than the remaining tendon in the Achilles tendon (Astrom & Westlin 1994b), consistent with greater amounts of fibrocartilage in this area.

Vascular supply to the tendon can arise from the musculotendinous junction and the bone–tendon junction, via the peri tissue structures, and not across the structural borders (Benjamin & Ralphs 1995, O'Brien 1997). In addition, in longer tendons, vessels can enter the surrounding connective tissue from adjacent arterioles (Schatzker & Branemark 1969). These peritendinous vessels then enter the tendon through the continuum with the endotendon (Archambault et al 1995, O'Brien 1992).

It is assumed that the metabolic demands of tendon remain low in exercise, due to the low number of cells (Kjaer et al 2000). It appears that these metabolic demands of the tendon are met by the blood supply in the active state (Boushel et al 2000). Thus speculation that normal tendons have critical areas of poor vascularity due to vascular and tendon anatomy, and that these areas are consequently more likely to develop pathology seems unlikely.

Critical areas have been reported to exist in the tendons of tibialis posterior at the medial malleolus and insertional areas of the supraspinatus tendon. These areas of tendon are more cartilaginous and will be less vascular than fibrous tendon due to their fibrocartilage structure (Vogel et al 1993). There is clear evidence that the vascular supply of the Achilles tendon is adequate throughout its length. In a study of cadaver Achilles tendons, there was no variation in the number of blood vessels at any point along the length of the tendon (Ahmed et al 1998). Similarly, the recorded blood flow at the midpoint, insertion and musculotendinous junction of normal Achilles tendon showed good correlation of flow between sites (Astrom & Westlin 1994b). These studies suggest that the blood supply at rest is not compromised at a particular point of the Achilles tendon.

Nerve supply

Tendons have a rich, almost exclusively afferent nerve supply that mediates proprioception (O'Brien 1997). Encapsulated and nonencapsulated nerve endings in tendon include type I Ruffini corpuscles, pressure receptors (stretch sensitive), type II Paccinian corpuscles, type III Golgi tendon organs (mechanoreceptors) and type IV free nerve endings (pain) (O'Brien 1997). Most afferent nerve endings are near the muscle–tendon junction (Kirkendall & Garrett 1997). Hence, the nerve supply of the midtendon may be minimal and pain sensitivity to early pathological processes may be compromised.

Tendon structures

The enthesis and myotendinous junction are two important structures of tendon.

Enthesis

Tendon insertion into bone (the enthesis) is a point of change in tissue flexibility from tendon to bone. Two types of enthesis have been described: the fibrocartilaginous enthesis and the fibrous enthesis. Fibrous enthesis occurs when the superficial tendon inserts into the periosteum and occurs in metaphyseal and diaphyseal attachments (Benjamin & Ralphs 1996).

The fibrocartilaginous enthesis is a transitional zone where tendon graduates to bone through the sequence of layers, from normal tendon to fibrocartilage, through mineralized fibrocartilage and finally bone. This transition occurs within a variable distance (200–400 μm to several millimeters) (Benjamin & Ralphs 1998) and the thickness may be related to the amount of movement and load that occurs between the bone and tendon.

The unmineralized fibrocartilage region has rows of rounded cells between bundles of type II collagen. Unlike tendon cells, these cells do not have connective arms to other cells (Benjamin & Ralphs 1998), hence there is no communication between bone and tendon cells. A distinct border (the blue line) separates mineralized from unmineralized fibrocartilage (Ferretti et al 1985). The blue line is composed of densely packed, randomly oriented collagen of various diameters that are continuous with both the mineralized and unmineralized fibrocartilage (O'Brien 1997).

The enthesis allows a gradual change in mechanical properties from the flexible tendon to the rigid bone. The fibrocartilage controls bending of fibers and distributes force to the bone (Kraushaar & Nirschl 1999). The more bending of fibers that occurs in a tendon due to load, the more fibrocartilage is present at the enthesis. The enthesis also protects the tendon insertion from narrowing when the tendon is stretched, thus restricting the decrease in cross-sectional area (Benjamin & Ralphs 1998).

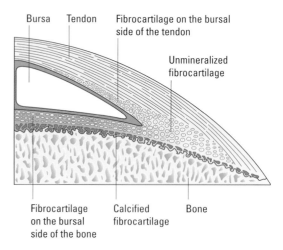

Figure 3.3 • Normal tendon enthesis.

It is important to consider other structures associated with fibrocartilaginous tendon insertions, including bursae and cartilaginous adaptations on both apposing bone and tendon (Fig. 3.3). This has been termed the 'enthesis organ' by Benjamin et al (2004). Hence the presentation of a bursitis at a tendon attachment (gluteus medius, tibial patellar tendon attachment) is likely reflective of an enthesis problem rather than an isolated bursitis, and should be treated as such. The Achilles tendon insertion and the effect of calcaneal shape on the enthesis structures has been well described by Rufai et al (1995). Diagnoses such as Haglund's deformity are merely variation of enthesis anatomy that predispose an individual to pathology and pain.

Myotendinous junction

The myotendinous junction is also a specialized anatomical area that allows transmission in force as well as the change in tissue flexibility and size. Because of these tissue changes it is a common site of injury, usually termed a muscle strain (Clancy 1990). The amount of folding increases the surface area by tenfold. At this junction, the tendon bundles are invaginated, but separate from the muscle sarcomeres by an aponeurosis. Similar to the bone–tendon junction, the connective tissue of muscle and tendon blend together. As tendon collagen extends into the muscle at the musculotendinous junction, it provides more extensive attachment of tendon to muscle (O'Brien 1997) There may be some structural differences in the myotendinous junctions between type 1 and type 2 muscle fibers (Kvist et al 1991).

Biomechanical properties of tendons

Tendons act as springs to store energy in locomotion and as a result, the elastic properties of tendon are essential in athletic function. At the same time, tendons must transfer force efficiently to bone with minimal energy loss. Thus, the mechanical response of tendon to load is variable due in part to the variation in tendon shape, size, and structure.

The mechanical properties of tendons can be expressed in terms of tensile stress and strain. Stress at any point in the tendon can be calculated by dividing the total tensile load of the tendon by the cross-sectional area at that point. Thus the thinnest part of the tendon will be under the most stress. Strain is the amount the tendon stretches under load when compared to its unloaded length.

The relationship between stress and strain is well described by the stress–strain curve (Fig. 3.4). In normal tendon, the initial load absorption is seen in the 'toe' region of the curve and represents tendon 'uncrimping'. The linear portion of the curve occurs between 2 and 4% strain and this slope represents the stiffness of the tendon. These two regions account for the normal physiological range of the tendon. Pathological load on tendon begins at approximately 4% strain when collagen failure begins. Initially crosslinks break down, but eventually fibers, fibrils and fascicles rupture, and this is represented by the plateau in the curve. At approximately 8–10% strain, the tendon fails completely. However, ultimate strain levels vary in tendons and individuals and may occur between 8 and 30% strain (Gelberman et al 1988).

It is critical to remember that the physiological magnitude of force produced by the muscle is normally well below that required to rupture a tendon unless it is weakened by other factors (Ker 2002). Most importantly the presence of tendon pathology has been shown to be negatively correlated with tensile strength, and underlying painful or pain-free pathology nearly always exists in tendons that rupture (Sano et al 1997). The absence of pain prior to rupture does not indicate the absence of pathology, with more than 60% of ruptured tendons pain free prior to rupture, but all have underlying pathology (Kannus & Józsa 1991).

Normal tendon reacts differently depending on the amount and rate of load application. At low tensile loads the tendon has high extensibility, while at higher tensile loads this extensibility is reduced (Gelberman et al 1988). The rate of load application also influences tendon properties, with quicker load application resulting in both greater tendon stiffness and ability to withstand load (Benjamin & Ralphs 1996). Larger tendons can withstand larger loads and longer tendons have greater absolute elongation before rupture (Fyfe & Stanish 1992).

Tendons are viscoelastic, mainly due to the presence of ground substance (Schatzmann et al 1998). Stress relaxation and creep are viscoelastic time-dependent behaviors of normal tendons. Stress relaxation, the decrease in force needed to maintain tendon length over time, is important in sport when constant and repetitive loads are applied.

Creep is the gradual lengthening of tendon under constant load. Cyclic loading of tendon in athletic participation may cause creep, and thus may lead to failure of part or all of the tendon at lower loads (Selvanetti et al 1997). An alternative opinion is that cyclic loading in sports 'softens' the tendon and decreases the potential of fatigue failure (Woo & Tkach 1990). Both these reactions to loading are possible and the tendon response may depend on the rate of loading, the immediate biomechanical history of the tendon and the condition of the tendon.

Tendons therefore resist tensile loads well, but only to a certain limit. This limit is determined by the size and shape of the tendon, and is affected by disease and non-tensile forces. Repeated loading has been investigated in animal tendons and may improve the mechanical properties of tendon. Improvement may be due to morphological change of tendon (e.g. increased cross-sectional area) but mechanical loading may also improve the quality of the tendon without a change in structure. In humans, cross-sectional area of runners' tendons are greater than controls, but cause or effect is not known (Rosager et al 2002).

Physiology of normal tendons

Tendons are physiologically and metabolically active, capable of adapting to a range of stimuli including change in load. Mechanical load is transmitted into the cell through cytoskeleton connectivity to the extracellular matrix by integrins, and induces change in the cell response. Hence, the cell responds to the extrinsic strain of the tightly packed extracellular environment and sets intrinsic strain to match. Any change in the extracellular matrix will change the internal environment of the cell.

Load is critical for tendon to maintain normal morphology. Longer term immobilization and/or rest from all tendon load will cause deterioration in tendon morphology. It has been hypothesized that areas within tendons may not be loaded optimally, and the resultant low load environment can cause tendon change. This has been termed stress-shielding (Almekinders et al 2003, Orchard & Cook 2004). In animal models, induced stress-shielding has been shown to induce changes not unlike that seen in pathological tendon (Majima et al 2003). The concept of stress shielding is feasible, as the parts of the patellar

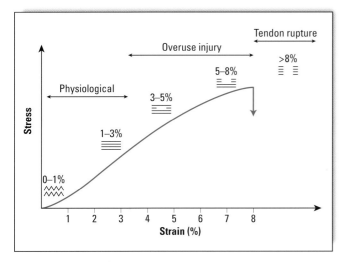

Figure 3.4 • Stress–strain curve for tendon. (Reproduced from Khan et al 1998 Patellar tendinopathy: some aspects of basic science and clinical management. British Journal of Sports Medicine 32:346–355, with permission from the BMJ Publishing Group.)

and Achilles tendon that succumbs to pathology (the posterior fibers) are under the least strain, conversely, those under most strain seem to maintain normal morphology (Almekinders et al 2002, Lyman et al 2004). Restressing the tendon recovers some but not all of the original tendon morphology and mechanical properties (Yamamoto et al 1996).

Exercise increases collagen synthesis, the size and number of fibrils, and consequently tensile strength (Kannus et al 1997, O'Brien 1997). If load is regularly applied to tendon, there is an increase in collagen turnover initially and then a net increase in collagen production if the exercise is maintained for several weeks (Kjaer et al 2005). Much of the newly manufactured collagen is destroyed before becoming incorporated into collagen fibrils and turnover may not reflect greater collagen quantity (Canty & Kadler 2002). Whether this further translates into larger tendon dimensions is unknown; however, human cross-sectional studies (Rosager et al 2002) and animal longitudinal studies suggest that it may. However, a nine month running intervention in humans did not change Achilles tendon cross-sectional area (Hansen et al 2003).

The physiological response of tendons to exercise in humans has been measured in the peritendon in the Achilles tendon. Peritendinous blood flow in humans has been shown to increase 2.5- to 4-fold in the Achilles peritendinous space during muscle exercise (Langberg et al 1998). The tendon response to exercise has been reported to be an increase in blood flow in tendons by up to seven times (Kjaer 2004). Peritendinous blood flow appears to be regulated by prostaglandin, especially COX-2 isoforms. COX-2 medication was shown to reduce blood flow by approximately 40% (Langberg et al 2003). In addition, the glucose uptake of tendons has been shown to increase up to two times that of rest, and this is independent of muscle uptake (Clark et al 2000). This supports an independent regulation of blood flow to tendons from that of muscle (Kallioloski et al 2005).

Other changes seen in the peritendinous region of the Achilles tendon during exercise include increased metabolic activity, change in matrix stimulants and degraders, increased prostaglandins and increased type I collagen formation (Kjaer et al 2000). In addition, it has been shown that inflammatory mediators, cytokines and lactate were increased (Langberg et al 1999a, 2002)

Most effects of exercise on tendon appear to border on the pathological, with collagen fiber changes, tenocyte activation and alterations in ground substance. It has been suggested that to effect a change in tendon strength there must be a period of transient weakness (Archambault et al 1995). This period provides a model for overuse tendinopathies, if load is reapplied before adaptation occurs (Fig. 3.5). The time frame of transient weakness and adaptation to load is not known, making clinical application impossible. There is some evidence that the collagen in tendon responds slowly to load and that the maximal response may be more than 72 hours after a bout of exercise (Langberg et al 1999b). It is unclear if repeat loading before maximal adaptation has a negative effect on tendon. This may have implications for training schedules of both athletes with normal tendons and those with tendon pathology and that greater time between tendon loading may be important.

There appears to be a fine line between load that stimulates positive cellular response and load that triggers a degradative response in tendons (Frank & Hart 1990). It has been suggested that the increase in inflammatory mediators in the peritendon

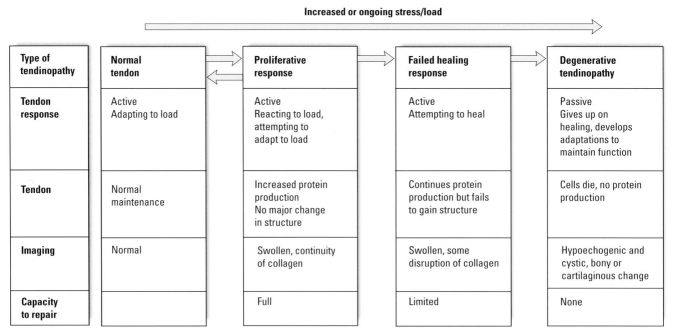

Figure 3.5 • Hypothesized relationship between pathology states described in tendon.

during and after exercise is a stimulant to increased collagen formation along an undefined pathway (Kjaer et al 2000). The relationship between these changes in the peritendon and what occurs in the tendon itself have been demonstrated in animal tendons where long term peritendon inflammation induced intratendinous pathology (Khan et al 2005).

Tendon pathology

Knowledge and understanding of tendon pathology is improving as better technology allows more sophisticated research. Historically, inflammation was accepted as the pathology of both acute and overuse tendon injury, and the term for tendon inflammation was tendinitis. The histopathology of overuse tendon injury at end stage disease, however, repeatedly shows little or no evidence of inflammation (Benazzo et al 1996, Ferretti et al 1983, Khan et al 1996).

There is a dearth of controlled, randomized prospective studies on all aspects of tendon disease (Almekinders & Temple 1998), particularly those studies that examine the early stages of tendinopathy and the repair process of overuse tendinopathy.

Nomenclature

Many different terms are used to describe tendinopathy (Almekinders & Temple 1998, Astrom & Rausing 1995), even the spelling varies from author to author. The terms used to describe tendon pathology (Khan et al 1999a, Maffulli et al 1998) must encompass pathology states as well as clinical status.

The term tendinosis was first used in the 1970s (Puddu et al 1976) to describe the noninflammatory tendon pathology reported at the end stage of the disease, and the term has been used interchangeably with the term degeneration. However, the terminology of degeneration suggests that a decrease in cellularity and function is involved (Leadbetter 1992). As tendinopathy is mainly hypercellular, and has an increase in tissue function, the term degeneration may not be the most applicable.

Failed healing response has also been used to describe the state of tendinopathy and this appears to be the most fitting concept. Clancy (1989) suggested that several factors may contribute to a tendon's failure to heal. These include diminished vascularity, decreased cellularity, lack of reparative cell migration, disease and autoimmune or hereditary factors.

An adaptive response to load could be termed a proliferative tendon response, and under conditions of load could lead to failed healing. Additional tendon load and/or stress in this state could be the stimulus for the local tendon repair process to completely fail: a degenerative condition.

These three pathology states may in fact be a state of increased damage due to an ongoing loading environment over and above that which the tendon can tolerate. As each state is probably associated with a decreased loading capacity, maintained loading may move a tendon to the next stage (Fig. 3.5).

Nature of tendon pathology

Although it is unclear what process initiates tendon pathology, the disease process is consistent, and there are four aspects of tendinopathy that are found in most types of tendinopathy: changes in tenocyte function, collagen degradation, vascular ingrowth and ground substance proliferation. All of these changes are critical components of tendon pathology and are discussed in the following section.

Tenocytes

In tendinopathy, there may be an increase or decrease in cell numbers and activity (Fig. 3.6). Tenocytes that are activated are stimulated into an active, blastic state by signals from the surrounding matrix such as shear forces that stimulate mechanoreceptors on the cell surface, or from self-produced stimulants

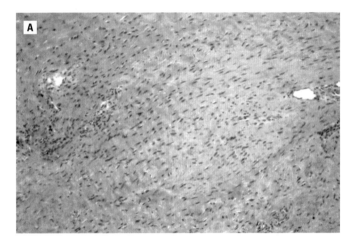

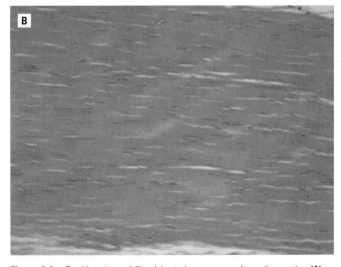

Figure 3.6 • Proliferation of fibroblasts in an area of tendinopathy **(A)**. The large number of cells in this area contrasts to normal tendon with sparse distribution of cells **(B)**. (Reproduced with the permission of Sally F. Bonar.)

such as growth factors (Postlethwaite 1989). These cells become more rounded and the nucleus more prominent and numerous and increased structures for protein synthesis such as Golgi apparatus and rough endoplasmic reticulum (Astrom & Rausing 1995).

Some areas of tendon are associated with tenocyte degeneration and death, not activation. The cell nucleus and organelles fail and the tenocyte is not capable of tendon repair (Józsa et al 1982). Investigations into cell death as a central feature of tendinopathy have focused on cell necrosis as a result in injury and apoptosis (programmed cell death). Apoptosis has been shown to occur after tendon rupture (Yuan et al 2002), and after high mechanical stress (Scott et al 2005), but the role of cell death in the development of tendon pathology is not known.

Extracellular matrix

Collagen

Collagen degradation is pivotal to the pathological process in tendons. It is described in all studies reporting tendon pathology and repair. The collagen is no longer tightly bundled and dense in network and loses its regular crimp, periodicity and birefringence under polarized light (Khan et al 1999a). These descriptions indicate there is a breakdown of the tightly packed collagen bundles of normal tendon, with a consequent loss of tissue and tendon strength. Apart from specific descriptions of transverse fiber disruption seen in tendon rupture, most descriptions of collagen changes allude to longitudinal disruption of the collagen.

Ground substance

The increase in ground substance is a central feature of tendinopathy and is the main component of the 'mucoid', 'cystic' and 'hyaline' appearance of pathology described in the literature (Astrom & Rausing 1995). Preliminary work in human patellar tendon has shown the increase to be three times that of normal tendon (Parkinson, unpublished data). The increase in ground substance has been suggested to be the primary response of activated cells to mechanical overload, secondarily affecting the collagen formation and crosslinks (Cook et al 2004a, Scott 1988). This is in contrast to the usual description of tendon reaction to overload, which is reported to have a primary effect on collagen.

Apart from an increase in ground substance, there may be a change in proteoglycans in the pathological state. The amount of large proteoglycan aggrecan is increased, changing the small to large proteoglycan ratio (Corps et al 2005). Aggrecan is the ground substance of cartilaginous tissue (Benazzo et al 1996).

Neurovascular structures

Neovascularization has been well documented as an important component of tendon pathology. It is closely related to collagen fiber degeneration and may be stimulated by hypoxia (Astrom & Rausing 1995). New vessels are generally considered to be an ingrowth of blood vessels, although Kraushaar & Nirschl

(1999) suggest they are the result of local metaplasia rather than ingrowth from an extrinsic source.

The new vessels in tendon pathology are reported to be thick walled, with an irregular distribution (Astrom & Rausing 1995, Leadbetter 1992), and thought to be compromised with obliterative and thrombotic vascular changes. The neovascularization does not appear to be associated with areas of improved repair (Kraushaar & Nirschl 1999).

Direct measurement of vascularity in Achilles tendinopathy, however, showed increased blood flow, with no evidence of local deficiency of vascular supply (Astrom & Westlin 1994a). Similarly, evidence of both arteriole and venous blood flow has been shown by Doppler ultrasound (US) in tendons diagnosed with tendinosis (Ohberg et al 2001). Imaging studies of tendinopathic tendons consistently report the majority have visible neovascularization (Cook et al 2004b, Khan et al 2003) (Fig. 3.7).

It has been shown that the vascularity is accompanied by neural ingrowth. In pathological tendon, nerve fibers may be found near tendon neovascularization. Biopsies have shown nerve structures closely related to the vessels (Bjur et al 2005). Studies have shown substance P nerves in the vascular wall, and CGRP (calcitonin gene-related peptide) nerves close to the vascular wall (Bjur et al 2005, Ljung et al 2004). Also, the neurokinin-1-receptor, which is known to have a high affinity for substance P, has been found in the vascular wall (Forsgren et al 2005).

Other pathology

The previous section describes the histopathology of basic tendinopathy; however, it encompasses more than this simple entity. Variations in tendinopathy exist, with slight differences in histopathological appearance. These variations include all the vascular, cellular, collagen and ground substance alterations as described in the previous section.

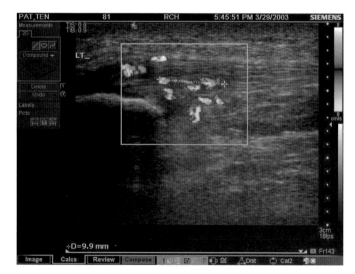

Figure 3.7 • Ultrasound imaging using color Doppler of patellar tendon showing infiltration with large-diameter vessels. Normal tendon will contain no visible vessels on Doppler ultrasound.

The names for these variations include hypoxic, mucoid, myxoid, lipoid and calcific tendinopathy (Järvinen et al 1997). It is unclear how or why tendon pathology varies in different tendons in the body and between individuals, and the causative factors underlying each type of pathology are unknown (Kannus 1997).

All these types of tendon pathology may be found in the same tendon, even in close proximity to each other. They are all found in ruptured tendons and appear to have an etiological role in tendon weakness and rupture (Kannus & Józsa 1991). In a series of 891 tendon ruptures, hypoxic change was the most common histopathology (Kannus & Józsa 1991). In the same study, only one-third of unruptured tendons in subjects of similar age and activity levels demonstrated histopathological changes.

Calcification in tendons is usually found in areas of pathology and is described as part of the process of tendon damage and repair. Formation of bone is reported to be in response to the application of both tensile and compressive loads. In the rotator cuff, however, calcifying tendinopathy can occur in areas of normal tendon. This process appears to be a cell-mediated response and is associated with specific human leukocyte antigen (HLA) tissue typing (A1) (Sengar et al 1987). This type of often resolving tendinopathy has rarely been reported in other tendons. The same authors reported no association between this HLA typing and rotator cuff rupture (Sengar et al 1989).

Inflammation

Inflammation is the initial response of all tissues to injury, and is also the start of the reparative process. Usually in acute injury the initiating damage is vascular disruption; however, other stimuli such as ischemia, and mechanical loading can also initiate inflammation (Scott et al 2004). Thus, it is well accepted that inflammation occurs in a tendon after macrotrauma such as tenotomy and tendon rupture, and that changes in tendon tissue that have aspects of a typical inflammatory response may occur after other stimuli. These stimuli may cause an inflammation via neuropepide release. This neurogenically mediated inflammation is likely to exist in tendons (Hart et al 1995).

Inflammation in tendons may be apparent around intratendinous calcification and at the site of steroid injection (Leadbetter 1992, Selvanetti et al 1997). It is also apparent in rheumatoid arthritis, gout, seronegative arthropathies and septic tendinopathies (Selvanetti et al 1997). Nirschl (1990) reported that inflammatory cells may be seen in tissues in close proximity to the tendon although absent from the tendon itself. Most investigators agree that inflammatory pathology affects peritendinous tissues (paratenonitis, peritendinitis, tenosynovitis, tenovaginitis) (Kvist 1994). The inflammatory response to tendon injury may be mediated by age, gender, disease and individual, perhaps genetically determined, factors.

Structural changes in tendon pathology

Enthesopathies

Musculotendinous overuse affects the enthesis, as can metabolic, endocrine and inflammatory disease (Benjamin & Ralphs 1996). All these stimulants cause the transitional bone–tendon zone to become abnormally organized. Pathology of the enthesis includes abnormalities in the fibrocartilage (thickening, mineralization and myxomatosis) (Benjamin & Ralphs 1995, Ferretti et al 1985, Selvanetti et al 1997, Uhthoff & Matsumoto 2000), the mineralized fibrocartilage (cystic cavities) (Ferretti et al 1985) and the tendon (decreased cellularity, calcification) (Selvanetti et al 1997). The pathology at endstage disease is identical to that seen in mid-tendon pathology (Maffulli et al 2004).

Enthesis failure often occurs at the subchondral bone, suggesting that the actual tendon attachment is not the area of weakness (Benjamin & Ralphs 1998). This is supported by studies of the mechanical properties of tendons that suggest the insertional regions of normal tendons withstand high strain without rupture (Wren et al 2001).

Paratenonitis

Paratenonitis commonly occurs where a tendon rubs over a bony protuberance or abuts another structure, but can occur anywhere along the length of a tendon. The term has been proposed as an umbrella term for the separate entities of peritendinitis, tenosynovitis and tenovaginitis. Examples include paratenonitis of the abductor pollicis longus and extensor pollicis longus (De Quervain disease), and of the flexor hallucis longus as it passes the medial malleolus of the tibia (Almekinders 1998).

Paratenonitis is characterized clinically by acute edema and hyperemia of the paratenon with infiltration of inflammatory cells. Fibrinous exudate fills the tendon sheath after hours to a few days, and causes the 'crepitus' that can be felt on clinical examination. In chronic paratenonitis, fibroblasts appear along with a perivascular lymphocytic infiltrate. Peritendinous tissue becomes macroscopically thickened and new connective tissue adhesions occur (Järvinen et al 1997). Myofibroblasts (cells with cytoplasmic myofilaments) also appear and make up about 20% of the noninflammatory cells. These cells are capable of active contraction, indicating that scarring and shrinkage associated with paratenonitis is an active cell-mediated process (Järvinen et al 1997). Blood vessels proliferate, and marked inflammatory changes are seen in more than 20% of the arteries (Kvist et al 1992). Thus, inflammatory cells are found in both the cellular elements of the peritendon and the vascular ingrowth.

Long-term peritendon inflammation has been shown to lead to intratendinous change (Khan et al 2005). As imaging modalities show very little peritendon change especially in tendons that have minimal peritendon tissue, it is possible that inflammation in the peritendon is largely undetected.

Tendon pain

The source of pain in pathological tendon tissue is not clearly understood. There are many theories about the cause of tendinopathic pain, and an increasing body of evidence that suggests a neurovascular or biochemical rather than structural cause of pain (Khan et al 2000).

Collagen disruption (either transverse or longitudinal) is not the source of pain in the tendon. The removal of large chunks of collagen (e.g. in the harvesting of tendon tissue for ligament reconstruction) rarely results in tendon pain. Similarly, there is poor correlation between imaging changes after tendon surgery and symptoms (Khan et al 1999b). Both these observations suggest that collagen damage is not a source of pain.

The concept that intact collagen surrounding tendinopathy is overloaded and that it is the source of pain is also partly rebutted by the above discussion. This model suggests that tendons with greater areas of tendinopathy should be more painful, as there is less intact tissue sustaining greater load. Imaging studies have shown that there is little correlation between the amount of collagen disruption and pain, with large areas demonstrated as being asymptomatic on ultrasound, and tendons with normal imaging having symptoms (Cook et al 1998, 2000a).

Although collagen disruption per se may not be the source of tendon pain, the tendon reaction to collagen damage may create a biochemical environment that stimulates nociceptors. Theoretically, cellular and extracellular debris, minor collagens and proteoglycans have been suggested as the source of nociceptor stimulation.

Other possible mechanisms for tendon pain include irritation of the surrounding (and usually well-innervated) structures (fat pad in the knee, subacromial bursa in the shoulder) and increased intratendinous pressure (Johnson et al 1996). These remain theories only, and further investigation is required.

By using methods like microdialysis, cDNA-arrays and PCR, and ultrasonography combined with color Doppler, there is now new and potentially important information about the biochemical and neurovascular sources of painful tendons. Tendon pathology has associated neovascularization, and several studies have linked increased tendon vascularity to greater tendon pain (Cook et al 2004b, 2005). The relationship, however, is not absolute and the amount of vascularity may merely reflect increased neural ingrowth.

Neural substances such as glutamate (Alfredson et al 1999), lactate and substance P (Gotoh et al 1998) have been shown in tendon pathology and are known to increase nociception. Receptors to substance P (Ljung et al 1999) and NMDAR receptors have been shown associated with tendon vessels. Glutamate, a well-known neurotransmitter and very potent modulator of pain in the central nervous system is found in high levels in painful tendons and not in normal tendons (Alfredson et al 2001). However, glutamate levels were not altered from baseline after an exercise program that abolished pain (Alfredson & Lorentzon 2003), suggesting that glutamate does not directly contribute to pain but may act by enhancing other neuropeptides.

The role of these pain modulators in tendon pain is enhanced by the findings of a local neural ingrowth (Bjur et al 2005). Biopsies taken from an area with tendinosis with neovascularization showed nerve structures in close relation to the vessels (Bjur et al 2005), and studies have shown substance P nerves in the vascular wall, and CGRP nerves close to the vascular wall (Bjur et al 2005, Ljung et al 2004). Also, the neurokinin-1-receptor, which is known to have a high affinity for substance P, has been found in the vascular wall (Forsgren et al 2005).

The source of tendon pain is a clinically critical aspect of tendinopathy as treatment for tendinopathy is primarily directed at decreasing pain. Further research in this area is underway, and pharmaceutical, not physical intervention may prove efficacious.

Physiology of tendon pathology

Tendon cells appear to be in a constant state of response to load, and shape their extracellular matrix to suit the loading environment. Minor disruption of this process may lead to a cascade of change in the extracellular matrix, changing load capacity and starting a cycle of matrix damage and load sensitivity.

The endstage of the pathology cycle is neovascularization, and the greatest stimulus for new blood vessels is hypoxia. The role of hypoxia in the development of pathology has not been clarified, but increased levels of lactate have been shown in abnormal tendons, suggesting anaerobic metabolism (Alfredson et al 2002). In addition, hypoxia stimulates the production of type III collagen (Mehm et al 1988, Rempel & Abrahamsson 2001), suggesting that hypoxia could drive several changes seen in tendon pathology. In addition, rotator cuff tendinopathy has been reported to have fewer vessels than normal tendon (Biberthaler et al 2003); however, it is unclear if this drives the hypoxia or is a result of cartilaginous metaplasia. Imaging studies suggest that the supraspinatus has compressive forces acting on it through most ranges of movement and this could result in cartilaginous change (Bey et al 2002).

In pathological tendon, change in tendon milieu has been quantified by imaging both immediately and over the long term. After a single bout of eccentric exercise the tendon volume and signal both increased (Shalabi et al 2004a). Eccentric exercise in the Achilles tendons over a 12-week period has been shown to decrease tendon volume and intratendinous signal. Change in pain correlated with change in signal, although the strength of the relationship was not reported (Shalabi et al 2004b).

Tendon repair

Soft tissue healing is usually sufficient to maintain function; however, repair of tendons is never complete (Frank et al 1999). Tendons appear to have the capacity to repair adequately, as both endogenous tenocytes and extrinsic cells originally from outside the tendon can migrate to the tendon damage and contribute to the repair process. There is some debate about the relative contributions of the intrinsic and extrinsic cells to tendon repair, and studies have indicated that the tendon is capable of healing without immigration of extrinsic cells (Kraushaar & Nirschl 1999). The type and site of the injury may determine which repair process is initiated (Gelberman et al 1988). Repair is influenced by age, tendon vascularity, gender, nutrition, hormones, activity and disease (Hart et al 1995, Leadbetter 1992).

Clancy (1989) considered that the poor healing response in tendon is due in part to reparative cells failing to migrate to the site of injury. Alternatively, the poor healing response

(Leadbetter 1992) may partly be explained by the inability of tenocytes to repair tendon quickly and adequately enough. There are, however, many chemotactic signals that stimulate the migration of cells to the injury site, including several that are produced without vascular damage. Tendon microtrauma should therefore produce a healing response with or without vascular disruption (Postlethwaite 1989).

Type III collagen is the collagen produced in repairing tendon after both acute and overuse tendon injury (Maffulli et al 2000), and considered by some authors to be a 'tendon patch' (Archambault et al 1995). It is smaller than type I collagen and forms a looser reticular network rather than the long thick bundles of type I (Józsa et al 1984). This collagen was also more easily denatured experimentally, indicating that crosslinks were weaker than in type I collagen. It has been hypothesized that this smaller diameter collagen may be, in part, responsible for the decrease in tendon strength associated with pathology (Archambault et al 1995, Williams et al 1984).

Post injury, type III collagen is reportedly replaced by type I collagen at a variable point in time and the tendon becomes stiffer and stronger as the replacing type I collagen matures (O'Brien 1997). In a study of equine tendon type III collagen comprised 20–30% of scarred tendon, and was still apparent up to 14 months after injury (Williams et al 1980, 1984). The time frame for maturation and repair are unknown, and thus application to clinical practice is impossible.

Macrotraumatic repair

Tendon repair research has evaluated models of tendon rupture and experimental tenotomy (Hart et al 1995). These studies have indicated that tendon requires three stages for repair: cell proliferation, collagen synthesis and collagen realignment (El Hawary et al 1997). The complete process includes inflammation, epitenon thickening, fibroblast proliferation, cell activation, vascular ingrowth, matrix and collagen production and remodeling (Gelberman et al 1988, Leadbetter 1992).

Microtraumatic repair

Overuse tendon injuries 'lack the ordered and timely triphasic reparative response' of acute injury (Selvanetti et al 1997). Very little, however, has been written on the repair of overuse tendon injury especially in human tendons (Clancy 1989, El Hawary et al 1997), where experimental design and ethical considerations limit investigation.

There are several factors that contribute to the quality of tendon healing response, including the type and intensity of the injury, individual factors and treatment. Overloaded tendon has been called a tissue that has a failed healing response, defined as either an inadequate or extravagant inflammatory process response (Clancy 1989, Hart et al 1995). This may be associated with a failure of the alignment and cross-linking of collagen (Kraushaar & Nirschl 1999).

There may be a cyclic relationship between normal tendon, pathology and repair. What is often reported as pathology may in fact represent tendon repair (Fredberg & Bolvig 1999). The distinction between repair and pathology may be important, as the presence of reparative signs such as type III collagen and tenocyte activity are a positive tendon response.

Do tendons repair completely and return to their original state? Although the theory of tendon repair describes the eventual replacement of type III collagen with type I collagen, it appears that there is less than perfect replacement, and consequently repair. Repaired tendons may only return to 70–80% of their original strength (Leadbetter 1993). However, longitudinal imaging studies have demonstrated that about 7% of tendons abnormal at baseline revert to a normal appearance at follow-up, suggesting that at the very least some abnormal tendons can normalize (Cook et al 2000b, 2000c, Fredberg & Bolvig 2002).

The future direction of tendon repair is to further explore critical factors in the tendons' response to injury. This includes investigation into tenocyte control systems, chemical signals for tendon maturation and collagen stimulation (Kraushaar & Nirschl 1999). Similarly, investigations in ligament tissue have suggested that altering the cellularity and altering cellular expression may offer improvement in the repair process (Frank et al 1999). This tissue engineering is in its embryonic stages, but may turn our current passive approach to tendon injury to more active interventions.

Growth factors

A superfamily of growth, differentiation and morphogenic factors exists in human cells, with each cell making and responding to some of these factors (Sanzone & Einhorn 1998). Growth factors are necessary for normal tissue repair, as load without growth factors may lead to cell death and matrix degradation (Banes et al 1995).

Many growth factors have been reported in tendon repairs; however, most have only been investigated in acutely injured tendon and their presence and action in overuse tendinopathy has not been established. In addition the role of growth factors such as vascular endothelial growth factor (VEGF) is currently under investigation as the role of neovascularization in tendinopathy becomes clearer.

Cells from both ligament and tendon have been shown to be responsive to several growth factors (Sanzone & Einhorn 1998). Growth factors act both embryogenically and as an intrinsic part of tissue repair, and have been shown to attract macrophages and tenoblasts to tissue injury (Jann et al 1999, Sporn & Roberts 1989), influence the differentiation of connective tissue cells into tendon forming cells (Sanzone & Einhorn 1998) and control extracellular matrix degradation (Robins 1988). Growth factors offer an exciting potential therapy after tissue damage, and tendons in particular would benefit from agents that can facilitate repair.

Summary

Tendon injury, although common, has been the subject of limited investigation. Although recovery from acute tendon injury highlights the similarity of tendon repair to other tissue, it is evident from the resistant nature of overuse tendinopathy to treatment that direct application of this knowledge may not be appropriate. From this chapter it is evident that both the process of injury and the process to repair are poorly understood in overuse tendinopathy.

Physiotherapeutic intervention in tendinopathy is primarily based on clinical experience, and studies investigating the effect of treatment are lacking. Therefore, studies improving the understanding of the disease and repair process and the most effective treatment are needed.

References

Ahmed I, Lagoloulos M, McConnell P et al 1998 Blood supply of the Achilles tendon. Journal of Orthopaedic Research 16:591–596

Alfredson H, Lorentzon R 2003 Intratendinous glutamate levels and eccentric training on chronic Achilles tendinosis: a prospective study using microdialysis technique. Knee Surgery, Sports Traumatology, Arthroscopy 11:196–199

Alfredson H, Thorsen K, Lorentzon R 1999 In situ microdialysis in tendon tissue: high levels of glutamate, but not protoglandin E_2 in chronic Achilles tendon pain. Knee Surgery, Sports Traumatology, Arthroscopy 7:378–381

Alfredson H, Forsgren S, Thorsen K et al 2001 In vivo microdialysis and immunohistochemical analyses of tendon tissue demonstrated high amounts of free glutamate and glutamate receptors, but no signs of inflammation, in Jumper's knee. Journal of Orthopaedic Research 19:881–886

Alfredson H, Bjur D, Thorsen K et al 2002 High intratendinous lactate levels in painful chronic Achilles tendinosis. An investigation using microdialysis technique. Journal of Orthopaedic Research 20:934–938

Almekinders L C 1998 Tendinitis and other chronic tendinopathies. Journal of American Academy of Orthopedic Surgery 6:157–164

Almekinders L, Temple J 1998 Etiology, diagnosis, and treatment of tendonitis: an analysis of the literature. Medicine and Science in Sports and Exercise 30:1183–1190

Almekinders L C, Banes A J, Ballenger C A 1993 Effects of repetitive motion on human fibroblasts. Medicine and Science in Sports and Exercise 25:603–607

Almekinders L C, Vellema J H, Weinhold P S 2002 Strain patterns in the patellar tendon and the implications for patellar tendinopathy. Knee Surgery, Sports Traumatology, Arthroscopy 10:2–5

Almekinders L C, Weinhold P S, Maffulli N 2003 Compression etiology in tendinopathy. Clinics in Sports Medicine 22:703–710

Archambault J M, Wiley J P, Bray R C 1995 Exercise loading of tendons and the development of overuse injuries. A review of the current literature. Sports Medicine 20:77–89

Astrom M, Rausing A 1995 Chronic Achilles tendinopathy. A survey of surgical and histopathologic findings. Clinical Orthopaedics 316:151–164

Astrom M, Westlin N 1994a Blood flow in chronic Achilles tendinopathy. Clinical Orthopaedics 308:166–172

Astrom M, Westlin N 1994b Blood flow in the normal Achilles tendon assessed by laser Doppler flowmetry. Journal of Orthopaedic Research 12:246–252

Banes A J, Hu P, Xiao H et al 1995 Tendon cells of the epitenon and internal tendon compartment communicate mechanical signals through gap junctions and respond differentially to mechanical load and growth factors. In: Gordon S L, Blair S J, Fine L J (eds) Repetitive motion disorders of the upper extremity. American Academy of Orthopaedic Surgeons, Park Ridge, IL, p 231–245

Banks R A, TeKoppele J M, Oostingh G et al 1999 Lysylhydroxylation and non-reducible crosslinking of human supraspinatus tendon collagen: changes with age and in chronic rotator cuff tendinitis. Annals of Rheumatic Diseases 58:35–41

Benazzo F, Stennardo G, Valli M 1996 Achilles and patellar tendinopathies in athletes: pathogenesis and surgical treatment. Bulletin (Hospital for Joint Diseases) 54:236–240

Benjamin M, Ralphs J 1995 Functional and developmental anatomy of tendons and ligaments. In: Gordon S L, Blair S J, Fine L J (eds) Repetitive motion disorders of the upper extremity. American Academy of Orthopaedic Surgeons, Park Ridge, IL, p 185–203

Benjamin M, Ralphs J 1996 Tendons in health and disease. Manual Therapy 1:186–191

Benjamin M, Ralphs J R 1998 Fibrocartilage in tendons and ligaments: an adaptation to compressive load. Journal of Anatomy 193:481–494

Benjamin M, Moriggl B, Brenner E et al 2004 The 'enthesis organ' concept. Why enthesopathies may not present as focal insertional disorders. Arthritis and Rheumatism 50:3306–3313

Bey M, Song H, Wehrli F et al 2002 Intratendinous strain fields of the intact supraspinatus tendon: the effect of glenohumeral joint position and tendon region. Journal of Orthopaedic Research 20:869–874

Biberthaler P, Weidemann E, Nerlich A et al 2003 Microcirculation associated with degenerative rotator cuff lesions. Journal of Bone and Joint Surgery (Am) 85-A:475–480

Bjur D, Alfredson H, Forsgren S 2005 The innervation pattern of the human Achilles tendon: studies of the normal and tendinosis tendon with markers for general and sensory innervation. Cell and Tissue Research 320:201–206

Boushel R, Langberg H, Green S et al 2000 Blood flow and oxygenation in peri-tendinous tissue and calf muscle during dynamic exercise. Journal of Physiology 524:305–313

Canty E, Kadler K 2002 Collagen fibril biosynthesis in tendon: a review and recent highlights. Comparative Biochemistry and Physiology A 133:979–985

Clancy W 1989 Failed healing responses. In: Leadbetter W B, Buckwalter J A, Gordon S (eds) Sports-induced inflammation: clinical and basic science concepts. American Orthopedic Society for Sports Medicine, Park Ridge, IL

Clancy W G J 1990 Tendon trauma and overuse injuries. In: Leadbetter W B, Buckwalter J A, Gordon S (eds) Sports-induced inflammation: clinical and basic science concepts. American Orthopedic Society for Sports Medicine, Park Ridge, IL, p 609–618

Clark M, Clerk L, Newman J et al 2000 Interaction between metabolism and flow in tendon and muscle. Scandinavian Journal of Medicine and Science in Sports 10:338–345

Cook J L, Khan K M, Harcourt P R et al 1998 Patellar tendon ultrasonography in asymptomatic active athletes reveals hypoechoic regions: a study of 320 tendons. Clinical Journal of Sports Medicine 8:73–77

Cook J, Coleman B, Khan K et al 2000a Patellar tendinopathy in junior basketball players: a controlled clinical and ultrasonographic study of 268 tendons in players aged 14–18 years. Scandinavian Journal of Medicine and Science in Sports 10:216–220

Cook J L, Khan K M, Kiss Z S et al 2000b Asymptomatic hypoechoic regions on patellar tendon US do not foreshadow symptoms of jumper's knee: a 4 year followup of 46 tendons. Scandinavian Journal of Science and Medicine in Sports 11:321–327

Cook J L, Kiss Z S, Khan K M et al 2000c Prospective imaging study of asymptomatic patellar tendinopathy in elite junior basketball players. Journal of Ultrasound in Medicine 19:473–479

Cook J L, Feller J, Bonar S F et al 2004a Abnormal tenocyte morphology is more prevalent than collagen disruption in asymptomatic athletes' patellar tendons: Is this the first step in the tendinosis cascade? Journal of Orthopaedic Research 24:334–338

Cook J L, Malliaras P, Luca J D et al 2004b Neovascularisation and pain in abnormal patellar tendons of active jumping athletes. Clinical Journal of Sports Medicine 14:296–299

Cook J L, Malliaras P, Luca J D et al 2005 Vascularity and pain in the patellar tendon of adult jumping athletes: a 5 month longitudinal study. British Journal of Sports Medicine 39:458–461

Corps A, Robinson A, Movin T et al 2006 Increased expression of aggrecan and biglycan mRNA in Achilles tendinopathy. Rheumatology: 45:291–294

Cribb A M, Scott J E 1995 Tendon response to tensile stress: an ultrastructural investigation of collagen:proteoglycan interactions in stressed tendon. Journal of Anatomy 187:423–428

El Hawary R, Stanish W D, Curwin S L 1997 Rehabilitation of tendon injuries in sport. Sports Medicine 24:347–358

Ferretti A, Ippolito E, Mariani P et al 1983 Jumper's knee. American Journal of Sports Medicine 11:58–62

Ferretti A, Puddu G, Mariani P et al 1985 The natural history of jumper's knee: patellar or quadriceps tendinitis. International Orthopaedics 8:239–242

Forsgren S, Danielsson S, Alfredson H 2005 Vascular NK-1R receptor occurrence in normal and chronic painful Achilles and patellar tendons. Studies on chemically unfixed as well as fixed specimens. Regulatory Peptides 126:173–181

Frank C, Shrive N, Hiraoka H et al 1999 Optimisation of the biology of soft tissue repair. Journal of Science and Medicine in Sport 2:190–210

Frank C B, Hart D A 1990 Cellular response to loading. In: Leadbetter W B, Buckwalter J A, Gordon S (eds) Sports-induced inflammation: clinical and basic science concepts. American Orthopedic Society for Sports Medicine, Park Ridge, IL

Fredberg U, Bolvig L 1999 Jumper's knee. Scandinavian Journal of Medicine and Science in Sports 9:66–73

Fredberg U, Bolvig L 2002 Significance of ultrasonographically detected asymptomatic tendinosis in the patellar and Achilles tendons of elite soccer players. American Journal of Sports Medicine 30:488–491

Frost H M 1990 Skeletal structural adaptations to mechanical usage (SATMU): 4. Mechanical influences on intact fibrous tissue. Anatomical Record 226:433–439

Fyfe I, Stanish WD 1992 The use of eccentric training and stretching in the treatment and prevention of tendon injuries. Clinics in Sports Medicine 11:601–624.

Gelberman R, Goldberg V, An K-N et al 1988 Tendon. In: Woo S L-Y, Buckwalter J A (eds) Injury and repair of the musculoskeletal soft tissues. American Academy of Orthopedic Surgeons, Park Ridge, IL, p 5–40

Giori N J, Beaupre G S, Carter D R 1993 Cellular shape and pressure may mediate mechanical control of tissue composition in tendons. Journal of Orthopaedic Research 11:581–591

Gotoh M, Hamada K, Yamakawa H et al 1998 Increased substance P in subacromial bursa and shoulder pain in rotator cuff disease. Journal of Orthopaedic Research 16:618–621

Gross M T 1992 Chronic tendonitis: pathomechanics of injury, factors affecting the healing response, and treatment. Journal of Orthopaedic and Sports Physical Therapy 16:248–261

Hansen P, Aagaard P, Kjaer M et al 2003 Effect of habitual running in human Achilles tendon load-deformation properties and cross-sectional area. Journal of Applied Physiology 95:2375–2380

Hart D A, Frank C B, Bray R C 1995. Inflammatory processes in repetitive motion and overuse syndromes: potential role of neurogenic mechanisms in tendons and ligaments. In: Gordon S L, Blair S J, Fine L J (eds) Repetitive motion disorders of the upper extremity. American Academy of Orthopaedic Surgeons, Park Ridge, IL, p 247–262

Hess G P, Cappiello W K, Poole R M et al 1989 Prevention and treatment of overuse tendon injuries. Sports Medicine 8:371–384

Jann H, Stein L, Slater D 1999 In vitro effects of epidermal growth factor or insulin-like growth factor on tenoblast migration on absorbable suture material. Veterinary Surgery 28:268–278

Järvinen M, Józsa L, Kannus P et al 1997 Histopathological findings in chronic tendon disorders. Scandinavian Journal of Medicine and Science in Sports 7:86–95

Johnson D P, Wakeley C J, Watt I 1996 Magnetic resonance imaging of patellar tendonitis. Journal of Bone and Joint Surgery (Br) 78-B:452–457

Józsa L, Kannus P 1997 Human tendons. Human Kinetics, Champaign, IL

Józsa L, Bálint B J, Demel Z 1982 Hypoxic alterations of tenocytes in degenerative tendonopathy. Archives of Orthopaedic and Traumatic Surgery 99:243–246

Józsa L, Réffy A, Bálint B J 1984 Polarisation and electron microscope studies on the collagen of intact and ruptured human tendons. Acta Histochemica 74:209–215

Józsa L, Kannus P, Bálint J B et al 1991 Three-dimensional ultrastructure of human tendons. Acta Anatomica 142:306–312

Kallioloski K, Langberg H, Ryberg A et al 2005 The effect of dynamic knee-extension exercise on patellar tendon and quadriceps femoris muscle glucose uptake in humans studied by positron emission tomography. Journal of Applied Physiology 99:1189–1192

Kannus P 1997 Etiology and pathophysiology of tendon ruptures in sports. Scandinavian Journal of Medicine and Science in Sports 7:107–112

Kannus P, Józsa L 1991 Histopathological changes preceding spontaneous rupture of a tendon. Journal of Bone and Joint Surgery (Am) 73A:1507–1525

Kannus P, Józsa L, Natri A et al 1997 Effects of training, immobilization and remobilization on tendons. Scandinavian Journal of Medicine and Science in Sports 7:67–71

Ker R F 2002 The implications of the adaptable fatigue quality of tendons for their construction, repair and function. Comparative Biochemistry and Physiology A 133:987–1000

Khan K M, Bonar F, Desmond P M et al 1996 Patellar tendinosis (jumper's knee): findings at histopathologic examination, US and MR imaging. Radiology 200:821–827

Khan K M, Cook J L, Bonar S F et al 1999a Histopathology of common overuse tendon conditions: update and implications for clinical management. Sports Medicine 6:393–408

Khan K M, Visentini P J, Kiss Z S et al 1999b Correlation of US and MR imaging with clinical outcome after open patellar tenotomy: prospective and retrospective studies. Clinical Journal of Sports Medicine 9:129–137

Khan K, Cook J, Maffulli N et al 2000 Where is the pain coming from in tendinopathy? It may be biochemical, not only structural, in origin. British Journal of Sports Medicine 34:81–83

Khan K M, Forster B B, Robinson J et al 2003 Are ultrasound and magnetic resonance imaging of value in assessment of Achilles tendon disorders? A two year prospective study. British Journal of Sports Medicine 37:149–154

Khan M H, Li Z, Wang J 2005 Repeated exposure of tendon to prostoglandin-E2 leads to localised tendon degeneration. Clinical Journal of Sport Medicine 15:28–33

Kirkendall D T, Garrett W E 1997 Function and biomechanics of tendons. Scandinavian Journal of Medicine and Science in Sports 7:62–66

Kjaer M 2004 Role of extracellular matrix in adaptation of tendon and skeletal muscle to mechanical loading. Physiology Review 84:649–698

Kjaer M, Langberg H, Skovgaard D et al 2000 In vivo studies of peritendinous tissue in exercise. Scandinavian Journal of Medicine and Science in Sports 10:326–331

Kjaer M, Langberg H, Miller B et al 2005 Metabolic activity and collagen turnover in human tendon in response to physical activity. Journal of Musculoskeletal and Neuronal Interaction 5:41–52

Kraushaar B, Nirschl R 1999 Tendinosis of the elbow (tennis elbow). Clinical features and findings of histological, immunohistochemical, and electron microscopy studies. Journal of Bone and Joint Surgery (Am) 81A:259–278

Kvist M 1994 Achilles tendon injuries in athletes. Sports Medicine 18:173–201

Kvist M, Józsa L, Kannus P et al 1991 Morphology and histochemistry of the myotendineal junction of the rat calf muscle. Acta Anatomica 141:199–205

Kvist M, Józsa L, Järvinen M 1992 Vascular changes in the ruptured Achilles tendon and its paratenon. International Orthopaedics 16:377–382

Langberg H, Bulow J, Kjaer M 1998 Blood flow in the peritendinous space of the human Achilles tendon during exercise. Acta Physiologica Scandinavia 163:149–153

Langberg H, Skovgaard D, Karamouzis M et al 1999a Metabolism and inflammatory mediators in the peritendinous space measured by microdialysis during intermittent isometric exercise in humans. Journal of Physiology 515:919–927

Langberg H, Skovgaard D, Petersen L J et al 1999b Type I collagen synthesis and degradation in peritendinous tissue after exercise determined by microdialysis in humans. Journal of Physiology 521:299–306

Langberg H, Olesen J L, Gemmer C et al 2002 Substantial elevation of interleukin-6 concentration in peritendinous tisses, in contrast to muscle, following prologed exercise in humans. Journal of Physiology 542:985–990

Langberg H, Boushel R, Skovgaard D et al 2003 Cyclo-oxygenase-2 mediated prostoglandin release regulates blood flow in connective tissue during mechanical loading in humans. Journal of Physiology 551:683–689

Leadbetter W 1992 Cell matrix response in tendon injury. Clinics in Sports Medicine 11:533–578

Leadbetter W B 1993 Tendon overuse injuries: diagnosis and treatment. In: Renstrom P A F H (ed) Sports injuries. Basic principles of prevention and care. Oxford Press, London, p 449–476

Ljung B, Forsgren S, Friden J 1999 Substance P and calcitonin gene-related peptide expression at the extensor carpi radialis brevis muscle origin: implications for the etiology of tennis elbow. Journal of Orthopaedic Research 17:554–559

Ljung B, Alfredson H, Forsgren S 2004 Neurokinin 1-receptors and sensory neuropeptides in tendon insertions at the medial and lateral epicondyles of the humerus. Studies on tennis elbow and medial epicondylalgia. Journal of Orthopaedic Research 22:321–327

Lyman J, Weinhold P, Almekinders L 2004 Strain behaviour of the distal Achilles tendon. American Journal of Sports Medicine 32:457–461

Maffulli N, Khan K M, Puddu G 1998 Overuse tendon conditions. Time to change a confusing terminology. Arthroscopy 14:840–843

Maffulli N, Ewen S, Waterston S et al 2000 Tenocytes from ruptured and tendinopathic Achilles tendons produce greater quantities of type III collagen than tenocytes from normal Achilles tendon. American Journal of Sports Medicine 28:499–505

Maffulli N, Testa V, Capasso G et al 2004 Similar histopathological picture in males with Achilles and patellar tendinopathy. Medicine and Science in Sports and Exercise 36:1470–1475

Majima T, Yasuda K, Tsuchida T et al 2003 Stress shielding of patellar tendon: effect on small diameter collagen fibrils in a rabbit model. Journal of Orthopaedic Science 8:836–841

Mehm W J, Pimsler M, Becker R L et al 1988 Effect of oxygen on in vitro fibroblast cell proliferation and collagen biosynthesis. Journal of Hyperbaric Medicine 3:227–234

Nirschl R P 1990 Patterns of failed healing in tendon injury. In: Leadbetter W B, Buckwalter J A, Gordon S (eds) Sports-induced inflammation: clinical and basic science concepts. American Orthopedic Society for Sports Medicine, Park Ridge, IL, p 577–585

O'Brien M 1992 Functional anatomy and physiology of tendons. Clinics in Sports Medicine 11:505–520

O'Brien M 1997 Structure and metabolism of tendons. Scandinavian Journal of Medicine and Science in Sports 7:55–61

Ohberg L, Lorentzon R, Alfredson H 2001 Neovascularisation in Achilles tendons with painful tendinosis but not in normal tendons: an ultrasonographic investigation. Knee Surgery, Sports Traumatology, Arthroscopy 9:233–238

Orchard J, Cook J L, Halpin N 2004 Stress shielding as a cause of insertional tendinopathy: the operative technique of limited adductor tenotomy supports this theory. Journal of Science and Medicine in Sport 7:424–428

Postlethwaite A E 1989 Failed healing responses in connective tissue and a comparison of medical conditions. In: Leadbetter W B, Buckwalter J A, Gordon S (eds) Sports-induced inflammation: clinical and basic science concepts. American Orthopedic Society for Sports Medicine, Park Ridge, IL

Puddu G, Ippolito E, Postacchini F 1976 A classification of Achilles tendon disease. American Journal of Sports Medicine 4:145–150

Rempel D, Abrahamsson S O 2001 The effects of reduced oxygen tension on cell proliferation and matrix synthesis in synovium and tendon explants from the rabbit carpal tunnel: an experimental study in vitro. Journal of Orthopaedic Research 19:143–148

Robins S P 1988 Functional properties of collagen and elastin. Baillière's Clinical Rheumatology 2:1–36

Rosager S, Aagaard P, Dyhre-Poulsen P et al 2002 Load-displacement properties of the human triceps surae aponeurosis and tendon in runners and non-runners. Scandinavian Journal of Medicine and Science in Sports 12:90–98

Rufai A, Ralphs J R, Benjamin M 1995 Structure and histopathology of the insertional region of the human Achilles tendon. Journal of Orthopaedic Research 13:585–593

Sano H, Ishii H, Yeadon A et al 1997 Degeneration of the insertion weakens the tensile strength of the supraspinatus tendon: a comparative mechanical and histologic study of the bone–tendon complex. Journal of Orthopaedic Research 15:719–726

Sanzone A G, Einhorn T A 1998 The use of bone morphogenic proteins to heal fractures, articular cartilage defects, and ligament and tendon injuries. Sports Medicine and Arthroscopy Review 6:118–123

Sarasa-Renedo A, Chiquet M 2005 Mechanical signals regulating extracellular matrix gene expression in fibroblasts. Scandinavian Journal of Medicine and Science in Sports 25:223

Schatzker J, Branemark P 1969 Intravital observations on the microvascular anatomy and microcirculation of the tendon. Acta Orthopaedica Scandinavia 126 (suppl):S1–S23

Schatzmann L, Brunner P, Staubli H U 1998 Effect of cyclic preconditioning on the tensile properties of human quadriceps tendons and patellar ligaments. Knee Surgery, Sports Traumatology, Arthroscopy 6:56–61

Scott A, Khan K M, Cook J L et al 2004 What do we mean by the term 'inflammation'? A contemporary basic science update for sports medicine. British Journal of Sports Medicine 38:372–380

Scott A, Khan K, Heer J et al 2005 High strain mechanical loading rapidly induces tendon apoptosis: an ex vivo rat tibialis anterior model. British Journal of Sports Medicine 39:e25

Scott J E 1988 Proteoglycan–fibrillar collagen interactions. Journal of Biochemistry 252:313–323

Scott J E 1995 Extracellular matrix, supramolecular organisation and shape. Journal of Anatomy 187:250–269

Selvanetti A, Cippola M, Puddu G 1997 Overuse tendon injuries: basic science and classification. Operative Techniques in Sports Medicine 5:110–117

Sengar D P S, McKendry R J, Uhthoff H K 1989 Lack of association between HLA and rotator cuff rupture. Tissue Antigens 34:205–206

Sengar J, McKendy R, Uhthoff H 1987 Increased frequency of HLA-A1 in calcifying tendinitis. Tissue Antigens 29:173–174

Shalabi A, Kristoffersen-Wiberg M, Aspelin P et al 2004a Immediate Achilles tendon response after strength training evaluated by MRI. Medicine and Science in Sports and Exercise 36:1841–1846

Shalabi A, Kristoffersen-Wilberg M, Svensson L et al, 2004b Eccentric training of the gastrocnemius–soleus complex in chronic Achilles tendinopathy results in decreased tendon volume and intratendinous signal as evaluated by MRI. American Journal of Sports Medicine 32:1286–1296

Shirakura K, Ciarelli M J, Arnoczky J H et al 1995 Deformation induced calcium signaling in tenocytes in situ. Presented at Combined Orthopaedic Research Societies Meeting, San Diego, CA

Sporn M B, Roberts A B 1989 Transforming growth factor-β. Multiple actions and potential clinical applications. Journal of the American Medical Association 262:938–941

Uhthoff H K, Matsumoto F 2000 Rotator cuff tendinopathy. Sports Medicine and Arthroscopy Review 8:56–68

Vogel K 2004 What happens when tendons bend and twist? Proteoglycans. Journal of Musculoskeletal and Neuronal Interaction 4:202–203

Vogel K G, Paulsson M, Heinegard D 1984 Specific inhibition of type I and type II collagen fibrillogenesis by the small proteoglycan of tendon. Journal of Biochemistry 223:587–597

Vogel K, Ordog A, Olah J 1993 Proteoglycans in the compressed region of human tibialis posterior tendon and in ligaments. Journal of Orthopaedic Research 11:68–77

Vogel K G, Meyers A B 1999 Proteins in the tensile region of adult bovine deep flexor tendon. Clinical Orthopaedics and Related Research 367 (suppl):344–355

Williams I F, Heaton A, McCullagh K G 1980 Cell morphology and collagen types in equine tendon scar. Research in Veterinary Science 28:302–310

Williams I F, McCullagh K G, Silver I A 1984 The distribution of types I and III collagen and fibronectin in the healing equine tendon. Connective Tissue Research 12:211–227

Woo S-L Y, Tkach L V 1990 The cellular and matrix response of ligaments and tendons to mechanical injury. In: Leadbetter W B, Buckwalter J A, Gordon S (eds) Sports-induced inflammation: clinical and basic science concepts. American Orthopedic Society for Sports Medicine, Park Ridge, IL p 198–204

Wren T A L, Yerby S A, Beaupre G S et al 2001 Mechanical properties of the human Achilles tendon. Clinical Biomechanics 16:245–251

Yamamoto N, Hayashi K, Kutiyama H et al 1996 Effects of restressing on the mechanical properties of stress-shielded patellar tendons in rabbits. Journal of Biomechanical Engineering 118:216–220

Yuan J, Murrell G A C, Wei A Q et al 2002 Apoptosis in rotator cuff tendonopathy. Journal of Orthopaedic Research 20:1372–1379

Ligament

Gabriel YF Ng

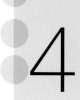

CHAPTER CONTENTS

Introduction 42

Development of body tissues 42

Structure and biochemistry of ligament 42

Ligament morphology 44

Biomechanics 45

Factors affecting ligament strength 47

Ligament injury and repair 48

Effects of immobilization and exercise 52

New direction in ligamentous repair 54

Summary 54

Introduction

The musculoskeletal system of the human body provides the morphological framework and machinery for movement. Muscles and nerves are the power generators whereas bones, cartilage, joint capsules and ligaments provide the structural strength to withstand forces imposed onto the body.

Injuries from sport or exercise often involve more than one structure and type of tissue. Understanding the organization and function of the body tissues can enhance the design of rehabilitation programs and help athletes return to their pre-injury levels of sport performance and physical activity.

Development of body tissues

Human life begins from the instance when a sperm fertilizes an egg. The first 7 weeks of life is the embryonic stage, and then starting from week 8 until birth is the fetal stage (White et al 1991). At the beginning of week 4 of embryonic life, there is the formation of neural tissue and somite, which continue to develop into muscles and mesenchyme. Mesenchyme is the precursor of connective tissues such as bones, cartilage and ligaments.

Basically, the human body contains four distinct types of tissues: epithelial, nervous, muscle, and connective (Whiting & Zernicke 1998). Ligament is classified as a form of connective tissue.

Structure and biochemistry of ligament

The word 'ligament' is derived from a Latin word *ligare* which means 'binding' (Dye & Dilworth Cannon 1988). As early as 3000 BC, in the Smith Papyrus, joint sprains began to be described and around 400 BC, Hippocrates described treatments for ligament injuries. Although in 100 BC, Hegator provided the first anatomical definition of ligament, the first correct description of ligament was provided by Galen in 130 AD (Snook 1983). Prior to this stage, ligaments were generally considered to be something similar to nerves but with a vague contractile function. In 1830, Schleiden and Schwann discovered cells and long fibers in dense connective tissues and then 20 years later, Rudinger and Hilton further discovered nerves in ligaments and postulated the ligament–muscle feedback system (Frank & Shrive 1994).

Ligament is classified as a form of dense regular connective tissue largely consisting of collagen (Whiting & Zernicke 1998).

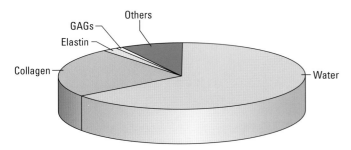

Figure 4.1 • Approximate chemical composition of normal skeletal ligaments by weight. Collagen represents nearly three-quarters of their dry weight. Two-thirds of their total weight is made up of water.

In general, there are at least two subgroups of ligaments: (1) skeletal ligaments in joints, and (2) suspensory ligaments in the abdominal organs (Frank et al 1985). The majority of skeletal ligaments are anatomically distinct, dense, relatively avascular, but homogeneous in appearance. At the microscopic level, ligaments comprise individual fibers running parallel to each other. Along the fibers are some scattered, long, thin fibroblasts that produce and maintain the surrounding matrix (Amiel et al 1984, Murray & Spector 1999).

According to Frank & Shrive (1994), the major functions of skeletal ligaments include:

- Attachment of articulating bones to one another across a joint
- Guidance of joint movements
- Maintenance of joint congruency
- Action as position sensors for joints.

Tendons and ligaments were often considered to be similar structures and they were both regarded as dense parallel connective tissues (Copenhaver et al 1971, Ham 1974). Initially, the literature on 'ligaments' and 'tendons' used the terms synonymously (Clayton et al 1968, O'Donoghue et al 1961). However, biochemical analysis of ligaments and tendons by Amiel et al (1984) revealed strong similarities and yet subtle differences between these structures. Ligaments contain approximately two-thirds of water by weight. The remaining one-third of dry weight is a constituent of collagen, elastin, glycosaminoglycans (GAGs), fibroblasts and other biochemical substances (Fig. 4.1) (Kasser 1996). In general, ligaments are more metabolically active than tendons. Ligaments have more protein but less total collagen content, and have a higher percentage of type III collagen and GAGs than do tendons.

Collagen

Collagen is the major constituent of the extracellular matrix of all connective tissues, and makes up approximately 80% of the dry weight of ligaments (Amiel et al 1984, Woo et al 1994). Collagen is a form of secretory protein containing three α-chains entangled in a triple-helical manner, and the biosynthetic events are similar between all collagen polypeptides (Olsen 1991). The basic collagen molecule is the tropocollagen which aggregates into a collagen fibril in a specific quarter staggering pattern that has most mechanical and biochemical stability (Gross 1974, Hodge & Petruska 1963).

There are at least 18 types of collagen identified in the body. Each type differs from one another by the types of α-chains that make up the tropocollagen. In general, the amino acids that make up an α-chain follow the sequence of glycine-x-y, where in most cases, x is proline, y is hydroxyproline, and this sequence repeats itself. The number of each collagen type essentially reflects the chronological order in which they were discovered. Each type of collagen has its unique characteristics and location throughout the body. In general, collagen is involved in cell attachment and differentiation, chemotactic reaction and immunopathological processes (Linsenmayer 1991).

Despite the different types of collagen in the body, types I, II and III may be regarded as most pertinent to sports physical therapists due to their abundance in the musculoskeletal system. Type I collagen constitutes about 90% of the total collagen in the body and is found in ligaments, tendons, bones and fascia. Type II collagen is found in hyaline cartilage and nucleus pulposus of the intervertebral disk, and consists of fine fibrils that are dispersed in the ground substance. Type III collagen is mostly found in skin and blood vessels (Eyre 1980).

Collagen provides strength to the tissues. The ability to form covalent intramolecular and intermolecular crosslinks is a key determination of the tensile strength and resistance to chemical enzymatic breakdown of collagen (Bailey et al 1974, Eyre 1980, Knott & Bailey 1998, Mechanic 1974, Patterson-Kane et al 1997, Tanzer 1973) (Fig. 4.2). Crosslinks are formed by enzymatic reactions between the amino acids lysine and hydroxylysine (Amiel & Kleiner 1988). The most prevalent intermolecular crosslinks include hydroxylysinonorleucine (HLNL), dihydroxylysinonorleucine (DHLNL) and the more complex combinations of histidinohydroxymerodesmosine (HHMD). These are labeled as reducible crosslinks due to the presence of a double bond.

Besides reducible crosslinks, there are also nonreducible crosslinks that do not contain a double bond. In older people, less reducible crosslinks are found in connective tissues, suggesting an age-related transformation of reducible to the more stable nonreducible crosslinks (Patterson-Kane et al 1997, Tanzer 1976). Hydroxypyridinoline (HP) has been identified as a type of non-reducible crosslink (Fujimoto 1977, Fujimoto & Moriguchi 1978). Frank et al (1994) and Ng et al (1996a) have respectively demonstrated a positive relationship between HP crosslink density and the mechanical strength of healing medial collateral ligament tissue and anterior cruciate ligament (ACL) graft in rabbits and goats.

Proteoglycans

Proteoglycans are important constituents of the extracellular matrix. Collagen fibrils resist tensile loading and proteoglycans resist compressive loading (Scott 1988). Proteoglycans are large molecules comprising a core protein, covalently linked to numerous GAG side chains that are polysaccharides of repeating disaccharide units. The GAGs contain a high density of

A

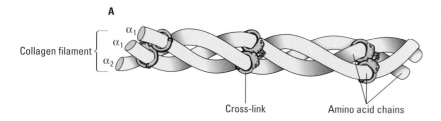

Collagen filament

α_1
α_1
α_2

Cross-link   Amino acid chains

B

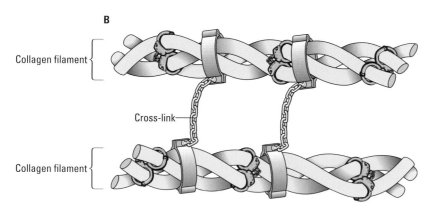

Collagen filament

Cross-link

Collagen filament

Figure 4.2 • Collagen bonding increases tensile strength. **A:** Weak intramolecular crosslinks form between amino acid chains within one collagen filament. **B:** Stronger intermolecular crosslinks form from one collagen filament to another. (Reproduced from Hardy M A 1989 The biology of scar formation. Physical Therapy 69:1014–1024, with permission of the American Physical Therapy Association.)

negative charges that repel each other, thus enabling the proteoglycans to extend through a larger volume than they do when uncharged. These negatively charged GAG molecules interact electrostatically with a variety of positively charged molecules such as water. The affinity of proteoglycans to water determines the viscosity of interstitial fluids and maintains the proper homeostatic environment for the cells and the surrounding matrix (Hardingham & Fosang 1992, Wight et al 1991).

Proteoglycans usually constitute about 1% of the ligament's dry weight (Amiel et al 1990, Frank & Shrive 1994). Studies of the relationships between proteoglycan and collagen reveal that some small size proteoglycans limit collagen fibrillogenesis through interaction between the proteoglycans' core protein and the surface of the collagen fibrils. Therefore, the size of collagen fibrils remains small when there are excessive small size proteoglycans (Pogany et al 1994, Vogel et al 1984, Vogel & Trotter 1987).

Elastin

Elastin is an extremely hydrophobic protein characterized by a high degree of reversible extensibility with small forces (Mecham & Heuser 1991). Most ligaments contain less than 5% of elastin by dry weight, but this may be important for the elasticity of the ligaments (Arnoczky et al 1993, Buckwalter & Cooper 1987). An exception is the ligamentum flavum in the spine which contains twice as much elastin than collagen, thus this ligament exhibits almost perfect elasticity when subject to loading (Kirby et al 1989, Nachemson & Evans 1968).

Other non-collagen proteins

There are some non-collagen proteins in the extracellular matrix that are present in small quantities but that are vital for wound healing should the tissue be injured. For example,

thrombospondin is involved in the early organization of the extracellular matrix to initiate the healing process (Bornstein et al 2000, Chen et al 2000, Miller & McDevitt 1991, Raugi et al 1987). Tenascin induces cell migration so as to facilitate the deployment of fibroblasts to the wound site for collagen synthesis (Jones & Jones 2000, Koukoulis et al 1991, Sakakura & Kusano 1991). Recent reports have also demonstrated tenascin to be involved in nerve regeneration (Guntinas-Lichius et al 2005, Ogawa et al 2005). Fibronectin has the roles of chemattraction of fibroblasts, cell adhesion and wound contraction (Grinnell et al 2006, McDonald 1988, Tani et al 2001); laminin attracts neutrophils that are important for preventing bacterial infection (Gugssa et al 2000, Kleinman et al 1985, Nakashima et al 2005). Therefore, these non-collagen proteins form the defense and repair network so as to enable the ligament to repair itself after injury and regain the normal functional strength.

Ligament morphology

The structural arrangements of collagen in ligaments and tendons are very similar. The collagen of the midsubstance of these structures is hierarchically arranged in ascending orders of tropocollagen, microfibrils, subfibrils, fibrils and fibers (Fig. 4.3). Tropocollagen molecules of about 1.5 nm in diameter are tightly packed in groups of five, forming microfibrils of approximately 3.5 nm in diameter. The microfibrils group into subfibrils, which aggregate to form fibrils of 50–500 nm. The fibrils further aggregate to form fibers of 50–300 μm in diameter, which become the smallest unit of collagen that can be seen using a light microscope (Frank & Shrive 1994).

When ligaments are viewed under a polarized light microscope, a distinct feature of accordion-like, wavy undulation

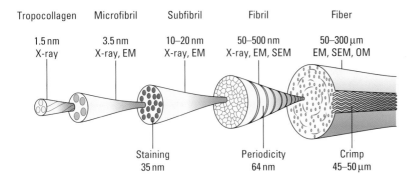

Tropocollagen	Microfibril	Subfibril	Fibril	Fiber
1.5 nm	3.5 nm	10–20 nm	50–500 nm	50–300 μm
X-ray	X-ray, EM	X-ray, EM	X-ray, EM, SEM	EM, SEM, OM

Staining
35 nm

Periodicity
64 nm

Crimp
45–50 μm

Figure 4.3 • Schematic illustration depicting the hierarchical structure of collagen in ligament midsubstance. EM = electron microscope; SEM = scanning EM; OM = optical microscope. (Modified from Kastelic et al 1978 with the permission of Connective Tissue Research. Copyright 1978 from the Multicomposite Structure of Tendon by J Kastelic et al. Reproduced by permission of Taylor & Francis, Inc., http://www.routledge-ny.com.)

of cells and matrix can be seen, which is known as ligament 'crimp' (Dale et al 1972, Dale & Baer 1974, Minns et al 1973, Murray & Spector 1999, Patterson-Kane et al 1997, Yahia & Drouin 1989). Crimp is a unique feature in parallel arranged connective tissues. It provides a buffer against mechanical loading, such that any rapid external load will stretch out the wavy undulation of the ligament without damaging its fibers (Dale et al 1972, Diamant et al 1972, Oakes 1994, Viidik 1980).

The crimp patterns are tissue specific and relatively little is known about the factors that determine and maintain the collagen crimp. There are a number of hypotheses, however, suggesting the factors that maintain collagen crimp. Among these hypotheses, the collagen–proteoglycan interaction is most widely accepted (Viidik 1980). Shah et al (1977) demonstrated that elongation of crimp was due to straightening of the crimp period but the crimp angle remained constant. This finding suggests that the crimp junction, where collagen fibrils are acutely angulated to each other, is stiffer than the components that make up the crimp period.

The insertion of ligament to bone provides another mechanical buffer. An early study by Cooper & Misol (1970) reported that skeletal ligaments are not simply cemented to bones by Sharpey's fibers. Most ligaments insert to bones by gradual transition through layers of fibrocartilage and mineralized fibrocartilage. This layered arrangement of tissues with different mechanical strength can prevent stress concentrations so that the forces can be distributed over a large area.

At the ultrastructural level, Parry and co-workers (Parry & Craig 1977, 1979, Parry et al 1978a, 1978b) pioneered the analyses of connective tissues using transmission electron microscopy for different animal tissues at various ages. They quantified the collagen fibril diameter profiles of the tissues and, based on their findings, proposed an association between collagen fibril size and mechanical properties of the tissues.

More recently, a number of investigators have studied the ultrastructural morphology of both normal ligaments and tendons, and tissues under repair (Chapman 1989, Frank et al 1989, 1992, 1997, Fung et al 2003a, 2003b, Fung & Ng 2004, Matthew & Moore 1991, Neurath & Stofft 1992, Ng 1995, Ng et al 2004a, Postacchini & De Martino 1980). Findings confirmed that normal adult ligaments and tendons have bimodal distributions of collagen fibril diameter. For ligaments under repair, a more homogeneous distribution of small collagen

fibrils exists in the early phase of repair, but the fibrils gradually enlarge over time (Frank et al 1992, 1997, Ng 1995, Oakes et al 2000, Postacchini & De Martino 1980), possibly due to the influence of mechanical loading to the healing tissues.

Biomechanics

Ligaments are viscoelastic structures with unique mechanical properties. The ability of a ligament to withstand tensile loading often determines its level of competence (Woo et al 1990). Understanding the mechanical behavior of a ligament is important to determine its functional safety limit. Often, when a ligament is loaded to failure, the degree of damage is related to both the magnitude and rate that the load is applied (Nordin et al 2001).

Like other soft connective tissues, the biomechanical properties of ligaments can be considered from the structural and material perspectives. Structural properties are the physical properties of a ligament that are dependent on its size, shape and alignment to the external force. Material properties refer to the physical properties of the substances that make up the ligament per se, irrespective of their geometrical shapes or dimensions.

Load–deformation characteristics

A common way to analyze the biomechanical properties of ligaments is to subject a specimen to tensile loading under a constant rate of elongation with a material testing machine. The ligament is deformed until failure. The concomitant load and elongation data during the test will enable the construction of a load–deformation curve (Fig. 4.4). There are four typical regions in the curve that correspond to different geometrical alignment and integrity of the collagen fibers of the ligament.

The first region (I) is the toe-phase, which is characterized by a disproportionate increase in elongation with a small load. This is the region where the force is mostly absorbed by the collagen crimp. The wavy, crimp pattern will become straighter as the load progresses (Diamant et al 1972, Hirsch 1974, Viidik et al 1965). The other reason for the nonlinear deformation is the heterogeneous distribution of the collagen fibers. Some fibers that are oriented parallel to the axis of loading may take up the load earlier than others, thus resulting in a stepwise recruitment of the collagen to withstand the load (Frank & Shrive 1994). The elongation is usually expressed as strain, which is defined as the percentage elongation over the original length. At the end of toe-phase, the strain has been reported to be approximately 4% (Diamant et al 1972, Haut & Little 1972, Viidik 1973), which is well within the functional safety limit of ligaments.

The second region (II) is the linear region in which the ligament follows more or less a linear fashion of elongation in response to loading. In this phase, the collagen fibers are stretched and become more parallel to each other. The slope in this region is defined as the stiffness (N/mm), signifying the resistance of a ligament to elongating against tensile loading. Theoretically, if the load is removed in the linear region, the ligament should return to its original length without any permanent damage. Practically, however, towards the end of the linear region, some collagen fibers will fail (presumably those recruited first), resulting in pathological irreversible damage to

the ligament. The severity of such damage is similar to a clinical grade 2 ligament tear where severe pain is evident and where an athlete cannot continue with a sporting activity (Oakes 1994).

When the linear region is surpassed, major disruption of collagen fiber bundles occurs (region III). The ligament loses stiffness unpredictably as more and more fiber bundles fail, and the force will be redistributed to the remaining fibers, thus increasing the likelihood of these fibers breaking. It only takes a small amount of additional elongation before all the fibers fail, resulting in total rupture of the ligament (region IV) (Frank & Shrive 1994).

The highest point in the load–deformation curve is the ultimate tensile strength, and the area covered by the curve reflects the energy absorption capacity of the ligament. The tensile stiffness, ultimate tensile strength and energy absorption capacity are dependent on the physical size of the ligament. When a ligament is separated longitudinally into two halves, each half will only demonstrate 50% of its original stiffness and strength. In order to compare the mechanical properties of the materials that make up the ligament, the load needs to be converted to stress (MPa) by dividing it by the cross-sectional area of the ligament, and elongation converted to strain by dividing it by the original length. The resultant stress–strain curve represents the material properties of the ligament substance, and the slope of this curve represents the Young's modulus (Table 4.1).

From the functional perspective, it is of limited interest for clinicians to study the ultimate tensile strength or total energy absorption capacity of a ligament, because in most of our daily activities, we only use about 30% of the full potential strength of our ligaments (Viidik 1980). Furthermore, the upper limit of physiological strain to ligaments is in the vicinity of 5% or less (Fung 1981), which is well below the ultimate strain of most ligaments in the body.

Viscoelastic behavior

Ligaments exhibit viscoelastic (time- or history-dependent) properties as a result of the complex interaction between the collagen fibers with its surrounding matrix (Nordin et al 2001). When a ligament is loaded and unloaded in successive manner, the load–deformation curve will shift to the right with each loading/unloading cycle instead of following the same path. This phenomenon is known as 'hysteresis' (Fig. 4.5), a process resulting from internal energy loss to heat during the loading/unloading cycles (Woo et al 1990). Hysteresis has important therapeutic

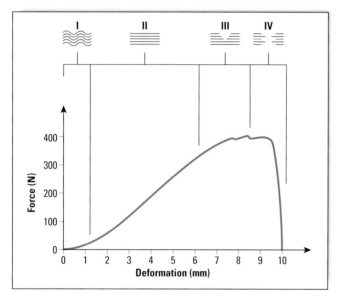

Figure 4.4 • A typical force–deformation curve for ligament. **I** = toe region; **II** = linear region; **III** = region of microfailure; **IV** = failure region. At the top are schematic representations of fibers going from crimped (I) through recruitment (II) to progressive failure (III and IV). (From Frank C B, Shrive N G 1994 Ligament. In: Nigg B M, Herzog W (eds) Biomechanics of the musculo-skeletal system. © 1994 John Wiley & Sons Limited. Reproduced with permission.)

Table 4.1 Comparison of structural and material properties with different dimensions of the same tissue. By reducing the cross-sectional area to 50%, structural stiffness is halved but Young's modulus remains the same

Original size	Force	Stress	Elongation	Strain	Stiffness	Young's modulus
Length = l Area = A	F	$F/A = \sigma$	δl	$\delta l/l \times 100\% = \varepsilon$	$F/\delta l$	σ/ε
Length = l Area = 0.5A	F	$F/0.5A = 2\sigma$	$2\delta l$	$2\delta l/l \times 100\% = 2\varepsilon$	$F/2\delta l$	$2\sigma/2\varepsilon = \sigma/\varepsilon$

implications such as during traction because the deformation is the desired effect of the treatment procedure. Hysteresis however, can also be a manifestation of pathological deformation resulting from repetitive microtrauma (Garde 1988).

Ligament specimens that have been subjected to the freeze–thaw preparation procedure exhibit larger hysteresis than fresh specimens in the first few cycles of loading (Woo et al 1986). At a low temperature of testing, ligament specimens show a decrease in the area of the hysteresis loop (Woo et al 1987a). Another significant implication of hysteresis for physical therapists is that during ligament stress testing, it is important to precondition the ligament with a few cyclic loading and unloading trials so as to dissipate the energy of hysteresis and obtain more repeatable test results.

When a ligament is subject to a constant load over time, it exhibits 'creep' behavior such that the elongation increases gradually before reaching a plateau. Conversely, when a ligament is subject to constant elongation over time, it exhibits the 'load-relaxation' characteristic (Fig. 4.6) (Fung et al 2002, Ng et al 1995, 1996b, 2003, See et al 2004).

The significance of creep and load-relaxation for physical therapists is demonstrated during stretching. In order to stretch the joint effectively, the force must be sustained for a period of time in a constant manner so that the ligaments and other soft tissues creep (Alter 1996). A study by Bandy & Irion (1994) demonstrated that stretching for 30 s produced the optimum results. No extra benefit was shown with longer than 30 s of stretch, probably because soft tissues creep most significantly in the initial 30 s of loading (Lee & Evans 1994).

With a stiff joint, pain will be elicited during stretching. If the joint is held at the end of the range and maintained in that position, the pain may decrease over time due to load-relaxation (Alter 1996, Etnyre & Abraham 1984). Such load-relaxation will render the stretching to be more tolerable by the patient before the therapist progresses further with larger stretching force.

Besides stretching, there are other clinical implications of the viscoelastic behavior of ligaments, in particular during exercises involving constant and repetitive ligamentous strains, such as jogging (Woo et al 1981, 1982). Cyclic load-relaxation will happen such that loading to joint tissues will decrease in order to protect the ligaments from overload failure. The repetitive constant loading to the joint will lead to ligament creep, resulting in a temporary increase in ligament stress immediately after exercises (Sailor et al 1995). With adequate rest, creep disappears and the ligament will return to its original length (Badtke et al 1993, Eklund & Corlett 1984, Wilby et al 1987).

Factors affecting ligament strength

Most ligaments in the body demonstrate the typical load–deformation curve discussed above. The exact biomechanical properties of each ligament, however, are unique. There are certain internal and external factors affecting the strength of ligaments. These factors include structural components, the

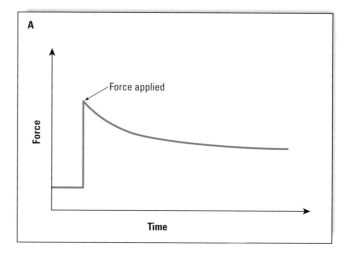

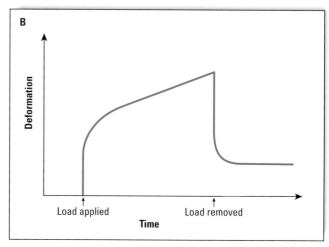

Figure 4.6 • Schematic force-relaxation **(A)** and creep-elongation **(B)** curve for ligaments. (From Frank C B, Shrive N G 1994 Ligament. In: Nigg B M, Herzog W (eds) Biomechanics of the musculo-skeletal system. © 1994 John Wiley & Sons Limited. Reproduced with permission.)

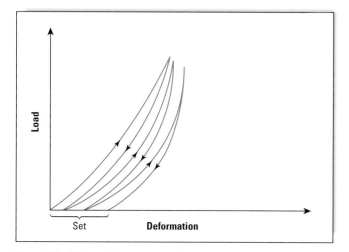

Figure 4.5 • Schematic representation of hysteresis.

subject's age, strain rate, and loading direction. Each of these will be discussed in the following sections.

Structural components

The strength of a ligament largely depends on the type and quantity of its collagen fibers. An anatomical study by Ramsey (1966) revealed that elastic fibers constitute more than two-thirds of the dry weight of ligamentum flavum. A later study by Nachemson & Evans (1968) demonstrated a very distinct biomechanical behavior of this ligament. It is almost perfectly elastic with an unusually high strain value of 70% before failure in young subjects (Fig. 4.7).

The decrease in electromyographic (EMG) activities of back muscles during trunk flexion movement was considered to be associated with energy stored in ligamentum flavum that provided passive support to the upper trunk (Kippers & Parker 1984, Ng & Walter 1995, Steventon & Ng 1995). Furthermore, the elastic nature of this ligament also has a protective function, such that it will not buckle into the spinal canal and impinge onto the spinal cord with trunk movements (Bogduk & Twomey 1987).

Age

In considering the factor of age, the processes of maturation and aging should be considered separately. Oakes & Parker (1981) reported an increase in the mean collagen fibril diameter in rat ACL from birth to about 7 weeks, and then a plateau afterwards. Larson & Parker (1982) found that the ultimate tensile strength of ACL changed in a similar pattern to the collagen fibril diameter, demonstrating an increase from birth to maturity, and then a leveling off. Woo et al (1990) compared the biomechanical properties of medial collateral ligament (MCL) in both skeletally immature and mature rabbits. They found that all skeletally immature specimens failed by tibial avulsion, whereas the mature specimens failed in the MCL substance regardless of the loading rate. These findings suggest that both the ligament substance and insertion site increased in strength with maturation, but the gain in strength is higher in the insertion than the ligament.

With aging, however, Noyes & Grood (1976) found that the human femur–ACL–tibia complex from donors aged between 16 and 26 years had higher ultimate tensile strength and stiffness than that from donors aged between 48 and 86 years by a factor of 2 to 3. Similar findings have also been reported by Woo & Adams (1990) where the linear stiffness and ultimate tensile strength both decreased with aging independent of the direction of loading.

The change in biomechanical properties with age is likely to be mediated by the increase in quantity and quality of crosslinks and collagen content with maturation, and the decrease of these with aging (Viidik et al 1982).

Strain rate

Studies of the bone–ligament–bone complex have revealed that the structures responded differently at different strain rates. At strain rates of less than 100% per second, most failures occurred in the insertions with bony avulsion, whereas at strain rates of 100% or higher per second, the failures occurred in the midsubstance of the ligaments (Crowninshield & Pope 1976, Haut 1983, Noyes et al 1974a). Besides the location of failure, the ultimate tensile strength and energy absorption capacity of the ligaments also increased with strain rate regardless of age of the subjects (Woo et al 1990).

Loading direction

Ligament such as the ACL has its longitudinal axis oriented at an angle to the bones. Previous studies have shown that with loading applied along the longitudinal axis of the tibia, the ultimate tensile strength of the ACL decreased with knee flexion, but when the load was applied along the ACL axis, no such change occurred (Figgie et al 1986, Woo et al 1987b).

Woo & Adams (1990) compared the direction of loading on 14 pairs of femur–ACL–tibia specimens with one leg tested along the tibial axis and the other tested along the ACL axis. They found higher ultimate strength and stiffness, but lower maximum strain to failure in the ACL when the load was applied along the ligament axis. The mode of failure was also different such that midsubstance failure was produced with ACL axial loading but tibial insertion failure was produced with tibial axial loading. It was suggested that during tibial axial loading, the load was not evenly distributed to the collagen fiber bundles (Woo & Adams, 1990). Some fibers may take up more load than others, which tends to 'peel off' the insertion thus affecting the structural properties.

Ligament injury and repair

The mechanisms of injury can be classified into seven categories (Leadbetter 1994):

1. Contact or direct trauma
2. Dynamic loading
3. Repetitive overuse

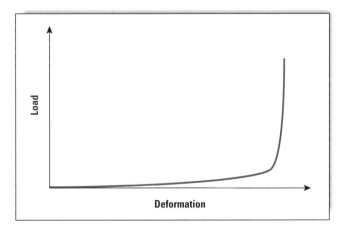

Figure 4.7 • Load–deformation characteristics of ligamentum flavum.

4. Structural vulnerability

5. Poor flexibility

6. Muscle imbalance

7. Rapid growth.

In sports medicine, the principal mechanism of injury is related to mechanical loading as characterized by the magnitude, location, direction, duration, frequency, variability and rate of the load (Whiting & Zernicke 1998).

Injury to a ligament will compromise its joint stabilizing function and ability to control movements (Allen & Harner 1996, Kannus & Järvinen 1987, Parolie & Bergfeld 1986). Injury can also reduce the proprioceptive function of ligaments and lengthen the ligament–muscle reflex time (Beard et al 1994, Borsa et al 1997, Friden et al 1996, 1997, Lam et al 2002, Wu et al 2001a, 2001b). Ligamentous injury can happen with a single dose of loading that surpasses the ligament's maximum tolerance, or from cumulative overloads (repetitive sprains) with insufficient time to recover, such that these chronic insults can set the stage for an acute ligamentous rupture (DiGiovanni et al 2000, Griffith et al 2001).

Knowing the extent of injury is of paramount importance for sports physical therapists in determining the management of athletes' injuries. Minor ligament sprains may only cause some annoyances without functional loss, but if ignored and with repeated loading, these minor injuries can progress to more severe ones. Increasing the severity of sprains will cause more functional loss and require a longer time to heal. In the cases of total rupture of some ligaments, the results can be catastrophic or even fatal, such as rupturing the annular ligament of the atlantoaxial joint in the cervical spine.

Every ligament injury is unique despite similarities in the biomechanical events and subsequent biological responses. Clinically, it is customary to grade the severity of ligament injury with some clinical classifications. The most typical is a three-level classification system that quantifies the structural involvement, signs and functional loss (Leadbetter 1994) (Table 4.2).

Healing after injury is ligament-specific. Some ligaments, such as the MCL, have good healing potential, whereas others, such as the ACL, have a poor chance of healing in the case of total rupture without surgical intervention (Clancy et al 1988, Frank et al 1985, Hefti et al 1991, O'Donoghue et al 1971). Generally, the biological responses following ligamentous injury can be summarized into three phases: (1) bleeding and inflammation, (2) active repair with proliferation of bridging materials and (3) remodeling (Frank 1996). The cellular activities and timing of each of these phases is depicted in Fig. 4.8.

Oakes (1991) reviewed the literature on the clinical aspects of soft tissue repair and concluded that the acute management of a ligamentous injury will have a significant effect on the outcome

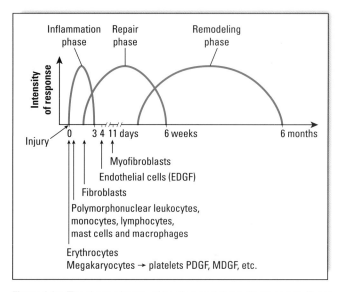

Figure 4.8 • The three phases of healing and the cells involved. (From Oakes B W 1992 The classifications of injuries and mechanisms of injury repair and healing. In: Bloomfield J, Fricker P A, Fitch K D (eds) Textbook of science and medicine in sport, p 201, 209. Blackwell Scientific Publications, reproduced with permission.)

Table 4.2 Classification of ligament injury. (Reproduced with permission from Leadbetter W B 1994 Soft tissue athletic injury. In: Fu F H, Stone D A (eds) Sports injuries: mechanisms, prevention, treatment. Williams and Wilkins, Baltimore, p 733–780)

Grade	Severity	Degree	Structural involvement	Examination	Performance deficit
1	Mild	First	Negligible	No visible injury Locally tender only Joint stable	Minimal to a few days
2	Moderate	Second	Partial	Visible swelling Marked tenderness ± stability	Up to 6 weeks (may be modified by protective bracing)
3	Severe	Third	Complete	Gross swelling Marked tenderness Antalgic posture Unstable	Indefinite, minimum of 6–8 weeks

of rehabilitation. If the injury is not managed appropriately in the early phase with adequate RICE (rest, ice, compression and elevation), the result will be uncontrolled bleeding and edema, causing abnormal arrangement of collagen fibers and a resultant scar that will become hypertrophic and painful (Fig. 4.9).

In the repair phase, water content remains high. The rate of collagen synthesis reaches its peak at about 3 weeks after injury (Amiel et al 1987). Studies incorporating quantitative collagen fibril analysis have indicated that early mobilization in the first 3 weeks could be detrimental to collagen orientation, but after this time frame, mobilization could increase the tensile strength of the repairing ligament (Oakes 1992).

The remodeling phase of ligament healing starts from week 6 and continues to week 26 or even up to 1 year. The water content of the ligament returns to normal while total collagen content remains slightly increased. The scar tissues continue to mature slowly and approximate the properties of the normal tissues. In a study of ACL repair in goat tissue with a 3-year follow-up period, Ng et al (1996b) induced a surgical transection injury to the posterolateral bundle of the ligament and kept the anteromedial bundle intact as an internal splint. It was found that the repair tissue attained 75% of the normal ultimate tensile strength at 1 year. At 3 years, the strength even surpassed that of the normal ligament by 28%. The structural stiffness of

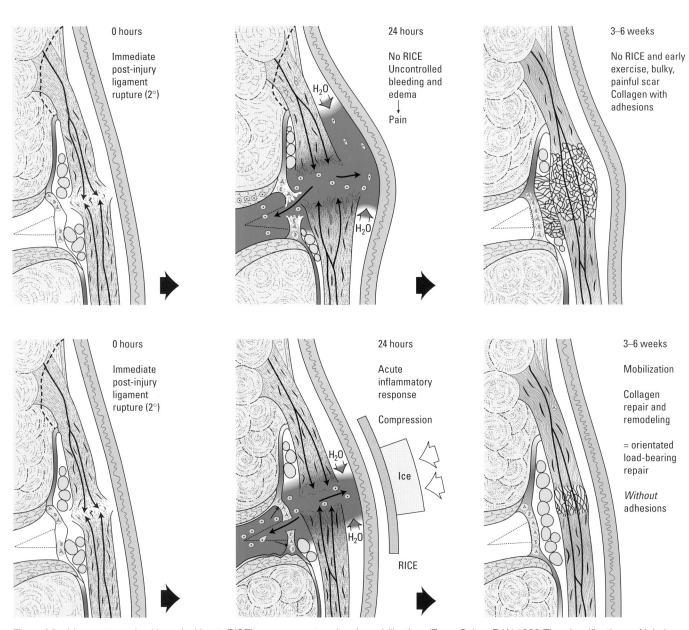

Figure 4.9 • Ligament repair with and without 'RICE' management and early mobilization. (From Oakes B W 1992 The classifications of injuries and mechanisms of injury repair and healing. In: Bloomfield J, Fricker P A, Fitch K D (eds) Textbook of science and medicine in sport. pp 201, 209. Blackwell Scientific Publications (www.blackwell-science.com), reproduced with permission.)

the ligament also improved with time and achieved 97% of the normal value at 3 years. The rate of improvement of Young's modulus, however, did not parallel the stiffness as it only achieved 72% of the normal value at 3 years. Examination of the repair tissue with transmission electron microscopy, however, revealed that most of the collagen fibrils at 3 years were small at a size of less than 100 nm in diameter, with very few large fibrils scattered in the matrix. Furthermore, the cross-sectional area of the repair bundle increased by about 50% at 3 years (Ng 1995).

The research findings of Ng and his colleagues (Ng 1995, Ng et al 1996b) indicate two important points. First, under favorable conditions, such as a clean wound and an incomplete rupture with close approximation of the ruptured ends, healing of the ACL is possible. With enough time, the repair tissue can simulate the structural properties of a normal ligament. This has also been supported by other researchers using different animal models and ligaments (Chimich et al 1991, Hefti et al 1991). Second, the material properties of the repaired ACL remain inferior to the normal tissue even at 3 years. The good ultimate tensile strength and stiffness of the repair ligament is due to hypertrophy of the scar. Despite the hypertrophic scar increasing the structural strength, it will occupy more space, especially for intra-articular ligaments. It is possible that the large intra-articular scar tissue impinges on other structures of the joint, thus leading to degenerative changes in the longer term (Kannus & Järvinen 1987).

Regarding the question of whether ligament repair could be facilitated by electrophysical modalities, Fung et al (2002, 2003b) recently studied the effect of therapeutic laser on MCL repair using a rat model. They found that a single high dose of GaAlAs laser applied at the time of injury significantly improved the strength and collagen morphology of the repairing ligament at 3 and 6 weeks after injury. These studies highlighted the positive responses of ligament injury to the biostimulation of laser even at the very early stage of the injury/repair process. More recently, Ng et al (2004a, 2004b) compared the effects of a single high dose of laser with multiple low doses of laser on ligament repair in rats and found that multiple doses of laser applications were more effective in improving the strength and ultrastructural collagen morphology of the repairing ligament over a 3-week period. The implications of these studies were that injured ligaments respond positively to the biostimulatory effect of therapeutic laser and that multiple applications would be more beneficial than single application at the early stage of injury, which was more coherent with the natural biological sequence of the ligament repair process.

Ligament grafts

Ligament grafting, in particular, ACL grafts, have attracted much attention in clinical and basic science research in the past two decades. The following discussion will focus on the biological, biomechanical and rehabilitation aspects of ACL autograft.

Since the first reported case of ACL graft by Hey Groves (1917), the surgical procedures, postoperative management and rehabilitation have made significant advancement. Generally,

ACL reconstruction will be the preferred choice of management for the following patient groups: (1) young and athletic people, (2) chronic cases with knee instability and episodes of giving way and (3) combined ligamentous and meniscal injuries (Anderson et al 2001, Ejerhed et al 2003, Herrington et al 2005, Noyes & Barber-Westin 1997, Renstrom & Lynch 1998, Veltri & Warren 1994a, 1994b).

There is evidence in the literature to suggest that ACL reconstruction should not be performed in the acute phase due to increased risk of arthrofibrosis (Shelbourne et al 1991, Wasilewski et al 1993). The surgical repair should be delayed for 2–3 weeks, and during that period the patient should receive an aggressive rehabilitation program to improve the range of motion and resolve swelling. The success of an ACL graft depends on the mechanical response of the graft tissue and surgical procedures (Renstrom & Lynch 1998). The selection of graft has been a subject of interest for a long time. Currently, three main types of grafts are used:

1. Bone–patellar tendon–bone autograft
2. Quadrupled semitendinosus autograft
3. Bone–patellar tendon–bone allograft (Table 4.3).

Oakes (1988) studied the collagen remodeling mechanisms of ACL grafts in patients requiring arthroscopic intervention because of joint stiffness, meniscal or cartilage problems at 9 months to 6 years postsurgery. Biopsies were taken from the graft and analyzed with transmission electron microscopy. His results indicated a predominance of small diameter collagen fibrils not arranged in an orderly manner.

Table 4.3 Comparison of different ACL grafts

Graft type	Advantages	Disadvantages
Bone–PT–bone autograft	Good initial strength Does not trigger immune response	Disturbs extensor mechanism Predisposes to anterior knee pain
Quadrupled semitendinosus autograft	Does not affect knee extension mechanism Does not trigger immune response	Low ultimate tensile strength High failure rate reported May lead to hamstring weakness
Bone–PT–bone allograft	No risk of donor site morbidity Availability of larger grafts Shorter operation time and smaller incision with improved cosmesis	Potential risk of disease transmission Risk of immunological response of the recipient Higher cost

Bone–PT–bone = bone–patellar tendon–bone

In a study of ACL–patella tendon autograft in goats (Ng 1995), it was found that most of the endogenous large collagen fibrils (greater than 100nm diameter) in the original patellar tendon graft disappeared as early as 6 weeks after surgery. The collagen fibril sizes remained small throughout the first year. At 3 years, there were some large fibrils repopulating and scattering inside the graft, but the packing density and orientations of the collagen fibrils were still inferior to the normal tissues (Fig. 4.10).

Ng et al (1995, 1996a) studied the biomechanical strength and biochemical crosslink density of the ACL graft at different time intervals and found the rate of load-relaxation in the graft to be significantly faster than normal at less than 1 year. After the first year, however, the load-relaxation rate slowed down. The ultimate strength and stiffness of the graft dropped in the initial 3 months and then gradually improved, but only achieving 43 and 48%, respectively, of the normal values at 3 years. In these studies, there was a concomitant change in hydroxypyridinium crosslinks density in the graft, which was significantly correlated with the Young's modulus of the graft.

The studies of ACL graft carried out by Ng and his colleagues (Ng et al 1995, 1996a) revealed that graft remodeling is a long and continuing process. Considering the long time (3 years) involved in these studies, and the persistent lower than normal biomechanical performance of the grafts in these time periods, the implication is that the grafts may never achieve the properties of normal tissues. The findings are in agreement with other animal studies that showed the ultimate tensile strength at 1 or 2 years after reconstruction was less than 50% of the normal value (Renstrom & Lynch 1998). In contrast, a biomechanical study with a human ACL graft revealed that the graft achieved 87% of ultimate tensile strength of the control value at 8 months after surgery (Beynnon et al 1997). The discrepancy between this human study and previous animal studies could be due to interspecies difference or success of the rehabilitation program in humans after ACL reconstruction. However, the Beynnon et al study only involved one subject and the strength of the normal ACL of that subject was 1015N, which was substantially lower than the normal value of 1730N to 2160N reported in the literature (Noyes et al 1984, Woo et al 1991). Therefore, caution must be exercised in interpreting the result of that single case human study.

Effects of immobilization and exercise

Ligaments are sensitive to training and disuse. The original work in this area was carried out by Noyes et al (1974b) as a part of the US Air Force experiments on the effect of long-term immobilization on ligaments. It was demonstrated that in primates, 8 weeks of cast immobilization of the lower limb resulted in substantial loss of strength in the ACL. With a reconditioning program, it took close to 1 year for the ligament to attain 91% ultimate tensile strength and 98% stiffness of the normal value.

From the metabolic perspective, Amiel et al (1983) analyzed the collagen turnover rate of rabbit MCL following 12 weeks of knee immobilization. They found that the collagen mass of MCL decreased by about 30% due to degradation of the collagen. In a later study, Amiel et al (1985) further demonstrated a close relationship between joint stiffness (as induced by immobilization) and decrease in GAGs of the joint tissues. Similar findings of ligament atrophy with immobilization were also reported by Woo et al (1987c), who demonstrated that an enforced exercise program could hasten the return of mechanical properties of the ligaments (Fig. 4.11).

The evidence in the literature clearly demonstrates that prolonged immobilization is detrimental to ligaments. The effects of immobilization are reversible but the effects of reconditioning took a longer time to show than that of immobilization. Exercise programs, however, can hasten the recovery following immobilization.

The beneficial effects of exercise on ligaments have been thoroughly investigated by several researchers (Andrews & O'Neill 1994, Cabaud et al 1980, Larsen & Parker 1982, Tipton et al 1970, 1975, Woo et al 2000). The early work of Tipton et al (1970) revealed that the MCL of dogs that had been subjected to 6 weeks of strenuous exercise training were significantly stronger and stiffer than those of the control group. Oakes & Parker (1981) studied the collagen fibril diameters of ACL and posterior cruciate ligaments of rats after 4 weeks of treadmill running and swimming. They found that the exercised rats had a higher number of collagen fibrils per unit area than the control rats. Interestingly, Oakes & Parker (1981) found a decrease in mean fibril diameter in the exercised rats, and they explained this phenomenon as related to the change in the type of GAGs in response to loading, which mediated the collagen fibril size. Andrews & O'Neill (1994) reported that pelvic exercise is useful in shortening the duration and lowering the intensity of ligament pain during pregnancy.

Ng & Maitland (2001) compared the anteroposterior laxity, stiffness, and rate of change of stiffness in the knee joints of athletes involved in basketball, running, swimming and of sedentary control subjects during an instrumented KT-2000 anterior drawer test. It was found that swimmers had the lowest laxity and highest stiffness in their knees followed by the basketball athletes, runners and then the control subjects (Table 4.4). This could be due to the different kinetic loading of these sports to the knees and to the response of the joint structures to loading. If this response also happens in ligaments under repair, it will have implications for the choice of rehabilitation exercises for subjects after ligament injuries.

Exercise may not always produce beneficial effects on ligaments. In the study by Burroughs & Dahners (1990), they examined the effect of the dosage of exercise on rats with different severity of injury to the MCL, ACL and medial joint capsule. Burroughs & Dahners (1990) measured the tensile strength of the repairing ligaments and laxity of the knee joint, and found that exercise had a beneficial effect on the healing MCL that had no associated ACL injury. For the knee joints that demonstrated severe instability with combined injuries of the MCL, ACL and the medial joint capsule, laxity in the joint deteriorated and no increase in tensile strength of the repairing

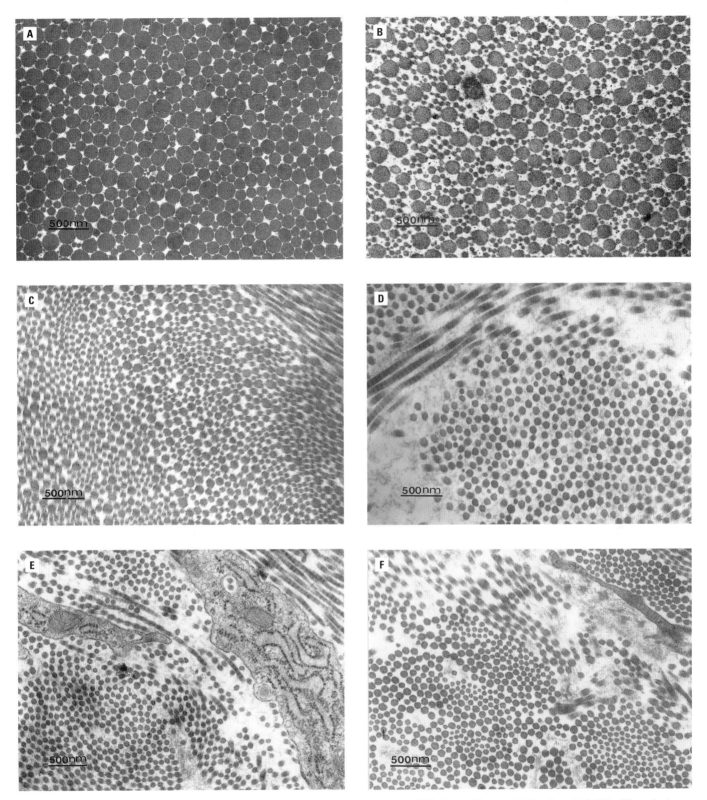

Figure 4.10 • Transverse sections through collagen fibrils of **A** normal patellar tendon (PT) of goat; **B** normal ACL of goat; **C** ACL–PT graft at 6 weeks; **D** ACL–PT graft at 12 weeks; **E** ACL–PT graft at 24 weeks; **F** ACL–PT graft at 1 year; **G** ACL–PT graft at 3 years. Magnification at × 20 000. The collagen fibril size remained small in the graft at all time points. Some large fibrils repopulated the graft at 3 years, but the orientation of the fibrils is still not parallel even at 3 years.

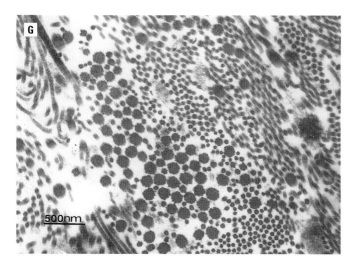

Figure 4.10 • (Continued)

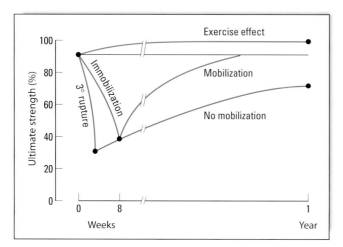

Figure 4.11 • The effects of immobilization, remobilization and exercise on strength of ligament. After only 8 weeks of immobilization, ligament strength decreased substantially, and it takes months to recover. The rate of recovery is faster with mobilization than without mobilization. (Reproduced with permission from Woo S L-Y, Gomez M A, Sites T J et al 1987 The biomechanical and morphological changes in the medial collateral ligament of the rabbit after immobilization and remobilization. Journal of Bone and Joint Surgery (Am) 69A:1200–1211. Copyright owned by Journal of Bone and Joint Surgery.)

ligaments was found with exercise training. Therefore, rehabilitation exercise programs should be carefully planned and monitored for athletes with severe joint instability.

New direction in ligamentous repair

Besides the traditional western approaches to ligamentous repair, herbal medications have been used for a long time in

Table 4.4 Means and (standard deviation) of anteroposterior laxity and stiffness of the knee joint of athletes in different sports measured by KT-2000 knee arthrometer. (Reprinted from Ng G Y F, Maitland M E 2001 Relationship of kinetic demands of athletic training and knee joint laxity. Physical Therapy in Sport 2:66–70, by permission of the publisher Churchill Livingstone)

	Basketball	Running	Swimming	Control
Laxity (mm)	6.4 (2.29)	7.3 (2.08)	5.9 (2.30)	7.8 (2.40)
Stiffness (N/mm)	47.5 (23.09)	45.2 (23.09)	57.8 (32.37)	37.9 (15.90)

eastern therapeutics. The clinical effects of herbal treatments have been documented, but the scientific bases of these have not been well addressed. Recently, Fung & Ng (2004, 2005) investigated a composite topical herbal formula for MCL repair in rats and found positive outcomes in terms of biomechanical and ultrastructural morphology at 3 and 6 weeks after injury. They further examined the combined effect of topical herbal application and therapeutic laser, and found that the effect was better than either treatment alone with biomechanical testing (Fung et al 2005). These findings highlight the complementary nature of eastern and western therapeutics. It is not known however, which herbal ingredient(s) in the composite formula was responsible for the therapeutic effects of the herbal treatment. Further studies are warranted to examine the active components of herbal formulas for ligament repair and whether these components could further augment the therapeutic effects of other physiotherapeutic treatments, so as to establish more scientific bases for an east-meets-west approach in ligament repair.

Summary

Ligaments are classified as dense connective tissue and the main organic constituent in most ligaments is collagen. The collagen determines the biomechanical strength and viscoelastic properties. Ligaments are important passive restraining structures for joints. Injuries to ligaments are common in sport and exercise and in the case of total rupture, the consequence can be debilitating if it is left untreated or mismanaged. Like many other body tissues, most ligaments are capable of repairing themselves after injury, but the whole process of remodeling for the repaired tissue may take 6–12 months, and the strength of the scar is persistently inferior to the normal tissue. For some ligaments, such as the ACL, active repair may not happen with total rupture, and surgical reconstruction is indicated. Some physical modalities such as therapeutic laser have been shown to augment ligament healing.

Prolonged immobilization weakens ligament and it takes a considerable time of reconditioning exercise in order to regain the functional strength. Ligaments respond to mechanical loading by synthesizing collagen, and thus increase strength. Too much loading, however, is not beneficial to ligaments, particularly in an unstable joint. It is therefore important that rehabilitation exercise programs should be strategically designed in order to induce the appropriate amount of loading to ligament according to the stage and timing of repair.

Chinese herbal applications could facilitate ligament healing, although there is a need to study the science underpinning the therapeutic effects of such Chinese therapeutics so that a new approach of combining eastern and western therapies for ligament repair can be developed.

References

Allen A A, Harner C D 1996 When your patient injures the posterior cruciate ligament. Journal of Musculoskeletal Medicine 13:44–55

Alter M J 1996 Science of flexibility, 2nd edn. Human Kinetics, Champaign, IL, p 113–126

Amiel D, Kleiner J B 1988 Biochemistry of tendon and ligament. In: Nimni M E, Olsen B (eds) Collagen. Biotechnology, vol III. CRC Press, Cleveland, OH, p 223–253

Amiel D, Akeson W H, Harwood F L et al 1983 Stress deprivation effect on the metabolic turnover of the medial collateral ligament collagen: a comparison between nine and 12-week immobilization. Clinical Orthopaedics and Related Research 172:265–270

Amiel D, Frank C B, Harwood F L et al 1984 Tendons and ligaments: a morphological and biochemical comparison. Journal of Orthopaedic Research 1:257–265

Amiel D, Frey C, Woo S L-Y et al 1985 Value of hyaluronic acid in the prevention of contracture formation. Clinical Orthopaedics and Related Research 196:306–311

Amiel D, Frank C B, Harwood F L et al 1987 Collagen alteration in medial collateral ligament healing in a rabbit model. Connective Tissue Research 16:357–366

Amiel D, Billings Jr E, Akeson W H 1990 Ligament structure, chemistry and physiology. In: Daniel D, Akeson W, O'Connor J (eds) Knee ligaments structure, function, injury, and repair. Raven Press, New York, p 77–91

Anderson AF, Snyder RB, Lipscomb AB 2001 Anterior cruciate ligament reconstruction: a prospective randomized study of three surgical methods. American Journal of Sports Medicine 29:272–279

Andrews C M, O'Neill L M 1994 Use of pelvic tilt exercise for ligament pain relief. Journal of Nurse-Midwifery 39:370–374

Arnoczky S P, Matyas J R, Buckwalter J A et al 1993 Anatomy of the anterior cruciate ligament. In: Jackson D W, Arnoczky S P, Frank C B et al (eds) The anterior cruciate ligament current and future concepts. Raven Press, New York, p 5–22

Badtke G, Bittmann F, Lazik D 1993 Changes in the vertebral column in the course of the day. International Journal of Sports Medicine 14:159

Bailey A J, Robins S P, Balian G 1974 Biological significance of the intermolecular crosslinks of collagen. Nature 251:105–109

Bandy W D, Irion J M 1994 The effect of time on static stretch on the flexibility of the hamstring muscles. Physical Therapy 74:845–850

Beard D J, Kyberd P J, O'Connor J J et al 1994 Reflex hamstring contraction latency in anterior cruciate ligament deficiency. Journal of Orthopaedic Research 12:219–228

Beynnon B D, Risberg M A, Tjomsland O et al 1997 Evaluation of knee joint laxity and the structural properties of the anterior cruciate ligament graft in the human: a case report. American Journal of Sports Medicine 25:203–206

Bogduk N, Twomey L T 1987 Clinical anatomy of the lumbar spine. Churchill Livingstone, Melbourne, p 35–36

Bornstein P, Armstrong L C, Hankenson K D et al 2000 Thrombospondin 2, a matricellular protein with diverse function. Matrix Biology 19:557–568

Borsa P A, Lephart S M, Irrgang J J et al 1997 The effects of joint position and direction of joint motion on proprioceptive sensibility in anterior cruciate ligament-deficient athletes. American Journal of Sports Medicine 25:336–340

Buckwalter J A, Cooper R R 1987 The cells and matrices of skeletal connective tissues. In: Albright, Brand (eds) The scientific basis of orthopaedics. Appleton and Lange, Norwalk, CT, p 1–29

Burroughs P, Dahners L E 1990 The effect of enforced exercise on the healing of ligament injuries. American Journal of Sports Medicine 18:376–378

Cabaud H E, Chatty A, Gildengorin V et al 1980 Exercise effects on the strength of the rat anterior cruciate ligament. American Journal of Sports Medicine 8:79–84

Chapman J A 1989 The regulation of size and form in the asssembly of collagen fibrils in vivo. Biopolymers 28:1367–1382

Chen H, Herndon M E, Lawler J 2000 The cell biology of thrombospondin: 1. Matrix Biology 19:597–614

Chimich D, Frank C, Shrive N et al 1991 The effects of initial end contact on medial collateral ligament healing: a morphological and biomechanical study in a rabbit model. Journal of Orthopaedic Research 9:37–47

Clancy W G, Ray J, Zoltan D 1988 Acute tear of the anterior cruciate ligament. Surgical versus conservative treatment. Journal of Bone and Joint Surgery (Am) 70A:1483–1488

Clayton M L, Miles J S, Abdulla M 1968 Experimental investigations of ligamentous healing. Clinical Orthopaedics and Related Research 61:146–153

Cooper R R, Misol S 1970 Tendon and ligament insertion. A light and electron microscopic study. Journal of Bone and Joint Surgery (Am) 52A:1–20

Copenhaver W M, Bunge R P, Bune M B 1971 Bailey's textbook of histology, 16th edn. Williams and Wilkins, Baltimore, MA, p 125–127.

Crowninshield R D, Pope M H 1976 The strength and failure characteristics of rat medial collateral ligaments. Journal of Trauma 16:99–105

Dale W C, Baer E 1974 Fibre-buckling in composite systems: a model for the ultrastructure of uncalcified collagen tissues. Journal of Material Science 9:369–382

Dale W C, Baer E, Keller A et al 1972 On the ultrastructure of mammalian tendon. Experientia 28:1293–1295

Diamant J, Keller A, Baer E et al 1972 Collagen, ultrastructure and its relation to mechanical properties as a function of ageing. Proceedings of the Royal Society of London (Biology) 180:293–315

DiGiovanni B F, Fraga C J, Cohen B E et al 2000 Associated injuries found in chronic lateral ankle instability. Foot and Ankle International 21:809–815

Dye S F, Dilworth Cannon W D 1988 Anatomy and biomechanics of the anterior cruciate ligament. Clinics in Sports Medicine 7:715–725

Ejerhed L, Kartus J, Sernert N et al 2003 Patellar tendon or semitendinosus tendon autografts for anterior cruciate ligament reconstruction? A prospective randomized study with a two-year follow-up. American Journal of Sports Medicine 31:19–25

Eklund J A E, Corlett E N 1984 Shrinkage as a measure of the effect of load on the spine. Spine 9:189–194

Etnyre B, Abraham L 1984 Effects of three stretching techniques on the motor pool excitability of the human soleus muscle. In: Roll W (ed) Abstracts of research papers 1984. American Alliance of Health, Physical Education, and Recreation. Reston, VA, p 90

Eyre D R 1980 Collagen: molecular diversity in the body's protein scaffold. Science 207:1315–1322

Figgie H E, Bahniuk E H, Heiple K G et al 1986 The effects of tibial-femoral angle on the failure mechanics of the canine anterior cruciate ligament. Journal of Biomechanics 19:89–91

Frank C B 1996 Ligament injuries: pathophysiology and healing. In: Zachazewski J E, Magee D J, Quillen W S (eds) Athletic injuries and rehabilitation. Saunders, Philadelphia, PA, p 9–26

Frank C B, Shrive N G 1994 Ligament. In: Nigg B M, Herzog W (eds) Biomechanics of the musculo-skeletal system. John Wiley, Chichester, p 106–132

Frank C B, Amiel D, Woo S L-Y et al 1985 Normal ligament properties and ligament healing. Clinical Orthopaedics and Related Research 196:15–25

Frank C B, Bray D F, Rademaker A et al 1989 Electron microscopic quantification of collagen fibril diameters in the rabbit medial collateral ligament: a baseline for comparison. Connective Tissue Research 19:11–25

Frank C B, McDonald D, Bray D R et al 1992 Collagen fibril diameters in the healing adult rabbit medial collateral ligament. Connective Tissue Research 27:251–263

Frank C B, Eyre D, Shrive N 1994 Hydroxypyridinium cross-link deficiency in ligament scar. Transactions of the 40th Annual Meeting of Orthopaedics Research Society, New Orleans. 13:3

Frank C B, McDonald D, Shrive N 1997 Collagen fibril diameters in the rabbit medial collateral ligament scar: a longer term assessment. Connective Tissue Research 36:261–269

Friden T, Roberts D, Zatterstrom R et al 1996 Proprioception in the nearly extended knee. Measurements of position and movement in healthy individuals and in symptomatic anterior cruciate ligament injured patients. Knee Surgery, Sports Traumatology and Arthroscopy 4:217–224

Friden T, Roberts D, Zatterstrom R et al 1997 Proprioception after an acute knee ligament injury: a longitudinal study on 16 consecutive patients. Journal of Orthopaedic Research 15:637–644

Fujimoto D 1977 Isolation and characterization of a fluorescent material in bovine Achilles tendon collagen. Biochemical and Biophysical Research Communication 74:1124–1129

Fujimoto D, Moriguchi T 1978 Pyridinoline, a non-reducible cross-link of collagen. Journal of Biochemistry 83:863–867

Fung D T C, Ng G Y F 2004 Effects of herbal application on the ultrastructural morphology of repairing medial collateral ligament in a rat model. Connective Tissue Research 45:122–130

Fung D T C, Ng G Y F 2005 Herbal remedies improve the strength of repairing ligament in a rat model. Phytomedicine 12:93–99

Fung D T C, Ng G Y F, Leung M C P et al 2002 Therapeutic low energy laser improves the mechanical strength of repairing medial collateral ligament. Lasers in Surgery and Medicine 31:91–96

Fung D T C, Ng G Y F, Leung M C P et al 2003a Investigation of the collagen fibril distribution of the medial collateral ligament in a rat knee model. Connective Tissue Research 44:2–11

Fung D T C, Ng G Y F, Leung M C P et al 2003b Effects of a therapeutic laser on the ultrastructural morphology of repairing medial collateral ligament in a rat model. Lasers in Surgery and Medicine 32:286–293

Fung D T C, Ng G Y F, Leung M C P 2005 Combined treatment of therapeutic laser and herbal application improves the strength of repairing ligament. Connective Tissue Research 46:125–130

Fung Y C B 1981 Biomechanics: mechanical properties of living tissues. Springer Verlag, New York, p 222

Garde R E 1988 Cervical traction: the neurophysiology of lordosis and the rheological characteristics of cervical curve rehabilitation. In: Harrison D D (ed) Chiropractic: the physics of spinal correction. Sunnyvale, CA, p 535–659

Griffith J F, Roebuck D J, Cheng J C et al 2001 Acute elbow trauma in children: spectrum of injury revealed by MR imaging not apparent on radiographs. American Journal of Roentgenology 176:53–60

Grinnell F, Rocha L B, Iucu C et al 2006 Nested collagen matrices: a new model to study migration of human fibroblast populations in three dimensions. Experimental Cell Research 312:86–94

Gross J 1974 Collagen biology: structure, degradation, and disease. Harvey Lecture 6(B):351–432

Gugssa A, Balan K V, Macias C et al 2000 Fibronectin/fibroblast growth factor/cell matrix signaling pathways and reciprocal membrane integration may be the regulators of cell growth and apoptosis in Trypanosoma musculi in co-cultures with fibroblasts. Journal of Submicroscopic Cytology and Pathology 32:281–296

Guntinas-Lichius O, Angelov D N, Morellini F et al 2005 Opposite impacts of tenascin-C and tenascin-R deficiency in mice on the functional outcome of facial nerve repair. European Journal of Neuroscience 22:2171–2179

Ham A W 1974 Histology, 6th edn. JB Lippincott, Philadelphia, PA, p 374–377

Hardingham T E, Fosang A J 1992 Proteoglycans: many forms and many functions. FASEB Journal 6:861–870

Hardy M A 1989 The biology of scar formation. Physical Therapy 69:1014–1024

Haut R C 1983 Age-dependent influence of strain rate on the tensile failure of rat-tail tendon. Journal of Biomechanical Engineering 105:296–299

Haut R C, Little R W A 1972 A constitutive equation for collagen fibers. Journal of Biomechanics 5:423–430

Hefti F L, Kress A, Fasel J et al 1991 Healing of the transected anterior cruciate ligament in the rabbit. Journal of Bone and Joint Surgery (Am) 73A:373–383

Herrington L, Wrapson C, Matthews M et al 2005 Anterior cruciate ligament reconstruction, hamstring versus bone-patella tendon-bone grafts: a systematic literature review of outcome from surgery. Knee 12:41–50

Hey Groves E W 1917 Operation for the repair of the crucial ligaments. Lancet 2:674–675

Hirsch G 1974 Tensile properties during tendon healing. Acta Orthopaedica Scandinavica Supplementum 153:1–145

Hodge A J, Petruska J A 1963 Recent studies with the electron microscope on ordered aggregates of the tropocollagen molecule. In: Ramachandran G (ed.) Aspects of protein structure. Academic Press, New York, p 289–301

Jones P L, Jones F S 2000 Tenascin-C in development and disease: gene regulation and cell formation. Matrix Biology 19:581–596

Kannus P, Järvinen M 1987 Conservatively treated tears of the anterior cruciate ligament: Long-term results. Journal of Bone and Joint Surgery (Am) 69A:1007–1012

Kasser J 1996 Orthopaedic knowledge update 5: home study syllabus. American Academy of Orthopaedic Surgeons, Park Ridge, IL

Kastelic J, Galeski A, Baer E 1978 The multicomposite structure of tendon. Connective Tissue Research 6:11–23

Kippers V, Parker A W 1984 Posture related to myoelectric silence of erectores spinae during trunk flexion. Spine 9:740–745

Kirby M C, Sikoryn T A, Hukins D W L et al 1989 Structure and mechanical properties of the longitudinal ligaments and ligamentum flavum of the spine. Journal of Biomedical Engineering 11:192–196

Kleinman J K, Cannon F B, Laurie G W et al 1985 Biological activities of laminin. Journal of Cell Biochemistry 27:235–242

Knott L, Bailey A J 1998 Collagen cross-links in mineralizing tissues: a review of their chemistry, function, and clinical relevance. Bone 22:181–187

Koukoulis G K, Gould V E, Bhattacharyya A et al 1991 Tenascin in normal, reactive, hyperplastic and neoplastic tissues: biologic and pathologic implications. Human Pathology 22:636–643

Lam R Y H, Ng G Y F, Chien E P 2002 Does wearing a functional knee brace affect hamstring reflex time on subjects with anterior cruciate ligament deficiency during muscle fatigue? Archives of Physical Medicine and Rehabilitation 83:1009–1012

Larson N, Parker A W 1982 Physical activity and its influence on the strength and elastic stiffness of knee ligaments. In: Howell M L, Parker A W (eds) Sports medicine: medical and scientific aspects of elitism in sport, vol 8. Australian Sports Medicine Federation, Brisbane, p 63–73

Leadbetter W B 1994 Soft tissue athletic injury. In: Fu F H, Stone D A (eds) Sports injuries: mechanisms, prevention, treatment. Williams and Wilkins, Baltimore, MA, p 733–780

Lee R, Evans J 1994 Towards a better understanding of spinal posteroanterior mobilisation. Physiotherapy 80:68–73

Linsenmayer T F 1991 Collagen. In: Hay E D (ed) Cell biology of extracellular matrix, 2nd edn. Plenum Press, New York, p 7–44

McDonald J A 1988 Fibronectin: a primitive matrix. In: Clark R A F, Henson P M (eds) The molecular and cellular biology of wound repair. Plenum Press, New York, p 405–435

Matthew C A, Moore M J 1991 Regeneration of rat extensor digitorum longus tendon: the effect of a sequential partial tenotomy on collagen fibril formation. Matrix 11:259–268

Mecham R P, Heuser J E 1991 The elastic fiber. In: Hay E (ed) Cell biology of extracellular matrix, 2nd edn. Plenum Press, New York, p 79–109

Mechanic G L 1974 An automated scintillation counting system for continuous analysis: cross-links of (3H)NaBH4 reduced collagen. Analytical Biochemistry 61:349–354

Miller R R, McDevitt C A 1991 Thrombospondin in ligament, meniscus and intervertebral disc. Biochimica et Biophysica Acta 111:85–88

Minns R J, Soden P D, Jackson D S 1973 The role of the fibrous components and ground substance in the mechanical properties of biological tissues: a preliminary investigation. Journal of Biomechanics 6:153–165

Murray M M, Spector M 1999 Fibroblast distribution in the antero-medial bundle of the human anterior cruciate ligament: the presence of alpha-smooth muscle actin-positive cells. Journal of Orthopaedic Research 17:18–27

Nachemson A L, Evans J H 1968 Some mechanical properties of the third human lumbar interlaminar ligament (ligament flavum). Journal of Biomechanics 1:211–220

Nakashima Y, Kariya Y, Yasuda C et al 2005 Regulation of cell adhesion and type VII collagen binding by the beta 3 chain short arm of laminin-5: effect of its proteolytic cleavage. Journal of Biochemistry 138:539–552

Neurath M F, Stofft E 1992 Collagen ultrastructure in ruptured cruciate ligaments. An electron microscopic investigation. Acta Orthopaedica Scandinavica 63:507–510

Ng C O Y, Ng G Y F, See E K N et al 2003 Therapeutic ultrasound improves strength of Achilles tendon repair in rats. Ultrasound in Medicine and Biology 29:1501–1506

Ng G Y F 1995 A long term study of the biomechanical and biological changes of the ACL-PT autograft and ACL repair after hemi-transection injury in a goat model. Thesis, Department of Anatomy, Monash University, Australia

Ng G Y F, Maitland M E 2001 Relationship of kinetic demands of athletic training and knee joint laxity. Physical Therapy in Sport 2:66–70

Ng G, Walter K 1995 Ageing does not affect flexion relaxation of erector spinae. Australian Journal of Physiotherapy 41:91–95

Ng G Y, Oakes B W, Deacon O W et al 1995 Biomechanics of patellar tendon autograft for reconstruction of the anterior cruciate ligament in the goat: three-year study. Journal of Orthopaedic Research 13:602–608

Ng G Y F, Oakes B W, Deacon O W et al 1996a Long-term study of the biochemistry and biomechanics of anterior cruciate ligament-patellar tendon autografts in goats. Journal of Orthopaedic Research 14:851–856

Ng G Y F, Oakes B W, McLean I D et al 1996b The long-term biomechanical and viscoelastic performance of repairing anterior cruciate ligament after hemitransection injury in a goat model. American Journal of Sports Medicine 24:109–117

Ng G Y F, Fung D T C, Leung M C P et al 2004a An ultrastructural comparison of medial collateral ligament repair after single or multiple applications of GaAlAs laser in rats. Lasers in Surgery and Medicine 35:317–323

Ng G Y F, Fung D T C, Leung M C P et al 2004b Comparison of single and multiple applications of GaAlAs laser on rat medial collateral ligament repair. Lasers in Surgery and Medicine 34:285–289

Nordin M, Lorenz T, Campello M 2001 Biomechanics of tendons and ligaments. In: Nordin M, Frankel V (eds) Basic biomechanics of the musculoskeletal system, 3rd edn. Lippincott Williams and Wilkins, Philadelphia, PA, p 102–125

Noyes F R, Barber-Westin S D 1997 A comparison of results in acute and chronic anterior cruciate ligament ruptures of arthroscopically assisted autogenous patellar tendon reconstruction. American Journal of Sports Medicine 25:460–471

Noyes F R, Grood E S 1976 The strength of the anterior cruciate ligament in humans and rhesus monkeys: age-related and species-related changes. Journal of Bone and Joint Surgery (Am) 58A:1074–1082

Noyes F R, De Lucas J L, Torvik P J 1974a Biomechanics of anterior cruciate ligament failure: an analysis of strain rate sensitivity and mechanisms of failure in primates. Journal of Bone and Joint Surgery (Am) 56A:236–253

Noyes F R, Torvik P J, Hyde W B et al 1974b Biomechanics of ligament failure: 2. An analysis of immobilization, exercise and reconditioning effects in primates. Journal of Bone and Joint Surgery (Am) 56A:1406–1418

Noyes F R, Butler D L, Grood E et al 1984 Biomechanical analysis of human ligament grafts used in knee-ligament repairs and reconstructions. Journal of Bone and Joint Surgery (Am) 66A:344–352

Oakes B W 1988 Ultrastructural studies on knee joint ligaments: quantitation of collagen fibre populations in exercised and control rat cruciate ligaments and in human anterior cruciate ligament grafts. In: Woo S L-Y, Buckwalter J (eds) Injury and repair of the musculoskeletal tissues, Section 2. American Academy of Orthopaedic Surgeons, Illinois, p 66–82

Oakes B W 1991 Clinical aspects of soft tissue repair. Sports Training, Medicine and Rehabilitation 2:279–283

Oakes B W 1992 The classification of injuries and mechanisms of injury, repair and healing. In: Bloomfield J, Fricker P A, Fitch K D (eds) Textbook of science and medicine in sport. Blackwell Scientific, Oxford, p 200–217

Oakes B W 1994 Tendon-ligament basic science. In: Harries M, Williams C, Stanish W D et al (eds) Oxford textbook of sports medicine. Oxford University Press, New York, p 493–511

Oakes B W, Parker A W 1981 Normal joint changes in collagen fibre populations in young rat cruciate ligaments in response to an intensive one month's exercise program. In: Russo P, Gass G (eds) Human adaptation. Cumberland College of Health Sciences, Sydney, p 223–230

Oakes B W, Deacon O W, Ng G Y et al 2000 Two biological determinants of anterior cruciate ligament graft strength. Book of abstract of 2000 Pre-Olympic Congress for International Congress on Sport Science, Sports Medicine and Physical Education, Brisbane, p 89–90

O'Donoghue D H, Rockwood C A, Zaricznyj B et al 1961 Repair of knee ligaments in dogs: I. The lateral collateral ligament. Journal of Bone and Joint Surgery (Am) 43A:1167–1178

O'Donoghue D H, Frank G R, Jeter G L et al 1971 Repair and reconstruction of the anterior cruciate ligament in dogs: factors influencing long term results. Journal of Bone and Joint Surgery (Am) 53A:710–718

Ogawa K, Ito M, Takeuchi K et al 2005 Tenascin-C is upregulated in the skin lesions of patients with atopic dermatitis. Journal of Dermatological Science 40:35–41

Olsen B R 1991 Collagen Biosynthesis. In: Hay E (ed.) Cell biology of extracellular matrix, 2nd edn. Plenum Press, New York, p 177–220

Parolie J M, Bergfeld J A 1986 Long-term results of non-operative treatment of isolated posterior cruciate ligament injuries in the athlete. American Journal of Sports Medicine 14:35–38

Parry D A D, Craig A S 1977 Quantitative electron microscope observations of the collagen fibrils in rat-tail tendon. Biopolymers 16:1015–1031

Parry D A D, Craig A S 1979 Electron microscope evidence for an 80Å unit in collagen fibrils. Nature 282:213–214

Parry D A D, Craig A S, Barnes G R G 1978a Tendon and ligament from the horse: an ultrastructural study of collagen fibrils and elastic fibres as a function of age. Proceedings of Royal Society of London (Biology) 203:293–303

Parry D A D, Barnes G R G, Craig A S 1978b A comparison of the size distribution of collagen fibrils in connective tissues as a function of age and a possible relation between fibril size distribution and mechanical properties. Proceedings of Royal Society of London (Biology) 203:305–321

Patterson-Kane J C, Parry D A, Birch H L et al 1997 An age-related study of morphology and cross-link composition of collagen fibrils in the digital flexor tendons of young thoroughbred horses. Connective Tissue Research 36:253–260

Pogany G, Hernandez D J, Vogel K G 1994 The in vitro interaction of proteoglycans with type I collagen is modulated by phosphate. Archives of Biochemistry and Biophysics 313:102–111

Postacchini F, De Martino C 1980 Regeneration of rabbit calcaneal tendon maturation of collagen and elastic fibers following partial tenotomy. Connective Tissue Research 8:41–47

Ramsey R H 1966 The anatomy of the ligamenta falva. Clinical Orthopaedics and Related Research 44:129–140

Raugi G J, Olerud J E, Gown A M 1987 Thrombospondin in early human wound tissue. Journal of Investigative Dermatology 89:551–554

Renstrom Per A F H, Lynch S A 1998 An overview of anterior cruciate ligament management. In: Chan K M, Fu F, Maffulli N (eds) Controversies in orthopedic sports medicine. Williams and Wilkins, Hong Kong, p 5–22

Sailor M E, Keskula D R, Perrin D H 1995 Effect of running on anterior knee laxity in collegiate-level female athletes after anterior cruciate ligament reconstruction. Journal of Orthopaedic and Sports Physical Therapy 21:233–239

Sakakura T, Kusano I 1991 Tenascin in tissue perturbation repair. Acta Pathologica Japonica 41:247–258

Scott J E 1988 Proteoglycan-fibrillar collagen interactions. Biochemical Journal 252:313–323

See E K N, Ng G Y F, Ng C O Y et al 2004 Running exercises improve the strength of a partially ruptured Achilles tendon. British Journal of Sports Medicine 38:597–600

Shah J S, Jayson M I V, Hampson W G J 1977 Low tension studies of collagen fibres from ligaments of the human spine. Annals of the Rheumatic Diseases 36:139–145

Shelbourne K D, Wickens J H, Mollabashy A et al 1991 Arthrofibrosis in acute anterior cruciate ligament reconstruction: the effect of timing of reconstruction and rehabilitation. American Journal of Sports Medicine 19:332–336

Snook G A 1983 A short history of the anterior cruciate ligament and the treatment of tears. Clinical Orthopaedics and Related Research 172:11–13

Steventon C, Ng G 1995 Effect of trunk flexion speed on flexion relaxation of erector spinae. Australian Journal of Physiotherapy 41:241–243

Tani N, Matsumoto K, Ota I et al 2001 Effects of fibronectin cleaved by neuropcin on cell adhesion and migration. Neuroscience Research 39:247–251

Tanzer M L 1973 Crosslinking of collagen. Science 180:561–566

Tanzer M L 1976 Cross-linking. In: Ramachandran G N, Reddi A H (eds) Biochemistry of collagen. Plenum Press, New York, p 137

Tipton C M, James S L, Mergner W et al 1970 Influence of exercise on the strength of the medial collateral knee ligament of dogs. American Journal of Physiology 218:894–902

Tipton C M, Matthes R D, Maynard J A et al 1975 The influence of physical activity on ligaments and tendons. Medicine and Science in Sports 7:165–175

Veltri D M, Warren R F 1994a Anatomy, biomechanics, and physical findings in posterolateral knee instability. Clinics in Sports Medicine 13:599–614

Veltri D M, Warren R F 1994b Operative treatment of posterolateral instability of the knee. Clinics in Sports Medicine 13:615–627

Viidik A 1973 Functional properties of collagenous tissues. International Review of Connective Tissue Research 6:127–215

Viidik A 1980 Interdependence between structure and function in collagenous tissues. In: Biology of collagen. Academic Press, New York, p 257–278

Viidik A, Sandqvist L, Magi M L 1965 Influence of postmortem storage on tensile strength characteristics and histology of rabbit ligaments. Acta Orthopaedica Scandinavica Supplementum 79:1–38

Viidik A, Danielsen C C, Oxlund H 1982 On fundamental and phenomenological models, structure and mechanical properties of collagen, elastic and glycosaminoglycan complexes. Biorheology 19:437–451

Vogel K G, Trotter J A 1987 The effect of proteoglycans on the morphology of collagen fibrils formed in vitro. Collagen Related Research 7:105–114

Vogel K G, Paulsson M, Heinegard D 1984 Specific inhibition of type I and type II collagen fibrillogenesis by the small proteoglycan of tendon. Biochemical Journal 223:587–597

Wasilewski S A, Covall D J, Cohen S 1993 Effect of surgical timing on recovery and associated injuries after anterior cruciate ligament reconstruction. American Journal of Sports Medicine 21:338–342

White D R, Widdowson E M, Woodard H Q et al 1991 The composition of body tissues (II). Fetus to young adult. British Journal of Radiology 64:149–159

Whiting W C, Zernicke R F 1998 Biomechanics of musculoskeletal injury. Human Kinetics, Champaign, IL, p 15–40, 87–136

Wight T N, Heinegard D K, Hascall V C 1991 Proteoglycans structure and function. In: Hay E (ed) Cell biology of extracellular matrix, 2nd edn. Plenum Press, New York, p 45–78

Wilby J, Linge K, Reilly T et al 1987 Spinal shrinkage in females: circadian variation and the effects of circuit weight-training. Ergonomics 30:47–54

Woo S L-Y, Adams D J 1990 The tensile properties of human anterior cruciate ligament (ACL) and ACL graft tissues. In: Daniel D, Akeson W, O'Connor J (eds) Knee ligaments structure, function, injury, and repair. Raven Press, New York, p 279–289

Woo S L-Y, Gomez M A, Akeson W H 1981 The time and history dependent viscoelastic properties of the canine medial collateral ligament. Journal of Biomechanical Engineering 103:293–298

Woo S L-Y, Gomex M A, Woo Y-K et al 1982 Mechanical properties of tendons and ligaments: I. Quasi-static and nonlinear viscoelastic properties. Biorheology 19:385–396

Woo S L-Y, Orlando C A, Camp J F et al 1986 Effects of postmortem storage by freezing on ligament tensile behavior. Journal of Biomechanics 19:399–404

Woo S L-Y, Lee T Q, Gomez M A et al 1987a Temperature dependent behavior of the canine medial collateral ligament. Journal of Biomechanical Engineering 109:68–71

Woo S L-Y, Hollis J M, Roux R D et al 1987b Effects of knee flexion on the structural properties of the rabbit femur-anterior cruciate ligament-tibia complex (FATC). Journal of Biomechanics 20:557–563

Woo S L-Y, Gomez M A, Sites T J et al 1987c The biomechanical and morphological changes in the medial collateral ligament of the rabbit after immobilization and remobilization. Journal of Bone and Joint Surgery (Am) 69A:1200–1211

Woo S L-Y, Young E P, Kwan M K 1990 Fundamental studies in knee ligament mechanics. In: Daniel D, Akeson W, O'Connor J (eds) Knee ligaments structure, function, injury, and repair. Raven Press, New York, p 115–134

Woo S L-Y, Hollis M, Adams D et al 1991 Tensile properties of the human femur-ACL-tibia complex. Effect of specimen age and orientation. American Journal of Sports Medicine 19:217–225

Woo SL-Y, An K N, Arnoczky S P et al 1994 Anatomy, biology, and biomechanics of tendon, ligament, and meniscus. In: Simon S R (ed) Orthopaedic basic science. American Academy of Orthopaedic Surgeons, Park Ridge, IL, p 89–126

Woo SL-Y, Vogrin T M, Abramowitch S D 2000 Healing and repair of ligament injuries in the knee. Journal of the American Academy of Orthopaedic Surgeons 8:364–372

Wu G K H, Ng G Y F, Mak A F T 2001a Effects of knee bracing on the functional performance of patients with anterior cruciate ligament reconstruction. Archives of Physical Medicine and Rehabilitation 82:282–285

Wu G K H, Ng G Y F, Mak A F T 2001b Effects of knee bracing on the sensori-motor function of subjects with ACL reconstruction. American Journal of Sports Medicine 29:641–645

Yahia L H, Drouin G 1989 Microscopical investigation of canine anterior cruciate ligament and patellar tendon: collagen fascicle morphology and architecture. Journal of Orthopaedic Research 7:243–251

Bone

Pekka Kannus and Kim Bennell

CHAPTER CONTENTS

Introduction 59

Bone anatomy. 59

Bone physiology. 60

Biomechanics of bone. 62

Structural properties of bone 62

How physical activity generates load on bone 63

Bone's response to local mechanical loading 64

Clinical bone conditions 64

Summary 76

Introduction

Bone is a unique tissue with the principal responsibility of supporting loads that are imposed on it. Fractures occur when the load exceeds bone strength. Acute fractures result from a single injurious load, while stress fractures are due to the accumulation of microdamage with repeated loading. Osteoporotic fractures occur in bone that is weakened due to low bone mass and microarchitectural deterioration. Physical therapists working in the area of sport and exercise are often involved in the prevention, diagnosis and rehabilitation of fractures. This chapter will firstly describe bone as an organ and tissue and then review how bone responds to mechanical loads. This will be followed by a discussion of the principles of prevention and treatment of acute, stress and osteoporotic fractures and the role that physical therapists play in this area.

Bone anatomy

Bone constituents

Bone consists of an organic component (20–25% of the wet weight of bone), an inorganic component (65–70% of the wet weight) and a water component (10% of the wet weight) (Wang 2005).

Organic matrix

The organic matrix determines the structure and the mechanical and biochemical properties of bone. About 90% of the organic matrix is made up of type I collagen and about 8% is composed of proteoglycans and numerous non-collagenous proteins. The remaining 2% consists of bone cells (Einhorn 1996, Wang 2005).

Collagen

Collagen is a protein that consists of three polypeptide chains of about 1000 amino acids each and wound together in a helix pattern by cross-links of hydrogen bonding. Each molecule is aligned with the next in parallel order to form a collagen microfibril and fibril. The fibrils are then grouped to form the collagen fiber (Einhorn 1996).

Non-collagenous proteins

Non-collagenous proteins make up only a small proportion of bone by weight but have great biological significance. Many of these proteins play a role in the metabolic processes of bone such as formation and resorption (Einhorn 1996).

Cells

Bone cells arise from different cell lines and carry out various functions. Osteoblasts are derived from local bone marrow mesenchymal cells and are located on all active bone surfaces. Their main function is to synthesize and secrete the organic matrix of bone. Once osteoblasts stop forming bone, they may either remain on the bone surface where they are known as bone-lining cells or they may surround themselves with matrix and become osteocytes. The main role of bone-lining cells is to contract and secrete enzymes that remove the thin layer of osteoid covering the mineralized matrix. This allows osteoclasts to attach to bone and begin resorption (Buckwalter et al 1995).

Osteocytes comprise more than 90% of the bone cells in the mature human skeleton. They are connected to other bone cells by numerous cytoplasmic projections that travel in channels (canaliculi) through mineralized matrix (Boivin et al 1990). These interconnections may allow the cells to sense deformation of bone by mechanical loads and to coordinate the remodeling process (described later under the heading of modeling and remodeling).

Osteoclasts are derived from extraskeletal, hematopoietic stem cells. They are large, motile, multinucleated cells found on bone surfaces undergoing resorption. To resorb the bone matrix, osteoclasts bind to the bone surface and create an acidic environment by secreting protons and enzymes (Peck & Woods 1988). The acid environment digests the non-collagenous link between hydroxyapatite crystals and collagen (Khan et al 2001).

Inorganic component

The inorganic component of bone consists mainly of platelike crystals of hydroxyapatite which itself is composed of calcium and phosphate. The chemical formula of the hydroxyapatite is $Ca_{10}(PO_4)_6(OH)_2$. These crystals are found in and around collagen fibers and give bone its strength.

Macroscopic and microscopic appearance

On the macroscopic level, the skeleton consists of two parts, the axial and the appendicular skeletons. The axial skeleton includes vertebrae, the pelvis, and other flat bones such as the skull and scapula. The appendicular skeleton includes all the long bones. Each long bone consists of two wider extremities (epiphyses), an essentially cylindrical shaft in the middle (diaphysis), and a zone between them (metaphysis) where remodeling of bone takes place during growth and development. In this way, bone can be described as an organ (Khan et al 2001).

Bone can also be described as tissue at the microscopic level. There are two types of bone tissue: woven bone and lamellar bone. Woven bone is considered immature bone with collagen arranged randomly. At birth, it makes up all the bone in the body; in later years it is found at sites of fracture healing or in response to extreme mechanical loads (Forwood & Burr 1993).

Lamellar bone is the name given to bone that eventually replaces woven bone. By the age of 4 years, most of the skeleton is lamellar bone. The collagen fibers arrange themselves along lines of principal force.

Anatomically, both woven and lamellar bone can be organized into compartments as either cortical or trabecular bone. Cortical bone forms the external part of long bones and is made up of dense, calcified tissue. The diaphysis of a long bone encloses the medullary cavity. Toward the metaphysis or epiphysis, cortical bone is thinner and the medullary cavity is replaced by cancellous or trabecular bone, which is characterized by an inner network of thin calcified trabeculae.

An important difference between cortical and trabecular bone is in the way the bone matrix and cellular elements are arranged. Calcium takes up 80–90% of cortical bone volume but only 15–25% of trabecular bone volume (Khan et al 2001). The trabecular arrangement permits bone marrow, blood vessels and connective tissues to be in contact with bone. The main function of cortical bone is for structure and protection (Khan et al 2001).

Haversian bone is the most complex type of cortical bone. It consists of blood vessels that are circumferentially surrounded by lamellae of bone. This arrangement of cortical bone around a vessel is called an osteon. Osteons are usually aligned with the long axis of bone. They are the major structural units of cortical bone and are connected to one another by Volkmann's canals that run at right angles to the osteon (Buckwalter et al 1995).

Bone physiology

It is well accepted that bone adapts its structure and function to applied loads but can be injured if load exceeds strength. The areas of bone physiology that will be discussed include mechanotransduction (the mechanism whereby loading influences bone cell function) and the processes of modeling, remodeling and fracture repair.

Mechanotransduction

It is not fully understood how bone responds to mechanical loads but it has been suggested that the response is controlled by a 'mechanostat' that endeavors to keep bone strain at an optimal level by adjusting bone structure (Frost 1983, Frost 2003, Turner 1999). It is thought that bone strains resulting from mechanical loading are transduced into a cellular signal. Osteocytes have been proposed as the bone cells responsible for sensing strain and transmitting signals (Aarden et al 1994) The cellular signals are then compared with the optimal strain for that region. If the signal falls within the optimal strain range, no adaptive response will occur and a state of remodeling or modeling equilibrium ensues. However, if the strains are above or below the optimal range, a state of overuse or disuse is perceived. This results in an appropriate response with net bone gain or loss in order to readjust bone strains (Fig. 5.1). Also, many other factors such as hormones, and diet and lifestyle

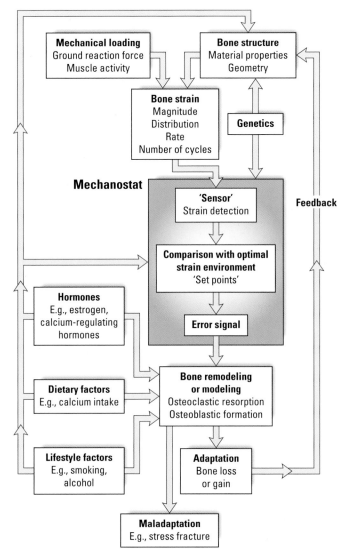

Figure 5.1 • Schematic diagram of a mechanism for bone adaptation to mechanical loads.

Remodeling is a continuous, sequential process of breakdown and repair of microscopic cavities in bone. Remodeling occurs on both periosteal and endosteal surfaces within cortical bone and on the surface of trabeculae. Both osteoclasts and osteoblasts are involved in remodeling, organized into discrete packets called basic multicellular units (Frost 1991).

Remodeling occurs in five stages: (i) quiescence, (ii) activation, (iii) resorption, (iv) reversal and (v) formation (Parfitt 1988). A small area of bone surface is converted from rest to activity by an initiating stimulus, which may be hormonal, chemical or physical. Osteoclast precursors are then recruited to the bone surface where they fuse to form multinucleated osteoclasts. These cells form a cavity by resorbing bone. A 1–2 week interval between termination of the resorptive processes and commencement of formation is known as the reversal phase. During this time, the bone site is weakened. Therefore continued mechanical loading during the reversal phase could result in microdamage accumulation and the beginning of a stress fracture (Brukner & Bennell 1997).

Repair of the resorption cavity is performed by osteoblasts and occurs in two stages: matrix synthesis and mineralization. First, a layer of type I collagen bone matrix, known as an osteoid seam, is deposited. After 5–10 days of maturation, the new matrix begins to mineralize with crystals of hydroxyapatite deposited within and between the collagen fibrils (Parfitt 1988).

A key feature of remodeling is that damaged tissue is replaced with an equal amount of new bone tissue in the healthy skeleton. In the aging and osteoporotic skeleton, however, the balance between the amount of bone resorbed and formed is shifted in favor of resorption, so that insufficient bone is formed to refill the resorption cavity (Parfitt 1988). A net loss of bone results, and eventually bone strength and integrity are compromised.

Fracture repair

Unlike many other tissues, bone repairs by regeneration. Primary bone healing occurs when there is direct and intimate contact between the bone ends. New bone grows directly across the bone ends to unite the fracture. The healing process involves osteoclastic bone resorption followed by osteoblastic new bone formation (Sheikh 2000a).

Secondary fracture healing represents mineralization and bony replacement of a cartilage matrix. The three main stages of fracture healing which may overlap include the inflammatory phase (10%), the reparative phase (40%) and the remodeling phase (70%) (Sheikh 2000a) (Table 5.1).

Inflammation is characterized by hematoma formation and the migration of inflammatory mediator cells to the injured site (Andrew et al 1994). These cells remove tissue debris and release growth factors and chemotactic agents which attract mesenchymal cells, fibroblasts and endothelial cells to the site of injury (Einhorn 1998). These cells divide and differentiate to produce a connective tissue matrix into which neovascularization takes place (Glowacki 1998).

Reparation is performed by two cellular cascades. One is associated with chondrogenesis while the other is associated

factors affect the remodeling, modeling and structure of bone and thus the mechanostat or mechanosensitivity of the system (Fig. 5.1) (Järvinen et al. 2003, Järvinen et al. 2005).

Modeling and remodeling

Bone modeling and remodeling are the processes that lead to changes in bone geometry and mass. Bone modeling is an organized bone cell activity that allows bone growth and adjusts bone strength through the strategically placed, non-adjacent activity of osteoblasts and osteoclasts (Frost 1990). Modeling improves bone strength not only by adding mass, but also by expanding the outer (periosteal) and inner (endocortical) diameters of bone (Khan et al 2001).

Table 5.1 Stages of fracture healing

Healing phase	Duration	Events
Inflammatory	1–2 weeks	Formation of fracture hematoma Invasion by inflammatory cells
Reparative	Several months	Differentiation of mesenchymal cells Callus matrix laid down by chondroblasts and fibroblasts Mineralization of soft callus by osteoblasts to form woven bone
Remodeling	Months to years	Replacement of immature woven bone with mature lamellar bone by osteoclasts and osteoblasts Reforming of medullary cavity

with osteogenesis. These two processes initially combine to form a bridge, known as the primary or provisional callus, which spans and surrounds the fracture site. The completion of this process results in clinical union. Following union, osteogenesis predominates with the cartilage formed during primary callus formation being replaced with new bone in a process of endochondral ossification (Einhorn 1998). The cartilage of the soft callus is invaded with blood vessels, chondroclasts and osteoblasts. Chondroclasts degrade the cartilage matrix until only thin spicules of cartilage remain, forming cavities into which osteoblasts migrate. The osteoblasts line the cavities and begin producing new compact bone matrix rich in type I collagen. This results in the formation of the secondary or definitive callus and consolidation of the fracture clinically.

The final stage of bone repair is remodeling, performed by osteoclasts and osteoblasts. This stage may take months to years to complete. Remodeling functions to replace mineralized cartilage with cancellous bone, replace cancellous bone with new compact bone, replace callus between the ends of bone and remove any callus in the marrow cavity thereby restoring cavity continuity (Frost 1989).

Biomechanics of bone

The key mechanical function of the skeleton is to allow effective movement of the body. Bones have to be strong enough to resist fracture. This depends on both its intrinsic material properties (mass, density, stiffness and strength) and its structural properties or gross geometric characteristics (size, shape, cortical thickness, cross-sectional area and trabecular architecture) (Carter et al 1976, Currey 2001, Currey 2003, Forwood 2001). Factors that affect skeletal strength and design include genetics, physical activity, hormones and dietary factors (Khan et al 2001). Of these, the mechanical loading activity of bone is vitally important (Moisio et al 2004, Ruff et al 2006).

Material properties of bone

The organic and inorganic components of bone (discussed previously) determine its material properties. The organic component, primarily type I collagen, provides tensile strength. Abnormal collagen matrix leaves bone brittle, irrespective of the amount of bone mineral present. The inorganic component, mineral, resists compressive forces. Functional tests under controlled conditions using a defined volume of bone can be used to measure the material behavior of bone as a tissue. When a load, or 'stress' is applied, the bone is deformed. This deformation is referred to as 'strain'.

Stress and strain

Stress, the force applied per unit area (pascal, newton per square meter), can be classified into three basic types: compression, tension and shear (Wang 2005). Alone or in combination, these three basic stress types produce four types of load on bone: compression, tension, bending and torsion (Wang 2005). Strain describes the deformation of a material without regard to its structural geometry and refers to the percentage change in bone length. Strain is greatest at the point of highest loading and dissipates along the length of the long bone (Nordin & Frankel 1989). For example, during walking or running, the highest measurable strain would occur at the calcaneus and distal tibia. In addition, during locomotion, the greatest strain is generated at the cortex under compression.

The intrinsic material properties of bone include the concepts of stiffness and strength. The amount of force required to deform a structure is termed its stiffness and is represented by the slope of the stress–strain curve (see Fig. 5.2). The strength of the structure can be defined as the load at the yield or failure points, or as the ultimate load, depending on the circumstances. Strength is an intrinsic property of bone and is independent of its size (Khan et al 2001).

Bone mineral mass

Bone mass is a determinant of bone material properties; the distribution of bone mass and bone geometry are connected to bone strength and stiffness. Further, the strength and stiffness of bone is a function of density. Although bone mass is only one component of overall bone strength (Mosekilde 1993), it does explain more than 80% of that variable (Johnston & Slemenda 1993). Because bone mass is highly correlated with dual energy X-ray absorptiometry (DXA) results, this technique is used to measure bone mass and give an estimate of fracture risk in humans (Cummings et al 1993, Martin 1991). DXA technology and its clinical implications are discussed further in the section on osteoporosis.

Structural properties of bone

Geometric characteristics of bone include size, shape, cortical thickness, cross-sectional area and trabecular architecture.

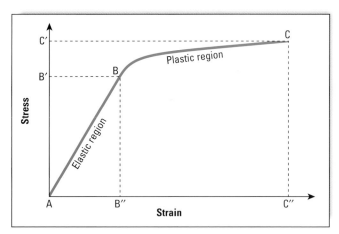

Figure 5.2 • Stress–strain curve for a cortical bone sample tested in tension. Yield point (B): point past which some permanent deformation of the bone sample occurred. Yield stress (B′): load per unit area sustained by the bone sample before plastic deformation took place. Yield strain (B″): amount of deformation withstood by the sample before plastic deformation occurred. The strain at any point in the elastic region of the curve is proportional to the stress at that point. Ultimate failure point (C): the point past which failure of the sample occurred. Ultimate stress (C′): load per unit area sustained by the sample before failure. Ultimate strain (C″): amount of deformation sustained by the sample before failure. (Reproduced from Nordin M, Frankel VH 1989 Basic biomechanics of the musculoskeletal system, 2nd edn, Lea & Febiger with the permission of Lippincott Williams & Wilkins.)

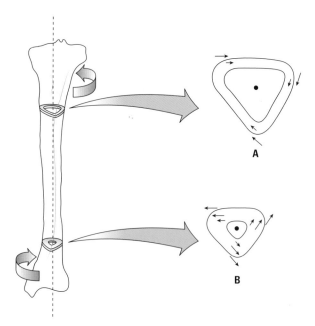

Figure 5.3 • Distribution of shear stress in two cross-sections of a tibia subjected to torsional loading. The proximal section **(A)** has a higher moment of inertia than does the distal section **(B)** because more bony material is distributed away from the neutral axis. (Reproduced from Nordin M, Frankel V H 1989 Basic biomechanics of the musculoskeletal system, 2nd edn, Lea and Febiger with the permission of Lippincott Williams and Wilkins, copyright Lippincott Williams and Wilkins.)

Appendicular bone adapts to mechanical loads by endocortical resorption and periosteal apposition of bone tissue. This increases bone diameter, cortical thickness or both, and thus provides greater resistance to loading.

For tension and compression loads, the strength of a bone is proportional to the bone cross-sectional area. Hence, a larger bone is more resistant to fracture as it distributes the internal forces over a larger surface area resulting in lower stresses (Hayes & Gerhart 1985). With respect to bending loads, both the cross-sectional area and the distribution of bone tissue around a neutral axis are important geometrical features. The area moment of inertia is the index that takes into account these two factors in bending. A larger area moment of inertia means that the bone tissue is distributed further away from the neutral axis (the axis where the stresses and strains are zero) and is more efficient in resisting bending (Fig. 5.3).

The length of a bone also influences its strength in bending. The longer the bone, the greater the magnitude of the bending moment caused by the application of a force. For this reason, the long bones of the lower extremity are subjected to high bending moments and hence high tensile and compressive stresses (Nordin & Frankel 1989).

The mechanical competence of whole bone can be characterized by the deformation it undergoes during loading. Deformation is characteristically measured and plotted as a load–deformation curve. This is similar to the stress–strain curve but it is used to assess whole bone. Generally, a linear relationship exists between the imposed load and the amount of bone deformation until the bone reaches its yield point. Prior to reaching this point, the bone is in its elastic region (if unloaded, it would return to its original shape). That is, applied forces in this region cause only temporary deformation. Beyond the yield point, the slope of the curve plateaus; the area beneath this part of the curve is called the plastic region. It marks the point at which permanent deformation occurs and, in extreme cases, the point at which local fractures or other damage may result. If the load continues to increase, failure load may be reached, and the structure may fail completely (Khan et al 2001).

How physical activity generates load on bone

The skeleton is subjected to forces produced by gravity (weight-bearing), by muscles and by other external factors. Effects of gravity and muscle action on bone are closely connected to and difficult to separate from each other since in vertical position gravity always activates antigravity muscles.

Bone tissue is an anisotropic material which means that its behavior varies depending on the direction of the applied load. In general, bone tissue can handle the greatest loads in a longitudinal direction (i.e. compressive forces), the direction of habitual loading, and lesser loads when they are applied across the bone surface (i.e. bending, shear or impacting forces). None of this is straightforward, as the degree of anisotropy varies with the anatomical region (cortical or trabecular bone) and with the magnitude and direction of the mechanical load (Khan et al 2001).

During physical activity, contact with the ground generates forces within the body. Without muscle activity, ground reaction forces (GRFs) are transmitted from the foot and along the lower limbs to the hips through a series of action–reaction forces (a system of three rigid links). Forces applied to bone, however, are primarily the result of muscular contraction. Therefore, with the additional influence of muscles and lever arms, GRFs vary. For example, running generates GRFs around 2–3 times body weight (Cavanagh & LaFortune 1980), whereas jumping and landing activities can be clearly higher at up to 12–22 times body weight (Heinonen et al 2001, McNitt-Gray 1991) (Fig. 5.4).

Bone's response to local mechanical loading

The skeleton's response to a load depends on the strain magnitude, rate, distribution and cycles in the target bone (Khan et al 2001). Much of what we know about the influence of functional

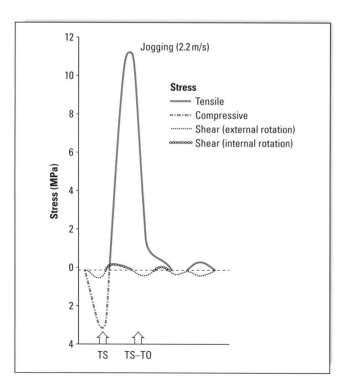

Figure 5.4 • Calculated stresses on the anteromedial cortex of a human adult tibia during running. TS = toe-strike; TO = toe-off. (Reproduced from Nordin M, Frankel V H 1989 Basic biomechanics of the musculoskeletal system, 2nd edn, Lea and Febiger with the permission of Lippincott Williams and Wilkins, copyright Lippincott Williams and Wilkins.)

loads on bone comes from research with animal models where the applied load can be precisely controlled.

Strain magnitude

Strain magnitude can be defined as the amount of percentage change in bone length under mechanical loading. Early work using the turkey ulna clearly showed that bone formation increased with larger strain magnitudes (Rubin & Lanyon 1985). Activities that elicit high peak forces (or high strain magnitude) may have a greater effect on bone mass than activities associated with a large number of loading cycles (Whalen et al 1988).

Strain rate

Strain rate, the rate at which strain develops and releases, determines bone's adaptive response. Higher strain rates are most effective for a maximal adaptive bone response (Turner et al 1995). Umemura et al (1995) compared jump training with running training in rats and found that jumping was associated with a higher strain rate and magnitude, and was more effective than running for eliciting a positive bone response.

Strain distribution

Strain distribution refers to the way strain is distributed across a section of bone. It has been hypothesized that unusual strains of uneven distribution are more likely to stimulate osteogenesis than repetitive strains that result from everyday activity (Lanyon 1984).

Strain cycles

Strain cycles denote the number of load repetitions that change bone dimensions at a given magnitude. Although a minimum number of loading cycles is required for a positive bone response, the number of strain cycles appears to be less important than strain magnitude or strain rate (Lanyon 1987, Rubin & Lanyon 1984, Umemura et al 1997). Appropriate rest periods between the loading cycles also appear important for a good bone response (Robling et al 2002, Turner & Robling 2005). Mechanical loading presents a potent osteogenic stimulus to bone cells, but bone cells desensitize rapidly to mechanical stimulation. Resensitization must occur before the cells can transduce future mechanical signals effectively. Experiments show that mechanical loading protocols are more osteogenic if the load cycles are divided into several discrete bouts, separated by several hours, than if the cycles are applied in a single uninterrupted bout (Robling et al 2002, Turner & Robling 2005).

Clinical bone conditions

Acute fractures

Acute fractures are caused either by direct trauma such as a car hitting a pedestrian or by indirect trauma such as a fall onto an outstretched hand resulting in a fracture of the humerus. The principles of fracture management involve:

1. Reduction – manipulating the bone to its correct anatomical position. Reduction may be achieved under anesthesia, by continuous traction (closed) or surgically (open).

2. Immobilization – holding the bone in the correct reduced position. Various devices are used to achieve different degrees of fixation including casts, external fixation, slings, plates, rods, screws and pins.

3. Rehabilitation – returning the person to as full function as possible after the trauma.

The physical therapies are important in the rehabilitation of patients with fractures and commence as soon as the fracture has been reduced. The main consideration affecting treatment is the stage of healing and thus it is important that the therapist liaises with the patient's medical practitioner (Atkinson et al 2005).

Healing times

Healing times vary depending on the location and severity of the fracture, associated injuries and patient characteristics such as age, smoking status and medical conditions (Sheikh 2000b). There are two major time points relevant to fracture healing and it is important to establish where along the continuum of fracture healing the patient lies as this will influence rehabilitation:

1. Union – the partial repair of bone when the initial callus forms around the bone ends so that there is minimal movement. On X-ray, the fracture line will still be visible. Full bone maturity has not been reached so full weightbearing cannot be undertaken and some form of external support is usually still needed. This can be reduced as healing moves from union to consolidation (Atkinson et al 2005).

2. Consolidation – the bone is fully repaired and there is no movement at the fracture site. No fracture line can be seen on X-ray and bone trabeculae cross where the fracture previously was. Full function can now commence (Atkinson et al 2005).

The approximate union and consolidation times in normal adult bone are shown in Table 5.2. Healing times for children are generally half that of adults.

Rehabilitation of acute fractures

Physical therapy in fracture rehabilitation is dictated by a number of factors including the stage of fracture healing, the type of fracture, the immobilization device used and the patient's weightbearing status. Following initial fracture management, the physical therapist must ensure that the patient understands the rehabilitation process and is educated as to steps to reduce the risk of complications. Exercises can be given to maintain the range of motion of joints that are not immobilized and

techniques employed to reduce inflammation and swelling and minimize pain.

When the fracture is stable and united, mild overpressures can be applied to joints next to the fracture site, and exercises can be commenced to regain the range of motion at joints proximal and distal to the fracture site and to strengthen muscles that attach to the injured bone. The amount of resistance and weightbearing can be progressively increased. It is important that at all times the patient does not experience pain at the actual fracture site (Atkinson et al 2005).

Despite rehabilitation, post-traumatic osteoporosis around the fracture site is a common finding (Fig. 5.5). For this reason, rehabilitation of acute bone fractures should be intense and last over a long period.

Stress fractures

Stress fractures are overuse bone injuries that result from the accumulation of microdamage that is not adequately repaired by the remodeling process. This section will provide a general overview of the assessment and treatment of stress fractures.

Table 5.2 Approximate union and consolidation times in normal adult bone (reproduced with permission from Atkinson et al 1999)

Fracture site	Union time (weeks)	Consolidation time (weeks)
Proximal third of humerus	3	6
Distal third of radius/ulna	6	12
Proximal third of femur	4–6	8–12
Distal third of femur	6	12
Proximal third of tibia	6–8	12–16
Distal third of tibia	8–10	16–20

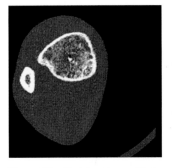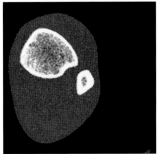

Figure 5.5 • Peripheral quantitative computed tomographic (pQCT) images reveal clear post-traumatic cortical and trabecular bone loss at the right distal tibia (left panel) a year after a surgically treated tibial shaft fracture. The structure and bone density at the contralateral limb are normal (right panel). (Courtesy of Dr. Harri Sievänen, Tampere, Finland.)

Diagnosis

When assessing the patient presenting with a possible stress fracture, there are four questions that need to be answered:

1. Is the pain bony in origin?
2. If so, which bone is involved?
3. At what stage in the continuum of bone stress is this injury?
4. What factors have predisposed this individual to a stress fracture?

To obtain answers to these questions a thorough history, precise examination, and appropriate use of imaging techniques are used.

History

The patient generally reports a history of insidious onset of activity-related pain. Initially the pain will usually be described as a mild ache occurring with exercise, but the pain may well become more severe or occur at an earlier stage of exercise if the patient continues. The pattern of pain differs from that of overuse soft tissue injuries, as it tends to get worse with exercise rather than decreasing after a period of warm-up.

The presence of predisposing factors needs to be determined from the history (Table 5.3). Therefore a training or activity history is essential. In particular, note should be taken of recent changes in activity level such as increased quantity of training, increased intensity of training, changes in surface, equipment (especially shoes) and technique. A full dietary history should be taken and particular attention paid to the possible presence of eating disorders and weight loss. Females should be asked about their menstrual history, including age of menarche and subsequent menstrual status.

A history of previous similar injury or any other musculoskeletal injury should be obtained. It is essential to obtain a brief history of the patient's general health and medication usage to ensure that there are no factors that may influence bone health. It is also important to obtain an understanding of the patient's work and sporting commitments (Brukner et al 1999).

Physical examination

On physical examination, the most obvious feature is localized bony tenderness. This is easier to determine in bones that are relatively superficial, but may be absent in stress fractures of the shaft or neck of femur. Occasionally, redness and swelling may be present at the site of the stress fracture. There may also be palpable periosteal thickening, especially in a long-standing fracture. Percussion of long bones may result in the production of pain at a point distant from the percussion.

Joint range of motion is usually unaffected except in situations where the stress fracture is close to the joint surface, such as a stress fracture of the neck of femur. Specific stress fractures may be associated with specific clinical tests. Examples of these are the hop test for stress fractures in the groin region

Table 5.3 Risk factor assessment in a patient presenting with a stress fracture

Risk factor	Variables
Training	Type Volume Intensity Surface Changes in training
Footwear	Type Age of shoe Use of insoles
Lower limb alignment	Foot type Tibial torsion Knee varus/valgus Femoral anteversion Leg length
Muscle length and joint range	Flexibility of calf, hamstrings, hip flexors Range of ankle dorsiflexion, hip internal/external rotation
Menstrual status	Current and past menstrual patterns Use of the oral contraceptive pill Sex hormonal levels if irregular
Bone density – dual energy X-ray absorptiometry (DXA)	If amenorrheic or multiple stress fracture history
Dietary intake	Calcium Energy Other nutrients influencing absorption of calcium or bone health (e.g. protein, fiber) Presence of eating disorder

(Brukner et al 1999) and hip extension while standing on the contralateral leg used in the diagnosis of stress fractures of the pars interarticularis of the spine (Brukner et al 1999).

The physical examination must also take into account the potential predisposing factors, and in all stress fractures involving the lower limb a full biomechanical examination must be performed. Any evidence of leg length discrepancy, malalignment (especially excessive subtalar pronation), muscle imbalance, weakness or lack of flexibility should be noted (Brukner et al 1999) (Table 5.3).

Imaging

Imaging plays an important role in supplementing clinical examination of stress fractures. In some cases a clinical diagnosis of stress fracture is sufficient. However, if the diagnosis is uncertain, or in the case of serious or elite athletes who wish to continue training if at all possible and require more specific knowledge of their condition, there are various imaging techniques available.

Radiography Radiography has poor sensitivity but high specificity in the diagnosis of stress fractures. The classic radiographic abnormalities seen in a stress fracture are new periosteal bone formation, a visible area of sclerosis, the presence of callus or a visible fracture line. If any of these radiographic signs are present, the diagnosis of stress fracture can be confirmed (Santi et al 1989).

Unfortunately, in the majority of stress fractures there is no obvious radiographic abnormality. The abnormalities on radiography are unlikely to be seen unless symptoms have been present for at least 2–3 weeks. In certain cases, they may not become evident for up to 3 months, and in a percentage of cases, never become abnormal (Meurman & Elfving 1980).

Isotopic bone scan (scintigraphy) The triple phase bone scan is highly sensitive for diagnosing stress fractures (Prather et al 1977) and changes may be seen as early as 7 hours after bone injury. A stress fracture appears as a sharply marginated or fusiform area of increased uptake involving one cortex, or occasionally extending the width of the bone in the third phase of the bone scan (Roub et al 1979) (Fig. 5.6). However, bone scintigraphy lacks specificity because other non-traumatic lesions such as tumor (especially osteoid osteoma) can also produce localized increased uptake. It is therefore vitally important to correlate the bone scan appearance with the clinical features.

The sensitivity of bone scintigraphy can be further increased by the use of single photon emission computer tomography (SPECT). Bone SPECT is most helpful in complex areas of the skeleton with overlapping structures that may obscure pathology such as the skull, pelvis and spine. It is particularly useful in the detection of stress fractures of the pars interarticularis in the spine.

Computerized tomography Computerized tomography (CT) may be useful in differentiating those conditions with increased uptake on bone scan that may mimic stress fracture. CT scans are particularly valuable in imaging fractures where this may be important in treatment such as the navicular bone (Kiss et al 1993). CT scanning may also be valuable in detecting fracture lines as evidence of stress fracture in long bones (e.g. metatarsal and tibia) where plain radiography is normal and isotope bone scan shows increased uptake. CT scanning will enable the clinician to differentiate between a stress fracture that will be visible on CT scan and a stress reaction. Particularly in elite athletes, this may considerably affect their rehabilitation program and their forthcoming competition program (Fig. 5.7).

Magnetic resonance imaging Magnetic resonance imaging (MRI), while not imaging cortical bone as well as CT scan, has certain advantages in the imaging of stress fractures. Specific MRI characteristics of stress fracture include new bone formation and fracture lines, and marrow and periosteal hemorrhage and edema. These changes are best seen if the MRI is performed within 3 weeks of symptoms (Lee & Yao 1988). Although CT scan visualizes bone detail, another advantage of MR imaging is in distinguishing stress fractures from a suspected bone tumor or infectious process.

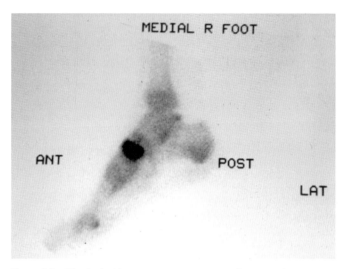

Figure 5.6 • The typical bone scan appearance of a stress fracture.

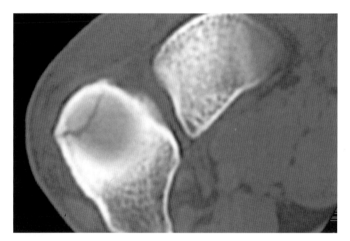

Figure 5.7 • The CT appearance of a stress factor of the navicular.

Treatment

The actual time from diagnosis of a stress fracture to full return to sport or physical activity depends on a number of factors including the site of the fracture, the length of the symptoms, and the severity of the lesion (stage in the spectrum of bone stress). Most stress fractures with a relatively brief history of symptoms will heal without complication or delay and permit return to sport within the 4–8 week range. However there is a group of stress fractures that require additional treatment and special consideration. These are listed separately, later in the chapter.

While there are many subtleties involved in the treatment of stress fractures, the primary treatment is modified (most frequently reduced) activity. During the phase of modified activity, a number of important issues are attended to, including modification of risk factors, maintenance of muscular strength and fitness, pain management, investigation of bone health and prescription of orthotic devices. The treatment of stress fractures can be divided into two phases: Phase I is the early treatment using modified activity and Phase II is the period from the reintroduction of physical activity to full return to sport.

Phase I

Pain management Pain is seldom severe but can be a problem even with normal walking. Mild analgesics can be used as well as physical therapy modalities (e.g. ice, interferential, electrical stimulation). Practitioners often suggest non-steroidal anti-inflammatory drugs (NSAIDs) but there is some speculation that the mode of action of some may slow or prevent repair of the stress fracture as they reduce the bone remodeling process (Burr 2001). In some cases where activities of daily living are painful, it may be necessary for the patient with a stress fracture to be non-weightbearing or partial weightbearing on crutches for a period of up to 10 days.

Muscle strengthening Skeletal muscle plays an important role in stress fracture development. At some regions, bone load is increased by muscular force, while at others, it is reduced as muscles absorb energy (Scott & Winter 1990). In endurance sports, it is possible that even low levels of muscular fatigue can affect the total impact load to bone, particularly in the lower extremity. Following fatiguing exercise, bone strain, particularly strain rate, has been shown to increase (Fyhrie et al 1998, Yoshikawa et al 1994). Some studies have shown that reduced muscle strength (Hoffman et al 1999) and smaller muscle size (Bennell et al 1996, Milgrom 1989) predispose to stress fractures in athletes and military recruits. While there are no studies that have evaluated the role of muscle strengthening in the treatment of stress fractures, it is logical to include a specific strengthening program because of the important role of muscles in shock absorption, and to help counteract the effects of detraining. Muscle strengthening programs are usually prescribed for a period of 6–12 weeks and can begin immediately after diagnosis of the stress fracture. It is important, however, that the exercises do not cause pain at the stress fracture site.

Maintaining fitness Maintenance of fitness during periods of forced inactivity due to injury is a major concern to coaches and athletes. Inactivity has marked detrimental effects on the cardiovascular system as well as the metabolic and morphological characteristics of skeletal muscle.

Non-loading activities that maintain fitness are those that use as many large muscle groups as possible without over-loading the bone. The most common methods of maintaining fitness are cycling, swimming, deep water running, rowing and stairmaster activities. For muscular strength, upper and lower body weight programs can usually be prescribed without risk. These workouts should as much as possible mimic the athlete's normal training program in both duration and intensity.

Modification of risk factors As with any overuse injury, it is not sufficient to merely treat the stress fracture itself. Stress fractures represent the result of incremental overload. Subtle adjustments to the modifiable factors that contribute to the total load are an essential component of the management of an athlete with a stress fracture. However, it should be pointed out that there have been few controlled trials to evaluate the effectiveness of risk factor modification in reducing stress fracture development or recurrence.

Training Controlled trials in the military showed that the reduction of high impact activities, such as running and jumping, was associated with a decrease in stress fracture incidence, whereas the reduction of marching distance had no effect (Giladi et al 1985a, Scully & Besterman 1982). Other studies have shown that training interventions, such as the inclusion of rest periods (Scully & Besterman 1982, Worthen & Yanklowitz 1978), elimination of running and marching on concrete (Greaney et al 1983, Reinker & Ozburne 1979), and pre-entry physical conditioning (Milgrom et al 2000, Shaffer et al 1999), may also reduce stress fracture risk in the military.

While there are few data relating to athletes, it is imperative to obtain a detailed training history to try and identify any training parameters that may have contributed to an individual's stress fracture. Athletes should be encouraged to keep an accurate training log book and to monitor responses to training. Coaches need to be reminded that training regimens for athletes should be individualized.

Footwear and insoles A recent Cochrane review concluded that the use of insoles inside the boots of military recruits during their initial training appears to reduce the number of stress fractures and/or stress reactions of bone (Rome et al 2005). There is insufficient evidence to determine the best design of such insoles but comfort and tolerability should be considered. Whether the results can be generalized to the sporting population is not clear.

Another important contributing factor to stress fracture development may be inadequate training shoes. These shoes may be inappropriate for the particular foot type of the individual, may have general inadequate support/shock absorption, or may be worn out. In a randomized trial, training in basketball shoes compared with normal military boots was associated with a significant reduction in the incidence of stress fractures in the foot but not in overall stress fractures (Milgrom et al 1992).

Biomechanical abnormalities Intrinsic biomechanical abnormalities are thought to contribute to the development of overuse injuries in general and stress fractures in particular. The structure of the foot will partly determine how much force is absorbed by the bones in the foot and how much force is transferred to proximal bones during ground contact. The high arched (pes cavus) foot is more rigid and may be less able to absorb shock, resulting in more force passing to the tibia and femur. The low arched (pes planus) foot is more flexible, allowing stress to be absorbed by the musculoskeletal structures of the foot. Stress fractures are also often associated with prolonged pronation or hyperpronation, which can induce a great amount of torsion on the tibia and may exacerbate muscle fatigue as the muscles have to work harder to control the excessive motion, especially at toe-off. Theoretically, either foot type could predispose to a stress fracture but results of studies have been conflicting (Brosh & Arcan 1994, Giladi et al 1985b, Montgomery et al 1989, Simkin et al 1989).

Since there is evidence to show that a leg length discrepancy increases the likelihood of stress fractures in both military (Friberg 1982) and athletic (Bennell et al 1996, Brunet et al 1990) populations, a heel raise should be provided if necessary. Other alignment features to be investigated include the presence of genu varum, valgum, or recurvatum, Q angle, and tibial torsion. Of these, only an increased Q angle has been found in association with stress fractures (Cowan et al 1996) although this is not a universal finding (Montgomery et al 1989, Winfield et al 1997).

A thorough biomechanical assessment is an essential part of both treatment and prevention of stress fractures. Until the contribution of biomechanical abnormalities to stress fracture risk is clarified through scientific research, correction of such abnormalities should be attempted, if possible.

Muscle flexibility and joint range of motion The role of flexibility is difficult to evaluate as flexibility encompasses a number of characteristics including active joint mobility, ligamentous laxity and muscle length. Of the numerous variables that have been assessed in relation to stress fractures (Bennell et al 1996, Ekenman et al 1996, Giladi et al 1987, Hughes 1985, Milgrom et al 1994, Montgomery et al 1989, Winfield et al 1997), only increased range of hip external rotation (Giladi et al 1991, Giladi et al 1987, Milgrom et al 1994) and decreased range of ankle dorsiflexion (Hughes 1985) have been associated with stress fracture development, and even these findings have been inconsistent.

The difficulty in assessing the role of muscle and joint flexibility in stress fractures may relate to a number of factors including the relatively imprecise methods of measurement, the heterogeneity of these variables, and the fact that both increased and decreased flexibility may be contributory. Until better evidence is available to the contrary, it is worth prescribing stretches if muscle flexibility and joint range are found to be restricted in the athlete who presents with a stress fracture.

Menstrual status Women with stress fractures should be questioned about their current and past menstrual status. There is evidence to show that menstrual disturbances increase the risk of stress fracture (Barrow & Saha 1988, Bennell et al 1996, Carbon et al 1990, Tomten 1996, Winfield et al 1997) and lead to premature bone loss particularly at trabecular sites (Gremion et al 2001, Hetland et al 1993, Jonnavithula et al 1993, Myburgh et al 1993, Robinson et al 1995). Lower bone density in women may be associated with a greater risk of stress fractures although results from studies are mixed (Bennell et al 1995, 1996, Carbon et al 1990, Cline et al 1998, Frusztajer et al 1990, Girrbach et al 2001, Grimston et al 1991, Lauder et al 2000, Myburgh et al 1990). If menstrual disturbances are present, the athlete should be referred to a medical practitioner for review.

Dietary intake Dietary surveys of various sporting groups often reveal inadequate intakes of nutrients that are important for skeletal health (Ronsen et al 1999, Ziegler et al 1999). However, there is currently little evidence to support low calcium intake as a risk factor for stress fractures in otherwise healthy athletic (Bennell et al 1996, Carbon et al 1990, Frusztajer et al 1990, Grimston et al 1991, Kadel et al 1992, Warren et al 1991) or military (Cline et al 1998) populations. In the only controlled trial, calcium supplementation of 500 mg daily had no significant effect on stress fracture incidence in male military recruits (Schwellnus & Jordaan 1992).

Athletes report a greater frequency of disordered eating patterns than the general population, especially those in sports emphasizing leanness and/or those competing at higher levels (Picard 1999). Low caloric intake has been hypothesized as one of the mechanisms for menstrual disturbances in sportswomen (Zanker & Swaine 1998). Disordered eating (often seen as weight loss), amenorrhea and osteopenia often occur simultaneously in athletic females, a syndrome that has been referred to as the 'female athlete triad' (Otis et al 1997) (see also Chapter 12). Abnormal and restrictive eating behaviors do seem to increase the likelihood of fracture in women (Bennell et al 1995, Bennell et al 1996, Frusztajer et al 1990, Nattiv et al 1997).

Healthy eating habits should be promoted in all individuals. If one is concerned about dietary intake in those presenting with a stress fracture, nutritional counseling should be recommended.

Bracing The use of a pneumatic air brace may assist with stress fracture healing in the leg and reduce the time taken to return to sport (Batt et al 2001, Dickson & Kichline 1987, Gillespie & Grant 2000, Rome et al 2005, Slayter 1995, Swenson et al 1997, Whitelaw et al 1991). It has been proposed that the brace may act by shifting a portion of the weightbearing load from the tibia to the soft tissue, which results in less impact loading (Swenson et al 1997). It is also suggested that the brace facilitates healing at the fracture site by compressing the soft tissue, thereby increasing the intravascular hydrostatic pressure and shifting fluid and electrolytes from the capillary space to the interstitial space (Swenson et al 1997). This theoretically enhances the piezo-electric effect and enhances osteoblastic bone formation.

Phase II

When normal, day-to-day ambulation is pain free, then resumption of the impact loading activities can begin. The rate of resumption of activity is individual and should be modified according to symptoms and physical findings. The time to return to sport is variable depending on a number of factors such as the site of stress fracture, the person's age, competitive level and time to diagnosis (Benazzo et al 1992).

There are no studies that have compared different return-to-sport programs. However, since healing bone is weaker, a progressive increase in load is needed so that the bone will adapt with increases in strength. For lower limb stress fractures where running is the aggravating activity, a program that involves initial brisk walking increased by 5–10 min per day up to a length of 45 min is recommended (Brukner et al 1999). Once this is achieved without pain, slow jogging for increasing periods within the 45-min walk is recommended. Once the 45-min goal is achieved, the pace can be increased, initially at half pace then gradually increasing to full pace striding. Once full sprinting is achieved free of pain, functional activities such as hopping, skipping, jumping, twisting and turning can be introduced gradually. A typical program for an uncomplicated lower limb stress fracture resuming activity after a period of initial rest and activities of daily living is shown in Table 5.4. This pattern of reintroduction of activity can be followed for other sports.

It is not uncommon for the patient to experience pain at some point during the reintroduction of activity. This is, by no means, an indication of a return of the stress fracture. In each instance, the activity should be discontinued, followed by several days of modified rest, and then training should resume at a level lower than that at which the pain occurred. Progress should be monitored clinically by the presence or absence of symptoms and local signs. It is not necessary to monitor progress by radiography, scintigraphy, CT or MRI since radiological healing often lags behind clinical healing. Only in cases of clearly delayed clinical healing, imaging can be considered.

When training resumes it is important to allow adequate recovery time after hard sessions or hard weeks of training. This can be accommodated by developing micro- and macrocycles. Alternating hard and easy training sessions is a microcycle adjustment but graduating the volume of work or alternating harder and easier sessions can also be done weekly or monthly. In view of the history of stress fracture, it is advisable that some form of cross training (e.g. swimming and cycling for a runner), be introduced to reduce the stress on the previously injured area and reduce the likelihood of a recurrence (Brukner et al 1999).

Surgery Surgery is virtually never required in the management of the routine stress fracture. In the case of a displaced stress fracture (e.g. neck of femur) or established non-union (e.g. anterior cortex of tibia, navicular, sesamoids, fifth metatarsal), however, surgery may be required.

Stress fractures requiring specific treatment While the majority of stress fractures will heal without complications in a relatively short time frame (and with relative rest), there are a number of stress fractures with a tendency to develop complications, such as delayed or non-union, and which require specific additional treatment, such as cast immobilization or surgery. These are shown in Box 5.1. While it is beyond the scope of this chapter to cover the treatment of these in detail,

readers are referred to other reviews in this area (Brukner et al 1999, Brukner & Bennell 1997, Egol & Frankel 2001).

Osteoporosis and associated factors

Osteoporosis is a metabolic bone disorder characterized by low bone mass and microarchitectural deterioration leading to skeletal fragility and increased fracture risk (Consensus Development Conference 1993). Physical therapists have a role to play in this condition through exercise prescription, education and strategies to maximize function, reduce the risk of falls and manage pain.

Bone mineral density (BMD) and falls are two major determinants of the risk of fracture (Kannus et al 2005, Lespessailles et al 1998, Petersen et al 1996). An individual's peak bone mass is reached around the late teens and early 20s (Bailey 1997, Haapasalo et al. 1996a, Young et al 1995). A slow rate of bone loss then starts in both sexes, and superimposed on this is an accelerated loss of bone in women at the menopause when estrogen production ceases (Fig. 5.8).

Approximately 60–80% of the interindividual variation in peak bone mass can be explained by genes (Zmuda et al 1999). Other determinants include hormones, mechanical loading,

---

Box 5.1 Stress fractures that require specific treatment

Neck of femur
Pars interarticularis of the spine
Patella
Anterior cortex, mid-shaft tibia
Medial malleolus
Talus
Navicular
5th metatarsal
2nd metatarsal (base)
Sesamoid

Table 5.4 Activity program following uncomplicated lower limb stress fracture following period of rest and ADL (taken from Brukner P, Bennell K, Matheson G 1999 Stress fractures. Blackwell Science, p 101, with permission)

	Day 1 (min)	Day 2 (min)	Day 3 (min)	Day 4 (min)	Day 5 (min)	Day 6 (min)	Day 7 (min)
Week 1	Walk 5	Walk 20	Walk 25	Walk 30	Walk 35	Walk 40	Walk 45
Week 2	Walk 20 Jog 5 Walk 15	Walk 15 Jog 15 Walk 15	Walk 15 Jog 20 Walk 15	Walk 10 Jog 25 Walk 10	Walk 5 Jog 30 Walk 10	Walk 5 Jog 35 Walk 5	Jog 45
Week 3	Jog 45 Stride 10	Jog 45 Stride 10	Jog 45 Stride 15	Jog 45 Stride 15	Jog 45 Sprint 0	Jog 45 Sprint 10	Jog 45 Sprint 15
Week 4	Add functional activities Gradually increase all week						
Week 5	RESUME FULL TRAINING						

nutrition, body composition and lifestyle factors such as smoking and alcohol intake. Physical therapists need to be aware of risk factors for osteoporosis as well as medical conditions and pharmacological agents that predispose to secondary osteoporosis (Box 5.2).

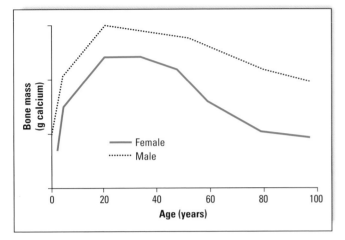

Figure 5.8 • Changes in bone density with age in men and women. (Reproduced with permission from Bennell et al 2000.)

Box 5.2 Risk factors for osteoporosis and medical conditions predisposing to secondary osteoporosis (reproduced with permission from Bennell et al 2000)

Risk factors for osteoporosis

- A family history of osteoporosis/hip fracture
- Postmenopausal without hormone replacement therapy
- Late onset of menstrual periods
- A sedentary lifestyle
- Inadequate calcium and Vitamin D intake
- Cigarette smoking
- Excessive alcohol
- High caffeine intake
- Amenorrhea – loss of menstrual periods
- Thin body type
- Caucasian or Asian race

Medical conditions predisposing to secondary osteoporosis

- Anorexia nervosa
- Rheumatological conditions (e.g. rheumatoid arthritis, ankylosing spondylitis)
- Endocrine disorders (e.g. Cushing's syndrome, primary hyperparathyroidism, thyrotoxicosis)
- Malignancy
- Gastrointestinal disorders (malabsorption, liver disease, partial gastrectomy)
- Certain drugs (corticosteroids, heparin)
- Immobilization (paralysis, prolonged bed rest, functional impairment)
- Congenital disorders (Turner's syndrome, Kleinfelter's syndrome)

A greater propensity to falling will increase the risk of fracture considerably (Kannus et al 2005, Parkkari et al 1999). Many risk factors for fall initiation have been identified. These can be classified into intrinsic factors (e.g. poor eyesight, reduced balance, reduced lower limb strength) and extrinsic factors, such as home hazards, multiple drug use and inappropriate footwear (Lord et al 1991, 1994).

Measurement of bone density

Dual energy X-ray absorptiometry (DXA) is currently the technique of choice to measure a real bone density (g/cm^2) and diagnose osteoporosis (Blake & Fogelman 1998). It has excellent measurement precision, is relatively fast and inexpensive, is widely available and uses only a small amount of radiation. As a planar measure, however, its accuracy is of concern, and it cannot reveal the three-dimensional geometry of bones well.

Physical therapists need to be able to interpret DXA scans as the results can guide patient management (Fig. 5.9). The most useful BMD scores are the Z- and T-scores. The Z-score compares the person's BMD with that of an age-matched group (calculated as the deviation from the mean result for the age- and sex-matched group divided by the standard deviation of the group). This score indicates whether one is losing bone more rapidly than one's peers. The T-score is similarly defined but uses the deviation from the mean peak bone density of a young, healthy sex-matched group. The World Health Organization has defined bone mass clinically based on T-scores (World Health Organization 1994) and has categorized it into normal, osteopenia, osteoporosis and established osteoporosis (Table 5.5). DXA-derived BMD scores have been shown clinically to predict fracture risk relatively well (Cummings et al 1993).

Signs and symptoms of osteoporosis

Low bone density per se is asymptomatic and many individuals are unaware that they have osteopenia or osteoporosis until a fracture occurs. The common fracture sites are the hip, vertebrae and wrist and less commonly the ribs, pelvis, ankle and upper arm (Sanders et al 1999). Vertebral compression fractures can cause loss of height and this may occur suddenly or gradually over time. A common clinical sign of advanced spinal osteoporosis is thoracic kyphosis or the 'dowager's hump'. This may be due to anterior wedge fractures of the vertebral bodies (Ensrud et al 1997) but muscle weakness and pain may also contribute (Cutler et al 1993). Postural changes may cause patients to complain of a 'pot belly' with a bulging stomach and concertina-like skin folds. These changes also result in less space within the thorax and abdominal region and increased intra-abdominal pressure. This can cause shortness of breath and reduced exercise tolerance, hiatus hernia, indigestion, heartburn and stress incontinence (Larsen 1998). Some patients complain of spinal pain due to fractures but not all fractures are symptomatic (Ross 1997).

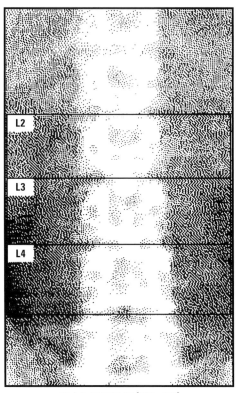

27 July 1999 15:40 [119 × 106]
Hologic QDR–1000/W (S/N 822)
Lumbar spine V4.62

Total BMD CV for L1–L4 1.0%			
CF	0.999	1.063	1.000
Region	Area (cm²)	BMC (g)	BMD (g/cm²)
L2	12.31	7.87	0.639
L3	14.21	9.76	0.687
L4	17.70	13.26	0.749
Total	44.23	30.90	0.699

Region	BMD	T (30.0)		Z	
N/A					
L2	0.639	−3.53	62%	−2.18	73%
L3	0.687	−3.61	63%	−2.19	74%
L4	0.749	−3.33	67%	−1.87	78%
L2–L4	0.699	−3.46	65%	−2.05	76%

♦ Age and sex matched
T = peak bone mass
Z = age matched

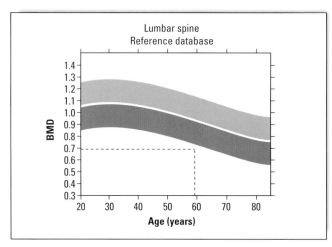

BMD(L2–L4) = 0.699 g/cm²

Figure 5.9 • Results from a DXA scan of the lumbar spine of a 59-year-old woman showing the absolute bone density as well as T- and Z-scores. Since she has a T-score of −3.46 for the L2–4 she is considered to have osteoporosis at this site. A Z-score of −2.05 indicates that she also has lower bone density compared with her peers.

Physical therapy assessment

A complete subjective and objective assessment is needed but the choice of questions and procedures depends on several factors including the age of the patient, severity of the condition, DXA results, coexisting pathologies, functional status and reasons for consultation. Specific questioning for osteoporosis is shown in Table 5.6. There are a number of reliable and standardized measurement tools that can be used to gain a more accurate assessment of the patient's needs. These are summarized in Table 5.7.

Table 5.5 Diagnostic criteria for osteoporosis (reproduced with permission from Bennell et al 2000)

Classification	DXA result
Normal	BMD greater than 1 s.d. below the mean of young adults (T-score above −1)
Osteopenia	BMD between 1 and 2.5 s.d. below the mean of young adults (T-score −1 to −2.5)
Osteoporosis	BMD more than 2.5 s.d. below the mean of young adults (T-score below −2.5)
Severe or established	BMD more than 2.5 s.d. below the mean of osteoporosis of young adults plus one or more fragility fractures

s.d. – standard deviation

Table 5.6 Relevant questions for subjective assessment in the area of bone health (reproduced with permission from Bennell et al 2000)

Category	Specific questions
DXA results	Date performed T- and Z-scores Amount of change with serial scans
Family history of osteoporosis	Which family member? Which sites?
Fracture status	Site When? Related to minimal trauma?
Falls history	Number of falls in past year Mechanism of falls Associated injuries Risk factors (e.g. eyesight, home hazards)
Medical history	Particularly with relation to risk factors including ovariectomy, eating disorder, endocrine disorder
Medication	Current or past, especially long-term steroids, hormone replacement therapy, bisphosphonates
Menstrual history	Age of onset of periods Ever had ≤8 periods per year and number of years? Menopausal status including age at menopause and number of years since menopause
Smoking habits	Number of cigarettes per day and number of years smoked currently or in past
Diet	Dietary restrictions, such as vegetarianism, low fat Sources of daily calcium – yoghurt, cheese, milk Calcium supplementation – type and daily dose Amount of caffeine Number of glasses of alcohol per week
Exercise status	Amount and type of activity during youth Current exercise – type, intensity, duration, frequency Interests and motivational factors Exercise tolerance and shortness of breath
Posture	Noticed any loss of height? Difficulty lying flat in bed? Number of pillows needed Any activities encouraging bad posture?
Musculoskeletal problems and functional status	Pain, weakness, poor balance, incontinence Functional limitations
Social history	Occupation – full time/part time Hobbies Family

Physical therapy management

Physical therapy management will vary depending on assessment findings, particularly the patient's age, DXA results and functional status. The aims of treatment should be clearly established so that appropriate management can be instigated.

Exercise prescription for bone loading

While regular exercise influences bone material and structural properties, and reduces the risk of falling (Kannus et al 2005), it is not well known whether exercise reduces fracture rates which is the ultimate goal. The fact that there are only two relatively small randomized controlled trials to answer this question (Korpelainen et al 2006, Sinaki et al 2002) reflects inherent methodological difficulties. However, large-scale epidemiological studies suggest that physical activity is associated with a lower risk of fracture in both men and women (Feskanich et al 2002, Joakimsen et al 1999, Kujala et al 2000, Nordström et al 2005, Paganini-Hill et al 1991).

The skeletal effects of exercise at different ages It is presently thought that exercise in childhood and adolescence produces much higher gains in bone mass than does exercise in adulthood (Bass et al 1998, Bradney et al 1998, Conroy et al 1993, Heinonen et al 2000, Kannus et al 1995, McKay et al 2000, Morris et al 1997, Wang 2005). In addition, it appears that childhood exercise stimulates the bone modeling process, expanding the bone size to produce a larger, possibly stronger bone (Bradney et al 1998, Haapasalo et al 1996b, Wang 2005). This phenomenon is generally not possible once growth has ceased.

Exercise in adulthood is important to conserve bone and to minimize bone loss with age (Bonaiuti et al 2002, Kelley et al 2000, Wolff et al 1999). In adulthood, exercise must be continued in order to maintain exercise-induced BMD levels (Dalsky et al 1988). Attrition rates from exercise are high, even in supervised clinical trials (Bassey & Ramsdale 1994, Kerschan

Table 5.7 Summary of outcome measurements that can be used to design and evaluate physical therapy programs for the prevention and treatment of osteoporosis

Variable	Measurement
Pain	• 10 cm visual analog scale • McGill Pain Questionnaire (Melzack 1975) • Daily analgesic use
Function and aerobic capacity	• Timed up and go (Podsiadlo & Richardson 1991) Time taken to rise from a chair, walk a distance of 3 m and return to sit down • Timed 6 m walk test (Hageman & Blanke 1986), time taken to walk 6 m at normal walking pace • Adapted shuttle walk (Singh et al 1994)
Self-reported function and health-related quality of life	• SF-36 questionnaire (Ware & Sherbourne 1992) • Osteoporosis Functional Disability Questionnaire (Helmes et al 1995) • Quality of Life questionnaire of the European Foundation for Osteoporosis (QUALEFFO) (Lips et al 1999)

Balance	• Balancing on one leg or in stride standing – eyes open/closed, on hard surface/foam (Shumway-Cook & Horak 1986)
	  Longest duration that the person can balance
	• Step test (Hill et al 1996)
	  Number of times that the person can place the foot onto and off a step (7.5 cm or 15 cm high) in 15 s
	• Functional reach (Duncan et al 1990)
	  Measure the distance that the person can reach forward in standing with the arm outstretched

Muscle strength	• Main muscles of interest include the quadriceps, ankle dorsiflexors, scapula retractors, trunk extensors, hip extensors and abdominals • Isometric, isotonic or isokinetic methods • Often assess 1 or 3 repetition maximum (1 or 3 RM) Determine the heaviest weight that the person can lift on one or three occasions • Grip strength using a hand held dynamometer
Posture and range of motion	• Measuring the distance of the tragus of the ear to the wall with the patient standing back against the wall to determine thoracic and cervical posture • Range of shoulder elevation

et al 1998). This reinforces the importance of developing strategies to improve adherence and encourage life-long participation in physical activity.

What types of exercise are best for improving bone strength? In humans, high impact exercises which generate ground reaction forces greater than twice body weight are more osteogenic than low-impact exercises (Bassey & Ramsdale 1994, Heinonen et al 1996, 1998, Nikander et al 2005, 2006).

Since lean mass (Flicker et al 1995, Young et al 1995) and muscle strength (Madsen et al 1993) are positively correlated with bone density, weight training has been advocated for skeletal health (Gleeson et al 1990, Hartard et al 1996, Lohmann et al 1995, Snow-Harter et al 1992). Loss of muscle mass and strength with age is well documented (Harries & Bassey 1990, Rutherford & Jones 1992). Progressive weight training even in the frail elderly can lead to large strength gains (Fiatarone et al 1990). In a unilateral exercise study, Kerr et al (1996) compared two strength-training regimens that differed in the number of repetitions and the weight lifted. The strength program (high loads, low repetitions) significantly increased bone density at the hip and forearm sites whereas the endurance program (low loads, high repetitions) had no effect. Walking is frequently recommended in clinical practice to maintain skeletal integrity but generally the results of walking trials have not demonstrated significant effects on densitometry-derived bone density (Ebrahim et al 1997, Hatori et al 1993, Humphries et al 2000, Martin & Notelovitz 1993). This may relate to the fact that walking imparts relatively low magnitude, repetitive, and customary strain to the skeleton. While walking has numerous health benefits, some of which may influence fracture risk, it should not be prescribed as the exercise of choice for skeletal loading in healthy ambulant individuals. Whether walking is effective in those with restricted mobility is yet to be researched.

Non-weightbearing activities such as cycling and swimming do not stimulate bone adaptation despite increases in muscle strength (Orwoll et al 1989, Rico et al 1993, Taaffe et al 1995). This suggests that these activities do not generate sufficient strain to reach the threshold for bone adaptation.

Exercise dosage The exact exercise dose required for maximal skeletal effects is not yet known. For an elderly or previously sedentary population, exercise should be gradually introduced to minimize fatigue and prevent soreness (Forwood & Larsen 2000). Exercise should be performed 2–3 times per week. Animal studies suggest that this is as effective for bone as daily loading (Raab-Cullen et al 1994).

For aerobic exercise, sessions should last between 15 and 60 min. The average conditioning intensity recommended for adults without fragility fractures is between 70 and 80% of their functional capacity. Individuals with a low functional capacity may initiate a program at 40–60% (Forwood & Larsen 2000).

Adults commencing a weight-training program may perform a few weeks of familiarization (Kerr et al 1996) followed by a single set of 8–10 repetitions at an intensity of 40–60% of 1 repetition maximum (RM). This can be progressed to 80%, even in the very elderly (American College of Sports Medicine 1998, Fiatarone et al 1994). Programs should include 8–10 exercises involving the major muscle groups. Supervision, particularly in the beginning, and attention to safe lifting technique is paramount.

Periodic progression of exercise dosage is needed, otherwise bone adaptation will cease. Increasing the intensity or weightbearing is more effective than increasing the duration of the exercise. A periodic increase in a step-like fashion may be better than progression in a linear fashion (Forwood & Larsen 2000). Nevertheless, there comes a point where gains in bone mass will slow and eventually plateau.

Clinical recommendations for exercise prescription In children and adolescents, the goal is to maximize peak bone mass and strength. A variety of weightbearing, high-impact activities should be encouraged as part of the physical education curriculum in schools and during extracurricular sport and play. Odd impacts (i.e. dynamic loading of bone from atypical or unusual directions) also seem effective for bone (Nikander et al 2005, 2006). In the premenopausal adult years, the emphasis is on structured exercise to load bone. This could involve high-impact activities and weight training. A healthy lifestyle should be promoted and, in females, attention paid to adequate diet and regular menstrual cycles. In the older adult years, a variety of exercise modes are needed to target clinically relevant hip, spine and forearm sites. Progressive weight training and low-impact exercise are appropriate given that high-impact loading may be injurious. Other activities for balance, posture, and aerobic fitness could include a fast walking program, cycling, swimming and specific exercises.

While exercise should be directed at improving or maintaining bone strength, in osteoporotic and older patients, the exercise focus shifts from specifically loading bone to preventing falls and improving function (Kannus et al 2005). Factors that will influence the choice of exercise program include bone density levels, patient's age, previous fractures, co-morbid musculoskeletal or medical conditions, lifestyle, interests and current fitness level. Exercises to avoid in osteoporotic patients include high-impact loading, abrupt or explosive movements, trunk flexion, twisting movements, and dynamic abdominal exercises.

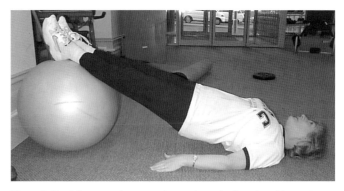

Figure 5.10 • Hip extension exercises using a ball assist with trunk and pelvic stability. (Reproduced with permission from Bennell et al 2000.)

Posture and flexibility

In patients with osteopenia or osteoporosis, treatment should aim to minimize the flexion load on the spine, promote extended posture and improve chest expansion. Land or water exercises can be designed to encourage diaphragmatic breathing, strengthen the hip, back and neck extensors and scapula retractors, and stretch the major upper and lower limb muscles (Bravo et al 1997, Chartered Society of Physiotherapy 1999). Postural re-education and dynamic stabilization for the trunk and limb girdles are particularly important to normalize mechanical forces (Figs 5.10 and 5.11). Stronger back extensors have been shown to be related to smaller thoracic kyphosis and reduced risk of spinal fractures (Sinaki et al 1996, 2002). Patients can be advised to spend time lying in a prone or prone-on-elbows position to stimulate thoracic extension. Postural taping (Fig. 5.12) or bracing may be required to assist with maintenance of correct posture and for pain relief. Advice can be given about correct ways to lift as well as correct posture during standing, lying, sitting and bending.

Falls reduction

In elderly individuals or where falls risk factors have been identified, treatment should be directed towards reducing falls and their consequences. Patients who report multiple falls may benefit from referral to a falls clinic or to medical specialists for further evaluation and multifaceted interventions (McMurdo et al 2000, Tinetti et al 1994). Exercise programs can address functional impairments in elderly individuals (Bravo et al 1997, Kronhed & Moller 1998, Lord 1996, McMurdo & Rennie 1993, Morganti et al 1995, Nelson et al 1994, Simmons & Hansen 1996) and there is strong high-quality evidence that regular strength and balance training can reduce the risk of falling (Carter et al 2001, Kannus et al 2005). Consideration should also be given to home hazard modification, withdrawal of extensive psychotropic medication, vitamin D and calcium supplementation, cataract surgery and, in appropriate patients, prescription of antislip devices, gait aids and external hip protectors (Kannus et al 2000, 2005, McKiernan 2005, Parkkari et al 1995, 1997).

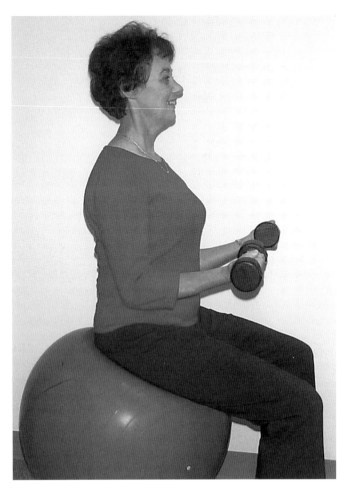

Figure 5.11 • Upper limb exercises can be performed while sitting on a ball to increase dynamic stability and trunk control. (Reproduced with permission from Bennell et al 2000.)

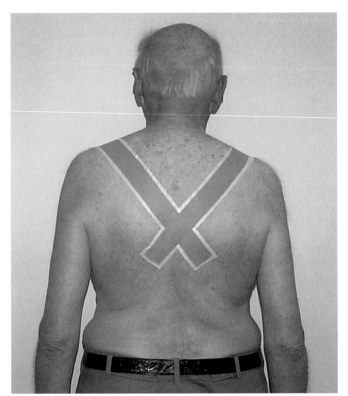

Figure 5.12 • Taping may be used to facilitate thoracic extension and improve posture. (Reproduced with permission from Bennell et al 2000.)

Education

A large part of the physical therapist's role is to provide osteoporosis education and to empower the individual to take control of the condition. In many cases, patients may be anxious and require reassurance and advice about safe activities. Physical therapists should continually update their knowledge about self-help groups, community programs and reputable gymnasiums and exercise classes in the local area. Osteoporosis organizations are found in many countries and provide a range of useful services and resources.

Summary

Bone injuries will be encountered by physical therapists working in a variety of settings. Acute fractures are due to a single load that exceeds bone strength while stress fractures result from the repeated application of lower loads. Osteoporotic fractures are usually caused by falls and occur in a bone weakened due to low bone density, cortical and trabecular thinning and microarchitectural deterioration. Rehabilitation following acute fractures must be guided by a number of factors including the stage of healing, the type of fracture, the method of fixation, associated injuries and the age of the patient. Stress fracture management involves modified rest, pain relief, lower limb strengthening, attention to risk factors and a program of

Pain-relieving techniques

Exercise has been shown to reduce back pain and improve psychological wellbeing in postmenopausal women with osteopenia (Bravo et al 1996, Preisinger et al 1996) and with established osteoporosis (Malmros et al 1998).

Hydrotherapy may be beneficial due to the heat and unloading effects (Bravo et al 1997), and is particularly useful for building patient confidence prior to commencing a land-based exercise program. Other pain-relieving techniques include ice, hot packs, soft tissue massage, transcutaneous electrical nerve stimulation (TENS), interferential therapy and shortwave diathermy. Gentle spinal mobilization can be performed even in patients with osteoporosis and osteopenia, provided care is taken and techniques that are well short of end range used. However, forceful joint manipulation is contraindicated. To deal more positively with chronic pain, cognitive and behavioral strategies or relaxation techniques may be employed by the physical therapist (see Chapter 9).

graduated return to activity. Prevention of stress fractures is an additional aim of physical therapists working with athletes. Identified risk factors in women include low bone density, a later than usual age of menarche, less lean mass, disordered patterns of eating and leg length discrepancy. From a physical therapy perspective, prevention of osteoporotic fractures focuses on regular weightbearing activity that is commenced in childhood and continued throughout life. Management of the older individual with osteoporosis includes education, pain-relieving techniques (if appropriate) and exercises designed to improve posture, balance, range of motion and lower limb strength.

References

Aarden E M, Burger E H, Nijweide P J 1994 Function of osteocytes in bone. Journal of Cell Biochemistry 55:287–299

American College of Sports Medicine 1998 Position stand on exercise and physical activity for older adults. Medicine and Science for Sports and Exercise 30:992–1008

Andrew J G, Andrew S M, Freemont A J et al 1994 Inflammatory cells in normal human fracture healing. Acta Orthopaedica Scandinavica 65:462–466

Atkinson K, Coutts F, Hassenkamp A 1999 Physiotherapy in orthopaedics. Churchill Livingstone, Edinburgh

Atkinson K, Coutts F, Hassenkamp A 2005 Physiotherapy in orthopaedics: a problem solving approach, 2nd edn. Churchill Livingstone, Edinburgh

Bailey D A 1997 The Saskatchewan pediatric bone mineral accrual study: bone mineral acquisition during the growing years. International Journal of Sports Medicine 18 (suppl 3):S191–S194

Barrow G W, Saha S 1988 Menstrual irregularity and stress fractures in collegiate female distance runners. American Journal of Sports Medicine 16:209–216

Bass S, Pearce G, Bradney M et al 1998 Exercise before puberty may confer residual benefits in bone density in adulthood: studies in active prepubertal and retired female gymnasts. Journal of Bone and Mineral Research 13:500–507

Bassey E J, Ramsdale S J 1994 Increase in femoral bone density in young women following high impact exercise. Osteoporosis International 4:72–75

Batt M E, Kemp S, Kerslake R 2001 Delayed union stress fractures of the anterior tibia: conservative management. British Journal of Sports Medicine 35:74–77

Benazzo F, Barnabei G, Ferrario A et al 1992 Stress fractures in track and field athletes. Journal of Sports Traumatology and Related Research 14:51–65

Bennell K L, Malcolm S A, Thomas S A et al 1995 Risk factors for stress fractures in female track-and-field athletes: a retrospective analysis. Clinical Journal of Sports Medicine 5:229–235

Bennell K L, Malcolm S A, Thomas S A et al 1996 Risk factors for stress fractures in track and field athletes: a 12 month prospective study. American Journal of Sports Medicine 24:810–818

Bennell K, Khan K, McKay H 2000 The role of physiotherapy in the prevention and treatment of osteoporosis. Manual Therapy 5:198–213

Blake G M, Fogelman I 1998 Applications of bone densitometry for osteoporosis. Endocrinology and Metabolism Clinics of North America 27:267–288

Boivin G, Anthoine-Terrier C, Obrant K J 1990 Transmission electron microscopy of bone tissue. Acta Orthopaedica Scandinavica 61:170–180

Bonaiuti D, Cranney A, Iovine R et al 2002 Exercise for preventing and treating osteoporosis in postmenopausal women. The Cochrane Database of Systematic Reviews 2:CD000333

Bradney M, Pearce G, Naughton G et al 1998 Moderate exercise during growth in prepubertal boys – changes in bone mass, size,

volumetric density, and bone strength: a controlled prospective study. Journal of Bone and Mineral Research 13:1814–1821

Bravo G, Gauthier P, Roy P M et al 1996 Impact of a 12-month exercise program on the physical and psychological health of osteopenic women. Journal of the American Geriatrics Society 44:756–62

Bravo G, Gauthier P, Roy P et al 1997 A weight-bearing, water-based exercise program for osteopenic women: its impact on bone, functional fitness, and well-being. Archives of Physical Medicine and Rehabilitation 78:1375–1380

Brosh T, Arcan M 1994 Toward early detection of the tendency to stress fractures. Clinical Biomechanics 9:111–116

Brukner P D, Bennell K L 1997 Stress fractures. Critical Reviews in Physical and Rehabilitation Medicine 9:151–190

Brukner P, Bennell K, Matheson G 1999 Stress fractures. Blackwell Science Asia, Melbourne

Brunet M E, Cook S D, Briuker M R et al 1990 A survey of running injuries in 1505 competitive and recreational runners. Journal of Sports Medicine and Physical Fitness 30:307–315

Buckwalter J A, Glimcher M J, Cooper R R et al 1995 Bone biology. Journal of Bone and Joint Surgery (Am) 77A:1256–1275

Burr D 2001 Pharmaceutical treatments that may prevent or delay the onset of stress fractures. In: Burr D B, Milgrom C (eds) Musculoskeletal fatigue and stress fractures. CRC Press, Boca Raton, FL, p 259–270

Carbon R, Sambrook P N, Deakin V et al 1990 Bone density of elite female athletes with stress fractures. Medical Journal of Australia 153:373–376

Carter D R, Hayes W C, Schurman D J 1976 Fatigue life of compact bone: 11. Effects of microstructure and density. Journal of Biomechanics 9:211–218

Carter N, Kannus P, Khan K M 2001 Exercise in the prevention of falls in older people: a systematic literature review examining the rationale and the evidence. Sports Medicine 31:427–438

Cavanagh P R, LaFortune M A 1980 Ground reaction forces in distance running. Journal of Biomechanics 13:397–406

Chartered Society of Physiotherapy 1999 Physiotherapy guidelines for the management of osteoporosis. Chartered Society of Physiotherapy, London

Cline A D, Jansen G R, Melby C L 1998 Stress fractures in female army recruits: implications of bone density, calcium intake, and exercise. Journal of the American College of Nutrition 17:128–135

Conroy B P, Kraemer W J, Maresh C M et al 1993 Bone mineral density in elite junior olympic weight lifters. Medicine and Science in Sports and Exercise 25:1103–1109

Consensus Development Conference 1993 Diagnosis, prophylaxis and treatment of osteoporosis. American Journal of Medicine 94:646–650

Cowan D N, Jones B H, Frykman P N et al 1996 Lower limb morphology and risk of overuse injury among male infantry trainees. Medicine and Science in Sports and Exercise 28:945–952

Cummings S R, Black D M, Nevitt M C et al 1993 Bone density at various sites for prediction of hip fractures. Lancet 341:72–75

Currey J D 2001 Bone strength: what are we trying to measure? Calcified Tissue International 68:205–210

Currey J D 2003 How well are bones designed to resist fracture? Journal of Bone and Mineral Research 18:591–598

Cutler W B, Friedmann E, Genovese-Stone E 1993 Prevalence of kyphosis in a healthy sample of pre- and postmenopausal women. American Journal of Physical Medicine and Rehabilitation 72:219–225

Dalsky G P, Stocke K S, Ehansi A A et al 1988 Weight-bearing exercise training and lumbar bone mineral content in postmenopausal women. Annals of Internal Medicine 108:824–828

Dickson T B, Kichline P D 1987 Functional management of stress fractures in female athletes using a pneumatic leg brace. American Journal of Sports Medicine 15:86–89

Ebrahim S, Thompson P, Baskaran V et al 1997 Randomized placebo-controlled trial of brisk walking in the prevention of postmenopausal osteoporosis. Age and Ageing 26:253–260

Egol K A, Frankel V H 2001 Problematic stress fracture. In: Burr D B, Milgrom C (eds) Musculoskeletal fatigue and stress fractures. CRC Press, Boca Raton, FL, p 305–319

Einhorn T A 1996 The bone organ system: form and function. In: Marcus R, Feldman D, Kelsey J (eds) Osteoporosis. Academic Press, San Diego, CA, p 3–22

Einhorn T A 1998 The cell and molecular biology of fracture healing. Clinical Orthopaedics and Related Research 355 (suppl):S7–S21

Ekenman I, Tsai-Fellander L, Westblad P et al 1996 A study of intrinsic factors in patients with stress fractures of the tibia. Foot and Ankle International 17:477–482

Ensrud K E, Black D M, Harris F et al 1997 Correlates of kyphosis in older women. Journal of the American Geriatrics Society 45:682–687

Feskanich D, Willett W, Colditz G 2002 Walking and leisure-time activity and risk of hip fracture in postmenopausal women. Journal of the American Medical Association 288:2300–2306

Fiatarone M, Marks E, Ryan N et al 1990 High-intensity training in nonagenarians. Journal of the American Medical Association 263:3029–3034

Fiatarone M A, O'Neill E F, Ryan N D et al 1994 Exercise training and nutritional supplementation for physical frailty in very elderly people. New England Journal of Medicine 330:1769–1775

Flicker L, Hopper J L, Rodgers L et al 1995 Bone density determinants in elderly women: a twin study. Journal of Bone and Mineral Research 10:1607–1613

Forwood M R 2001 Mechanical effects on the skeleton: are there clinical implications? Osteoporosis International 12:77–83

Forwood M R, Burr D B 1993 Physical activity and bone mass: exercises in futility? Bone and Mineral 21:89–112

Forwood M, Larsen J 2000 Exercise recommendations for osteoporosis: a position statement for the Australian and New Zealand Bone and Mineral Society. Australian Family Physician 29:761–764

Friberg O 1982 Leg length asymmetry in stress fractures. A clinical and radiological study. Journal of Sports Medicine 22:485–488

Frost H M 1983 A determinant of bone architecture. The minimum effective strain. Clinical Orthopaedics and Related Research 175:286–292

Frost H M 1989 The biology of fracture healing: an overview for clinicians. Part I. Clinical Orthopaedics and Related Research 248:283–293

Frost H M 1990 Structural adaptations to mechanical usage (SATMU): redefining Wolff's Law. Anatomical Records 226:403–422

Frost H M 1991 Some ABCs of skeletal pathophyiology: 6. The growth/modeling/remodeling distinction. Calcified Tissue International 49:301–302

Frost H M 2003 Bone's mechanostat: a 2003 update. Anatomical Record 275A:1081–1101

Frusztajer N T, Dhuper S, Warren M P et al 1990 Nutrition and the incidence of stress fractures in ballet dancers. American Journal of Clinical Nutrition 51:779–783

Fyhrie D P, Milgrom C, Hoshaw S J et al 1998 Effect of fatiguing exercise on longitudinal bone strain as related to stress fracture in humans. Annals of Biomedical Engineering 26:660–665

Giladi M, Milgrom C, Danon Y et al 1985a The correlation between cumulative march training and stress fractures in soldiers. Military Medicine 150:600–601

Giladi M, Milgrom C, Stein M et al 1985b The low arch, a protective factor in stress fractures. A prospective study of 295 military recruits. Orthopaedic Review 14:709–712

Giladi M, Milgrom C, Stein M et al 1987 External rotation of the hip. A predictor of risk for stress fractures. Clinical Orthopaedics and Related Research 216:131–134

Giladi M, Milgrom C, Simkin A et al 1991 Stress fractures: identifiable risk factors. American Journal of Sports Medicine 19:647–652

Gillespie W J, Grant I 2000 Interventions for preventing and treating stress fractures and stress reactions of bone of the lower limbs in young adults. Cochrane Database of Systematic Reviews 2: CD000450

Girrbach R T, Flynn T W, Browder D A et al 2001 Flexural wave propagation velocity and bone mineral density in females with and without tibial bone stress injuries. Journal of Orthopaedic and Sports Physical Therapy 31:54–62

Gleeson P, Protas E, LeBlanc A et al 1990 Effects of weight lifting on bone mineral density in premenopausal women. Journal of Bone and Mineral Research 5:153–158

Glowacki J 1998 Angiogenesis in fracture repair. Clinical Orthopaedics and Related Research 355 (suppl):S82–S89

Greaney R B, Gerber R H, Laughlin R L et al 1983 Distribution and natural history of stress fractures in US marine recruits. Radiology 146:339–346

Gremion G, Rizzoli R, Slosman D et al 2001 Oligo-amenorrheic long-distance runners may lose more bone in spine than in femur. Medicine and Science in Sports and Exercise 33:15–21

Grimston S K, Engsberg J R, Kloiber R et al 1991 Bone mass, external loads, and stress fractures in female runners. International Journal of Sport Biomechanics 7:293–302

Haapasalo H, Kannus P, Sievanen H et al 1996a Development of mass, density, and estimated mechanical characteristics of bones in Caucasian females. Journal of Bone and Mineral Research 11:1751–1760

Haapasalo H, Sievanen H, Kannus P et al 1996b Dimensions and estimated mechanical characteristics of the humerus after long-term tennis loading. Journal of Bone and Mineral Research 11:864–872

Harries U J, Bassey E J 1990 Torque-velocity relationships for the knee extensors in women in their 3rd and 7th decades. European Journal of Applied Physiology 60:187–190

Hartard M, Haber P, Ilieva D et al 1996 Systematic strength training as a model of therapeutic intervention. American Journal of Physical Medicine and Rehabilitation 75:21–28

Hatori M, Hasegawa A, Adachi H et al 1993 The effects of walking at the anaerobic threshold level on vertebral bone loss in postmenopausal women. Calcified Tissue International 52:411–414

Hayes W C, Gerhart T N 1985 Biomechanics of bone: applications for assessment of bone strength. Bone and Mineral Research 3:259–294

Heinonen A, Kannus P, Sievanen H et al 1996 Randomised, controlled trial of effect of high-impact exercise on selected risk factors for osteoporotic fractures. Lancet 348:1343–1347

Heinonen A, Oja P, Sievanen H et al 1998 Effect of two training regimens on bone mineral density in healthy perimenopausal women: a randomised, controlled trial. Journal of Bone and Mineral Research 13:483–490

Heinonen A, Sievanen H, Kannus P et al 2000 High-impact exercise and bones of growing girls: a 9-month controlled trial. Osteoporosis International 11:1010–1017

Heinonen A, Sievänen H, Kyröläinen H et al 2001 Mineral mass, size and estimated mechanical strength of the lower limb bones of triple jumpers. Bone 29:279–285

Hetland M L, Haarbo J, Christiansen C et al 1993 Running induces menstrual disturbances but bone mass is unaffected, except in amenorrheic women. American Journal of Medicine 95:53–60

Hoffman J R, Chapnik L, Shamis A et al 1999 The effect of leg length on the incidence of lower extremity overuse injuries during military training. Military Medicine 164:153–156

Hughes L Y 1985 Biomechanical analysis of the foot and ankle for predisposition to developing stress fractures. Journal of Orthopaedic and Sports Physical Therapy 7:96–101

Humphries B, Newton R U, Bronks R et al 2000 Effect of exercise intensity on bone density, strength, and calcium turnover in older women. Medicine and Science in Sports and Exercise 32:1043–1050

Järvinen TL, Kannus P, Sievänen H 2003 Estrogen and bone: a reproductive and locomotive perspective. Journal of Bone and Mineral Research 18:1921–1931

Järvinen TLN, Sievänen H, Jokihaara J et al 2005 Revival of bone strength: the bottom line. Journal of Bone and Mineral Research 20:717–720

Joakimsen R M, Fonnebo V, Magnus J H et al 1999 The Truomso study: physical activity and the incidence of fractures in a middle-aged population. Journal of Bone and Mineral Research 13:1149–1157

Johnston J, Slemenda C 1993 Determinants of peak bone mass. Osteoporosis International 3 (suppl 1):S54–S55

Jonnavithula S, Warren M P, Fox R P et al 1993 Bone density is compromised in amenorrheic women despite return of menses: a 2-year study. Obstetrics and Gynecology 81:669–674

Kadel N J, Teitz C C, Kronmal R A 1992 Stress fractures in ballet dancers. American Journal of Sports Medicine 20:445–449

Kannus P, Haapasalo H, Sankelo M et al 1995 Effect of starting age of physical activity on bone mass in the dominant arm of tennis and squash players. Annals of Internal Medicine 123:27–31

Kannus P, Parkkari J, Niemi S et al 2000 Prevention of hip fracture in elderly people with use of a hip protector. New England Journal of Medicine 343:1506–1513

Kannus P, Sievänen H, Palvanen M et al 2005 Prevention of falls and consequent injuries in elderly people. Lancet 366:1885–1893

Kelley G A, Kelley K S, Tran Z V 2000 Exercise and bone mineral density in men: a meta-analysis. Journal of Applied Physiology 88:1730–1736

Kerr D, Morton A, Dick I et al 1996 Exercise effects on bone mass in postmenopausal women are site-specific and load-dependent. Journal of Bone and Mineral Research 11:218–225

Kerschan K, Alacamlioglu Y, Kollmitzer J et al 1998 Functional impact of unvarying exercise program in women after menopause. American Journal of Physical Medicine and Rehabilitation 77:326–332

Khan K, McKay H, Kannus P et al 2001 Physical activity and bone health. Human Kinetics, Champaign, IL

Kiss Z A, Khan K M, Fuller P J 1993 Stress fractures of the tarsal navicular bone: CT findings in 55 cases. American Journal of Roentgenology 160:111–115

Korpelainen R, Keinänen-Kiukaanniemi S, Heikkinen J et al 2006 Effect of impact exercise on bone mineral density in elderly women with low BMD: a population-based randomized controlled 30-month intervention. Osteoporosis International 17:109–118

Kronhed A, Moller M 1998 Effects of physical exercise on bone mass, balance skill and aerobic capacity in women and men with low bone mineral density, after one year of training: a prospective study. Scandinavian Journal of Medicine and Science in Sports 8:290–298

Kujala U M, Kaprio J, Kannus P et al 2000 Physical activity and osteoporotic hip fracture risk in men. Archives of Internal Medicine 160:705–708

Lanyon L E 1984 Functional strain as a determinant for bone remodeling. Calcified Tissue International 36 (suppl 1):S56–S61

Lanyon L E 1987 Functional strain in bone tissue as an objective, and controlling stimulus for adaptive bone remodelling. Journal of Biomechanics 20:1083–1093

Larsen J 1998 Osteoporosis. In: Sapsford R, Bullock-Saxton J, Markwell S (eds) Women's health. A textbook for physiotherapists. WB Saunders, London, p 412–453

Lauder T D, Dixit S, Pezzin L E et al 2000 The relation between stress fractures and bone mineral density: evidence from active-duty army women. Archives of Physical Medicine and Rehabilitation 81:73–79

Lee J K, Yao L 1988 Stress fractures: MR imaging. Radiology 169:2217–2220

Lespessailles E, Jullien A, Eynard E et al 1998 Biomechanical properties of human os calcanei: relationships with bone density and fractal evaluation of bone microarchitecture. Journal of Biomechanics 31:817–824

Lohmann T, Going S, Pamenter R et al 1995 Effects of resistance training on regional and total bone mineral density in premenopausal women: a randomized prospective study. Journal of Bone and Mineral Research 10:1015–1024

Lord S 1996 The effects of a community exercise program on fracture risk factors in older women. Osteoporosis International 6:361–367

Lord S R, Clark R D, Webster I W 1991 Physiological factors associated with falls in an elderly population. Journal of the Geriatrics Society 39:1194–1200

Lord S R, Sambrook P N, Gilbert C et al 1994 Postural stability, falls and fractures in the elderly: results from the Dubbo Osteoporosis Epidemiology Study. Medical Journal of Australia 160:684–691

McKay H A, Petit M A, Schutz R W et al 2000 Augmented trochanteric bone mineral density after modified physical education classes: a randomized school-based exercise intervention study in prepubescent and early pubescent children. Journal of Pediatrics 136:156–162

McKiernan F E 2005 A simple gait-stabilizing device reduces outdoor falls and nonserious injurious falls in fall-prone older people during the winter. Journal of the American Geriatrics Society 53:943–947

McMurdo M, Rennie L 1993 A controlled trial of exercise by residents of old people's homes. Age and Ageing 22:11–15

McMurdo M E T, Millar A M, Daly F 2000 A randomized controlled trial of fall prevention strategies in old peoples' homes. Gerontology 46:83–87

McNitt-Gray J 1991 Kinematics and impulse characteristics of drop landings from three heights. International Journal of Sports Biomechanics 7:201–223

Madsen O R, Schaadt O, Bliddal H et al 1993 Relationship between quadriceps strength and bone mineral density of the proximal tibia and distal forearm in women. Journal of Bone and Mineral Research 8:1439–1444

Malmros B, Mortenson L, Jensen M B et al 1998 Positive effects of physiotherapy on chronic pain and performance in osteoporosis. Osteoporosis International 8:215–221

Martin D, Notelovitz M 1993 Effects of aerobic training on bone mineral density of postmenopausal women. Journal of Bone and Mineral Research 8:931–936

Martin R B 1991 Determinants of the mechanical properties of bones. Journal of Biomechanics 24:79–88

Meurman K O A, Elfving S 1980 Stress fracture in soldiers: a multifocal bone disorder. Radiology 134:483–487

Milgrom C 1989 The Israeli elite infantry recruit: a model for understanding the biomechanics of stress fractures. Journal of the Royal College of Surgeons Edinburgh 34 (6 suppl):S18–S22

Milgrom C, Finestone A, Shlamkovitch N et al 1992 Prevention of overuse injuries of the foot by improved shoe shock attenuation. A randomized, prospective study. Clinical Orthopaedics 281:189–192

Milgrom C, Finestone A, Shlamkovitch N et al 1994 Youth is a risk factor for stress fracture. A study of 783 infantry recruits. Journal of Bone and Joint Surgery (Br) 76:20–22

Milgrom C, Simkin A, Eldad A et al 2000 Using bone's adaptation ability to lower the incidence of stress fractures. American Journal of Sports Medicine 28:245–251

Moisio K C, Hurwitz D E, Sumner D R 2004 Dynamic loads are determinants of peak bone mass. Journal of Orthopaedic Research 22:339–345

Montgomery L C, Nelson F R T, Norton J P et al 1989 Orthopedic history and examination in the etiology of overuse injuries. Medicine and Science in Sports and Exercise 21:237–243

Morganti C M, Nelson M E, Fiatarone M et al 1995 Strength improvements with 1 yr of progressive resistance training in older women. Medicine and Science in Sports and Exercise 27:906–912

Morris F L, Naughton G A, Gibbs J L et al 1997 Prospective ten-month exercise intervention in premenarcheal girls: positive effects on bone and lean mass. Journal of Bone and Mineral Research 12:1453–1462

Mosekilde L 1993 Vertebral structure and strength in vivo and in vitro. Calcified Tissue International 53 (suppl 1):S121–S126

Myburgh K H, Hutchins J, Fataar A B et al 1990 Low bone density is an etiologic risk factor for stress fractures in athletes. Annals of Internal Medicine 113:754–759

Myburgh K H, Bachrach L K, Lewis B et al 1993 Low bone mineral density at axial and appendicular sites in amenorrheic athletes. Medicine and Science in Sports and Exercise 25:1197–1202

Nattiv A, Puffer J C, Green G A 1997 Lifestyles and health risks of collegiate athletes: a multi-center study. Clinical Journal of Sport Medicine 7:262–272

Nelson M, Fiatarone M, Morganti C et al 1994 Effects of high-intensity strength training on multiple risk factors for osteoporotic fractures: a randomized controlled trial. Journal of the American Medical Association 272:1909–1914

Nikander R, Sievanen H, Heinonen A et al 2005 Femoral neck structure in adult female athletes subjected to different loading modalities. Journal of Bone and Mineral Research 20:520–528

Nikander R, Sievanen H, Uusi-Rasi K et al 2006 Loading modalities and bone structures at nonweight-bearing upper extremity and weight-bearing lower extremity: a pQCT study of adult female athletes. Bone 39(4):886–894.

Nordin M, Frankel V H 1989 Basic biomechanics of the musculoskeletal system. Lea and Febiger, Philadelphia, PA

Nordström A, Karlsson C, Nyquist et al 2005 Bone loss and fracture risk after reduced physical activity. Journal of Bone and Mineral Research 20:202–207

Orwoll E S, Ferar J, Oviatt S K et al 1989 The relationship of swimming exercise to bone mass in men and women. Archives of Internal Medicine 149:2197–2200

Otis C L, Drinkwater B, Johnson M et al 1997 American College of Sports Medicine position stand. The female athlete triad. Medicine and Science in Sports and Exercise 29:I–X

Paganini-Hill A, Chao A, Ross R K et al 1991 Exercise and other factors in the prevention of hip fracture: the Leisure World study. Epidemiology 2:16–25

Parfitt A M 1988 Bone remodeling: relationship to the amount and structure of bone, and the pathogenesis and prevention of fractures. In: Riggs B L, Melton III L J (eds) Osteoporosis: etiology, diagnosis, and management. Raven Press, New York, p 45–93

Parkkari J, Kannus P, Heikkila J et al 1995 Energy-shunting external hip protector attenuates the peak femoral impact force below the theoretical fracture threshold: an in vitro biomechanical study under falling conditions of the elderly. Journal of Bone and Mineral Research 10:1437–1442

Parkkari J, Kannus P, Heikkila J et al 1997 Impact experiments of an external hip protector in young volunteers. Calcified Tissue International 60:354–357

Parkkari J, Kannus P, Palvanen M et al 1999 Majority of hip fractures occur as a result of a fall and impact on the greater trochanter of the femur: a prospective controlled hip fracture study with 206 consecutive patients. Calcified Tissue International 65:183–187

Peck W A, Woods W L 1988 The cells of bone. In: Riggs B L, Melton III L J (eds) Osteoporosis: etiology, diagnosis, and management. Raven Press, New York, p 1–44

Petersen M M, Jensen N C, Gehrchen P M et al 1996 The relation between trabecular bone strength and bone mineral density assessed by dual photon and dual energy X-ray absorptiometry in the proximal tibia. Calcified Tissue International 59:311–314

Picard C L 1999 The level of competition as a factor for the development of eating disorders in female collegiate athletes. Journal of Youth and Adolescence 28:583–594

Prather J L, Nusynowitz M L, Snowdy H A et al 1977 Scintigraphic findings in stress fractures. Journal of Bone and Joint Surgery (Am) 59:869–874

Preisinger E, Alacamlioglu Y, Pils K et al 1996 Exercise therapy for osteoporosis: results of a randomised, controlled trial. British Journal of Sports Medicine 30:209–212

Raab-Cullen D M, Akhter M P, Kimmel D B et al 1994 Bone response to alternate-day mechanical loading of the rat tibia. Journal of Bone and Mineral Research 9:203–211

Reinker K A, Ozburne S 1979 A comparison of male and female orthopaedic pathology in basic training. Military Medicine 144:532–536

Rico H, Revilla M, Hernandez E R et al 1993 Bone mineral content and body composition in postpubertal cyclist boys. Bone 14:93–95

Robinson T L, Snow-Harter C, Taaffe D R et al 1995 Gymnasts exhibit higher bone mass than runners despite similar prevalence of amenorrhea and oligomenorrhea. Journal of Bone and Mineral Research 10:26–35

Robling A G, Hinant F M, Burr D B et al 2002 Improved bone structure and strength after long-term mechanical loading is greatest if loading is separated into short bouts. Journal of Bone and Mineral Research 17:1545–1554

Rome K, Handoll HHG, Ashford R 2005 Interventions for preventing and treating stress fractures and stress reactions of bone of the lower limbs in young adults. Cochrane Database of Systematic Reviews 2: CD000450

Ronsen O, Sundgot-Borgen J, Maehlum S 1999 Supplement use and nutritional habits in Norwegian elite athletes. Scandinavian Journal of Medicine and Science in Sports 9:28–35

Ross P D 1997 Clinical consequences of vertebral fractures. American Journal of Medicine 103(2A):30S–43S

Roub L W, Gumerman L W, Hanley E N et al 1979 Bone stress: a radionuclide imaging perspective. Radiology 132:431–438

Rubin C T, Lanyon L E 1984 Regulation of bone formation by applied dynamic loads. Journal of Bone and Joint Surgery (Am) 66:397–402

Rubin C T, Lanyon L E 1985 Regulation of bone mass by mechanical strain magnitude. Calcified Tissue International 37:411–417

Ruff C, Holt B, Trinkaus E 2006 Who's afraid of the Big Bad Wolff: 'Wolff's law' and bone functional adaptation. American Journal of Physical Anthropology 129:484–498

Rutherford O M, Jones D A 1992 The relationship of muscle and bone loss and activity levels with age in women. Age and Ageing 21:286–293

Sanders K M, Nicholson G C, Ugoni A M et al 1999 Health burden of hip and other fractures in Australia beyond 2000: projections based on the Geelong Osteoporosis Study. Medical Journal of Australia 170:467–470

Santi M, Sartoris D J, Resnick D 1989 Diagnostic imaging of tarsal and metatarsal stress fractures: Part 11. Orthopaedic Review 18:178–185

Schwellnus M P, Jordaan G 1992 Does calcium supplementation prevent bone stress injuries? A clinical trial. International Journal of Sport Nutrition 2:165–174

Scott S H, Winter D A 1990 Internal forces at chronic running injury sites. Medicine and Science in Sports and Exercise 22:357–369

Scully T J, Besterman G 1982 Stress fracture: a preventable training injury. Military Medicine 147:285–287

Shaffer R A, Brodine S K, Almeida S A et al 1999 Use of simple measures of physical activity to predict stress fractures in young men undergoing a rigorous physical training program. American Journal of Epidemiology 149:236–242

Sheikh B 2000a Bone healing. In: Hoppenfeld S, Murthy V (eds) Treatment and rehabilitation of fractures. Lippincott Williams and Wilkins, Philadelphia, PA, p 1–6

Sheikh B 2000b Determining when a fracture has healed. In: Hoppenfeld S, Murthy V L (eds) Treatment and rehabilitation of fractures. Lippincott Williams and Wilkins, Philadelphia, PA, p 7–10

Simkin A, Leichter I, Giladi M et al 1989 Combined effect of foot arch structure and an orthotic device on stress fractures. Foot and Ankle 10:25–29

Simmons V, Hansen P D 1996 Effectiveness of water exercise on postural mobility in the well elderly: an experimental study on balance enhancement. Journal of Gerontology 51:M233–M238

Sinaki M, Ito E, Rogers J W et al 1996 Correlation of back extensor strength with thoracic hyphosis and lumbar lordosis in estrogen-deficient women. American Journal of Physical Medicine and Rehabilitation 75:370–374

Sinaki M, Itoi E, Wahner H W et al 2002 Stronger back muscles reduce the incidence of vertebral fractures: a prospective 10 year follow-up of postmenopausal women. Bone 30:836–841

Slayter M 1995 Lower limb training injuries in an army recruit population. PhD thesis, University of Newcastle

Snow-Harter C, Bouxsein M L, Lewis B T et al 1992 Effects of resistance and endurance exercise on bone mineral status of young women: a randomized exercise intervention trial. Journal of Bone and Mineral Research 7:761–769

Swenson E J, DeHaven K E, Sebastianelli W J et al 1997 The effect of a pneumatic leg brace on return to play in athletes with tibial stress fractures. American Journal of Sports Medicine 25:322–328

Taaffe D R, Snow-Harter C, Connolly D A et al 1995 Differential effects of swimming versus weight-bearing activity on bone mineral status of eumenorrheic athletes. Journal of Bone and Mineral Research 10:586–593

Tinetti M, Baker D, McAvay G et al 1994 A multifactorial intervention to reduce the risk of falling among elderly people living in the community. New England Journal of Medicine 331:822–827

Tomten S E 1996 Prevalence of menstrual dysfunction in Norwegian long-distance runners participating in the Oslo marathon games. Scandinavian Journal of Medicine and Science in Sport 6:164–171

Turner C H 1999 Toward a mathematical description of bone biology: the principle of cellular accommodation. Calcified Tissue International 65:466–471

Turner C H, Robling A G 2005 Exercise for improving bone strength. British Journal of Sports Medicine 39:188–189

Turner C H, Owan I, Takano Y 1995 Mechanotransduction in bone: role of strain rate. American Journal of Physiology 269: E438–E442

Umemura Y, Ishiko T, Tsujimoto H et al 1995 Effects of jump training on bone hypertrophy in young and old rats. International Journal of Sports Medicine 16:364–367

Umemura Y, Ishiko T, Yamauchi T et al 1997 Five jumps per day increase bone mass and breaking force in rats. Journal of Bone and Mineral Research 12:1480–1485

Wang Q J 2005. Bone growth in pubertal girls. Academic thesis, Studies in sport, physical education and health 110. University of Jyväskylä, Finland, p 1–75.

Warren M P, Brooks-Gunn J, Fox R P et al 1991 Lack of bone accretion and amenorrhea: evidence for a relative osteopenia in weight bearing bones. Journal of Clinical Endocrinology and Metabolism 72:847–853

Whalen R T, Carter D R, Steele C R 1988 Influence of physical activity on the regulation of bone density. Journal of Biomechanics 21:825–837

Whitelaw G P, Wetzler M J, Levy A S et al 1991 A pneumatic leg brace for the treatment of tibial stress fractures. Clinical Orthopedic and Related Research 270:302–305

Winfield A C, Bracker M, Moore J et al 1997 Risk factors associated with stress reactions in female marines. Military Medicine 162:698–702

Wolff I, van Croonenborg J J, Kemper H C G et al 1999 The effect of exercise training programs on bone mass: a meta-analysis of published controlled trials in pre- and postmenopausal women. Osteoporosis International 9:1–12

World Health Organization 1994 The World Health Organization assessment of fracture risk and its application to screening for osteoporosis. Report of WHO Study Group

Worthen B M, Yanklowitz B A D 1978 The pathophysiology and treatment of stress fractures in military personnel. Journal of the American Podiatric Medical Association 68:317–325

Yoshikawa T, Mori S, Santiesteban A J et al 1994 The effects of muscle fatigue on bone strain. Journal of Experimental Biology 188:217–233

Young D, Hopper J L, Nowson C A et al 1995 Determinants of bone mass in 10- to 26-year-old females: a twin study. Journal of Bone and Mineral Research 10:558–567

Zanker C L, Swaine I L 1998 Relation between bone turnover, oestradiol, and energy balance in women distance runners. British Journal of Sports Medicine 32:167–171

Ziegler P J, Nelson J A, Jonnalagadda S S 1999 Nutritional and physiological status of US national figure skaters. International Journal of Sport Nutrition 9:345–360

Zmuda J M, Cauley J A, Ferrell R E 1999 Recent progress in understanding the genetic susceptibility to osteoporosis. Genetic Epidemiology 16:356–367

Nerves

6

Robert J. Nee, David S. Butler and Michel W. Coppieters

CHAPTER CONTENTS

Introduction 82
Relevant functional anatomy and physiology 83
Neurodynamics 88
Pathodynamics 92
Summary 96

Introduction

Nervous system function is often conceptualized in terms of the generation, transmission and processing of impulses related to motor control and nociception (see Chapters 8 and 9). Health care practitioners may less commonly appreciate how chemical communication enables the nervous system to monitor and influence the health of musculoskeletal tissues. Compounds from the periphery are carried within afferent axons to dorsal root ganglia and inform cell bodies about the health of innervated structures. The cell bodies respond by producing neuropeptides that are transported back to the periphery to enhance tissue health (Rempel et al 1999). In situations where musculoskeletal tissues are injured, cell bodies manufacture different neuropeptides that contribute to the inflammatory response necessary for healing (i.e. neurogenic inflammation) (Costigan & Woolf 2000, Sluka 1996, Weinstein 1991).

The length of an axon can be 10000 to 15000 times the diameter of the cell body (Rempel et al 1999). In more clinically conceivable terms, major sensory axons within the femoral nerve are about 0.5 m long (Schwartz 1995), and tibial nerve axons may be over 1 m in length as they course from the spine to terminal branches in the foot (Butler 2000). Because of this unique structure, neural tissues possess biomechanical properties that facilitate maintenance of electrochemical communication as neurons bend, glide and stretch in concert with body movement (Rempel et al 1999, Shacklock 1995a, Topp & Boyd 2006). Electrochemical and biomechanical functions of the nervous system are interdependent, and their interaction in healthy and injured neural tissues has been referred to as neurodynamics and pathodynamics, respectively (Shacklock 1995a).

Sometimes sport or exercise activities place excessive mechanical demands on neural structures, leading to symptoms associated with injury to the connective or impulse conducting tissues of the nervous system (Asbury & Fields 1984, Baron 2000, Butler 2000, Greening & Lynn 1998, Hall & Elvey 1999, Nee & Butler 2006, Rempel et al 1999). A review of relevant functional anatomy and physiology provides a foundation for describing how the nervous system normally adapts to mechanical loads (neurodynamics) and for discussing the processes involved in neural tissue injury (pathodynamics). An understanding of these concepts can assist those working in the physical therapies in providing appropriate exercise and rehabilitation for their clients.

Relevant functional anatomy and physiology

Peripheral nerves

Axons within peripheral nerves are arranged into bundles called fascicles. Each fascicle is surrounded by a perineurial sheath composed of 6–15 layers of connective tissue contingent upon the fascicular diameter (Lundborg 1988, Matloub & Yousif 1992, Sunderland 1990) (Fig. 6.1). Although the primary orientation of connective tissue fibers is longitudinal, the inclination changes slightly between successive layers of the perineurium (Matloub & Yousif 1992). The laminated architecture enables the perineurial sheath to function as a viscoelastic tube. Because of this viscoelasticity, the perineurial tube is able to change dimensions and maintain pressures in the fascicle that are within physiological limits regardless of the length of the nerve (Kwan et al 1992, Millesi et al 1995, Sunderland 1990). Since the interior of a fascicle is labeled the endoneurial space (Millesi et al 1995), this intrafascicular pressure is referred to as endoneurial fluid pressure (Lundborg 1988).

Besides preserving a constant mechanical environment for enclosed nerve fibers, the perineurium controls the biochemical milieu within the fascicle. The innermost connective tissue lamellae of the perineurial sheath create a metabolically active diffusion barrier that permits only certain chemicals and ions to come in contact with neural tissues (Lundborg 1988, Lundborg & Dahlin 1992, Matloub & Yousif 1992, Rempel et al 1999). For example, chemicals associated with edema around a fascicle or infection around a nerve trunk do not come in contact with the intrafascicular environment (Lundborg 1988). The perineurial diffusion barrier works bidirectionally. Therefore, if mechanical or chemical stimuli cause endoneurial inflammation followed by intrafascicular edema, the resultant increase in endoneurial fluid pressure persists because the perineurium does not allow the inflammatory exudate to escape (Lundborg 1988, Lundborg & Dahlin 1992, Lundborg et al 1983, Murphy 1977). Mechanical perturbation from surgical dissection of nerve fascicles or from experimentally sustained compression does not alter function of the perineurial diffusion barrier (Lundborg 1988).

Structures within the endoneurial space rely on the optimal mechanical and biochemical environment regulated by the perineurium. In addition to axons, the endoneurial space accommodates Schwann cells, blood vessels, interstitial fluid and a connective tissue network known as the endoneurium (Matloub & Yousif 1992, Rempel et al 1999) (Fig. 6.1). Schwann cells are glial cells that provide nutritional support for peripheral nerve fibers and contribute to saltatory conduction of impulses (Bear et al 2001, Matloub & Yousif 1992). They are also a source of proinflammatory cytokines that participate in the inflammatory response exhibited by injured neural tissues (Watkins & Maier 2004). A chain of Schwann cells envelops a single axon in a myelin sheath designed for high-speed transmission of impulses. In the case of unmyelinated axons, a chain of Schwann cells surrounds several axons to insulate them from the endoneurial space (Bear et al 2001, Matloub & Yousif 1992). Endoneurial connective tissue provides a scaffolding through which a capillary network courses to supply blood to nerve fibers and associated Schwann cells (Lundborg 1988). This connective tissue scaffolding becomes specialized to form an endoneurial tubule around each myelinated axon or group of unmyelinated axons (Sunderland 1990).

Integrity of endoneurial tubules plays an important role in the movement capabilities of nerve fibers. Axons follow an undulated course within the endoneurium, and lengthening of a nerve trunk causes these undulations to straighten, effectively lengthening axons with minimal to no increase in endoneurial pressure (Millesi et al 1995, Sunderland 1990). Conversely, shortening of a nerve trunk causes the undulations to increase, enabling axons to adapt without being unduly compressed (Millesi et al 1995). This mechanism for accommodating change in length is lost when the endoneurial network is compromised, or when the perineurium is not able to function as a viscoelastic tube as previously discussed (Millesi et al 1995).

Just as axons follow an undulating path within the endoneurial space, each fascicle takes a tortuous course within the nerve

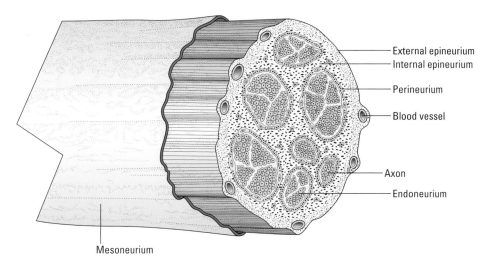

Figure 6.1 • Peripheral nerve connective tissue sheaths. (Reproduced with permission from Butler 1991.)

External epineurium
Internal epineurium

Perineurium

Blood vessel

Axon

Endoneurium

Mesoneurium

trunk (Sunderland 1990). Fascicles repeatedly unite and divide along the length of a nerve to create fascicular plexuses. These plexuses enable the nerve trunk to adapt to changes in length, but also permit gliding between fascicles as nerves are twisted, compressed or lengthened during joint movement (Millesi et al 1995, Rempel et al 1999, Sunderland 1990). Fascicular gliding is possible due to the internal epineurium, a loose connective tissue incorporated between fascicles (Millesi et al 1995, Sunderland 1990) (Fig. 6.1). The internal epineurium also acts as a cushion to protect fascicles from compressive forces (Lundborg & Dahlin 1992, Sunderland 1990). Because they are adept at sheltering nerve fibers from mechanical loads, fascicular plexuses and internal epineurial tissues are well developed in portions of nerve trunks susceptible to injury (Lundborg & Dahlin 1992, Matloub & Yousif 1992, Rydevik et al 1984, Sunderland 1990). Examples of such locations include areas where nerves cross joints or pass through osseous (e.g. intervertebral foramen), osteoligamentous (e.g. carpal tunnel) or fibrous (e.g. arcade of Frohse) tunnels.

The external epineurium is the connective tissue layer wrapping around the internal epineurium and fascicles to separate them from neighboring structures (Matloub & Yousif 1992, Millesi et al 1995, Rempel et al 1999, Sunderland 1990) (Fig. 6.1). During limb movements, peripheral nerves exhibit a significant amount of sliding relative to surrounding tissues (Coppieters et al 2006, Dilley et al 2003, Hough et al 2000, McLellan & Swash 1976, Ugbolue et al 2005, Wilgis & Murphy 1986, Wright et al 1996, 2001, 2005). This excursion is facilitated by additional connective tissue enveloping the nerve trunk referred to as the mesoneurium or paraneurium (Lundborg 1988, Millesi et al 1995, Sunderland 1990) (Fig. 6.1). If the mesoneurium becomes fibrotic, it can shrink and adhere to the external epineurium or adjacent non-neural structures, thereby impairing mobility of the nerve trunk (Millesi et al 1995).

Nerve root complexes

Neural tissues undergo significant changes in connective tissue morphology and physiology as they pass through the intervertebral foramen (IVF) (McCabe & Low 1969, Parke & Watanabe 1985, Rydevik et al 1984, Yoshizawa et al 1991). This area of transition is appropriately termed the nerve root complex (Rauschning 1997) (Fig. 6.2). At the external aspect of the IVF, nerve fibers from the extremities are grouped into a ventral ramus while those from the posterior aspect of the spine and trunk are collected within a dorsal ramus. These rami merge to form a spinal nerve that enters the foramen and divides into sensory and motor roots. Nerve fibers in sensory and motor roots track proximally through the IVF and spinal canal to reach their destinations within the spinal cord (Bogduk 1997, Rydevik et al 1984). As they approach the spinal cord, sensory and motor nerve fibers display intradural connections between adjacent segments (Tanaka et al 2000), contradicting the common perception that nerve roots within each foramen are associated with a single spinal cord level. An enlargement of each sensory root contains the cell bodies of afferent nerve

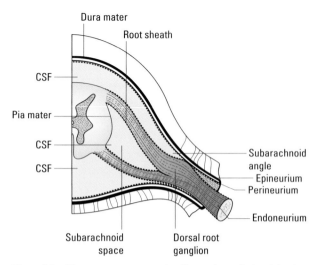

Figure 6.2 • The nerve root complex illustrating relationships between the connective tissues and neural elements. Note how tensile forces are taken away from the roots by the split perineurium and the dura. CSF = cerebrospinal fluid. (Reproduced from Haller F R, Low F N 1971 The fine structure of the peripheral nerve sheath in the subarachnoid space in the rat and other laboratory animals. American Journal of Anatomy 131:1–19 with the permission of the American Journal of Anatomy.)

fibers passing through a particular IVF, and this enlargement is referred to as the dorsal root ganglion (DRG). The DRG has a variable location within each cervical or lumbar foramen (Jenis & An 2000, Kikuchi et al 1994, Tanaka et al 2000, Yabuki & Kikuchi 1996), and this structure warrants special mention as its mechanosensitivity and neurochemistry appear to play a significant role in radicular pain syndromes (Devor & Seltzer 1999, Hanai et al 1996, Hasue 1993, Igarashi et al 2005, Nakamura & Myers 2000, Takebayashi et al 2001, Yabuki et al 2001). Additionally, connective tissue changes described below seem to take place just proximal to the DRG (McCabe & Low 1969, Olmarker & Rydevik 1991, Yoshizawa et al 1991).

Connective tissue layers of nerve trunks do not link exactly with meningeal layers of the spinal canal (Haller & Low 1971, McCabe & Low 1969, Murphy 1977, Olmarker & Rydevik 1991, Yoshizawa et al 1991) (Fig. 6.2). Peripheral nerve endoneurium encompasses nerve fibers in a connective tissue network that is continuous throughout the nerve root complex and eventually merges with pia mater (Murphy 1977, Olmarker & Rydevik 1991, Sunderland 1974, Yoshizawa et al 1991). In contrast to nerve trunks, fascicles in sensory and motor roots run parallel to one another and are not enclosed in a durable perineurial sheath (Beel et al 1986, McCabe & Low 1969, Murphy 1977, Olmarker & Rydevik 1991, Yoshizawa et al 1991). A more delicate connective tissue derived from pia mater encircles each nerve root fascicle and has been labeled fascicular pia by Parke & Watanabe (1985). The same authors used the term radicular pia to describe the open mesh configuration of pial tissue that surrounds each nerve root (Fig. 6.3). The delicate and porous

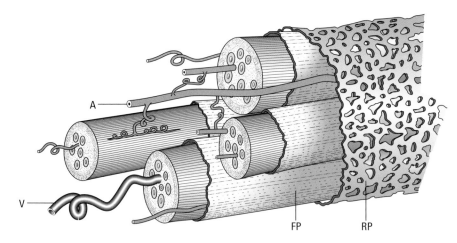

Figure 6.3 • The intrinsic blood supply to a nerve root illustrating the coiled configuration of intraneural vessels. A = arteriole, FP = fascicular pia, RP = radicular pia, V = venule. (Reproduced with permission from Butler 1991.)

nature of these sheaths enables percolation of cerebrospinal fluid (CSF) to provide over 50% of the nutrition for sensory and motor roots (Rydevik et al 1990).

Since the perineurium is not present in sensory or motor roots, its structure must terminate somewhere in the region of the DRG. Perineurial tissue forms a tight capsule around each DRG (Murphy 1977, Olmarker & Rydevik 1991, Rydevik et al 1984, Rydevik et al 1989), contributing to the inherent mechanosensitivity of this structure (Howe et al 1977, Sugawara et al 1996). Proximal to the DRG, however, outer layers of perineurium merge with dura and arachnoid mater, while inner layers apparently meld with previously described fascicular and radicular pial sheaths (Haller & Low 1971, McCabe & Low, 1969, Murphy 1977, Olmarker & Rydevik 1991, Yoshizawa et al 1991) (Fig. 6.2). This separation of perineurial layers facilitates transmission of mechanical loads to stronger dural tissues, sparing delicate nerve roots that exhibit 90% less tensile strength than peripheral nerves (Beel et al 1986, Butler 1991). Concurrently, diffusion barrier mechanisms are maintained due to perineurial continuity with dura and arachnoid mater, preserving the biochemical environment of nerve root fascicles (Butler 1991).

Sensory and motor roots have minimal internal epineurium (Beel et al 1986, Murphy 1977, Rydevik et al 1984, Stodieck et al 1986, Sunderland 1990). This lack of fascicular cushioning, combined with the aforementioned parallel fascicular alignment and absence of perineurium, leads to concern that nerve roots are susceptible to mechanical injury (Murphy 1977, Rydevik et al 1984, Stodieck et al 1986, Sunderland 1990). However, under normal circumstances, anatomical features of the nerve root complex protect neural tissues from mechanical loads (Butler 1991, Sunderland 1974).

Nerve roots occupy only 30 to 40% of the space available within cervical and lumbar foramina (Jenis & An 2000, Sunderland 1974, Tanaka et al 2000), allowing ample room for adaptations to changes in foraminal dimensions known to occur with spinal movement (Fujiwara et al 2001, Kitagawa et al 2004, Muhle et al 2001, Nuckley et al 2002, Yoo et al 1992). Adipose tissue and circulating CSF provide an additional safeguard against undesirable mechanical forces (Jenis & An 2000, Louis 1981, Rydevik et al 1984, Sunderland 1974). At the

proximal portion of the IVF, the external epineurium links with arachnoid, dural, and epidural tissues to form a dural sleeve around each pair of sensory and motor roots (Bogduk 1997, Olmarker & Rydevik 1991, Sunderland 1974, Yoshizawa et al 1991) (Fig. 6.2). Neural tissues glide independently within the protective container of this dural sleeve as the entire nerve root complex moves within the IVF (Smith et al 1993, Sunderland 1974). These sleeves also shield enclosed nerve roots from tensile loads by acting as plugs when limb movement pulls neural structures distal and lateral into the foramina (Smith et al 1993, Sunderland 1974). Attachments of dural sleeves to cervical and lumbar foramina assist this plugging mechanism in attenuating mechanical forces associated with nerve root movement (Caglar et al 2004, Grimes et al 2000, Kraan et al 2005, Moses & Carman 1996, Smith et al 1993). The previously described link between perineurium and dura is another anatomical element that deflects tensile forces away from fragile sensory and motor roots. Finally, major brachial and lumbosacral plexuses protect neural structures by preventing concentration of tensile loads at any single nerve root complex (Kleinrensink et al 2000).

Neuromeningeal structures

The length of the spinal canal is 5–9 cm longer in flexion than extension (Louis 1981, Rossitti 1993). Lateral flexion requires canal shortening on the concave side and lengthening on the convex side (Rossitti 1993). Neuromeningeal structures must accommodate these changes. Since spinal cord tissues have six times less collagen content than mechanically delicate nerve roots (Stodieck et al 1986), durable connective tissue meninges and contained CSF offer require protection against mechanical forces produced by head, trunk and limb movement.

The dura mater is the outermost meningeal layer and possesses the greatest mechanical strength (Butler 1991, Runza et al 1999) (Figs 6.4, 6.5 and 6.6). Organization of collagen and elastin fibers changes between different layers of dural tissue. Inner layers appear to have a more longitudinal orientation, while outer layers exhibit a multidirectional arrangement to form a viscoelastic cylinder around the spinal cord and CSF (Nakagawa et al 1994, Runza et al 1999). In spite of differences

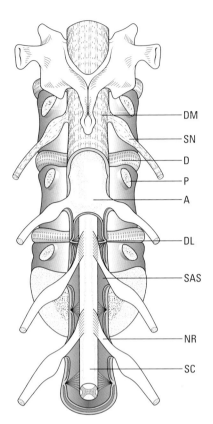

Figure 6.4 • Diagram of the spinal canal, meninges and spinal cord with the posterior vertebral arch removed. A = arachnoid, D = disk, DL = denticulate ligament, DM = dura mater, NR = nerve root complex, P = pedicle (cut), SAS = subarachnoid space, SC = spinal cord, SN = spinal nerve. (Reproduced with permission from Butler 1991.)

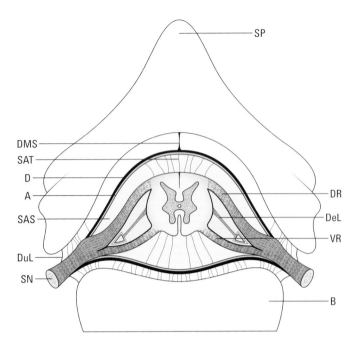

Figure 6.5 • Diagrammatic cross-section of the cord and spinal canal illustrating intradural and extradural connections. A = arachnoid, B = body, D = dura, DuL = dural ligament, DeL = denticulate ligament, DMS = dorsomedian septum, DR = dorsal root, SAS = subarachnoid space, SAT = subarachnoid trabeculae, SN = spinal nerve, SP = spinous process, VR = ventral root. (Reproduced with permission from Butler 1991.)

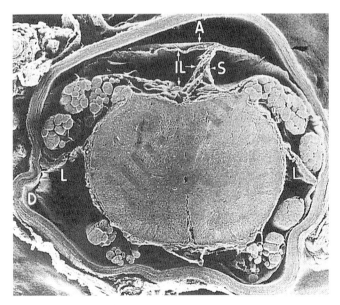

Figure 6.6 • Scanning electron micrograph of the lumbar spinal cord of a 15-month-old child. L = denticulate ligaments, D = dura (note the layers), A = arachnoid, S = dorsal septum, IL = intermediate leptomeningeal layer. Note also the nerve root fascicles dispersed around the spinal cord. (Reproduced from Nicholas D S, Weller R O 1988 The fine anatomy of the human spinal meninges. Journal of Neurosurgery 69: 276–282 with the permission of the Journal of Neurosurgery.)

between layers, the dominant fiber orientation is longitudinal, accounting for superior mechanical strength in this direction (Rossitti 1993, Runza et al 1999). Distribution of elastin within the dura correlates with mobility requirements. Compared to anterior dura, posterior dural tissue is further removed from the axis of motion for spinal flexion and extension. Consequently, posterior dura undergoes more displacement during sagittal plane movement and possesses more elastin to meet these mobility demands (Louis 1981, Nakagawa et al 1994, Rossitti 1993). The elastin content in posterior dural tissues is highest in the cervical and lumbar regions, because these portions of the vertebral canal have the most sagittal plane mobility (Louis 1981, Nakagawa et al 1994, Rossitti 1993).

Pia mater is the innermost meningeal layer consisting of a connective tissue mesh separating CSF from spinal cord tissues (Nicholas & Weller 1988). A continuous lateral projection of pia mater forms the origin of a dentate ligament on each side of the spinal canal (Rossitti 1993). These ligaments become serrated to pierce the arachnoid and attach to the dura between the dural sleeves (Nicholas & Weller 1988, Rossitti 1993) (Fig. 6.4). Serrations of the dentate ligaments exhibit a superolateral orientation in the upper cervical spine, a transverse arrangement in the remainder of the cervical region, and a progressively inferolateral alignment in the thoracic and lumbar regions (Rossitti 1993).

The dura mater, pia mater and dentate ligaments form a functional unit that shields the spinal cord from mechanical loads accompanying movement (Rossitti 1993). Head, trunk and limb motion create tension in the dura because of dural attachments to the skeleton at the cranial sutures, the foramen magnum, the coccyx via the filum terminale, the intervertebral foramina via the dural sleeves, and other margins of the spinal canal via meningovertebral ligaments and the dorsomedian septum (Breig & Marions 1963, Rossitti 1993, Wadhwani et al 2004) (Fig. 6.5). These tensile forces are transmitted through serrations of the dentate ligaments to the pia mater for optimal positioning of the cord within the spinal canal (Rossitti 1993). Optimal positioning may involve any combination of axial, anteroposterior or lateral displacement of the cord so it can follow the shortest path through the vertebral canal (Louis 1981, Muhle et al 1998, Rossitti 1993). The varied orientation of dentate ligament attachments enables this mechanism of force transmission to move the spinal cord without generating significant mechanical stress within the delicate neural tissues (Rossitti 1993). Similar events enable the spinal cord to adapt to mechanical loads imposed by limb movements (Sunderland 1974).

CSF assists positioning of the cord within the spinal canal. The arachnoid mater is the intermediate meningeal layer that holds CSF within the subarachnoid space (Figs 6.5 and 6.6). CSF is contained under slight pressure to act as a hydraulic cushion protecting the spinal cord (Butler 1991, Louis 1981). Arachnoid trabeculae and an intermediate leptomeningeal layer are thought to optimize the cushioning effect of CSF by dampening any pressure waves caused by body movement (Nicholas & Weller 1988) (Fig. 6.6).

Spinal cord tissues possess intrinsic anatomical properties for adapting to movement of the vertebral column. In a neutral position, neurons and glia are arranged into folds and spirals, analogous to the undulating course of axons within the endoneurium of nerve trunks and nerve roots (Murphy 1977, Rossitti 1993). These folds are increased posteriorly during spinal extension, enabling cord structures to adjust to a shorter vertebral canal. Conversely, with vertebral flexion these undulations unwind so cord tissues lengthen without detrimental increases in mechanical stress (Louis 1981, Murphy 1977, Rossitti 1993) (Fig. 6.7). Different spinal cord tracts may also accommodate asymmetrical displacement associated with sagittal and frontal plane movements by sliding against each other (Louis 1981, Rossitti 1993, Yuan et al 1998), comparable to fascicular gliding in nerve trunks and nerve roots. These adaptive processes are most evident in the mobile cervical and lumbar regions (Louis 1981, Rossitti 1993).

Innervation of neural connective tissue

Considering the mechanical abilities of the nervous system, it follows that neural connective tissues should be innervated to enhance their capacity for protecting fragile nerve fibers.

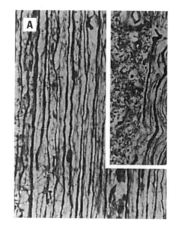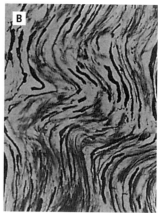

Figure 6.7 • Strain behavior of a segment of human spinal cord taken from the area of the anterior median fissure and the anterior white commissure (×525). **A:** No undulations are present when cord tissues are lengthened by spinal flexion. **B:** Nerve fibers fold on themselves as they shorten with spinal extension. (Reproduced from Breig A 1978, with the permission of Almqvist and Wiksell International.)

Peripheral nerve connective tissue innervation

Endoneurial, perineurial and epineurial connective tissues are innervated by local axon branches called nervi nervorum (Asbury & Fields 1984, Bove & Light 1997, Hromada 1963). Autonomic fibers from nearby perivascular plexuses also innervate these connective tissue sheaths (Hromada 1963, Lincoln et al 1993, Thomas & Olsson 1984). Nervi nervorum possess nociceptive capabilities (Bove & Light 1997, Hromada 1963, Sauer et al 1999), and they contain neuropeptides that mediate the inflammatory response exhibited by nerve trunks exposed to irritating mechanical or chemical stimuli (Sauer et al 1999, Triano & Luttges 1982, Zochodne 1993).

Meningeal innervation

Studies addressing meningeal innervation have focused on the dura mater. Sinu-vertebral nerves innervate the ventral, lateral and posterolateral aspects of the dura within the spinal canal, and they also innervate the dural sleeves of nerve root complexes (Cuatico et al 1988, Edgar & Nundy 1966, Groen et al 1988, Kallakuri et al 1998). These nerves originate from the ventral ramus just distal to the DRG, and they merge with sympathetic fibers from the gray ramus communicantes or sympathetic ganglion prior to entering the spinal canal through the intervertebral foramina (Butler 1991, Edgar & Nundy 1966). Once inside the spinal canal, sinu-vertebral nerves branch to span four or more spinal segments and form a plexus that innervates dural tissues (Butler 1991, Edgar & Nundy 1966, Groen et al 1988) (Fig. 6.8). Spinal dura innervation is most richly developed in the mobile cervical and lumbar regions (Cuatico et al 1988), and although some controversy exists (Kumar et al 1996), it appears that this innervation has a nociceptive function (Kallakuri et al 1998).

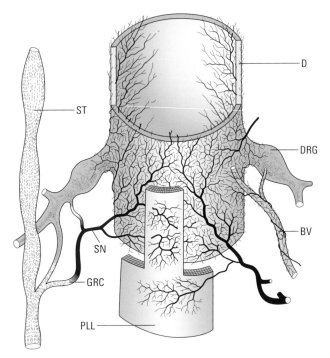

Figure 6.8 • Diagram of the ventral aspect of the dura illustrating the sinu-vertebral nerve plexus. BV = blood vessel, D = dura, DRG = dorsal root ganglion, GRC = gray ramus communicantes, PLL = posterior longitudinal ligament, SN = sinu-vertebral nerve, ST = sympathetic trunk. (Reproduced with permission from Butler 1991.)

The arachnoid and pia mater are collectively known as the leptomeninges (Nicholas & Weller 1988). Their pattern of innervation is less clear, but authors have reported the presence of neural structures in these meningeal tissues (Bridge 1959, Jänig & Koltzenburg 1990). Additionally, mechanoreceptors located in pial ligaments that attach to the anterior spinal artery may provide a mechanism for detecting tensile forces (Parke & Whalen 1993).

Axoplasm and blood flow – the link between mechanics and physiology

Recalling the unique architecture of neurons, a mechanism of intraneuronal communication must exist so that these cells can function within a mechanically dynamic setting. This cellular communication is accomplished through axoplasmic transport (Dahlin & Lundborg 1990, Devor 1991, Lundborg 1988, Lundborg & Dahlin 1992, Rempel et al 1999). Retrograde axoplasmic transport provides the cell body with chemical feedback concerning the status of the axon and surrounding tissues. This feedback enables the genetic machinery of the cell body to direct production of neurotransmitters and other materials necessary for synaptic function, impulse transmission and structural health of the axon (Devor & Seltzer 1999, Lundborg 1988, Lundborg & Dahlin 1992, Rempel et al 1999). The cell body also produces ion channels that are embedded in the axolemma and determine

neuron excitability (Bear et al 2001, Butler 2000, Costigan & Woolf 2000, Devor & Seltzer 1999, Koester & Siegelbaum 1995). Anterograde axoplasmic transport ferries all products from the cell body to appropriate destinations within the neuron (Bear et al 2001, Butler 2000, Dahlin & Lundborg 1990, Lundborg 1988, Lundborg & Dahlin 1992, Rempel et al 1999).

Axoplasm in mammals is five times more viscous than water (Haak et al 1976). Additionally, axoplasm exhibits thixotrophic properties, meaning it flows better when kept moving (Baker et al 1977, Shacklock 1995a). Describing axoplasm as 'nerve juice' that needs movement can be a useful strategy in educating clients rehabilitating from neural tissue injuries (Butler 2000).

Bidirectional axoplasmic transport is a process that requires a continuous energy supply. Neural connective tissues also need nutritional support to maintain their viscoelastic properties. Therefore, vascular anatomy is designed to deliver adequate blood flow to meet the energy demands of the nervous system during all postures and movements (Lundborg 1988, Rempel et al 1999). External vascular systems feeding neural structures exhibit a coiled or pig-tailed configuration so that blood flow is not impaired during movement of peripheral nerves or spinal nerve roots. This coiled architecture also exists within intraneural vessels so that normal fascicular gliding does not inhibit circulation (Dommisse 1994, Lundborg 1988, Parke & Watanabe 1985, Rempel et al 1999) (Fig. 6.3). In addition, intraneural vascular networks possess several anastomoses that allow the direction of blood flow to change in response to any local circulatory deficits imposed by mechanical loads associated with sport or exercise activities (Kobayashi et al 2000, Lundborg 1988, Parke & Watanabe 1985, Rempel et al 1999) (Fig. 6.9). Besides being mobile, intraneural vasculature protects neural tissues from harmful chemical stimuli. Endoneurial vessels possess a blood–nerve barrier that works in concert with the perineurial diffusion barrier to provide nerve fibers with an optimal chemical environment (Lundborg 1988, Rempel et al 1999).

Axoplasmic flow and intraneural circulation exemplify the theory of neurodynamics. These two physiological processes are vital to the physical health and function of neural tissues and, as will be discussed in subsequent sections, mechanical forces associated with daily or athletic activities can influence 'nerve juice' and blood flow.

Neurodynamics

Shacklock (1995a) defined neurodynamics as the interaction between the mechanics and physiology of the nervous system. The following sections highlight some basic 'rules' of neurodynamics that have clinical relevance for examination and management of neural tissue injuries.

The neural container and mechanical interface

The concepts of a 'neural container' (Shacklock 1995a) and a 'mechanical interface' (Butler 1991) assist in understanding how

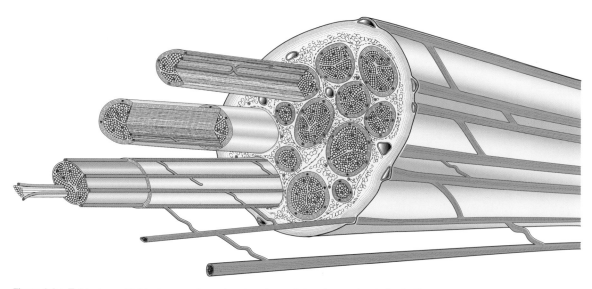

Figure 6.9 • Extrinsic and intrinsic vascular networks of a peripheral nerve trunk illustrating numerous anastomoses between vessels. (Reproduced with permission from Butler 1991.)

body movements affect neural tissues. The body can be considered to be the container of the nervous system, and within this container musculoskeletal tissues form a mechanical interface with neural structures (Shacklock 1995a). Examples of interfacing structures where neural tissues may be prone to injury are the intervertebral foramina, the scalenes, the carpal tunnel, the anterior aspect of the sacroiliac joint (Atlihan et al 2000), the piriformis, the fibular head and the tarsal tunnel. As the body or container moves, interfacing musculoskeletal tissues change dimensions and exert mechanical forces on neural structures (Shacklock 1995a). Consequently, management of neural tissue injuries should ensure that musculoskeletal structures of the neural container function at an optimal level, thereby minimizing physical forces on adjacent neural tissues (Butler 2000, Hall & Elvey 1999, Shacklock 2005).

Relationship of nerve structures to joint axes

Neural tissue mobility during trunk and limb movement is dictated by the spatial relationship between nerve structures and the axes of joint motion (Beith et al 1995, Millesi et al 1995, Shacklock 1995a, Topp & Boyd 2006). Previous discussion in this chapter addressed how neuromeningeal structures are affected by sagittal and frontal plane motions of the spinal column. Neurodynamic tests biased toward various peripheral nerves have evolved from clinical application of nerve geography. For example, the median nerve can be challenged mechanically by combining shoulder abduction, elbow extension and wrist extension because it passes caudal to the glenohumeral joint and ventral to the axes of motion at the elbow and wrist (Byl et al 2002, Dilley et al 2003, Kenneally et al 1988, Kleinrensink et al 1995, 2000, Lewis et al 1998). In contrast, assessment of the mechanosensitivity of the ulnar

nerve needs to incorporate elbow flexion with wrist extension since this structure courses dorsal to the axis of motion at the elbow and ventral to the wrist joint (Buehler & Thayer 1988, Butler 2000, Byl et al 2002, Pechan 1973, Wright et al 2001). In the lower extremities, the tibial branch of the sciatic nerve is challenged by hip flexion, knee extension and ankle dorsiflexion (Beith et al 1995, Coppieters et al 2006), while the peroneal branch can be loaded by ankle plantar flexion and inversion rather than dorsiflexion (Butler 2000, Mauhart 1990, Pahor & Toppenberg 1996).

Because of their three-dimensional structure, neural tissues are not displaced in a uniform manner during joint motion (Millesi et al 1995). With cervical flexion, the posterior portion of the cervical spinal cord is subjected to more displacement than the anterior portion (Yuan et al 1998). A peripheral nerve may have a diameter of 1 cm or more, therefore, portions of the nerve at a greater perpendicular distance from the joint axis will be displaced more than parts nearer the axis of motion (Millesi et al 1995, Topp & Boyd 2006). As discussed previously, gliding between fascicles enables neural structures to adapt to asymmetrical displacement (Millesi et al 1995, Rossitti 1993).

Strain, excursion and tensile stress

Neural containers in the spinal canal and extremities change in length during movement. Previous sections of this chapter have described how movement of the vertebral column alters the length of the spinal canal. Limb movement changes the length of neural containers surrounding peripheral nerves. Zoch et al (1991) measured the container for the median nerve with the shoulder in 90° abduction. When comparing a position of elbow and wrist flexion to one of elbow and wrist extension, the distance from the upper border of the latissimus dorsi muscle to the wrist increased by approximately 10 cm. In the lower

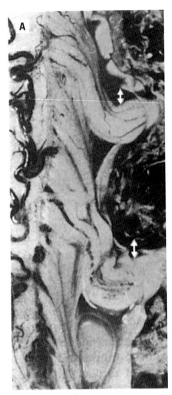
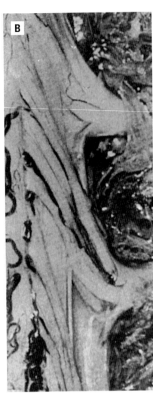

Figure 6.10 • Normal deformation of the dura, cord and nerve roots in the cervical canal in a cadaver due to sagittal plane movement of the cervical spine. A total laminectomy has been performed, and the dura opened and retracted although still able to transmit tensile forces. In **A** the cervical spine is in extension, the nervous system is slack, the root sleeves have lost contact with the pedicles (lower arrows) and the nerve roots have separated from the inner surfaces of the sleeves (upper arrows). In **B** the cervical spine has been flexed, and the nervous system including the dura has been stretched and moved in relation to surrounding structures. Note that the root sleeves have come in contact with the pedicles and the nerve roots now contact the inner surface of the sleeves. Note also the change in shape of blood vessels. (Reproduced from Breig A 1978, with the permission of Almqvist & Wiksell International.)

extremity, Beith et al (1995) found that combined motions of 90° hip flexion, 90° knee extension and 20° ankle dorsiflexion increased the length of the neural container for the sciatic, tibial and medial plantar nerves by 9–12 cm. Nerve structures adapt to these changes in the container with a combination of strain, excursion and tensile stress (Beith et al 1995, Byl et al 2002, Coppieters et al 2006, Dilley et al 2003, McLellan & Swash 1976, Millesi et al 1995, Shacklock 1995a, Smith et al 1993, Wilgis & Murphy 1986, Wright et al 1996, 2001, 2005).

Strain is defined as the percentage change in length of a structure relative to its original length (Rodgers & Cavanagh 1984). As discussed previously, axons take an undulatory course through all portions of the nervous system, folding and unfolding as neural tissues undergo strain (Louis 1981, Millesi et al 1995,

Rossitti 1993, Sunderland 1990). This mechanism for adapting to length changes is dependent on the viscoelastic tubes created by the endoneurium, perineurium and dura (Millesi et al 1995, Runza et al 1999). Nerve trunks and neuromeningeal structures are also able to fold and unfold at a macroscopic level (Fig. 6.10), because intraneural connective tissues facilitate gliding between fascicles (Louis 1981, Millesi et al 1995, Shacklock 1995a, Sunderland 1990, Wright et al 1996). This macroscopic folding, or 'wrinkle effect' (Wright et al 1996), further contributes to the strain behavior of neural tissues, particularly when they need to shorten. Examples include folding of the neuromeningeal structures on the concave side of a laterally flexed spinal column (Breig 1978), wrinkling of the median nerve at a flexed elbow (Wright et al 1996) and undulations forming in the ulnar nerve as the elbow is extended (Byl et al 2002).

Once neural tissues have unfolded to the point where their undulations are eliminated, they respond to continued lengthening of the neural container by sliding (Shacklock 1995a, Topp & Boyd 2006). Excursion or sliding of neural tissues relative to interfacing structures has been documented within the spinal canal (Louis 1981, Rossitti 1993), the intervertebral foramina (Kenneally et al 1988, Smith et al 1993, Sunderland 1974) and the extremities (Coppieters et al 2006, Dilley et al 2003, McLellan & Swash 1976, Millesi et al 1995, Wilgis & Murphy 1986, Wright et al 1996, 2001, 2005). Recalling previous sections on relevant neuroanatomy, this sliding is facilitated by mesoneurium surrounding peripheral nerve trunks.

Excursion does not only take place along the longitudinal axis of each neural structure. Neuromeningeal tissues slide in anteroposterior and lateral directions during movement of the spinal column (Breig 1978, Louis 1981, Rossitti 1993). Nerve root complexes move in a cephalocaudal direction within the intervertebral foramina during spinal (Breig & Marions 1963, Louis 1981) (Fig. 6.10) and limb movement (Kenneally et al 1988, Smith et al 1993, Sunderland 1974). Transverse sliding has also been observed in peripheral nerves. Greening et al (1999) demonstrated that the median nerve moves radially and posteriorly within the carpal tunnel during wrist flexion, and Ugbolue et al (2005) found that isolated movement of the metacarpophalangeal joint of the index or middle fingers caused small and irregular transverse displacement of the median nerve at the wrist. The superficial branch of the peroneal nerve exhibits a significant amount of transverse excursion when palpated on the dorsum of the foot (Butler 2000).

When sliding mechanisms have been exhausted, additional strain in neural tissues is associated with reductions in cross-sectional area of the nerve trunk and concomitant increases in intraneural pressure or tensile stress (Driscoll et al 2002, Kwan et al 1992, Millesi et al 1995, Shacklock 1995a). Tensile stress is defined as the force per unit of cross-sectional area generated within a structure subjected to a tensile load (Rodgers & Cavanagh 1984). The viscoelastic behavior of biological tissues is often characterized by stress–strain curves. Nerve structures in situ appear capable of undergoing significant strain with development of relatively minimal tensile stress (Kwan et al 1992). One notable exception is the ulnar nerve at the elbow.

During combined shoulder abduction, elbow flexion and wrist extension, the ulnar nerve at the elbow undergoes at least 15% strain (Wright et al 2001) and develops a 4-fold increase in tensile stress (Pechan & Julis 1975).

A mechanical model has been proposed that may partially explain the viscoelastic properties that nerve structures exhibit during tensile loading (Georgeu et al 2005, Walbeehm et al 2004). The perineurium, endoneurium and axons form a pressurized neural core that is surrounded by a connective tissue sheath comprised of the internal and external epineurium (Walbeehm et al 2004). As the tensile load increases, the architecture of the connective tissue sheath converts this tensile load into a modest compressive force. The normal positive pressure within the neural tissue core is able to resist this modest compressive force and protect the neural elements from damage (Walbeehm et al 2004). The interface between the pressurized neural core and connective tissue sheath is thought to be located within the inner layers of the perineurium, and this 'core–sheath interface' is the first place to fail when the nerve trunk is placed under tensile load (Georgeu et al 2005). While this mechanical model has been confirmed in animal studies of principally monofascicular nerves, it is hypothesized that similar mechanisms contribute to the viscoelastic behavior of multifascicular nerves (Georgeu et al 2005). When the cooperative mechanism between the pressurized neural tissue core and connective tissue sheath has been altered by injury or fibrosis to the endoneurium, perineurium or epineurium, viscoelasticity of the nerve trunk is compromised as the same amount of limb movement leads to detrimental increases in strain and tensile stress (Beel et al 1984, Boyd et al 2005, Millesi et al 1995).

Non-uniform mechanics and order movement

Strain, excursion and tensile stress develop within neural tissues in a non-uniform fashion (Millesi et al 1995, Shacklock 1995a). For example, the median nerve accumulates more stress per unit of strain in areas where it has more branches (Millesi et al 1995). Phillips et al (2004) found that segments of rat median and sciatic nerves that cross joints are more compliant during tensile loading than segments of these same nerve trunks located between joints. Flexion of the entire spinal column causes dural strain of 15% at L1–2, but approximately 30% at L5 (Louis 1981). It has been proposed that the non-uniform mechanics of neural tissues are due to differences in fascicular plexuses and connective tissue content at different points along a nerve (Grewal et al 1996, Shacklock 1995a). Since Phillips et al (2004) could not find consistent differences in fascicular arrangement or connective tissue content that explained the variations in compliance between the joint and non-joint segments of rat peripheral nerves, an explanation for the non-uniform mechanics of neural tissues may vary for different regions of the body (Topp & Boyd 2006). Other factors that may contribute to the non-uniform mechanics of neural tissues include the unique kinematic properties of each joint complex a nerve crosses, regional limitations in excursion

because of attachments to the neural container, nerve branching and exposure to a variety of forces from different interfacing structures such as bone, muscle and fascia (Butler 2000, Grewal et al 1996, Shacklock 1995a).

Neural tissues are subjected to different mechanical loads depending on the type and combination of movements (Butler 2000, Shacklock 1995a). If the cervical spine is flexed in isolation, neural structures in the lumbar region undergo cranial displacement relative to surrounding vertebrae (Breig & Marions 1963). When the entire spine is flexed, however, neural tissues in the upper lumbar region move in a caudal direction relative to corresponding vertebral segments (Louis 1981). Shoulder abduction from 90 to 110° causes proximal excursion of the median nerve at the elbow, while wrist extension from 0 to 60° causes the median nerve to slide distally within the cubital fossa (Wright et al 1996).

Mimicking a neurodynamic test for the median nerve, Coppieters et al (2001, 2002) showed that elbow extension is significantly reduced when preceded by contralateral cervical side-bending, wrist extension, lateral rotation of the shoulder and/or shoulder girdle depression. Johnson & Chiarello (1997) demonstrated that knee extension in a slump sit position is reduced when preceded by neck flexion, and further decreased when preceded by a combination of neck flexion, ankle dorsiflexion and hip medial rotation. The addition of sensitizing maneuvers (e.g. ankle dorsiflexion) has also been shown to alter the mobility and/or symptom response during straight leg raise (Boland & Adams 2000, Butler 1991). In vivo studies utilizing ultrasound imaging have confirmed that the amount of excursion of a nerve relative to its surrounding structures depends on the position of neighboring joints (Dilley et al 2003). Health care practitioners have long noticed that the sequence of joint movement alters the symptom response and range of motion available during a neurodynamic test (Butler 2000), and this observation may be related to the aforementioned differences in loading when a nerve is successively challenged at different joints.

There are two key points for clinical application of the above information. First, the greatest mechanical challenge for a segment of neural tissue is thought to occur when the joint adjacent to the nerve is loaded first during the testing sequence. The development of strain, excursion and tensile stress will spread to other portions of the neural tissue tract as more joint complexes participate in the movement (Shacklock 1995a). Second, even though the diagnostic value of altering the test sequence needs to be determined by further validation studies, neurodynamic examination should be modified to replicate the order of movement utilized by clients during symptomatic sport or exercise activities (Butler 2000, Shacklock 2005).

The mechanical continuum

A fundamental principle of neurodynamics is appreciating that the nervous system forms a tissue continuum throughout the body, and this mechanical continuity should be evident from previous discussion on neuroanatomy. The most dramatic example of neural tissue continuity is the aforementioned ability of neck flexion to alter knee extension mobility in a slump sit position (Johnson & Chiarello 1997), but similar continuity exists in the extremities. Movement of the wrist and fingers affects median and ulnar neural tissues at the elbow and upper arm (Dilley et al 2003, Kleinrensink et al 1995, 2000, McLellan & Swash 1976, Wilgis & Murphy 1986, Wright et al 1996, 2001). When the ankle is positioned in dorsiflexion, subsequent movement into hip flexion with the knee extended causes proximal excursion and increase in strain of the tibial nerve at the tarsal tunnel (Coppieters et al 2006). Ipsilateral straight leg raise can increase tensile stress in a median nerve already placed in a mechanically loaded position (Lewis et al 1998).

The implication of this tissue continuum is that mechanical events in one part of the nervous system will have an impact on remote areas along the neural tissue tract (Butler 2000, Shacklock 1995a). Loss of excursion in one segment of a nerve can cause detrimental increases in tensile stress or intraneural pressure in other areas (Wright et al 1996, 2001). Clinically, peripheral neurogenic syndromes in the carpal tunnel and tarsal tunnel may often be related to concomitant problems in the cervical and lumbar nerve roots (Mackinnon 1992, Sammarco et al 1993, Upton & McComas 1973). The hypothesis that injury in one site of a nerve can predispose remaining areas of the same nerve to injury is referred to as 'double or multiple crush' (Mackinnon 1992, Upton & McComas 1973). Animal models provide a pathophysiological explanation for 'double crush' by showing that impairment in axoplasmic flow at one site predisposes the remainder of the nerve to further entrapment injury (Mackinnon 1992). Pathological changes at each 'crush' site may be minor and localized to those fascicles affected most by injurious mechanical forces (Mackinnon 1992, Novak & Mackinnon 1998). These minor changes may not be detected electrodiagnostically (Mackinnon 1992, Novak & Mackinnon 1998), which may explain why electrodiagnostic studies have both denied (Bednarik et al 1999) and supported (Golovchinsky 1998) the 'double crush' hypothesis. In spite of somewhat conflicting information in the literature, physical therapists should be cognizant of the neural tissue continuum and examine along the entire tissue tract in clients with neural injuries (Butler 2000, Novak & Mackinnon 1998).

The impact of mechanical forces on physiology

Mechanical forces from sport and exercise activities can alter intraneural circulation and axoplasmic flow. A clear relationship exists between nerve strain and intraneural circulation (Ogata & Naito 1986, Rempel et al 1999). Blood flow in peripheral nerves slows at 6 to 8% strain (Ogata & Naito 1986), and nerve conduction may also be compromised (Wall et al 1992). These values of strain occur in peripheral nerves during daily movement of extremity joints (Byl et al 2002, Coppieters et al 2006, Wright et al 1996, 2001, 2005), but anastomoses between intraneural vessels enable nerves to recover from temporary deficits in circulation and nerve conduction (Kobayashi et al 2000, Lundborg 1988, Parke & Watanabe 1985, Rempel et al 1999) (Fig. 6.9).

Neural tissues are also subjected to external compression by movement of interfacing structures. Extraneural pressure can be increased by events such as narrowing of the IVF, wrist motion that increases carpal tunnel pressure or by muscle contraction (Farmer & Wisneski 1994, Fujiwara et al 2001, Mazurek & Shin 2001, Muhle et al 2001, Novak & Mackinnon 1998, Nuckley et al 2002, Shacklock 1995a). External compression alters nerve function in a direct dose–response relationship (Lundborg & Dahlin 1992, Novak & Mackinnon 1998, Rempel et al 1999), and extraneural pressures as low as 20 to 40 mmHg can impair axoplasmic transport, blood flow and nerve conduction (Dahlin & McLean 1986, Rempel et al 1999, Rydevik et al 1981). As with the development of strain, these levels of compression occur during daily activities (Mackinnon 1992, Novak & Mackinnon 1998, Shacklock 1995a), but as long as the magnitude and duration of compression are not excessive, their effects on neural structures are completely reversible (Butler 1991, Dahlin & McLean 1986). Recall that anatomical features enable nerve root complexes and nerve trunks to recover from compressive loads. Adipose tissue, dural sleeves and CSF safeguard nerve root complexes (Jenis & An 2000, Louis 1981, Rydevik et al 1984, Sunderland 1974), while fascicular plexuses and internal epineurium protect nerve trunks (Lundborg & Dahlin 1992, Sunderland 1990).

Clinical examination

Given the multiple forces imposed by interfacing structures and the non-uniform mechanics of the neural tissue continuum, a series of base neurodynamic tests summarized by Butler (2000) and Shacklock (2005) have been proposed to examine the movement capabilities of the nervous system. These limb and trunk movements can reproduce the tensile, compressive and friction forces placed on neural tissues during sport or exercise activities. Sustained manual compression and isometric muscle contraction may be additional clinical methods for imparting mechanical loads onto neural structures (Mazurek & Shin 2001, Novak & Mackinnon 1998, 2005).

Pathodynamics

Even though the nervous system is well designed to tolerate mechanical forces associated with body postures and movements, protective mechanisms in neural tissues sometimes fail, leading to symptoms of nerve injury (Novak & Mackinnon 1998, Shacklock 1995a) (Box 6.1).

Venous congestion, intraneural edema, fibrosis and myelin changes

A summary of the processes related to the production of symptoms in neural tissue injury can be seen in Fig. 6.11. Compromise in intraneural circulation appears to be the first step in the pathophysiological cascade of nerve injury. Compressive, tensile, friction or vibration stimuli that exceed the physical capacities of neural tissues will induce venous congestion, thereby impeding intraneural circulation and axoplasmic flow (Greening & Lynn 1998, Hasue 1993, Kobayashi et al 2000, Rempel et al 1999). Resulting hypoxia causes an inflammatory response in nerve trunks and DRGs, leading to subperineurial edema and increased endoneurial fluid pressure (Hasue 1993, Kobayashi et al 2000, Lundborg & Dahlin 1992, Novak & Mackinnon 1998, Olmarker & Rydevik 2001, Parke & Whalen 2002, Rempel et al 1999, Yabuki et al 2001). Neuropeptides released from mechanically irritated nervi nervorum and proinflammatory mediators produced by immune cell activation contribute to this inflammatory response (Gazda et al 2001, Sauer et al 1999, Watkins & Maier 2004). Endoneurial edema persists because, as discussed previously, the perineurial diffusion barrier does not allow the inflammatory exudate to escape.

Persistent endoneurial edema leads to intraneural fibrosis, decreasing the viscoelastic properties of neural connective tissues (Beel et al 1984, Millesi et al 1995, Novak & Mackinnon 1998, Rempel et al 1999). Bearing in mind the concept of a mechanical continuum, localized restrictions in nerve strain or sliding can cause detrimental increases in tensile stress at other segments of the neural tissue tract, potentially leading to additional injury (Bove & Light 1997, Hunter 1991, Wilgis & Murphy 1986, Wright et al 1996, 2001). The ability to tolerate external compression may also be decreased because of internal epineurial fibrosis and impairment of fascicular gliding. Additionally, fibrotic changes may affect the external epineurium and mesoneurium, further compromising nerve excursion and neural biomechanics (Bove & Light 1997, Greening & Lynn 1998, Millesi et al 1995). Transverse excursion of the median nerve is reduced in patients with carpal tunnel syndrome

(Greening et al 1999, Erel et al 2003), but conflicting reports exist as to whether longitudinal sliding of the median nerve is altered in this patient population (Erel et al 2003, Valls-Sole et al 1995). Anatomical anomalies limiting excursion of the superficial peroneal nerve were found in a surgical study of eight patients with superficial peroneal neuralgia after ankle sprains (Johnston & Howell 1999).

After intraneural fibrosis, myelin and axon changes occur along a continuum. Initially, only thinning of myelin takes place, followed by segmental demyelination with progression to diffuse demyelination and axonal degeneration in more severe nerve injury (Hasue 1993, Novak & Mackinnon 1998, Rempel et al 1999). Greater amount and duration of endoneurial edema is directly correlated with more significant degradation in myelin content and axon structure (Rempel et al 1999). It has been hypothesized that these changes are related to impairment in bidirectional axoplasmic flow and altered function of the cell body (Dahlin et al 1987). The severity of impairment in nerve conduction measured by electrodiagnostic studies can indicate the amount of myelin and axon damage (Novak & Mackinnon 1998, Rempel et al 1999).

The inflammatory response exhibited by neural tissues does not have to be the result of direct mechanical overload. Inflammatory processes in neighboring structures produce chemical stimuli that can induce an inflammatory reaction in nerve structures (Bove & Light 1997). A common example is that inflammatory processes associated with exposed nucleus pulposus produce chemical stimuli that inflame the nerve root complex, leading to radicular pain without mechanical compression (Gifford 2001, Murata et al 2005, Olmarker & Rydevik 2001, Takebayashi et al 2001).

Increased mechanosensitivity

It is important to remember that symptoms of neural tissue injury are not due solely to changes in nerve conduction (Box 6.1). Daily activities, clinical examination of the neural container, neurodynamic tests and nerve palpation may evoke symptoms indicative of increased mechanosensitivity in injured neural tissues (Gifford & Butler 1997, Hall & Elvey 1999, Nee & Butler 2006). Enhanced mechanosensitivity associated with nerve injury can be explained by increased nociceptive input from innervated connective tissues, and from abnormal impulse generating sites within impulse conducting tissues (Baron 2000, Devor & Seltzer 1999, Gifford & Butler 1997, Hall & Elvey 1999, Hasue 1993) (Fig. 6.11).

Innervated connective tissues

Nervi nervorum and sinu-vertebral nerves supplying nerve sheaths and dura have a nociceptive function (Bove & Light 1997, Hromada 1963, Kallakuri et al 1998, Sauer et al 1999). Once neural connective tissues are inflamed, these nociceptors become sensitized to mechanical or chemical stimuli, contributing to the enhanced mechanosensitivity observed in nerve injuries (Baron 2000, Bove & Light 1997, Devor & Seltzer 1999,

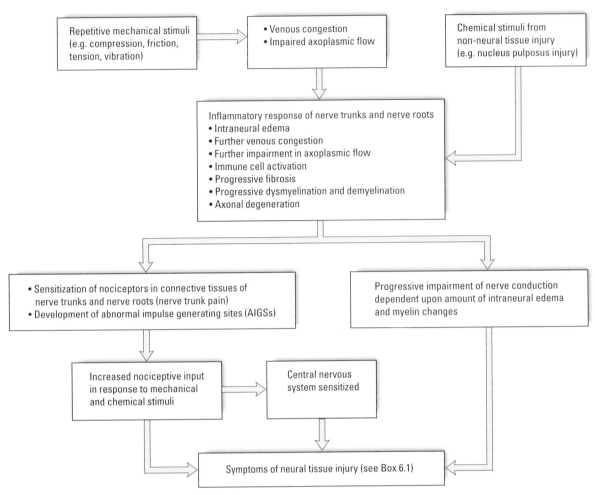

Figure 6.11 • Summary of processes related to the production of symptoms of neural tissue injury. (Compiled from Hassue 1993, Bove & Light 1997, Greening & Lynn 1998, Gifford 2001.)

Dilley et al 2005, Gifford & Butler 1997, Hall & Elvey 1999). When intraneural fibrosis has compromised the extensibility of neural connective tissues, already sensitized nociceptors will be subjected to more intense mechanical stimulation, because fibrotic connective tissues can no longer efficiently attenuate compressive, tensile, friction and vibration loads associated with sport or exercise activities (Bove & Light 1997, Butler 2000). Consequently, normally asymptomatic movements may remain sensitive. Increased nociceptive activity from nervi nervorum has been referred to as nerve trunk pain (Asbury & Fields 1984), and this pain may be perceived as having a deep aching quality (Asbury & Fields 1984, Bove & Light 1997, Bove et al 2005, Hall & Elvey 1999).

Abnormal impulse generating sites

An injured segment of peripheral nerve may develop the ability to repeatedly generate its own impulses (Devor & Seltzer 1999). These injured areas are referred to as abnormal impulse generating sites (AIGSs), because axons that normally just transmit impulses become capable of initiating them. The main features of AIGSs are mechanosensitivity and spontaneous firing (Butler 2000, Devor & Seltzer 1999).

Earlier discussion in this chapter alluded to the ensemble of ion channels that insert into the axon membrane and determine neuron excitability. Constant remodeling of ion channels normally occurs so that an afferent neuron maintains an appropriate level of sensitivity to surrounding stimuli (Bear et al 2001, Costigan & Woolf 2000, Devor & Seltzer 1999, Koester & Siegelbaum 1995). Nerve injury alters the gene expression within the cell body (Baron 2000, Costigan & Woolf 2000). Consequently, the type and number of ion channels in the axon membrane changes so that neurons are more easily excited by mechanical and chemical input (Baron 2000, Devor & Seltzer 1999, Gifford 1998, Harden 2005). Ion channels insert into areas of the axon membrane not covered by myelin; therefore, dorsal root ganglia, areas of myelin thinning and areas of segmental demyelination provide opportunities for abnormal accumulation of mechanosensitive and chemosensitive ion channels (Amir & Devor 1993, Calvin et al 1982, Chen & Devor 1998, Devor & Seltzer 1999, England et al 1998, Liu et al 2000, Tal & Eliav 1996, Wall & Gutnick 1974). Presumably, ion channels are evenly spread along unmyelinated fibers.

With an abnormal accumulation of ion channels, the type and number of channels determines which stimuli will evoke symptoms. Normally innocuous lengthening, pinching or friction forces become capable of eliciting symptoms in situations where concentrations of mechanosensitive channels are increased (Devor & Seltzer 1999, Gifford 1998, Gifford & Butler 1997). Nerve ischemia induced by repetitive movement or sustained positioning may create an exaggerated response from AIGSs packed with ischemosensitive channels (Devor & Seltzer 1999, Gifford 2001). Inflammatory chemicals from injured neural or non-neural tissues can stimulate chemosensitive channels (Butler 2000, Devor & Seltzer 1999).

Adrenaline (epinephrine) and noradrenaline (norepinephrine) also become capable of stimulating AIGSs (Baron 2000, Devor & Seltzer 1999, Greening & Lynn 1998, Hasue 1993, Shacklock 1995a). Presence of adrenosensitive channels provides a partial explanation for the observation that emotional stress can exacerbate symptoms of nerve injury (Butler 2000, Gifford 2001). Van Meeteren et al (1997) found that rats exposed to chronic intermittent stress recovered more slowly from sciatic nerve crush injury. Therefore, adrenoreceptors may influence healing of nerve tissues, and education that decreases patient apprehension may assist recovery (Butler 2000, Butler & Moseley 2003).

Abnormal impulse generating sites exhibit spontaneous activity, because the ensemble of ion channels places the axon membrane near the threshold for firing (Devor & Seltzer 1999). Therefore, patients experiencing nerve injuries may report that symptoms sometimes occur without any type of stimulus (Gifford 2001, Gifford & Butler 1997). Axonal mechanosensitivity and spontaneous discharge secondary to neural inflammation appear to develop primarily in A-delta and C fibers that innervate deep structures (Bove et al 2003), and this may provide a partial explanation for the aforementioned observation that peripheral neural tissue pain may often be described as deep in nature (Bove et al 2005).

Recovery and relevance of neural pathology

Reports from animal studies of nerve injury indicate that neuropathic pain behavior and histological findings usually resolve in approximately 6–8 weeks (Lindenlaub & Sommer 2000). But when symptoms persist at 15 weeks, intraneural pathology is still present (Lindenlaub & Sommer 2000). Extraneural fibrosis adhering to interfacing structures may also be present 15 weeks after experimental nerve injury (Greening & Lynn 1998). Pathology does not always correlate with symptoms. Neary & Ochoa (1975) showed that 50% of cadavers have neural connective tissue and nerve fiber changes, particularly at vulnerable sites such as the ulnar nerve at the elbow, but in life these subjects never complained of pain in these areas.

A variety of issues contribute to the inconsistent relationship between neural pathology and pain. Pain is a complex biopsychosocial phenomenon that is only partly influenced by nerve injury (see Chapter 9). Additionally, increased nociceptive input from nerve injury causes changes in central nervous system processing (Baron 2000, Costigan & Woolf 2000, Devor & Seltzer 1999, Harden 2005, Mannion & Woolf 2000, Woolf 2004). In neurogenic pain states, the central nervous system becomes sensitized and may process normally innocuous stimuli as painful (Doubell et al 1999, Mannion & Woolf 2000, Shacklock 1999, Zusman 1992) (Fig. 6.11). This sensitization results in potentially false positive responses to physical tests, including neurodynamic tests (Butler 2000, Gifford 2001, Zusman 1992). Although the patient reports pain during the test, the neural tissues may be relatively normal. The pain response is simply due to altered processing in the central nervous system. Physical therapists need to consider these issues when interpreting symptomatic responses to neurodynamic and other physical examination tests (Butler 2000, Gifford & Butler 1997, Shacklock 1999, Zusman 1992).

In spite of the inconsistent relationship between nerve pathology and pain, several case reports have illustrated the successful integration of neurodynamics in the assessment and treatment of various disorders, such as lateral epicondylalgia (Ekstrom & Holden 2002), cubital tunnel syndrome (Coppieters et al 2004), cervicobrachial pain (Cleland et al 2005, Cowell & Phillips 2002), heel pain (Meyer et al 2002, Shacklock 1995b) and lumbar-lower extremity pain (Cleland et al 2004, George 2002, Klingman 1999). In addition, a limited number of clinical trials have investigated the effectiveness of a treatment regime that includes interventions aimed at restoring normal neural biomechanics. Although a comprehensive review is beyond the scope of this chapter, some of these clinical trials will be briefly discussed.

In a retrospective study, Rozmaryn et al (1998) found that a program of nerve and tendon gliding exercises reduced the rate of carpal tunnel surgery to 43%, compared to a surgical rate of 71% in patients who did not utilize the gliding exercises. Symptom improvement was maintained in the majority of cases over an average follow-up period of 23 months. Two randomized trials on patients with carpal tunnel syndrome showed that neural mobilization techniques were more beneficial than no treatment but were not superior to mobilization of the carpal bones (Tal-Akabi & Rushton 2000) or splinting (Akalin et al 2002). A cervical lateral glide technique has been shown in two randomized trials to be beneficial for patients with neurogenic cervicobrachial pain when used in isolation (Coppieters et al 2003a, 2003b) or when combined with other exercises (Allison et al 2002).

Although these studies suggest that patients with a variety of symptoms and conditions may benefit from inclusion of neural tissue mobilization techniques, clinicians should keep in mind that these techniques may not be appropriate for many patient populations. For example, Scrimshaw & Maher (2001) demonstrated that nerve mobilization techniques provided no additional benefit when routinely added to the standard postoperative care in patients who had undergone lumbar discectomy, laminectomy or fusion. Given the limited number of clinical trials that have been conducted and the fact that single case studies cannot be generalized to the larger population, it is clear that additional clinical research is necessary to determine which groups of patients with signs of increased neural tissue mechanosensitivity would most likely benefit from neural tissue mobilization techniques. These future studies also need to identify specific treatment parameters that would be most effective.

Summary

Neural tissues are well designed to tolerate mechanical forces associated with sport and exercise activities. When these mechanical forces exceed the physical capacities of the nervous system, symptoms of nerve injury occur. Neurogenic symptoms result from changes in neural connective tissues and impulse conducting tissues, as well as from changes in central nervous system processing (Fig. 6.11). Knowledge of neurodynamics and pathodynamics will enable clinicians to develop appropriate strategies for intervention when rehabilitating clients experiencing neural tissue injury.

References

Akalin E, El O, Peker O et al 2002 Treatment of carpal tunnel syndrome with nerve and tendon gliding exercises. American Journal of Physical Medicine and Rehabilitation 81:108–113

Allison G, Nagy B, Hall T 2002 A randomized clinical trial of manual therapy for cervico-brachial pain syndrome: a pilot study. Manual Therapy 7:95–102

Amir R, Devor M 1993 Ongoing activity in neuroma afferents bearing retrograde sprouts. Brain Research 630:283–288

Asbury A K, Fields H L 1984 Pain due to peripheral nerve damage: an hypothesis. Neurology 34:1587–1590

Atlihan D, Tekdemir I, Ates Y et al 2000 Anatomy of the anterior sacroiliac joint with reference to lumbosacral nerves. Clinical Orthopaedics and Related Research 376:236–241

Baker P, Ladds M, Rubinson K 1977 Measurement of the flow properties of isolated axoplasm in a defined chemical environment. Journal of Physiology 269:10–11

Baron R 2000 Peripheral neuropathic pain: from mechanisms to symptoms. Clinical Journal of Pain 16 (2 suppl):S12–S20

Bear M, Connors B, Paradiso M 2001 Neuroscience: exploring the brain. Lippincott Williams and Wilkins, Baltimore, MD

Bednarik J, Kadanka Z, Vohanka S 1999 Median nerve neuropathy in spondylotic cervical myelopathy: double crush syndrome. Journal of Neurology 246:541–545

Beel J A, Groswald D E, Luttges M W 1984 Alterations in the mechanical properties of peripheral nerve following crush injury. Journal of Biomechanics 17:185–193

Beel J, Stodieck L, Luttges M 1986 Structural properties of spinal nerve roots: biomechanics. Experimental Neurology 91:30–40

Beith I D, Robins E J, Richards P R 1995 An assessment of the adaptive mechanisms within and surrounding the peripheral nervous system, during changes in nerve bed length resulting from underlying joint movement. In: Shacklock M O (ed) Moving in on pain. Butterworth-Heinemann, Sydney, p 194–203

Bogduk N 1997 Clinical anatomy of the lumbar spine and sacrum. Churchill Livingstone, New York

Boland R, Adams R 2000 Effects of ankle dorsiflexion on range and reliability of straight leg raising. Australian Journal of Physiotherapy 46:191–200

Bove G M, Light A R 1997 The nervi nervorum: missing link for neuropathic pain? Pain Forum 6:181–190

Bove G M, Ransil B, Lin H et al 2003 Inflammation induces ectopic mechanical sensitivity in axons of nociceptors innervating deep tissues. Journal of Physiology 90:1949–1955

Bove G M, Zaheen A, Bajwa Z 2005 Subjective nature of lower limb radicular pain. Journal of Manipulative and Physiological Therapeutics 28:12–12

Boyd B S, Puttlitz C, Gan J et al 2005 Strain and excursion in the rat sciatic nerve during a modified straight leg raise are altered after traumatic nerve injury. Journal of Orthopaedic Research 23:764–770

Breig A 1978 Adverse mechanical tension in the central nervous system. Almqvist and Wiksell, Stockholm

Breig A, Marions O 1963 Biomechanics of the lumbosacral nerve roots. Acta Radiologica 1:1141–1160

Bridge C J 1959 Innervation of spinal meninges and epidural structures. Anatomical Record 133:533–561

Buehler M J, Thayer D T 1988 The elbow flexion test. Clinical Orthopaedics and Related Research 233:213–216

Butler D S 1991 Mobilisation of the nervous system. Churchill Livingstone, Melbourne

Butler D S 2000 The sensitive nervous system. Noigroup, Adelaide

Butler D S, Moseley G L 2003 Explain pain. Noigroup Publications, Adelaide

Byl C, Puttlitz C, Byl N et al 2002 Strain in the median and ulnar nerves during upper-extremity positioning. Journal of Hand Therapy (Am) 27:1032–1040

Caglar Y S, Dolgun H, Ugur H C et al 2004 A ligament in the lumbar foramina: inverted Y ligament. Spine 29:1504–1507

Calvin W H, Devor M, Howe J F 1982 Can neuralgias arise from minor demyelination? Spontaneous firing, mechanosensitivity, and afterdischarge from conduction axons. Experimental Neurology 75:755–763

Chen Y, Devor M 1998 Ectopic mechanosensitivity in injured sensory axons arises from the site of spontaneous electrogenesis. European Journal of Pain 2:165–178

Cleland J, Hunt G, Palmer S 2004 Effectiveness of neural mobilization in the treatment of a subject with lower extremity peripheral neurogenic pain: a single-case design. Journal of Manual and Manipulative Therapy 12:143–152

Cleland J, Whitman J, Fritz J et al 2005 Manual physical therapy, cervical traction, and strengthening exercises in patients with cervical radiculopathy: a case series. Journal of Orthopaedic and Sports Physical Therapy 35:802–811

Coppieters M, Stappaerts K, Everaert D et al 2001 Addition of test components during neurodynamic testing: effect on range of motion and sensory responses. Journal of Orthopaedic and Sports Physical Therapy 31:226–237

Coppieters M, Van de Velde M, Stappaerts K 2002 Positioning in anesthesiology: toward a better understanding of stretch-induced perioperative neuropathies. Anesthesiology 97:75–81

Coppieters M, Stappaerts K, Wouters L et al 2003a Aberrant protective force generation during neural provocation testing and the effect of treatment in patients with neurogenic cervicobrachial pain. Journal of Manipulative and Physiological Therapeutics 26:99–106

Coppieters M, Stappaerts K, Wouters L et al 2003b The immediate effects of a cervical lateral glide treatment technique in patients with neurogenic cervicobrachial pain. Journal of Orthopaedic and Sports Physical Therapy 33:369–378

Coppieters M, Bartholomeeusen K, Stappaerts K 2004 Incorporating nerve-gliding techniques in the conservative treatment of cubital tunnel syndrome. Journal of Manipulative and Physiological Therapeutics 27:560–568

Coppieters M, Alshami A, Babri A et al 2006 Strain and excursion of the sciatic, tibial and plantar nerves during a modified straight leg raising test. Journal of Orthopaedic Research 24:1885–1889

Costigan M, Woolf C 2000 Pain: molecular mechanisms. Journal of Pain 1 (3 suppl):35–44

Cowell I M, Phillips D R 2002 Effectiveness of manipulative physiotherapy for the treatment of a neurogenic cervicobrachial pain syndrome: a single case study – experimental design. Manual Therapy 7:31–38

Cuatico W, Parker J C, Pappert E et al 1988 An anatomical and clinical investigation of spinal meningeal nerves. Acta Neurochirurgica 90:139–143

Dahlin L, McLean W G 1986 Effects of graded experimental compression on slow and fast axonal transport in rabbit vagus nerve. Journal of Neurological Science 72:19–30

Dahlin L, Lundborg G 1990 The neurone and its response to peripheral nerve compression. Journal of Hand Surgery (Br) 15:5–10

Dahlin L, Nordborg C, Lundborg G 1987 Morphological changes in nerve cell bodies induced by experimental graded compression. Experimental Neurology 95:611–621

Devor M 1991 Neuropathic pain and injured nerve: peripheral mechanisms. British Medical Bulletin 47:619–630

Devor M, Seltzer Z 1999 Pathophysiology of damaged nerves in relation to chronic pain. In: Wall P D, Melzack R (eds) Textbook of pain, 4th edn. Churchill Livingstone, Edinburgh, p 129–164

Dilley A, Lynn B, Greening J et al 2003 Quantitative in vivo studies of median nerve sliding in response to wrist, elbow, shoulder and neck movements. Clinical Biomechanics 18:899–907

Dilley A, Lynn B, Pang S J 2005 Pressure and stretch mechanosensitivity of peripheral nerve fibres following local inflammation in the nerve trunk. Pain 117:462–472

Dommisse G F (ed) 1994 The blood supply of the spinal cord and the consequences of failure, 2nd edn. Churchill Livingstone, Edinburgh.

Doubell T P, Mannion R, Woolf C J 1999 The dorsal horn: state dependent sensory processing, plasticity and the generation of pain. In: Wall P D, Melzack R (eds) Textbook of pain, 4th edn. Churchill Livingstone, Edinburgh, p 165–181

Driscoll P J, Glasby M A, Lawson G M 2002 An in vivo study of peripheral nerves in continuity: biomechanical and physiological responses to elongation. Journal of Orthopaedic Research 20:370–375

Edgar M A, Nundy S 1966 Innervation of the spinal dura mater. Journal of Neurology, Neurosurgery, and Psychiatry 29:530–534

Ekstrom R, Holden K 2002 Examination of and intervention for a patient with chronic lateral elbow pain with signs of nerve entrapment. Physical Therapy 82:1077–1086

England J D, Happel L T, Liu Z P et al 1998 Abnormal distributions of potassium channels in human neuromas. Neuroscience Letters 255:37–40

Erel E, Dilley A, Greening J et al 2003 Longitudinal sliding of the median nerve in patients with carpal tunnel syndrome. Journal of Hand Surgery (Br) 28:439–443

Farmer J, Wisneski R 1994 Cervical spine nerve root compression: an analysis of neuroforaminal pressures with varying head and arm positions. Spine 19:1850–1855

Fujiwara A, An H, Lim T et al 2001 Morphologic changes in lumbar intervertebral foramen due to flexion–extension, lateral bending and axial rotation. Spine 26:876–882

Gazda L, Milligan E, Hansen, M et al 2001 Sciatic inflammatory neuritis (SIN): behavioral allodynia is paralleled by peri-sciatic proinflammatory cytokine and superoxide production. Journal of the Peripheral Nervous System 6:111–129

George S 2002 Characteristics of patients with lower extremity symptoms treated with slump stretching: a case series. Journal of Orthopaedic and Sports Physical Therapy 32:391–398

Georgeu G A, Walbeehm E T, Tillett R et al 2005 Investigating the mechanical shear-plane between core and sheath elements of peripheral nerves. Cell and Tissue Research 320:229–234

Gifford L 1998 Pain. In: Pitt-Brooke J, Reid H, Lockwood J et al (eds) Rehabilitation of movement. WB Saunders, London, p 196–232

Gifford L 2001 Acute low cervical nerve root conditions: symptom presentations and pathobiological reasoning. Manual Therapy 6:106–115

Gifford L, Butler D 1997 The integration of pain sciences into clinical practice. Journal of Hand Therapy 10:86–95

Golovchinsky V 1998 Double crush syndrome in lower extremities. Electromyography and Clinical Neurophysiology 38:115–120

Greening J, Lynn B 1998 Minor peripheral nerve injuries: an underestimated source of pain? Manual Therapy 3:187–194

Greening J, Smart S, Leary R et al 1999 Reduced movement of the median nerve in carpal tunnel during wrist flexion in patients with non specific arm pain. Lancet 354:217–218

Grewal R, Xu J, Sotereanos D G et al 1996 Biomechanical properties of peripheral nerves. Hand Clinics 12:195–204

Grimes P, Massie J, Garfin S 2000 Anatomic and biomechanical analysis of lower lumbar foraminal ligaments. Spine 25:2009–2014

Groen G J, Baljet B, Drukker J 1988 The innervation of the spinal dura mater: anatomy and clincial implications. Acta Neurochirurgica 92:39–46

Haak R A, Kleinhaus F W, Ochs S 1976 The viscosity of mammalian nerve axoplasm measured by electron spin resonance. Journal of Physiology 263:115–137

Hall T, Elvey R 1999 Nerve trunk pain: physical diagnosis and treatment. Manual Therapy 4:63–73

Haller F R, Low F N 1971 The fine structure of the peripheral nerve sheath in the subarachnoid space in the rat and other laboratory animals. American Journal of Anatomy 131:1–20

Hanai F, Matsui N, Hongo N 1996 Changes in responses of wide dynamic range neurons in the spinal dorsal horn after dorsal root or dorsal root ganglion compression. Spine 21:1408–1415

Harden R 2005 Chronic neuropathic pain: mechanisms, diagnosis, and treatment. Neurologist 11:111–122

Hasue M 1993 Pain and the nerve root: an interdisciplinary approach. Spine 18:2053–2058

Hough A, Moore A, Jones M 2000 Measuring longitudinal nerve motion using ultrasonography. Manual Therapy 5:173–180

Howe J F, Loeser J D, Calvin W H 1977 Mechanosensitivity of dorsal root ganglia and chronically injured axons: a physiological basis for radicular pain of nerve root compression. Pain 3:25–41

Hromada J 1963 On the nerve supply of the connective tissue of some peripheral nervous system components. Acta Anatomica 55:343–351

Hunter J M 1991 Recurrent carpal tunnel syndrome, epineural fibrous fixation, and traction neuropathy. Hand Clinics 7:491–504

Igarashi T, Yabuki S, Kikuchi S et al 2005 Effect of acute nerve root compression on endoneurial fluid pressure and blood flow in rat dorsal root ganglia. Journal of Orthopaedic Research 23:420–424

Jänig W, Koltzenburg M 1990 Receptive properties of pial afferents. Pain 45:300–309

Jenis L, An H 2000 Spine update: lumbar foraminal stenosis. Spine 25:389–394

Johnson E K, Chiarello C M 1997 The slump test: the effects of head and lower extremity position on knee extension. Journal of Orthopaedic and Sports Physical Therapy 26:310–317

Johnston E C, Howell S J 1999 Tension neuropathy of the superficial peroneal nerve: associated conditions and results of release. Foot and Ankle International 20:576–580

Kallakuri S, Cavanaugh J M, Blagoev D C 1998 An immunohistochemical study of innervation of lumbar spinal dura and longitudinal ligaments. Spine 23:403–411

Kenneally M, Rubenach H, Elvey R 1988 The upper limb tension test: the SLR of the arm. In: Grant R (ed) Physical therapy of the cervical and thoracic spine. Churchill Livingstone, New York, p 167–194

Kikuchi S, Sato K, Konno S et al 1994 Anatomic and radiographic study of dorsal root ganglia. Spine 19:6–11

Kitagawa F, Fujiwara A, Kobayashi N et al 2004 Morphologic changes in the cervical neural foramen due to flexion and extension: in vivo imaging study. Spine 29:2821–2825

Kleinrensink G J, Stoeckart R, Vleeming A et al 1995 Mechanical tension in the median nerve. The effects of joint positions. Clinical Biomechanics 10:240–244

Kleinrensink G J, Stoeckart R, Mulder P G H et al 2000 Limb tension tests as tools in the diagnosis of nerve and plexus lesions. Clinical Biomechanics 15:9–14

Klingman R 1999 The pseudoradicular syndrome: a case report implicating double crush mechanisms in peripheral nerve tissue of the lower extremity. Journal of Manual and Manipulative Therapy 7:81–91

Kobayashi S, Yoshizawa H, Nakai S 2000 Experimental study on the dynamics of lumbosacral nerve root circulation. Spine 25:298–305

Koester J, Siegelbaum S 1995 Ion channels. In: Kandel E, Schwartz J, Jessell T (eds) Essentials of neural science and behavior. Appleton and Lange, Norwalk, CT, p 115–131

Kraan G A, Delwel E J, Hoogland P et al 2005 Extraforaminal ligament attachments of human lumbar nerves. Spine 30:601–605

Kumar R, Berger R, Dunsker S, Keller J 1996 Innervation of the spinal dura: myth or reality. Spine 21:18–26

Kwan M K, Wall E J, Massie J et al 1992 Strain, stress and stretch of peripheral nerve. Acta Orthopaedica Scandinavica 63:267–272

Lewis J, Ramot R, Green A 1998 Changes in mechanical tension in the median nerve: possible implications for the upper limb tension test. Physiotherapy 84:254–261

Lincoln J, Milner P, Appenzeller O et al 1993 Innervation of normal human sural and optic nerves by noradrenaline and peptide containing nervi vasorum and nervorum: effect of diabetes and alcoholism. Brain Research 632:48–56

Lindenlaub T, Sommer C 2000 Partial sciatic nerve transection as a model of neuropathic pain: a qualitative and quantitative neuropathological study. Pain 89:97–106

Liu X, Eschenfelder S, Blenk K H et al 2000 Spontaneous activity of axotomised afferent neurons after L5 spinal nerve injury in rats. Pain 84:309–318

Louis R 1981 Vertebroradicular and vertebromedullar dynamics. Anatomia Clinica 3:1–11

Lundborg G 1988 Intraneural microcirculation. Orthopedic Clinics of North America 19:1–12

Lundborg G, Dahlin L B 1992 The pathophysiology of nerve compression. Hand Clinics 8:215–227

Lundborg G, Myers R, Powell H 1983 Nerve compression injury and increased endoneurial fluid pressure: a 'miniature compartment syndrome'. Journal of Neurology, Neurosurgery and Psychiatry 46:1119–1124

McCabe J, Low F 1969 The subarachnoid angle: an area of transition in peripheral nerve. Anatomical Record 164:15–34

Mackinnon S E 1992 Double and multiple 'crush' syndromes. Hand Clinics 8:369–390

McLellan D L, Swash M 1976 Longitudinal sliding of the median nerve during movements of the upper limb. Journal of Neurology, Neurosurgery, and Psychiatry 39:566–570

Mannion R, Woolf C 2000 Pain mechanisms and management: a central perspective. Clinical Journal of Pain 16 (3 suppl):S144–S156

Matloub H, Yousif N 1992 Peripheral nerve anatomy and innervation pattern. Hand Clinics 8:201–214

Mauhart D 1990 The effect of chronic ankle inversion sprains on the plantarflexion/inversion straight leg raise test. Australian Journal of Physiotherapy 36:277

Mazurek M, Shin A 2001 Upper extremity peripheral nerve anatomy. Clinical Orthopaedics and Related Research 383:7–20

Meyer J, Kulig K, Landel R 2002 Differential diagnosis and treatment of subcalcaneal heel pain: a case report. Journal of Orthopaedic and Sports Physical Therapy 32:114–124

Millesi H, Zoch G, Riehsner R 1995 Mechanical properties of peripheral nerves. Clinical Orthopaedics and Related Research 314:76–83

Moses A, Carman J 1996 Anatomy of the cervical spine: implications for the upper limb tension test. Australian Journal of Physiotherapy 42:31–35

Muhle C, Wiskirchen J, Weinert D et al 1998 Biomechanical aspects of the subarachnoid space and cervical cord in healthy individuals examined with kinematic magnetic resonance imaging. Spine 23:556–567

Muhle C, Resnick D, Ahn J et al 2001 In vivo changes in the neuroforaminal size at flexion–extension and axial rotation of the cervical spine in healthy persons examined using kinematic magnetic resonance imaging. Spine 26:E287–E293

Murata Y, Rydevik B, Takahashi K et al 2005 Incision of the intervertebral disc induces disintegration and increases permeability of the dorsal root ganglion capsule. Spine 30:1712–1716

Murphy R 1977 Nerve roots and spinal nerves in degenerative disk disease. Clinical Orthopaedics and Related Research 129:46–60

Nakagawa H, Mikawa Y, Watanabe R 1994 Elastin in the human posterior longitudinal ligament and spinal dura: a histologic and biochemical study. Spine 19:2164–2169

Nakamura S I, Myers R R 2000 Injury to dorsal root ganglia alters innervation of spinal cord dorsal horn lamina involved in nociception. Spine 25:537–542

Neary D, Ochoa R W 1975 Sub-clinical entrapment neuropathy in man. Journal of the Neurological Sciences 24:283–298

Nee R J, Butler D 2006 Management of peripheral neuropathic pain: integrating neurobiology, neurodynamics, and clinical evidence. Physical Therapy in Sport 7:36–49

Nicholas D S, Weller R O 1988 The fine anatomy of the human spinal meninges. Journal of Neurosurgery 69:276–282

Novak C B, Mackinnon S E 1998 Nerve injury in repetitive motion disorders. Clinical Orthopaedics and Related Research 351:10–20

Novak C B, Mackinnon S E 2005 Evaluation of nerve injury and nerve compression in the upper quadrant. Journal of Hand Therapy 18:230–240

Nuckley D J, Konodi M A, Raynak G C et al 2002 Neural space integrity of the lower cervical spine: effect of normal range of motion. Spine 27:587–595

Ogata K, Naito M 1986 Blood flow of peripheral nerve: effects of dissection, stretching and compression. Journal of Hand Surgery (Br) 11:10–14

Olmarker K, Rydevik B 1991 Pathophysiology of sciatica. Orthopedic Clinics of North America 22:223–234

Olmarker K, Rydevik B 2001 Selective inhibition of tumor necrosis factor alpha prevents nucleus pulposus-induced thrombus formation, intraneural edema, and reduction of nerve conduction velocity. Spine 26:863–869

Pahor S, Toppenberg R 1996 An investigation of neural tissue involvement in ankle inversion sprains. Manual Therapy 1:192–197

Parke W W, Watanabe R 1985 The intrinsic vasculature of the lumbosacral spinal nerve roots. Spine 10:508–515

Parke W W, Whalen J L 1993 The pial ligaments of the anterior spinal artery and their stretch receptors. Spine 18:1542–1549

Parke W W, Whalen J L 2002 The vascular pattern of the human dorsal root ganglion and its probable bearing on a compartment syndrome. Spine 27:347–352

Pechan J 1973 Ulnar nerve manoeuvre as a diagnostic aid in pressure lesions in the cubital region. Ceskoslovenska Neurologie 36:13–19

Pechan J, Julis F 1975 The pressure measurement in the ulnar nerve: a contribution to the pathophysiology of cubital tunnel syndrome. Journal of Biomechanics 8:75–79

Phillips J B, Smit X, De Zoysa N et al 2004 Peripheral nerves in the rat exhibit localized heterogeneity of tensile properties during limb movement. Journal of Physiology 557:879–887

Rauschning W 1997 Anatomy and pathology of the cervical spine. In: Frymoyer J W (ed) The adult spine: principles and practice, 2nd edn. Lippincott-Raven, Philadelphia, PA

Rempel D, Dahlin L, Lundborg G 1999 Pathophysiology of nerve compression syndromes: response of peripheral nerves to loading. Journal of Bone and Joint Surgery (Am) 81A:1600–1610

Rodgers M, Cavanagh P 1984 Glossary of biomechanical terms, concepts, and units. Physical Therapy 64:1886–1902

Rossitti S 1993 Biomechanics of the pons-cord tract and its enveloping structures: An overview. Acta Neurochirurgica 124:144–152

Rozmaryn L, Dovelle S, Rothman E et al 1998 Nerve and tendon gliding exercises and the conservative management of carpal tunnel syndrome. Journal of Hand Therapy 11:171–179

Runza M, Pietrabissa R, Mantero S et al 1999 Lumbar dura mater biomechanics: experimental characterization and scanning electron microscopy observations. Anesthesia and Analgesia 88:1317–1321

Rydevik B, Lundborg G, Bagge U 1981 Effects of graded compression on intraneural blood flow. An in-vivo study on rabbit tibial nerve. Journal of Hand Surgery (Am) 6:3–12

Rydevik B, Brown M, Lundborg G 1984 Pathoanatomy and pathophysiology of nerve root compression. Spine 9:7–15

Rydevik B, Myers R, Powell H 1989 Pressure increase in the dorsal root ganglion following mechanical compression: closed compartment syndrome in nerve roots. Spine 14:574–576

Rydevik B, Holm S, Brown M et al 1990 Diffusion from cerebrospinal fluid as a nutritional pathway for spinal nerve roots. Acta Physiologica Scandinavica 138:247–248

Sammarco G J, Chalk D E, Feibel J H 1993 Tarsal tunnel syndrome and additional nerve lesions in the same limb. Foot and Ankle 14:71–77

Sauer S K, Bove G M, Averbeck B et al 1999 Rat peripheral nerve components release calcitonin gene-related peptide and prostaglandin E2 in response to noxious stimuli: evidence that the nervi nervorum are nociceptors. Neuroscience 92:319–325

Schwartz J 1995 The neuron. In: Kandel E, Schwartz J, Jessell T (eds) Essentials of neural science and behavior. Appleton and Lange, Norwalk, CT, p 45–55

Scrimshaw S, Maher C 2001 Randomized controlled trial of neural mobilization after spinal surgery. Spine 26:2647–2652

Shacklock M O 1995a Neurodynamics. Physiotherapy 81:9–16

Shacklock M O 1995b Application of neurodynamics. In: Shacklock M O (ed) Moving in on pain. Butterworth-Heinemann, Sydney, p 123–131

Shacklock M O 1999 Central pain mechanisms: a new horizon in manual therapy. Australian Journal of Physiotherapy 45:83–92

Shacklock M O 2005 Clinical neurodynamics: a new system of musculoskeletal treatment. Elsevier Butterworth Heinemann, Edinburgh

Sluka K 1996 Pain mechanisms involved in musculoskeletal disorders. Journal of Orthopaedic and Sports Physical Therapy 24:240–254

Smith S, Massie J, Chesnut R et al 1993 Straight leg raising: anatomical effects on the spinal nerve root without and with fusion. Spine 18:992–999

Stodieck L S, Beel J A, Lutges M W 1986 Structural properties of spinal nerve roots: protein composition. Experimental Neurology 91:41–51

Sugawara O, Atsuta Y, Iwahara T et al 1996 The effects of mechanical compression and hypoxia on nerve roots and dorsal root ganglia. Spine 21:2089–2094

Sunderland S 1974 Meningeal-neural relations in the intervertebral foramen. Journal of Neurosurgery 40:756–763

Sunderland S 1990 The anatomy and physiology of nerve injury. Muscle and Nerve 13:771–784

Takebayashi T, Cavanaugh J, Ozaktay A et al 2001 Effect of nucleus pulposus on the neural activity of dorsal root ganglion. Spine 26:940–945

Tal M, Eliav E 1996 Abnormal discharge originates at the site of nerve injury in experimental constriction neuropathy in the rat. Pain 64:511–518

Tal-Akabi A, Rushton A 2000 An investigation to compare the effectiveness of carpal bone mobilization and neurodynamic mobilization as methods of treatment for carpal tunnel syndrome. Manual Therapy 5:214–222

Tanaka N, Fujimoto Y, An H et al 2000 The anatomic relation among the nerve roots, intervertebral foramina, and the intervertebral discs of the cervical spine. Spine 25:286–291

Thomas P K, Olsson Y 1984 Microscopic anatomy and function of the connective tissue components of peripheral nerve. In: Dyck P J, Thomas P K, Lambert E H et al (eds) Peripheral neuropathy, 2nd edn. Saunders, Philadelphia, PA, p 97–120

Topp K S, Boyd B S 2006 Structure and biomechanics of peripheral nerves: nerve responses to physical stresses and implications for physical therapist practice. Physical Therapy 86:92–109

Triano J, Luttges M 1982 Nerve irritation: a possible model of sciatic neuritis. Spine 7:129–136

Ugbolue U C, Hsu W H, Goitz R J et al 2005 Tendon and nerve displacement at the wrist during finger movements. Clinical Biomechanics 20:50–56

Upton A R M, McComas A J 1973 The double crush in nerve entrapment syndromes. Lancet 18:359–361

Valls-Sole J, Alvarez R, Nunez M 1995 Limited longitudinal sliding of the median nerve in patients with carpal tunnel syndrome. Muscle and Nerve 18:761–767

van Meeteren N L, Brakee J H, Helders P J et al 1997 Functional recovery from sciatic nerve crush lesion in the rat correlates with individual differences in responses to chronic intermittent stress. Journal of Neuroscience Research 48:524–532

Wadhwani S, Loughenbury P, Saomes R 2004 The anterior dural (Hofmann) ligaments. Spine 29:623–627

Walbeehm E T, Afoke A, de Wit T et al 2004 Mechanical functioning of peripheral nerves: linkage with the 'mushrooming' effect. Cell and Tissue Research 316:115–121

Wall E J, Massie J B, Kwan M K et al 1992 Experimental stretch neuropathy. Journal of Bone and Joint Surgery (Br) 74B:126–129

Wall P D, Gutnick M 1974 Ongoing activity in peripheral nerves: the physiology and pharmacology of impulses originating from a neuroma. Experimental Neurology 43:580–593

Watkins L, Maier S 2004 Neuropathic pain: the immune connection. Pain Clinical Updates 13:1–4

Weinstein J 1991 Neurogenic and nonneurogenic pain and inflammatory mediators. Orthopedic Clinics of North America 22:235–246

Wilgis E, Murphy R 1986 The significance of longitudinal excursion in peripheral nerves. Hand Clinics 2:761–766

Woolf C 2004 Dissecting out mechanisms responsible for peripheral neuropathic pain: implications for diagnosis and therapy. Life Sciences 74:2605–2610

Wright T W, Glowczewski F, Wheeler D et al 1996 Excursion and strain of the median nerve. Journal of Bone and Joint Surgery (Am) 78A:1897–1903

Wright T W, Glowczewski F, Cowin D et al 2001 Ulnar nerve excursion and strain at the elbow and wrist associated with upper extremity motion. Journal of Hand Surgery (Am) 26:655–662

Wright T W, Glowczewskie F, Cowin D et al 2005 Radian nerve excursion and strain at the elbow and wrist associated with upper-extremity motion. Journal of Hand Surgery (Am) 30:990–996

Yabuki S, Kikuchi S 1996 Positions of dorsal root ganglia in the cervical spine: an anatomic and clinic study. Spine 21:1513–1517

Yabuki S, Onda A, Kikuchi S et al 2001 Prevention of compartment syndrome in dorsal root ganglia caused by exposure to nucleus pulposus. Spine 29:870–875

Yoo J U, Zou D, Edward W T et al 1992 Effect of cervical spine motion on the neuroforaminal dimensions of human cervical spine. Spine 17:1131–1136

Yoshizawa H, Kobayashi S, Hachiya Y 1991 Blood supply of nerve roots and dorsal root ganglia. Orthopedic Clinics of North America 22:195–211

Yuan Q, Dougherty L, Margulies S S 1998 In vivo human spinal cord deformation and displacement in flexion. Spine 23:1677–1683

Zoch G, Reihsner R, Beer R et al 1991 Stress and strain in peripheral nerves. Neuro-Orthopedics 10:73–82

Zochodne D W 1993 Epineurial peptides: a role in neuropathic pain? Canadian Journal of Neurological Sciences 20:69–72

Zusman M 1992 Central nervous system contribution to mechanically produced motor and sensory responses. Australian Journal of Physiotherapy 38:245–253

Cartilage

Stefano Zaffagnini, Marc Safran and Elizaveta Kon

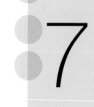

CHAPTER CONTENTS

Introduction 100

Anatomy 100

Biomechanics 102

Cartilage lesions classification 102

Treatment options 104

Conservative treatment 106

Rehabilitation 107

Future development 108

Summary 108

Introduction

Cartilage is an important tissue found in many places around the human body. It has several purposes (depending on the type of cartilage) including providing a smooth surface for the movement of articulating bones within joints, and providing a framework upon which bone deposition can begin. This chapter will outline the anatomy and biomechanics of cartilage, present classification systems to describe cartilage lesions and discuss a variety of treatment options for damaged cartilage, including both reparative and regenerative techniques, and conservative treatment options.

Anatomy

The simple homogeneous appearance of cartilage at gross and light microscopic levels hides a highly ordered complex structure that gives cartilage properties unmatched by any available substitute. Cartilage consists of cells (i.e. chondrocytes) embedded in an abundant extracellular matrix. Unlike the situation in parenchymal tissue, chondrocyte cells contribute relatively little to the total volume of cartilage, usually 10% or less (Hamerman et al 1970, Stockwell 1978). The important functional properties of cartilage, including stiffness, durability and distribution of load, depend on the extracellular matrix. The cartilage matrix is not homogeneous, nor does it consist primarily of collagen. The largest component of the matrix is water, and an elaborate framework of macromolecules including collagens, proteoglycans and noncollagenous proteins organizes and maintains water in the matrix.

Tissue fluid contributes 60 to 80% of the wet weight of cartilage and consists of water with dissolved gases, small proteins and metabolites (Linn & Sokoloff 1965, Maroudas & Schneiderman 1987). Because the cells rely on diffusion of nutrients and metabolites through the matrix rather than on a vascular supply, chondrocyte function also depends on the interaction of the tissue fluid and the matrix macromolecules. Details of the interaction between the tissue fluid and the matrix molecules remain uncertain, but since the tissue fluid can exchange with water outside the tissue, and small solutes can move freely in the cartilage tissue fluid, the water must be loosely bound to the molecular framework in a way that maintains the hydration of the tissue but still allows exchange with fluid outside the tissue (Torzilli et al 1982).

The structural macromolecules contribute 20 to 40% of the wet weight of cartilage and include collagens, proteoglycans and noncollagenous proteins or glycoproteins. In most cartilage, collagen contributes about 50% of the tissue's dry weight, proteoglycans contribute 30 to 35% and noncollagenous proteins and glycoproteins contribute about 15 to 20% (Buckwalter 1983). Collagen forms the fibrillar meshwork that gives cartilage its tensile strength and form (Kempson 1980).

The principal collagen of articular cartilage, type II, forms the characteristic cross-banded fibrils seen by electron microscopy and accounts for 90 to 95% of the total cartilage collagen. Cartilage also contains at least two quantitatively minor collagens, types IX and XI. In addition, Apone and associates (1987) reported the presence of types V and VI collagens within articular cartilage. The function and interrelationships of the quantitatively minor collagens remain unclear but it has been suggested that they may contribute to the formation and stability of the type II collagen fibril meshwork (Mayne & Irwin 1986).

Type II collagen is normally found in tissues with higher proteoglycan and water contents, suggesting that type II has specific properties that allow it to establish an ordered relationship with proteoglycans, thus helping to create and maintain a highly hydrated matrix.

Proteoglycans form the major macromolecule of cartilage ground substance. They have multiple forms, including large aggregating proteoglycans that exist as individual monomers or as aggregates containing multiple monomers, large nonaggregating proteoglycans and small nonaggregating proteoglycans (Hascall 1977, Heinegard & Paulson 1984).

The glycosaminoglycans, chondroitin sulfate and keratan sulfate, constitute about 95% of the molecule and protein contributes about 5%. The protein core filament consists of three regions: the hyaluronic acid-binding region, the keratan sulfate-rich region and the chondroitin sulfate-rich region (Heinegard & Alexsson 1977).

In the matrix, most of the aggregating proteoglycan monomers associate with hyaluronic acid filaments and link proteins to form aggregates. Hyaluronic acid forms the backbone of the aggregate, and may range in length from several hundred nanometers with a few associated monomers to more than 10 000 nm with more than 300 monomers (Hardingham & Muir 1973). The importance of aggregate formation is not entirely clear. It may help anchor monomers within the matrix, prevent their displacement, organize and stabilize the relationship between proteoglycan monomers and type II collagen fibrils and help control the flow of water through the matrix (Mow et al 1984a). Because of their ability to interact with tissue fluid, proteoglycans help to give cartilage its stiffness, compression and resilience, and durability as a joint surface.

Evidence indicates that the structure and composition of aggregating cartilage proteoglycans change with age (Buckwalter et al 1985). With increasing age, the keratan sulfate and protein content of monomers increases, the chondroitin sulfate content decreases, chondroitin sulfate chains become shorter, average monomer size decreases and the variability in monomer size increases (Buckwalter et al 1985). In addition, link proteins may fragment, the concentration of functional link protein decreases, aggregates become smaller, the proportion of monomers that aggregate decreases, hyaluronate filament length decreases and the proportion of hyaluronic acid-binding region fragments of the protein core may increase with age (Buckwalter & Roughly 1987, Plaas & Sandy 1984). These changes may be caused by age-related alterations in chondrocyte synthetic function, by degradation of proteoglycans in the matrix or by a combination of the two.

Although less is known about noncollagenous proteins than about either collagens or proteoglycans, they form a significant component of the macromolecular framework. It appears that at least some of these molecules help organize and maintain the macromolecular structure of the matrix and the relationship between the chondrocytes and the matrix. The material properties of cartilage depend on its extracellular matrix but the existence and maintenance of the matrix depends on chondrocytes. Changes in matrix composition such as a decrease in proteoglycan content, the loss of type II collagen and an increase or decrease in hyaluronic acid concentration alter chondrocyte synthetic function. The matrix may also transmit mechanical signals to chondrocytes through changes in tension on the cell membrane, or it may act as an electromechanical transducer. During formation of articular cartilage, chondrocytes proliferate rapidly and synthesize large volumes of matrix. With maturation, these processes slow and the cell numerical density decreases.

Articular cartilage is often described in terms of its layers or zones: the superficial zone, the middle or transition zone, the deep or radial zone and the zone of calcified cartilage. Within these layers or zones, distinct matrix regions or compartments can be identified, including the pericellular matrix, the territorial matrix and the interterritorial matrix (Poole et al 1984, Schenk et al 1986).

The thinnest of the zones, the superficial zone, forms the gliding surface of the joint. Directly adjacent to the joint lies a thin cell-free layer of matrix. It consists primarily of fine fibrils with little polysaccharide. This most superficial layer presumably corresponds to the thin, clear film that can be mechanically stripped from articular cartilage, and it also probably represents the 'lamina splendens', so named because phase-contrast studies of articular cartilage sections show a conspicuous bright layer at the articular surface.

The transitional (middle) zone occupies several times the volume of the superficial zone. The cells become more spherical and fill their cytoplasm with endoplasmic reticulum, golgi membranes, mitochondria, glycogen and occasionally intracytoplasmic filaments. The collagen fibrils of this zone are larger than those of the superficial zone.

The deep (radial) zone usually forms the largest part of articular cartilage. The cells resemble the spheroidal cells in the transitional zone, but tend to arrange themselves in an almost columnar pattern perpendicular to the joint surface. This zone contains the largest collagen fibrils of articular cartilage and has the highest proteoglycan content as well as the lowest water content.

The zone of calcified cartilage separates the softer hyaline cartilage from the stiffer subchondral bone. Collagen fibrils of the radial zone penetrate directly into the calcified cartilage.

The differences in matrix composition and organization among zones reflect differences in mechanical function. The superficial zone primarily resists shearing forces, the transitional zone allows the change in orientation of collagen fibrils from the superficial zone to the radial zone and the radial zone primarily helps to resist and distribute compressive loads. The zone of calcified cartilage provides a transition in material properties between hyaline cartilage and bone, as well as anchors the hyaline cartilage to the bone.

Biomechanics

In diarthrodial joints, articular cartilage serves as a wear-resistant (Lipshitz et al 1980), smooth (Clarke 1971), near-frictionless (Mann & McCutchen 1997) and load-bearing (Ahmed 1983, Ahmed & Burke 1983) surface. The composition and physico-chemical properties of articular cartilage (Maroudas 1975), the ultrastructural organization of the collagen network (Poole et al 1984) and molecular organization of collagen and proteoglycans (Nimni 1974) all have profound influences on the intrinsic mechanical properties of the extracellular matrix as well as on fluid transport and diffusional properties of the tissue (Mow et al 1980, 1984b).

The tensile properties of articular cartilage have been determined in a number of studies (e.g. Akizuki et al 1986, 1987). These studies have shown that adult articular cartilage is highly inhomogeneous, that is, there is a pronounced variation of tensile stiffness and strength with depth. Specimens from the superficial zone have much higher stiffness and failure stresses than those of the deeper zones (Akizuki et al 1986, Poole et al 1984). These tensile characteristics are consistent with collagen composition data and our understanding of the ultrastructural organization of cartilage.

Articular cartilage is anisotropic, meaning that its material properties are different for tissue specimens obtained from different orientations relative to the joint surface (Akizuki et al 1986, Woo et al 1980). It is thought that this anisotropy is related to the varying collagen fibril arrangements within the planes parallel to the articular surface. In tension, this anisotrophy is usually described with respect to the direction of the articular surface 'split lines' pattern (Mow et al 1984a).

When an external load is applied to the cartilage, there is an instantaneous deformation caused primarily by a change in the proteoglycan molecular domain. This external load can also cause the interstitial fluid pressure in the porous solid matrix to exceed the Donnan osmotic swelling pressure; consequently, the interstitial fluid begins to flow and exudation occurs (Mow & Rosenwasser 1991).

Collagen and proteoglycan, as well as the organization of the collagen and proteoglycan matrix, contribute to the tensile properties of the matrix (Akizuki et al 1987). The shear stiffness of articular cartilage must also be derived from its collagen content or from the collagen–proteoglycan interaction (Mow et al 1984b). Disruption of the collagen network may be a key factor leading to the development of osteoarthritis. Also, loosening of the collagen network is generally believed to be responsible for the increased swelling, and thus water content, and loss of proteoglycans in osteoarthritic cartilage (Mankin & Thrasher 1975). Also Milentijevic & Torzilli (2005) and Milentijevic et al (2005) have shown that after impact, cell death from the superficial layer is the start of the degradation process of osteoarthritis. In other words, loss of the lamina splendans may be all that is necessary to begin the progressive and irreversible process of degenerative arthritis.

In summary, collagen and proteoglycan macromolecules interact to form a porous, composite, fiber-reinforced matrix possessing all the essential mechanical characteristics of a solid swollen with water and able to resist the stresses and strain of joint articulation. A strong correlation between cartilage component interactions and the material and mechanical properties of normal articular cartilage has been demonstrated.

The intrinsic compressive modulus, Ha, is approximately 0.8 MPa for both human and bovine cartilage (Woo et al 1987). These coefficients are intrinsic material properties of the porous collagen–proteoglycan solid matrix.

Under physiologic loading conditions, excessive stress levels are difficult to maintain in cartilage since stress relaxation rapidly attenuates the stress. This must necessarily lead to the rapid spreading of the contact area in the joint during articulation.

Articular cartilage also exhibits viscoelastic behavior under tension (Simon et al 1984, Woo et al 1987). This viscoelastic behavior is attributable to both the internal friction associated with the molecular motion of collagen and proteoglycan (Woo et al 1987) and the flow of the interstitial fluid (Simon et al 1984).

With normal compressive physiologic loading, articular cartilage undergoes surface compaction with the lubricating fluid being exuded through this compacted region near the surface. As described above, however, fluid redistribution within the articular cartilage occurs with time to relieve the stress in this compact region. This process of stress regulation takes place quite quickly; the stress may decrease by 63% within two to five seconds (Mow et al 1980, 1984b). If, however, loads are applied so quickly that there is insufficient time for internal fluid redistribution to relieve the compacted region, the high stresses produced in the collagen–proteoglycan matrix may produce damage. This phenomenon could well explain why Radin et al (1984) and Radin & Paul (1971) found dramatic articular cartilage damage with repeated impact loads. Thus, failure of cartilage occurs as an imbalance between biomechanical wear rates and the ability of the chondrocytes to maintain the extracellular matrix.

Cartilage lesions classification

A number of classifications have been used to evaluate the severity of cartilaginous lesions, in order to choose the most

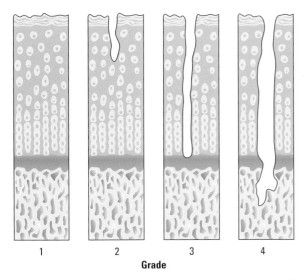

Figure 7.1 • The Outerbridge Morphological Classification. Grade 1: the articular surface is swollen, soft and edematous, and is covered with vesicles. Grade 2: includes non-full-depth lesions, with superficial fissurations that do not reach the subchondral bone. The lesions are never larger than 1.5 cm. Grade 3: the lesions reach the subchondral bone and are larger than 1.5 cm in diameter. Grade 4: there are full-depth cartilage erosions that include the subchondral bone, exposing it.

Table 7.1 The Outerbridge Morphological Classification (Outerbridge 1961)

Grade 1	The articular surface is swollen, soft and edematous, and is covered with vesicles
Grade 2	Includes non-full-depth lesions, with superficial fissurations that do not reach the subchondral bone. The lesions are never larger than 1.5 cm
Grade 3	The lesions reach the subchondral bone and are larger than 1.5 cm in diameter
Grade 4	There are full-depth cartilage erosions that include the subchondral bone, exposing it

efficient and adequate method of intervention, and thus restore a good articular function – improving the patients' quality of life and, more importantly, preventing the progressive degeneration towards early arthrosis.

Pathogenic cause classification

As many conditions can lead to chondropathies, the pathogenic cause classification divides these conditions into four principal groups: the osteochondral dystrophies, the osteochondroses, the osteonecroses and the arthrosynovites. The latter can be divided into septic (caused by bacteria, fungi, viruses and parasites) and aseptic (traumatic, inflammatory, degenerative, metabolic and tumoral) causes.

Morphological classifications

Morphological classifications suggest that a cartilaginous lesion develops in a step-by-step sequence whereby repeated trauma leads to swelling of the cartilage with a progressive increase in the diameter of the collagen fibers and eventual changes in the relationships between the collagen fibers and the proteoglycans. The most frequently used morphological classification is the Outerbridge Classification (Outerbridge 1961), which divides the cartilaginous lesions into four grades (Fig. 7.1, Table 7.1).

Some authors have proposed other classifications based on morphological changes such as the International Cartilage Repair

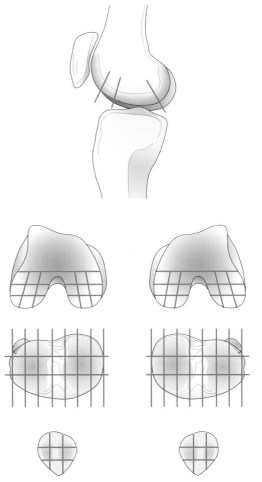

Figure 7.2 • Classification of the articular cartilage lesions based on their site and their extension, using a subdivision into quadrants.

Society (ICRS) (Brittberg 2000) and Noyes–Stabler (Noyes & Stabler 1989) criteria. Aspects that must be taken into consideration other than the lesions' grade are the site and the extent of the lesion. A precise subdivision in quadrants allows an exact representation of the site of the lesion (Fig. 7.2).

Treatment options

Many authors (Browne & Branch 2000, Minas 2001, Ochi et al 2002) suggest that articular cartilage does not regenerate. The regeneration capacity of cartilage is limited due to its isolation from systemic regulation, and its lack of vasculature and nerve supply (Buckwalter & Mankin 1997a, 1997b, Ochi et al 2002, Sgaglione et al 2002). The interaction between the cells, collagen framework, aggrecan and fluid constitute the complex biomechanical nature of hyaline cartilage making it difficult to replace or reproduce. This is probably the reason why operative management such as the use of continuous passive motion or arthroscopic lavage has shown low capacity to heal a cartilage defect (Sgaglione et al 2002).

A great variety of surgical options have been proposed for the treatment of partial or full-thickness cartilage lesions. They can be divided into reparative, reconstructive and regenerative techniques, but first, we will discuss the factors required for cartilage healing.

Factors required for cartilage healing

As stated above, cartilage has a poor capacity to heal, partly due to its lack of blood and nerve supply, low cellularity, complex architecture, low cellular turnover and isolation from systemic regulation. As a result, it also has a poor capacity for regeneration and has continued to be a source of scientific investigation into optimizing repair or regenerative techniques. The basics of cartilage healing is grounded on the presence of cells, having a matrix to attach to, having the correct environment of signal mediators and growth factors and, lastly, the appropriate mechanical environment.

Of the factors required for healing of cartilage, cells are needed first and foremost. These cells ideally are chondrocytes themselves, but may also be mesenchymal stem cells, the precursors to chondrocytes. How the cells respond to factors such as growth factors and similar cytokines, and the response to mechanical stimuli, will be affected. The cell specific factors include number, density, age, phenotype and cellular response to cues. Thus, having cells only will not result in repair or restoration of articular cartilage. The environment in which the cells exist is also crucial. This includes a matrix or bed for the cells to attach to. Then a variety of different signal mediators are needed to allow for proliferation, differentiation and production of extracellular matrix and proteins. The interaction between the cells and signal mediators, in particular the timing and number, is critical for appropriate growth, differentiation and phenotypic expression. The interplay of these different cytokines and cellular mediators with the cell receptors is very complex and still being studied. Lastly, there is the environment to which the cells are subjected – specifically, the mechanical stresses of compression, shear and the amount and timing of such. Much work has been done in this area, beginning with the work of Salter et al (1980) on the role of continuous passive motion (CPM) on cartilage defects and healing in rabbit chondral defects. Research has shown that cartilage responds differently to different forces, including a positive response to intermittent compression forces (Adams 2006, Mizuno et al 2002, Schumann et al 2006).

Recent work has attempted to augment the normal response of cartilage to injury. Research has focused on adding matrix to injured areas to serve as a scaffold for mesenchymal stem cells (Hoemann et al 2005), growing chondrocytes ex vivo and reintroduced (e.g. autologous chondrocyte implantation (ACI), MACI, Hyaff, Neocart) with and without matrices to support them (Grigolo et al 2005, Marcacci et al 2005a), and introducing growth factors directly or through the advent of gene therapy or viral vectors (Brower-Toland et al 2001, Caplan 2000, Carlberg et al 2001, Gelse et al 2003, Goodrich 2002, Palmer et al 2002, Trippel et al 2004). A combination of gene therapy with other techniques has also been attempted in the laboratory and will likely be required to solve this difficult problem (Chen et al 2003, Grande et al 2003).

Reparative techniques

Reparative techniques are directed to the recruitment of bone marrow cells to obtain potential cartilage precursors. Many marrow stimulation techniques have been developed to allow stem cell migration from the marrow cavity to the fibrin clot of the defect (Peterson et al 2000); however, these treatment options such as abrasion, drilling and microfracture produce a predominantly fibrous repair tissue, with mostly type I collagen fibers and an unorganized matrix (Peterson et al 2000, 2002) which lacks the biomechanical and viscoelastic characteristics of normal hyaline cartilage (Ochi et al 2002, Peterson et al 2000).

Steadman et al (2003a) reported encouraging results after 11 years follow-up from microfracture technique. However, patients may have had to adjust their activity level to that of their 'good' knee function, and the authors stressed the importance of a meticulous postoperative program that includes the use of CPM and 8 weeks of restricted weight bearing. This technique is simple but the repair tissue response can be unpredictable and variable. It also still remains unclear which stress is optimal for cartilage regeneration. Nehrer et al (1999) has frequently found fibrous soft, spongiform tissue combined with central degeneration in the defect. Moreover, clinical failure has been observed at a mean time of 21 months after treatment.

Techniques for repairing cartilage defects have been partially successful in reducing pain and increasing mobility (Steadman et al 2003b). However, the failure rate is quite high and no well-established solution to this problem has yet been found.

Reconstructive techniques

Reconstructive techniques are based on the autologous or homologous osteochondral unit transfer (with underlying bone), in order to capitalize on bone-to-bone healing, since the cartilaginous cup itself does not bond to the recipient bone or cartilage and maintains the normal tidemark of bone–cartilage integration. Osteochondral graft insertion is a promising procedure because it is single-stage and guarantees an immediate reliable tissue transfer of a viable osteochondral unit.

Autologous osteochondral grafting

Various ways of using autografts for osteochondral defect reconstruction have been advocated. They differ in donor site, methods of application and fixation of the grafts (Ahmad et al 2001, Duchov et al 2000, Jerosch et al 2000). An autologous osteochondral graft can be applied by arthroscopic or open surgery, according to the size of the articular defect and the surgical approach options (Bobic 1996, Hangody et al 1997a, Marcacci et al 1999, Matsusue et al 1993).

Osteochondral autograft transfer proposed by Hangody et al (1998) can be used in symptomatic unipolar grade IV distal femoral condyle lesions with a size between 1 and 2.5 cm in diameter. Many authors have reported encouraging results in small to medium sized full-thickness chondral lesions. Hangody & Fules (2003) reported 91% good and excellent clinical results at medium- to long-term follow-up, and other authors (Berlet et al 1999, Bobic 1996, Imhoff et al 1999, Jakob et al 2002, Laprell & Peterson 2001, Marcacci et al 2005a, Maynou et al 1998, Pearce et al 2001) have also shown encouraging results in 80–90% of patients with short- to medium-term follow-up.

Osteochondral autograft transfer is technically demanding and the location of the donor site and the size of the harvested grafts play a key role. The complete coverage of the defect and the mechanical stability of the plugs mean that the possibility to restore a congruent level with the healthy cartilage is critical and difficult to achieve (Koh et al 2004, 2006). Moreover there is a significant limitation of graft availability that severely reduces the possibility to use this procedure.

Osteochondral allograft

Fresh and deep-frozen allografts are widely used for treatment of large and deep osteochondral lesions. The most important survivorship studies (Beaver et al 1992, Gross et al 2005, Shasha et al 2002) have shown 75–95% of graft survival at 5 years after transplantation; however, this decreases to 63–65% at 14–15 years follow-up. Other authors have reported a lower rate of success and report variable success rates that greatly differed depending on the patient's age, the grade of joint destruction and the defect etiology (Garrett 1986, McDermott et al 1985, Meyers et al 1989). Most hypothesize that the high failure rate is due to an immune response of the host to allogenic bone (Phipatanakul et al 2004). Some investigators have suggested that clinically successful osteochondral allograft can 'buy time' for patients who have disabling pain that has not been relieved by other surgical procedures and for those who are too young for total knee replacement (Meyers et al 1989). Our opinion is that this type of treatment should not be recommended to the young active patient.

Regenerative techniques

Autologous chondrocytes transplantation

The use of autologous chondrocyte transplantation was initiated in the 1980s. Several studies have shown the ability to stimulate chondrocyte reproduction in vitro (Brittberg et al 2001), and animal studies have demonstrated the production of hyaline-like repair tissue when cultured chondrocytes were implanted (Peterson et al 2002).

The first clinical report (Brittberg et al 1994) showed highly satisfactory results with biopsy samples demonstrating hyaline-like cartilage. Since being introduced in Sweden, autologous chondrocyte implantation (ACI) has gained increasing acceptance as a technique to restore articular cartilage lesions. Researchers have reported encouraging early clinical results, especially for femoral condylar chondral lesions (Peterson et al 2002).

Peterson et al (2002) has shown durability of the early results obtained with the ACI technique: after 2 years, 50 of 61 patients had good to excellent results. At 5 to 11 years follow-up 51 of 61 patients had satisfactory results. The biomechanical evaluation of the grafted area by means of indentation probe demonstrated treated lesion stiffness to be 90% or more of normal cartilage. The outcome of this study has demonstrated that 84 to 91% of patients were able to achieve good to excellent results and return to an active lifestyle.

According to most authors (Buckwalter & Mankin 1997b, Minas 2001, Peterson et al 2000, 2002, Sgaglione et al 2002) ACI is a safe, effective and reproducible treatment that should be considered a viable option for young patients (with cartilage lesions greater than $2\,cm^2$) who want to resume an active lifestyle and restore a so-called 'normal cartilage'. However, these good results have to be weighed against the number of problems that can be observed with the standard ACI methods (Wood et al 2006). Such problems include the difficulty in handling a delicate liquid suspension of chondrocytes during surgery, the need to make a hermetic periosteum seal using sutures, the requirement of a second open surgery operation, the very long rehabilitation period and possible complications related to the use of a periosteal flap. In the original ACI technique, the liquid chondrocyte suspension was difficult to handle during surgery. The suspension has no structural integrity, and requires a patch to hold the cells in position within the defect that is to be treated; a periosteal flap is typically used. The surgical technique of suturing the periosteal flap is long, tedious and often very difficult. Recent prospective studies (Browne & Branch 2000, Knutsen et al 2004) have not completely clarified the better performance of the ACI technique compared to other procedures used for cartilage repair. Knutsen et al (2004), in particular, reported similar results using microfracture or traditional ACI techniques at 2 years follow-up. The surgical technique is long, technically demanding and requires a large joint exposure. These factors increase the morbidity of the ACI method and carry with it a high risk of joint stiffness and arthrofibrosis. Micheli et al (2001) and Anderson et al (2003) have shown a re-operation rate up to 42% due to joint stiffness. Further, the maintenance of chondrocyte phenotype during a prolonged monolayer culture is critical. In fact, chondrocytes tend to loose their ability to form matrix and produce mainly collagen type I (Ochi et al 2002).

Second-generation autologous chondrocyte transplantation

In an attempt to avoid the aforementioned technical problems associated with ACI, new cell-based tissue engineering technologies that create cartilage-like tissue using a three-dimensional culture system have been developed. This second-generation cartilage repair strategy aims to reduce morbidity, improve cell culture biology and ultimately improve clinical results. The in-vitro three-dimensional cartilage regeneration is performed with chondrocytes seeded onto a bioresorbable polymeric scaffold. Actually there are several scaffolds (polymeric, collagen, hyaluronan) proposed for clinical application. Our clinical experience is based on the utilization of a scaffold entirely based on the benzylic ester of hyaluronic acid (HYAFF® 11, Fidia Advanced Biopolymers Laboratories, Padova, Italy); it consists of a network of 20 μm-thick fibers with interstices of variable sizes, which has been demonstrated to be an optimal physical support to allow cell–cell contact, cluster formation and extracellular matrix deposition (Brun et al 1999, Grigolo et al 2001, 2002). The cells harvested from the patient are expanded and then seeded onto the scaffold to create the tissue-engineered product Hyalograft C®. Seeded on the scaffold the cells are able to redifferentiate and to retain a chondrocytic phenotype even after a long period of in vitro expansion in monolayer culture (Aigner et al 1998, Campoccia et al 1998, Pavesio et al 2003).

We have started to use Hyalograft C to treat symptomatic cartilage lesions. HYAFF possesses handling characteristics that can be implanted using mini-open (limited arthrotomy) or arthroscopic techniques (Marcacci et al 2002, 2005a) (Fig. 7.3): the use of either of these methods is largely dependent upon the location of the defect. The HYAFF scaffold is hydrophilic, and if the patch is correctly positioned inside a prepared defect, a tensioactive pressure facilitates a natural fixation of the patch that does not require the use of fibrin glue, sutures or a periosteal cover. By eliminating the need for a periosteal cover, an arthroscopic implant procedure that simplified this two-stage procedure was developed (Marcacci et al 2002). This approach reduces morbidity and improves upon the original ACI cell based repair technique.

Conservative treatment

The direct effect of repetitive impact torsional loading on articular cartilage during exercise or sport, especially in the presence of abnormal alignment or muscle weakness, elevates the risk for subsequent joint degeneration (Buckwalter & Lane 1997). Early osteoarthritis in young athletes has been associated with severe anterolateral knee instability (Grahm & Fairclough 1998, Roos

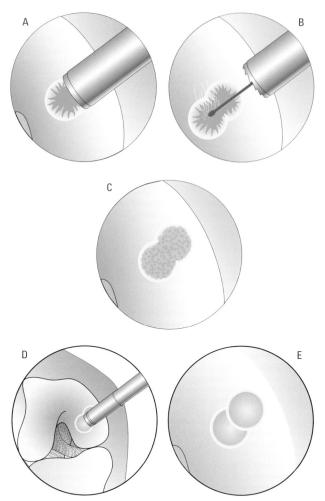

Figure 7.3 • Operative technique of second-generation autologous chondrocyte transplantation. **A:** With the sharp edge of delivery system the sizing and mapping of the lesion is performed. **B:** With a low-profile and slow-speed drill, preparation of the area is performed avoiding lesion of the subchondral bone. **C:** Prepared surface of the chondral lesion after drilling. **D:** The tamp is pushed in the delivery system to precisely plug the stamp in the defect. **E:** Complete coverage of the defect by two implanted patches after irrigation removal from the joint.

1998), but impact loading can also produce structural damage and osteoarthritic like changes (Levin et al 2001).

Traumatic insults of sufficient magnitude may also release cartilage fragments that can be responsible not only for the chondral defect, but also for a secondary inflammatory reaction (Howell et al 1983). This joint inflammation contributes to the cartilage degeneration mediated by the action of proteases and inflammatory cytokines.

The number of athletes with acute injuries to the joints and those with subacute or chronic joint pain has grown (Centers for Disease Control and Prevention 2002). Presently a narrow spectrum of satisfactory nonoperative treatment regimes is available for such patients. However, conservative treatment must still be the initial treatment choice for most patients with cartilage lesions considering the variable and inconsistent results of operative treatment modalities. For example, Dozin et al (2005) compared ACI with mosaicplasty, and found that 47% of the recruited patients healed after 6 months without any surgical treatment. Knutsen et al (2004) found no clinical and histological differences at 2 years follow-up between ACI and microfracture technique for the treatment of cartilage defects. These studies confirm that many unknown variables regulate the inflammatory and repair response of the joint after a cartilage injury, and it is unclear what factors exist that can restore normal function or determine a severe loss of function.

Conservative treatment should assist or provide an environment to improve or enhance the biological response by correct mechanical stimuli or correct pharmacological support with the aim of inducing healing of cartilage and reduction of symptoms. The therapeutic modalities that can be used for conservative treatment include physical therapy, medication, infiltration and magnetic fields. Many rehabilitation protocols limit weight bearing on the chondral injured knee for a certain period of time; however, no evidence based medicine studies have demonstrated a detrimental effect of a physiologic level of impact loading (Donohue et al 1983). On the contrary, normal loading of the knee positively influences the metabolic activity of articular cartilage (DePalma et al 1966) and allows for better regulation of matrix metabolism (Sah et al 1989). Caution should be noted, however, as strenuous activity can significantly deteriorate the cartilage (Jurvelin et al 1990, Säämänen 1989). Marder et al (2005) reported no difference in clinical outcome between patients undergoing weight bearing or non weight-bearing rehabilitation following microfracture surgery.

Water rehabilitation exercises are fundamental in allowing movement while also adding positive pressure on the lower body. This type of exercise is effective in reducing ground reaction forces while also facilitating gait (Eastlack et al 2005).

Another therapeutic modality that could have an important impact in the future treatment and prevention of articular cartilage injuries is the use of magnetic fields. It has been shown (Fini et al 2005) that the use of magnetic fields in vitro contribute to the reduction of articular cartilage inflammation and the subchondral bone injury. Moreover it reduces the catabolic effect of inflammatory cytokines on the articular chondrocytes and increases the metabolic activity of chondrocytes by increasing proteoglycan synthesis (Aaron & Plaas 1987, Aaron et al 1987). Despite the efficacy demonstrated in in vitro studies, prospective and randomized studies are needed to validate the use of magnetic fields in a clinical environment. This modality may be useful in chronic cases to reduce inflammation in athletes, to prevent the catabolic response of repetitive microtrauma or even after a surgical procedure to enhance the healing capacity of articular cartilage. The methodologies described are now some of the more advanced therapies used to conservatively treat articular cartilage lesions.

There continues to be a tremendous quest for knowledge of the biological behavior of the chondrocyte and its metabolism that could allow for a better, more research-based method of treatment to improve the conservative and surgical treatment options proposed.

Rehabilitation

It is beyond the scope of this chapter to detail the rehabilitation of each different cartilage surgical procedure; thus only a review of the general concepts will be provided. Some aspects of rehabilitation have also been outlined in section above.

As with all rehabilitation, an individualized approach is important, and certainly this is true with articular cartilage treatments. There are several individual specific variables that may influence the outcome of the treatment. These include the exact location of the lesion, whether it is surrounded by normal cartilage (contained) or not, its size, depth and the integrity of the surrounding and opposing articular cartilage. The quality of each individual's articular cartilage is the result of several factors, including the patient's age, height, weight, body mass index, extremity alignment, general health, nutrition and history of previous or concomitant injuries (meniscal or ligamentous) or surgery (Cohen et al 1998).

An important principle of articular cartilage rehabilitation involves creating an environment that facilitates the healing process while avoiding potentially deleterious forces to the repair site. Knowledge of the healing and maturation process following different articular cartilage repair procedures (Brittberg et al 1994, 1996, Peterson et al 2000, 2002) can ensure that excessive forces or other factors are not introduced too early to disrupt the healing.

The four biological phases of the cartilage maturation process are the proliferation, transitional, remodeling and maturation phases (Brittberg et al 1994, 1996, Frisbie et al 2003, Hangody et al 1997b, Nam et al 2004, Peterson et al 2000, 2002). The duration of each phase will vary depending on the lesion, patient and the specifics of the surgery discussed previously; however, the concepts of each phase are consistent.

The first phase of cartilage healing, the proliferation phase, requires protection of the repair and typically involves the first 4 to 6 weeks following surgery (Brittberg et al 1994, 1996, Frisbie et al 2003, Hangody et al 1997b, Nam et al 2004, Peterson et al 2000, 2002). Two of the most important aspects of rehabilitation of articular cartilage procedures, especially in this protective phase, are weight-bearing restrictions and range of motion (ROM) limitations. Complete unloading and immobilization, however, have been shown to have a detrimental effect on healing articular cartilage, resulting in proteoglycan loss and gradual weakening (Behrens et al 1989, Haapala et al 2000, Vanwanseele et al 2002). Therefore, controlled weight bearing (pool therapy or platform unloading) and ROM are essential to facilitate healing, prevent degeneration, nourish healing cartilage and limit the formation of adhesions. This gradual progression has been shown to stimulate matrix production and improve the tissue's mechanical properties (Buckwalter & Mankin 1997a, 1997b, Kim et al 1991, Salter 2004, Salter et al 1980, Williams et al 1994).

The second phase, known as the transition phase, usually occurs from weeks 4 through 12 postsurgery (Brittberg et al 1994, 1996, Frisbie et al 2003, Hangody et al 1997b, Nam et al 2004, Peterson et al 2000, 2002). The repair tissue is generally maturing and gaining strength. During this phase, the rehabilitation progresses, including progression from partial to full weight bearing while full ROM and soft tissue flexibility are achieved. The rehabilitation program will gradually progress with regard to strengthening activities as the patient's weight bearing status returns to normal.

The remodeling phase is the third phase of cartilage healing and usually takes place 3 to 6 months postoperation (Brittberg et al 1994, 1996, Frisbie et al 2003, Hangody et al 1997b, Nam et al 2004, Peterson et al 2000, 2002). During this phase there is a continuous remodeling of tissue into a more organized structure (Brittberg et al 1994, 1996, Frisbie et al 2003, Hangody et al 1997b, Nam et al 2004, Peterson et al 2000, 2002) that is increasing in strength and durability. As the tissue becomes firmer, and, ideally, integrated, rehabilitation is generally progressed to include more functional training activities. Low to moderate impact activities such as bicycle riding, golfing and recreational walking are usually begun.

The fourth and final phase, described as the maturation phase, begins somewhere between 4 and 6 months, and can last up to 18 months postsurgery (Brittberg et al 1994, 1996, Frisbie et al 2003, Hangody et al 1997b, Nam et al 2004, Peterson et al 2000, 2002). It is during this phase that the repair tissue reaches its full maturation and the patient can return to full preinjury activities as tolerated. The duration of this phase varies based on several factors such as lesion size and location, and the specific surgical procedure performed. Most procedures are designed to restore basic function to the individual rather than for a return to high-impact sport and exercise activities. Thus, while impact-loading activities can be gradually introduced, there is significant controversy about whether a patient should return to these activities after surgical intervention for chondral loss, especially if the lesion is large or unconstrained. Nonetheless, return to competitive sport has been reported for microfracture (Gudas et al 2005, Steadman et al 2003a), osteochondral autologous transplantation (OATS) (Gudas et al 2005, Lahav et al 2006, Marcacci et al 2005b) and ACI (Mithofer et al 2005a, 2005b) procedures with good results. However, long-term outcomes are pending and the consequences to the athletes are a potential concern.

Future development

The future of the treatment for cartilage defects will probably focus on less invasive and more accurate surgical procedures that may allow a complete restoration of healthy hyaline cartilage in severe defects. The treatment of small lesions, and even more importantly the prevention of this pathology, especially in young sport and exercise participants, we believe will move towards a complete noninvasive approach such as medication.

A number of research studies have shown how several pharmacological modalities reduce the cartilage degeneration in an osteoarthritis model or after trauma. In the future, matrix metalloproteinase (MMP) inhibitors and aggrecanose inhibitors (Brewster et al 2001) may substitute the treatment modalities that are in use today. Delivery methods, the dose of medication and the quality of tissue obtained will also need to be addressed. To maintain the perfect environment for a normal joint function we will need to develop an algorithm that takes into account time, magnitude and frequency of pharmacological agents in order to achieve the perfect solution.

Summary

Cartilage is a complex structure that is very difficult to match with artificial substitutes. The main function of cartilage is to load-bear and reduce friction in joint articulation. Options for repair of cartilage lesions are under constant investigation, and are often hampered by the lack of blood and nerve supply and its complex architecture. Autologous osteochondral grafting and autologous chondrocyte implantation are two of the methods most commonly used; however, conservative treatment should also be considered.

Acknowledgments

The chapter was developed in collaboration with Giordano Giovanni, MD, Marcheggiani Muccioli Giulio Maria, MD, and Silvia Bassini, Laboratorio di Biomeccanica, Istituti Ortopedici Rizzoli, Bologna, Italy.

References

Aaron R K, Plaas A A K 1987 Stimulation of proteoglycan synthesis in articular chondrocyte cultures by a pulsed electromagnetic field. Transactions of the Orthopaedic Research Society 12:273

Aaron R K, Ciomber D M, Jolly G 1987 Modulation of chondrogenesis and chondrocyte differentiation by pulsed electromagnetic fields. Transactions of the Orthopaedic Research Society 12:272

Adams M A 2006 The mechanical environment of chondrocytes in articular cartilage. Biorheology 43:537–545

Ahmed A M 1983 A pressure distribution transducer for in-vitro static measurements in synovial joints. Journal of Biomechanical Engineering 105:309–314

Ahmed A M, Burke D L 1983 In-vitro measurement of static pressure distribution in synovial joints: I. Tibial surface of the knee. Journal of Biomechanical Engineering 105:216–225

Ahmad C S, Cohen Z A, Levine W N et al 2001 Biomechanical and topographic considerations for autologous osteochondral grafting in the knee. American Journal of Sports Medicine 29:201–206

Aigner J, Tegeler J, Hutzler P et al 1998 Cartilage tissue engineering with novel nonwoven structured biomaterial based on hyaluronic acid benzyl ester. Journal of Biomedical Materials Research 42:172–181

Akizuki S, Mow V C, Muller F et al 1986 Tensile properties of human knee joint cartilage: I. Influence of ionic conditions, weight bearing, and fibrillation on the tensile modulus. Journal of Orthopaedic Research 4:379–392

Akizuki S, Mow V C, Muller F et al 1987 Tensile properties of human knee joint cartilage: II. Correlations between weight bearing and tissue pathology and the kinetics of swelling. Journal of Orthopaedic Research 5:172–186

Anderson A F, Fu F H, Bert R M et al 2003 A controlled study of autologous chondrocyte implantation versus microfracture for articular cartilage lesions of the femur. Proceedings of the 70th American Academy of Orthopaedic Surgeons Annual Meeting, New Orleans, LA

Apone S, Wu J J, Eyre D R 1987 Collagen heterogeneity in articular cartilage: identification of five genetically distinct molecular species. Transactions of the Orthopaedic Research Society 12:109

Beaver R J, Mahomed M, Backstein D et al 1992 Fresh osteochondral allografts for post-traumatic defects in the knee. Journal of Bone and Joint Surgery (Br) 74B:105–110

Behrens F, Kraft EL, Oegema T R Jr 1989 Biochemical changes in articular cartilage after joint immobilization by casting or external fixation. Journal of Orthopaedic Research 7:335–343

Berlet G C, Mascia A, Miniaci A 1999 Case Report. Treatment of unstable osteochondritis dissecans lesions of the knee using autogenous osteochondral grafts (Mosaicplasty). Arthroscopy 15:312–316

Bobic V 1996 Arthroscopic osteochondral autograft transplantation in anterior cruciate ligament reconstruction: a preliminary clinical study. Knee Surgery and Sports Traumatology and Arthroscopy 3:262–264

Brewster M, Lewis E J, Wilson K L et al 2001 Ro 32-3555, an orally active collagenase selective inhibitor, prevents structural damage in the STR/ORT mouse model of osteoarthritis. Arthritis and Rheumatism 44:343–350

Brittberg M 2000 Clinical evaluation of cartilage defects and repair. Proceeding of the 3rd Symposium of International Cartilage Repair Society, Cartilage and Cartilage Repair in the New Millennium, Göteborg, Sweden

Brittberg M, Lindahl A, Ohlsson C et al 1994 Treatment of deep cartilage defects in the knee with autologous chondrocyte transplantation. New England Journal of Medicine 331:889–895

Brittberg M, Nilsson A, Lindahl A et al 1996 Rabbit articular cartilage defects treated with autologous cultured chondrocytes. Clinical Orthopaedics and Related Research 326:270–283

Brittberg M, Tallheden T, Sjogren-Jansson B et al 2001 Autologous chondrocytes used for articular cartilage repair: an update. Clinical Orthopaedics and Related Research 391 (suppl):S337–348

Brower-Toland B D, Saxer R A, Goodrich L R et al 2001 Direct adenovirus-mediated insulin-like growth factor I gene transfer enhances transplant chondrocyte function. Human Gene Therapy 12:117–129

Browne J E, Branch T P 2000 Surgical alternatives for treatment of articular cartilage lesions. Journal of the American Academy of Orthopaedic Surgeons 8:180–189

Brun P, Abatangelo G, Radice M et al 1999 Chondrocyte aggregation and reorganization into three-dimensional scaffolds. Journal of Biomedical Materials Research 46:337–346

Buckwalter J A 1983 Articular cartilage. In: American Academy of Orthopaedic Surgeons instructional course lectures, XXXII. CV Mosby, St Louis, MO, p 349–370

Buckwalter J A, Lane N E 1997 Athletics and osteoarthritis. American Journal of Sports Medicine 25:873–881

Buckwalter J A, Mankin H J 1997a Articular cartilage. Journal of Bone and Joint Surgery (Am) 79A:600–611

Buckwalter J A, Mankin H J 1997b Articular cartilage: II. Degeneration and osteoarthrosis, repair, regeneration, and transplantation. Journal of Bone and Joint Surgery (Am) 79A:612–632

Buckwalter J A, Roughley P J 1987 Age-related changes in human articular cartilage proteoglycans. Transactions of the Orthopaedic Research Society 12:152

Buckwalter J A, Kuettner K E, Thonar E J M 1985 Age-related changes in articular cartilage proteoglycans: electron microscopic studies. Journal of Orthopaedic Research 3:251–257

Campoccia D, Doherty P, Radice M et al 1998 Semisynthetic resorbable materials from hyaluronan esterification. Biomaterials 19:2101–2127

Caplan A I 2000 Mesenchymal stem cells and gene therapy. Clinical Orthopaedics and Related Research 379 (suppl):S67–S70

Carlberg A L, Pucci B, Rallapalli R et al 2001 Efficient chondrogenic differentiation of mesenchymal cells in micromass culture by retroviral gene transfer of BMP-2. Differentiation 67:128–138

Centers for Disease Control and Prevention 2002 Nonfatal sports- and recreation-related injuries treated in emergency departments: United States, July 2000–June 2001. Journal of the American Medical Association 288:1977–1979

Chen G, Sato T, Ushida T 2003 Redifferentiation of dedifferentiated bovine chondrocytes when cultured in vitro in a PLGA-collagen hybrid mesh. Federation of European Biochemical Societies Letters 542:95–99

Clarke I C 1971 Surface characteristics of human articular cartilage: a scanning electron microscope study. Journal of Anatomy 108:23–30

Cohen B, Lai W M, Mow V C 1998 Composition and dynamics of articular cartilage: structure, function, and maintaining healthy state. Journal of Orthopaedic and Sports Physical Therapy 28:203–215

DePalma A F, McKeever C D, Subin D K 1966 Process of repair of articular cartilage demonstrated by histology and autoradiography with tritiated thymidine. Clinical Orthopaedics and Related Research 48:229–242

Donohue J M, Buss D, Oegema T R Jr, et al 1983 The effects of indirect blunt trauma on adult canine articular cartilage. Journal of Bone and Joint Surgery (Am) 65A:948–957

Dozin B, Malpeli M, Cancedda R et al 2005 Comparative evaluation of autologous chondrocyte implantation and mosaicplasty: a multi-centered randomized clinical trial. Clinical Journal of Sports Medicine 15:220–226

Duchov J, Hess T, Kohn D 2000 Primary stability of press-fit-implanted osteochondral grafts. Influence of graft size, repeated insertion, and harvesting technique. American Journal of Sports Medicine 28:24–27

Eastlack R K, Hargens A R, Groppo E R et al 2005 Lower body positive-pressure exercise after knee surgery. Clinical Orthopaedics and Related Research 431:213–219

Fini M, Riaversi G, Torricelli P et al 2005 Pulsed electromagnetic fields reduce knee osteoarthritic lesion progression in the aged Dunkin Hartley guinea pig. Journal of Orthopaedic Research 23:899–908

Frisbie D D, Oxford J T, Southwood L et al 2003 Early events in cartilage repair after subchondral bone microfracture. Clinical Orthopaedics and Related Research 407:215–227

Garrett J C 1986 Treatment of osteochondral defects of the distal femur with fresh osteochondral allografts: a preliminary report. Arthroscopy 2:222–226

Gelse K, von der Mark K, Aigner T et al 2003 Articular cartilage repair by gene therapy using growth factor-producing mesenchymal cells. Arthritis and Rheumatism 48:430–441

Goodrich L R 2002 Enhanced early healing of articular cartilage with genetically modified chondrocytes expressing insulin-like growth factor-I. Veterinary Surgery 31:482

Grahm G P, Fairclough J A 1998 Early osteoarthritis in young sportsmen with severe anterolateral instability of the knee. Injury 19:247–248

Grande D A, Mason J, Light E et al 2003 Stem cells as platforms for delivery of genes to enhance cartilage repair. Journal of Bone and Joint Surgery (Am) 85A (suppl 2):111–116

Grigolo B, Roseti L, Fiorini M et al 2001 Transplantation of chondrocytes seeded on a hyaluronan derivative (HYAFF®11) into cartilage defects in rabbits. Biomaterials 22:2417–2424

Grigolo B, Lisignoli G, Piacentini A et al 2002 Evidence for redifferentiation of human chondrocytes grown on a hyaluronan-based biomaterial (HYAFF®11). Biomaterials 23:1187–1195

Grigolo B, Roseti L, De Franceschi L et al 2005 Molecular and immunohistological characterization of human cartilage two years following autologous cell transplantation. Journal of Bone and Joint Surgery (Am) 87A:46–57

Gross A E, Shasha N, Aubin P 2005 Long-term follow-up of the use of fresh osteochondral allografts for posttraumatic knee defects. Clinical Orthopaedics and Related Research 435:79–87

Gudas R, Kalesinskas R J, Kimtys V et al 2005 A prospective randomized clinical study of mosaic osteochondral autologous transplantation versus microfracture for the treatment of osteochondral defects in the knee joint in young athletes. Arthroscopy 21:1066–1075

Haapala J, Arokoski J, Pirttimaki J et al 2000 Incomplete restoration of immobilization induced softening of young beagle knee articular cartilage after 50-week remobilization. International Journal of Sports Medicine 21:76–81

Hamerman D, Rosenberg L C, Schubert M 1970 Diarthrodial joints revisited. Journal of Bone and Joint Surgery (Am) 52A:725–774

Hangody L, Fules P 2003 Autologous osteochondral mosaicplasty for the treatment of full-thickness defects of weight-bearing joints: ten years of experimental and clinical experience. Journal of Bone and Joint Surgery (Am) 85A (suppl 2):25–32

Hangody L, Kish G, Karapati Z et al 1997a Arthroscopic autogenous osteochondral mosaicplasty for the treatment of femoral condylar articular defects. A preliminary report. Knee Surgery and Sports Traumatology and Arthroscopy 5:262–267

Hangody L, Kish G, Karpati Z 1997b Autogenous osteochondral graft technique for replacing knee cartilage defects in dogs. Orthopaedics International 5:175–181

Hangody L, Kish G, Karpati Z et al 1998 Mosaicplasty for the treatment of articular cartilage defects: application in clinical practice. Orthopedics 21:751–756

Hardingham T E, Muir H 1973 Binding of oligosaccharides of hyaluronic acid to proteoglycans. Biochemistry Journal 135:905–908

Hascall V C 1977 Interaction of cartilage proteoglycans with hyaluronic acid. Journal of Supramolecular Structure 7:101–120

Heinegard D, Alexsson I 1977 Distribution of keratan sulfate in cartilage proteoglycans. Journal of Biological Chemistry 252:1971–1979

Heinegard D, Paulson M 1984 Structure and metabolism of proteoglycans. In: Piez K A, Reddi A H (eds) Extracellular matrix biochemistry. Elsevier, New York, p 277–328

Hoemann C D, Hurtig M, Rossomacha E et al 2005 Chitosan-glycerol phosphate/blood implants improve hyaline cartilage repair in ovine microfracture defects. Journal of Bone and Joint Surgery (Am) 87A:2671–2686

Howell D S, Pita J C, Woessner J F 1983 Which comes first: crystals, necrosis or inflammation. Journal of Rheumatology 10 (suppl 9): 59–61

Imhoff A B, Ottl G M, Burkart A et al 1999 Autologous osteochondral transplantation on various joints. Orthopade 28:33–44

Jakob R P, Franz T, Gautier E et al 2002 Autologous osteochondral grafting in the knee: indications, results and reflections. Clinical Orthopaedics and Related Research 401:170–184

Jerosch J, Filler T, Peuker E 2000 Is there an option for harvesting autologous osteochondral grafts without damaging weight-bearing areas in the knee joint? Knee Surgery and Sports Traumatology and Arthroscopy 8:237–240

Jurvelin J, Kiviranta I, Säämänen A-M et al 1990 Indentation stiffness of canine knee articular cartilage: influence of strenuous joint loading. Journal of Biomechanics 23:1239–1246

Kempson G E 1980 The mechanical properties of articular cartilage. In: Sokoloff L (ed) The joints and synovial fluid, vol 2. Academic Press, New York, p 177–238

Kim H K, Moran M E, Salter R B 1991 The potential for regeneration of articular cartilage in defects created by chondral shaving and subchondral abrasion. An experimental investigation in rabbits. Journal of Bone and Joint Surgery (Am) 73A:1301–1315

Knutsen G, Engebretsen L, Ludvigsen T C et al 2004 Autologous chondrocyte implantation compared with microfracture in the knee. A randomized trial. Journal of Bone and Joint Surgery (Am) 86A:455–464

Koh J L, Wirsing K, Lautenschlager E et al 2004 The effect of graft height mismatch on contact pressure following osteochondral grafting: a biomechanical study. American Journal of Sports Medicine 32:317–320

Koh J L, Kowalski A, Lautenschlager E 2006 The effect of angled osteochondral grafting on contact pressure: a biomechanical study. American Journal of Sports Medicine 34:116–119

Lahav A, Burks RT, Greis P E et al 2006 Clinical outcomes following osteochondral autologous transplantation (OATS). Journal of Knee Surgery 19:169–173

Laprell H, Peterson W 2001 Autologous osteochondral transplantation using the diamond bone cutting system (DBCS): 6–12 years' follow-up of 35 patients with osteochondral defects at the knee joint. Archives of Orthopaedic and Trauma Surgery 121:248–253

Levin A, Burton-Wurster N, Chen C T et al 2001 Intercellular signaling as a cause of cell death in clinically impacted cartilage explant. Osteoarthritis and Cartilage 9:702–711

Linn F C, Sokoloff L 1965 Movement and composition of interstitial fluid of cartilage. Arthritis and Rheumatism 8:481–494

Lipshitz H, Etheredge R 3rd, Glimcher M J 1980 In vitro studies of the wear of articular cartilage: III. The wear characteristics of chemical modified articular cartilage when worn against a highly polished characterized stainless steel surface. Journal of Biomechanics 13:423–436

McDermott A G P, Langer F, Pritzker K P H et al 1985 Fresh small-fragment osteochondral allografts. Clinical Orthopaedics and Related Research 197:96–102

Mankin H J, Thrasher A Z 1975 Water content and binding in normal and osteoarthritic human cartilage. Journal of Bone and Joint Surgery (Am) 57A:76–80

Mann R W, McCutchen C W 1997 Comment on 'A theoretical solution for the frictionless rolling contact of cylindrical biphasic articular cartilage layers'. Journal of Biomechanics 30:99

Marcacci M, Kon E, Zaffagnini S et al 1999 Use of autologous grafts for reconstruction of osteochondral defects of the knee. Orthopedics 22:595–600

Marcacci M, Zaffagnini S, Kon E et al 2002 Arthroscopic autologous chondrocyte transplantation: technical note. Knee Surgery and Sports Traumatology and Arthroscopy 10:154–159

Marcacci M, Berruto M, Brocchetta D et al 2005a Articular cartilage engineering with Hyalograft C: 3-year clinical results. Clinical Orthopaedics and Related Research 435:96–105

Marcacci M, Kon E, Zaffagnini S et al 2005b Multiple osteochondral arthroscopic grafting (mosaicplasty) for cartilage defects of the knee: prospective study results at 2-year follow-up. Arthroscopy 21:462–470

Marder R A, Hopkins G Jr, Timmerman L A 2005 Arthroscopic microfracture of chondral defects of the knee: a comparison of two postoperative treatments. Arthroscopy 21(2):152–158

Maroudas A 1975 Biophysical chemistry of cartilaginous tissues with special reference to solute and fluid transport. Biorheology 12:233–248

Maroudas A, Schneiderman R 1987 'Free' and 'exchangeable' or 'trapped' and 'non-exchangeable' water in cartilage. Journal of Orthopaedic Research 5:133–138

Matsusue Y, Yamamuro T, Hama H 1993 Case report. Arthroscopic multiple osteochondral transplantation to the defect in the knee associated with anterior cruciate ligament disruption. Arthroscopy 9:318–321

Mayne R, Irwin M H 1986 Collagen types in cartilage. In: Kuettner K E, Schleyerbach R, Hascall V C (eds) Articular cartilage biochemistry. Raven Press, New York, p 23–38

Maynou C, Mestdagh H, Beltrand E et al 1998 Resultats a long term de l'autogreffe osteo-cartilagineuse de voisinage dans les destructions cartilagineuses etendues du genou. A propos de 5 cas. Acta Orthopaedica Belgica 64:193–200

Meyers M H, Akeson W, Convery F R 1989 Resurfacing of the knee with fresh osteochondral allografts. Journal of Bone and Joint Surgery (Am) 71A:704–713

Micheli L J, Browne J E, Erggelet C 2001 Autologous chondrocyte implantation of the knee: multicenter experience and minimum 3-year follow-up. Clinical Journal of Sports Medicine 11:223–228

Milentijevic D, Torzilli P A 2005 Influence of stress rate on water loss, matrix deformation and chondrocyte viability in impacted articular cartilage. Journal of Biomechanics 38:493–502

Milentijevic D, Rubel I F, Liew A S et al 2005 An in vivo rabbit model for cartilage trauma: a preliminary study of the influence of impact stress magnitude on chondrocyte death and matrix damage. Journal of Orthopaedic Trauma 19:466–473

Minas T 2001 Autologous chondrocyte implantation for focal chondral defects of the knee. Clinical Orthopaedics and Related Research 391 (suppl):S349–361

Mithofer K, Minas T, Peterson L et al 2005a Functional outcome of knee articular cartilage repair in adolescent athletes. American Journal of Sports Medicine 33:1147–1153

Mithofer K, Peterson L, Mandelbaum B R et al 2005b Articular cartilage repair in soccer players with autologous chondrocyte transplantation: functional outcome and return to competition. American Journal of Sports Medicine 33:1639–1646

Mizuno S, Tateishi T, Ushida T et al 2002 Hydrostatic fluid pressure enhances matrix synthesis and accumulation by bovine chondrocytes in three-dimensional culture. Journal of Cell Physiology 193:319–327

Mow V C, Rosenwasser M 1991 Articular cartilage: Biomechanics. In: Woo S L-Y, Buckwalter J A (eds) Injury and repair of the musculo-skeletal soft tissues. American Academy of Orthopaedic Surgeons, Rosemont, IL, p 427–463

Mow V C, Kuei S C, Lai W M et al 1980 Biphasic creep and stress relaxation of articular cartilage in compression: theory and experiments. Journal of Biomechanical Engineering 102:73–84

Mow V C, Mak A F, Lai W M et al 1984a Viscoelastic properties of proteoglycan subunits and aggregates in varying solution concentrations. Journal of Biomechanics 17:325–338

Mow V C, Holmes M H, Lai W M 1984b Fluid transport and mechanical properties of articular cartilage: a review. Journal of Biomechanics 17:377–394

Nam E K, Makhsous M, Koh J et al 2004 Biomechanical and histological evaluation of osteochondral transplantation in a rabbit model. American Journal of Sports Medicine 32:308–316

Nehrer S, Spector M, Minas T 1999 Histologic analysis of tissue after failed cartilage repair procedures. Clinical Orthopaedics and Related Research 365:149–162

Nimni M E 1974 Collagen: Its structure and function in normal and pathological connective tissues. Seminars in Arthritis and Rheumatism 4:95–150

Noyes F R, Stabler C L 1989 A system for grading articular cartilage lesions at arthroscopy. American Journal of Sports Medicine 17:505–513

Ochi M, Uchio Y, Kawasaki K et al 2002 Transplantation of cartilage-like tissue made by tissue engineering in the treatment of cartilage defects of the knee. Journal of Bone and Joint Surgery (Br) 84B:571–578

Outerbridge R E 1961 The etiology of chondromalacia patellae. Journal of Bone and Joint Surgery (Br) 43B:752–757

Palmer G, Pascher A, Gouze E et al 2002 Development of gene-based therapies for cartilage repair. Critical Reviews of Eukaryotic Gene Expression 12:259–273

Pavesio A, Abatangelo G, Borrione A et al 2003 Hyaluronan-based scaffolds (Hyalograft C) in the treatment of knee cartilage defects: preliminary clinical findings. Novartis Foundation Symposium 249:203–217; discussion 229–233, 234–238, 239–241

Pearce S G, Hurtig M B, Clarnette R et al 2001 An investigation of 2 techniques for optimizing joint surface congruency using multiple cylindrical osteochondral autografts. Arthroscopy 17:50–55

Peterson L, Minas T, Brittberg M et al 2000 Two- to 9-year outcome after autologous chondrocyte transplantation of the knee. Clinical Orthopaedics and Related Research 374:212–234

Peterson L, Brittberg M, Kiviranta I et al 2002 Autologous chondrocyte transplantation. Biomechanics and long-term durability. American Journal of Sports Medicine 30:2–12

Phipatanakul W P, Vande Vord P J, Teitge R A et al 2004 Immune response in patients receiving fresh osteochondral allografts. American Journal of Orthopaedics 33:345–348

Plaas A H K, Sandy J D 1984 Age-related decrease in the link-stability of proteoglycan aggregates formed by articular chondrocytes. Biochemistry Journal 220:337–340

Poole C A, Flint M H, Beaumont B W 1984 Morphological and functional interrelationships of articular cartilage matrices. Journal of Anatomy 138:113–138

Radin E L, Paul I L 1971 Response of joints to impact loading: I. In vitro wear. Arthritis and Rheumatology 14:356–362

Radin E L, Martin R B, Burr D B et al 1984 Effects of mechanical loading on the tissues of the rabbit knee. Journal of Orthopaedic Research 2:221–234

Roos H 1998 Are there long term sequelae from soccer? Clinical Sports Medicine 17:819–831

Säämänen A-M 1989 Articular cartilage proteoglycans and joint loading. A study in young rabbits and dogs. Thesis. Publications of the University of Kuopio Medical School Original Production 7:1–67

Sah R L, Kim Y J, Doong J H et al 1989 Biosynthetic response of cartilage explants to dynamic compression. Journal of Orthopaedic Research 7:619–636

Salter R B 2004 Continuous passive motion: from origination to research to clinical application. Journal of Rheumatology 31:2104–2105

Salter R B, Simmonds D F, Malcolm B W et al 1980 The biological effect of continuous passive motion on the healing of full-thickness defects in articular cartilage. An experimental investigation in the rabbit. Journal of Bone and Joint Surgery (Am) 62A:1232–1251

Schenk R K, Eggli P S, Hunziker E B 1986 Articular cartilage morphology. In: Kuettner K E, Schleyerbach R, Hascall V C (eds) Articular cartilage biochemistry. Raven Press, New York, p 3–22

Schumann D, Kujat R, Nerlich M et al 2006 Mechanobiological conditioning of stem cells for cartilage tissue engineering. Biomedical Materials Engineering 16 (4 suppl):S37–52

Sgaglione N A, Miniaci A, Gillogly S D et al 2002 Update on advanced surgical techniques in the treatment of traumatic focal articular cartilage lesions in the knee. Arthroscopy 18 (2 suppl 1):9–32

Shasha N, Aubin P P, Cheah H K et al 2002 Long-term clinical experience with fresh osteochondral allografts for articular knee defects in high demand patients. Cell Tissue Bank 3:175–182

Simon B R, Coats R S, Woo S L-Y 1984 Relaxation and creep quasilinear viscoelastic models for normal articular cartilage. Journal of Biomechanical Engineering 106:159–164

Steadman J R, Briggs K K, Rodrigo J J et al 2003a Outcomes of microfracture for traumatic chondral defects of the knee: average 11-year follow-up. Arthroscopy 19:477–484

Steadman J R, Miller B S, Karas S G et al 2003b The microfracture technique in the treatment of full-thickness chondral lesions of the knee in National Football League players. Journal of Knee Surgery 16:83–86

Stockwell R A 1978 Chondrocytes. Journal of Clinical Pathology 12 (suppl):7–13

Torzilli P A, Rose D E, Dethmers D A 1982 Equilibrium water partition in articular cartilage. Biorheology 19:519–537

Trippel S B, Ghivizzani S C, Nixon A J 2004 Gene-based approaches for the repair of articular cartilage. Gene Therapy 11:351–359

Vanwanseele B, Lucchinetti E, Stussi E 2002 The effects of immobilization on the characteristics of articular cartilage: current concepts and future directions. Osteoarthritis and Cartilage 10:408–419

Williams J M, Moran M, Thonar E J et al 1994 Continuous passive motion stimulates repair of rabbit knee articular cartilage after matrix proteoglycan loss. Clinical Orthopaedics and Related Research 304:252–262

Woo S L-Y, Simon B R, Kuei S C et al 1980 Quasi linear viscoelastic properties of normal articular cartilage. Journal of Biomechanical Engineering 102:85–90

Woo S L-Y, Mow V C, Lai W M 1987 Biomechanical properties of articular cartilage. In: Skalak R, Chien S (eds) Handbook of bioengineering. McGraw-Hill, New York, p 4.1–4.44

Wood J J, Malek M A, Frassica F J et al 2006 Autologous cultured chondrocytes: adverse events reported to the United States Food and Drug Administration. Journal of Bone and Joint Surgery (Am) 88A:503–507

Concepts in managing sport and exercise injuries

8	Motor control	115
9	Pain	133
10	Exercise-based conditioning and rehabilitation	149
11	Psychology of injury and rehabilitation	171
12	Screening for sport and exercise participation	190
13	Clinical outcomes in sport and exercise physical therapies	206
14	Electrophysical agents in sport and exercise injury management	220
15	Prevention of injury	236

Motor control

Paul W. Hodges

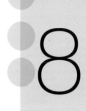

CHAPTER CONTENTS

Introduction 115

Factors to consider in motor control. 115

Changes in motor control in musculoskeletal
injury and pain. 121

Motor learning in the management of sports-related
injuries. 126

Application of motor control and motor learning
in physical therapy of sports- and exercise-related
injuries – low back pain 129

Summary 130

Introduction

Many factors influence movement of the body. These include not only the biomechanical properties of bone, articulations and muscle, but also the controller, the system which must determine the requirements for movement and stability and generate appropriate strategies of muscle activity to effectively move the body and limbs, and control the relationship to the environment and between segments. An important consideration for sport and exercise is that injury and pain may affect the accuracy of the control system. Alternatively, inadequate function of the controller may contribute to the etiology of dysfunction and injury. The aim of this chapter is to consider the theory and application of motor control and motor learning as it applies to physical therapies for the management of sport- and exercise-related injury and pain, with reference to the elements of the neuromotor control system (receptors, controller), control strategies and how motor learning techniques can be used clinically to deal with changes in the control system when people have musculoskeletal pain.

Factors to consider in motor control

In order to understand and develop strategies for application of motor learning to physical therapy management of sport- and exercise-related injuries, it is essential to understand how movement is coordinated by the central nervous system (CNS). Performance of coordinated movement involves control of an appropriate sequence of movements of the limbs and trunk by an organized sequence of muscle activity. Furthermore, this coordinated pattern must be matched to environmental demands and be able to compensate for predictable or unpredictable disturbances that may interfere with the movement. For the CNS to meet the demands of sport and physical exercise, the coordination of these parameters must be streamlined. Numerous theories have been presented for the control of movement. This section will discuss the factors that must be addressed by the motor control system, provide a brief introduction to the major contemporary theories of motor control, and consider a specific example of motor control regarding postural and joint stability. Many theories of motor control have been presented in the literature, some from an anatomical basis and others from a behavioral point of view. This summary will focus on the behavioral approach.

Control strategies

The CNS has a variety of strategies available for the control and coordination of movement. These strategies incorporate two basic systems of control that are derived from mechanical engineering. The first depends on sensory feedback (i.e. closed-loop strategies) and the second, controlled centrally, is largely independent of sensory feedback (i.e. open-loop strategies) (Fig. 8.1) (Schmidt & Lee, 1999). Each system requires a controller and effector organs (muscles). In both systems, the controller generates the movement command to drive the muscles for movement. In the closed-loop system, the control of the movement is continually updated and modified on the basis of feedback. In contrast, for open-loop control all aspects of the movement are preplanned and the movement is performed without consideration of feedback. This may occur because the feedback is not needed or is too slow to make adjustments to the movement.

Closed-loop control – sensory control of movement

In a closed-loop system, the command to move is generated in a similar manner to an open-loop system (see below); however, the intended movement is compared against feedback regarding the status of the body and its relationship to the environment. If the feedback differs from the intended movement, an error command is generated to correct the movement performance. In this way, sensory feedback is used to mold and correct movement performance.

Clearly, this system requires effective systems for detecting the state of the environment, and the position and movements of the body segments. A variety of receptors are available including the visual system, auditory information, vestibular apparatus and proprioceptors. The following section provides

a review of the main receptor classes and their contribution to movement control.

Receptors

Endogenous information about movement and position of body segments is provided by mechanoreceptors ranging from free nerve endings to specialized receptor organs located in muscle, joints and skin (Fig. 8.2). Each of these receptor types provides afferent input that is useful for movement control.

Muscle spindles

Muscle spindles are the most complex of the mechanoreceptors and consist of sensory and contractile components that lie parallel to muscle fibers so that they are stretched with the muscle. The sensory component has two main types of sensory endings, bag and chain fibers. These endings are sensitive to length and/or velocity of lengthening. The contractile component of the muscle spindle provides a mechanism for the CNS to control its sensitivity and to adapt the spindle to changes in muscle length. The contractile component of the muscle spindle is innervated by a special class of motorneurons, called gamma-motorneurons. It is considered that alpha- and gamma-motorneurons are coactivated during muscle contraction. Many studies have confirmed that the input from muscle spindles is critical for the perception of movement, yet stimulation of single muscle afferents does not result in conscious perception.

Golgi tendon organs

Golgi tendon organs are located in the tendon, in series with the muscle fibers. These receptors provide an inhibitory input to the alpha-motorneurons and were originally proposed to influence motorneurone excitability only during strong contractions to prevent damage to the muscles. However, each receptor is attached to a small population of muscle fibers and is sensitive to small forces to provide discrete detection of tension in different parts of the muscle. Thus, these receptors are likely to provide an important contribution to feedback during movement.

Joint receptors

Joint receptors are encapsulated receptors (Ruffini endings and Pacinian corpuscles) situated in the joint capsule. The

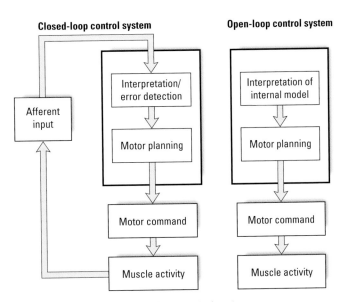

Figure 8.1 • Open- and closed-loop control systems.

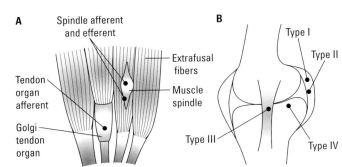

Figure 8.2 • Location and types of muscle and joint receptors.

contribution of these receptors to perception of movement and movement control has often been considered to be limited. While some receptors are activated at specific ranges of motion, the majority fire at the end of range when the joint capsule is stretched. Other joint structures such as the ligaments also contain receptors which may contribute to proprioception. It is known that stimulation of receptors in the anterior cruciate ligament modulates activity of muscles surrounding the knee (Johansson et al 1991).

Skin receptors

There are several types of tactile receptors that are distributed in the layers of the skin. These receptors include Pacinican corpuscles, Mesiner corpuscles, Merkel cells and Ruffini endings, and provide important tactile information. For example, input from the cutaneous receptors is important for the perception of movement of large and small joints such as those of the hand (Collins et al 2000). Furthermore, information derived from these receptors is critical for the coordination of grip force (Johansson et al 1991) and studies have shown a relationship between firing of afferent neurons and the motor-unit action potentials in the muscles of the wrist and hand (McNulty et al 1999).

Vestibular apparatus

The vestibular apparatus involves the saccule and utricle, which detect the position of the head with respect to gravity, and the semicircular canals, which provide information of acceleration of the head around the three major axes. The major function of the vestibular apparatus is to provide information about movements of the head. Integration of vestibular information and proprioceptive information from the neck and trunk allow the interpretation of the position of the body relative to gravity.

Visual system

The visual system provides information regarding not only the position and movement of the body, but also the interaction between the body and environment or objects. As such, vision provides an important contribution to closed-loop control.

Auditory system

Although hearing does not play a major role in movement control, auditory information may provide useful feedback from environmental factors and issues such as success of performance. For instance, professional golfers can interpret the quality of a golf swing from the sound made when the ball is hit. There may also be more specific contributions such as feedback of the accuracy of movements involved in tasks, such as speech or foot contacts during running.

Closed-loop control mechanisms

Closed-loop control operates at a variety of levels, from simple monosynaptic reflexes to complex, fine motor tasks involving coordinated finger movements. The complexity of information processing involved in these different levels is clearly different and each is important to consider.

At the more basic end of the spectrum, closed-loop control may operate at the reflex level. The most basic of these is the monosynaptic stretch reflex. When muscle spindles are stretched, the afferent impulse from the receptor region of the spindles excites the alpha-motorneurons in the same muscle, resulting in contraction. This simple response is inflexible and represents a basic mechanism for the motor system to correct an error (i.e. to resist an imposed stretch). These responses are short in latency, and involve the time for transmission of the action potential along the afferent (sensory) and efferent (motor) nerves and a single synapse. In a sporting context, this aspect of movement control is likely to be important. For example, when the ankle is inverted, the body requires a rapid response of the peroneal muscles to overcome the inversion strain. Even these most rapid responses, however, may not be fast enough to prevent damage to joint structures.

More complex than the simple stretch reflex, are the long-loop reflexes that involve information processing at higher levels of the CNS, including transcortical mechanisms. These responses have a longer latency than the simple stretch reflex, are more flexible and can be modified voluntarily. Due to their flexibility, these responses are thought to have a greater role in error correction.

Another response group is the triggered responses. These responses are faster than a voluntary reaction time but involve a more complex and widespread response than is initiated via simple reflex mechanisms. For example, when the support surface on which a person is standing is rapidly moved, such as that which would occur when standing in a boat, a complex interplay of several body segments is initiated in order to maintain the equilibrium of the body. These responses have been shown to be too fast to be voluntary, but are task and context specific, and inconsistent with stretch reflexes.

The most complex level of closed-loop control is the fine control of long duration tasks that require accuracy. In these tasks, the sensory information may be used unconsciously or consciously to provide feedback of performance and to continually modulate movement performance. However, even during these goal-directed tasks sensory information may be used at a subconscious level to modulate muscle activity.

Problems of closed-loop control

Even the fastest reflex responses involve a delay from stimulus to response. Thus, it has been argued that this system is unable to adequately meet the demands necessary to overcome the effects of external forces. For instance, the impact from a force applied to the posterior tibia may be sufficient to injure the anterior cruciate ligament (ACL) before any reflex response could be initiated. More important is the consideration that the latency required to make corrections for an error involves delays in the order of hundreds of milliseconds. This delay is required to receive and interpret afferent information and then generate appropriate responses. Thus, with rapid movements there is little time to provide information, apart from feedback that indicates that the movement has been completed or that the goal has been achieved. On this basis it may be considered that closed-loop mechanisms are most appropriate for slow movements that need constant regulation for accuracy. Clearly, other mechanisms must exist.

Open-loop control – centrally controlled movement

In contrast to the closed-loop control of movement, open-loop control implies that all aspects of the movement performance are preplanned by the CNS and that the movement occurs without modification by sensory feedback. Movements that are likely to fit into this category are ballistic and repetitive movements that are common in sport and exercise. Basic evidence that this type of control exists comes from studies of humans and animals with de-afferented limbs. In these cases, limb movement can occur in a manner that is almost indistinguishable from that of a limb with a full complement of sensory input, except for fine, controlled movements of the fingers that appear slightly clumsy (Taub & Berman 1968).

To reconcile these observations, a range of coordinative mechanisms have been described that would allow movement to be controlled without the need for feedback. In animals, the presence of central pattern generators (CPG) has been confirmed (Grillner 1981). A CPG is a collection of neurons that may control a repetitive function such as locomotion or respiration. These neuron groups can control the alternating contraction of muscles to perform the movement, and while they can be modified by afferent feedback, they can function independently of feedback. The existence of CPGs has not been confirmed in humans.

Another organizational theory that has been proposed to explain the central control of movement is the motor program. Motor programs involve a memory-based mechanism whereby a generalized motor program is stored as an abstract representation of a group of movements that are retrieved when a movement is performed (Schmidt & Lee 1999). This theory argues that the CNS stores details of invariant features of a movement (e.g. order of events, relative timing, relative force). This information is accessed, with selected task duration and muscles, when the movement is performed. While this theory is popular, there are several problems. For instance, there are problems associated with the retention of large amount of information that would need to be stored to cover the full complement of movement possibilities. Furthermore, there is the problem of the number of degrees of freedom. This issue was highlighted by Bernstein (1967) who argued that there are too many components that need to be controlled concurrently. For even the simplest movements of the hand, motion of each joint between the fingertip and the floor requires consideration. This is compounded when considering all of the muscles that are available to control each joint and the motor units within each muscle. As suggested by Bernstein (1967), this is an enormous problem for the CNS in view of the resources required to individually control the large number of muscles and joints. A system is needed that can reduce processing demands, for instance, by grouping degrees of freedom together.

Another model of movement control has been presented to reconcile some of these difficulties in movement control: the dynamic pattern theory (Kelso 1984). The dynamic pattern theory suggests that there is no central representation of all components of the movement; instead, the organization of the muscle contractions and joint movement is coordinated by environmental invariants and limb dynamics. Central to this theory is the idea that movements are attracted to steady-state behaviors, and movements follow the principles of nonlinear dynamics. In other words, if a particular variable is changed systematically, the system may move between separate stable states. A familiar example to illustrate this point is the transition from walking to running. In the dynamic pattern theory, it is argued that at slower speeds the movements of the arm and legs are 'attracted' to a coordinated pattern that is walking, yet at faster speeds the pattern changes, in part for reasons of efficiency. Thus, coordinated movement is self-organized according to the characteristics of limb behavior and environmental constraints.

Thus, the contemporary theories of motor control vary in the level of emphasis placed on the different, centrally or environmentally driven aspects of movement performance. Currently, the debate continues regarding these theories. Movement, in reality, is likely to be coordinated by a hybrid of these possibilities.

Movement and stability – motor control of postural and joint stability

To this point, movement has been considered as a sequence of movements to achieve a goal. One issue that underlies achievement of any movement goal is the coordination of movement and stability. All movements involve a complex interaction of movement and stability (Massion 1992) and movement occurs in conjunction with a subtle background of postural adjustments. Movement perturbs stability as a result of the interaction between internal and external forces. These forces include the reactive moments from limb movements, changes in the influence of gravity on the body as a result of the modification of the position of the center mass with movement, and the interaction with objects and the environment (e.g. catching a ball). Even a simple action, such as a movement of a limb, changes the position of the center of mass, and is associated with reactive moments that are equal in amplitude but opposite in direction to the forces producing the moment. Thus, the CNS not only has to deal with coordination of muscle activity to perform the movement but must also counteract the disturbance to postural stability. Conversely, no posture is purely static. For example, even static posture involves some component of movement, of which at least one component is actively controlled. For example, breathing produces a cyclical movement of the trunk (Gurfinkel et al 1971). Although this perturbation presents a challenge to the stability of the body, this movement is compensated by a coordinated sequence of movements of the trunk and lower limbs so that little, if any, movement is detected in forces recorded at the ground (Hodges et al 2002). When considering the complex nature of movement there is often considerable argument about which parts of a performance of the task are 'movement-related' and which are purely 'posture-related'. As many issues of relevance to sport and physical exercise relate to control of posture and joint stability, it is important to consider the normal control of these elements of movement control.

It should be noted that the stability involves control of the body at a number of different levels. The relationship between the body and the environment (i.e. postural equilibrium) must be controlled. In addition the stability of joints must be maintained. This includes the control of the relationship between adjacent segments of the body and the control of translations and rotations. Although these components require individual consideration they are interdependent. For instance, maintenance of postural equilibrium requires movement between adjacent body regions. Strategies must be available to control stability at each level and it is accepted that motor control strategies for each involve both closed- and open-loop processes, including reflex responses, and complex feedback mediated responses, such as triggered responses and feedforward strategies that precede a predictable challenge to stability at each of the interdependent levels. In a basic sense, a division can be made between predictable and unpredictable perturbations. However, in reality most movement involves a combination of these.

Control of postural equilibrium

Reflexes have long been regarded as the cornerstones of postural control. While it is clear that short-latency stretch reflexes may help maintain postural stability by maintenance of muscle length, the situation is likely to be more complex. For example, when the floor is tilted to stretch the calf muscles, it would be expected that this would generate a stretch reflex in the homonymous muscles. However, if this was initiated, the response would tend to increase the perturbation and lead to a loss of balance. Instead, the response of the calf muscles is restricted and a more appropriate response is generated that involves multiple segments (Nashner 1977). Considerable research has been devoted to investigation of these 'triggered' responses, which involve multiple segments. Balance is perturbed in many of these studies by movement of the support surface. Two main strategies have been identified that involve either ankle movement ('ankle strategy') or hip movement ('hip strategy'), depending on the context and the support surface characteristics (Horak & Nashner 1986).

What sensory information is used to initiate these triggered responses to maintain the equilibrium of the body? All sensory modalities including vestibular, somatosensory and visual information may be involved. On this basis, clinical assessment techniques have been developed with the aim of interpreting the specific contribution of each modality by removing or minimizing the input from one sensory modality or by providing conflicting information (Horak 1987). Recent studies have confirmed that vestibular input provides little contribution in quiet stance, as this system is not sensitive enough to detect small changes (Fitzpatrick et al 1996). Thus, in quiet stance, vision and proprioceptive information are the most critical.

The contribution of stretch reflexes to the maintenance of balance, however, has also been considered in terms of maintaining muscle stiffness (Winter et al 1998). Muscle stiffness is the property of muscles to act like springs; in other words, it is the ratio of length change to force change. When a muscle is stiff, it takes large amounts of force for it to lengthen. Thus, if antagonist muscles on either side of a joint have high stiffness, then increased force is required to move the joint. In terms of postural control, the stiffness of the ankle muscles may resist falling. It is the stretch reflex, and the control of the gamma-motorneurons which control the sensitivity of the sensory component of the muscle spindles, that control this system.

If a challenge to the body is predictable, then the CNS has the opportunity to deal with the perturbation in advance of the movement. For example, if a limb is moved, the CNS can predict the effect that this movement will have on the body and plan a sequence of muscle activity to overcome this perturbation. This type of strategy depends on the ability of the CNS to predict the interaction between body segments, and the body and its environment. Theoretically, this is thought to involve an 'Internal System of Body Dynamics' which is an abstract construct built up over a lifetime of movement experience (Gahéry & Massion 1981). Using this model, the CNS is able to determine how torques and inertias of adjacent and distant segments may interact, and how this will affect the external forces acting on the body. Several possibilities could explain the organization of the movement and postural parts of the task. In general, the postural activity could exist as a part of the motor command for movement or the postural part could be organized separately, but in parallel with the movement command. Several studies have investigated this question and are generally in support of the idea that movement and stability are controlled by parallel processes (Massion 1992).

It is important to consider that both processes may act concurrently and the outcome of feedforward processes (open loop control) may be molded by later feedback-mediated (closed loop control) processes. In general, feedforward- and feedback-mediated responses closely match the demands of the task and are scaled to the amplitude of the perturbing forces and the context of the perturbation. As such, postural adjustments represent a finely tuned component of human movement.

Control of joint stability

Joint stability is dependent on multiple factors that include the passive, active and control systems. Although the passive structures that surround a joint provide support, particularly towards the end of range, a major contributor to joint control is the active/muscle system. Yet the active contribution that muscles provide to stability is dependent on the controller, the CNS (Panjabi 1992). The mechanisms described above for the control of postural equilibrium also apply to the control of joint stability with contributions from open- and closed-loop systems. Reflex responses have been extensively investigated. For instance, short-latency responses of the trunk muscles are initiated in response to the unexpected addition of a load, such as dropping a load in a bucket held in the hands (Wilder et al 1996). Similarly, short-latency responses of the peroneal muscles contribute to the maintenance of the position of the ankle in response to inversion (Hopper et al 1998). More complex triggered responses are also involved. For instance, activity of the neck and trunk muscles precedes movement of these segments when the support surface is moved. This suggests that these responses are triggered by input from distal afferents (Keshner 1990). Biomechanical and in vivo data indicate that reflex control of muscle stiffness (as outlined in the previous section) also contributes to the control of joint stability. It is argued that reflex responses are too slow and that joint stability may be maintained by modulation of muscle stiffness. The stretch reflex may provide an important contribution to this control. Notably the control of stiffness may also be affected by other sensory inputs; for instance knee muscle activity, and therefore stiffness, is modulated in response to afferent input from the ACL (Johansson et al 1991).

Joint stability is also maintained in an open-loop feedforward manner. Two typical examples include the anticipatory reduction in activity of the biceps muscle to maintain the position of the forearm when a person removes a mass from their own hand (Hugon et al 1982), and the activity of the trunk muscles in advance of movement of an upper or lower limb to overcome the perturbation to the trunk from limb movement (Fig. 8.3) (Hodges & Richardson, 1997). An additional finding from these trunk muscle studies was that the activity of trunk muscles may contribute to different elements of control of the spine. Activity of the superficial muscles was linked to the direction of perturbation to the orientation of the spine. This suggests a contribution to control of the alignment of the spine and the control of buckling, whereas the activity of the deep muscles occurred in a nondirectional specific manner, which is consistent with a contribution to stiffening of the intervertebral segments (i.e. intersegmental stability). This has been confirmed in biomechanical studies (Hodges et al 2003).

Problems for the control of postural equilibrium and joint stability

Although postural adjustments provide a precise compensation for perturbation to postural equilibrium and joint stability, their control requires special consideration. For example, postural adjustments themselves may perturb balance. For instance, the change in lower leg muscle activity that precedes arm movements would cause the person to fall over if it occurred too early. Thus, the temporal and spatial organization of the postural responses needs to be perfectly matched to the actual or predicted perturbation. Another complication is that the requirements for control of joint stability and postural control may be contradictory. For example, the body may need to change the position of the spine in order to overcome a challenge to equilibrium. Thus, the CNS must balance the requirements for stability and equilibrium (Hodges et al 1999). Further complicating the control of movement and stability is the requirement for muscles to perform multiple functions concurrently. For

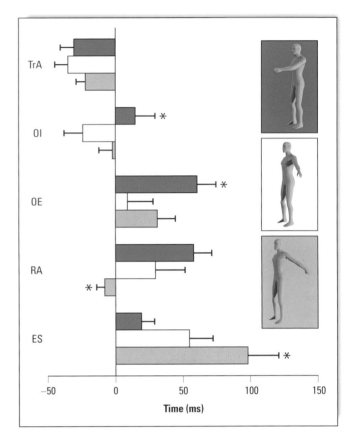

Figure 8.3 • Feedforward control of trunk stability. Rapid arm movement is associated with a sequence of trunk muscle activity that varies between directions of limb movement. Data in this figure are presented relative to the onset of the deltoid muscle which flexes the arm. The onset of activity of many of the muscles varies between movement directions and is linked to the control of the alignment of the spine. The deep muscle, transversus abdominis, is controlled separately and does not vary with movement direction. It is thought that the CNS uses this muscle to control intersegmental motion. (Adapted from Hodges & Richardson 1996.)

example, many trunk muscles are also involved in tasks such as respiration, and when posture is challenged the CNS needs to be able to integrate the postural and respiratory functions. Whether this integration occurs at spinal or higher centers has not been determined.

Characteristics of the muscle control system

Another issue in motor control that requires consideration is the selection of muscles for movement and stability. To this point, discussion has focused on strategies for control of movement, but it is necessary to consider the selection of muscles. An important consideration is the redundancy in the muscle system (i.e. multiple muscle are available to achieve a goal). Many muscles cross the joints and may be capable of performing similar

Local muscles 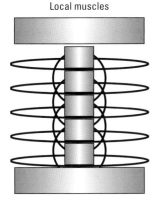 Global muscles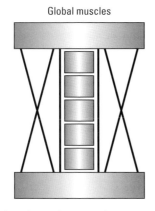

Figure 8.4 • Local and global muscles. Local muscles cross few segments and control intersegmental motion. Global muscles cross several segments and have moment arms sufficient to generate torques. (Adapted from Bergmark 1989.)

functions. It has been proposed by several authors, however, that there may be functional differentiation in the muscle system. A basic division is between muscles that perform functions based on their specific contribution to control of motion and stability (e.g. Bergmark 1989, Goff 1972, Janda 1978, Sahrman, 2002). Notably, Bergmark (1989) presented a model for the trunk that may be extrapolated to the other regions of the body. This model identified muscles as either 'local' or 'global', based on anatomical characteristics (Fig. 8.4). The local muscles are those that cross one or a few segment/s and that have a limited moment arm to move the joint, but ideal anatomy to maintain joint stability. In contrast, the global muscles cross several joints, with a larger moment arm to generate torque at the joint. While simple division of muscles into groups is likely to oversimplify the complex control of spinal motion and stability, it provides a useful definition to consider clinically, as it contributes to our understanding of why the CNS uses different strategies to control the different muscle groups. In basic sense it can be considered that deeper muscles that are closer to a joint, have a lesser moment arm to generate torque at the joint, but contribute to control of joint stiffness. Conversely, larger more superficial muscles that may cross more than one joint and are distant from a joint axis generate greater torque, and in co-contraction with antagonist muscles can also contribute to joint stiffness, but with different mechanical properties.

Changes in motor control in musculoskeletal injury and pain

When pain and injury occur, the strategies used by the CNS to control movement and/or posture and stability may be compromised. The mechanism for these changes is poorly understood but may be due to changes at many levels of the CNS. This section will review some of the ways in which motor control may be affected by pain and injury, and consider possible mechanisms for these changes.

It is possible to consider the changes in motor control in view of the theories outlined in the previous section. Changes have been identified in both open- and closed-loop type components of movement control and in terms of both the 'stability' and 'movement' components of coordinated movement. The implications of each of these will differ in terms of motor learning as a component of rehabilitation. The following section presents a variety of the motor control changes to illustrate the changes that occur in each component of the motor control system.

Changes in sensory control of movement – closed-loop control problems

Deficits in the sensory control of movement have been identified, including changes in sensory feedback, abnormal reflex responses and inaccurate coordination of movement. From behavioral studies of human movement, it is difficult to determine the exact component or components of the system that are responsible for the change in motor control. For instance, if the amplitude of activity of a muscle is increased during a pointing task, it is difficult to determine whether the change results from inaccurate feedback from the periphery, inaccurate interpretation of normal feedback or inability to initiate an appropriate command. The following sections deal with several specific instances in which changes in elements of the closed-loop system may be implicated.

Sensory deficits

The basis of closed-loop control is accurate feedback from movement. Deficits in sensation are amongst the most commonly identified deficits in motor control identified in association with musculoskeletal pain and injury. These have been recognized in two major ways: first, by measurement of the acuity for detection of movement, such as the smallest movement that can be accurately detected; and second, by the ability to accurately copy a position or return to a position of a limb after it has been demonstrated with the same or opposite limb. Using these methods, studies have identified: decreased acuity to spinal motion in low back pain (Taimela et al 1999); decreased acuity to ankle movement in the inversion/eversion direction (Garn & Newton 1988), but not plantarflexion or dorsiflexion following ankle sprain (Refshauge et al 2000); decreased acuity to shoulder motion with shoulder instability (Warner et al 1996); increased threshold to perception of vibration (indicating decreased sensory function) following ankle sprain (Bullock-Saxton 1994); and impaired ability to accurately reposition with low back pain (Brumagne et al 2000), ankle sprain and knee osteoarthritis (Garsden & Bullock-Saxton 1999).

Due to the importance of sensory information to closed-loop control of movement, deficits such as those outlined above may lead to impaired movement control at a number of levels. For instance, decreased acuity may lead to delayed reflex responses as a result of increased time to reach the threshold for movement detection. More complex changes are also possible, such as impaired coordination during voluntary movement due to inaccurate feedback from movement. This inaccurate feedback may lead to faulty error detection and correction. Another possibility is that inaccurate feedback may lead to development of a faulty internal model of body dynamics. In this case, the CNS may generate commands that are inaccurate for performance of the required movement. An additional possibility is that the muscle spindle sensitivity may be altered by pain (Pedersen et al 1997).

The reason for sensory feedback to change with injury and pain may be multifactorial. For example, it may be due to injury to joint, muscle or cutaneous receptors. Alternatively, it may be due to changes in interpretation of the afferent input, such as the potential for afferent input to be misinterpreted as nociceptive in hyperalgesia. In addition, changes in muscle activity may affect sensory acuity. Muscle activity is known to augment acuity (Gandevia et al 1992); thus any change in activation may adversely affect movement sensation. Furthermore, many

muscles, particularly deep muscles close to the joints, have extensive attachments to joint structures and contraction is likely to affect sensation. Finally, several studies have argued that sensory acuity may be reduced by fatigue (Carpenter et al 1998); thus decreased muscle endurance with injury or pain may lead to impaired sensory acuity.

Reflex changes

Changes in a variety of reflex responses have been identified in musculoskeletal pain syndromes. These changes include delayed reaction time of the peroneal muscle response to ankle inversion in ankle sprain (Lofvenberg et al 1995), delayed onset of activity of the erector spinae to trunk loading (Magnusson et al 1996) and delayed offset of activity of the oblique abdominal and thoracolumbar erector spinae muscles of the trunk in response to unloading in chronic low back pain (Fig. 8.5)

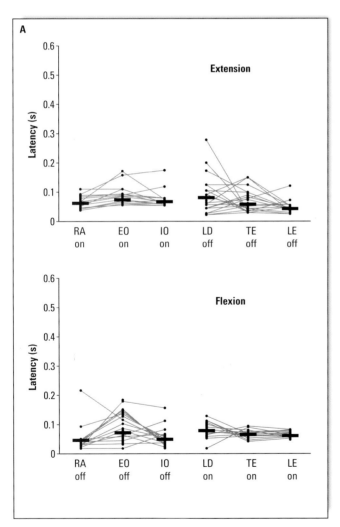
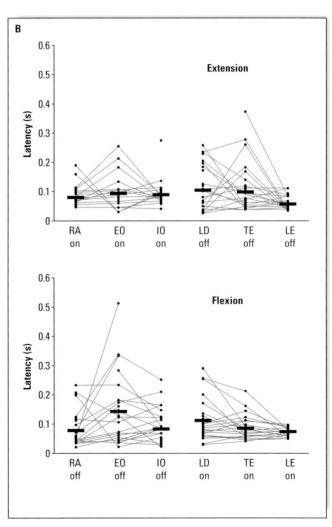

Figure 8.5 • When a mass attached to the front (extension) or back (flexion) of the trunk is suddenly removed, the trunk muscles must reduce their activity to maintain the upright position of the trunk. When people have low back pain the offset of the external oblique abdominal and thoracic erector spinae muscles is delayed. **A:** Healthy controls. **B:** Low back pain patients. (Reproduced from Radebold et al 2000 with the permission of Lippincott Williams and Wilkins.)

(Radebold et al 2000). Others, however, have failed to find changes in reflex responses of the erector spinae, elicited by a muscle tap, with experimentally induced pain.

Changes in reflex responses may be due to altered sensory input (see the section on sensory deficits above) and changes in motorneuron excitability may be the result of descending drive or spinal mechanisms (see the section on Changes in Motorneuron Excitability – Reflex Inhibition below). In addition, it has been suggested that reflex responses may be delayed by slowed conduction velocity in the motor axons (Kleinrensink et al 1994). This later mechanism is unlikely to be altered by motor learning.

Movement coordination

Although it is difficult to identify the exact site for changes in motor control from behavioral studies of human movement, several examples have been identified in the literature. For example, studies have identified impaired control of the trajectory of arm movement in a pointing task when vision is occluded in people with shoulder instability (Forwell & Carnahan 1996), and changes in amplitude and time onset of muscle activity of serratus anterior and upper trapezius in shoulder impingement during arm elevation (Ludewig & Cook 2000). In addition, slow

reaction time has been identified in low back pain (Luoto et al 1995). This latter finding has been associated with musculoskeletal injuries in a variety of sports (Taimela & Kujala 1992).

Many reasons could be hypothesized for these changes (Fig. 8.6). Again, sensory deficits may be responsible (see the section on Sensory Deficits above). In addition, it has been argued that changes may arise due to an inability to ignore unnecessary information, and the effect that this would have on limited attention resources (Luoto et al 1999). The effects may also occur as a result of fear or stress (Moseley et al 2004a, 2004b). Changes may also be due to alterations in cortical excitability (Valeriani et al 1999), motorneuron excitability (see the section on Changes in Motorneuron Excitability – Reflex Inhibition below) or delayed transmission in the CNS. However, there is considerable debate regarding the nature of these changes as evidence of increased or decreased excitability has been reported at each of these sites. Alternatively, effects may be due to the direct or indirect influence of pain on planning of motor responses (Derbyshire 1997). For instance, the strategy of muscle activation may be changed to protect the part from further pain and injury. This response, however, may be associated with increased activity of antagonist muscles and decreased activity of agonist muscles to reduce movement velocity and

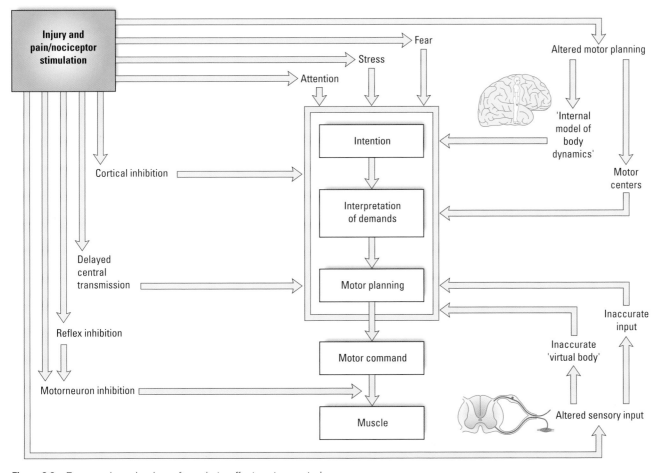

Figure 8.6 • Proposed mechanisms for pain to affect motor control.

displacement which has been described as the 'pain adaptation' model by Lund et al (1991). Alternatively the strategy may involve co-contraction to increase joint stiffness and stability (for a review see Hodges & Cholewicki 2006).

Control of posture and joint stability

Joint stability

A number of changes in motor control in musculoskeletal pain can be directly associated with impairments in the control of joint stability. These changes include changes in reflex responses of the erector spinae (see above), and changes in timing and amplitude of muscle activity during ongoing functional movements (i.e. closed-loop control). For example, changes in the time of activation of the medial and lateral vastii muscles have been identified during stair-stepping tasks in people with patellofemoral pain syndrome. Although there has been considerable disagreement regarding whether or not impaired activity of the medial vastii (vastus medialis obliquus) leads to abnormal tracking of the patella and pain (Powers et al 1996), recent studies have identified delayed activity of this muscle in comparison to the lateral vastii, when stepping onto and off a step (Fig. 8.7) (Cowan et al 2001). Consistent with this observation, coordination of firing of motor units in the medial and lateral vasti muscles is reduced in patellofemoral pain (Mellor & Hodges 2005). In addition, reduced amplitude of multifidus activity (a muscle considered to provide a critical contribution

to spinal stability) has been identified during functional tasks in people with low back pain (Lindgren et al 1993). Although these changes imply impaired muscle activity, other studies provide evidence of augmented activity, such as sustained activity of the erector spinae muscles at the end of the range of spinal flexion, a point at which these muscles are normally inactive, in people with low back pain (Shirado et al 1995). This has been replicated by experimental pain (Zedka et al 1999).

As outlined above, it has been argued that one response of the nervous system to pain is to reduce movement by a combination of augmentation or impairment of muscle activity. This somewhat simplistic view has gained some support in the literature. One interpretation of the results presented here is that the activation of the multisegmented global muscles, such as the erector spinae, may be modified to reduce the overall motion of the joints, by either reducing their activity as an agonist activation during movement, or by co-contraction to make a segment rigid. In contrast, a relatively consistent response of the system is to reduce the activation of the deep local muscles, which may compromise the fine-tuning of segmental control.

Postural control

Several studies have investigated parameters of ongoing closed-loop control of posture in people with low back pain. These studies have identified impairments of balance when standing on one (Luoto et al 1998) or two legs (Byl & Sinnott 1991) or sitting (Radebold et al 2001). Furthermore, an increased risk of low back pain or recurrence of pain has been identified for people with poor performance in a test of standing balance (Takala & Viikari-Juntura 2000). Although it is not possible to determine the mechanism for these changes, they may be due to sensory deficits or changes in information processing or motor planning. These changes indicate a general reduction of the accuracy of the postural control system in these patients; hence, the relationship to increased risk of re-injury.

Changes in motor planning – open-loop control problems

Feedforward strategies

The major factors that have implicated changes in the open-loop control of movement are changes in feedforward strategies. As mentioned above, these strategies are preplanned by the nervous system and represent the pattern of muscle activity initiated by the CNS in advance of movement. Several studies have investigated onset of muscle activity in association with rapid limb movements. These studies have identified delayed onset of activity of the deep abdominal muscle, transversus abdominis, with arm and leg movements in people with chronic low back pain (Hodges & Richardson 1996), delayed activity of the deep cervical flexor muscles in neck pain (Falla et al 2004), activity of the rotator cuff muscles in shoulder pain (Hess et al 2005) and similar change in the patterns of activation of the scapula muscles has been identified in association with shoulder movement in people with shoulder impingement (Wadsworth & Bullock-Saxton 1997). Similar changes in feedforward strategies

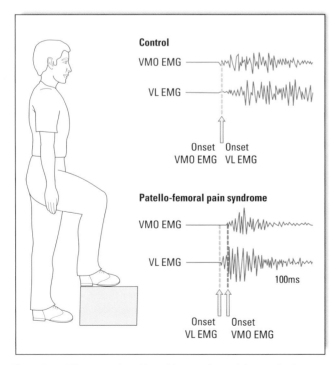

Figure 8.7 • When people with no history of patellofemoral pain step up onto a step the onsets of the medial and lateral vastii occur simultaneously. However, when patellofemoral pain is present the onset of VMO occurs before that of VL. (Adapted from Cowan et al 2001.)

have been replicated when pain is induced by the injection of hypertonic saline into the paraspinal muscles (Fig. 8.8) (Hodges et al 2001). These changes are associated with impaired motor planning rather than changes in excitability or transmission of the command in the CNS (Hodges 2001).

The possible mechanisms for changes in feedforward responses are similar to those outlined above for changes in closed-loop control of movement. However, the changes must occur in motor planning as these responses are initiated in advance of movement, and therefore in advance of sensory feedback from the movement. Despite the open-loop nature of the responses, sensory deficits may influence the quality of movement control as accurate sensory input is required to develop the internal model of body dynamics that is built up by movement experience. If the internal model is based on inaccurate sensory input open loop control of movement is likely to be compromised.

Changes in motorneuron excitability – reflex inhibition

A factor that may influence motor control, and therefore the output of the motor system, irrespective of whether open- or closed-loop systems are involved, is changes in the excitability of the spinal motorneurons. Although there is considerable debate whether motorneuron excitability is directly affected by pain, there is some evidence that motorneuron excitability may be reduced as a result of injury to joint structures (i.e. reflex inhibition). The mechanism for reflex inhibition is generally considered to involve inhibition of the alpha-motorneuron as a result of afferent input from effusion (Stokes & Young 1984) or injury to joint structures (Ekholm et al 1960). For example, when effusion is present in the knee, the motorneuron excitability of quadriceps muscles is reduced (Spencer et al 1984). In general it is regarded that reflex inhibition leads to inhibition

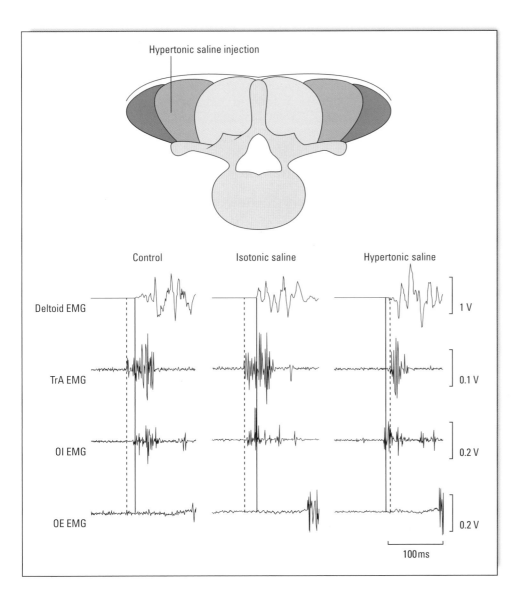

Figure 8.8 • Change in trunk muscle with low back pain. When people have experimental pain induced by injection of hypertonic saline into the paraspinal muscles, the onset of EMG of transversus abdominis is delayed relative to the onset of the muscle responsible for arm movement when the arm is moved rapidly in response to a light. (Adapted from Hodges et al 2001a.)

of extensor muscles (Ekholm et al 1960), although some data suggest that specific muscles may be more susceptible to the effects of reflex inhibition, such as the oblique fibers of vastus medialis which become inhibited with lower volumes of knee joint effusion than the other vasti muscles. Reflex inhibition has also been used as an explanation for the rapid atrophy of multi-fidus in people with acute low back pain (Hides et al 1994). Recently it has been confirmed that multifidus muscles atrophy rapidly after injury to spinal structures including the interverte-bral disc (Hodges et al 2006b). Although the excitability of the motorneurons has not been directly measured this is a likely mechanism to explain the rapid changes in muscle size.

Pain or changes in motor control – which comes first?

There is considerable debate in the literature regarding the sequence of changes in motor control and pain (Fig. 8.9). Several possibilities have been outlined above that suggest that injury and pain may affect motor control. Furthermore, many of the control changes that are observed in clinical popula-tions may be replicated in healthy subjects by experimentally induced pain (Hodges et al 2006b, Zedka et al 1999). Thus there is strong evidence that pain and injury may be responsible for the changes in motor control; however, it is also possible that changes in motor control lead to pain. Several authors have argued that poor joint control leads to microtrauma and even-tual injury (Farfan 1973, Panjabi 1992) and this may be due to poor motor control. Consistent with this proposal, recent data suggest that changes in the control of the trunk muscles are associated with the development of low back pain in a sport-ing population (Cholewicki et al 2005). However, it is unclear what factors are responsible for the changes in control prior to pain and injury. In summary, it is likely that motor control changes are both a cause and result of pain and injury and that the mechanisms are likely to be multifactorial. Regardless of the initial event, the cyclic nature of this relationship suggests that a goal of intervention must be to break the cycle through a combination of strategies to reduce pain, facilitate healing and optimize motor control.

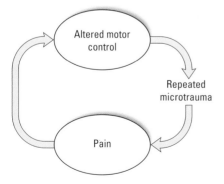

Figure 8.9 • Possible cycle of pain, injury and motor control changes.

Motor learning in the management of sports-related injuries

The overwhelming evidence that motor control is compro-mised in pain and injury makes it clear that rehabilitation of sports-related injuries must include consideration of control and coordination of movement and stability. Fortunately, the nervous system has considerable potential for plasticity and learning. Motor learning refers to the acquisition and refine-ment of movement and coordination that leads to a perma-nent change in movement performance. Irrespective of the skill being trained, motor learning is characterized by several goals including improvement of motor performance (increased precision, decreased error), improved performance consist-ency (decreased variability), persistence of improvements (continued improvement over time leading to permanent improvement) and the adaptability of the skill to a variety of environments (novel contexts, decreased feedback, changes in physical or personal characteristics). Numerous motor learn-ing strategies have been presented in the literature to achieve these goals. This section provides an overview of the stages of motor learning and several contemporary strategies for training specific motor skills that are applicable to the clinical situation for the management and prevention of injuries and pain. For a more comprehensive review, refer to Magill (2001), Schmidt & Lee (1999) and Shumway-Cooke & Woollacott (1995).

Stages of motor learning

Several authors have presented sequential models of the stages of motor learning. One popular model, first presented by Fitts & Posner (1967), considers that learning involves three main stages: the *cognitive, associative* and *autonomous* phases. In the *cognitive* phase, the focus is on cognitively oriented problems. All elements of the movement performance are organized con-sciously with attention to feedback, movement sequence, per-formance and instruction during repetition and practice. This phase is characterized by frequent, large errors and variabil-ity. Animal studies have identified increased size of the hand area of the sensory cortex during the cognitive phase of motor learning of a task involving interpretation of sensory informa-tion from the hand (Recanzone et al 1992). The second stage is the *associative* phase, in which the fundamentals of the movement have been acquired and the cognitive demands are reduced. The focus moves from simple elements of perform-ance of the task to consistency of performance, success and refinement. Correspondingly, the frequency and size of errors are reduced. The final stage of motor learning, the *autonomous* stage, is achieved after considerable practice and experience. The task becomes habitual or automatic and the requirement for conscious intervention is reduced. Although the features of each stage are distinct, it is important to consider that there is a smooth transition between stages and it may not be obvious when a person moves between phases.

Other models of motor learning have similar features to this three-stage process with differences in the emphasis placed on elements of the progression of learning. Gentile (1987) divides learning into two phases based on the goal of the learner. In the first phase, the goal of the learner is to 'get the idea' of the task. The second phase involves fixation or diversification of the skill, that is, improved consistency in stable environments and improved transfer to new contexts. Irrespective of the specific features of each model the basic elements of motor learning are similar.

Strategies for motor learning

Practice of parts and/or practice of the whole

There has been considerable debate in the literature regarding whether it is more optimal to train motor skills by practicing a whole movement, or with practice of essential components of the skill with later integration of the components into the complete skill. While both methods are likely to result in changes to skill performance, it is likely that specific types of skill are more amenable to each method. It has been argued that movements with simple organization (i.e. tasks composed of several elements that are independent) and high complexity (i.e. many elements) are amenable to practice of parts of the skill (Naylor & Briggs 1963). In contrast, movements with complex organization (i.e. tasks composed of a sequence of skills in which performance of one is dependent on performance of another) and low complexity (i.e. few elements) are best trained with practice of the whole task (Naylor & Briggs 1963).

In whole-task practice, it is possible to develop the spatial and temporal relationship of the independent elements of the task. However, when a skill is trained in parts, the attention demand is reduced to allow attention to be focused on a single element. At a later stage, it is important to perform the interdependent parts of a task together. This approach is ideal when there are a few discrete elements of a skilled task that are problematic and require training or refinement. Several techniques have been described for part-task training. These include *segmentation* and *simplification* (Magill 2001). In the *segmentation* approach, the task is broken up into smaller parts to be practiced as independent units, and then the practiced elements are integrated together progressively to practice the complete skill. In the *simplification* approach the movement or its parts are simplified to increase the ease of movement performance. *Simplification* may be achieved by changing parameters such as reduction of the attention demands, reduction of speed of the task or using additional strategies to augment the performance (Fig. 8.10) (e.g. application of tape over the patella to change the timing of the vastii, reduction of swelling to reduce reflex inhibition, positioning to decrease load, improved sensory acuity to improve accuracy of feedback). Alternatively, a person can practice the whole task, but attend to a specific part of the task. In this way, a part practice environment can be integrated into whole practice. This latter approach may be facilitated by augmentation of the level of feedback (see below) of the movement element that is being addressed.

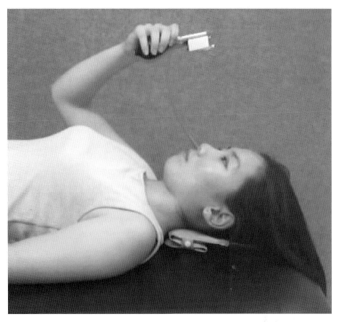

Figure 8.10 • Simplification. Simplification of a task can take many forms. Here the performance of the control exercise for the upper cervical flexors in a patient with neck pain is simplified by modification of the position of the patient. In the supine position the gravitational load is reduced, making it easier for the subject to perform the task in a precise manner. Additional feedback of the task is provided with a pressure cuff placed under the cervical spine.

Instruction versus demonstration

Two major ways to teach a skill or part of a task are demonstration and instruction. The precise nature of instructions varies and may include information of the goal, the steps in task performance or errors. Demonstration may involve visual information by showing the task or another form of feedback, such as kinesthetic information (e.g. moving the learner through a required range of motion or electrical stimulation of a muscle contraction). An essential component of both techniques is accurate analysis of the movement and identification of the elements to be trained or refined.

It has been argued that instruction or demonstration may lead to better improvement, depending on the task being performed. For example, it has been argued that demonstration is better for tasks in which a new pattern of coordination is being trained, rather than an adaptation of a pattern that has already been learnt (Magill & Schoenfelder-Zohndi 1996). The aim of demonstration fits with Gentile's goal for the first stage of motor learning to 'give the idea' of the task (Gentile 1987). If demonstration is selected as the technique for training a skill, this can be done either by demonstrating a skilled performance or allowing the learner to observe practice by an unskilled person. Additional improvement may be achieved if the learner is cued to the important elements of the skilled performance during the demonstration. Verbal instruction is one of the most common techniques for training a motor skill. Several important factors require consideration. First, the complexity of instruction needs to match the attention capacity of the learner; instruction will be most effective if the minimum instruction is given. Second, some types of information may hinder learning. Third, verbal instruction can be used for two purposes: to cue attention to a specific element, or to cue the patient to initiate an action.

Feedback

An important element of motor learning is the provision of augmented feedback. Feedback can be generally divided into two main types: knowledge of performance and knowledge of results. Put simply, feedback that provides knowledge of performance relates to ongoing sensory/perceptual information provided during the movement, whereas knowledge of results provides feedback on the outcome of the movement. Each of the sensory systems, including visual, auditory, proprioceptive and vestibular information, may be utilized to provide each form of feedback. This feedback may be intrinsic (naturally occurring) or augmented/enhanced in some way (e.g. electromyographic biofeedback or ultrasound imaging to increase awareness of muscle contraction, verbal feedback of quality of performance, video replay of performance). Thus, augmented feedback may be provided during the task or upon its completion and may be used to encourage and motivate achievement of the goal of a task or used to refine its performance. In general, feedback may be particularly important if the intrinsic information is not sufficient (e.g. when sensory acuity is impaired or due to lack of experience). If intrinsic information is sufficient, augmentation of the feedback may enhance the development of the skill.

Three issues require further consideration. First, should feedback of correct or incorrect aspects of performance be given? In general, feedback of errors leads to skill improvement, whereas feedback of correct elements is motivational; both may be beneficial. Second, should feedback provide qualitative or quantitative information? For example, qualitative information of speed of contraction or quantitative information of the number of seconds to complete the task could be provided. Although it may be assumed that quantitative feedback may be optimal, as it provides the most precise information, others argue that qualitative information provides an easier to interpret form of feedback in the early stages of learning. Third, there are several situations in which feedback may compromise motor learning, for example, if a learner becomes dependent on the feedback that is not available during natural performance. This may occur if the intrinsic feedback is limited or complex. In this case, the learner may substitute the augmented feedback for the intrinsic feedback and may not learn to use the intrinsic feedback. In general, it is important to be certain that augmented feedback is accurate and that mechanisms are in place to ensure that learners will be able to progress to using available intrinsic feedback. It is generally accepted that it is better not to provide feedback on every trial to avoid dependence.

As discussed earlier, augmented feedback may be provided in a variety of different ways. These include verbal feedback, providing descriptive information about an error or information

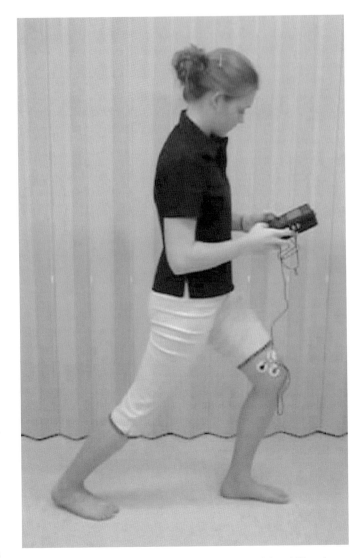

Figure 8.11 • Augmented feedback. In order to provide additional feedback of contraction of vastus medialis obliquus, EMG biofeedback electrodes are placed over VMO of a patient with patellofemoral pain syndrome. Dual-channel EMG could provide additional feedback of the relative activity of the medial and lateral vastii.

on how to improve the performance, visual feedback using mirrors, video, etc., and enhanced kinesthetic information using biofeedback of muscle activity with electromyography (EMG) (Fig. 8.11), ultrasound or palpation of contraction, movement kinematics or force output. All forms may be beneficial, but it is important to consider whether the learner is capable of using the selected feedback and the stage of learning.

Transfer of training

An important component of skill learning is that the performance of the skill can be transferred to different conditions in which the environment, personal characteristics or predictability are changed. In order to optimize transfer, it is considered essential to sequentially progress the task from easy to more complex situations. Transfer occurs when there are similarities in performance between tasks. In other words, specificity of practice is required to ensure transfer between environments. If the aim is to transfer a skilled movement to functional tasks, then it is necessary to progress to function. More specifically, it may be necessary to replicate sensory characteristics (e.g. limitation of visual feedback), environmental contexts (e.g. unstable surfaces, distractions) and personal contexts (e.g. anxiety, fatigue) to ensure that the elements of the skill can be transferred to specific contexts. A specific example of training transfer relates to bilateral transfer in which it is easier to learn a particular skill with one limb if it has already been learnt with the other (see Magill 2001).

Variability of practice

A goal of motor learning is that the trained task can be utilized under a variety of conditions. One method to facilitate this consistency of response is to vary environmental and personal contexts during practice (Schmidt & Lee 1999). Variability of practice aims to improve the performance of the task and enhance the ability to perform the task in novel environments. Progression may be provided by starting with practice in closed repeatable environments and progressing to complex open environments with increased levels of unpredictability.

Dosage

The ability of motor learning to change performance is influenced by the distribution of practice. Factors to consider are the frequency of training and the interval between practice sessions. Massed practice refers to few, longer sessions of practice, whereas distributed practice refers to more frequent, shorter sessions. In the literature, it is generally agreed that shorter practice sessions result in greater improvements in performance. Massed practice may lead to poorer retention and poorer performance outcome (Baddeley & Longman 1978). However, for short discrete tasks, massed practice may have additional benefits.

Mental practice

An additional tool that may lead to improvements in motor performance is mental practice (see Chapter 11). This strategy involves mental rehearsal of the task without actually moving. While it can lead to additional benefits, it is best when combined with physical practice.

Sensory learning

In addition to and in conjunction with training movement performance, strategies can be utilized to train sensation or the use of sensation to aid movement performance. A spectrum of strategies have been described in the literature that range from tasks aimed at improving sensory acuity (e.g. balance board training, joint repositioning) to training a learner to use visual or other sensory information to aid movement control. These strategies may be of critical importance when training an individual in the use of intrinsic feedback to guide movement as

they would allow for accurate error detection and withdrawal of augmented feedback.

Application of motor control and motor learning in physical therapy of sports- and exercise-related injuries – low back pain

This section will illustrate the implementation of motor learning strategies for musculoskeletal pain. One region of the body that has received extensive attention in relation to the motor control system and pain is lumbar spine pain. The spine is inherently unstable and is dependent on the contribution of muscle for its control. Obviously, the muscular contribution to stability is dependent on an efficient motor control system that can detect the status of stability and that is able to generate appropriate responses to maintain stability in the face of predictable and unpredictable challenges. It has been argued by several authors that changes in motor control may predispose to back pain (Cholewicki et al 2005), be caused by back pain (Hodges et al 2003) and cause recurrence of back pain (Hides et al 2001, Hodges & Richardson 1996, Panjabi 1992).

While there are many ways to investigate motor control of the spine, and many have been considered above, one aspect that has been investigated extensively is the problem of coordination of mobility and stability. To test this control, studies have investigated the control of the trunk muscles in association with rapid limb movements. This task provides a window to investigate one aspect of the motor control mechanism and is particularly relevant to sport as it involves a predictable and rapid limb movement. In this task, several studies have shown that there are changes in the pattern of muscle activity that is initiated prior to the onset of the movement (i.e. feedforward postural strategy) (Hodges & Richardson 1996). This change primarily involves a delay in the onset of activity of transversus abdominis, the deepest of the abdominal muscles, which has been shown to augment stability of the lumbar spine and sacroiliac joints (Hodges et al 2003, Hodges et al 2005, Snijders et al 1995). Evidence from other tasks suggests that activity of the more superficial trunk muscles, such as the obliquus externus abdominis, may be increased (for a review see van Dieen et al 2003), although the pattern of changes in superficial muscle activity varies between individuals (Hodges et al 2006a). On the basis of this and other evidence, clinical strategies have been developed that rely on the principles of motor learning to retrain motor control (see Richardson et al 1999). A key issue that requires consideration is whether the adaptation in motor control is positive or negative, and, thus, whether it should be augmented or corrected. For instance it could be argued that the increased activity of the more superficial muscles of the trunk acts to stabilize and protect the spine from further pain and injury (van Dieen et al 2003), and in this case it may be argued that the strategy should be increased, rather than corrected. On the other hand, it may be argued that although these strategies could be appropriate in an acute situation, they may not be ideal to maintain in the long term as these strategies are associated with increased spinal load (due to increased co-contraction of superficial muscles) and less ideal control of intervertebral motion (due to decreased control of the deeper muscles) (Hodges & Cholewicki 2006). In reality it is likely the both alternatives may be correct, but dependent on the presentation of the patient.

A key element of motor control training in low back pain is the identification of the specific elements of motor control that are problematic (i.e. reduced tonic activity and delayed activation of the deep intrinsic spinal muscles, increased activity of the more superficial muscles). In line with motor learning theory, outlined above, the training program involves segmentation and simplification (Fig. 8.12). First, movement is broken into parts and the deep muscle activation is trained as a *part* of the movement. The specific components that need to be trained are identified through precise assessment. At the same time any overactivity of the superficial muscles is evaluated and discouraged. Second, the performance of this maneuver is simplified by positioning the patient to increase the ease of learning the skilled contraction of the deeper muscles. Techniques to reduce or enhance activation of muscles involved in this task, and feedback of contraction, are augmented by palpation, observation or, in special cases, visualization of contraction with ultrasound imaging (Hides et al 1996). Part training is progressed by decreasing augmented feedback, training intrinsic feedback, improving performance and consistency, and changing the context of contraction by modifying body posture and environment. Once the performance of this movement element is improved, the program progresses to integrate other parts of the movement performance, such as the incorporation of the activation of other trunk muscles and the practice of a variety of functional tasks, including those that are pain provocative. This final stage of whole practice is progressed via practice in contexts of increasing complexity, such as exercise on unstable surfaces and open environments.

There is evidence from randomized controlled clinical trials that this approach is clinically beneficial (Ferreira et al 2006, O'Sullivan et al 1997, Stuge et al 2004). Furthermore, recent data confirm that the coordination of the deep and superficial muscles can be restored by this intervention (Tsao & Hodges 2007), and clinical outcome is linked to the change in motor control strategy. Thus, there is preliminary evidence that the motor relearning strategy can lead to changes in the preplanned postural component associated with movement of the limbs.

Summary

Motor control and motor learning are important elements in the management of pain and injury associated with sport and physical activity. Recent research has highlighted the incidence and extent of deficits in motor control that are present in the sporting population. Increasing numbers of clinical trails have been conducted to investigate the efficacy of motor learning techniques in the treatment of pain and reduction of injury recurrence. Future work is likely to lead to further developments in this field.

References

Baddeley A D, Longman D J A 1978 The influence of length and frequency of training session on the rate of learning to type. Ergonomics 21:627–635

Bergmark A 1989 Stability of the lumbar spine. a study in mechanical engineering. Acta Orthopedica Scandinavica 60:1–54

Bernstein N 1967 The co-ordination and regulation of movements. Pergamon Press, Oxford

Brumagne S, Cordo P, Lysens R et al 2000 The role of paraspinal muscle spindles in lumbosacral position sense in individuals with and without low back pain. Spine 25:989–994

Bullock-Saxton J E 1994 Local sensation changes and altered hip muscle function following severe ankle sprain. Physical Therapy 74:17–28

Byl N N, Sinnott P L 1991 Variations in balance and body sway in middle-aged adults: subjects with healthy backs compared with subjects with low back dysfunction. Spine 16:325–330

Carpenter J E, Blasier R B, Pellizzon G G 1998 The effects of muscle fatigue on shoulder joint position sense. American Journal of Sports Medicine 26:262–265

Cholewicki J, Silfies S, Shah R et al 2005 Delayed trunk muscle reflex responses increase the risk of low back pain injuries. Spine 30:2614–2620

Collins D F, Refshauge K M, Gandevia S C 2000 Sensory integration in the perception of movements at the human metacarpophalangeal joint. Journal of Physiology 529:505–515

Cowan S, Bennell K, Hodges P et al 2001 Delayed onset of electromyographic activity of vastus medialis obliquus relative to vastus lateralis in subjects with patellofemoral pain syndrome. Archives of Physical Medicine and Rehabilitation 82:183–189

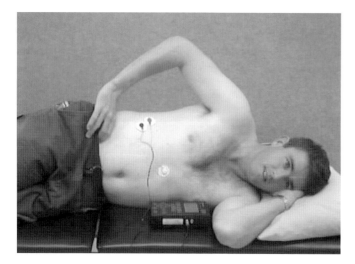

Figure 8.12 • Simplification, segmentation and augmented feedback are combined to optimize the performance of the coordinated contraction of the deep abdominal muscles in a patient with low back pain. Here the patient is performing a part task (deep muscle control) in preparation for functional training. The task is simplified by the position of the patient to reduce load. Feedback is augmented by use of tactile feedback of contraction from the fingers and EMG of the superficial abdominal muscles to reduce overactivity. The task is further simplified by having the patient perform a contraction of the pelvic floor muscle, which has been shown to trigger activation of the deep abdominal muscles.

Derbyshire S W, Jones A K, Gyulai F et al 1997 Pain processing during three levels of noxious stimulation produces differential patterns of central activity. Pain 73:431–445

Ekholm J, Eklund G, Skoglund S 1960 On reflex effects from knee joint of cats. Acta Physiologica Scandinavica 50:167–174

Falla D, Jull G, Hodges PW 2004 Feedforward activity of the cervical flexor muscles during voluntary arm movements is delayed in chronic neck pain. Experimental Brain Research 157:43–48

Farfan H F 1973 Mechanical disorders of the low back. Lea and Febiger, Philadelphia, PA

Ferreira P H, Ferreira M L, Maher C G et al 2006 Specific stabilisation exercise for spinal and pelvic pain: a systematic review. Australian Journal of Physiotherapy 52:79–88

Fitts P M, Posner M I 1967 Human performance. Brooks/Cole, Belmont, CA

Fitzpatrick R, Burke D, Gandevia S C 1996 Loop gain of reflexes controlling human standing measured with the use of postural and vestibular disturbances. Journal of Neurophysiology 76:3994–4008

Forwell L A, Carnahan H 1996 Proprioception during manual aiming in individuals with shoulder instability and controls. Journal of Orthopaedic and Sports Physical Therapy 23:111–119

Gahéry Y, Massion J 1981 Co-ordination between posture and movement. Trends in Neurosciences 4:119–202

Gandevia S C, McCloskey D I, Burke D 1992 Kinaesthetic signals and muscle contraction. Trends in Neurosciences 15:62–65

Garn S N, Newton R A 1988 Kinesthetic awareness in subjects with multiple ankle sprains. Physical Therapy 68:1667–1671

Garsden L R, Bullock-Saxton J E 1999 Joint reposition sense in subjects with unilateral osteoarthritis of the knee. Clinical Rehabilitation 13:148–155

Gentile A M 1987 Skill acquisition: action, movement and neuromuscular processes. In: Carr J H, Shephard R B, Gordon J et al (eds) Movement and science: foundations for physical therapy in rehabilitation. Aspen Publishers, Gaithersburg, MD, p 93–154

Goff B 1972 The application of recent advances in neurophysiology to Miss M. Rood's concept of neuromuscular facilitation. Physiotherapy 58:409–415

Grillner S 1981 Control of locomotion in bipeds, tetrapods, and fish. In: Brookhart M, Mountcastle V B (eds) Handbook of physiology: the nervous system. Motor control, vol ii, part 2. American Physiological Society, Washington, DC, p 1179–1235

Gurfinkel V S, Kots Y M, Paltsev E I et al 1971 The compensation of respiratory disturbances of erect posture of man as an example of the organisation of interarticular interaction. In: Gelfard I M, Gurfinkel V S, Formin S V et al (eds) Models of the structural functional organization of certain biological systems. MIT Press, Cambridge, MA, p 382–395

Hess S A, Richardson C, Darnell R et al 2005 Timing of rotator cuff activation during shoulder external rotation in throwers with and without symptoms of pain. Journal of Orthopaedic and Sports Physical Therapy 35:812–820

Hides J A, Stokes M J, Saide M et al 1994 Evidence of lumbar multifidus muscle wasting ipsilateral to symptoms in patients with acute/subacute low back pain. Spine 19:165–177

Hides J A, Richardson C A, Jull G A et al 1996 Ultrasound imaging in rehabilitation. Australian Journal of Physiotherapy 41:187–193

Hides J A, Jull G A, Richardson C A 2001 Long term effects of specific stabilizing exercises for first episode low back pain. Spine 26:243–248

Hodges P 2001 Changes in motor planning of feedforward postural responses of the trunk muscles in low back pain. Experimental Brain Research 141:261–266

Hodges P W, Cholewicki J 2006 Functional control of the spine. In: Vleeming A, Mooney V & Stoeckart R (eds) Movement, stability and lumbopelvic pain. Churchill Livingstone, Edinburgh, p 547–573

Hodges P W, Richardson C A 1996 Inefficient muscular stabilisation of the lumbar spine associated with low back pain: a motor control evaluation of transversus abdominis. Spine 21:2640–2650

Hodges P W, Richardson C A 1997 Feedforward contraction of transversus abdominis is not influenced by the direction of arm movement. Experimental Brain Research 114:362–370

Hodges P W, Cresswell A G, Thorstensson A 1999 Preparatory trunk motion accompanies rapid upper limb movement. Experimental Brain Research 124:69–79

Hodges P, Moseley G, Gabrielsson A et al 2001 Acute experimental pain changes postural recruitment of the trunk muscles in pain-free humans. Society for Neuroscience Abstracts 27 (304):13

Hodges P, Gurfinkel V S, Brumagne S et al 2002 Coexistence of stability and mobility in postural control: evidence from postural compensation for respiration. Experimental Brain Research 144:293–302

Hodges P, Kaigle Holm A, Holm S, et al 2003 Intervertebral stiffness of the spine is increased by evoked contraction of transversus abdominis and the diaphragm: in vivo porcine studies. Spine 28:2594–2601.

Hodges P W, Eriksson A E M, Shirley D et al 2005 Intra-abdominal pressure increases stiffness of the lumbar spine. Journal of Biomechanics 38(9):1873–1880.

Hodges P, Cholewicki J, Coppieters M et al 2006a Trunk muscle activity is increased during experimental back pain, but the pattern varies between individuals. International Society for Electrophysiology and Kinesiology, Torino, Italy

Hodges P W, KaigleHolm A, Hansson T et al 2006b Rapid atrophy of the lumbar multifidus follows experimental disc or nerve root injury. Spine 31(25): 2926–2933.

Hopper D, Allison G, Fernandes N et al 1998 The reliability of the peroneal latency in normal ankles. Clinical Orthopaedics and Related Research 350:159–165

Horak F B 1987 Clinical measurement of postural control in adults. Physical Therapy 67:1881–1885

Horak F, Nashner L M 1986 Central programming of postural movements: adaptation to altered support-surface configurations. Journal of Neurophysiology 55:1369–1381

Hugon M, Massion J, Weisendanger M 1982 Anticipatory postural changes induced by active unloading and comparison with passive unloading in man. Pflügers Archives 393:292–296

Janda V 1978 Muscles, central nervous motor regulation and back problems. In: Korr I M (ed) The neurobiologic mechanisms in manipulative therapy. Plenum Press, New York, p 27–41

Johansson H, Sjolander P, Sojka P 1991 A sensory role for the cruciate ligaments. Clinical Orthopaedics and Related Research 268:161–178

Kelso J A S 1984 Phase transitions and critical behaviour in human bimanual coordination. American Journal of Physiology: Regulatory, Integrative, and Comparative Physiology 15:R1000–1004

Keshner E A 1990 Controlling stability of a complex movement system. Physical Therapy 70:844–854

Kleinrensink G J, Stoeckart R, Meulstee J et al 1994 Lowered motor conduction velocity of the peroneal nerve after inversion trauma. Medicine and Science in Sports and Exercise 26:877–883

Lindgren K A, Sihvonen T, Leino E et al 1993 Exercise therapy effects on functional radiographic findings and segmental electromyographic activity in lumbar spine instability. Archives of Physical Medicine and Rehabilitation 74:933–939

Lofvenberg R, Karrholm J, Sundelin G et al 1995 Prolonged reaction time in patients with chronic lateral instability of the ankle. American Journal of Sports Medicine 23:414–417

Ludewig P M, Cook T M 2000 Alterations in shoulder kinematics and associated muscle activity in people with symptoms of shoulder impingement. Physical Therapy 80:276–291

Lund J P, Donga R, Widmer C G et al 1991 The pain-adaptation model: a discussion of the relationship between chronic musculoskeletal pain and motor activity. Canadian Journal of Physiology and Pharmacology 69:683–694

Luoto S, Hurri H, Alaranta H 1995 Reaction time in patients with chronic low back pain. European Journal of Physical Medicine and Rehabilitation 5:47–50

Luoto S, Aalto H, Taimela S et al 1998 One-footed and externally disturbed two-footed postural control in patients with chronic low back pain and healthy control subjects. A controlled study with follow-up. Spine 23:2081–2089

Luoto S, Taimela S, Hurri H et al 1999 Mechanisms explaining the association between low back trouble and deficits in information processing. A controlled study with follow-up. Spine 24:255–261

McNulty P A, Turker K S, Macefield V G 1999 Evidence for strong synaptic coupling between single tactile afferents and motoneurones supplying the human hand. Journal of Physiology 518:883–893

Magill R A 2001 Motor learning: concepts and applications. McGraw-Hill, New York

Magill R A, Schoenfelder-Zohndi B 1996 A visual model and knowledge of performance as sources of information for learning a rhythmic gymnastics skill. International Journal of Sport Psychology 27:7–22

Magnusson M, Aleksiev A, Wilder D et al 1996 Sudden load as an aetiologic factor in low back pain. European Journal of Physical Medicine and Rehabilitation 6:74–81

Massion J 1992 Movement, posture and equilibrium: interaction and coordination. Progress in Neurobiology 38:35–56

Mellor R, Hodges P W 2005 Motor unit synchronization is reduced in anterior knee pain. Journal of Pain 6:550–558

Moseley G L, Nicholas M K, Hodges P W 2004a Does anticipation of back pain predispose to back trouble? Brain 127:2339–2347

Moseley G L, Nicholas M K, Hodges P W 2004b Pain differs from non-painful attention-demanding or stressful tasks in its effect on postural control patterns of trunk muscles. Experimental Brain Research 156:64–71

Nashner L M 1977 Fixed patterns of rapid postural responses among leg muscles during stance. Experimental Brain Research 30:13–24

Naylor J, Briggs G 1963 Effects of task complexity and task organisation on the relative efficiency of part and whole training methods. Journal of Experimental Psychology 65:217–244

O'Sullivan P B, Twomey L T, Allison G T 1997 Evaluation of specific stabilizing exercise in the treatment of chronic low back pain with radiologic diagnosis of spondylolysis or spondylolisthesis. Spine 22:2959–2967

Panjabi M M 1992 The stabilizing system of the spine: I. Function, dysfunction, adaptation, and enhancement. Journal of Spinal Disorders 5:383–389

Pedersen J, Sjolander P, Wenngren B I et al 1997 Increased intramuscular concentration of bradykinin increases the static fusimotor drive to muscle spindles in neck muscles of the cat. Pain 70:83–91

Powers C, Landel R, Perry J 1996 Timing and intensity of vastus muscle activity during functional activities in subjects with and without patellofemoral pain. Physical Therapy 76:946–955

Radebold A, Cholewicki J, Panjabi M M et al 2000 Muscle response pattern to sudden trunk loading in healthy individuals and in patients with chronic low back pain. Spine 25:947–954

Radebold A, Cholewicki J, Polzhofer G K et al 2001 Impaired postural control of the lumbar spine is associated with delayed muscle response times in patients with chronic idiopathic low back pain. Spine 26:724–730

Recanzone G H, Merzenich M M, Jenkins W M et al 1992 Topographic reorganization of the hand representation in cortical area 3b owl monkeys trained in a frequency-discrimination task. Journal of Neurophysiology 67:1031–1056

Refshauge K M, Kilbreath S L, Raymond J 2000 The effect of recurrent ankle inversion sprain and taping on proprioception at the ankle. Medicine and Science in Sports and Exercise 32:10–15

Richardson C A, Jull G A, Hodges P W et al 1999 Therapeutic exercise for spinal segmental stabilisation in low back pain: scientific basis and clinical approach. Churchill Livingstone, Edinburgh

Sahrman S 2002 Diagnosis and treatment of movement impairment syndromes. Mosby, St Louis, MO

Schmidt R A, Lee T D 1999 Motor control and learning: a behavioural emphasis. Human Kinetics, Champaign, IL

Shirado O, Ito T, Kaneda K et al 1995 Flexion-relaxation phenomenon in the back muscles. A comparative study between healthy subjects and patients with chronic low back pain. American Journal of Physical Medicine and Rehabilitation 74:139–144

Shumway-Cooke A, Woollacott M H 1995 Motor control. Williams and Wilkins, Baltimore, MD

Snijders C J, Vleeming A, Stoeckart R et al 1995 Biomechanical modelling of sacroiliac joint stability in different postures. Spine: State of the Art Reviews 9:419–432

Spencer J D, Hayes K C, Alexander I J 1984 Knee joint effusion and quadriceps reflex inhibition in man. Archives of Physical Medicine and Rehabilitation 65:171–177

Stokes M, Young A 1984 The contribution of reflex inhibition to arthrogenous muscle weakness. Clinical Science 67:7–14

Stuge B, Laerum E, Kirkesola G et al 2004 The efficacy of a treatment program focusing on specific stabilizing exercises for pelvic girdle pain after pregnancy: a randomized controlled trial. Spine 29:351–359

Taimela S, Kujala U M 1992 Reaction times with reference to musculoskeletal complaints in adolescence. Perceptual and Motor Skills 75:1075–1082

Taimela S, Kankaanpaa M, Luoto S 1999 The effect of lumbar fatigue on the ability to sense a change in lumbar position. a controlled study. Spine 24:1322–1327

Takala E, Viikari-Juntura E 2000 Do functional tests predict low back pain? Spine 2:2126–2132

Taub E, Berman A J 1968 Movement and learning in the absence of sensory feedback. In: Freedman S J (ed) The neurophysiology of spatially oriented behaviour. Dorsey Press, Homewood, IL, p 173–192

Tsao H, Hodges PW 2007 Immediate changes in feedforward postural adjustments following voluntary motor training. Experimental Brain Research, in press.

Valeriani M, Restuccia D, Di Lazzaro V et al 1999 Inhibition of the human primary motor area by painful heat stimulation of the skin. Clinical Neurophysiology 110:1475–1480

van Dieen J H, Selen L P, Cholewicki J 2003 Trunk muscle activation in low-back pain patients, an analysis of the literature. Journal of Electromyography and Kinesiology 13:333–351

Wadsworth D J, Bullock-Saxton J E 1997 Recruitment patterns of the scapular rotator muscles in freestyle swimmers with subacromial impingement. International Journal of Sports Medicine 18:618–624

Warner J J, Lephart S, Fu F H 1996 Role of proprioception in pathoetiology of shoulder instability. Clinical Orthopaedics 330:5–39

Wilder D G, Aleksiev A R, Magnusson M L et al 1996 Muscular response to sudden load. A tool to evaluate fatigue and rehabilitation. Spine 21:2628–2639

Winter D A, Patla A E, Prince F et al 1998 Stiffness control of balance in quiet standing. Journal of Neurophysiology 80:1211–1221

Zedka M, Prochazka A, Knight B et al 1999 Voluntary and reflex control of human back muscles during induced pain. Journal of Physiology 520:591–604

Pain

Gregory S. Kolt

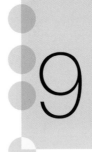

CHAPTER CONTENTS

Introduction 133

Mechanisms of pain 133

Theoretical perspectives of pain 134

Experience of pain 136

Assessment of pain 138

Management of pain 142

Summary 145

Introduction

Involvement in sport, exercise and other forms of physical activity carries with it a risk of injury and resultant pain. Pain in sport can be associated with routine performance of sport skills (e.g. tackles in contact sports, or the extreme physical demands of endurance activities), minor postexercise soreness, sudden severe injury, chronic pathologies or even some usual components of treatment and rehabilitation.

Pain is a debilitating and pervasive obstacle to effective injury rehabilitation in athletes (Taylor & Taylor 1998). As pain is often not well understood, physical therapists tend to spend too little time educating athletes about pain and the myriad of ways it can affect them, and how they can manage it within the confines of their rehabilitation and training programs. Pain, and the physiological and psychological responses it evokes, can greatly inhibit rehabilitation progress if not dealt with adequately.

The experience of pain by athletes varies greatly, as does the way pain is communicated in behaviors. As a result, measurement and quantification of pain is difficult, and, at best, it can be relatively scaled, qualified or described. This difficulty in quantification makes the study of pain processes a challenge. However, an understanding of the biological and psychological mechanisms of the pain process and their interdependence is required.

Practitioners involved in the physical therapies as they relate to sport and exercise play an integral role in assisting athletes in coping with and managing pain. Therefore, a thorough knowledge of the biopsychology of pain, pain theories, the meaning of pain to athletes and pain management strategies is essential for physical therapists in designing appropriate interventions.

This chapter will provide practitioners involved in the physical therapies with a background on the mechanisms of pain, theories of pain, methods used in the assessment of pain and the management of pain. It should be noted that it is not the aim of this chapter to provide a detailed complex discussion of the neurophysiological aspects of pain.

Mechanisms of pain

The most common definition of pain in the musculoskeletal literature has been that adopted by the International Association for the Study of Pain (IASP), which is that pain is an unpleasant sensory and emotional experience associated with actual or potential tissue damage or described in terms of such damage

(IASP 1986). This definition is widely accepted for research and clinical purposes, as it acknowledges that pain is a psychological, as well as physical, experience. The IASP (1986) definition will be used to describe the phenomenon of pain throughout this chapter.

Nociceptors

The sensation, transmission and perception of pain are the function of the nociceptive system of the nervous network. The process of nociception involves four processing components: transduction, transmission, modulation and perception (Heil & Fine 1999). Transduction involves the translation of noxious stimuli into electrical activity at the sensory nerve endings. During transmission, the transduced electrical impulses are propagated throughout the sensory nervous system. Within the modulation phase, the nociceptive transmission is modified by several neural influences, including central, cortical, and peripheral sensory inputs. The fourth process, perception, describes the cognitive-emotional experience of pain from the resultant transduction, transmission and modulation (Heil & Fine 1999).

The nociceptive system normally has a threshold of excitation too high to be stimulated by normal innocuous stimuli, but becomes activated through strong, intense, potentially damaging stimuli. Once experiencing pain, however, lesser or more innocuous stimuli can activate the system and lead to the perception of pain (Wright & Zusman 2004). Noxious stimuli are carried predominantly by small myelinated alpha-delta (A-δ) fibers and unmyelinated C fibers.

There are three main types of nociceptors: unimodal, bimodal and polymodal. The unimodal nociceptors (predominantly A-δ) are mechanosensitive or thermosensitive, and respond to sharp mechanical pressure or tissue temperatures of 45°C or more respectively. The bimodal nociceptors (mainly A-δ mechanoheat receptors) also respond to mechanical and thermal stimulation, or a combination of both (Campbell & Meyer 1986). The majority of receptors are polymodal (C fibers), and react to mechanical, thermal or chemical stimulation. While these polymodal receptors respond to a variety of stimuli, they can become differentially senstitized to particular sensations (Wright & Zusman, 2004). The three categories of nociceptors apply at the cutaneous level and deeper levels (e.g. joint structures) (Charman 1994).

Spinal cord

The unmyelinated C fibers unite forming a single nerve fiber that enters the peripheral nerve sheath before reaching the dorsal root ganglion. The A-δ fibers travel as individual myelinated fibers to the dorsal root ganglion. As both of these fiber types enter the dorsal root of the spinal cord, they separate, with the myelinated fibers forming the dorsomedial bundle and the unmyelinated fibers forming the anterolateral bundle (Fig. 9.1) (Fitzgerald 1989).

There are several ascending nociceptive pathways or tracts that transmit pain sensations from the spinal cord to the brain

(Smith 1976). In particular, the lateral and anterior spinothalamic tracts of the spinal cord receive the axons that have crossed into the gray commissure and transport the impulses to the thalamus where they terminate (Mehler 1962). The spinothalamic tract carries sharp, discriminatory and spatial pain stimuli, predominantly of A-δ origin. There are also several more diffuse ascending pathways that carry multisynaptic unmyelinated and thinly myelinated fibers (Charman 1994).

Theoretical perspectives of pain

To implement pain management strategies, an understanding of the theoretical perspectives of pain is important. The most widely accepted theoretical conceptualization of pain and the role that psychological factors play in the experience of pain is the gate control theory of pain (Melzack 1986, Melzack & Wall 1965). Other theories to be discussed in this section are the neuromatrix theory (Melzack 1999) and the parallel processing model of pain distress (Leventhal & Everhart 1979)

Gate control theory of pain

The gate control theory of pain views pain from a neurophysiological perspective, and conceptually, it is still the most comprehensive and relevant of all pain theories for understanding

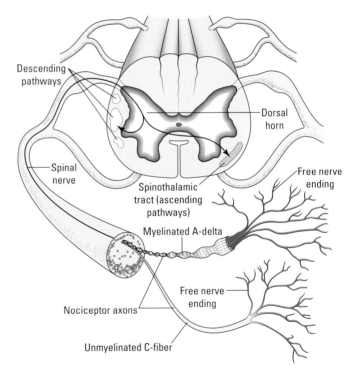

Figure 9.1 • The spinal cord and peripheral nociceptors. Pain transmission fibers from the periphery enter the central nervous system via the dorsal root and synapse within the dorsal horns of the spinal cord. (Reproduced from Heil 1993 with the permission of Human Kinetics and Perry G, Fine M D.)

the cognitive aspects of pain (Weisenberg 1999). The primary assumption in the gate control theory is that the substantia gelatinosa of the dorsal horns of the spinal cord contains a neural mechanism that acts as a pain gate (Melzack 1990, 1998, Melzack & Wall 1965). This gate controls (increases or

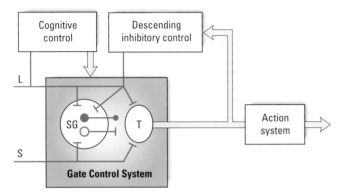

Figure 9.2 • Schematic representation of the gate control theory of pain mechanisms: L = large-diameter fibers; S = small-diameter fibers. The fibers project to the substantia gelatinosa (SG) and first central transmission (T) cells. The inhibitory effect exerted by the SG on the afferent fiber terminals is increased by activity in L fibers and decreased by activity in S fibers. (Reprinted with permission from Melzack R 1998 Psychological aspects of pain. Implications for neural blockade. In: Cousins M J, Bridenbaugh P S (eds) Neural blockade in clinical anesthesia and management of pain, 3rd edn. Lippincott-Raven, St Louis, MO.)

decreases) the flow of nerve impulses from peripheral nerves of the central nervous system (CNS) using the reciprocal activity of the large-diameter A-δ and the small-diameter A-δ and C fibers, and the influence from the cortex via the descending pyramidal and extrapyramidal tracts. When the amount of information that passes through the gate exceeds a critical level, the neural mechanisms responsible for pain experience and control are activated. The A-δ fibers can depolarize the intermedullary afferent terminals and close the gate. Thus, the effectiveness of the excitatory synapses is lowered and the experience of pain is decreased (Fig. 9.2).

Melzack (1998) suggested three neurophysiologic dimensions that can interact to influence the pattern of responses that characterize pain: the sensory-discriminative dimension that provides perceptual information on the magnitude, location and spatiotemporal aspects of the noxious stimuli; the motivational-affective dimension which is influenced by reticular and limbic structure activity; and the cognitive dimension which uses past pain experiences to help predict the possible outcomes of a variety of responses (Brown et al 2002).

Neuromatrix theory

The neuromatrix theory of pain (Melzack 1999, 2001) suggests that patterns of nerve impulses generated by the widely distributed neural network called the 'body-self neuromatrix' produces a 'neurosignature'. The neuromatrix (Fig. 9.3) is thought to be produced by both genetic and sensory influences, with the neurosignature pattern influenced by sensory inputs

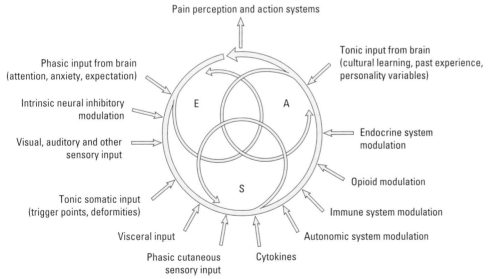

Figure 9.3 • The body-self neuromatrix, which comprises a widely distributed neural network that includes somatosensory, limbic and thalamo-cortical components, is schematically depicted as a circle containing smaller parallel networks that contribute to the sensory-discriminative (S), affective-motivational (A) and evaluative-cognitive (E) dimensions of pain experience. The synaptic architecture of the neuromatrix is determined by genetic and sensory influences. The 'neurosignature' output of the neuromatrix – patterns of nerve impulses of varying temporal and spatial dimensions – is produced by neural programs genetically built into the neuromatrix and determines the particular qualities and other properties of the pain experience and behavior. (Reprinted from Melzack R 1999 From the gate to the neuromatrix. Pain Supplement 6:S121–S126 with permission from Elsevier.)

and by cognitive events such as psychological stress (Melzack 1999). In a clinical setting the neuromatrix theory is very useful given its consideration of pain as a multidimensional experience, and not simply as a sensation related to injury, inflammation or other tissue pathology. Figure 9.3 shows the range of factors that contribute to the neuromatrix output responsible for the sensory, affective and cognitive dimensions of pain and pain behavior.

Parallel processing model of pain distress

The parallel processing model of pain distress suggests that pain can be processed along two pathways: informational or emotional, focusing on the psychosocial influences that affect the pain experience (Leventhal & Everhart 1979). The informational pathway focuses on issues such as location of pain, cause of pain and the sensory characteristics of the pain. The emotional pathway in this model produces particular emotional responses to pain (e.g. distress, avoidance, fear) and a generalized state of arousal. It is apparent that, from their historical experiences of pain, individuals develop schemata that include both informational and emotional components of painful events. Thus, when subsequent episodes of pain occur, the experience of the pain will be determined by aspects of the pain schemata activated (Taylor & Taylor 1998). The main function of these schemata in the processing of pain is in the selection of what people attend to when experiencing pain (Leventhal & Everhart 1979). Their research showed that when people focus on informational elements of pain, they experience significantly less pain than when they focus on its emotional aspects. This information has important clinical implications for implementing pain management techniques.

Experience of pain

Descriptions of pain

It has been suggested that three different forms of pain can be distinguished on a temporal basis (Melzack & Dennis 1980), and that each of these is associated with distinct affective states (Craig 1999). These forms of pain are phasic, acute and chronic. In addition, Crue (1983) described subacute pain and recurrent acute pain. It should be noted that pain is not always the immediate consequence of injury; in fact, substantial proportions of people report that pain emerged some time after the injury itself (Wall 1979).

Phasic pain

Phasic pain is of short duration and suggests an immediate impact of injury onset (Craig 1999). This usually involves reflexive withdrawal, protective movements and non-verbal and expressive behaviors that are recognizable as pain to onlookers (Craig et al 2001). The main biological function of phasic pain may be to trigger recuperative behavior rather than to indicate physical danger (Weisenberg 1999). This initial reaction to physical injury is subject to modulation dependent on the biological, physical and social context in which it occurs.

Acute pain

Acute pain is caused by tissue damage (and usually associated with a well-defined cause) and comprises a phasic state as well as a continued tonic state that persists until healing takes place (Craig 1999). It has been suggested that acute pain, biochemically, is similar to an anxiety state, such that excessive activity of the sympathetic nervous system is evident, and feelings of anxiety and fear surface (Elton 1995). Weisenberg (1999) reported that the contradictory findings regarding the pain–anxiety relationship could be due to inconsistencies in pain definitions between studies, a variable response bias due to people's willingness to complain of pain when anxious, and the moderating role that attention has on both pain and anxiety (Crombez et al 1998, 2002). The other complicating factor in examining the pain–anxiety relationship is that of causality; that is, do high levels of anxiety impact on pain perception, or do pain levels affect anxiety?

From a clinical perspective, while physical therapists typically report anxiety to be linked to acute pain, it is also recognized as an integral part of the emotional reactions to chronic pain.

Chronic pain

In chronic pain, the tonic component that begins after the phasic component is over can persist long after healing of the injurious event. Heil (1993) summarized chronic pain well by describing it as long-lasting and constant, persisting long after the initial injury, and comprising physical, psychological and social components. Some researchers and professional organizations have adopted a rather simplistic approach to describing chronic pain. The American Medical Association (1988) described chronic pain as a syndrome in which pain has persisted beyond the normal time of healing, while the IASP (1986) refers to chronic pain as one which is constant or recurring in nature, and that has endured for longer than 3 months. Cocchiarella & Andersson (2000) described chronic pain as an evolving process where injury causes one pathogenic mechanism, which in turn can produce others, to the point where the causes of pain can change over the course of the chronic pain episode. Despite semantic differences in definitions, chronic pain involves a prolonged time course, with the likelihood of anxiety, depression and social dysfunction increasing, the longer the pain persists (Craig 1999).

The difficulty in deciding when acute pain becomes chronic is a dilemma faced by all physical therapy practitioners. Although the term 'chronic pain' suggests an obligate temporal difference, more than just the length of time from onset distinguishes these two types of pain. It has been reported that acute pain can lead to CNS changes in the dorsal horn that outlast the nociceptive input from the periphery (Loeser 1996). The affective responses to perceived noxious stimuli may be related to individual genetics, past pain experiences, mood or interpretation of the meaning of pain to generate and perpetuate long-term pain (Shipton 1999).

A particular aspect of chronic pain is depression (Craig 1999), which may range from minor to clinical depression. Symptoms such as depressed mood, sleep disturbances, concentration difficulties, loss of interest and appetite changes are common in chronic pain (Sullivan et al 1995). Despite attempts to explain the causal relationship between depression and pain, no definitive model is evident. Examples of suggested theoretical explanations include biomedical theories, psychodynamic theories, and those based on past experiences. For example, Eich et al (1990) suggested that pain, by increasing unpleasant effect, promotes access to memories and thoughts of previous unpleasant events. The negative cognitions, in turn, intensify the negative affect and perpetuate pain. Biomedical theories suggest that pain and depression share common biological systems (Bair et al 2003). In an extensive review of the literature Bair et al (2003) suggested that higher levels of pain are often associated with more depressive symptoms and worse depression outcomes, and that depression in patients with pain is related to a greater number of pain complaints and increased impairment.

Subacute pain

Subacute pain is similar to acute pain in relation to etiological and nociceptive mechanisms, and refers to pain that is evident regularly but not on a constant basis (e.g. daily pain for several weeks) (Crue 1983).

Recurrent acute pain

Recurrent acute pain has been described as the acute exacerbation of peripheral tissue pathology resulting from an underlying chronic pathology entity (e.g. degenerative joint or disk disease) (Crue 1983). Recurrent acute pain, unlike acute or chronic pain refers to discrete acute episodes that return over time. For example, daily pain for several weeks can be classified as subacute pain, whereas several time-limited pain episodes over months or years fits the description of recurrent acute pain (Thienhaus & Cole 2002). The reason for distinguishing between the various types of pain is to adopt the most beneficial management approach.

Classification of pain

Due to the subjective nature of pain, and the wide variety of physical and psychological presentations, classifying pain is complex. Without an accepted and commonly used method of classifying pain, communication between practitioners is difficult. The IASP (1986) developed a pain classification system based on descriptive lists of pain syndromes. In this classification system, a five-axis coding scheme is used to describe various aspects of pain:

- Axis I indicates the region of the pain (e.g. cervical region, lower limbs)
- Axis II indicates the organ system involved (e.g. musculoskeletal system and connective tissue; nervous system)

- Axis III indicates the temporal characteristics and pattern of occurrence of the pain (e.g. single episode, limited duration; continuous or nearly continuous, nonfluctuating)
- Axis IV relates to the patient's statement of pain intensity and duration since onset (e.g. mild with a duration of 1 month or less; medium with a duration of 1 month or less)
- Axis V indicates the presumed etiology (e.g. trauma, operation, burns, inflammatory)

Use of the IASP classification for chronic pain potentially gives the practitioner vital information on the definition, anatomical location, main features, associated symptoms, laboratory findings, usual course and potential complications for most pain problems. The system summarizes information on the physical and social disabilities, pathology, diagnostic criteria and differential diagnoses for chronic pain conditions. Although the IASP system is detailed and provides specific definitions to encourage consistency of pain description, it is currently not in wide use (Thienhaus & Cole 2002), and research is required to determine its psychometric properties (Turk & Okifuki 2001). Readers are referred to the original source (IASP 1986) for further information about the use of this complex pain classification system.

Pain thresholds and tolerance

The way in which people experience pain is usually related to individual pain thresholds. There are several thresholds to pain, and distinguishing between them for clinical purposes is essential (Melzack & Wall 2004). *Sensation threshold* (or lower threshold) refers to the lowest stimulus value at which a sensation is reported. *Pain perception threshold* is the lowest stimulus at which a person reports that the stimulation feels painful. *Pain tolerance* (upper threshold) is the lowest stimulus level at which a person withdraws from the stimulus. *Encouraged pain tolerance* is the level at which the person withdraws from the stimulus after encouragement to tolerate higher levels of stimulation (Melzack & Wall 2004). According to Charman (1994) research has repeatedly shown that the majority of people have a uniform sensation threshold to recognize different stimuli. As stimulus intensity increases, most people will indicate that they initially perceive sensation at a common baseline level. It is the pain perception and pain tolerance thresholds that differ between people (Charman 1994).

The work of several researchers (e.g. Feuerstein & Beattie 1995, Melzack & Wall 2004) has led to the recognition that there is a multitude of factors (e.g. attention, anxiety, social reinforcement) that can influence an individual's perception of pain. Therefore, pain is more currently seen as consisting of sensory, affective, evaluative, cognitive and behavioral elements (Sim & Waterfield 1997). This recognition helps explain the diversity of experiences and individual differences in pain severity.

Despite the large literature on the physical causes and treatment of injury in sport and exercise, there is a dearth of literature that has focused on the ability of athletes to tolerate and cope with the pain associated with injury and rehabilitation. Pain and discomfort are characteristics of most sport injury rehabilitation programs, and can interrupt, or in some cases terminate, treatment (Fisher & Hoisington 1993, Pen & Fisher 1994). As athletes differ in their ability to cope with and/or tolerate pain (Manning & Fillingim 2002, Ord & Gijsbers 2003, Paparizos et al 2005), their adherence to rehabilitation programs may also differ. Being able to manage pain is, therefore, integral to successful completion of sport injury rehabilitation regimens. Meyers et al (2001), from a review of the literature, reported that a strong relationship between level of pain and physical/psychological dysfunction exists. Further to this, Jensen et al (2001) reported that better perceived control over pain was related to less catastrophizing over pain. It could be concluded, therefore, that an athlete's attitude towards pain, and the strategies used to cope with pain, can affect both sport performance and adherence to prescribed rehabilitation (Crossman 1997, Meyers et al 1993, Pen & Fisher 1994).

There is evidence that athletes have higher pain tolerance levels than non-athletes (Manning & Fillingim 2002, Ord & Gijsbers 2003, Paparizos et al 2005, Tajet-Foxell & Rose 1995). Differences in pain tolerance have even been found among different sports (Egan 1988). Paparizos et al (2005) compared pain perception and catastrophizing in high-skilled ballet dancers, low-skilled ballet dancers and non-dancers and found that those with higher-level dance skills had a higher pain tolerance than the others. Manning & Fillingim (2002) examined athletes from a variety of sports and found that they had a higher tolerance for several types of pain compared with non-athletes. Similarly, Ord & Gijsbers (2003) reported higher pain tolerance for a group of competitive rowers than for a control group. Of note, is that although pain tolerance is consistently coming out as higher in athletes than non-athletes, pain threshold is not showing such differences. Several explanations have been suggested for higher pain tolerance in athletes than non-athletes. First, compared to non-athletes, athletes have a greater exposure to physical training and increased fitness, resulting in higher levels of circulating endogenous opioids. The second explanation relates to psychological factors. As suggested by Tajet-Foxell & Rose (1995), athletes, as part of their physical training and performance, explore boundaries in relation to extreme physical activity and pain experience, giving a perception of control over the pain–physical activity interface. Further, there is a tendency of athletes to control noxious stimuli (e.g. play through an injury) and to compete against themselves with a task (e.g. pain) task (Manning & Fillingim 2002).

Evidence also exists to show that males demonstrate higher pain thresholds and tolerance than do females to some types of pain (Jackson et al 2005), and that this is also the case with athletes (Koltyn et al 1998, Manning & Fillingim 2002, Tajet-Foxell & Rose 1995). When discussing pain tolerance, it is important to consider the sociocultural aspects of the sport and exercise environment. Wiese-Bjornstal & Shaffer (1999) referred to an attitude found commonly in sport that relates to 'acting tough' in the face of pain and injury and the unwillingness to seek out medical treatment for fear of being labeled 'weak'. In addition, the 'culture of risk' in sport (as described by Frey 1991)

suggests that sport produces role pressures, and in some cases monetary inducements, to play with pain and injuries. Other cultural values inherent in sport link pain tolerance to the demonstration of masculine character, and view pain as being 'part of the game' and 'for the good of the team' (Frey 1991). These cultural values have also spread to the increasing number of females participating in competitive sport (Wiese-Bjornstal & Shaffer 1999).

Pain tolerance levels should be carefully considered when planning and implementing rehabilitation programs for athletes. Evidence exists for a positive association between pain tolerance and adherence to sport injury rehabilitation (Byerly et al 1994, Fields et al 1995, Fisher et al 1988); that is, those able to tolerate pain better tend to adhere more rigidly to their rehabilitation regimens. From the practitioner's viewpoint, a study by Fisher et al (1993) reported that athletic trainers believed an injured athlete's ability to accept pain was important in treatment adherence.

It is also important to look more broadly than at the rehabilitation tasks themselves. Two recent studies focused on asking physical therapists what they believe differentiated athletes who cope successfully with injury from those who cope less successfully (Francis et al 2000, Ninedek & Kolt 2000). Interestingly, having a high pain tolerance was not perceived as important by physical therapists in either of the investigations (Francis et al 2000, Ninedek & Kolt 2000) or by professional athletes (Francis et al 2000) in coping with sport-related injury. It could be that, despite evidence summarized by Brewer (1998) indicating that adherence to injury rehabilitation is linked to pain tolerance levels, when the broader issues of coping with injury are considered, the impact of pain tolerance is diluted.

Assessment of pain

A large number of pain assessment methods are suggested in the literature, including several which are more commonly used in relation to sport and exercise injuries. Making pain tangible through the use of assessment tools ensures that pain is understood as important information that can facilitate rehabilitation (Taylor & Taylor 1998).

To effectively evaluate rehabilitation aimed at reducing pain is a challenge, as practitioners and researchers predominantly use patients' subjective interpretations of their pain to gauge or measure such changes (McDowell & Newell 1996). So that meaningful inferences can be drawn from pain measurement, the assessment on which pain measurements have been based must exhibit validity, reliability and responsiveness (Sim & Arnell 1993). Validity refers to the ability of an instrument to measure what it purports to measure, thereby allowing meaningful information to be gained from the data. Reliability relates to the extent to which an instrument yields the same measurement on repeated uses, either by the same practitioner (intra-observer reliability), or by different practitioners (inter-observer reliability). Responsiveness refers to the capability of detecting small gradations of change that will be of clinical importance.

Measurement tools that assess the degree and quality of pain during rehabilitation include pain drawings (Ransford et al 1976), verbal rating scales, numerical rating scales, visual analog scales (Huskisson 1983), the McGill Pain Questionnaire (Melzack 1975), the Short-Form McGill Pain Questionnaire (Melzack 1987), the Sport Inventory for Pain (Meyers et al 1992), the Descriptor Differential Scale (Gracely & Kwilosz 1988), the Brief Pain Inventory (Cleeland 1989) and the Pain Anxiety Symptoms Scale (McCracken et al 1992), just to mention a few. It is not the intent of this chapter to provide a review of each of these pain measures, but to highlight some of the more commonly used tools and their application to pain in sport.

Verbal and numerical rating scales

The verbal rating scale (VRS) and numerical rating scale (NRS) are two of the more commonly used (Bolton & Wilkinson 1998) and extensively reviewed (Sim & Waterfield 1997) pain measures.

The VRS typically consists of a series of verbal pain descriptors that are ordered from least to most intense (e.g. no pain, mild, moderate, severe) (Jensen & Karoly 1991). This scale is scored by allocating a value of zero to the least intense descriptor, a value of 1 to the next intense descriptor word, etc. A problem in using this scale is that it lacks responsiveness (Sim & Waterfield 1997).

The NRS usually comprises a series of numbers (e.g. 0 to 10 or 0 to 100) anchored by words such as 'no pain' and 'extreme pain'. Patients choose the number that best reflects their intensity of pain (Fig. 9.4). Although this scale has the advantage of being simple, clear and efficient, and therefore is easy to use in a clinical setting, it has been suggested that it lacks validity, as it represents only a single pain element (e.g. intensity).

The reliability of VRSs and NRSs has been demonstrated to be adequate (Lara-Munoz et al 2004, Melzack & Katz 1999). Responses given on measures like these do not reflect the complexity of the pain experience as well as multidimensional pain measures might.

Visual analog scales

The visual analog scale (VAS) most commonly takes the form of a 10 cm horizontal line which is anchored at each end with terms representing the minimum score (e.g. 'no pain') on the left and the maximum score (e.g. 'worst ever pain') on the right (Fig. 9.5). Patients rate their pain by placing a vertical mark on the 10 cm line which corresponds to the level of pain intensity they are experiencing. A score is subsequently derived by measuring the distance in millimeters between this mark and the left-hand end of the scale. Although the reliability of the VAS has been shown to be high when repeatedly used on the same individual (Bijur et al 2001, Bowsher 1994), its content validity is questionable, mainly due to its ability to measure only a single aspect of pain (Sim & Waterfield 1997). As VASs have a large number of points that can be marked to reflect pain intensity, their responsiveness is high.

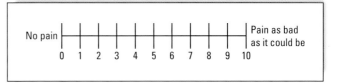

Figure 9.4 • A numerical rating scale. The patient is instructed to mark the numbered vertical line as appropriate.

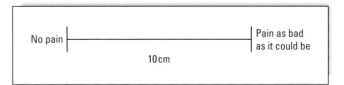

Figure 9.5 • A visual analog scale for pain intensity.

The advantages of using VASs include their favorable psychometric properties, ease and brevity of administration and scoring, minimal intrusiveness and conceptual simplicity (Melzack & Katz 1999, Price & Harkins 1987).

VASs have also been used to measure aspects of pain aside from simply intensity. For example, to measure pain affect, the patient could be asked to rate the unpleasantness of the pain experience with anchors of 'not bad at all' to 'the most unpleasant feeling imaginable' (Price et al 1987).

McGill Pain Questionnaire

The McGill Pain Questionnaire (MPQ) (Melzack 1975) is a multidimensional measure that has the ability to describe the diverse dimensions of pain. It provides valuable information on the sensory, affective and evaluative dimensions of pain experience and is able to discriminate among different pain problems (Reading 1984). The MPQ has become a widely used clinical and research tool. The MPQ (Fig. 9.6) contains 20 subclasses of 78 adjectives divided among four dimensions: sensory, affective, evaluative and miscellaneous. Patients choose one word in each category to describe their present pain. Separate scores can be obtained for each of these four dimensions in addition to a total score (Pain Rating Index, PRI). In addition to the lists of pain descriptors, the MPQ contains line drawings of the body to record spatial distribution of the pain and words that describe the temporal properties of the pain. The final component of the MPQ is the Present Pain Intensity (PPI) scale, a number–word combination that provides an indication of the pain intensity at the time of completion of the questionnaire. The MPQ is designed to provide quantitative indices of the subjective pain experience. It is a widely used tool in both research and clinical settings and has been translated into several languages. The reliability and validity of the MPQ have been extensively researched and shown to be sound (see Melzack & Katz 2001). As the MPQ usually takes 5–10 minutes to administer (Melzack 1987), many practitioners and researchers have sought a shortened version for more regular use.

McGill Pain Questionnaire

Patient's name _____ Date _____ Time _____ am/pm

PRI: S _____ A _____ E _____ M _____ PRI(T) _____ PPI _____
    (1–10)   (11–15)   (16)   (17–20)   (1–20)

1 FLICKERING	11 TIRING	BRIEF	RHYTHMIC	CONTINUOUS
QUIVERING	EXHAUSTING	MOMENTARY	PERIODIC	STEADY
PULSING	12 SICKENING	TRANSIENT	INTERMITTENT	CONSTANT
THROBBING	SUFFOCATING			
BEATING				
POUNDING				

1 FLICKERING
  QUIVERING
  PULSING
  THROBBING
  BEATING
  POUNDING

2 JUMPING
  FLASHING
  SHOOTING

3 PRICKING
  BORING
  DRILLING
  STABBING
  LANCINATING

4 SHARP
  CUTTING
  LACERATING

5 PINCHING
  PRESSING
  GNAWING
  CRAMPING
  CRUSHING

6 TUGGING
  PULLING
  WRENCHING

7 HOT
  BURNING
  SCALDING
  SEARING

8 TINGLING
  ITCHY
  SMARTING
  STINGING

9 DULL
  SORE
  HURTING
  ACHING
  HEAVY

10 TENDER
  TAUT
  RASPING
  SPLITTING

11 TIRING
  EXHAUSTING

12 SICKENING
  SUFFOCATING

13 FEARFUL
  FRIGHTFUL
  TERRIFYING

14 PUNISHING
  GRUELLING
  CRUEL
  VICIOUS
  KILLING

15 WRETCHED
  BLINDING

16 ANNOYING
  TROUBLESOME
  MISERABLE
  INTENSE
  UNBEARABLE

17 SPREADING
  RADIATING
  PENETRATING
  PIERCING

18 TIGHT
  NUMB
  DRAWING
  SQUEEZING
  TEARING

19 COOL
  COLD
  FREEZING

20 NAGGING
  NAUSEATING
  AGONIZING
  DREADFUL
  TORTURING

PPI
0 NO PAIN
1 MILD
2 DISCOMFORTING
3 DISTRESSING
4 HORRIBLE
5 EXCRUCIATING

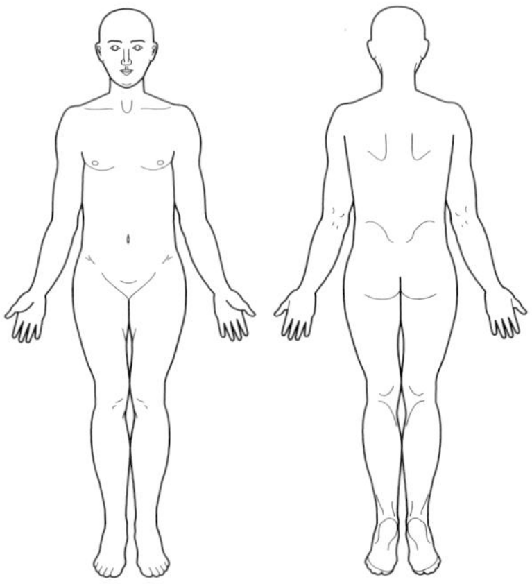

E = EXTERNAL

I = INTERNAL

COMMENTS:

Figure 9.6 • McGill Pain Questionnaire. The descriptors fall into four major groups: sensory, 1–10; affective, 11–15; evaluative, 16; and miscellaneous, 17–20. The rank value for each descriptor is based on its position in the word set. The sum of the rank values is the pain rating index (PRI). The present pain intensity (PPI) is based on a scale of 0–5. (Reproduced with permission from Melzack 1975.)

Short-form McGill Pain Questionnaire
Ronald Melzack

Patient's name _____ Date _____

	NONE	MILD	MODERATE	SEVERE
THROBBING	0) ___	1) ___	2) ___	3) ___
SHOOTING	0) ___	1) ___	2) ___	3) ___
STABBING	0) ___	1) ___	2) ___	3) ___
SHARP	0) ___	1) ___	2) ___	3) ___
CRAMPING	0) ___	1) ___	2) ___	3) ___
GNAWING	0) ___	1) ___	2) ___	3) ___
HOT-BURNING	0) ___	1) ___	2) ___	3) ___
ACHING	0) ___	1) ___	2) ___	3) ___
HEAVY	0) ___	1) ___	2) ___	3) ___
TENDER	0) ___	1) ___	2) ___	3) ___
SPLITTING	0) ___	1) ___	2) ___	3) ___
TIRING-EXHAUSTING	0) ___	1) ___	2) ___	3) ___
SICKENING	0) ___	1) ___	2) ___	3) ___
FEARFUL	0) ___	1) ___	2) ___	3) ___
PUNISHING-CRUEL	0) ___	1) ___	2) ___	3) ___

No pain |————————————————| Worst possible pain

PPI
0 NO PAIN ___
1 MILD ___
2 DISCOMFORTING ___
3 DISTRESSING ___
4 HORRIBLE ___
5 EXCRUCIATING ___

Figure 9.7 • The Short-Form McGill Pain Questionnaire. The first descriptors represent the sensory dimension of pain experience and the last three represent the affective dimension. Each descriptor is ranked on an intensity scale of 0 = none, 1 = mild, 2 = moderate, 3 = severe. The present pain intensity (PPI) of the standard long-form McGill Pain Questionnaire and the visual analog scale are also included to provide overall pain intensity scores. (Reproduced with permission from Melzack 1987.)

Short-Form McGill Pain Questionnaire

The Short-Form McGill Pain Questionnaire (SFMPQ) (Melzack 1987) was developed for use when the time taken to obtain information on pain is limited, and when more information than intensity is required. The SFMPQ (Fig. 9.7) incorporates elements of the MPQ but allows for a more rapid and simple acquisition of pain data. The SFMPQ has three components: a descriptive component, the PPI and a VAS. The main component of the SFMPQ contains 15 descriptors (11 sensory and 4 affective) which are rated on an intensity scale where 0 = none,

1 = mild, 2 = moderate and 3 = severe. The second component, the PPI is the same as that used in the MPQ. The third component is a VAS anchored by the terms 'no pain' and 'worst possible pain'. The PPI and VAS are included to provide indices of overall pain intensity.

The SFMPQ has been shown to be correlated highly with the sensory, affective and total PRI scores of the MPQ (Melzack 1987), and is highly sensitive to clinical changes brought about by various therapies (see Melzack & Katz 2001). The SFMPQ also has high content validity (Melzack & Katz 2001), and the inclusion of a VAS (not a component of the original MPQ) has been reported to enhance the test–retest reliability of the SFMPQ beyond that of the MPQ (Bowsher 1994).

Sport inventory for pain

The pain assessment instruments discussed so far in this chapter have not been developed specifically for pain that is associated with sport and exercise injury. One questionnaire focused on sport is the Sport Inventory for Pain (SIP) (Meyers et al 1992). Although not aimed at pain intensity, the SIP was developed to identify and predict an athlete's ability to cope with pain. The SIP is a 25-item questionnaire comprising five pain subscales: coping (a measure of direct coping responses), cognitive strategies used in the face of pain, avoidance (the tendency to avoid pain-producing responses), catastrophizing (the tendency to be overwhelmed by pain) and body awareness (a measure of response style). Although it has been reported that the SIP subscales demonstrated satisfactory test–retest reliability and internal consistency (Meyers et al 1992), more recent research has challenged the integrity of the SIP. It was found that the SIP had an unstable factor structure (Bartholomew et al 1998b), and that the validity of the instrument and reliabilities of the individual subscales were poor (Bartholomew et al 1998a). Further research is clearly needed if sport-specific pain measures are to be developed.

Management of pain

The management of pain is complex and usually consists of several forms of therapy being used concurrently. Typically, approaches such as physical therapy, pharmacological therapy and cognitive-behavioral techniques are methods of choice. The complex nature of the pain experience, which can be moderated by various forms of psychosocial input, makes selection of appropriate approaches difficult. It is important, however, to focus more broadly than on the presenting signs and symptoms. Consideration of the impact of pain on the athlete, and the sport and non-sport aspects of their lives, is integral to successful rehabilitation.

Some guiding principles for managing pain will be presented that focus on the physical, pharmacological and cognitive-behavioral approaches. Readers are referred to Weiner (2002) for a detailed account of pain management.

Physical rehabilitation therapies

The majority of patients that consult physical therapists do so, predominantly, because of a pain complaint. Rarely does a patient present complaining of poor biomechanics in their running technique. Rather, they will present with lower limb pain that, upon assessment, is linked to poor biomechanical sequencing. Thus, the physical therapist is required to attend to both the presenting pain, and the underlying cause of that pain.

There are several rehabilitation therapies that are used to manage pain. These include electrophysical agents, manual techniques and interventions that change movement patterns thought to provoke pain.

Electrophysical agents

Several electrophysical agents can provide an analgesic effect. As outlined in Chapter 14, there are several uses for transcutaneous electrical nerve stimulation (TENS), ultrasound, interferential stimulation, laser, cryotherapy, superficial heat and high-voltage galvanic stimulation in managing pain. It should be considered, however, that available evidence is limited to support the use of these modalities in pain relief (Ellis 1998).

One of the electrophysical agents more commonly used to manage pain is TENS. When used for pain relief, TENS involves a high-frequency current administered to the skin. This current selectively activates large-diameter, non-noxious fibers (A-β) and inhibits second-order nociceptive transmission neurons within the CNS. Research on the efficacy of TENS in reducing pain of both an acute and chronic nature has been the topic of several systematic reviews (e.g. Carroll et al 2001, Khadilkar et al 2005, Milne et al 2001, Osiri et al 2001) and produced conflicting findings (see Sluka & Walsh 2003). TENS can also be applied using high-intensity, low-frequency currents (acupuncture-like TENS). This form of TENS results in endorphin release within the CNS, and is often used to stimulate trigger points or acupuncture points. Research has shown that longer duration pain relief can be obtained from this form of TENS than when using the more traditional high frequency TENS (Johnson 1998).

The use of ultrasound therapy in managing pain is also common in physical therapy settings. The efficacy of ultrasound, when used for therapeutic purposes is still relatively unknown. Research that has addressed its effects has generally been poorly designed and has relied on small sample sizes, therefore making conclusions regarding efficacy difficult (van der Windt et al 1999). A systematic review of the therapeutic effects of ultrasound (Robertson & Baker 2001) showed little clinical efficacy. An adaptation of ultrasound therapy in physical therapy settings is phonophoresis, where a pharmacological agent (e.g. an analgesic) is used as a coupling medium and transferred to the superficial tissues via the thermal effect and acoustic streaming of the ultrasound (Baumert 1999, Shin & Choi 1997). Baumert (1999) advocated that higher concentration pharmacological agents (e.g. 10% hydrocortisone) have been shown to produce the best results.

Interferential stimulation has also been suggested as a pain management therapy. Interferential stimulation involves two alternating medium-frequency currents applied to the skin simultaneously. At the point where the two currents intersect, wave interference occurs, and it has an effect on pain similar to that of TENS. Although interferential current is suggested to provide greater analgesic effects than other forms of electrical stimulation, research does not support this assertion (Taylor et al 1987).

The use of laser has been increasing in physical therapy settings. It has been suggested that cold (or soft) lasers of varying intensity may, among other effects (e.g. elevation of blood cortisol levels), reduce pain. As for many electrophysical agents, the research investigating the efficacy of laser therapy has shown conflicting findings (Bingol et al 2005, Ozkan et al 2004, Tascioglu et al 2004).

Other modalities (although not classified as electrophysical agents) that are used extensively in physical therapy to manage pain are cryotherapy and superficial heat. Cryotherapy involves the application of ice or cold to the painful area, having the effect of decreasing conduction velocities of both motor and sensory nerves, reducing the rate of firing of muscle spindle afferents and decreasing acetylcholine levels. In general, cryotherapy seems to be effective in reducing pain (Bleakley et al 2004). The application of superficial heat, among other effects, can produce also analgesia (Lehman & Delateur 1990).

Manual techniques

A major component of physical therapy management involves manual techniques. Such techniques involve various combinations of soft tissue massage, joint and soft tissue mobilization, and joint manipulation. Soft tissue massage is commonly used in pain management (Hernandez-Reif et al 2001, Leivadi et al 1999, Weerapong et al 2005) due to its effects of decreasing excessive tissue tension associated with activated mechanical nociceptors, and by aiding the removal of the chemical substances in soft tissue that activate chemical nociceptors. Soft tissue massage can also, according to the gate control theory of pain, reduce pain by stimulating the large, rapidly conducting nerve fibers through selectively closing the gate against the smaller pain fiber input (Arnheim & Prentice 2000). The evidence to support or refute the effects of massage within sport, however, is insufficient to make any definitive statements (Moraska 2005).

Manual techniques that address myofascial trigger points are commonly used in pain management. The initial stimulation of trigger points results in impulses being sent to the CNS causing muscle contraction and vasoconstriction. The resulting increased vascular permeability and ischemia changes the extracellular environment and increases the sensitivity of nociceptors in the area (Travell & Simons 1998). Treatment from a trigger point perspective should focus on all active and latent trigger points thought to contribute to the pain. It should also be noted that trigger points can develop secondary to the actual injurious event, simply as a result of the adaptive postures adopted (Travell & Simons 1998). For a detailed approach to managing pain through myofascial trigger points, refer to Travell & Simons (1983) and Simons et al (1998).

Exercise

Exercise can play an important role in the management of long-term or chronic pain, with several studies having shown that exercise reduces pain associated with musculoskeletal, nervous, respiratory and cardiovascular disorders (see review by Smidt et al 2005). Carabelli et al (1998) suggested that exercise programs for pain management should include all major components of physical fitness: cardiorespiratory endurance, muscular strength, muscular endurance, flexibility and body composition.

Exercise programs should initially address stretching, with chronic pain patients, to return muscles back to normal resting length (Carabelli et al 1998). Such stretches should focus on the muscles which, through postural changes during the pain episode, have become shortened. It should be remembered that painful stimuli could cause prolonged excitation of the spinal reflex causing continued muscle contraction (Carabelli et al 1998). In more recent times, aquatic therapy or hydrotherapy has been used as a medium to achieve many of the exercise program components. The buoyancy of the water aids the low-impact needs of many people with chronic pain. Exercise in suitably heated hydrotherapy facilities can also provide the additional benefits that superficial heat is capable of in terms of pain management (see above).

Not only does exercise provide physiological effects that can be beneficial to pain, but there may also be possible psychological mechanisms of exercise that assist pain. An early hypothesis by Bahrke & Morgan (1978) suggested that exercise distracts people from stressful stimuli (e.g. pain). Another hypothesis relates to self-efficacy theory; that is, people assess their self-efficacy in physical activities by using levels of fatigue, fitness and pain. Therefore, as fitness increases through appropriate exercise, feelings of pain and fatigue will reduce, and self-efficacy should be increased resulting in a further desire to continue exercise (Petruzzello et al 1991). Other important effects of exercise in pain management include the reduction of stress that is so often associated with pain (Salmon 2001), and the promotion of relaxation (Shephard 1997).

Pharmacological agents

Some form of pharmacological intervention is usually an integral and necessary component of pain management. While Chapter 29 provides details on the various forms of pharmacological agents that can reduce pain, this section will briefly describe some general principles of the use of such agents. The three common groups of drugs used in pain management in sport and exercise are analgesics, non-steroidal anti-inflammatory drugs (NSAIDs) and corticosteroids.

Analgesics are often used in the acute stage of soft tissue injuries to reduce pain. The most common forms of analgesics currently used are aspirin, paracetamol and codeine. It should be noted, however, that the use of aspirin compounds in acute injuries is contraindicated due to their ability to inhibit platelet aggregation, which can therefore increase the bleeding associated with the injury. Paracetamol has no effect on inflammation and serves as an analgesic and antipyretic. Codeine is used in circumstances where a stronger analgesic is needed.

NSAIDs work to reduce inflammation by inhibiting cyclo-oxygenase and reducing the production of prostaglandins, thromboxane and prostacyclins, all mediators of the inflammatory response (Buchanan 2000). In addition, NSAIDs have multiple other functions at a cellular level, including decreasing granulocyte and monocyte migration and phagocytosis, and displacing an endogenous anti-inflammatory peptide from plasma proteins (Buchanan 2000). Despite the widespread clinical use of NSAIDs for musculoskeletal injuries, Paoloni & Orchard (2006) suggested that at best, NSAIDs have a mild effect on relieving symptoms and are potentially deleterious to tissue healing. They can, however, produce modest inhibition of the initial inflammatory response for injuries such as strains and contusions (Almekinders 1999), and thus, be used in the early stage of injury.

Corticosteroids and their use in the treatment of sports injuries are controversial (Nichols 2005). They work by inhibiting both prostaglandin and leukotriene synthesis by blocking the action of phospholipase enzyme, which converts phospholipids in cell membranes to arachidonic acid (Buchanan 2000). Corticosteroids can be administered orally, by local injection or by iontophoresis. The main concern with corticosteroids is with local injection and their effect on inhibiting collagen synthesis and tissue repair. Refer to Chapter 29 for an overview of the side effects and contraindications of corticosteroid use.

Cognitive therapies

Physical therapists are becoming increasingly aware of psychosocial factors that influence injury, and are enhancing their management skills by adding a psychological dimension. Due to the nature of their work, physical therapists are in an ideal situation to provide some form of basic psychological assistance to aid the injury rehabilitation process (Kolt 2000, Ninedek & Kolt 2000). Given that pain, and particularly chronic pain, has psychosocial elements, knowledge of managing pain from a cognitive perspective is imperative. Pain management approaches based on psychophysiology explore the relation between mental events and neuromuscular activity, whereby stress leads to autonomic arousal, muscle tension and vascular changes, with a resultant influence on pain (Smith et al 2001).

The majority of psychological approaches to pain management focus around cognitive-behavioral techniques (CBTs), that is, techniques that address the patient's cognitions (thought processes) and behaviors. The techniques used include those that are aimed at reducing pain, those that address a patient's focus on their pain, and those that teach people to cope with pain. As will be evident in the following description of some relevant CBTs, there is a strong emphasis on educating patients about their pain and injury.

The cognitive-behavioral approach to managing pain is based around five assumptions (Turk & Okifuji 1999). First, individuals are active processors of information and not passive reactors. Second, thoughts can elicit and influence mood, affect physiological processes, can serve as an impetus for behavior and can have social consequences; conversely, mood, physiological changes, environmental factors and behavior can influence thought processes. Third, behavior is reciprocally determined by both the individual and environment factors. Fourth, individuals can learn more adaptive ways of thinking, feeling and behaving. Finally, individuals should be active and collaborative in changing their maladaptive thoughts, feelings and behaviors.

Taylor & Taylor (1998) categorized the non-physical and non-psychological pain management strategies as either pain reduction or pain focusing techniques. The pain reduction techniques are those that act on the nociceptive aspects of the pain, thus decreasing the amount of pain that is felt (e.g. muscle relaxation techniques). The pain focusing techniques are those that involve directing attention onto (association) or away from (dissociation) the pain as a way of reducing the pain (Taylor & Taylor 1998). Examples of pain focusing techniques include external focus, pleasant imagery and hypnosis.

A brief summary follows of some CBTs and other psychological techniques that can be useful in the management of pain; some techniques could fall into either category. Note, however, that as suggested earlier in the chapter, the management of pain usually works best with several forms of therapy being used concurrently.

Reconceptualizing the pain

An essential feature of cognitive-behavioral treatment is for the patient to be able to reconceptualize the pain from being vague, undifferentiated and overwhelming to being addressable, manageable and controlled. This is achieved largely through education of the patient on the basis and causes of pain, and the treatment and rehabilitation program. Reconceptualization allows the patient to change their view of pain from one that is predominantly sensory in nature to a more multifaceted view with cognitive, affective and socioenvironmental factors considered as contributors to the experience of pain (Turk & Okifuji 1999). The overall aim of this approach is to provide patients with better control over their lives, even if the pain itself cannot be completely ameliorated.

Relaxation

Several forms of relaxation exist that achieve their function by various means. Given that pain can influence muscle tension that, in turn, restricts blood flow and further increases pain (Cousins & Phillips 1985), relaxation techniques that directly target muscle are often indicated. The most common form of muscular relaxation is progressive relaxation (Jacobson 1938). Progressive relaxation involves systematically relaxing major skeletal muscle groups by firstly recognizing muscle tension present (initially achieved by contracting the muscles), then by relaxing those muscles. The role of muscle contraction before relaxation is proposed so that the patient can become sensitive to muscle tension, and therefore learn to recognize the sensations of relaxed muscle. As the patients become more familiar with the technique, they may merely relax muscle groups from whatever condition they are in at rest, rather than having to contract muscle groups first. Although there has been some research support for progressive muscle relaxation techniques (de Paula et al 2002), there is still divided opinion regarding the value of muscle contraction before relaxation (Carroll & Seers 1998, Lucic et al 1991, O'Bannon et al 1987, Payne 2000). In using progressive relaxation on patients with pain, it is important to monitor the level of muscle contraction used in the exercise so that it does not aggravate pain symptoms.

Another commonly used relaxation technique is Benson's Relaxation Response (Benson 1975). This technique is based on the proposal that there are four common elements underlying the elicitation of a relaxation response. The first element is a quiet environment, which allows for the reduction of external distractions. The second is the adoption of a comfortable position to reduce undue muscular tension. The third is an object to dwell on, such as the repetition of a word. The fourth element is a passive attitude that includes emptying all other thoughts from one's mind, and letting distracting thoughts that do return pass on while returning to a focused state. Practically speaking, the Relaxation Response is based around transcendental meditation and involves focus on breathing, repetition of a word in time with breathing, and in more recent adaptations, imagery that focuses on an object that moves in time with the patient's breathing (Kolt & McConville 2000). The Relaxation Response works by reducing the sympathetic nervous system activity that can accentuate pain (Wallace et al 1971). The Relaxation Response also serves as a distraction, drawing focus away from the pain and onto the more pleasant feeling of relaxation. It also provides a greater sense of control of pain and a reduction in the negative emotions associated with the pain and injury (Taylor & Taylor 1998).

In general, further evidence is still required to be confident of the relationship between relaxation techniques and pain reduction (Carroll & Seers 1998). For a more detailed account of relaxation techniques refer to Payne (2004).

Imagery

Different forms of imagery have been used in the management of pain, and specifically by athletes during rehabilitation (Law et al 2006, Sordoni et al 2000). Such imagery generally serves a motivational and cognitive role (Hall et al 1998, Martin et al 1999). In general, imagery involves individuals imagining themselves in a relaxing environment (i.e. an environment that has a relaxing meaning to the individual), and focusing on how it feels to be in that environment. This form of imagery aims to distract the individual from the feeling of pain. From clinical experience, the more complex the imagined scene is, and the more detail the individual is asked to attend to (i.e. using not just the sense of vision but other senses such as tactile, auditory, etc.), the more they are distracted from their pain.

Specific types of imagery have also been developed. For example, in pain management imagery (Ievleva & Orlick 1999), individuals could imagine the pain being washed away or see cool colors soothing and reducing any inflammation and pain (e.g. seeing cool blue colors running through the painful area; imaging the pain leaving the body; imagining an ice-pack over the painful area). There is an increasing body of research suggesting that imagery can assist with pain and rehabilitation in athletes (Driediger et al 2006, Ievleva & Orlick 1999, Milne et al 2005). For a more detailed discussion of the use of imagery, refer to Taylor & Taylor (1997, 1998), Ievleva & Orlick (1999) and Hall (2001).

Association and dissociation

Association involves patients focusing their attention on the pain. It has been suggested that such techniques allow patients to use the pain as important information about the extent to which they can exert themselves in rehabilitation and how far they can extend the physical limits (Taylor & Taylor 1998). Heil (1993) suggested that association methods heighten body awareness, increase perceptions of control over pain and encourage a sense of emotional detachment by athletes. This emotional detachment, in turn, acts to separate the sensory aspects of pain from its physical manifestations. The initial association with the sensory aspects of pain produces an emotional dissociation, thereby diminishing the discomfort and perception of pain.

Dissociation, which involves directing a patient's attention away from the pain, can make pain more manageable (Fisher 1999). Such distractions could come from components of relaxation exercises, but could also come from activities like exercise, listening to music or imagining doing other sport activities that demand deployment of attention. It has been reported that dissociation strategies are more effective for increasing pain threshold than are associative strategies (Fisher 1999). Fisher (1999) also suggested that dissociative strategies might be better in preparing athletes to cope with pain before its onset rather than after pain is present. The obvious clinical implication of this strategy is to prepare patients for painful aspects of rehabilitation.

Self-efficacy

Self-efficacy refers to the conviction that one has to successfully execute the behavior required to produce a certain outcome (Bandura 1977). For example, in an athlete with injury and pain, self-efficacy would relate to their belief that they can do something about the pain. In relation to pain, the encouragement of higher levels of self-efficacy by the physical therapist should be an underlying aspect of all communications with injured athletes during rehabilitation. As self-efficacy is an important component of sport injury rehabilitation, it is covered in more detail in Chapter 11.

Summary

Dealing with pain from sport and exercise injuries is complex. As pain is a subjective experience, two people with the same presenting injury could experience pain in very different ways. As evidence exists that athletes may have different pain sensitivities and pain tolerance levels than non-athletes, rehabilitation programs must be made specifically to cater for these differences. An understanding of the mechanisms of pain and how pain can influence adherence to rehabilitation are integral to successful rehabilitation.

The management of pain in sport and exercise goes beyond simply injury. There are aspects of normal sport participation that can evoke pain. Therefore, the pain management techniques outlined in this chapter have their place in the clinic, at home, on the training ground and at competition. The predominant message from all the literature on pain management is that effective rehabilitation involves a combination of strategies utilizing both physical and psychosocial elements.

References

Almekinders L C 1999 Anti-inflammatory treatment of muscular injuries in sport. An update of recent studies. Sports Medicine 28:383–388

American Medical Association 1988 Guides to the evaluation of permanent impairment, 3rd edn. American Medical Association, Washington, DC

Arnheim D D, Prentice W E 2000 Principles of athletic training, 10th edn. McGraw Hill, New York

Bahrke M S, Morgan W P 1978 Anxiety reduction following exercise and meditation. Cognitive Therapy and Research 2:323–333

Bair M J, Robinson R L, Katon W et al 2003 Depression and pain comorbidity: a literature review. Archives of Internal Medicine 163:2433–2445

Bandura A 1977 Self-efficacy: toward a unifying theory of behavioral change. Psychological Review 84:191–215

Bartholomew J B, Brewer B W, Van Raalte J L et al 1998a A psychometric evaluation of the Sports Inventory for Pain. The Sport Psychologist 12:29–39

Bartholomew J B, Edwards S M, Brewer B W et al 1998b The Sports Inventory for Pain: a confirmatory factor analysis. Research Quarterly for Exercise and Sport 69:24–29

Baumert P W Jr 1999 Modalities in rehabilitation. In: Lillegard W A, Butcher J D, Rucker K S (eds) Handbook of sports medicine: a symptom-oriented approach, 2nd edn. Butterworth-Heinemann, Boston, MA

Benson H 1975 The relaxation response. William Morrow, New York

Bijur P E, Silver W, Gallagher E J 2001 Reliability of the visual analog scale for measurement of acute pain. Academic Emergency Medicine 8:1154–1157

Bingol U, Altan L, Yurtkuran M 2005 Low-power laser treatment for shoulder pain. Photomedicine and Laser Surgery 23:459–464

Bleakley C, McDonough S, MacAuley D 2004 The use of ice in the treatment of acute soft-tissue injury: a systematic review of randomized controlled trials. American Journal of Sports Medicine 32:251–261

Bolton J E, Wilkinson R A 1998 Responsiveness of pain scales; a comparison of three pain intensity measures in chiropractic patients. Journal of Manipulative and Physiological Therapeutics 21:1–7

Bowsher D 1994 Acute and chronic pain and assessment. In: Wells P E, Frampton V, Bowsher D (eds) Pain management by physiotherapy, 2nd edn. Butterworth-Heinemann, Oxford

Brewer B W 1998 Adherence to sport injury rehabilitation programs. Journal of Applied Sport Psychology 10:70–82

Brown S C, Glass J M, Park D C 2002 The relationship of pain and depression to cognitive function in rheumatoid arthritis. Pain 96:279–284

Buchanan W W 2000 Inflammation: its influences and consequences in athletes. In: Kumbhare D A, Basmajian J V (eds) Decision making and outcomes in sports rehabilitation. Churchill Livingstone, Edinburgh

Byerly P N, Worrell T, Gahimer J et al 1994 Rehabilitation compliance in an athletic training environment. Journal of Athletic Training 29:352–355

Campbell J N, Meyer R A 1986 Primary afferents and hyperalgesia. In: Yaksh T L (ed) Spinal afferent processing. Plenum Press, New York

Carabelli R A, Pertes S M, Koob K et al 1998 The role of exercise in the management of chronic pain. In: Weiner R S (ed) Pain management. A practical guide for clinicians, 5th edn, vol. 2. St Lucie Press, Florida

Carroll DE, Seers K 1998 Relaxation for the relief of chronic pain: a systematic review. Journal of Advanced Nursing 27:276–287

Carroll D, Moore R A, McQuay H J et al 2001 Transcutaneous electrical nerve stimulation (TENS) for chronic pain. Cochrane Database Systematic Review 3:CD003222

Charman R A 1994 Pain and nociception: mechanisms and modulation in sensory context. In: Boyling J D, Palastanga N (eds) Grieve's modern manual therapy, 2nd edn. Churchill Livingstone, Edinburgh

Cleeland C S 1989 Measurement of pain by subjective report. In: Chapman C R, Loeser J D (eds.) Advances in pain research and management, vol 12. Issues in pain management. Raven Press, New York, p 391–403

Cocchiarella L, Andersson G B J 2000 Guides to the evaluation of permanent impairment, 5th edn. American Medical Association

Cousins M J, Phillips G D 1985 Acute pain management. Clinics in Critical Care Medicine 8:82–117

Craig K D 1999 Emotions and psychobiology. In: Wall P D, Melzack R (eds) Textbook of pain, 4th edn. Churchill Livingstone, New York, p 331–343

Craig K D, Prkachin K M, Eckstein Grunau R 2001 The facial expression of pain. In: Turk D C, Melzack R (eds) Handbook of pain assessment, 2nd edn. Guilford Press, New York, p 153–169

Crombez G, Eccleston C, Baeyens F et al 1998 When somatic information threatens, catastrophic thinking enhances attentional interference. Pain 75:187–198

Crombez G, Eccleston C, Van den Broek A et al 2002 The effects of catastrophic thinking about pain on attentional interference by pain: no mediation of negative affectivity in healthy volunteers and in patients with low back pain. Pain Research and Management 7:31–39

Crossman J 1997 Psychological rehabilitation from sports injuries. Sports Medicine 23:333–339

Crue B L 1983 The neurophysiology and taxonomy of pain. In: Brena S F, Chapman S L (eds) Management of patients with chronic pain. Spectrum, New York

de Paula A A, de Carvalho E C, dos Santos C B 2002 The use of the 'progressive muscle relaxation' technique for pain relief in gynecology and obstetrics. Latin American Journal of Nursing 10:654–659

Driediger M, Hall C, Callow N 2006 Imagery use by injured athletes: a qualitative analysis. Journal of Sports Science 24:261–271

Egan S 1988 Acute pain tolerance amongst athletes. Physiotherapy in Sport 11:11–13

Eich E, Rachman S, Lopatka C 1990 Affect, pain, and autobiographic memory. Journal of Abnormal Psychology 99:174–178

Ellis B 1998 Transcutaneous electrical nerve stimulation for pain relief: recent research findings and implications for clinical use. Physical Therapy Reviews 3:3–8

Elton D 1995 Injury and pain. In: Zuluaga M, Briggs C, Carlisle J et al (eds) Sports physiotherapy. Applied science and practice. Churchill Livingstone, Edinburgh

Feuerstein M, Beattie P 1995 Biobehavioural factors affecting pain and disability in low back pain: mechanisms and assessment. Physical Therapy 75:267–280

Fields J, Murphey M, Horodyski M et al 1995 Factors associated with adherence to sport injury rehabilitation in college-age recreational athletes. Journal of Sport Rehabilitation 4:172–180

Fisher A C 1999 Counseling for improved rehabilitation adherence. In: Ray R, Wiese-Bjornstal D M (eds) Counseling in sport medicine. Human Kinetics, Champaign, IL

Fisher A C, Hoisington L L 1993 Injured athletes' attitudes and judgments toward rehabilitation adherence. Journal of the National Athletic Trainers Association 28:48–54

Fisher A C, Domm M A, Wuest D A 1988 Adherence to sports injury rehabilitation programs. Physician and Sportsmedicine 16(7):47–51

Fisher A C, Mullins S A, Frye P A 1993 Athletic trainers' attitudes and judgments of injured athletes' rehabilitation adherence. Journal of Athletic Training 28:43–47

Fitzgerald M 1989 The course and termination of primary afferent fibres. In Wall P D, Melzack R (eds) Textbook of pain, 2nd edn. Churchill Livingstone, Edinburgh

Francis S R, Andersen M B, Maley P 2000 Physiotherapists' and male professional athletes' views on psychological skills for rehabilitation. Journal of Science and Medicine in Sport 3:17–29

Frey J H 1991 Social risk and the meaning of sport. Sociology of Sport Journal 8:136–145

Gracely R H, Kwilosz D M 1988 The Descriptor Differential Scale: applying psychophysical principles to clinical pain assessment. Pain 35:279–288

Hall C R 2001 Imagery in sport and exercise. In: Singer R N, Hausenblas H A, Janelle C M (eds) Handbook of sport psychology, 2nd edn. John Wiley, New York

Hall C, Mack D, Pavio A et al 1998 Imagery use by athletes: development of the Sport Imagery Questionnaire. International Journal of Sport Psychology 29:73–89

Heil J 1993 Psychology of sport injury. Human Kinetics, Champaign, IL

Heil J, Fine P G 1999 Pain in sport: A biopsychological perspective. In: Pargman D (ed) Psychological bases of sport injuries, 2nd edn. Fitness Information Technology, Morgantown, WV

Hernandez-Reif M, Field T, Krasnegor J et al 2001 Lower back pain is reduced and range of motion increased after massage therapy. International Journal of Neuroscience 106:131–145

Huskisson E C 1983 Visual analogue scales. In: Melzack R (ed) Pain measurement and assessment. Raven, New York

Ievleva L, Orlick T 1999 Mental paths to enhanced recovery from a sports injury. In: Pargman D (ed) Psychological bases of sport injuries, 2nd edn. Fitness Information Technology, Morgantown, WV

International Association for the Study of Pain (IASP) 1986 Classification of chronic pain: descriptions of chronic pain syndromes and definitions of pain terms. Pain 27:S1–S225

Jackson T, Iezzi T, Chen H et al 2005 Gender, interpersonal transactions, and the perception of pain: an experimental analysis. Journal of Pain 6:228–236

Jacobson E 1938 Progressive relaxation. University of Chicago Press, Chicago

Jensen M P, Karoly P 1991 Control beliefs, coping efforts, and adjustments to chronic pain. Journal of Consulting and Clinical Psychology 59:431–438

Jensen M P, Turner J A, Romano J M 2001 Changes in beliefs, catastrophizing, and coping are associated with improvement in multidisciplinary pain treatment. Journal of Consulting and Clinical Psychology 69:655–662

Johnson M I 1998 Acupuncture-like transcutaneous electrical nerve stimulation (AL-TENS) in the management of pain. Physical Therapy Reviews 3:73–93

Khadilkar A, Milne S, Brosseau et al 2005 Transcutaneous electrical nerve stimulation for the treatment of chronic low back pain: a systematic review. Spine 30:2657–2666

Kolt G S 2000 Doing sport psychology with injured athletes. In: Andersen M B (ed) Doing sport psychology. Human Kinetics, Champaign, IL, p 223–236

Kolt G S, McConville L C 2000 The effects of a Feldenkrais Awareness Through Movement program on state of anxiety. Journal of Bodywork and Movement Therapies 4:216–220

Koltyn K F, Focht B C, Ancker J M et al 1998 The effect of time of day and gender on pain perception and selected psychological responses. Medicine and Science in Sports and Exercise 30:S5

Lara-Munoz C, De Leon S P, Feinstein A R et al 2004 Comparison of three rating scales for measuring subjective phenomena in clinical research: I. Use of experimentally controlled auditory stimuli. Archives of Medical Research 35:43–48

Law B, Driediger M, Hall C et al 2006 Imagery use, perceived pain, limb functioning and satisfaction in athletic injury rehabilitation. New Zealand Journal of Physiotherapy 34:10–16

Lehman J D, Delateur B J 1990 Therapeutic heat. In: Lehman J F (ed) Therapeutic heat and cold. Williams and Wilkins, Baltimore, MD

Leivadi S, Hernandez-Reif M, Field T et al 1999 Massage therapy and relaxation effects on university dance students. Journal of Dance Medicine and Science 3:108–112

Leventhal H, Everhart D 1979 Emotion, pain and physical illness. In: Izard C E (ed) Emotions in personality and psychopathology. Plenum, New York

Loeser J D 1996 Pain: concepts and management. 150 years on – a selection of papers presented at the 11th World Congress of Anaesthesiologists. Bridge, Rosebery, Australia

Lucic K S, Steffen J J, Harrigan J A et al 1991 Progressive relaxation training: muscle contraction before relaxation? Behavior Therapy 22:249–256

McCracken L M, Zayfert C, Gross R T 1992 The Pain Anxiety Symptoms Scale: development and validation of a scale to measure fear of pain. Pain 50:67–93

McDowell I, Newell C 1996 Measuring health: a guide to rating scales and questionnaires, 2nd edn. Oxford University Press, New York

Manning E L, Fillingim R B 2002 The influence of athletic status and gender on experimental pain responses. Journal of Pain 3:421–428

Martin K A, Moritz S E, Hall C R 1999 Imagery use in sport: a literature review and applied model. The Sport Psychologist 13:345–368

Mehler W R 1962 The anatomy of the so-called 'pain tract' in man: an analysis of the course and distribution of the ascending fibres of the fasciculus anterolateralis. In: French J D, Porter R W (eds) Basic research in paraplegia. Thomas, Springfield, IL

Melzack R 1975 The McGill Pain Questionnaire: major properties and scoring methods. Pain 1:277–299

Melzack R 1986 Neurophysiological foundations of pain. In: Sternbach R A (ed) The psychology of pain. Raven, New York

Melzack R 1987 The Short-Form McGill Pain Questionnaire. Pain 30:191–197

Melzack R 1990 The tragedy of needless pain. Scientific American 262:19–25

Melzack R 1998 Psychological aspects of pain. Implications for neural blockade. In Cousins M J, Bridenbaugh P O (eds) Neural blockade in clinical anesthesia and management of pain, 3rd edn. Lippincott-Raven, St Louis, MO, p 781–792

Melzack R 1999 From the gate to the neuromatrix. Pain 6 (suppl): S121–S126

Melzack R 2001 Pain and the neuromatrix in the brain. Journal of Dental Education 65:1378–1382

Melzack R, Dennis S G 1980 Phylogenic evolution of pain expression in animals. In: Kosterlitz H W, Terenius L Y (eds) Pain and society. Verlag Chemie, Weinheim

Melzack R, Katz J 1999 Pain measurement in persons with pain. In: Wall P D, Melzack R (eds) Textbook of pain, 4th edn. Churchill Livingstone, Edinburgh

Melzack R, Katz J 2001 The McGill Pain Questionnaire: appraisal and current status. In: Turk D C, Melzack R (eds) Handbook of pain assessment, 2nd edn. Guilford Press, New York, p 35–52

Melzack R, Wall P D 1965 Pain mechanisms: a new theory. Science 150:971–979

Melzack R, Wall P D 2004 The challenge of pain, 2nd edn. Penguin

Meyers M C, Bourgeois A E, Stewart S et al 1992 Predicting pain response in athletes: development and assessment of the Sports Inventory for Pain. Journal of Sport and Exercise Psychology 14:249–261

Meyers M C, Bourgeois A E, Murray N et al 1993 Comparison of psychological characteristics and skills of elite and sub-elite equestrian athletes. Medicine and Science in Sports and Exercise 25:S154

Meyers M C, Bourgeois A E, LeUnes A 2001 Pain coping response of collegiate athletes involved in high contact, high injury-potential sport. International Journal of Sport Psychology 32:29–42

Milne M, Hall C, Forwell L 2005 Self-efficacy, imagery use, and adherence to rehabilitation by injured athletes. Journal of Sport Rehabilitation 14:150–167

Milne S, Welch V, Brosseau L et al 2001 Transcutaneous electrical nerve stimulation (TENS) for chronic low back pain. Cochrane Database Systematic Review 2:CD003008

Moraska A 2005 Sports massage. A comprehensive review. Journal of Sports Medicine and Physical Fitness 45:370–380

Nichols A W 2005 Complications associated with the use of corticosteroids in the treatment of athletic injuries. Clinical Journal of Sports medicine 15:E370

Ninedek A, Kolt G S 2000 Sports physiotherapists' perceptions of psychological strategies in sport injury rehabilitation. Journal of Sport Rehabilitation 9:191–206

O'Bannon R M, Rickard H C, Runcie D 1987 Progressive relaxation as a function of procedural variations and anxiety level. International Journal of Psychophysiology 5:207–214

Ord P, Gijsbers K 2003 Pain thresholds and tolerances of competitive rowers and their use of spontaneous self-generated pain-coping strategies. Perceptual and Motor Skills 97:1219–1222

Osiri M, Welch V, Brosseau L et al 2001 Transcutaneous electrical nerve stimulation (TENS) for knee osteoarthritis. Cochrane Database Systematic Review

Ozkan N, Altan L, Bingol U et al 2004 Investigation of the supplementary effect of GaAs laser therapy on the rehabilitation of human digital flexor tendons. Journal of Clinical Laser Medicine and Surgery 22:105–110

Paoloni J A, Orchard J W 2006 The use of therapeutic medications for soft-tissue injuries in sports medicine. Medical Journal of Australia 184:198

Paparizos A L, Tripp D A, Sullivan M J L et al 2005 Catastrophizing and pain perception in recreational ballet dancers. Journal of Sport Behavior 28:35–50

Payne R A 2000 Relaxation techniques. A practical handbook for the health care professional, 2nd edn. Churchill Livingstone, Edinburgh

Payne R A 2004 Relaxation techniques. In: Kolt G S, Andersen M B (eds) Psychology in the physical and manual therapies. Churchill Livingstone, Edinburgh, p 111–124

Pen L J, Fisher C A 1994 Athletes and pain tolerance. Sports Medicine 18:319–329

Petruzzello S J, Landers D M, Hatfield B D et al 1991 A meta-analysis of the anxiety reducing effects of acute and chronic exercise: outcomes and mechanisms. Sports Medicine 11:143–182

Price D D, Harkins, S W 1987 Combined use of experimental pain and visual analogue scales in providing standardized measurement of clinical pain. Clinical Journal of Pain 3:1–8

Price D D, Harkins S W, Baker C 1987 Sensory-affective relationships among different types of clinical and experimental pain. Pain 28:297–307

Ransford A O, Cairns D, Mooney V 1976 The pain drawing as an aid to the psychologic evaluation of patients with low-back pain. Spine 1:127–134

Reading A E 1984 Testing pain mechanisms in persons with pain. In: Wall P D, Melzack R (eds) Textbook of pain. Churchill Livingstone, Edinburgh

Robertson V J, Baker K G 2001 A review of therapeutic ultrasound: effectiveness studies. Physical Therapy 81:1339–1350

Salmon P 2001 Effects of physical exercise on anxiety, depression, and sensitivity to stress: a unifying theory. Clinical Psychology Review 21:33–61

Shephard R J 1997 Exercise and relaxation in health promotion. Sports Medicine 23:211–217

Shin S M, Choi J K 1997 Effect of indomethacin phonophoresis on the relief of temporomandibular joint pain. Journal of Craniomandibular Practice 15:345–348

Shipton E A 1999 Pain. Acute and chronic, 2nd edn. Arnold, London

Sim J, Arnell P 1993 Measurement and validity in physical therapy research. Physical Therapy 73:102–115

Sim J, Waterfield J 1997 Validity, reliability and responsiveness in the assessment of pain. Physiotherapy Theory and Practice 13:23–37

Simons D G, Travell, J G, Simons L S, Cumings B D 1998 Myofascial pain and dysfunction. The trigger point manual, vol 1. Upper half of body. Lippincott Williams & Wilkins, Baltimore, MD

Sluka K A, Walsh D 2003 Transcutaneous electrical nerve stimulation: basic science mechanisms and clinical effectiveness. Journal of Pain 4:109–121

Smidt N, de Vet H C W, Bouter L M et al 2005 Effectiveness of exercise therapy: a best-evidence summary of systematic reviews. Australian Journal of Physiotherapy 51:71–85

Smith A L, Kolt G S, McConville J C 2001 The effect of the Feldenkrais Method on pain and anxiety in people experiencing chronic low back pain. New Zealand Journal of Physiotherapy 29:6–14

Smith M C 1976 Retrograde cell changes in human spinal cord after anterolateral cordotomies: location and identification after different periods of survival. Advances in Pain Research and Therapy 1:91–98

Sordoni C, Hall C, Forwell L 2000 The use of imagery by athletes during injury rehabilitation. Journal of Sport Rehabilitation 9:329–228

Sullivan M J L, Bishop S R, Pivak J 1995 The pain catastrophizing scale: development and validation. Psychological Assessment 7:524–532

Tajet-Foxell B, Rose F D 1995 Pain and pain tolerance in professional ballet dancers. British Journal of Sports Medicine 29:31–34

Tascioglu F, Armagan O, Tabak Y et al 2004 Low power laser treatment in patients with knee osteoarthritis. Swiss Medical Weekly 134:254–258

Taylor J, Taylor S 1997 Psychological approaches to sports injury rehabilitation. Aspen Publishers, Gaithersburg, MD

Taylor J, Taylor S 1998 Pain education and management in the rehabilitation from sports injury. The Sport Psychologist 12:68–88

Taylor K, Newton R A, Personius W J et al 1987 Effects of interferential current stimulation for treatment of subjects with recurrent jaw pain. Physical Therapy 67:346–350

Thienhaus O, Cole B E 2002 The classification of pain. In: Weiner R S (ed) Pain management. A practical guide for clinicians. CRC Press, Boca Raton, FL, p 27–36

Travell J G, Simons D G 1983 Myofascial pain and dysfunction. The trigger point manual. The lower extremities (vol 2). Williams and Wilkins, Baltimore, MD

Turk D C, Okifuji A 1999 A cognitive-behavioural approach to pain management. In: Wall P D, Melzack R (eds) Textbook of pain, 4th edn. Churchill Livingstone, London

Turk D C, Okifuji A 2001 Pain terms and taxonomies of pain. In: Loeser J D (ed) Bonica's management of pain, 3rd edn. Lippincott Williams & Wilkins, Philadelphia, PA, p 17–25

van der Windt P A, van der Heijden G J, van der Berg S G et al 1999 Ultrasound therapy for musculoskeletal disorders: a systematic review. Pain 81:257–271

Wall P D 1979 On the relation of injury to pain. Pain 6:253–264

Wallace R K, Benson J, Wilson A F 1971 A wakeful hypometabolic physiologic state. American Journal of Physiology 221:795–799

Weerapong P, Hume P A, Kolt G S 2005 The mechanisms of massage and effects on performance, muscle recovery and injury prevention. Sports Medicine 35:235–256

Weiner R S 2002 Pain management. A practical guide for clinicians, 6th edn. CRC Press, Boca Raton, FL

Weisenberg M 1999 Cognitive aspects of pain. In: Wall P D, Melzack R (eds) Textbook of pain, 4th edn. Churchill Livingstone, London

Wiese-Bjornstal D M, Shaffer S M 1999 Psychological dimensions of sport injury. In: Ray R, Wiese-Bjornstal D M (eds) Counseling in sports medicine. Human Kinetics, Champaign, IL

Wright A, Zusman M 2004 Neurophysiology of pain and pain modulation. In: Boyling J D, Jull G A (eds) Grieve's modern manual therapy. The vertebral column, 3rd edn. Churchill Livingstone, Edinburgh, p 155–171

Exercise-based conditioning and rehabilitation

10

Rafael F. Escamilla and Robbin Wickham-Bruno

CHAPTER CONTENTS

Introduction 149

Strength training. 149

Interval training 163

Endurance training 163

Stabilization 165

Summary 166

Introduction

This chapter will present evidence for the use of exercise in injury prevention and rehabilitation. Specific areas covered will include strength and plyometrics training, interval training, endurance training and stabilization training. Strength training has been shown to be effective in injury prevention and rehabilitation by increasing muscle, ligament and tendon strength and size. As well, strength training can increase bone strength and density, decrease the risk of osteoporosis, decrease risk of falling and subsequent injury, improve gait stability, walking speed and efficiency, increase stair climbing and chair raising ability, and increase balance. Plyometric training is helpful in enhancing muscle strength and power, which decreases an athlete's injury risk by allowing muscles and connective tissue to absorb more energy. Interval training allows a greater volume of work to be performed compared to continuous training. Endurance training is important in enhancing the cardio-vascular system, which improves overall function and enhances the rehabilitation process. Stabilization training is important in enhancing the core strength of the body.

Strength training

In discussing strength training it is important to consider the principles, types and systems of strength training, physiologic adaptations to strength training and research evidence for employing strength training for injury prevention and rehabilitation. Strength training is an important component in sport and exercise for training, injury prevention and rehabilitation. Research findings involving both males and females over a wide range of ages have shown that strength training, especially higher intensity training, is efficacious in minimizing injuries, maximizing performance and enhancing rehabilitation. The large literature in this area has demonstrated benefits of strength training that span several different areas of human function and health benefits, such as an increase in muscle size and strength, increased bone strength and density, decreased risk of falling, enhanced gait efficiency and activities of daily living and positive psychological effects (see Table 10.1). Somewhat surprisingly, cardiovascular effects have also been observed with strength training. For example, Tanasescu et al (2002) tracked nearly 45 000 men aged 40–75 over a 13-year period to assess amount, type and intensity of physical activity in relation to the risk of coronary artery disease (CAD). Strength training for 30 min or more per week was associated with a 23%

Table 10.1 Effects of strength training

Effect of strength training	Referenced evidence
Increase in muscle size, strength and power	Bemben et al (2000) Hagerman et al (2000) Porter (2001)
Acute and chronic adaptations in neuromuscular function	Hakkinen et al (2000) Kraemer et al (1996) del Olmo et al (2006)
Increase in bone strength and density, and a decrease in osteoporosis	Granhed et al (1987) Kerr et al (2001) Weaver et al (2001)
Increase in ligament and tendon strength and thickness	Fleck & Falkel (1986) Kannus et al (1997) Zernicke & Loitz (1992)
Increase in balance and decrease in risk of falling and subsequent injury	Gregg et al (2000) Hess & Woollacott (2005) Weiss et al (2000)
Increase in gait stability, walking speed and efficiency	Carmeli et al (2000) Scandalis et al (2001) Schlicht et al (2001)
Increase in stair climbing and chair raising ability	Brill et al (1998) Chandler et al (1998) Weiss et al (2000)
Increase in hormonal adaptations	Borst et al (2001) Gorostiaga et al (1999) Kraemer et al (1999)
Decrease in blood pressure	Martel et al (1999)
Decrease in glucose intolerance and insulin resistance	Ryan et al (2001) Yaspelkis (2006)
Decrease in body fat, increase in fat free mass and increase in basal metabolic rate	Byrne & Wilmore (2001) Hagerman et al (2000) Lemmer et al (2001)
Increase in positive mood and decrease in anxiety and tension	Beniamini et al (1997) Tsutsumi et al (1998) Tucker & Maxwell (1992)
Decrease in coronary heart disease	Tanasescu et al (2002)

risk reduction in CAD, with higher intensity training more effective than lower intensity training.

Physiologic adaptations to strength training

Research findings suggest that connective tissue growth is stimulated most effectively by moderate to higher intensity and volume (e.g. 3–5 sets of 8–12 repetitions) strength training (Stone 1988). This growth is further enhanced by using antigravity muscles and weight-bearing exercises (Stone 1988), especially for bone remodeling. As well, overtraining should be avoided as it can adversely affect connective tissue rejuvenation. While connective tissue weakens with disuse, strength training increases the maximum tensile strength in connective tissue and the amount of energy that can be absorbed prior to failure (Stone 1988), thus minimizing injury risk.

Strength training can alter the mechanical principles of muscle fascia, tendons, ligaments and bones by increasing both size and strength of these tissues (Zernicke & Loitz 1992). Several studies have shown that high intensity strength training increases bone strength by increasing bone mineral density, thereby reducing injury risk and providing a protection against bone weakening processes such as osteoporosis (Kerr et al 2001, Weaver et al 2001). One study reported extremely high bone mineral content in the lumbar vertebrae in world-class powerlifters who lifted extremely heavy loads during weight-bearing exercises (i.e. while performing the squat and deadlift exercises) and had very high annual training volumes (Granhed et al 1987). Although increases in bone strength occur at a much slower rate compared to increases in muscle strength (Conroy et al 1992), employing weight-bearing exercises in a strength training program will maximize bone remodeling and strength gains (Stone 1988).

While optimal intensity for strengthening ligaments and tendons is not clear, studies have shown an increase in the strength and size of tendons and ligaments due to exercise (Michna & Hartmann 1989, Stone 1988). Strength training in the elderly has been shown to help reverse the deteriorating effect of aging on tendon properties and function by increasing tendon stiffness (Maganaris et al 2004). It is currently unknown if strength training has beneficial effects in increasing the thickness of articular cartilage, although weight-bearing exercise has been shown to have this effect in articular cartilage tissue (Barneveld & van Weeren 1999). Since articular cartilage provides a cushion between bony surfaces of a joint, increasing articular cartilage thickness facilitates shock absorption, thereby decreasing injury potential (Barneveld & van Weeren 1999).

Strength training can also improve glucose transport in both normal and insulin-resistant skeletal muscle by enhancing the activation of the insulin signaling cascade and increasing GLUT-4 protein concentration (Yaspelkis 2006). These training-induced changes from resistance training improve the quality of the skeletal muscle and can occur independent of muscle hypertrophy.

During the initial several weeks of a new strength training program muscle strength is increased primarily by neural adaptations. These adaptations include increased efficiency in motor unit recruitment, discharge rate and synchronization, enhanced neural drive to muscles, increased neuromuscular coordination between muscles, decreased sensitivity in the golgi tendon organs (i.e. disinhibition) and motor learning effects (Hakkinen et al 2000, Kraemer et al 1996). Muscle hypertrophy and further strength increases occur sometime later, typically at least 4–8 weeks after a resistance training program begins.

Chronic neural adaptation has recently been shown to occur in long-term resistance training of greater than two years (del Olmo et al 2006). Long-term resistance training results in central nervous system adaptations that likely lead to an enhancement of muscle activation due to a greater number of motor units being recruited and an increased firing frequency in these motor units (del Olmo et al 2006).

Principles of strength training

When using overall strength training in sport and exercise it is important to understand the principles of progressive overload, specificity, reversibility, fitness and recovery.

Progressive overload principle

The basic premise of progressive overload is to progressively increase the load on the musculoskeletal system. Once muscles, tendons, ligaments and bones adapt to a given stimuli, additional loads must be placed on these structures for further adaptation to occur. This is often done by small increases in load and keeping the repetitions the same, or by larger increases in load and at the same time decreasing the number of repetitions performed. The overload principle can be manipulated by varying several factors discussed below. These include exercise intensity, rest intervals, exercise duration, exercise frequency, exercise mode and periodization.

Intensity

Training intensity is commonly synonymous with the amount of weight, load or resistance being lifted or overcome. The higher the load lifted, the higher the training intensity. Intensity is most commonly expressed in terms of a percentage of an individual's one repetition maximum (1 RM). Training studies have shown that strength is maximized by employing heavy resistance between approximately 80 and 95% of an individual's 1 RM (Bemben et al 2000, Hagerman et al 2000, Kraemer 1997, Stone et al 1981), which equates to training between a 3 RM (heaviest weight performed for three consecutive repetitions) and 8 RM. Therefore, it is common for strength training programs to employ multiple sets between 3 and 8 repetitions.

For individuals whose goal is to achieve strength without lifting such high percentages of 1 RM (e.g. individuals who want to minimize joint stress), a more moderate intensity of 70–80% of 1 RM, or approximately 8–12 repetitions, is also an effective means of developing musculoskeletal strength. Performing beyond 12 repetitions is considered low intensity training, which changes the emphasis from muscular strength to muscular endurance. Several studies have demonstrated that higher intensity strength training (approximately 80% 1 RM) is more effective in strength gains compared to lower intensity (40–60% 1 RM) strength training, even in older individuals (Fatouros et al 2005, Sullivan et al 2005, Taaffe et al 1996). For example, having both high (82% 1 RM) and low (55% 1 RM) intensity training groups consisting of elderly men (mean age of 71 ± 4) strength train for 24 weeks, Fatouros et al (2005) reported a 63–91% increase in upper and lower body strength in the high intensity group but only a 42–66% increase in upper and lower body strength in the low intensity group. In addition, Taaffe et al (1996) conducted a similar study using similar age women and training intensities over 52 weeks of strength training and reported a 59% increase in upper and lower body strength in the high intensity group, but only a 41% increase in upper and lower body strength in the low intensity group.

Training intensity can also be quantified and expressed as the power output generated while performing an exercise. Power is defined as work per unit time. Since Work = (Force)(Distance), and Speed = Distance/Time, then Power can be expressed as the product of force and speed as follows: Power = (Work/Time) = [(Force)(Distance)/Time] = (Force)(Speed). The highest power outputs recorded in sport activities occur in lifting maximum or near-maximum loads during the snatch and clean and jerk exercises during weightlifting competition (Garhammer 1993). These types of exercises are performed explosively generating high force and power outputs. Explosive training with moderate to heavy loads produce maximum fast twitch fiber recruitment, which is important since the peak power output of fast twitch fibers is about 4 times as great as in slow twitch fibers (Faulkner et al 1986). Explosive power training, especially combined with strength training, also increases motor unit synchronization and the rate of force development (Hakkinen & Hakkinen 1995).

When using free weights or machine weights as resistance, the number of repetitions that relate to a given percentage of 1 RM is highly variable depending on the exercise employed, the muscle group being worked (smaller muscles produce fewer repetitions for a given percentage of 1 RM and larger muscles produce higher repetitions for a given percentage of 1 RM) and the training level (trained or untrained) of the individual (Kraemer 1997). Nevertheless, for trained athletes the relationship between performing repetitions to failure and a percentage of one's 1 RM can be estimated as follows (Mayhew et al 1993):

10 RM	$\approx$ 74–76% 1 RM
9 RM	$\approx$ 76–78% 1 RM
8 RM	$\approx$ 79–81% 1 RM
7 RM	$\approx$ 81–83% 1 RM
6 RM	$\approx$ 84–86% 1 RM
5 RM	$\approx$ 86–88% 1 RM
4 RM	$\approx$ 89–91% 1 RM
3 RM	$\approx$ 92–94% 1 RM
2 RM	$\approx$ 94–96% 1 RM

In addition, an individual's 1 RM can be estimated by dividing the load employed while performing a given number of repetitions to failure by the corresponding percentage of their 1 RM at which they are training.

Volume

Training volume for any given exercise is determined by multiplying the total number of sets, repetitions and load (or resistance). For example, performing 3 sets of 8 repetitions of bench press with 100 kg has an exercise volume of 2400 kg (i.e. $3 \times 8 \times 100$). Typically, volume increases as intensity decreases, and volume decreases as intensity increases. For example, consider an athlete who has a 150 kg 1 RM bench press. Performing high intensity training for 4 sets of 4 repetitions at 90% of their 1 RM would yield an exercise volume of 2160 kg (i.e. $4 \times 4 \times [0.9 \times 150]$). If that same athlete performed 4 sets of 8 repetitions at a lower intensity of 80% of their 1 RM, this would yield an exercise volume of 3840 kg (i.e. $4 \times 8 \times [0.80 \times 150]$). In this example the lower training intensity of 80% 1 RM produced 78% greater volume compared to the higher training intensity of 90% 1 RM. Since the weight is being moved through a given distance, training volume is also a measure of the total mechanical work performed during an exercise or training session.

Rest intervals and recovery

Rest intervals refer to the total rest time between repetitions, sets and exercises for a given muscle group being worked. When training a specific muscle group, a 2–3 min rest interval between sets is common in strength training, often increasing with increasing intensities (e.g. 4–5 min rest interval for > 90% 1 RM training intensities) and decreasing with decreasing intensities (e.g. 1–2 min rest interval for 70–80% 1 RM training intensities and 30–60 s rest interval for 40–60% 1 RM training intensity). The increase in rest intervals with higher intensity training compared to lower intensity training is necessary in part due to the greater number of motor units recruited, a larger accumulation of lactate and to allow complete recovery when training with near maximal loads. Also, multi-muscle, multi-joint exercises (e.g. squat, powercleans, bench press), which require a large energy expenditure, require longer rest times than single-muscle, single joint exercises (e.g. leg extensions, leg curls, arm curls), which have a much lower energy expenditure.

In some exercises, such as the barbell squat, it is not uncommon to rest several seconds between repetitions when training with near maximal loads, allowing the muscles to briefly rest so they will be able to contract with greater force during each repetition. This type of training allows maximum loads to be performed for a greater number of repetitions than could otherwise be performed without the rest interval, increases the total work output accomplished during the set and maximizes strength gains.

Rest intervals are also needed between exercise sessions in order to allow time for muscle and connective tissue to repair and regenerate from training (Pincivero et al 1997). Compared to low intensity training, high intensity training causes more muscle and connective tissue damage and requires greater time to repair and regenerate (Stone 1988). Typically, 48–72 hours are needed between training sessions for muscle and connective tissue muscle to adequately recover (Stone 1988). Adequate rest and protein intake are two of the most common factors for muscle regeneration. Research has shown that a protein intake of 1.5–2 g/kg body mass is most effective in muscle regeneration after high intensity resistance training (Lemon 1998).

Larger muscle groups, such as the back and hip extensors, often require a longer rest period between training sessions compared to smaller muscle groups, especially those that move through a smaller range of motion (e.g. rectus abdominis, which may be trained daily with varying intensities and volume). A commonly employed rest interval protocol for any given muscle group is training on alternating days.

Duration

Training duration refers to the total quantity of time during resistance exercise, and will vary depending on the type of strength training that is being performed. As the number of exercises, repetitions, sets and rest intervals increase within a session, training duration will also increase. A typical strength training session lasts between 20 and 60 min. Training duration also refers to the number of weeks or months a given strength training program is adhered to. A strength training program typically will last 6–12 weeks before intensity, duration, frequency or mode are modified, which is in accordance with a periodization model (Stone 1990, Stone et al 1981).

Frequency

Training frequency refers to how often an athlete engages in a strength training program. It is often expressed as total number of training sessions per week. Although strength training once per week can build or maintain strength (McLester et al 2000, Taaffe et al 1999), several studies have shown that strength gains are maximized when training occurs 2–3 sessions per week (DeMichele et al 1997, McLester et al 2000, Pollock et al 1993). Despite the evidence that performing multiple strength training sessions per week is superior in producing strength gains when compared to performing a single strength training session each week, it should be emphasized that single weekly sessions are still efficacious. The single weekly strength training session, therefore, may be preferred by individuals who have time constraints and whose goals are not to maximize strength gains.

Several studies have shown that strength gains can be maintained with as little as one strength training session per week (Taaffe et al 1999), or one training session every 2–4 weeks (Tucci et al 1992), as long as high intensity training to failure is employed. From these data it can be deduced that the intensity of training is more important than duration or frequency of training in maintaining strength gains.

For high-level athletes and deconditioned individuals, it is not uncommon to split a larger training session involving several muscle groups into multiple shorter training sessions throughout the week involving only one or two muscle groups. This is referred to as split routine training. A large training session may also be split into multiple shorter training sessions throughout the day. An advantage of splitting a larger training session into multiple shorter sessions is to decrease the physiological and psychological fatigue that accompanies long sessions. A split routine allows an athlete to devote full effort and intensity for each muscle group. The same principles are true for a deconditioned individual training the entire body by performing 3 sets of 8 exercises three times per week. This individual may elect to perform 4 upper body exercises in the morning, and the remaining 4 lower body exercises in the evening, or perform 4 upper body exercises one day and the remaining 4 lower body exercises the following day.

Mode

The most common modes of strength training include resistance machines, free weights, body weight resistance and resistance from elastic bands. There are several different types of machines now available, such as the commonly used variable resistance machines (VRM) (which often employ a cam to vary the lever arm throughout the range of motion) and several types of isokinetic machines. For a detailed discussion of the advantages and disadvantages of free weights and machines refer to Haff (2000). Some advantages and disadvantages are shown in Box 10.1.

A potential advantage of VRM is that they attempt to match muscle torques that are generated throughout a range of motion. For example, the muscle torques generated by the elbow flexor muscles during an arm curl exercise begin small at full elbow extension (small muscle moment arms), progressively increase to maximum at 90° elbow flexion (large muscle moment arms) and then progressively decrease as the elbow continues to flex. This is referred to as an ascending–descending muscle torque curve. VRM attempt to match these curves by asymmetrically shaped cams in which the resistance moment arm varies throughout the range of motion. In effect, less resistance is offered at weaker joint positions and greater resistance is offered at stronger joint positions. Studies, however, have shown that some VRM do not effectively match muscle torque curves of the body throughout a given range of motion (Harman 1983, Johnson et al 1990).

Free weights are also very common for strength training, and include both barbells and dumbbells. Some advantages and disadvantages of free weights can be seen in Box 10.2.

Periodization

When muscles and connective tissues are given the same stimuli for a prolonged period of time, the strength gains exhibited in these tissues begin diminishing. To continue to stimulate muscles and connective tissues, training intensities, volumes and exercises must periodically be changed (Stone 1990). This is also important in preventing psychological staleness due to performing the same program for a prolonged period of time. Periodization is a system of training that varies training intensities and volumes throughout a year-long training cycle, referred to as a macrocycle (Stone 1990, Stone et al 1981). Periodized

training has been shown to produce superior strength and power gains compared to single-set or multi-set training with a constant repetition scheme (Kraemer 1997, Kraemer et al 1997, Kraemer et al 2000, Marx et al 2001, Stone et al 2000), even when the training sets and repetitions employed have not been to failure (Kraemer et al 1997). In addition, periodization training has been shown to increase physical performance abilities in athletes (Kraemer 1997, Kraemer et al 2000).

A typical macrocycle is broken down into 3–4 mesocycles (each 3–4 months in duration), and each mesocycle can in turn be broken down into 3–4 microcycles (each 3–4 weeks in duration). A common periodization pattern for the strength athlete involves beginning a training microcycle with higher volume and lower intensities, and progressively increasing intensity and decreasing volume (Stone et al 1981). For example, consider a 4-month mesocycle comprised of 4 microcycles of 4 weeks each. The initial 4-week microcycle could involve a higher training volume of 4 sets of 12 repetitions and a lower training intensity of 70% of 1 RM. This higher volume–lower intensity training microcycle, referred to as the preparatory phase (Stone et al 1981), will gradually allow the muscles and connective tissue to adapt to new stresses. Also, the first microcycle allows the athlete to adapt to performing new exercises that have recently not been performed, with an emphasis on proper lifting form and technique. As previously mentioned, the strength gains during this initial microcycle will primarily be due to neural factors. The second 4-week microcycle, referred to as the hypertrophy phase (Stone et al 1981), could involve training at 80% 1 RM

Box 10.1 Some advantages and disadvantages of machines

Advantages

- safe
- ease of use
- little knowledge of proper exercise form and technique is required
- a spotter for safety is not required
- little time to set up and change the weight is needed
- excellent muscle isolation

Disadvantages

- can be expensive
- often are heavy and bulky
- lack specificity to most movements that occur in sport due to largely single plane motion
- do not require balancing the weight while lifting through a range of motion
- do not allow for explosive training since many (e.g. the VRM) hinder acceleration
- may not offer an eccentric phase in the lift

Box 10.2 Free weight advantages and disadvantages

Advantages

- relatively easy to use
- offer numerous multi-joint, multi-muscle exercises
- inexpensive
- take up little space (especially dumbbells)
- are more sport-specific than machines since they allow the weight to accelerate and move in multiple planes
- require more muscle activity from synergists and stabilizers in order to balance the weight, and have a large energy expenditure compared to machines
- allow both concentric and eccentric muscle movements
- allow counter movements similar to sport activities
- provide range of motions and muscle activation patterns similar to what occurs in sport
- provide endless exercise variations that can be performed
- elicit greater proprioception and coordination development compared to machines

Disadvantages

- require a greater knowledge of proper exercise form and technique than VRMs
- require more time to set up and change weights than VRMs
- are not as safe as machines
- may require a spotter for safety

intensity and decreasing the training volume to 4 sets of 8 repetitions. The emphasis of this cycle is muscle hypertrophy, which research has shown to be effective when training occurs between approximately 8 and 10 RM (75–80% 1 RM) (Hakkinen et al 1998, Hurley et al 1995, McCall et al 1996, Narici et al 1996, Stone et al 1981). As muscles increase in size their potential for strength also increases, since the force a muscle can generate is directly proportional to that muscle's physiological cross-sectional area (Brand et al 1986, Delp et al 2001). Compared to younger individuals beyond puberty, muscle hypertrophy occurs to a lesser extent in the elderly, who instead experience a greater period of strength gains due to neural factors (Welle et al 1996). The third 4-week microcycle, referred to as the strength phase (Stone et al 1981), could involve training at an 85–90% 1 RM intensity and decreasing the training volume to 4 sets of 4–6 repetitions. The emphasis of this cycle is on muscle strength. Upper and lower extremity high intensity weight training studies have demonstrated significant increases in muscle strength when training between 2 and 12 RM (Hagerman et al 2000, Kraemer et al 2001, Rhodes et al 2000, Taaffe et al 1999). Many strength coaches, however, believe that strength is maximized using multiple sets per session, multiple sessions per week, and an intensity between 2 and 6 RM (approximately 85–95% 1 RM). This approach is supported by data from several strength training studies (Kraemer 1997, Stone et al 1981). The final 4-week microcycle, referred to as the power phase (Stone et al 1981), could involve training at a 90–95% 1 RM intensity and decreasing the training volume to 3–5 sets of 2–3 repetitions. The emphasis of this cycle is muscle power, which research has shown is maximized in select explosive exercises (i.e. clean and jerk, power cleans, snatch) while employing maximal or near maximal loads (Garhammer 1993).

Specificity principle (SAID)

Muscles and connective tissue adapt specifically to the demands placed on them. This is known as the Specific Adaptation to Imposed Demands (SAID) principle. For example, for muscles to hypertrophy, they have to be trained employing an optimal intensity for that specific adaptation, which as previously mentioned is approximately 70–80% 1 RM. Similarly, for muscles to maximally adapt to becoming stronger a higher intensity should be employed (approximately 80–95% 1 RM), and for bones to increase in density and become stronger weight bearing exercises should be used.

In addition to applying the SAID principle to muscle and connective tissues, the SAID principle also applies to exercise selections for sport-specific movements. An example of this is the squat movement, being specific to jumping in basketball. The squat is also sport specific for American football, since it develops the largest and most powerful muscles of the body (i.e. gluteals, quadriceps, hamstrings, erector spinae), which are important in both sprinting and jumping. In addition, an incline bench press follows a path that is more sport-specific to the shot-put compared to the flat bench press. Moreover, while the powerclean is a sport-specific movement to several positions in American football, it is not a sport specific movement for

overhand throwing and hitting in baseball, and could potentially have deleterious effects.

Reversibility principle

Strength gains are transient and reversible with disuse, with further losses in strength due to disuse occurring at a greater rate than gains in strength due to training (Bloomfield 1997). However, as previously outlined, strength gains can be maintained with as little as one strength training session per week (Taaffe et al 1999) as long as high intensity training is employed.

Fitness principle

Unfit individuals achieve strength gains at a faster rate than trained individuals, but also lose strength due to disuse at a faster rate than trained individuals (Bloomfield 1997). As discussed previously, the initial strength gains experienced by unfit individuals are largely due to neural factors such as increased neuromuscular coordination between muscles and decreased sensitivity in the golgi tendon organs.

Types of strength training

Isometric training

Isometric training occurs when tension develops in the muscle without a change in muscle length. Isometric training reached its peak popularity in the 1950s and 1960s largely due to the work of two Germans, Hettinger and Muller (Hettinger & Muller 1953). Several training studies (3–15 weeks in length) have shown moderate strength gains while performing multiple maximum isometric contractions 3–10 s in duration (Alway et al 1989, Carolan & Cafarelli 1992, Garfinkel & Cafarelli 1992). While isometric training is appropriate in rehabilitation settings in which joint movements are contraindicated, it is not as an effective form of strength training for athletes due to the static nature of the exercise compared to strength training through a range of motion that is more sport specific. However, isometric training is valuable in some sports, such as competitive powerlifting, that require high levels of strength in static or near static positions. For example, while performing the 1 RM deadlift exercise during powerlifting competition, the most difficult part of the lift (known as the 'sticking point') is when the upward moving barbell just passes the knees with the knees flexed approximately 20° and the hips flexed approximately 60° (Escamilla et al 2000). The 'sticking point' is often where a lifter fails in their attempt for a successful lift. Since at the 'sticking point' the barbell is very near a static position, isometric training with the body positioned in a similar manner may be helpful in developing the strength needed to move beyond the 'sticking point' and have a successful lift.

Dynamic training

Dynamic training involves both concentric (muscle shortening) and eccentric (muscle lengthening) muscle contractions in which joint motion occurs. The two most common modes of dynamic training are free weights and machines (Fig. 10.1 and 10.2). The use of free weights is referred to as dynamic constant

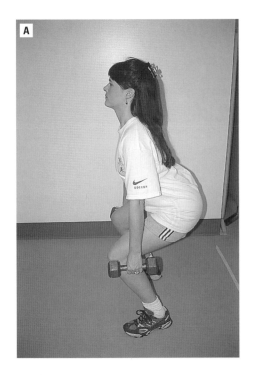

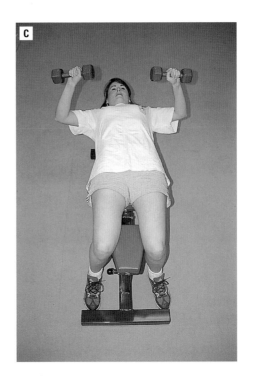

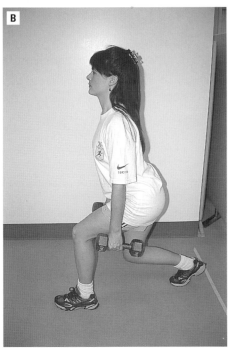

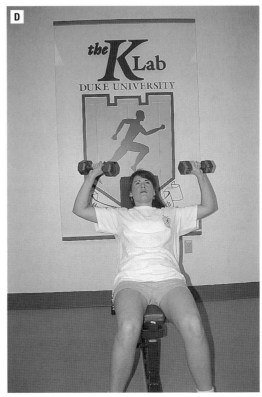

Figure 10.1 • Common free weight dumbbell exercises. **A:** Squat. **B:** Lunge. **C:** Bench press. **D:** Incline press.

external resistance training since the weight remains constant throughout a range of motion. The use of many machines (e.g. the VRM) is referred to as dynamic variable resistance training since the cam system employed in machines varies the resistance throughout a range of motion in an attempt to match the torque generating capabilities of muscle. The advantages and disadvantages of free weights and machines have been previously discussed. Several upper and lower extremity training studies

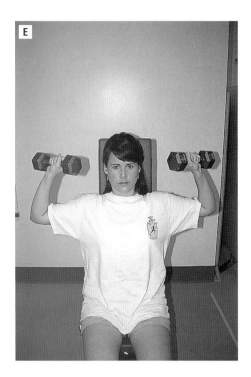

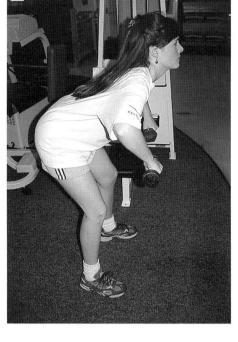

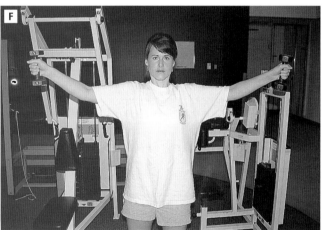

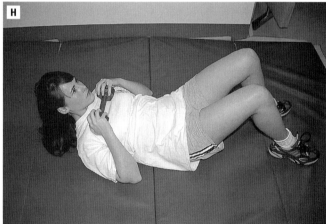

Figure 10.1 • (Continued) **E:** Shoulder press. **F:** Shoulder scaption. **G:** Bent over rowing. **H:** Crunchies.

involving both free weights and machines have shown significant strength increases while performing approximately 3–4 sets of 2–10 RM for 3–4 days per week for 10–20 weeks (Hagerman et al 2000, Kraemer 1997, Kraemer et al 1997, Kraemer et al 2001, Marx et al 2001, Rhodes et al 2000, Taaffe et al 1999). While strength training studies using both machines (Smith & Melton 1981) and free weights (Wathen & Shutes 1982) have shown increases in sport-specific movements (e.g. short sprints, vertical jumps), free weights appear to offer more optimal sport-specific strength gains compared to machines (Haff 2000).

Other common forms of dynamic training involve elastic bands, manual resistance from a partner and bodyweight exercises such as push-ups, pull-ups and sit-to-stand exercises. These exercises require no equipment to perform and can be done almost anywhere. It is common for children to start off with these exercises to build a strength base before advancing to machines and free weights. Bodyweight exercises, such as sit-to-stand, are appropriate during rehabilitation and strengthening, particularly for the elderly.

Eccentric training

Eccentric training, often referred to as negatives, involves eccentric muscle contractions only. To illustrate, consider the bench press exercise. In dynamic training, concentric contractions from the pectoralis major, triceps brachii and anterior deltoids result in the weight being pressed upward. During the downward phase of the bench press, these same muscles must now lengthen and

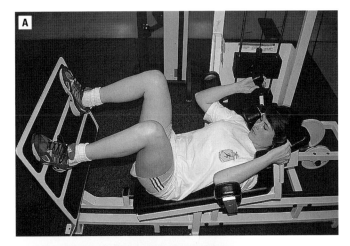

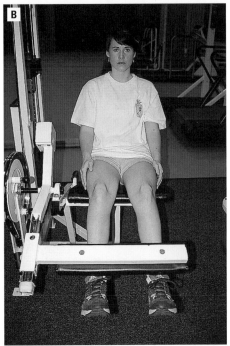

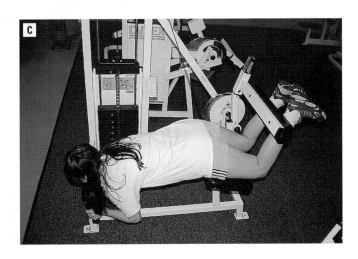

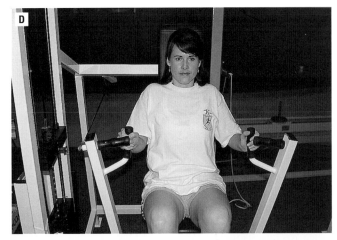

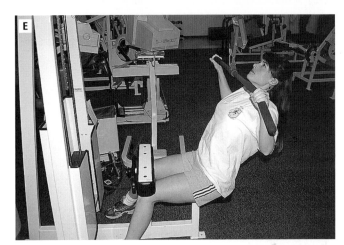

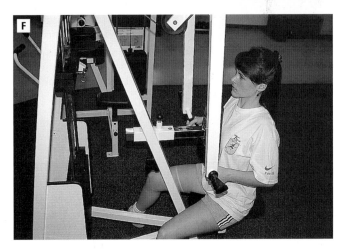

Figure 10.2 • Common machine weight exercises. **A:** Leg press.
B: Leg extension. **C:** Leg curls. **D:** Bench press. **E:** Pull downs.
F: Seated rows.

contract eccentrically to control the descent rate as the weight is lowered. Due to differences in muscle mechanics, peak tension during eccentric contraction is much greater than peak tension generated during concentric contractions (Gohner 1994). Hence, a much greater amount of weight can be lowered at a given rate compared to the amount of weight that can be raised at that same rate. This allows an individual to lower a weight in a controlled manner that is well in excess of the 1 RM. Athletes will often use spotters to help lift the weight up, and then they will lower the weight eccentrically. This entire process is then repeated for multiple repetitions and sets. Research has shown that eccentric training does result in strength gains similar to the strength gains in isometric, concentric and isokinetic training, and is most effective when used in combination with concentric contractions (Gohner 1994, Higbie et al 1996, Morrissey et al 1995, Tesch et al 1990). However, one undesirable effect of eccentric training is an excessive amount of muscle and connective tissue damage, which results in increased muscle soreness and an increased recovery period (Ebbeling & Clarkson 1989).

Isokinetic training

Isokinetic training involves moving through a range of motion at a constant speed. The harder an individual pushes or pulls against the machine, the greater the resistance that is accommodated by the machine, thereby producing an equal but opposite reaction force (torque) to the force or torque generated by the individual. This accommodation in resistance maintains a constant speed according to the speed setting on the machine. Most isokinetic machines generate speeds up to $300-500°/s$, allowing both concentric and eccentric contractions. Several isokinetic training studies have shown significant strength increases while performing approximately 1–5 sets of 5–15 repetitions between 60 and $120°/s$ for 3 days per week over 8–20 weeks (McCarrick & Kemp 2000, Mannion et al 1992, Narici et al 1996). A thorough review comparing the specificity and effectiveness of resistance training modes relative to different types of training (e.g. static versus dynamic, concentric versus eccentric, weight training versus isokinetic) was written by Morrissey et al (1995).

Plyometrics

Eastern European athletes dominated power sports in the 1972 Olympic Games, spurring widespread interest in their training techniques. The alleged training regimen used by Valeri Borzov, a Russian track and field medallist, was jump training (Wilt 1975). In 1966, Yuri Verkhoshanski, a prominent Russian track and field coach, described a depth jump training program used in conjunction with traditional strength training to improve power in high caliber athletes (Verkhoshanski 1966). Wilt (1975) called the technique plyometric exercise and specifically referred to activities using a quick stretch to facilitate force development in the subsequent shortening cycle. Thus, with little knowledge of how the new training augmented performance, the elite athletic world incorporated plyometric exercises (also called jump training, depth jump or stretch-shortening exercises) into training programs for power sports.

All motion requires force production. The ability to generate force is a measure of strength. The ability to develop force rapidly is a measure of power. Since most activities (e.g. throwing a ball, putting the shot, sprinting) require rapid force development, rehabilitation programs must include techniques to improve power. Plyometric exercises are one training tool focusing on increased power production. Some of the benefits of plyometric training include increased peak bone mineralization (Witzke & Snow 2000), increased musculotendinous stiffness (Spurrs et al 2003), increased running speed and efficiency (Rimmer & Sleivert 2000) and enhanced neuromuscular development and a decreased risk of knee ligament injury due to lower impact forces (Hewett et al 2005, Irmischer et al 2004). Most of the benefits of plyometric training reported in the literature involve the lower extremity, and there is relatively little research on upper extremity plyometrics.

Theories of force augmentation

Three theories explain the augmented muscle force production observed in plyometric exercises. First, the rapid stretch of the agonist muscle activates the muscle spindle causing an increase in the firing rate of the Ia sensory neurons associated with the intrafusal nuclear chain and bag fibers (Swash & Fox 1972). Increased firing of the Ia neurons results in increased firing of the agonist and synergist alpha motor neurons via a monosynaptic spinal reflex leading to increased muscle contraction force (Asmussen & Bonde-Petersen 1974, Bosco et al 1986).

The second theory proposes a decrease in golgi tendon organ (GTO) sensitivity to stretch. The GTO, located in the muscle tendon, is activated by tension within the muscle. The GTO provides a protective mechanism by inhibiting agonist force production when tension reaches a level that could be damaging to the muscle. Plyometric training is thought to desensitize the GTO which would ultimately lead to enhanced force production by removing the inhibition of the agonist (Bosco & Komi 1979).

A third theory is based on neuromuscular adaptation. Motor learning literature (see Chapter 8) states that acquisition of new skills progresses from cognitive to automatic (Higgins 1991). Performing jumping skills improves jumping as motor patterns are learned. With training, efficiency improves leading to improved performance. Furthermore, with jump training, transition time between the eccentric and concentric phases decreases, thereby enhancing the return of stored elastic energy (Toumi et al 2004, Voight 1992, Wilk et al 1993). This improved performance is seen after training even in the absence of changes in muscle cross sectional area (Chu 1992, Toumi et al 2004, Wilk et al 1993). Plyometric training has been shown to improve rebound time by minimizing the transition from eccentric to concentric contraction (Toumi et al 2004), to decrease reaction time between the neural impulse and muscle contraction (Wilk et al 1993) and to recruit more motor units (Chu 1992).

Training program considerations

Before plyometric training is implemented the athlete's age, body weight, strength relative to body weight, experience and current strength and speed training regimen must be considered. Because of the risk of growth plate injuries, it is recommended that skeletally immature athletes not perform drop jumps (LaChance 1995). Heavy athletes also should not perform drop jumps from a height greater than 18 inches due to the large impact forces associated with landing (Fowler et al 1997, Santos 1979). An adequate lower extremity strength base assessed by squatting with 1.5–2.5 times body weight is necessary before the highest level of plyometric training (drop jumps and weighted drop jumps) is attempted (Wathen 1993), or bench pressing 1–1.5 times body-weight for high intensity upper extremity plyometrics. Because there is also a speed component to plyometric training, an athlete should be able to squat or bench press 5 repetitions with 60% bodyweight in 5 s or less prior to initiating higher intensity lower or upper extremity plyometrics. Also, the athlete should have 2–4 weeks of strength and sprint training as a base before beginning a plyometric training program (Santos 1979). Finally, inexperienced athletes will need to progress more slowly than elite athletes to allow proper skill acquisition (Chu 1992).

Like all training programs the number of repetitions per training session, duration of the training session and frequency of training must be regulated to minimize the risk of injury. The plyometric program should begin with low intensity exercises and progressively increase to higher intensity exercise. Common lower extremity plyometric drills include vertical jumps in place, horizontal standing jumps, multiple hops and jumps, bounding drills, box jumps and depth jumps. Vertical and horizontal jumps are often used initially during lower intensity training, while box jumps and depth jumps are often used for higher intensity exercise, progressing from two-leg jumps to one-leg jumps (Fig. 10.3). Weighted jumps are the highest intensity level of lower extremity plyometric exercise and are appropriate only for highly trained strength and power athletes who demonstrate adequate strength and good technique on all other plyometric and weightlifting exercises. Upper extremity exercises using bodyweight can progress from lower intensity to higher intensity by gradually increasing the effects of gravity, such as progressing from inclined wall pushups to horizontal pushups to declined pushups. Medicine balls and rebound devices (e.g. plyoback) can also be used for multi-planar sport-specific upper extremity and trunk plyometrics, progressing from throwing lighter to heavier balls, softer to harder throws and two arm to one arm throws.

The total work (volume) done in a plyometric session is determined by the total number of contacts (repetitions) performed. Multiple sets of 6–12 contacts are common for higher intensity exercise (e.g. 6–12 consecutive jumps in place for 3–4 sets), while multiple sets of 12–20 contacts are common for lower intensity exercise. A common number of contacts performed per session is 80–100 for beginners just starting a plyometric program, 100–120 contacts for those with some experience in plyometric exercises and 120–140 contacts for those with extensive experience with plyometric exercises. The work:rest ratio between sets is dependent on intensity level and the energy system employed. For high intensity plyometrics the ATP-PC and glycolytic energy systems are employed, which requires greater rest periods between sets, such as 1:5 to 1:10 work:rest ratios, in order to allow adequate time to replenish these systems and for the neuromuscular system to fully recover. For low intensity plyometrics, 1:1 to 1:2 work:rest ratios are common.

High intensity plyometrics are often performed twice a week with at least 48–72 hours of rest for full recovery between sessions. This greater rest time is needed compared to more traditional strength training due to a greater amount of muscle damage and accompanying soreness (largely due to the rapid eccentric contractions and a high rate of force development). A higher frequency of training can be employed with lower intensity plyometrics. Plyometric training is typically performed intermediately (e.g. 6–16 weeks) throughout a periodization yearly regimen.

Common systems of strength training

Single-sets versus multi-sets

For a given exercise, single-set systems consist of performing a single set of repetitions to failure, while multi-set systems consist of performing multiple sets of repetitions to failure. While maximum strength gains occur while employing single or multiple sets of near maximum loads between 2 and 6 repetitions (Stone et al 1981), significant strength and power gains have been reported in many training studies involving both single-set and multi-set training between approximately 2 and 12 repetitions (see Table 10.2). However, multi-set training involving both a constant and

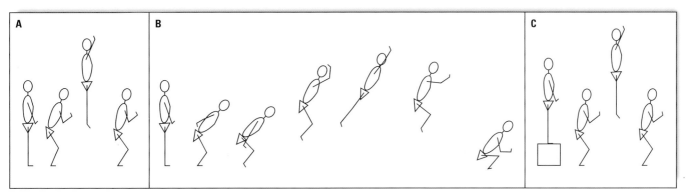

Figure 10.3 • Plyometric exercises. **A:** vertical jump. **B:** horizontal jump. **C:** depth jump.

Table 10.2 Examples of strength and power gain comparisons between single-set (SS) versus multiple set (MSC and MSV) training studies

Authors	Group	Strength and power training protocol per workout session	Sex	No.	Age (years)	Frequency (days/week)	Duration (weeks)	Training sets × RM	Strength or power testing protocol	Mean % strength increase* for SS, MSC and MSV	Result Difference between MSC/MSV
Borst et al (2001)	SS	7 MedX Ma circuit	M/F	11	35 ± 7	3	25	1 × 8–12	1 RM Ma knee extension +	30% SS*	S
	MSC	7 MedX Ma circuit	M/F	11	41 ± 7	3	25	3 × 8–12	1 RM Ma bench press	50% MSC*	
Hass et al (2001)	SS	9 MedX Ma circuit	M/F	21	40 ± 6	3	13	1 × 8–12	1 RM Ma knee extension	13% SS*	NS
	MSC	9 MedX Ma circuit	M/F	21	39 ± 7	3	13	3 × 8–12		12% MSC*	
									1 RM Ma leg curl	5% SS*	S
										10% MSC*	
									1 RM Ma chest press	11% SS*	NS
										10% MSC*	
									1 RM Ma overhead press	5% SS*	NS
										15% MSC*	
									1 RM Ma biceps curls	10% SS*	NS
										9% MSC*	
Kraemer (1997)	SS	9 Universal and Marcy Ma circuit	M	17	C	3	14	1 × 8–12	1 RM FW hang cleans	3% SS	S
	MSV	7–9 Ma and FW exercises	M	17	C	3	14	2–5 × 1–10		20% MSV*	
									1 RM Ma bench press	3% SS*	S
										11% MSV*	
									Peak power from maximum effort vertical jump	3% SS	S
										17% MSV*	
									Peak power from Wingate anaerobic cycle test	1% SS	S
										14% MSV*	
Kraemer (1997)	SS	10 Ma and FW exercises	M	22	C	3	24	1 × 8–12	1 RM Ma bench press	13% SS*	S
	MSV	8–13 Ma and FW exercises	M	22	C	4	24	2–4 × 3–15		29% MSV*	
									1 RM Ma leg press	8% SS*	S
										20% MSV*	
									Maximum effort vertical jump	7% SS*	S
										23% MSV*	
									Peak power from Wingate anaerobic cycle test	5% SS*	S
										55% MSV*	
Kraemer et al (1997)	SS	4 Ma and FW exercises	M	16	C	3	14	1 × 8–12	1 RM FW squat	12% SS*	Sss
	MSC	4 Ma and FW exercises	M	14	C	3	14	3 × 10		26% MSC*	Sss
	MSV	4 Ma and FW exercises	M	13	C	3	14	1–3 × 2–10		22% MSV*	

Study	Group	Training program	Sex	n	Age	Sessions	Weeks	Sets reps	Measurement	% change	
Kraemer (1997)	SS	10 Nautilus Ma circuit	M	20	C	3	10	1 3 8–12	1 RM Nautilus Ma bench press	4% SS / 13% MSC*	S
	MSC	10 Nautilus Ma circuit	M	20	C	3	10	3 3 8–12	1 RM Nautilus Ma leg press	3% SS / 19% MSC*	S
Marx et al (2001)	SS	10 Ma exercise circuit	F	12	236 5	3	24	1 3 8–12	1 RM Ma bench press	12% SS* / 47% MSV*	S
	MSV	7–12 Ma and FW exercises	F	12	236 4	4	24	2–4 3 3–15	1 RM Ma leg press	11% SS* / 32% MSV*	S
									Maximum effort vertical jump	10% SS* / 40% MSV*	S
									40 yard dash	1% SS / 6% MSV*	S
									Peak power from Wingate anaerobic cycle test	4% SS / 27% MSV*	S
Sanborn et al (2000)	SS	5 FW exercises	F	9	C	3	8	1 3 8–12	1 RM FW squat	24% SS* / 35% MSV*	NS
	MSV	5 FW exercises	F	8	C	3	8	3–5 3 2–10	Peak power from maximum effort vertical jump	0% SS / 11% MSV*	S
Schlumberger et al (2001)	SS	7 Ma exercises	F	9	296 9	2	6	1 3 6–9	1 RM Ma bench press	4% SS / 10% MS*	S
	MSC	7 Ma exercises	F	9	246 3	2	6	3 3 6–9	1 RM Ma knee extension	7% SS* / 16% MS*	S
Starkey et al (1996)	SS	MedX Dynamic Ma knee extension and flexion	M/F	18	346 10	3	14	1 3 8–12	MedX peak isometric knee extension	30% SS* / 27% MSC*	NS
	MSC	MedX Dynamic Ma knee extension and flexion	M/F	20	356 8	3	14	1 3 8–12	MedX peak isometric knee flexion	19% SS* / 18% MSC*	NS

SS = single-set; MSC = multiple sets using a constant number of repetitions and sets; MSV = multiple sets using a varied number of repetitions and sets; S = significant difference between SS and MSC or between SS and MSV; Sss = significantly greater than SS; NS = non-significant difference between SS and MSC or between SS and MSV; * = significant increase in strength gain due to SS, MSC or MSV training; C = college age; Ma = machine; FW = free weight varied number of repetitions and sets has been shown to be superior to single-set training in maximizing strength and power gains (Table 10.2), especially in athletes training for sport and employing periodization techniques (Kraemer 1997, Kraemer et al 2000). This is contrary to previous beliefs (Carpinelli & Otto 1998, Feigenbaum & Pollock 1999) that single-set training is just as effective as multi-set training in producing strength gains. It should be emphasized there has never been a strength training study that has shown that single-set training produces superior strength gains compared to multi-set training, but several recent strength training studies have shown that multi-set training produces superior strength and power gains compared to single-set training (Table 10.2). This implies that athletes who desire to maximize strength gains should employ a multi-set system of training. However, since single-set systems are effective in maintaining or producing strength gains, single-set training systems are an effective alternative for those who have limited time for resistance training and whose goal is not to maximize strength gains but rather build a functional strength base to enhance their activities of daily living (e.g. non-athletes, rehabilitation patients, elderly).

DeLorme – light to heavy

The DeLorme system of training is one in which the initial set starts out light, and progressively greater resistance is added in each subsequent set. The DeLorme system became popular in the 1950s and 1960s when DeLorme and colleagues reported significant strength gains during short-term training studies while performing 3 sets of 10 repetitions (DeLorme & Watkins 1948, DeLorme et al 1952). In the original DeLorme system the resistances employed were equal to 50% of the lifter's 10 RM for the first set, 66% of their 10 RM for the second set and 100% of their 10 RM for the third set. Variations of these training percentages may be employed when using the DeLorme system.

Oxford – heavy to light

The Oxford system of training is one in which the initial set starts out heavy, and progressively smaller resistance is employed in each subsequent set. Like the DeLorme system, the Oxford system became popular in the 1950s and 1960s. Several studies have reported significant strength gains using the Oxford technique (Leighton et al 1967, McMorris & Elkins 1954, Zinovieff 1951). The resistances employed in the Oxford technique are the same but in reverse order as the DeLorme system: the resistance is equal to 100% of the lifter's 10 RM for the first set, 66% of their 10 RM for the second set and 50% of their 10 RM for the third set. Variations of these training percentages may be employed when using the Oxford system.

Pyramid

The pyramid system combines the light-to-heavy and heavy-to-light systems, and is common both in powerlifting and weightlifting. A lifter can progress from light-to-heavy resistance on the way up the pyramid, and from heavy-to-light resistance on the way down the pyramid. Conversely, in an inverse pyramid a lifter can progress from heavy-to-light resistance on the way down the pyramid, and from light-to-heavy resistance on the way up the pyramid. An early study of the pyramid type system of training has been shown to be effective in building leg and trunk strength, as well as elbow and extension strength (Leighton et al 1967). More recent literature evaluating this system is lacking. A typical example employing a pyramid system for strength training is as follows:

Set 1: 10 RM
Set 2: 8 RM
Set 3: 5 RM
Set 4: 3 RM
Set 5: 5 RM
Set 6: 8 RM
Set 7: 10 RM

Super-set

The super-set system (Leighton et al 1967) is typically performed in one of two ways. Using the first method, a super-set involves performing one set each of multiple exercises (2–3) to work the same muscle group with little or no rest between exercises. In the second method, the super-set system involves performing with little or no rest one set of multiple exercises (2–3) that work muscle groups which have opposite muscle actions. Pairs of agonist–antagonist exercises are most common in this type of super-set, which allows the agonist muscle group to rest while the antagonist muscle group works (and vice versa). Super-set systems are common in bodybuilding, and have been shown to increase muscle strength (Leighton et al 1967). Due to the large number of repetitions performed and high exercise volume, this type of training also produces a higher level of muscular endurance and has a large energy expenditure (Kraemer et al 1987).

Circuit

The circuit system of training consists of performing multiple exercises (typically 8–12) using higher repetitions (typically 12–20) and lower intensities (40–60% or 1 RM) with minimal rest intervals between exercises (10–20 s) (Beckham & Earnest 2000, Green et al 2001, Haennel et al 1991, Todd et al 1992). This type of training is most beneficial for those individuals whose primary aim is to increase their cardiovascular fitness and muscular endurance (Beckham & Earnest 2000, Green et al 2001, Haennel et al 1991, Todd et al 1992). This approach is useful for people who are deconditioned, have excess body fat and need to lose weight and have cardiovascular issues (e.g. hypertension, cardiovascular disease). However, studies have shown that strength increases also occur with circuit training, especially for the deconditioned (Sparling et al 1990, Stewart 1989). Circuit training is also effective for individuals who need a supervised, structured program and have limited time to work out.

The circuit is commonly set up so an individual moves from one exercise to another in a timed sequence such as a 30 s exercise period followed by a 15 s rest interval. Following this format, a 12-exercise circuit would take approximately 10 min to perform. The circuit could be performed 2–3 times, thereby allowing 2–3 sets of each exercise to be performed in 20–30 min, which makes the circuit time efficient. A circuit is often set up to employ alternating upper and lower body exercises, or alternating muscle groups, thus allowing one muscle group to rest and recover while another muscle group is being worked. Also, multi-joint, multi-muscle exercises should comprise most of the exercises in the circuit since they have a greater energy expenditure and develop overall muscular strength and endurance to a greater extent compared to single-joint, single-muscle exercises (Beckham & Earnest 2000, Escamilla et al 2000). A circuit primarily consists of resistance machines rather than free weights since they are safer, easier to use and take minimal time to change resistance.

Interval training

Interval training typically involves moderate to high intensity exercise alternating with brief to moderate rest periods (Billat 2001). In general, higher intensity training uses greater recovery periods and is more anaerobic, whereas lower intensity training uses shorter recovery periods and is more aerobic. Circuit training is an example of interval resistance training, consisting of approximately 30 s of exercise and 15 s of rest and recovery. Circuit training involves lower intensities of exercise followed by shorter rest intervals. A common higher intensity example of interval training involves sprinting a certain distance followed by walking or jogging that same distance. For example, consider an athlete sprinting 40–50 m followed by slowly jogging or walking back to the starting line. In this example there is 5–10 s of higher intensity exercise followed by a 30–45 s recovery. This sequence is repeated multiple times. A primary advantage of interval training is that it allows a greater volume of work to be performed compared to continuous training. Interval training is more sport specific for many athletic movements; for example, a running back in American football typically runs at high intensity for a few seconds followed by 30–45 s of rest (Billat 2001).

Endurance training

Endurance is the ability to perform sustained activity. Increased resistance to fatigue is gained through aerobic or endurance training. Although daily life requires fatigue resistance for optimal performance, the focus of this section will be on the training adaptations resulting from sustained exercise of 20 min or more.

Measurement of aerobic fitness

A person's endurance or aerobic fitness can be measured by several different techniques. The 12 min run and timed 1.5 mile run have been used for general screening of aerobic fitness (Cooper 1968). A more precise measurement of aerobic fitness is the

Table 10.3 Maximal oxygen uptake for males

	Absolute VO$_2$max L min^{-1}	Relative VO$_2$max mL kg^{-1} min^{-1}
Sedentary	2–2.5	<30
Moderately trained	3–3.5	30–50
Well trained	4–4.5	50–70
Elite	>5	>70

treadmill or cycle ergometer test for maximal oxygen uptake (VO$_2$max) (Pollock et al 1976). VO$_2$max represents the maximum amount of oxygen used per unit time by the metabolically active tissues in the body. VO$_2$max is measured in liters of oxygen per minute (absolute VO$_2$max) or may be expressed relative to body weight (relative VO$_2$max). An individual's VO$_2$max is dependent on age (VO$_2$max declines from early adulthood to old age) (Paterson et al 1999, Trappe et al 1996), gender (males generally have a higher VO$_2$max than females) (Bouchard et al 1999), genetics (Bouchard et al 1999) and training status (aerobically fit individuals have a higher VO$_2$max than non-fit persons) (Ekblom et al 1968) (Table 10.3).

Maximal oxygen consumption or VO$_2$max is dependent on oxygen delivery to the cells and metabolic capacity of the tissues. This relationship is expressed in the Fick equation which relates oxygen uptake (VO$_2$) to cardiac output (CO) and arteriovenous oxygen difference (a-vO$_2$dif) as follows: VO$_2$ = CO × a-vO$_2$dif. To increase oxygen uptake CO, a-vO$_2$dif or both must increase.

Physiological adaptations to endurance training

Cardiovascular

With endurance training, several physiological adaptations occur to enhance cardiac output (CO), the product of heart rate (HR) and stroke volume (SV). During exercise, HR increases as workload and intensity increase due in part to an increase in circulating norepinephrine from the sympathetic nervous system (Schwarz & Kindermann 1990). As intensity continues to increase a maximum HR is achieved after which further increases in intensity produce no further increases in HR. With training, maximal HR is unchanged but occurs at a higher workload (Fig. 10.4A). Alternatively, HR at any submaximal intensity is lower after training (Wilmore et al 2001).

The second determinant of CO is SV. SV increases with increased workload due to an increase in myocardial contractility (force of contraction, inotropic effect) and an increase in venous return (Laughlin 1999) (Fig. 10.4B). Both contractility and venous return increase during exercise due to release of norepinephrine by the sympathetic nervous system (Schwarz & Kindermann 1990). Because contractility increases, more blood is ejected from the left ventricle during

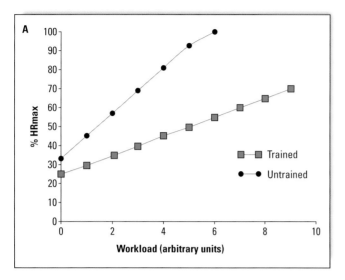

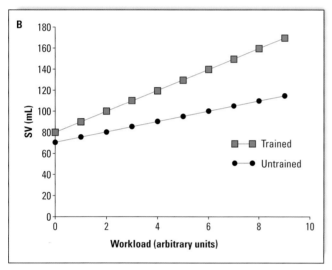

Figure 10.4 • Heart rate **(A)** and stroke volume **(B)** responses to increased workload in the trained and untrained state.

Muscle adaptations

Following endurance training, skeletal muscle undergoes characteristic changes. Progressive aerobic exercise leads to an increase in capillary density of the trained muscle mass (Gute et al 1996, Madsen & Holmskov 1995). The benefits of increased capillarity include decreased diffusion distance, increased red blood cell transit time and improved blood distribution. Temperature elevation and decreased pH in the active muscle facilitate oxygen unloading from hemoglobin (the Bohr effect). The combined effect of increased capillarity and enhanced oxygen unloading results in an increase in the a-vO$_2$dif. Current theory holds that the increase in CO and increase in a-vO$_2$dif contribute equally to the increased VO$_2$max observed after training (Laughlin 1999).

Other changes in muscle tissue with training include an increase in the size and number of mitochondria (Holloszy 1967, Suter et al 1995), increased activity of enzymes associated with carbohydrate and fat oxidation (Mole et al 1971, Svedenhag et al 1983) and improved glucose uptake (Greiwe et al 2000, Houmard et al 1995). Increased mitochondrial density reduces oxygen diffusion distance and increases the surface area for oxidation. Fully oxidizing carbohydrate (yielding 38 ATP per glucose molecule versus 2 ATP per glucose via glycolysis) has a glucose and glycogen sparing effect. Increased activity of enzymes involved in fat oxidation enhances breakdown of triglycerides, movement of fatty acids into mitochondria and beta oxidation. Use of fats as an energy source also has a glucose/glycogen sparing effect. Additionally, endurance training decreases the expression of fast glycolytic (type IIb) muscle fiber type (O'Neill et al 1999). With endurance training VO$_2$max increases 15–20% in both young and older adults (Levy et al 1998).

The less fit a person is prior to the start of an endurance training program (thus having greater potential for improvement), the larger the increase in VO$_2$max. However, a physiological maximum for the individual does exist beyond which further training does not elicit further increases in VO$_2$max.

Principles of endurance training

The American College of Sports Medicine has established guidelines for exercise to improve aerobic fitness. These guidelines state that 30 min of daily activity at a HR greater than 60% of the predicted maximum HR (220 – age) at least three times per week promotes aerobic fitness and health gains (American College of Sports Medicine 2000).

Endurance training is associated with decreased risk of coronary artery disease, stroke, non-insulin-dependent diabetes mellitus, hypertension, osteoporosis and colon, breast, cervical, ovarian and uterine cancers (American College of Sports Medicine 2000).

High-density lipoprotein cholesterol (the 'good' cholesterol) increases with endurance training while plasma triglyceride concentration decreases (Lindheim et al 1994, Schwartz et al 1992). Endurance training enhances insulin receptor sensitivity (Dela et al 1996, Houmard et al 1995) leading to improved glucose

systole. Sympathetic stimulation also causes vasoconstriction of the peripheral vessels leading to greater blood return during diastole. Stretch of the myocardium enhances overlap of myosin and actin myofilaments and greater force is generated in the subsequent contraction (Starling's Law of the Heart). Increased HR and SV at maximal exercise produce the elevated CO.

Oxygen uptake at the tissue level is determined by oxygen delivery and tissue extraction. Due to elevated CO, blood flow to the metabolically active skeletal muscles is increased. Muscle blood flow is increased more in trained muscle than untrained muscle (Delp 1995). Not only is a greater percentage of the CO going to the active muscle but the blood also has a greater oxygen carrying capacity as a result of increased red blood cell formation stimulated by erythropoietin (Bodary et al 1999). Adaptations in the muscle also provide improved oxygen extraction capacity at the tissue level (Roca et al 1992).

homeostasis. Systolic and diastolic blood pressure decreases with endurance training (Cononie et al 1991). Women participating in regular exercise, especially weightbearing, maintain or possibly increase bone mineral density reducing the risk of osteoporotic fractures (Chow et al 1987, Smith et al 1989).

Injury prevention during endurance training

Whether the goal of aerobic training is to improve fitness, decrease body fat or maximize athletic performance, certain training factors must be addressed to minimize the risk of injury. Common endurance training activities include swimming, cycling, rollerblading, cross country skiing, walking and running (with running associated with the highest rate of overuse injuries). Training errors (inappropriate footwear, hard irregular terrain, excessive mileage or rapid increase in mileage and speed) are responsible for a high percentage of injuries (Ballas et al 1997, Bovens et al 1989, Macera et al 1989). During the evaluation of an injured runner, it is important to assess the running shoes for signs of wear or breakdown as this will decrease the support and stability of the shoe. Likewise, total shoe mileage may provide insight into the cause of an injury. The runner should also be questioned about the surface on which he or she trains. Hill running (Clement & Taunton 1981), running on concrete (Macera et al 1989) and running on crowned streets (Bovens et al 1989) all contribute to an increased risk of injury but the strongest correlate with injury is weekly running frequency and distance (Bovens et al 1989, Macera et al 1989).

To minimize the risk of injury Ballas et al (1997) recommended increasing mileage slowly (no more than 10% increase per week), weekly running mileage less than 45 miles (72.5 km), running on a soft flat surface (rubber track, dirt path, etc.), alternating high intensity and low intensity workouts and changing running shoes every 500 miles (800 km). Because shock absorption in running shoes is decreased by 50% after 300 miles (500 km) (Cook et al 1990), it may be necessary to replace shoes before 500 miles of wear. For all participants in aerobic conditioning programs cross training is encouraged to balance muscle strength and flexibility as well as to reduce overuse injuries (Ballas et al 1997).

Endurance training in special populations

Children

Despite an increase in organized sports participation, the overall fitness level of youth in many developed countries is poor. Like adults, children who have a high daily activity level have a higher VO_2max than do sedentary children. Using adult guidelines for frequency, intensity and duration, endurance training programs can lead to increased VO_2max in children (Mahon & Vaccaro 1989, Mandigout et al 2001) although the magnitude of the increase may be smaller (Mahon & Vaccaro 1989) and require higher training intensity to achieve (Rowland 1992). Endurance training appears to have no effect on blood lipid levels in children (Rowland et al 1996) but does enhance bone deposition (Eliakim et al 1997). Regular physical activity during childhood enhances skill acquisition, muscle strength and endurance and weight management.

Older people

Many physiological changes occur with aging nearly all of which contribute to a decrease in functional independence (see Chapter 26). Endurance training in older adults (including those 80+ years old) improves cardiovascular function measured by VO_2max (Buchner et al 1997, Steinhaus et al 1990), decreases resting HR, decreases systolic blood pressure and results in fewer premature ventricular contractions (Steinhaus et al 1990). Participation in an endurance training program increases leg strength (Buchner et al 1997) and fat-free body mass (Wilmore et al 1999), while percentage in body fat decreases (Wilmore et al 1999). Despite increased fat-free mass, resting metabolic rate is unchanged with regular participation in an endurance training program (Wilmore et al 1998).

Endurance training in the elderly has other benefits besides reduced disease risk. These benefits include improved balance, cognition, perception of self-efficacy and decreased depression (American College of Sports Medicine 1998). Elderly clients should be encouraged to participate in moderate intensity exercise for at least 30 min three or more times per week. Increased frequency, duration and intensity lead to greater improvements in cardiorespiratory fitness. Individuals with orthopedic or balance disorders may find aquatic activities more suitable although the benefit of maintaining bone mass is lost due to the non-weight-bearing nature of this activity.

Stabilization

Core strength and stability are vital in many activities. Yet in spite of the important role the trunk plays in force production by the extremities, it is often overlooked during training to the detriment of optimal athletic performance. As an example, consider the baseball pitcher. The pitcher does not merely draw the arm back and throw the ball. Rather a wind-up phase in which the leg is raised initiates the pitching sequence and force generated in the legs is transferred through the trunk to the throwing arm (Fleisig et al 1999). If core strength is lacking, the energy generated in the legs is lost and the pitcher instead has to rely solely on the musculature of the upper extremity. Over time, the stress placed on the shoulder and elbow musculature causes injuries. A strong core allows force to be transferred from the legs to the arm smoothly and efficiently (Gambetta & Clark 1999).

Training the core muscles involves more than general abdominal exercises and back extensions. Rather than focusing on individual muscle groups, core training emphasizes combined flexion, extension and rotation movement patterns using sport-specific drills (Cook & Fields 1997). Training for maximum core stability is accomplished through daily workouts in which the movements are varied. Proper technique is the primary focus and should not be sacrificed for increased resistance or repetitions. Core training begins with low intensity, low volume workouts and gradually progresses to higher difficulty routines. Training involves utilizing opposing muscle groups equally (e.g. back extensors and abdominals, anterior chest and scapular muscles, hip flexors and extensors). Rotational movements should be performed to both sides to reduce muscle imbalances. Finally, training movements should replicate the movements required for the actual sport and exercise activity (Hedrick 2000).

Progression of core stability training programs encourages continued adaptations. Progression is accomplished beginning with simple movements and advancing to complex exercises only when the basic movements have been mastered. Training should progress from a controlled environment to an environment with distractions (e.g. uneven surface, varied timing), from static to dynamic conditions and from high level of support (lying) to low level of support (e.g. standing on one leg) (Gambetta & Clark 1999).

Summary

This chapter has focused on providing scientific rationale for the use of strength, plyometric, endurance, interval and stabilization training in injury prevention and rehabilitation. Research supports the use of plyometric, interval, endurance and stabilization training in injury prevention and rehabilitation. In addition, several research studies have reported that high intensity strength training results in several efficacious effects that enhance rehabilitation and prevent injuries. These include:

- An increase in muscle strength, size and power
- An increase in neuromuscular function
- An increase in bone strength and density with a concomitant decrease in osteoporosis
- An increase in tendon and ligament strength and thickness
- An increase in balance and decrease in risk of falling and subsequent injury
- An increase in gait stability, walking speed and efficiency
- An increase in chair rising and stair climbing
- An increase in hormonal adaptations
- A decrease in blood pressure, glucose intolerance and insulin resistance
- A decrease in body fat, and an increase in fat free mass and basal metabolic rate.

References

Alway S E, MacDougall J D, Sale D G 1989 Contractile adaptations in the human triceps surae after isometric exercise. Journal of Applied Physiology 66:2725–2732

American College of Sports Medicine 1998 American College of Sports medicine position stand. Exercise and physical activity for older adults. Medicine and Science in Sports and Exercise 30:992–1008

American College of Sports Medicine 2000 ACSM's Guidelines for Exercise Testing and Prescription. Lippincott Williams & Wilkins, Philadelphia, PA

Asmussen E, Bonde-Petersen F 1974 Storage of elastic energy in skeletal muscles in man. Acta Physiologica Scandinavica 91:385–392

Ballas M T, Tytko J, Cookson D 1997 Common overuse running injuries: diagnosis and management. American Family Physician 55:2473–2484

Barneveld A, van Weeren P R 1999 Conclusions regarding the influence of exercise on the development of the equine musculoskeletal system with special reference to osteochondrosis. Equine Vetrinary Journal 31:112–119

Beckham S G, Earnest C P 2000 Metabolic cost of free weight circuit weight training. Journal of Sports Medicine and Physical Fitness 40:118–125

Bemben D A, Fetters N L, Bemben M G et al 2000 Musculoskeletal responses to high- and low-intensity resistance training in early postmenopausal women. Medicine and Science in Sports and Exercise 32:1949–1957

Beniamini Y, Rubenstein J J, Zaichkowsky L D et al 1997 Effects of high-intensity strength training on quality-of-life parameters in cardiac rehabilitation patients. American Journal of Cardiology 80:841–846

Billat, L V 2001 Interval training for performance: a scientific and empirical practice. Special recommendations for middle- and long-distance running: II. Anaerobic interval training. Sports Medicine 31:75–90

Bloomfield S A 1997 Changes in musculoskeletal structure and function with prolonged bed rest. Medicine and Science in Sports and Exercise 29:197–206

Bodary P F, Pate R R, Wu Q F et al 1999 Effects of acute exercise on plasma erythropoietin levels in trained runners. Medicine and Science in Sports and Exercise 31:543–546

Borst S E, De Hoyos D V, Garzarella L et al 2001 Effects of resistance training on insulin-like growth factor-I and IGF binding proteins. Medicine and Science in Sports and Exercise 33:648–653

Bosco C, Komi P V 1979 Potentiation of the mechanical behavior of the human skeletal muscle through prestretching. Acta Physiologica Scandinavica 106:467–472

Bosco C, Tihanyi J, Latteri F et al 1986 The effect of fatigue on store and re-use of elastic energy in slow and fast types of human skeletal muscle. Acta Physiologica Scandinavica 128:109–117

Bouchard C, An P, Rice T, Skinner J S et al 1999 Familial aggregation of VO$_2$max response to exercise training: results from the HERITAGE Family Study. Journal of Applied Physiology 87:1003–1008

Bovens A M, Janssen G M, Vermeer H G et al 1989 Occurrence of running injuries in adults following a supervised training program. International Journal of Sports Medicine 10:S186–S190

Brand R A, Pedersen D R, Friederich J A 1986 The sensitivity of muscle force predictions to changes in physiologic cross-sectional area. Journal of Biomechanics 19:589–596

Brill P A, Probst J C, Greenhouse D L et al 1998 Clinical feasibility of a free-weight strength-training program for older adults. Journal of the American Board of Family Practice 11:445–451

Buchner D M, Cress M E, de Lateur B J et al 1997 A comparison of the effects of three types of endurance training on balance and other fall risk factors in older adults. Aging 9:112–119

Byrne H K, Wilmore J H 2001 The effects of a 20-week exercise training program on resting metabolic rate in previously sedentary, moderately obese women. International Journal of Sport Nutrition and Exercise Metabolism 11:15–31

Carmeli E, Reznick A Z, Coleman R et al 2000 Muscle strength and mass of lower extremities in relation to functional abilities in elderly adults. Gerontology 46:249–257

Carolan B, Cafarelli E 1992 Adaptations in coactivation after isometric resistance training. Journal of Applied Physiology 73:911–917

Carpinelli R N, Otto R M 1998 Strength training. Single versus multiple sets. Sports Medicine 26:73–84

Chandler J M, Duncan P W, Kochersberger G et al 1998 Is lower extremity strength gain associated with improvement in physical performance and disability in frail, community-dwelling elders? Archives of Physical Medicine and Rehabilitation 79:24–30

Chow R, Harrison J, Notarius C 1987 Effect of two randomized exercise programmes on bone mass of healthy postmenopausal women. British Medical Journal 295:1441–1444

Chu D 1992 Jumping into plyometrics. Human Kinetics, Champaign, IL

Clement D B, Taunton J E 1981 A guide to the prevention of running injuries. Australian Family Physician 10:156–164

Cononie C C, Graves J E, Pollock M L et al 1991 Effect of exercise training on blood pressure in 70- to 79-yr-old men and women. Medicine and Science in Sports and Exercise 23:505–11

Conroy B P, Kraemer W J, Maresh C M et al 1992 Adaptive responses of bone to physical activity. Medicine, Exercise, Nutrition and Health 1:64–74

Cook G, Fields K 1997 Functional training for the torso. Strength and Conditioning 19:14–19

Cook S D, Brinker M R, Mahlon P 1990 Running shoes: their relation to running injuries. Sports Medicine 10:1–8

Cooper K H 1968 A means of assessing maximal oxygen intake. Journal of the American Medical Association 203:135–138

del Olmo M F, Reimunde P, Viana O et al 2006 Chronic neural adaptation induced by long-term resistance training in humans. European Journal of Applied Physiology 96:722–728

Dela F, Mikines K, Larsen J et al 1996 Training-induced enhancement of insulin action in human skeletal muscle: the influence of aging. Journal of Gerontology 51 (4 suppl):B247–B252

DeLorme T L, Watkins A L 1948 Techniques of progressive resistance exercise. Archives of Physical Medicine 29:263–273

DeLorme T L, Ferris B G, Gallagher J R 1952 Effect of progressive exercise on muscular contraction time. Archives of Physical Medicine 33:86–97

Delp M D 1995 Effects of exercise training on endothelium-dependent peripheral vascular responsiveness. Medicine and Science in Sports and Exercise 27:1152–1157

Delp S L, Suryanarayanan S, Murray W M et al 2001 Architecture of the rectus abdominis, quadratus lumborum, and erector spinae. Journal of Biomechanics 34:371–375

DeMichele P L, Pollock M L, Graves J E et al 1997 Isometric torso rotation strength: effect of training frequency on its development. Archives of Physical Medicine and Rehabilitation 78:64–69

Ebbeling C B, Clarkson P M 1989 Exercise-induced muscle damage and adaptation. Sports Medicine 7:207–234

Ekblom B, Astrand P O, Saltin B et al 1968 Effect of training on circulatory response to exercise. Journal of Applied Physiology 24:518–528

Eliakim A, Raisz L G, Brasel J A et al 1997 Evidence for increased bone formation following a brief endurance-type training intervention in adolescent males. Journal of Bone Mineral Research 12:1708–1713

Escamilla R F, Francisco A C, Fleisig G S et al 2000 A three-dimensional biomechanical analysis of sumo and conventional style deadlifts. Medicine and Science in Sports and Exercise 32:1265–1275

Fatouros I G, Kambas A, Katrabasas I et al 2005 Strength training and detraining effects on muscular strength, anaerobic power, and mobility of inactive older men are intensity dependent. British Journal of Sports Medicine 39:776–780

Faulkner J A, Claflin D R, McCully K K 1986 Power output of fast and slow fibers from human skeletal muscle. In: Jones N L, McCartney N, McComas A J (eds) Human muscle power. Human Kinetics, Champaign, IL, p 38–39.

Feigenbaum M S, Pollock M L 1999 Prescription of resistance training for health and disease. Medicine and Science in Sports and Exercise 31:38–45

Fleck S J, Falkel J E 1986 Value of resistance training for the reduction of sports injuries. Sports Medicine 3:61–68

Fleisig G S, Barrentine S W, Zheng N et al 1999 Kinematic and kinetic comparison of baseball pitching among various levels of development. Journal of Biomechanics 32:1371–1375

Fowler N E, Lees A, Reilly T 1997 Changes in stature following plyometric drop-jump and pendulum exercises. Ergonomics 40:1279–1286

Gambetta V, Clark M 1999 Hard core training. Training and Conditioning 10:34–40

Garfinkel S, Cafarelli E 1992 Relative changes in maximal force, EMG, and muscle cross-sectional area after isometric training. Medicine and Science in Sports and Exercise 24:1220–1227

Garhammer J 1993 A review of power output studies of olympic and power lifting: methodology, performance prediction, and evaluation tests. Journal of Strength and Conditioning Research 7:76–89

Gohner U 1994 Experimental results on forced eccentric strength gains. International Journal of Sports Medicine 15 (1 suppl):S43–49

Gorostiaga E M, Izquierdo M, Iturralde P et al 1999 Effects of heavy resistance training on maximal and explosive force production, endurance and serum hormones in adolescent handball players. European Journal of Applied Physiology and Occupational Physiology 80:485–493

Granhed H, Jonson R, Hansson T 1987 The loads on the lumbar spine during extreme weight lifting. Spine 12:146–149

Green D J, Watts K, Maiorana A J et al 2001 A comparison of ambulatory oxygen consumption during circuit training and aerobic exercise in patients with chronic heart failure. Journal of Cardiopulmonary Rehabilitation 21:167–174

Gregg E W, Pereira M A, Caspersen C J 2000 Physical activity, falls, and fractures among older adults: a review of the epidemiologic evidence. Journal of the American Geriatrics Society 48:883–893

Greiwe J S, Holloszy J O, Semenkovich C F 2000 Exercise induces lipoprotein lipase and GLUT-4 protein in muscle independent of adrenergic-receptor signaling. Journal of Applied Physiology 89:176–181

Gute D, Fraga C, Laughlin M H et al 1996 Regional changes in capillary supply in skeletal muscle of high-intensity endurance-trained rats. Journal of Applied Physiology 81:619–626

Haennel R G, Quinney H A, Kappagoda C T 1991 Effects of hydraulic circuit training following coronary artery bypass surgery. Medicine and Science in Sports and Exercise 23:158–165

Haff G G 2000 Roundtable discussion: machines versus free weights. Strength and Conditioning 22:18–30

Hagerman F C, Walsh S J, Staron R S et al 2000 Effects of high-intensity resistance training on untrained older men: strength, cardiovascular, and metabolic responses. Journals of Gerontology. Series A, Biological Sciences and Medical Sciences 55:B336–346

Hakkinen K, Hakkinen A 1995 Neuromuscular adaptations during intensive strength training in middle-aged and elderly males and females. Electromyography and Clinical Neurophysiology 35:137–147

Hakkinen K, Newton R U, Gordon S E et al 1998 Changes in muscle morphology, electromyographic activity, and force production characteristics during progressive strength training in young and older men. Journals of Gerontology. Series A, Biological Sciences and Medical Sciences 53:B415–423

Hakkinen K, Alen M, Kallinen M et al 2000 Neuromuscular adaptation during prolonged strength training, detraining and re-strength-training in middle-aged and elderly people. European Journal of Applied Physiology 83:51–62

Harman E A 1983 Resistive torque analysis of 5 nautilus machines. Medicine and Science in Sports and Exercise 15:115

Hedrick A 2000 Training the trunk for improved athletic performance. Strength and Conditioning 22:50–61

Hess J A, Woollacott M 2005 Effect of high-intensity strength-training on functional measures of balance ability in balance-impaired older adults. Journal of Manipulative and Physiological Therapeutics 28:582–590

Hettinger R, Muller E 1953 Muskelleistung und Muskeltraining. Arbeits Physiologie 15:111–126

Hewett T E, Myer G D, Ford K R et al 2005. Biomechanical measures of neuromuscular control and valgus loading of the knee predict anterior cruciate ligament injury risk in female athletes: a prospective study. American Journal of Sports Medicine 33:492–501

Higbie E J, Cureton K J, Warren G L et al 1996 Effects of concentric and eccentric training on muscle strength, cross-sectional area, and neural activation. Journal of Applied Physiology 81:2173–2181

Higgins S 1991 Motor skill acquisition. Physical Therapy 71:123–139

Holloszy J O 1967 Biochemical adaptations in muscle. Effects of exercise on mitochondrial oxygen uptake and respiratory enzyme activity in skeletal muscle. Journal of Biological Chemistry 242:2278–2282

Houmard J, Hickey M, Tyndall G et al 1995 Seven days of exercise increase GLUT-4 protein content in human skeletal muscle. Journal of Applied Physiology 79:1936–1938

Hurley B F, Redmond R A, Pratley R E et al 1995 Effects of strength training on muscle hypertrophy and muscle cell disruption in older men. International Journal of Sports Medicine 16:378–384

Irmischer B S, Harris C, Pfeiffer R P et al 2004 Effects of a knee ligament injury prevention exercise program on impact forces in women. Journal of Strength and Conditioning Research 18:703–707

Johnson J H, Colodny S, Jackson D 1990 Human torque capability versus machine resistive torque for four Eagle resistive machines. Journal of Applied Sport Science Research 4:83–87

Kannus P, Jozsa L, Natri A et al 1997 Effects of training, immobilization and remobilization on tendons. Scandinavian Journal of Medicine and Science in Sports 7:67–71

Kerr D, Ackland T, Maslen B et al 2001 Resistance training over 2 years increases bone mass in calcium-replete postmenopausal women. Journal of Bone Mineral Research 16:175–181

Kraemer W J 1997 A series of studies – the physiological basis for strength in American football: fact over philosophy. Journal of Strength and Conditioning Research 11:131–142

Kraemer W J, Noble B J, Clark M J et al 1987 Physiologic responses to heavy-resistance exercise with very short rest periods. International Journal of Sports Medicine 8: 247–252

Kraemer W J, Fleck S J, Evans W J 1996 Strength and power training: physiological mechanisms of adaptation. Exercise and Sport Sciences Reviews 24:363–397

Kraemer W J, Stone M H, O'Bryant H S et al 1997 Effects of single vs. multiple sets of weight training: impact of volume, intensity, and variation. Journal of Strength and Conditioning Research 11:143–147

Kraemer W J, Hakkinen K, Newton R U et al 1999 Effects of heavy-resistance training on hormonal response patterns in younger vs. older men. Journal of Applied Physiology 87:982–992

Kraemer W J, Ratamess N, Fry A C et al 2000 Influence of resistance training volume and periodization on physiological and performance adaptations in collegiate women tennis players. American Journal of Sports Medicine 28:626–633

Kraemer W J, Mazzetti S A, Nindl B C et al 2001 Effect of resistance training on women's strength/power and occupational performances. Medicine and Science in Sports and Exercise 33:1011–1025

LaChance P 1995 Plyometric exercise. Strength and Conditioning 17:16–23

Laughlin M H 1999 Cardiovascular response to exercise. Advances in Physiology Education 22:S244–S259

Leighton J, Holmes D, Benson J et al 1967 A study of the effectiveness of ten different methods of progressive resistance exercise on the development of strength, flexibility, girth, and body weight. Journal of the Association for Physical and Mental Rehabilitation 21:78–81

Lemmer J T, Ivey F M, Ryan A S et al 2001 Effect of strength training on resting metabolic rate and physical activity: age and gender comparisons. Medicine and Science in Sports and Exercise 33:532–541

Lemon P W 1998 Effects of exercise on dietary protein requirements. International Journal of Sport Nutrition 8:426–447

Levy W C, Cerqueira M D, Harp G D et al 1998 Effect of endurance exercise training on heart rate variability at rest in healthy young and older men. American Journal of Cardiology 82:1236–1241

Lindheim S, Notelovitz M, Feldman E et al 1994 The independent effects of exercise and estrogen on lipids and lipoproteins in postmenopausal women. Obstetrics and Gynecology 83:167–172

McCall G E, Byrnes W C, Dickinson A et al 1996 Muscle fiber hypertrophy, hyperplasia, and capillary density in college men after resistance training. Journal of Applied Physiology 81:2004–2012

McCarrick M J, Kemp J G 2000 The effect of strength training and reduced training on rotator cuff musculature. Clinical Biomechanics 15 (1 suppl):S42–45

Macera C A, Pate R R, Powell K E et al 1989 Predicting lower-extremity injuries among habitual runners. Archives of Internal Medicine 149:256–258

McLester J R, Bishop P, Guilliams M E 2000 Comparison of 1 day and 3 days per week of equal-volume resistance training in experienced subjects. Journal of Strength and Conditioning Research 14:273–281

McMorris R O, Elkins E C 1954 A study of production and evaluation of muscular hypertrophy. Archives of Physical Medicine and Rehabilitation 35:420–426

Madsen K, Holmskov U 1995 Capillary density measurements in skeletal muscle using immunohistochemical staining with anti-collagen type IV antibodies. European Journal of Applied Physiology and Occupational Physiology 71:472–474

Mahon A D, Vaccaro P 1989 Ventilatory threshold and VO₂max changes in children following endurance training. Medicine and Science in Sports and Exercise 21:425–431

Maganaris C N, Narici M V, Reeves N D 2004 In vivo human tendon mechanical properties: effect of resistance training in old age. Journal of Musculoskeletal and Neuronal Interactions 4:204–208

Mandigout S, Lecoq A M, Courteix C et al 2001 Effect of gender in response to an aerobic training programme in prepubertal children. Acta Paediatrica 90:9–15

Mannion A F, Jakeman P M, Willan P L 1992 Effects of isokinetic training of the knee extensors on isometric strength and peak power output during cycling. European Journal of Applied Physiology and Occupational Physiology 65:370–375

Martel G F, Hurlbut D E, Lott M E et al 1999 Strength training normalizes resting blood pressure in 65- to 73-year-old men and women with high normal blood pressure. Journal of the American Geriatrics Society 47:1215–1221

Marx J O, Ratamess N A, Nindl B C et al 2001 Low-volume circuit versus high-volume periodized resistance training in women. Medicine and Science in Sports and Exercise 33:635–643

Mayhew J L, Ware J R, Prinster J L 1993 Using lift repetitions to predict muscular strength in adolescent males. National Strength and Conditioning Association Journal 15:35–38

Michna H, Hartmann G 1989 Adaptation of tendon collagen to exercise. International Orthopaedics 13:161–165

Mole P A, Oscai L B, Holloszy J O 1971 Adaptations of muscle to exercise. Increase in levels of palmityl-CoA synthase, carnitine palmityltransferase and palmityl CoA dehydrogenase and in the capacity to oxidize fatty acids. Journal of Clinical Investigation 50:2323–2330

Morrissey M C, Harman E A, Johnson M J 1995 Resistance training modes: specificity and effectiveness. Medicine and Science in Sports and Exercise 27:648–660

Narici M V, Hoppeler H, Kayser B et al 1996 Human quadriceps cross-sectional area, torque and neural activation during 6 months strength training. Acta Physiologica Scandinavica 157:175–186

O'Neill D S, Zheng D, Anderson W K et al 1999 Effect of endurance exercise on myosin heavy chain gene regulation in human skeletal muscle. American Journal of Physiology 276:R414–R419

Paterson D H, Cunningham D A, Koval J J et al 1999 Aerobic fitness in a population of independently living men and women aged 55–86 years. Medicine and Science in Sports and Exercise 31:1813–1820

Pincivero D M, Lephart S M, Karunakara R G 1997 Effects of rest interval on isokinetic strength and functional performance after short-term high intensity training. British Journal of Sports Medicine 31:229–234

Pollock M L, Bohannon R L, Cooper K H et al 1976 A comparative analysis of four protocols for maximal treadmill stress testing. American Heart Journal 92:39–46.

Pollock M L, Graves J E, Bamman M M 1993 Frequency and volume of resistance training: effect on cervical extension strength. Archives of Physical Medicine and Rehabilitation 74:1080–1086

Porter M M 2001 The effects of strength training on sarcopenia. Canadian Journal of Applied Physiology 26:123–141

Roca J, Agusti A G, Alonso A et al 1992 Effects of training on muscle O$_2$ transport at VO$_2$max. Journal of Applied Physiology 73:1067–1076

Rhodes E C, Martin A D, Taunton J E et al 2000 Effects of one year of resistance training on the relation between muscular strength and bone density in elderly women. British Journal of Sports Medicine 34:18–22

Rimmer E, Sleivert G 2000 Effects of a plyometric intervention program on sprint performance. Journal of Strength and Conditioning Research 14:295–301.

Rowland T W 1992 Trainability of the cardiorespiratory system during childhood. Canadian Journal of Sport Science 17:259–263

Rowland T W, Martel L, Vanderburgh P et al 1996 The influence of short-term aerobic training on blood lipids in healthy 10–12 year old children. International Journal of Sports Medicine 17:487–492

Ryan A S, Hurlbut D E, Lott M E et al 2001 Insulin action after resistive training in insulin resistant older men and women. Journal of the American Geriatrics Society 49:247–253

Santos J 1979 Jump training for speed and neuromuscular development. Track and Field Quarterly Review 79:59

Scandalis T A, Bosak A, Berliner J C et al 2001 Resistance training and gait function in patients with Parkinson's disease. American Journal of Physical Medicine and Rehabilitation 80:38–43

Schlicht J, Camaione D N, Owen S V 2001 Effect of intense strength training on standing balance, walking speed, and sit-to-stand performance in older adults. Journals of Gerontology. Series A, Biological Sciences and Medical Sciences 56:M281–286

Schwartz R S, Cain K C, Shuman W P et al 1992 Effect of intensive endurance training on lipoprotein profiles in young and older men. Metabolism 41:649–654

Schwarz R, Kindermann W 1990 B-endorphin, adrenocorticotropin hormone, cortisol and catecholamines during aerobic and anaerobic exercise. European Journal of Applied Physiology 61:165–171.

Smith E, Gilligan C, McAdam M et al 1989 Deterring bone loss by exercise. Calcified Tissue International 44:312–321

Smith M J, Melton P 1981 Isokinetic versus isotonic variable-resistance training. American Journal of Sports Medicine 9:275–279

Sparling P B, Cantwell J D, Dolan C M et al 1990 Strength training in a cardiac rehabilitation program: a six-month follow-up. Archives of Physical Medicine and Rehabilitation 71:148–152

Spurs R W, Murphy A J, Watsford M L 2003 The effects of plyometric training on distance running performance. European Journal of Applied Physiology 89:1–7

Steinhaus L A, Dustman R E, Ruhling R O et al 1990 Aerobic capacity of older adults: a training study. Journal of Sports Medicine and Physical Fitness 30:163–172

Stewart K J 1989 Resistive training effects on strength and cardiovascular endurance in cardiac and coronary prone patients. Medicine and Science in Sports and Exercise 21:678–682

Stone M H 1988 Implications for connective tissue and bone alterations resulting from resistance exercise training. Medicine and Science in Sports and Exercise 20 (5 suppl):S162–168

Stone M H 1990 Muscle conditioning and muscle injuries. Medicine and Science in Sports and Exercise 22:457–462

Stone M H, O'Bryant H, Garhammer J 1981 A hypothetical model for strength training. Journal of Sports Medicine and Physical Fitness 21:342–351

Stone M H, Potteiger J A, Pierce K C et al 2000 Comparison of the effects of three different weight-training programs on the one-repetition maximum squat. Journal of Strength and Conditioning Research 14:332–337

Sullivan D H, Roberson P K, Johnson, L E et al 2005 Effects of muscle strength training and testosterone in frail elderly males. Medicine and Science in Sports and Exercise 37:1664–1672

Suter E, Hoppeler H, Claassen H et al 1995 Ultrastructural modification of human skeletal muscle tissue with 6-month moderate-intensity exercise training. International Journal of Sports Medicine 16:160–166

Svedenhag J, Henriksson J, Sylven C 1983 Dissociation of training effects on skeletal muscle mitochondrial enzymes and myoglobin in man. Acta Physiologica Scandinavica 117:213–218

Swash M, Fox K 1972 Muscle spindle innervation in man. Journal of Anatomy 112:61–80

Taaffe D R, Pruitt L, Pyka G et al 1996 Comparative effects of high- and low-intensity resistance training on thigh muscle strength, fiber area, and tissue composition in elderly women. Clinical Physiology 16:381–392

Taaffe D R, Duret C, Wheeler S et al 1999 Once-weekly resistance exercise improves muscle strength and neuromuscular performance in older adults. Journal of the American Geriatrics Society 47:1208–1214

Tanasescu M, Leitzmann M F, Rimm E B et al 2002 Exercise type and intensity in relation to coronary heart disease in men. Journal of the American Medical Association 288:1994–2000

Tesch P A, Thorsson A, Colliander E B 1990 Effects of eccentric and concentric resistance training on skeletal muscle substrates, enzyme activities and capillary supply. Acta Physiologica Scandinavica 140:575–580

Todd I C, Wosornu D, Stewart I et al 1992 Cardiac rehabilitation following myocardial infarction. A practical approach. Sports Medicine 14:243–259

Toumi H, Best T M, Martin A et al 2004 Effects of eccentric phase velocity of plyometric training on the vertical jump. International Journal of Sports Medicine 25:391–398

Trappe S W, Costill D L, Vukovich M D et al 1996 Aging among elite distance runners: a 22-yr longitudinal study. Journal of Applied Physiology 80:285–290

Tsutsumi T, Don B M, Zaichkowsky L D et al 1998 Comparison of high and moderate intensity of strength training on mood and anxiety in older adults. Perceptual and Motor Skills 87:1003–1011

Tucci J T, Carpenter D M, Pollock M L et al 1992 Effect of reduced frequency of training and detraining on lumbar extension strength. Spine 17:1497–1501

Tucker L A, Maxwell K 1992 Effects of weight training on the emotional well-being and body image of females: predictors of greatest benefit. American Journal of Health Promotion 6:338–344, 371

Verkhoshanski Y 1966 Perspectives in the improvement of speed-strength preparation of jumpers. Track and Field 9:11–12

Voight M L 1992 Stretch-strengthening: an introduction toplyometrics. Orthopedic Physical Therapy Clinics of North America 1:243–252

Wathen D 1993 NSCA position paper: explosive/plyometric exercises. National Strength and Conditioning Association Journal 15:16–19

Wathen D, Shutes M 1982 A comparison of the effects of selected isotonic and isokinetic modalities, and programs on the acquisition of strength and power in collegiate football players. National Strength and Conditioning Association Journal 4:40–42

Weaver C M, Teegarden D, Lyle R M et al 2001 Impact of exercise on bone health and contraindication of oral contraceptive use in young women. Medicine and Science in Sports and Exercise 33:873–880

Weiss A, Suzuki T, Bean J et al 2000 High intensity strength training improves strength and functional performance after stroke. American Journal of Physical Medicine and Rehabilitation 79:369–376

Welle S, Totterman S, Thornton C 1996 Effect of age on muscle hypertrophy induced by resistance training. Journals of Gerontology. Series A, Biological Sciences and Medical Sciences 51:M270–275

Wilk K E, Voight M L, Keirns M A et al 1993 Stretch-shortening drills for the upper extremities: theory and clinical application. Journal of Orthopaedic and Sports Physical Therapy 17:225–239

Wilmore J H, Stanforth P R, Hudspeth L A et al 1998 Alterations in resting metabolic rate as a consequence of 20 wk of endurance training: the HERITAGE Family Study. American Journal of Clinical Nutrition 68:66–71

Wilmore J H, Despres J P, Stanforth P R et al 1999 Alterations in body weight and composition consequent to 20 wk of endurance training: the HERITAGE Family Study. American Journal of Clinical Nutrition 70:346–352

Wilmore J H, Stanforth P R, Gagnon J et al 2001 Heart rate and blood pressure changes with endurance training: the HERITAGE Family Study. Medicine and Science in Sports and Exercise 33:107–116

Wilt F 1975 Plyometrics: what it is and how it works. Athletic Journal 55b:76–91

Witzke KA, Snow CM 2000 Effects of plyometric jump training on bone mass in adolescent girls. Medicine and Science in Sports and Exercise 32:1051–1057

Yaspelkis B B 2006 Resistance training improves insulin signaling and action in skeletal muscle. Exercise and Sport Science Reviews 34:42–46

Zernicke R F, Loitz B J 1992 Exercise-related adaptations in connective tissue. In: Komi P V (ed) Strength and power in sport. Blackwell Scientific, Oxford, p 96–108.

Zinovieff A 1951 Heavy resistance exercise: the Oxford technique. British Journal of Physical Medicine 14:129–132

Psychology of injury and rehabilitation

11

Gregory S. Kolt and Britton W. Brewer

CHAPTER CONTENTS

Introduction 171
Psychological precursors to injury 172
Interventions to reduce injury vulnerability 173
Psychology of sport and exercise injury
rehabilitation. 174
Psychological responses to injury 178
Adherence to injury rehabilitation 180
Role of physical therapists in providing
psychological support for injured athletes 182
Cognitive-behavioral interventions for
injured athletes 183
Summary 185

Introduction

Participation in sport, exercise and physical activity has become a major public health priority due to rising obesity rates and the increase in non-communicable diseases related to a sedentary lifestyle. Participation in such activities, however, results in a greater potential for, and incidence of, physical injury. The costs involved in rehabilitating people injured through sport and exercise, the loss of sport and work participation time, interventions to reduce injury vulnerability, the risk of long-term injury and the consequential reduced quality of life are all public health concerns.

The extent of sport and exercise injuries varies across countries. For example, of the estimated 7 million annual sport and recreation injuries in the USA (Conn et al 2003), more than 2 million require hospital emergency room consultations (Burt & Overpeck 2001). Highlighting the problem further, Weaver et al (1999) suggested that in a single state in the USA, injuries sustained by high school athletes in 12 sports would produce medical costs of $10 million in the long term and a further $19 million of lost earnings. In Australia, 20% of child and adolescent and 18% of adult hospital emergency room consultations were related to sport injuries (Finch et al 1998). The cost of sport- and recreation-related injuries in Australia was recently estimated at $1.8 billion per annum (Medibank Private 2004). In the UK, sport- and exercise-related injuries accounted for 33% of all injuries reported in a population survey (Uitenbroek 1996).

The impact of sport and exercise injury is wide reaching. Not only are there the obviously detrimental effects on the financial, physical and performance aspects of individuals in sport, but also a psychological impact is often apparent. In the past, a principal focus of sport injury rehabilitation has been to return individuals to their prior level of functioning by treating their overt physical problems. More current literature, however, highlights the increasing trend toward managing athletes more holistically, with a greater emphasis on addressing the psychological consequences of injury and rehabilitation (Brewer et al 2002a, Francis et al 2000, Hemmings & Povey 2001, Kolt 2000, Ninedek & Kolt 2000). The purpose of this chapter is to discuss the psychological precursors to injury, the psychological responses to injury and the psychological factors that can influence rehabilitation from sport and exercise injury. The chapter will also focus on psychosocial approaches that can be used by physical therapists to complement their physical management programs.

Psychological precursors to injury

An increasing body of research over the past few decades has focused on psychosocial variables and their influence on injury vulnerability and resiliency. This research has considered a wide range of psychosocial factors including stress, anxiety, self-confidence, locus of control, attention, cognitive mood states, coping mechanisms, motivation and personality (Kirkby 1995, Williams & Andersen 1998).

Personality components were among the earlier variables researched in this area (e.g. Brown 1971, Govern & Koppenhaver 1965, Ogilvie and Tutko 1966), along with the stress caused by major life events (e.g. Bramwell et al 1975). Although this foundation work suggested that athletes' injuries were linked to factors such as life stress, fear of competition, hostility, masochism and masculinity, no theoretical framework was offered to explain the relationships.

In response to the lack of an underpinning theoretical model, Andersen & Williams (1988) developed a multicomponent theoretical model of stress and injury. This model suggested that most psychological variables, if they influence injury outcome, do so through a link with stress and a resulting stress response. The original stress–injury model was revised and refined over the following decade (Williams & Andersen 1998). This model (Fig. 11.1) is still viewed as the definitive explanation of the relationship between sports injury and psychological factors.

The majority of recent investigations into psychological variables and injury in sport have drawn upon the Williams & Andersen (1998) model of stress and athletic injury and its earlier version. Figure 11.1 shows that the model focuses on the stress response (the central portion of the model) and the three broad categories of variables hypothesized to influence this

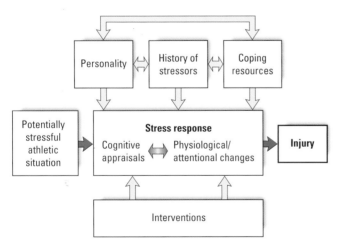

Figure 11.1 • The stress and injury model. (Copyright 1998 from Psychosocial antecedents of sport injury: review and critique of the stress and injury model by Williams J M, Andersen M B. Reproduced by permission of Taylor and Francis, Inc., http://www. routledge-ny.com.)

response: personality, history of stressors and coping resources. Following the concepts of Folkman & Lazarus (1985), the stress response is viewed as the way in which the cognitive and physiological elements of stressful situations interact. That is, the impact of a stressor is likely to be a function of the individual's appraisal of the extent of the stressor, the coping processes used by the individual and the perceptions of the resources that the individual has to manage the stressor. Applying this to a sports context, athletes continually appraise the demands of varying situations and their ability to meet those demands. When the demands of a particular situation outweigh the resources that the athlete has to respond to that situation, the stress response elevates.

The cognitive appraisal of demands and resources is connected bidirectionally to physiological and attentional responses (Williams & Andersen 1998). For example, a common somatic response to stress involves generalized muscle tension. This muscle tension can, in turn, lead to altered motor coordination and reduced flexibility, thus contributing to musculoskeletal injuries such as strains and sprains (Andersen & Williams 1988). Also relevant to this are the attentional changes related to stress. For example, narrowing of the visual field can occur during stress resulting in a failure to extract vital cues from the periphery and, thereby, increase the likelihood of injury (Andersen & Williams 1988). Also, under conditions of stress, attention can become distracted resulting in athletes attending to stimuli irrelevant to the task at hand and missing the more vital cues (Andersen & Williams 1988). In relation to the cognitive appraisal influence on the stress response, individuals will appraise the demands of a situation, the adequacy of their ability to meet those demands and the potential consequences of success or failure (Williams & Andersen 1998). From a cognitive perspective, it is the level of match or mismatch between the demands, the ability to meet those demands and the consequences of success or failure that will influence the stress response.

Three broad categories of variables influence the stress response: personality factors, history of stressors and coping resources, as identified in Fig. 11.1 (Williams & Andersen 1998). These variables can either act singly or in combination to influence the stress response, and ultimately, injury. The model indicates that an individual's history of stressors, personality factors and coping resources can influence the stress response either directly or through a moderating influence on each other.

There is substantial evidence to support Andersen & Williams' (1988) assertion that an individual's history of stressors (i.e. major life events, chronic daily problems and previous injuries) can have a substantial impact on the stress response and, thus, on injury. Reviews of the literature on life stress and injury provide excellent support for a relationship between these factors in a range of contact and non-contact sports (Williams & Roepke 1993, Williams & Andersen 1998). More recent research has found that sport-specific stressors may be more closely related to injury than stressors of a more general nature (Dunn et al 2001). A large majority of studies over the past 30 years have found some type of positive relationship between high life stress (both negative life stress, such as death of a close family member, or positive life stress, such as a competitive win at a major sports event) and injury in sport (e.g. Andersen & Williams 1999, Dunn et al 2001, Galambos et al 2005, Kolt & Kirkby 1996, Petrie 1993a, 1993b, Thompson & Morris 1994).

The history of stressors in the Williams & Andersen (1998) model includes daily hassles. The role of minor daily problems, irritations and changes in influencing the stress response has been less researched than life stress, with less conclusive evidence available. While the early studies failed to show any positive relationship between daily hassles and injury (e.g. Blackwell & McCullagh 1990), Fawkner et al (1999) found that athletes were more likely to incur an injury when they experienced significant increases in daily hassles in the week before and the week of the injury.

The final type of stressor described in the Williams & Andersen (1998) model relates to past injuries. Previous injury can affect future injury when athletes have not recovered enough physically to return to sport, but do so anyway. Also, if athletes return to sport when physically, but not psychologically, prepared problems could arise from negative self-evaluations regarding their ability to perform, given their injury and reduced training schedule during the rehabilitation process. Furthermore, according to Williams & Andersen (1998), fear of reinjury can, in itself, be a substantial stressor, and thus can increase the likelihood of injury. This aspect of the model, however, has only received limited support (Lysens et al 1984).

The second category of variables thought to influence the stress response is components of personality (e.g. locus of control, competitive trait anxiety, hardiness, achievement motivation and sensation seeking characteristics). Research of these variables has produced mixed findings and the literature in this area is too large to review in detail. However, it should be noted that positive links have been found to athletic injury for variables including locus of control, state anxiety, trait anxiety, negative state of mind, tough mindedness and defensive pessimism (see Williams & Andersen 1998).

The final component of the model consists of coping resources, which are thought to influence the stress response. Coping resources can include social support, stress management skills, other psychological coping skills and general coping behaviors, such as appropriate nutrition and sleep habits. There is significant evidence that coping resources are related to injury outcome or moderate the influence of life stress on injury vulnerability (Williams & Andersen 1998). For example, Andersen & Williams (1999) found that low levels of social support directly influenced stress responsivity, and hence injury vulnerability. Smith et al (1990a) also showed that coping resources can moderate the effect of stressors on psychological and physical outcomes.

Despite further research being required to verify certain aspects of the Williams & Andersen (1998) model of stress and injury, the evidence to date supports it as an explanation of injury occurrence that is useful in applied sport injury settings.

Interventions to reduce injury vulnerability

Although previous focus on injury prevention has been on physical, rather than psychosocial dimensions (Petitpas & Danish 1995), more recently, those involved in sports and exercise medicine have become increasingly aware of psychosocial influences (Francis et al 2000, Hemmings & Povey 2002, Jevon & Johnston 2003, McKenna et al 2002, Ninedek & Kolt 2000). Based on the evidence available supporting the relationship between stress and injury vulnerability in sport, it is reasonable to assume that interventions to reduce stress levels or modify the stress response in athletes might decrease the risk of injury. A growing body of research has supported this assumption.

In the earliest of the studies looking at sports injury prevention through psychological intervention, American football players who received a cognitive and biofeedback intervention reported that they experienced a decrease in minor injuries as a result of the intervention (DeWitt 1980); however, no preintervention injury data were available and no statistical comparisons were performed. May & Brown (1989) used imagery, attention control and other mental practice skills with US Olympic alpine skiers at the Calgary Olympic Games. Although they reported a reduced injury rate, increased confidence and enhanced self-control as a result of the intervention, they failed to employ a control group or statistical comparisons. A study where marathon runners were taught how to use appropriate attentional strategies (i.e. associative thought processes) over a 5-week period reported that heavy training could be facilitated without injury (Schomer 1990). However, this study did not use a control group either and did not use statistical procedures. Davis (1991) used a program of imagery of sports skills and progressive muscular relaxation with collegiate swimmers and football players and found a 52% reduction in swimming injuries and a 33% reduction in football injuries. These findings, however, were based on a problematic methodology where no control group or statistical analyses were used.

More sophisticated research methods have been used to investigate the role of stress management in injury prevention in five studies (Johnson et al 2005, Kerr & Goss 1996, Kolt et al 2004, Maddison & Prapavessis 2005, Perna et al 2003). Kerr & Goss (1996) provided a 16-session stress management program to 12 national and international level Canadian gymnasts over an 8-month period. The stress management program was based primarily on Meichenbaum's (1985) Stress Inoculation Training and included work on thought processes, self-talk, dealing with distractions, thought stopping, relaxation, imagery and preparation for competition. A further 12 gymnasts, matched according to sex, age and performance level, acted as a control group. It was found that the gymnasts who undertook the stress management intervention reported significantly lower levels of negative athletic stress from the mid-part of the season to the peak of the season. In relation to injury, although it appeared that the stress management group spent less time injured by the end of the 8-month intervention, the difference was not statistically significant. Notwithstanding this finding, Andersen & Stoove (1998), in commenting on the Kerr & Goss study, pointed out that Kerr & Goss probably showed a clinically significant effect in injury reduction from their stress management intervention, despite statistical significance not being achieved. That is, their failure to show a significant difference probably had more to do with the small sample size and resultant low power than the effectiveness of the intervention.

Kolt et al (2004) studied the effects of a 12-session stress management program on national and international level female gymnasts. The stress management program was based on that developed by Kerr & Goss (1996) and injury and stress data were collected longitudinally over 9 months. They found no differences on either injury or stress scores over the 9-month period, most likely due to the relatively small sample in the study. Less ambiguous findings were obtained by Perna et al (2003), who examined the effects of a cognitive behavioral stress management (CBSM) intervention on injury and illness in collegiate rowers in a randomized, controlled clinical trial. Relative to participants in the control group, rowers who received the CBSM intervention had significantly fewer days lost to injury and illness over the course of the competitive season. Treatment group participants also had only half as many health service visits as control group participants during the study period. Similar strong findings in support of the ability of CBSM interventions to reduce the occurrence of and time loss due to sport injuries were reported in a pair of randomized trials in which only athletes with psychological profiles indicating an increased risk for injury were studied (Johnson et al 2005, Maddison & Prapavessis 2005). Participants in the Johnson et al study were soccer players, and the intervention consisted of 6 to 8 mental skills training sessions. Players in the treatment group had significantly fewer injuries (as recorded by their coaches) over the 19-week competitive season than those in the control group. In the Maddison & Prapavessis study, rugby players served as participants. A 6-session CBSM intervention was implemented during a 4-week period prior to the competitive season. Players who received the intervention reported having significantly less time lost due to injury than their counterparts in the control group. It therefore appears that the salubrious effects of psychological interventions on sport injury outcomes generalize across multiple sports (e.g., gymnastics, rowing, soccer, rugby).

Sports medicine professionals are well placed to teach athletes ways of handling stressful events, reaching goals, and identifying and overcoming barriers (Shaffer & Wiese-Bjornstal 1999). Shaffer & Wiese-Bjornstal further suggested that the role of various psychological techniques in reducing injury can 'psychologically strengthen' athletes and can have an effect on minimizing injury occurrence. The techniques commonly recommended in such interventions include the teaching of coping mechanisms, relaxation techniques, imagery or cognitive rehearsal, positive self-talk (including the minimization of negative thoughts), social support and other general stress reduction methods (Ievleva & Orlick 1999, Shaffer & Wiese-Bjornstal 1999, Williams 2001). Smith et al (1990a) proposed that, from

an intervention perspective, resiliency to sport injuries could be increased by either increasing social support in athletes' lives or by instructing athletes in coping skills.

Psychology of sport and exercise injury rehabilitation

In addition to psychological factors playing a role in injury occurrence, more recent research has focused on the impact of psychological variables on the way athletes react to injury and the rehabilitation process that follows.

Models of psychosocial factors in injury rehabilitation

To put into perspective the psychological responses athletes have to injury and the consequent rehabilitation process, it is important to consider appropriate theoretical models. Not only do such theoretical explanations allow better-grounded research to take place, but they also allow physical therapists to interpret psychological reactions displayed by athletes in a broader and more meaningful sense. Two types of models have been reported in the literature: the biopsychosocial model (Brewer et al 2002a) and psychological models.

Biopsychosocial model

Both the medical and psychological perspectives need to be considered in order to fully examine psychological factors within the overall context of sport injury rehabilitation (Brewer 2002a). The most recent model of sport injury rehabilitation that has drawn on this combined structure is the biopsychosocial model of sport injury rehabilitation (Fig. 11.2) (Brewer et al 2002a). This model was developed by integrating the frameworks of existing models of sport injury rehabilitation (Flint 1998, Leadbetter 1994, Wiese-Bjornstal et al 1998) with more general models of health outcome (Cohen & Rodriguez 1995, Matthews et al 1997). The main components of the model are injury, sociodemographic factors, biological factors, psychological factors, social/contextual factors, intermediate biopsychological outcomes and sport injury rehabilitation outcomes. In this theoretical explanation, the characteristics of injury (e.g. type, course, severity, location and history) and sociodemographic factors (e.g. age, gender, race/ethnicity and socioeconomic status) are proposed to influence the biological, psychological and social/contextual factors. The three categories of factors resulting from injury can influence intermediate biopsychological outcomes (e.g. range of motion, strength, joint laxity, pain, endurance and recovery rate) and, in turn, affect rehabilitation outcomes. The psychological factors resulting from injury have a unique role in this model in that they have a direct bidirectional path to sport injury rehabilitation outcomes.

The biopsychosocial model described above has its advantage in proposing links between components of traditional psychological models and more medically focused models. By suggesting these links, however, it does not provide for the

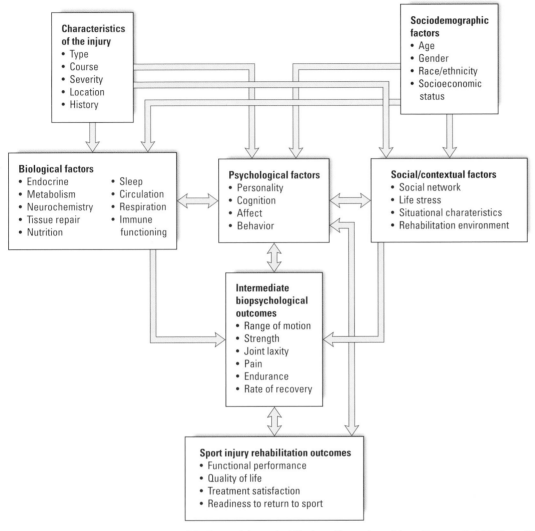

Figure 11.2 • The biopsychosocial model of sport injury rehabilitation. (Reproduced from Brewer et al 2002a with the permission of Fitness Information Technology.)

many interactions that can occur between specific psychological variables during the injury and rehabilitation process, relying instead on psychological models to perform this function.

Psychological models

It is important to consider the many psychological models that have been outlined in the literature. The grief response model and the cognitive appraisal model are two recognized models that can be applied to rehabilitation from a sport injury.

Grief response model

One of the commonly used models to explain psychological aspects of injury rehabilitation in sport and exercise is Kubler-Ross' (1969) grief response model. This model, initially developed to explain significant loss (e.g. death of a family member) suggests that individuals typically progress through five stages of grieving: denial, anger, bargaining, depression and acceptance.

This model has been applied to sport injury rehabilitation as a result of suggestions that injuries involve a loss of an aspect of the self (Gordon et al 1991, Macchi & Crossman 1996, Peretz 1970).

The grief response model indicates that each 'stage' is characterized by specific moods and behaviors, and that athletes will move through the various stages over the recovery and rehabilitation period. Initially, athletes may show *denial* of their injury, possibly rejecting the prognosis and refusing to accept the limitations placed upon them as a result of the injury. After denial, some athletes can experience *anger* and display extreme and abrupt emotional reactions (possibly towards someone or something considered responsible for the injury); often, such responses are irrational. Following anger, athletes can enter a *bargaining* stage (e.g. bargaining with sports medicine providers over rehabilitation and return to sport recommendations). The fourth stage of the grief response model is that of *depression*.

Table 11.1 Examples of typical thoughts and behaviors present at each stage of the grief response model as it relates to sport injury

Stage of reaction	Thoughts	Behaviors
1. Denial	'I can play my way through this injury. It won't stop me'	Continue to play or train with an injury
2. Anger	'Why did the coach make me play this new position?' 'Just my luck to get injured before the finals'	Storm away from training or a team meeting
3. Bargaining	'If I do all my exercises at home, maybe I can begin playing a week earlier than the physical therapist said I could. They really don't know what athletes go through'	Failure to follow medical advice regarding rest and rehabilitation activities
4. Depression	'I'm not getting anywhere with this exercise program. Why should I even bother with going to rehabilitation?'	Lack of motivation Lethargy Withdrawal from sport involvement
5. Acceptance	'I can now see that the physical therapist was right. I should continue to follow their instructions'	Positive self-talk Displaying commitment to the rehabilitation program Adhering to rehabilitation advice

Athletes can show depressive symptoms when the full realization of the extent of an injury is recognized; this can result in diminished motivation for rehabilitation, and engagement in counterproductive behaviors (Horsley 1995). *Acceptance* of the extent and implications of the injury characterize the final stage of this model. Table 11.1 shows examples of typical thoughts and behaviors present at each stage of the grief response model as it relates to sport or exercise injury.

Despite the early anecdotal support for stage models such as the grief response model (Astle 1986, Lynch 1988), more recent evidence has indicated that athletes do not typically progress through the injury period in a structured and staged manner (Brewer 1994). Athletes vary considerably in the way they react to and deal with injury and are influenced by both personal and situational factors (Brewer 1994, Wiese-Bjornstal et al 1998). Consequently, models that consider such individual differences, whilst also recognizing staged responses to grief, have been developed (Evans & Hardy 1999).

Cognitive appraisal models

Cognitive appraisal models are those that are based around stress, coping and emotional responsivity theories. In sport and exercise, several such theories have been proposed (e.g. Gordon 1986, Weiss & Troxel 1986). Weiss & Troxel (1986) reported a stress model based on the cognitive concept that people's experience of stress (i.e. that may arise from an injury) is a function of their thoughts about stressful situations. For example, a stressful situation (e.g. an injury) is cognitively appraised in relation to the situational and personal resources one has to deal with the situation, as well as the possible outcomes of the event. Then, an emotional response (comprising psychological and attentional components) follows the appraisal. The final stage of the stress process is the behavioral consequences that stem from the emotional responses. This stress process was summarized by Horsley (1995) (Fig. 11.3).

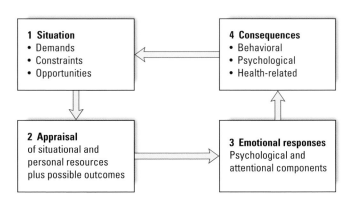

Figure 11.3 • The stress process as an example of a cognitive appraisal model of response to sport injury. (Reproduced with permission from Horsley 1995.)

The most developed cognitive appraisal model to date is the Integrated Model of Psychological Response to the Sport Injury and Rehabilitation Process (Wiese-Bjornstal et al 1998). This model (Fig. 11.4) contends that an athlete's response to a sports injury is influenced by both preinjury variables (personality, history of stressors, coping resources, preventative interventions) and postinjury variables. In relation to postinjury variables, the cognitive appraisal of the injury is proposed to influence behavioral responses (e.g. adherence to rehabilitation), emotional responses (e.g. tension, anger and depression) and the recovery outcomes (psychosocial and physical). The model indicates that both personal and situational factors can affect the cognitive appraisal or interpretation of the injurious event.

Although the interactional aspects of cognitive appraisal models have not been extensively researched, particular aspects of such models have been strongly supported (see review by Brewer 2001). Thus, cognitive appraisal models such as that of Wiese-Bjornstal et al (1998) appear to be the best framework

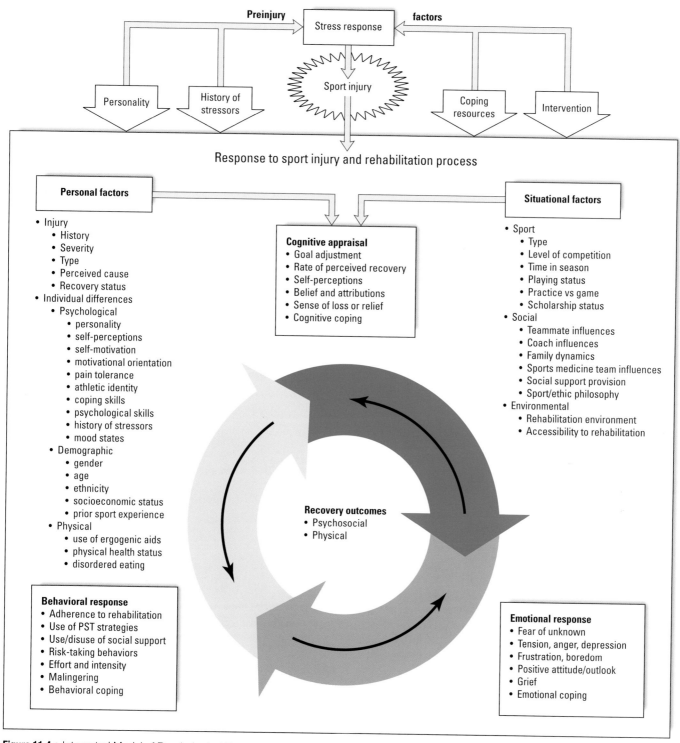

Figure 11.4 • Integrated Model of Psychological Response to the Sport Injury and Rehabilitation Process. (Copyright 1998 from An integrated model of response to sport injury: psychological and sociological dimensions by Wiese-Bjornstal D M, Smith A M, Shaffer S M, Morrey M A. Reproduced by permission of Taylor and Francis, Inc., http://www.routledge-ny.com.)

from which to view the psychological responses to sport injury and rehabilitation.

Psychological responses to injury

Participants in sport and exercise can display a variety of psychological reactions to injury. These responses range from those that are productive and improve the chance for more efficacious rehabilitation to those that are unproductive, causing problems for effective rehabilitation and return to activity. Although the focus for rehabilitation should be on the productive responses to injury, an understanding of the unproductive or maladaptive reactions to the injury process is paramount to the physical therapist and sports medicine practitioner. An important feature of psychological responses to athletic injury is their transient nature. In general, the temporal pattern of psychological responses proceeds from a negative to positive affect over time (McDonald & Hardy 1990, McGowan et al 1994, Smith et al 1990b, Smith et al 1993), although some support for oscillation between 'highs' and 'lows' during the rehabilitation period has been found (Pearson & Jones 1992).

In line with the cognitive appraisal explanations of the injury process described above, three categories of responses to injury will be discussed: cognitive responses, emotional responses and behavioral responses.

Cognitive responses to injury

Several cognitive responses have been linked with injury. These include changes in global and domain-specific self-esteem and self-confidence, and increases in negative thoughts and self-talk. Self-esteem appears to be the cognitive response that has been most extensively researched in relation to sport injury. Some studies have shown that global self-esteem decreases after injury (Leddy et al 1994) or differs as a result of injury status (i.e. injured or non-injured) (Kleiber & Brock 1992, Leddy et al 1994, McGowan et al 1994). Other studies have found no global self-esteem differences in relation to injury (Brewer & Petrie 1995, Smith et al 1993). When considering domain-specific self-esteem (i.e. self-esteem for particular sports activities), evidence exists that injured athletes report lower levels than non-injured athletes (Leddy et al 1994).

Some studies have looked at specific aspects of self-referent cognitive responses to injury (e.g. sport self-confidence and rehabilitation self-efficacy). For example, a study by Quinn & Fallon (1999) showed that sport self-confidence was high at the commencement of rehabilitation, decreased throughout rehabilitation, and increased again towards the end of the rehabilitation period for athletes with significant injuries (i.e. there was a mean recovery duration of 19.25 weeks). Also, the same group of athletes reported constant high levels of self-confidence in adhering to their rehabilitation programs. It is evident that domain-specific self-referent cognitions in response to injury are variable both between individuals and across periods of rehabilitation.

There appears to be three particular characteristics of the cognitive reactions of injured athletes: irrational and unrealistic beliefs, negative thought processes and unwarranted worry about problems beyond their control. Relating irrational thoughts of injured athletes back to the early work of Beck (1976), athletes could exaggerate the meaning of the injury (e.g. catastrophize the situation), ignore important aspects of the injury (e.g. physical restrictions as a result of the injury) and rely on unwarranted conclusions when evidence is lacking (e.g. assuming that they will never play sport again). These irrational thoughts and beliefs can influence emotions and subsequently self-esteem and confidence (Horsley 1995). The tendency of injured athletes to worry about things outside of their control can have the effect of channeling their focus away from things that they can control (e.g. rehabilitation tasks).

Emotional responses to injury

A large body of research has addressed the emotions, mood and affect of injured athletes. Depression, anger, confusion, fear and frustration appear to be common emotional responses to injury, particularly in the early phases of rehabilitation (Bianco et al 1999, Chan & Crossman 1988, Shelley & Sherman 1996, Smith et al 1990b, Tracey 2003, Udry et al 1997, Weiss & Troxel 1986). Qualitative studies have also shown that as rehabilitation is ending and return to sport is near, emotions related to fear of reinjury increase (Bianco et al 1999, Johnston & Carroll 1998). In relating these responses back to the model of Wiese-Bjornstal et al (1998), Brewer (2001) suggested it is important to consider that these emotional responses to injury seem to be influenced by several personal factors (e.g. age, previous injury experience) and situational factors (e.g. time of the season the injury occurred, rehabilitation progress).

Although it is usually considered that emotional disturbance linked to sport injury does not reach clinical levels (Heil 1993), epidemiological findings provide evidence that up to 27% of injured athletes do display clinically meaningful levels of emotional disturbance (Brewer 2001, Manuel et al 2002). At the extreme of the continuum, some athletes with severe depression consider attempting suicide (Smith & Milliner 1994). The majority of research indicates that, generally, negative emotions decrease and positive emotions increase as the rehabilitation period and recovery progress (Dawes & Roach 1997, Macchi & Crossman 1996, Miller 1998, Quinn & Fallon 1999). As mentioned earlier, however, negative emotions can increase again towards the end of the rehabilitation period with the prospect of returning to sporting activity and the associated fear of reinjury. This has been shown particularly with long-term rehabilitation from reconstructive knee surgery (Morrey et al 1999). More specifically, athletes who underwent reconstructive knee surgery showed high negative and low positive mood states around the time of the surgical intervention, which then progressed to more positive and less negative mood during the first few weeks postsurgery, returning to more negative and less positive as they were about to return to sporting activity.

Behavioral responses to injury

Cognitive and emotional responses to injury impact on the behaviors displayed by athletes during the rehabilitation period. Some of the primary behavioral responses to injury are adherence to rehabilitation and the use of coping mechanisms. The behaviors related to rehabilitation adherence will be covered in a later section of this chapter. Coping mechanisms, due to the dynamic and changing nature of rehabilitation programs, can change over the course of rehabilitation (Bianco et al 1999, Udry 1997). Athletes use a broad range of coping behaviors. For example, a study of skiers who had sustained major injuries that precluded further participation for the remainder of a competitive season found that using social support, distraction, avoiding others and isolating oneself, and 'driving through' (e.g. working hard towards rehabilitation goals) were the predominant coping behaviors used (Gould et al 1997). Udry (1997) reported that athletes recovering from knee surgery used instrumental coping behaviors (i.e. those aimed at dealing directly with a stressor) most commonly. It is interesting to note that athletes tend to prefer active (i.e. behaviors that involve their own input) rather than passive (i.e. behaviors that are reliant on others) coping strategies (Smith et al 1990b, Gould et al 1997). Albinson and Petrie (2003) presented evidence suggesting that athletes are most likely to use active behavioral coping strategies when they appraise their injuries as highly stressful and difficult to cope with.

A further behavioral response to injury involves malingering. Malingering behavior has been described by Rotella et al (1999) as an adjustment to negative circumstances that requires an external incentive for being injured. For example, athletes who are trying to avoid returning to sport after a significant injury may consciously exaggerate their symptoms. It has been suggested that athletes who repeatedly adopt this behavior might be doing so as a response to fear, requiring attention, or both (Rotella et al 1999). Reasons for malingering could include poor performance, an escape from the pressure of sport, personal realizations of limited ability and rationalization of loss of place in a team. Although no data on the prevalence of malingering in sport injury rehabilitation are available, physical therapists and other sports medicine practitioners should be aware of malingering as a behavior so that they can modify their approach to management accordingly.

Positive responses to injury

It should be noted, that on some occasions positive emotional benefits emerge from sport and exercise injuries. Udry et al (1997), based on interviews with injured elite athletes, reported an example of this. Of the athletes interviewed, 95% reported positive consequences of their injury that could be categorized into personal growth consequences, psychologically based performance enhancements and physical-technical development opportunities. The athletes reported that they learnt to be more empathic toward other injured athletes and developed skills and interests outside of their sport. They also indicated that they

Table 11.2 Summary of Udry's (1999) recommendations for facilitating positive consequences from athletic injuries

Recommendation for facilitating positive consequence from athletic injury	Comment
Recognize that deriving positive consequence takes effort	Injured athletes must not passively assume that positive consequences will occur; they will need to work on this
Recognize different problem-solving strategies can be used	A variety of techniques can be used. These include 'reversals' where a negative situation is converted to a positive one (or a less negative one) and 'extrications' where athletes voluntarily relinquish problematic roles
Recognize that reframing may not occur immediately	A considerable amount of time may be needed for athletes to counterbalance the negative aspects of their injuries
Avoid secondary victimization	Ensure that those who come into contact with injured athletes do not trivialize or minimize the experiences of the injured athlete
Acknowledge that positive consequences may extend beyond the individual athlete	Individuals whose lives are related to the injured athlete must often also work to counterbalance the negative impact of injury

became 'mentally tougher' and learned more about their psychological boundaries. Furthermore, they reported that they could spend time on the more physical (e.g., conditioning) and technical aspects of their sport. Similar findings have been obtained in several other qualitative studies (Ford & Gordon 1999, Rose & Jevne 1993, San Jose 2003, Tracey 2003).

The positive consequences of injury fit well with the Life Development Model (Danish et al 1995). According to the Life Development Model perspective, when people are faced with what are called 'critical life events' or 'turning points', they respond in several ways. Specifically, critical life events (e.g. major injuries) can lead to debilitation or decreased functioning, increased opportunities for growth or, in some individuals, no change at all.

It stands to reason that for rehabilitation practitioners and athletes to get the most out of the injury process, they should facilitate the positive consequences of such injuries. While recognizing that most athletes will not automatically derive such consequences from their injury, Udry (1999) suggested five particular recommendations for facilitating positive consequences from athletic injuries (Table 11.2).

Adherence to injury rehabilitation

There are many aspects of rehabilitation that require adherence by athletes. These include attendance at rehabilitation appointments, adherence to advice given by physical therapists and other sports medicine personnel (e.g. regarding rest or activity restriction), home- and clinic-based rehabilitation exercises, cryotherapy usage and adherence to advice given and changes made to rehabilitation during clinic appointments. Estimates of adherence to such rehabilitation behaviors range from 40 to 91% (Almekinders & Almekinders 1994, Daly et al 1995, Laubach et al 1996, Taylor and May 1996).

The assumption underlying most adherence research is that adherence to appropriate rehabilitation behaviors is related to rehabilitation outcome. Empirical support for this relationship has accrued, with a growing body of studies in which higher levels of adherence have been related to better sport injury rehabilitation outcomes (Alzate Saez de Heredia et al 2004, Brewer et al 2000a, 2004, Derscheid & Feiring 1987, Pizzari et al 2005, Treacy et al 1997).

Measurement of rehabilitation adherence

Given that adherence to sport injury rehabilitation involves a variety of behaviors over a number of settings, it is understandable that a range of adherence measures have been developed and used. Primarily, adherence measures have focused on attendance at clinic-based sessions, patient behavior during clinic sessions and home-based rehabilitation components.

Attendance at rehabilitation

Several researchers have used attendance at rehabilitation sessions as a measure of adherence (Brewer et al 2000a, 2004, Byerly et al 1994, Daly et al 1995, Fields et al 1995, Kolt & McEvoy 2003, Pizzari et al 2005, Udry 1997). Generally, attendance is calculated as a ratio of rehabilitation sessions attended to sessions scheduled. This simple measure, however, has been criticized on the basis that it only captures one aspect of rehabilitation and does not provide any information on what athletes do during rehabilitation sessions (Brewer 1998, Spetch & Kolt 2001). Also, attendance measures tend to be negatively skewed, as athletes usually attend the majority of scheduled rehabilitation appointments (Brewer 1998). Therefore, attendance measures should be used in conjunction with other adherence measures.

Adherence to clinic-based rehabilitation

Measuring patient behavior during rehabilitation sessions is important to physical therapists in their decision making regarding further rehabilitation. The Sport Injury Rehabilitation Adherence Scale (SIRAS) (Brewer et al 2000b) is the measure most commonly used in this area. The SIRAS can be used to rate the intensity with which participants complete rehabilitation exercises, the frequency of following practitioner instructions and advice and the receptivity to changes in the rehabilitation

1. Circle the number that best indicates the intensity with which this patient completed the rehabilitation exercises during today's appointment:

   minimum effort   1   2   3   4   5   maximum effort

2. During today's appointment, how frequently did this patient follow your instructions and advice?

   never   1   2   3   4   5   always

3. How receptive was this patient to changes in the rehabilitation program during today's appointment?

   very unreceptive   1   2   3   4   5   very receptive

Note: The Sport Injury Rehabilitation Adherence Scale can also be used with reference to adherence tendencies in general by using the present tense (without reference to "today's appointment")

Figure 11.5 • Sport Injury Rehabilitation Adherence Scale. (Reproduced with permission from Brewer et al 2000b.)

program during that day's appointment (Fig. 11.5). The SIRAS has been used extensively and its psychometric properties have been well documented (Brewer et al 2000b, 2002b, Kolt et al 2007).

The Sports Medicine Observation Code (SMOC) (Crossman & Roch 1991) is another instrument that can be used to measure clinic-based rehabilitation behavior. The SMOC allows practitioners to systematically code behavior into 13 categories (e.g. active rehabilitation, waiting, non-activity). These categories are grouped into productive behaviors (i.e. those behaviors which have a high probability of facilitating rehabilitation from injury), unproductive behaviors (i.e. those behaviors which have little or no potential of facilitating rehabilitation from injury) and concurrent behaviors (i.e. those behaviors which have a moderate potential of facilitating the rehabilitation process). Although not the original intent, the SMOC may be useful as a measure of adherence, as its productive behaviors score has been shown to correlate significantly with SIRAS scores (Kolt et al 2001).

Adherence to home-based rehabilitation

Measurement of adherence has also been applied to home-based rehabilitation (Almekinders & Almekinders 1994, Brewer 1998, Brewer et al 2000a, 2004, Kolt & McEvoy 2003, Pizzari et al 2005, Spetch & Kolt 2001). This method of assessment usually involves self-reporting and has been criticized for that reason (Dunbar-Jacob et al 1993, Meichenbaum & Turk 1987), in that it can include biased, distorted and inaccurate recall. Assessment of home-based rehabilitation can include single retrospective reports of adherence over the course of the home-based rehabilitation program or a daily home exercise adherence log or diary.

Researchers should focus on developing more objective assessment devices of home rehabilitation programs, as suggested by Brewer (1998). These could include, for example, home exercise programs administered by videotapes that contain electronic counters registering usage (Brewer et al 2004), embedding a motion sensor and counting device within an ankle exerciser (Belanger & Noel 1991) or using accelerometers to detect movement (Schlenk et al 2000). Brewer et al (2004) found that self-reports of home exercise completion in a postoperative ACL rehabilitation program overestimated adherence in relation to objective measurement of the same behavior.

Predictors of sport injury rehabilitation adherence

Personal factors, situational factors and cognitive and emotional responses to injury can all affect adherence to rehabilitation (Brewer 2001). This suggestion fits well with Wiese-Bjornstal et al's (1998) integrated model of psychological response to sport injury and rehabilitation (Fig. 11.4). Several personal factors have been positively correlated with sport injury rehabilitation adherence. These include pain tolerance (Byerly et al 1994, Fields et al 1995, Fisher at al 1988), health locus of control (Murphy et al 1999), task involvement (Duda et al 1989), self-motivation (Brewer et al 2000a, Duda et al 1989, Fields et al 1995, Fisher et al 1988) and tough-mindedness (Wittig & Schurr 1994).

As well as personal variables, several situational variables have been identified as positively related to sport injury rehabilitation adherence. These include a belief in the efficacy of the treatment (Brewer et al 2003, Duda et al 1989, Taylor & May 1996), rehabilitation scheduling convenience (Fields et al 1995, Fisher et al 1988), the importance or value of the rehabilitation to the athlete (Taylor & May 1996), perceived injury severity (Taylor & May 1996), perceived exertion during rehabilitation (Fisher et al 1988), social support for rehabilitation (Byerly et al 1994, Duda et al 1989, Finnie 1999) and comfort of the clinical environment (Fields et al 1995, Fisher et al 1988).

Cognitive and emotional responses to injury can have an impact on adherence levels, in addition to personal and situational variables, which are linked to adherence. For example, athletes who show high rehabilitation self-efficacy are more likely to adhere to rehabilitation programs (Brewer et al 2003, Milne et al 2005, Taylor & May 1996). Also, Daly et al (1995) reported that those athletes with a higher coping ability for their injuries tend to adhere better to rehabilitation regimens. Furthermore, Laubach et al (1996) indicated that athletes who attributed their recovery to stable and personally controllable factors adhered to higher levels than their counterparts who attributed their recovery to unstable factors that were outside of their control.

Enhancing sport injury rehabilitation adherence

Several strategies have been suggested to enhance adherence to sport injury rehabilitation. Given the range of cognitive, emotional and behavioral challenges faced by injured athletes (Kolt 2000),

it is not surprising that a multi-faceted approach to rehabilitation adherence has been suggested. Fisher et al (1993a), based on surveys of athletic trainers and athletes (Fisher & Hoisington 1993, Fisher et al 1993b), suggested that the key components to enhance adherence should be education, communication and rapport, social support, goal setting, treatment efficacy and tailoring, threats and scare tactics and athlete responsibility.

Education

Educating athletes on the nature of their injury, treatment rationale, realistic expectations and injury management have been recommended (Weiss & Troxel 1986). Despite this ideal, however, Webborn et al (1997) reported that 77% of injured athletes they interviewed misunderstood some aspect of their rehabilitation, and only 14% were given any written instructions. Also, Schneiders et al (1998), in a randomized controlled study, reported that patients who were given written exercise instructions adhered to 77% of their home exercise program compared to 38.1% for those who received verbal exercise instructions only. Similarly, Weeks et al (2002) documented the superiority of video instruction over still-photographic instruction in the acquisition, retention and motivation to perform common rehabilitation exercises.

Communication and rapport

Although no studies have been found that specifically examined the relationship between adherence and communication and rapport between practitioner and patient, several investigators have suggested that athletes who feel that medical professionals are genuinely interested in their wellbeing, and who are aware of the psychological manifestations relating to their injury, may be more highly motivated to adhere to programs (Byerly et al 1994, Duda et al 1989, Ford & Gordon 1993).

Social support

Approaches such as peer modeling and injury support groups have been recommended for use in sport injury rehabilitation (Flint 1991, Wiese et al 1991). Peer modeling involves linking a currently injured athlete with an athlete who has successfully rehabilitated (preferably from a similar injury). Injury support groups are useful in providing a forum for athletes to regularly voice concerns about their injury and rehabilitation. Such groups can provide mutual understanding and support and can help to motivate injured athletes (Weiss & Troxel 1986). Modeling has been shown to improve adherence to postsurgical knee rehabilitation (Flint 1991).

Goal setting and attainment

Considerable research has focused on goal setting as a strategy to enhance adherence (Fisher 1999). Correlational studies have shown that adherence to sport injury rehabilitation regimens is greater among those who report setting rehabilitation goals (Scherzer et al 2001). Experimental evidence indicates that goal setting can enhance adherence (Evans & Hardy 2002a, Penpraze & Mutrie 1999). The process of goal setting for injured athletes

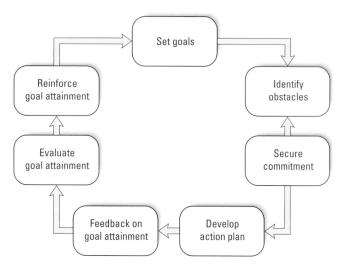

Figure 11.6 • Goal setting implementation process. (Reproduced from Burton D, Naylor S, Holliday B 2001 Goal setting in sport: investigating the goal effectiveness paradox. In Singer R N, Hausenblas H A, Janelle C M (eds) Handbook of sport psychology, 2nd edn. Copyright 2001 John Wiley & Sons, Inc. This material is used by permission of John Wiley & Sons, Inc.)

contains three important elements. First, athletes and physical therapists should work together to establish challenging yet realistic and positive goals for rehabilitation; it is paramount that these goals are recorded and measurable (Wiese & Weiss 1987). Second, to enhance a sense of control by athletes, strategies for achieving these goals should be negotiated by the athlete and the practitioner. Third, the agreed goals should be closely monitored, periodically evaluated and modified if necessary. See Fig. 11.6.

Treatment efficacy and tailoring

An athlete's perception of treatment efficacy is important to their belief that rehabilitation goals will be met; therefore, rehabilitation programs should be tailored to the needs of individual athletes. Duda et al (1989) argued that perceived treatment efficacy can have an important impact on adherence behaviors. Positive associations between belief in the efficacy of treatment and rehabilitation adherence have been documented in several studies (Brewer et al 2003, Duda et al 1989, Noyes et al 1987, Taylor & May 1996). Therefore, in fostering perceptions of treatment efficacy, physical therapists should ensure that athletes are capable of performing their rehabilitation tasks and identifying the context of their rehabilitation as meaningful and worthwhile. Of interest, is that complex rehabilitation programs (e.g. those that contain skills beyond the abilities of the patient) can lead to lower levels of adherence (Sluijs et al 1993).

Athlete responsibility

Athletes need to feel responsible for their own rehabilitation (Fisher et al 1993a). By having a sense of control over their rehabilitation programs, athletes can increase commitment and adherence to the behaviors required for successful rehabilitation.

This concept has been supported by Laubach et al (1996), who reported a positive relationship between personal control and rehabilitation adherence in a sample of athletes following knee surgery.

Threats and scare tactics

Increasing an athlete's perception of severity of an injury and susceptibility to poor rehabilitation, reinjury or more serious debilitation can enhance their ability to adhere to appropriate rehabilitation guidelines (Taylor & May 1996). However, one must be careful in using such tactics, as by using threats or ultimatums, practitioners risk losing respect or harming rapport with athletes (Fisher et al 1993a). This approach would usually be used as a last resort to improve adherence.

There are several other cognitive-behavioral approaches that have been suggested for enhancing rehabilitation adherence, but, like those described above, most have received little empirical support. These include imagery (Heil 1993, Weiss & Troxel 1986) and relaxation (Duda et al 1989, Weiss & Troxel 1986, Wiese & Weiss 1987). Scherzer et al (2001) found that self-reported use of imagery and positive self-talk during postoperative ACL rehabilitation was positively correlated with adherence to the rehabilitation program.

Role of physical therapists in providing psychological support for injured athletes

Physical therapists are suited to provide some form of psychological assistance to injured athletes (Driediger et al 2006, Francis et al 2000, Gordon et al 1998, Hemmings & Povey 2001, Kolt 2000, Ninedek & Kolt 2000, Pearson & Jones 1992). There are four main reasons for this suggestion (Kolt 2000). First, physical therapists are closely involved with injured athletes during rehabilitation and spend longer periods of time with athletes than most other health professionals. Athletes may be more likely, therefore, to raise psychological issues with them. Second, with the use of touch in physical therapy techniques (an integral aspect of physiotherapeutic skills), athletes are more likely to open up about psychosocial issues (Nathan 1999), making it beneficial to deal with them at the time, particularly if these issues are affecting recovery progress. Third, due to the psychological after-effects of injury, it appears reasonable that such issues are discussed concurrently with the physical aspects of rehabilitation so as to maximally benefit the psychological and physical rehabilitation processes. Finally, according to some research reports (e.g. Pearson & Jones 1992), injured athletes feel that physical therapists are in an ideal position to provide them with basic counseling and psychological support.

If physical therapists are to incorporate basic psychological techniques into their rehabilitation, their willingness and ability to deliver appropriate services must be established. From survey-based studies (Francis et al 2000, Hemmings & Povey 2002, Ninedek & Kolt 2000), physical therapists reported that having knowledge about setting realistic goals, using a positive and sincere communication style, understanding individual motivation, understanding stress and anxiety, encouraging positive self-thoughts, encouraging self-confidence and reducing depression were all important for them in dealing with injured athletes. Similar findings have been reported for athletic trainers (Wiese et al 1991). While not directly in the area of sport, Potter et al (2003a) interviewed physical therapists about the strategies they use to deal with 'difficult' patients. They concluded that further training in the area of communication and behavior modification techniques were a high priority.

Despite these findings, however, physical therapists have suggested that they were limited in their ability to deal with psychosocial aspects of the recovery process and desired further practical training in this area (Gordon et al 1991, Hemmings & Povey 2002). Potter et al (2003b), after seeking the opinion of patients, suggested that specific training in the area of communication skills would help ensure a more patient-centered approach to treatment and optimize the physical therapist–patient interaction. A possible goal for future research and education involves developing a standardized educational framework for sport injury rehabilitation personnel (Gordon et al 1998). Further research efforts could examine the effects of physical therapists actively implementing basic psychological intervention strategies on the recovery of injured athletes.

There appears to be adequate justification for physical therapists to play a more active role in managing some of the basic psychological consequences of sport and exercise injuries. It should be emphasized, however, that where more severe psychological difficulties are experienced, athletes should be referred to other professionals (e.g. psychologists, sport psychologists, psychiatrists) for further specialized intervention.

Clearly, qualified sport psychologists are the best-trained members of sports medicine teams to address athletes' post-injury emotional responses (Crossman 1997, Brewer et al 1991). However, access to a sport psychologist is often unavailable or limited in clinical settings (Gordon et al 1998, Larson et al 1996, Moulton et al 1997), and in circumstances where they are available, many athletes are reticent to accept formal psychological help (Pinkerton et al 1989). Some athletes view seeking psychological help as a sign of weakness and would rather endure the negative consequences of a problematic rehabilitation than request formal psychological assistance (Kolt 2000).

Cognitive-behavioral interventions for injured athletes

It is not the intent of this chapter to provide a detailed account of the many cognitive-behavioral techniques that can be of use to injured athletes during the rehabilitation program. Details on these techniques can be found in many sources (e.g. Crossman 2001, Heil 1993, Kolt 2000, Pargman 1999, Ray & Wiese-Bjornstal 1999, Taylor & Taylor 1997). However, this chapter provides a brief outline of certain cognitive-behavioral techniques that are of use to the physical therapist and other sports medicine practitioners in managing sport and exercise injuries.

Relaxation techniques

Several forms of relaxation exist that achieve their function by various means. Given that the stress and pain associated with injury can elicit muscle tension which, in turn, restricts blood flow and further increases pain (Cousins & Phillips 1985), relaxation techniques that directly target muscle are indicated in many circumstances. The most common form of muscular relaxation is progressive relaxation (Jacobson 1938). Progressive relaxation involves systematically relaxing major skeletal muscle groups by firstly recognizing muscle tension present (initially achieved by contracting the muscles), then by relaxing those muscles. The role of muscle contraction before relaxation is proposed in order to sensitize the individual to the recognition of muscle tension, so that the individual learns what the sensations of relaxed muscle are like. As the individual becomes more familiar with the technique, it may be possible to merely relax muscle groups from whatever condition they are in at rest, rather than having to contract muscle groups first. It should be noted that divided opinion exists regarding the value of muscle contraction before relaxation (Lucic et al 1991, O'Bannon et al 1987, Payne 2000). When using progressive relaxation on athletes with pain it is important to monitor that the level of muscle contraction used in the exercise does not aggravate pain symptoms.

Another commonly used relaxation technique is Benson's Relaxation Response (Benson 1975). As outlined in Chapter 9, this technique is based on the proposal that there are four common elements underlying the elicitation of a relaxation response. The first element is a quiet environment, which allows for the reduction of external distractions. The second is adopting a comfortable position to reduce undue muscular tension. The third is an object to dwell on, such as the repetition of a word. The fourth element is a passive attitude that includes emptying all other thoughts from one's mind, and letting distracting thoughts that do return pass on while returning to a focused state. Practically speaking, Benson's Relaxation Response is based around transcendental meditation and involves focus on breathing, repetition of a word in time with breathing and in more recent adaptations, imagery that focuses on an object that moves in time with the patient's breathing (Kolt & McConville 2000). Benson's Relaxation Response works predominantly by distracting or drawing focus away from the stressors associated with injury and rehabilitation. As it is not uncommon for an injured athlete to continually think about the negative consequences of their injury, Benson's Relaxation Response can distract them from this and allow a better focus on the rehabilitation activities. It can also provide a greater sense of control over pain, reduce the negative emotions associated with pain and injury (Taylor & Taylor 1998) and facilitate imagery interventions (Cupal & Brewer 2001). For a more detailed account of relaxation techniques refer to Payne (2000) or Payne (2004).

Cognitive rehearsal

The term cognitive rehearsal refers to cognitive-behavioral techniques such as mental rehearsal, visualization, mental practice and imagery, and is often used synonymously with these terms. The technique relates to practicing a skill in one's mind. As described by White & Hardy (1998), it involves a cognitive experience that mimics real experience. That is, it utilizes athletes' abilities to feel a movement, as well as hear the sounds and incorporate other senses in rehearsing an activity without actually experiencing the real thing. A more recent definition relevant to the broader health sciences describes imagery as a psychophysiological process, which is dynamic and quasi-real (Menzies & Gill Taylor 2004).

Cognitive rehearsal is used by athletes for several reasons. Athletes typically use this skill to improve a variety of performance-related issues, including technique, mental preparation, tactics and competitive performance (Vealey & Walter 1993). Only relatively recently, however, has cognitive rehearsal been considered as a tool to facilitate rehabilitation and return to sport following injury (Green 1992). Shaffer & Wiese-Bjornstal (1999) suggested using cognitive rehearsal as an adjunct to physical therapy so that athletes can achieve a specific mindset for maintaining a positive outlook, controlling stress, using positive and descriptive self-talk and sustaining belief in the rehabilitation process. They also suggested that using cognitive rehearsal enables athletes to develop a sense of control over the injured body part. Other important benefits of cognitive rehearsal during rehabilitation include coping with pain and keeping physical skills from deteriorating during periods of no physical practice (Richardson & Latuda 1995). In a recent investigation by Driediger et al (2006) injured athletes believed that imagery assisted in effective rehabilitation through cognitive, motivational and healing methods. The athletes reported they used imagery to learn and correctly execute rehabilitation exercises, and to assist in goal setting, to help maintain concentration, and to encourage a positive attitude (e.g. by imaging being fully recovered). As well, these athletes reported using imagery in several forms to control pain.

As described in Chapter 9, different forms of imagery (or cognitive rehearsal) have been used in the management of pain. Imagery of pleasant situations, guided by either the practitioner or by the patient, is an internal dissociative strategy shown to be effective in reducing pain in sport and medical settings (Whitmarsh & Alderman 1993). In general, imagery involves patients imagining themselves in a relaxing environment (i.e. an environment that has a relaxing meaning to the patient), and focusing on how it feels to be in that environment. As is evident, this form of imagery aims to distract the patient from the feeling of pain or from the other stressors associated with injury and abstinence from training. From clinical experience, the more complex the scene to be imaged, and the more detail that patients are asked to attend to (i.e. using not just the visual sense but the tactile and auditory senses as well), the more they are distracted from their pain.

Specific types of imagery have also been developed. For example, in pain management imagery (Ievleva & Orlick 1999), patients could imagine the pain being washed away or see cool colors soothing and reducing any inflammation and pain (e.g. seeing cool blue colors running through the painful area; imaging

the pain leaving the body; imagining an ice-pack over the painful area). In cognitive rehearsal based around sports skills, injured athletes can rehearse sport techniques to avoid skill level decline during rehabilitation (Hall 2001).

There is an increasing body of research suggesting that cognitive rehearsal can assist with pain and healing in athletes (Cupal & Brewer 2001, Ievleva & Orlick 1999) and with many other aspects of rehabilitation (Green 1999, Hall 2001, Newsom et al 2003, Taylor & Taylor 1997). For example, Cupal & Brewer (2001) found that athletes who received an intervention that combined relaxation and guided imagery had greater knee strength and reported less knee pain and reinjury anxiety 6 months after ACL reconstruction surgery than those who received no treatment or a placebo treatment.

Systematic desensitization

Systematic desensitization is the process of combining relaxation and imagery to overcome progressively stressful or fearful events (Shaffer & Wiese-Bjornstal 1999). For example, an athlete could image or visualize situations in which anxiety progressively heightens (e.g. returning for the first training session, returning to the first competitive event), and with each event being imaged (from least to most fear provoking), use relaxation to curb anxiety until it dissipates. This process is repeated until the list of anxiety producing situations has been dealt with. Despite the widespread use of this technique in sport settings, no research other than a single case study (Rotella & Campbell 1983) has investigated its use in rehabilitation.

Cognitive restructuring

Cognitive restructuring involves athletes reframing negative and irrational thoughts into more positive, rational thoughts. This involves athletes firstly recognizing their negative self-talk, and then replacing it with positive or productive comments. Ievleva & Orlick (1991) reported that injured athletes who healed faster were more likely to use self-talk that was positive and encouraging compared to their counterparts who healed at a slower rate. Cognitive restructuring has been based on the behavior change work of Ellis (1967).

Goal setting

Goal setting has been well recognized as an important part of rehabilitation (Evans & Hardy 2002a, 2002b, Shaffer & Wiese-Bjornstal 1999). As this is a skill that many athletes are accustomed to using, adapting it to the rehabilitation setting should not be difficult. It has been suggested by Danish et al (1993) that teaching goal setting is a means of empowerment that encourages athletes to take greater responsibility for their return to sport following injury. Research has documented the effectiveness of goal setting in improving sport injury rehabilitation processes and outcomes (Theodorakis et al 1997). For example, a 5-week goal setting intervention for injured athletes was related to higher levels of rehabilitation adherence and self-efficacy, and stronger perceptions of control in the rehabilitation setting (Evans & Hardy 2002a, 2002b). General principles of goal setting have been covered earlier in the chapter in relation to enhancing rehabilitation adherence. The goal setting process (Fig. 11. 6) has been well described by Burton et al (2001).

Social support

The role of social support in injury rehabilitation has been widely investigated (Brewer 2001). In this context, social support refers to the quantity, quality and type of interactions that athletes have with other people (Udry 1996). Richman et al (1993) described eight types of social support: listening support, emotional support, emotional challenge, task appreciation, task challenge, reality confirmation, material assistance and personal assistance. Social support providers in sports injury rehabilitation can include physical therapists, medical personnel, coaches, team-mates, friends, family members, significant others and sports administrators. Research has shown that, in general, injured athletes perceive family members and team-mates as better social support providers than medical professionals and coaches (although they do recognize that medical professionals and coaches are the most frequent providers of technical and informational support) (see reviews by Bianco & Eklund 2001 and Brewer 2001). A study of social support for injured adolescent athletes showed that higher levels of social support were associated with lower initial depressive symptoms postinjury (Manuel et al 2002). It should be noted that the need for different types of social support changes throughout the rehabilitation period and it appears that the need for emotional support decreases as rehabilitation progresses, with a possible need for increased emotional support as the athlete returns to sport participation (Johnston & Carroll 1998).

Summary

Research in the area of psychological aspects of injury and rehabilitation is growing, as is the integration of psychological and physical approaches to rehabilitation in clinical practice. Models of the psychological predictors of injury have been developed and increasingly researched over the past 20 years. Findings have indicated a strong relationship between stress and injury in sport (Williams & Andersen 1998). A more recent area of research is that of the psychology of sport injury rehabilitation. Although athlete adherence to sport injury rehabilitation programs has been addressed both clinically and with empirical research, the use of cognitive-behavioral techniques in rehabilitation is still based largely on anecdotal evidence. Extrapolating from research in other areas of health, it stands to reason that such techniques are potentially valuable to injured athletes.

If physical therapists and other sports medicine practitioners are to integrate basic psychological techniques into their rehabilitation programs, they must ensure that they seek appropriate training in these skills, and in how to combine a physical and psychological approach to rehabilitation.

References

Albinson C B, Petrie T 2003 Cognitive appraisals, stress, and coping: Preinjury and postinjury factors influencing psychological adjustment to athletic injury. Journal of Sport Rehabilitation 12:306–322

Almekinders L C, Almekinders S V 1994 Outcome in the treatment of chronic overuse sports injuries: a retrospective study. Journal of Orthopaedic and Sports Physical Therapy 19:157–161

Alzate Saez de Heredia R, Ramirez A, Lazaro I 2004 The effect of psychological response on recovery of sport injury. Research in Sports Medicine 12:15–31

Andersen M B, Stoove M A 1998 The sanctity of p < .05 obfuscates good stuff: a comment on Kerr and Goss. Journal of Applied Sport Psychology 10:168–173

Andersen M B, Williams J M 1988 A model of stress and athletic injury: prediction and prevention. Journal of Sport and Exercise Psychology 10:294–306

Andersen M B, Williams J M 1999 Athletic injury, psychosocial factors, and perceptual changes during stress. Journal of Sports Science 17:735–751

Astle S J 1986 The experience of loss in athletes. Journal of Sports Medicine and Physical Fitness 26:279–284

Beck A T 1976 Cognitive therapy and the emotional disorders. Penguin, London

Belanger A Y, Noel G 1990 Compliance to and effects of a home strengthening exercise program for adult dystrophic patients: a pilot study. Physiotherapy Canada 43:24–30

Benson H 1975 The relaxation response. William Morrow, New York

Bianco T, Eklund R C 2001 Conceptual considerations for social support research in sport and exercise settings: The case of sport injury. Journal of Sport and Exercise Psychology 23:85–107

Bianco T, Malo S, Orlick T 1999 Sport injury and illness: elite skiers describe their experiences. Research Quarterly for Exercise and Sport 70:157–169

Blackwell B, McCullagh P 1990 The relationship of athletic injury to life stress, competitive anxiety and coping resources. Athletic Training 25:23–27

Bramwell S T, Masuda M, Wagner N N et al 1975 Psychosocial factors in athletic injuries: development and application of the Social and Athletic Readjustment Rating Scale (SARRS). Journal of Human Stress 1:6–20

Brewer B W 1994 Review and critique of models of psychological adjustment to athletic injury. Journal of Applied Sport Psychology 6:87–100

Brewer B W 1998 Adherence to sport injury rehabilitation programs. Journal of Applied Sport Psychology 10:70–82

Brewer B W 2001 Psychology of sport injury rehabilitation. In: Singer R N, Hausenblas H A, Janelle C M (eds) Handbook of sport psychology, 2nd edn. John Wiley, New York

Brewer B W, Petrie T A 1995 A comparison between injured and uninjured football players on selected psychosocial variables. Academic Athletic Journal 10:11–18

Brewer B W, Van Raalte J L, Linder D E 1991 Role of the sport psychologist in treating injured athletes: a survey of sports medicine providers. Journal of Applied Sport Psychology 3:183–190

Brewer B W, Van Raalte J L, Cornelius A E et al 2000a Psychological factors, rehabilitation adherence, and rehabilitation outcome following anterior cruciate ligament reconstruction. Rehabilitation Psychology 45:20–37

Brewer B W, Van Raalte J L, Petitpas A J et al 2000b Preliminary psychometric evaluation of a measure of adherence to clinic-based sport injury rehabilitation. Physical Therapy in Sport 1:68–74

Brewer B W, Andersen M B, Van Raalte J L 2002a Psychological aspects of sport injury rehabilitation: toward a biopsychosocial approach. In: Mostofsky D I, Zaichkowsky L D (eds) Medical aspects of sport and exercise. Fitness Information Technology, Morgantown, WV

Brewer B W, Avondoglio J B, Cornelius A E et al 2002b Construct validity and interrater agreement of the Sport Injury Rehabilitation Adherence Scale. Journal of Sport Rehabilitation 11:170–178

Brewer B W, Cornelius A E, Van Raalte J L et al 2004 Rehabilitation adherence and anterior cruciate ligament outcome. Psychology, Health and Medicine 9:163–175

Brown R B 1971 Personality characteristics related to injury in football. Research Quarterly 42:133–138

Burt C W, Overpeck M D 2001 Emergency visits for sports-related injuries. Annals of Emergency Medicine 37:301–338

Burton D, Naylor S, Holliday B 2001 Goal setting in sport: investigating the goal effectiveness paradox. In: Singer R N, Hausenblas H A, Janelle C M (eds) Handbook of sport psychology, 2nd edn. John Wiley, New York

Byerly P N, Worrell T, Gahimer J et al 1994 Rehabilitation compliance in an athletic training environment. Journal of Athletic Training 29:352–355

Chan C S, Crossman H Y 1988 Psychological effects of running loss on consistent runners. Perceptual and Motor Skills 66:875–883

Cohen S, Rodriguez M S 1995 Pathways linking affective disturbance and physical disorders. Health Psychology 14:374–380

Conn J M, Annest J L, Gilchrist J 2003 Sports and recreation related injury episodes in the US population 1997–1999. Injury Prevention 9:117–123

Cousins M J, Phillips G D 1985 Acute pain management. Clinics in Critical Care Medicine 8:82–117

Crossman J 1997 Psychological rehabilitation from sports injuries. Sports Medicine 23:333–339

Crossman J (ed) 2001 Coping with sports injuries: psychological strategies for rehabilitation. Oxford University Press, Oxford

Crossman J, Roch J 1991 An observation instrument for use in sports medicine clinics. Journal of the Canadian Athletic Therapists Association April:10–13

Cupal D D, Brewer B W 2001 Effects of relaxation and guided imagery on knee strength, reinjury anxiety, and pain following anterior cruciate ligament reconstruction. Rehabilitation Psychology 46:28–43

Daly J M, Brewer B W, Van Raalte J L et al 1995 Cognitive appraisal, emotional adjustment, and adherence to rehabilitation following knee surgery. Journal of Sport Rehabilitation 4:23–30

Danish S J, Petitpas A J, Hale B D 1993 Life development interventions for athletes: life skills through sports. Counseling Psychologist 21:352–385

Danish S J, Petitpas A, Hale B D 1995 Psychological interventions: a life developmental model. In: Murphy S (ed) Sport psychology interventions. Human Kinetics, Champaign, IL

Davis J 1991 Sports injuries and stress management: an opportunity for research. The Sport Psychologist 5:175–182

Dawes H, Roach N K 1997 Emotional responses of athletes to injury and treatment. Physiotherapy 83:243–247

Derscheid G L, Feiring D C 1987 A statistical analysis to characterize treatment adherence of the 18 most common diagnoses seen at a sports medicine clinic. Journal of Orthopaedic and Sports Physical Therapy 9:40–46

DeWitt D J 1980 Cognitive and biofeedback training for stress reduction with university athletes. Journal of Sport Psychology 2:288–294

Driediger M, Hall C, Callow N 2006 Imagery use by injured athletes: a qualitative analysis. Journal of Sports Sciences 24:261–272

Duda J L, Smart A E, Tappe M L 1989 Predictors of adherence in the rehabilitation of athletic injuries: an application of personal investment theory. Journal of Sport and Exercise Psychology 11:367–381

Dunbar-Jacob J, Dunning E J, Dwyer K 1993 Compliance research in pediatric and adolescent populations: two decades of research. In: Krasnegor N A, Epstein L, Johnson S B et al (eds) Developmental aspects of health compliance behavior. Erlbaum, Hillsdale, NJ

Dunn E C, Smith R E, Smoll F L 2001 Do sport-specific stressors predict athletic injury? Journal of Science and Medicine in Sport 4:283–291

Durso-Cupal D 1998 Psychological interventions in sport injury prevention and rehabilitation. Journal of Applied Sport Psychology 10:103–123

Ellis A 1967 Rational-emotive psychotherapy. In: Arbuckle D S (ed) Counseling and psychotherapy: an overview. McGraw-Hill, New York

Evans L, Hardy L 1999 Psychological and emotional response to athletic injury: measurement issues. In: Pargman D (ed) Psychological bases of sport injury, 2nd edn. Fitness Information Technology, Morgantown, WV

Evans L, Hardy L 2002a Injury rehabilitation: a goal-setting intervention study. Research Quarterly for Exercise and Sport 73:310–319

Evans L, Hardy L 2002b Injury rehabilitation: a qualitative follow-up study. Research Quarterly for Exercise and Sport 73:320–329

Fawkner H J, McMurray N E, Summers J J 1999 Athletic injury and minor life events: a prospective study. Journal of Science and Medicine in Sport 2:117–124

Fields J, Murphey M, Horodyski M et al 1995 Factors associated with adherence to sport injury rehabilitation in college-age recreational athletes. Journal of Sport Rehabilitation 4:172–180

Finch C, Valuri G, Ozanne-Smith J 1998 Sport and active recreation injuries in Australia: evidence from emergency department presentations. British Journal of Sports Medicine 32:220–225

Finnie S B 1999 The rehabilitation support team: using social support to aid compliance to sports injury rehabilitation programs. Paper presented at the annual meeting of the Association for the Advancement of Applied Sport Psychology, Banff, Canada

Fisher A C 1999 Counseling for improved rehabilitation adherence. In: Ray R, Wiese-Bjornstal D M (eds) Counseling in sports medicine. Human Kinetics, Champaign, IL

Fisher A C, Hoisington L L 1993 Injured athletes' attitudes and judgments toward rehabilitation adherence. Journal of the National Athletic Trainers Association 28:48–54

Fisher A C, Domm M A, Wuest D A 1988 Adherence to sports injury rehabilitation programs. Physician and Sportsmedicine 16(7):47–51

Fisher A C, Mullins S A, Frye P A 1993a Athletic trainers' attitudes and judgements of injured athletes' rehabilitation adherence. Journal of Athletic Training 28:43–47

Fisher A C, Scriber K C, Matheny M L et al 1993b Enhancing athletic injury rehabilitation adherence. Journal of Athletic Training 28:312–318

Flint F A 1991 The psychological effects of modeling in athletic injury rehabilitation. Unpublished doctoral dissertation, University of Oregon

Flint F A 1998 Integrating sport psychology and sports medicine in research: the dilemmas. Journal of Applied Sport Psychology 10:83–102

Folkman S, Lazarus R S 1985 If it changes it must be a process: study of emotion and coping during three stages of a college examination. Journal of Personality and Social Psychology 48:150–170

Ford I W, Gordon S 1993 Social support and athletic injury: the perspective of sport physiotherapists. Australian Journal of Science and Medicine in Sport 25:17–25

Ford I W, Gordon S 1999 Coping with sport injury: resource loss and the role of social support. Journal of Personal and Interpersonal Loss 4:243–256

Francis S R, Andersen M B, Maley P 2000 Physiotherapists' and male professional athletes' views on psychological skills for rehabilitation. Journal of Science and Medicine in Sport 3:17–29

Galambos S A, Terry P C, Moyle G M et al 2005 Psychological predictors of injury among elite athletes. British Journal of Sports Medicine 39:351–354

Gordon S 1986 Sport psychology and the injured athlete: a cognitive-behavioral approach to injury response and injury rehabilitation. Science Periodical on Research and Technology in Sport March:1–10

Gordon S, Milios S, Grove J R 1991 Psychological aspects of the recovery process from sport injury: the perspective of sports physiotherapists. Australian Journal of Science and Medicine in Sport 23:53–60

Gordon S, Potter M, Ford I W 1998 Towards a psychoeducational curriculum for training sport-injury rehabilitation personnel. Journal of Applied Sport Psychology 10:140–156

Gould D, Udry E, Bridges D et al 1997 Stress sources encountered when rehabilitating from season-ending ski injuries. The Sport Psychologist 11:361–378

Govern J W, Koppenhaver R 1965 Attempt to predict athletic injuries. Medical Times 93:421–422

Green L 1992 The use of imagery in the rehabilitation of injured athletes. The Sport Psychologist 6:416–428

Green L B 1999 The use of imagery in the rehabilitation of injured athletes. In: Pargman D (ed) Psychological bases of sport injuries, 2nd edn. Fitness Information Technology, Morgantown, WV

Hall C R 2001 Imagery in sport and exercise. In: Singer R N, Hausenblas H A, Janelle C M (eds) Handbook of sport psychology, 2nd edn. John Wiley, New York

Heil J 1993 Psychology of sport injury. Human Kinetics, Champaign, IL

Hemmings B, Povey L 2002 Views of chartered physiotherapists on the psychological content of their practice: a preliminary study in the United Kingdom. British Journal of Sports Medicine 31:61–64

Horsley C 1995 Understanding and managing the injured athlete. In: Zuluaga M, Briggs C, Carlisle J et al (eds) Sports physiotherapy: applied science and practice. Churchill Livingstone, Melbourne

Ievleva L, Orlick T 1991 Mental links to enhanced healing: an exploratory study. The Sport Psychologist 5:25–40

Ievleva L, Orlick T 1999 Mental paths to enhanced recovery from a sports injury. In: Pargman D (ed) Psychological bases of sport injuries, 2nd edn. Fitness Information Technology, Morgantown, WV

Jacobson E 1938 Progressive relaxation. University of Chicago Press, Chicago

Jevon S M, Johnston L H 2003 The perceived knowledge and attitudes of governing body chartered physiotherapists towards the psychological aspects of rehabilitation. Physical Therapy in Sport 4:74–81

Johnson U, Ekengren J, Andersen M 2005 Injury in Sweden: helping soccer players at risk. Journal of Sport and Exercise Psychology 27:32–38

Johnston L H, Carroll D 1998 The provision of social support to injured athletes: a qualitative analysis. Journal of Sport Rehabilitation 7:267–284

Kerr G, Goss J 1996 The effects of a stress management program on injuries and stress levels. Journal of Applied Sport Psychology 8:109–117

Kirkby R J 1995 Psychological factors in sport injuries. In: Morris T, Summers J (eds) Sport psychology. Theories, applications and issues. John Wiley, Milton, Australia

Kleiber D A, Brock S C 1992 The effect of career-ending injuries on the subsequent well-being of elite college athletes. Sociology of Sport Journal 9:70–75

Kolt G S 2000 Doing sport psychology with injured athletes. In: Andersen M B (ed) Doing sport psychology. Human Kinetics, Champaign, IL, p 223–236

Kolt G S, Brewer B W, Pizzar T et al 2007 The Sport Injury Rehabilitation Adherence Scale: a reliable scale for use in clinical physiotherapy. Physiotherapy 93:17–22

Kolt G S, Kirkby R J 1996 Injury in Australian female competitive gymnasts: a psychological perspective. Australian Journal of Physiotherapy 42:121–126

Kolt G S, McConville L C 2000 The effects of a Feldenkrais Awareness Through Movement program on state anxiety. Journal of Bodywork and Movement Therapies 4:216–220

Kolt G S, McEvoy J F 2003 Adherence to rehabilitation in patients with low back pain. Manual Therapy 8:110–116

Kolt G S, Pizzari T, Schoo A M M et al 2001 The Sport Injury Rehabilitation Adherence Scale: a reliable and valid measure of clinic-based injury rehabilitation. In: Papaioannou A, Goudas M, Theodorakis Y (eds) Proceedings of the 10th World Congress of Sport Psychology (vol 4). Christodoulidi, Thessaloniki, Greece, p 144–146

Kolt G S, Hume P A, Smith P et al 2004 Effects of a stress management program on injury and stress of competitive gymnasts. Perceptual and Motor Skills 99:195–207.

Kubler-Ross E 1969 On death and dying. Macmillan, New York

Larson G A, Starkey C, Zaichkowsky L D 1996 Psychological aspects of athletic injuries as perceived by athletic trainers. The Sport Psychologist 10:37–47

Laubach W J, Brewer B W, Van Raalte J L et al 1996 Attributions for recovery and adherence to sport injury rehabilitation. Australian Journal of Science and Medicine in Sport 28:30–34

Leadbetter W B 1994 Soft tissue athletic injury. In: Fu F H, Stone D A (eds) Sports injuries: mechanisms, prevention, and treatment. Williams and Wilkins, Baltimore, MD

Leddy M H, Lambert M J, Ogles B M 1994 Psychological consequences of athletic injury among high-level competitors. Research Quarterly for Exercise and Sport 65:347–354

Lucic K S, Steffen J J, Harrigan J A et al 1991 Progressive relaxation training: muscle contraction before relaxation? Behavior Therapy 22:249–256

Lynch G P 1988 Athletic injuries and the practicing sport psychologist: practical guidelines for assisting athletes. The Sport Psychologist 2:161–167

Lysens R, Steverlynk A, Vanden Auweele Y et al 1984 The predictability of sports injuries. Sports Medicine 1:6–10

McDonald S A, Hardy C J 1990 Affective response patterns of the injured athlete: an exploratory analysis. The Sport Psychologist 4:261–274

McGowan R W, Pierce E F, Williams N et al 1994 Athletic injury and self-diminution. Journal of Sports Medicine and Physical Fitness 34:299–304

McKenna J, Delaney H, Phillips S 2002 Physiotherapists' lived experience of rehabilitating elite athletes. Physical Therapy in Sport 3:66–78

Macchi R, Crossman J 1996 After the fall: reflections of injured classical ballet dancers. Journal of Sport Behavior 19:221–234

Maddison R, Prapavessis H 2005 A psychological approach to the prediction and prevention of athletic injury. Journal of Sport and Exercise Psychology 27:289–310

Manuel J C, Shilt J S, Curl W W et al 2002 Coping with sports injuries: an examination of the adolescent athlete. Journal of Adolescent Health 31:391–393

Matthews K A, Shumaker S A, Bowen D J et al 1997 Women's Health Initiative: Why now? What is it? What's new. American Psychologist 52:101–116

May J R, Brown L 1989 Delivery of psychological services to the US alpine ski team prior to and during the Olympics in Calgary. The Sport Psychologist 3:320–329

Medibank Private 2004 Medibank Private sports injuries report. Medibank Private Limited, Melbourne

Meichenbaum D 1985 Stress inoculation training. Pergamon, New York

Meichenbaum D, Turk D C 1987 Facilitating treatment adherence: a practitioner's guidebook. Plenum, New York

Menzies V, Gill Taylor A 2004 The idea of imagination: an analysis of 'imagery'. Advances in Mind-Body Medicine 20:4–10

Miller W N 1998 Athletic injury: mood disturbances and hardiness of intercollegiate athletes [abstract]. Journal of Applied Sport Psychology 10 (suppl.):S127–S128

Milne M, Hall C, Forwell L 2005 Self-efficacy, imagery use, and adherence to rehabilitation by injured athletes. Journal of Sport Rehabilitation 14:150–167

Morrey M A, Stuart M J, Smith A M et al 1999 A longitudinal examination of athletes' emotional and cognitive responses to anterior cruciate ligament injury. Clinical Journal of Sport Medicine 9:63–69

Moulton M A, Molstad S, Turner A 1997 The role of athletic trainers in counseling collegiate athletes. Journal of Athletic Training 32:148–150

Murphy G C, Foreman P E, Simpson C A et al 1999 The development of a locus of control measure predictive of injured athletes' adherence to treatment. Journal of Science and Medicine in Sport 2:145–152

Nathan B 1999 Touch and emotion in manual therapy. Churchill Livingstone, London

NEISS data highlights 1998 Consumer Product Safety Review 3:4–6

Newsom J, Knight P, Balnave R 2003 Use of mental imagery to limit strength loss after immobilization. Journal of Sport Rehabilitation 12:249–258

Ninedek A, Kolt G S 2000 Sports physiotherapists' perceptions of psychological strategies in sport injury rehabilitation. Journal of Sport Rehabilitation 9:191–206

O'Bannon R M, Rickard H C, Runcie D 1987 Progressive relaxation as a function of procedural variations and anxiety level. International Journal of Psychophysiology 5:207–214

Ogilvie B C, Tutko T A 1966 Problem athletes and how to handle them. Pelham, London

Pargman D (ed) 1999 Psychological bases of sport injury, 2nd edn. Fitness Information Technology, Morgantown, WV

Payne R A 2000 Relaxation techniques. A practical handbook for the health care professional, 2nd edn. Churchill Livingstone, Edinburgh

Payne R A 2004 Relaxation techniques. In: Kolt G S, Andersen M B (eds) Psychology in the physical and manual therapies. Churchill Livingstone, Edinburgh, p 111–124

Pearson L, Jones G 1992 Emotional effects of sports injuries: implications for physiotherapists. Physiotherapy 78:762–770

Penpraze P, Mutrie N 1999 Effectiveness of goal setting in an injury rehabilitation programme for increasing patient understanding and compliance. British Journal of Sports Medicine 33:60

Peretz D 1970 Development, object-relationships, and loss. In: Schoenberg B, Carr A C, Peretz D et al (eds) Loss and grief: psychological management in medical practice. Columbia University Press, New York

Perna F M, Antoni M H, Baum A et al 2003 Cognitive behavioral stress management effects on injury and illness among competitive athletes: a randomized clinical trial. Annals of Behavioral Medicine 25:66–73

Petitpas A, Danish S J 1995 Caring for injured athletes. In: Murphy S M (ed) Sport psychology interventions. Human Kinetics, Champaign, IL

Petrie T A 1993a The moderating effects of social support and playing status on the life stress-injury relationship. Journal of Applied Sport Psychology 5:1–16

Petrie T A 1993b Coping skills, competitive trait anxiety, and playing status: moderating effects of the life stress-injury relationship. Journal of Sport and Exercise Psychology 15:261–274

Pinkerton R S, Hinz L D, Borrow J C 1989 The college student athlete: psychological considerations and interventions. Journal of American College Health 37:218–225

Pizzari T, Taylor N F, McBurney H et al 2005 Adherence to rehabilitation after anterior cruciate ligament reconstructive surgery: implications for outcome. Journal of Sport Rehabilitation 14:201–214

Potter M, Gordon S, Hamer P 2003a The difficult patient in private practice physiotherapy: a qualitative study. Australian Journal of Physiotherapy 49:53–61

Potter M, Gordon S, Hamer P 2003b The physiotherapy experience in private practice: the patients' perspective. Australian Journal of Physiotherapy 49:195–202

Quinn A M, Fallon B J 1999 The changes in psychological characteristics and reactions of elite athletes from injury onset until full recovery. Journal of Applied Sport Psychology 11:210–229

Ray R, Wiese-Bjornstal (eds) 1999 Counseling in sports medicine. Human Kinetics, Champaign, IL

Richardson P A, Latuda L M 1995 Therapeutic imagery and athletic injuries. Journal of Athletic Training 30:10–12

Richman J M, Rosenfeld L B, Hardy C J 1993 The Social Support Survey: a validation study of a clinical measure of the social support process. Research on Social Work Practice 3:288–311

Rose J, Jevne R F J 1993 Psychosocial processes associated with sport injuries. The Sport Psychologist 7:309–328

Rotella R J, Campbell M S 1983 Systematic desensitization: psychological rehabilitation of injured athletes. Athletic Training 18:140–142, 151

Rotella R J, Ogilvie B C, Perrin D H 1999 The malingering athlete: psychological considerations. In: Pargman D (ed) Psychological bases of sport injuries, 2nd edn. Fitness Information Technology, Morgantown, WV

San Jose A 2003 Injury of elite athletes: sport- and gender-related representations. International Journal of Sport and Exercise Psychology 1:434–459

Scherzer C B, Brewer B W, Cornelius A E et al 2001 Psychological skills and adherence to rehabilitation after reconstruction of the anterior cruciate ligament. Journal of Sport Rehabilitation 10:165–172

Schlenk EA, Dunbar-Jacob J, Sereika S et al 2000 Comparability of daily diaries and accelerometers in exercise adherence in fibromyalgia syndrome [abstract]. Measurement and Evaluation in Physical Education and Exercise Science 4:133–134

Schneiders A G, Zusman G, Singer K P 1998 Exercise therapy compliance in acute low back pain patients. Manual Therapy 3:147–152

Schomer H H 1990 A cognitive strategy training programme for marathon runners: ten case studies. South African Journal of Research in Sport, Physical Education and Recreation 13:47–78

Shaffer S M, Wiese-Bjornstal D M 1999 Effective intervention strategies in sports medicine. In: Ray R, Wiese-Bjornstal D M (eds) Counseling in sports medicine. Human Kinetics, Champaign, IL

Shelley G A, Sherman C P 1996 The sport injury experience: a qualitative case study [abstract]. Journal of Applied Sport Psychology 8 (suppl):S164

Sluijs E M, Kok G J, van der Zee J 1993 Correlates of exercise compliance in physical therapy. Physical Therapy 73:771–786

Smith A M, Milliner E K 1994 Injured athletes and the risk of suicide. Journal of Athletic Training 29:337–341

Smith A M, Scott S G, O'Fallon W M et al 1990b Emotional responses of athletes to injury. Mayo Clinic Proceedings 65:38–50

Smith A M, Stuart M J, Wiese-Bjornstal D M et al 1993 Competitive athletes: preinjury and postinjury mood state and self-esteem. Mayo Clinic Proceedings 68:939–947

Smith R E, Smoll F L, Ptacek J T 1990a Conjunctive moderator variables in vulnerability and resiliency research: life stress, social support and coping skills, and adolescent sport injuries. Journal of Personality and Social Psychology 58:360–369

Spetch L A, Kolt G S 2001 Adherence to sport injury rehabilitation: implications for sports medicine providers and researchers. Physical Therapy in Sport 2:80–90

Taylor A H, May S 1996 Threat and coping appraisal as determinants of compliance with sports injury rehabilitation: an application of protection motivation theory. Journal of Sports Sciences 14:471–482

Taylor J, Taylor S 1997 Psychological approaches to sports injury rehabilitation. Aspen, Gaithersburg, MD

Taylor J, Taylor S 1998 Pain education and management in the rehabilitation from sports injury. The Sport Psychologist 12:68–88

Theodorakis Y, Beneca A, Malliou P et al 1997 Examining psychological factors during injury rehabilitation. Journal of Sport Rehabilitation 6:355–363

Thompson N J, Morris R D 1994 Predicting injury risk in adolescent football players: the importance of psychological variables. Journal of Pediatric Psychology 19:415–429

Tracey J 2003 The emotional response to the injury and rehabilitation process. Journal of Applied Sport Psychology 15:279–293

Treacy S H, Barron O A, Brunet M E et al 1997 Assessing the need for extensive supervised rehabilitation following arthroscopic ACL reconstruction. American Journal of Orthopedics 26:25–29

Udry E 1996 Social support: exploring its role in the context of athletic injuries. Journal of Sport Rehabilitation 5:151–163

Udry E 1997 Coping and social support among injured athletes following surgery. Journal of Sport and Exercise Psychology 19:71–90

Udry E 1999 The paradox of injuries: unexpected positive consequences. In: Pargman D (ed) Psychological bases of sport injuries, 2nd edn. Fitness Information Technology, Morgantown, WV

Udry E, Gould D, Bridges D et al 1997 Down but not out: athlete responses to season-ending injuries. Journal of Sport and Exercise Psychology 19:229–248

Uitenbroek D G 1996 Sports, exercise, and other causes of injuries: results of a population survey. Research Quarterly for Exercise and Sport 67:380–385

Vealey R S, Walter S M 1993 Imagery training for performance enhancement and personal growth. In: Williams J M (ed) Applied sport psychology: personal growth to peak performance, 2nd edn. Mayfield, Mountain View, CA

Weaver N L, Marshall S W, Spicer R et al 1999 Cost of athletic injuries in 12 North Carolina high school sports [abstract]. Medicine and Science in Sports and Exercise 31 (suppl):S93

Webborn A D, Carbon R J, Miller B P 1997 Injury rehabilitation programs: what are we talking about? Journal of Sport Rehabilitation 6:54–61

Weeks D L, Brubaker J, Byrt J et al 2002 Videotape instruction versus illustrations for influencing quality of performance, motivation, and confidence to perform simple and complex exercises in healthy subjects. Physiotherapy Theory and Practice 18:65–73

Weiss M R, Troxel R K 1986 Psychology of the injured athlete. Athletic Training 21:104–109, 154

White A, Hardy L 1998 An in-depth analysis of the uses of imagery by high-level slalom canoeists and artistic gymnasts. The Sport Psychologist 12:387–403

Whitmarsh B G, Alderman R B 1993 Role of psychological skills training in increasing athletic pain tolerance. The Sport Psychologist 7:388–399

Wiese D M, Weiss M R 1987 Psychological rehabilitation and physical injury: implication for the sports medicine team. The Sport Psychologist 1:318–330

Wiese D M, Weiss M R, Yukelson D P 1991 Sport psychology in the training room: a survey of athletic trainers. The Sport Psychologist 5:15–24

Wiese-Bjornstal D M, Smith A M, Shaffer S M et al 1998 An integrated model of response to sport injury: psychological and sociological dimensions. Journal of Applied Sport Psychology 10:46–69

Williams J M 2001 Psychology of injury risk and prevention. In: Singer R N, Hausenblas H A, Janelle C M (eds) Handbook of sport psychology, 2nd edn. John Wiley, New York

Williams J M, Andersen M B 1998 Psychosocial antecedents of sport injury: review and critique of the stress and injury model. Journal of Applied Sport Psychology 10:5–25

Williams J M, Roepke N 1993 Psychology of injury and injury rehabilitation. In: Singer R N, Murphey M, Tennant L K (eds) Handbook of research on sport psychology. Macmillan, New York

Wittig A F, Schurr K T 1994 Psychological characteristics of women volleyball players: relationships with injuries, rehabilitation, and team success. Personality and Social Psychology Bulletin 20:322–330

Screening for sport and exercise participation

Lisa Casson Barkley and Michael J. Axe

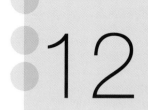

CHAPTER CONTENTS

Introduction 190

Target audience 190

Goals and objectives of screening examinations 191

How are preparticipation screening examinations done? 191

Determining clearance 201

Summary 204

Introduction

Every year, around the world, hundreds of thousands of athletes undergo preparticipation physical examinations or screenings prior to participating in organized sports and exercise. While their cost effectiveness and evidence of effectiveness as a screening tool has been debated (Bratton & Agerter 1995, Wingfield et al 2004), these examinations fulfill several important functions. They help to detect medical conditions that may prevent the athlete from safe participation, screen for general health and provide the opportunity for health education that can prevent future problems. A screening is an abbreviated preseason preparticipation physical examination designed to satisfy standards mandated in some countries, and to identify any significant health and medical problems. It includes reviewing the history, noting allergies, recording vital signs and cardiopulmonary status, and assessing the current condition of previous injuries. The major focus of this chapter is the medical aspects of preparticipation screening where evidence has shown a benefit (AAFP, AAP, AMSSM, AOSSM, AOASM 2004).

Target audience

Preparticipation physical exams are most commonly performed on athletes involved in organized athletic programs or on older people entering physical activity and sport programs. In some countries (e.g. the USA), middle school, high school and college/university athletes are mandated to take such preseason examinations. In several other countries, these examinations are increasingly used, particularly at elite and professional levels of sport. In Australia, medical screening is done with athletes at the elite and national level and not at the high school level (Brukner et al 2004). In Italy, Great Britain and the USA, athletes are required to have examinations at the younger age groups of participation (Batt et al 2004, Pigozzi et al 2003). The examination does, however, have a much broader target audience as athletic participation widens to all age groups. In the USA, for example, there has been a particularly significant increase in the number of athletes who participate at the youth level who are of preschool and elementary school age. As our world becomes more technologically advanced and less manual labor is required in our daily lives, medical professionals encourage participating in sport and exercise at a recreational level at all ages to maintain physical fitness and weight control. Furthermore, as medical advances allow individuals to live longer, more senior adults will be participating in sport and exercise pursuits.

Goals and objectives of screening examinations

Preparticipation screening examinations can fulfill the following goals and objectives, which can be beneficial to people involved in sport and exercise (AAFP, AAP, AMSSM, AOSSM, AOASM 1996, 2004):

- To detect medical conditions that may place an athlete at risk for injury or death.

- To detect medical and musculoskeletal conditions that will limit or prevent an athlete from participating safely in a particular sport. A detailed history and focused physical examination is the best defense currently available to detect conditions that may lead to sudden death or increased morbidity or mortality from existing medical conditions. This allows for proper rehabilitation and/or use of protective equipment that can correct abnormalities that may otherwise endanger the athlete and their competitors.

- To define sport and exercise activities that an athlete can participate in safely. If an athlete cannot play a chosen sport for a medical reason, it is very important to provide alternative activities.

- Provide general health screening on a limited basis. The preparticipation screening examination is not designed to replace regular health examinations. The reality is, however, that is does, especially in adolescent athletes who are generally healthy and would not otherwise enter the health care system. It has been reported that over 78% of athletes use the preparticipation examination as the only health maintenance contact (Carek & Futrell 1999). It is therefore important to use this examination as an opportunity to address global health needs. Also, since this exam is an important entry point into the health care system for many adolescents, attention must be placed on follow-up plans and referrals (AAFP, AAP ACSM, AMSSM, AOSSM, AOASM 2004).

- Counsel and educate athletes on sport and health related issues. This is especially important in adolescent athletes who may be starting to engage in high-risk behaviors, which can adversely affect their current and future health. It also helps foster an open relationship between the athlete and the medical staff, making it easier to discuss any future concerns or problems.

- Fulfill legal and/or insurance requirements in certain sectors and countries. Identifying and addressing health problems of athletes involved in organized sports programs may provide some degree of protection from liability of the athlete and the institution that sponsors the activity. It may also lead to lower insurance rates for institutions (Mac 1998).

How are preparticipation screening examinations done?

When to conduct examinations

Timing of examinations should allow for the opportunity to rehabilitate injuries that are identified, and/or to perform diagnostic testing and evaluation. The generally recommended time is 6–8 weeks before the start of the preseason or the start of an exercise program. If the examination is done too close to the start of the preseason or the exercise program, valuable time needed to diagnose or rehabilitate would be lost from the participation time. If the examination is done too far in advance, new problems or injuries can occur by the time the activity starts. For high school and college athletes in the USA, it is often necessary to perform exams at the end of the school year in May or June to accommodate school attendance schedules. If the exam has to be done further in advance, when the athletes return for practice there should be an update history carried out to make sure no new injuries or illness occurred in the interim (AAFP, AAP, ACSM, AMSSM, AOSSM, AOASM 2004).

The frequency of performing these examinations is not uniform. Different sports governing associations have varying requirements. Some countries have quite strong recommendations. For example, in the USA, the American Heart Association recommends a complete history and physical examination at the entrance to high school, with a repeat history and physical examination every 2 years for younger adolescents and every 2–3 years for older adolescents (AAFP, AAP, ACSM, AMSSM, AOSSM, AOASM 2004, Maron et al 1996a). A screening to include a history review, blood pressure measurement and injury assessment should occur in each intervening year. It has been suggested that college level and university athletes have a complete evaluation upon entrance to the school and a history screening and blood pressure measurement yearly during participation (Maron et al 1998). The exam should also be incorporated into the routine physical exam of children starting at age 6. This will allow for the opportunity for screening by the primary care provider and not require an additional examination (AAFP, AAP, ACSM, AMSSM, AOSSM, AOASM 2004).

Performing the examination

There are two recognized ways to perform examinations: individually or coordinated medical team exams. Both types of processing have advantages and disadvantages. Individual examinations are on a one-on-one basis with the athlete or exercise participant and the medical provider and physical therapist present. The advantages of this type of examination are: the personal attention, which facilitates the provision of health education and assessment of high-risk behavior; it allows for the development of a relationship between the athlete and the providers, which will lay the foundation for future communication; and confidentiality and privacy are easier to maintain. The disadvantages are: whether or not the medical provider has specific knowledge relating to the specific needs of athletes, which can lead to varying degrees of injury assessment; these examinations are also time consuming.

In the USA, school-based health centers are another location where individual examinations can be performed. These centers are established in some high schools and middle schools to improve access to care for adolescents. The centers provide multidisciplinary health care providers such as physicians, nurse practitioners, dietitians and social workers. The location in the school provides easier follow-up of identified problems, and helps establish relationships with the athletes.

Coordinated medical team examinations allow for more rapid processing of a large number of athletes. Athletes progress through several sites where different providers perform the different phases of the preparticipation examination. The advantages are that providers can be chosen for their expertise, improving the quality of that component of the examination. The typical stations include history review, vital signs, general medical evaluation, cardiopulmonary assessment, musculoskeletal evaluation and determination of medical clearance by senior medical personnel. The disadvantage is that there is little privacy, making it difficult to establish relationships with athletes and to discuss sensitive issues. Also, the exam areas are often noisy making it difficult to listen for heart murmurs and to hear systolic and diastolic blood pressure readings (Esquivel & McCormick 1987). It is therefore important to carefully consider the location of such exams to ensure that privacy and noise are reduced.

Preparticipation history

The history, as in most areas of health care, is the most important component of the preparticipation examination. Most conditions that predispose athletes to injury or death during athletic participation, if they can be identified at all, are detected in the history rather than on physical examination. Rifat et al (1995) reviewed 2574 preparticipation physical examinations and reported that the history indicated 88% of abnormal findings and 57% of restrictions from sport.

Self-report history

Self-report history forms provide a very useful and consistent means of obtaining the pertinent history and can be reviewed rapidly for areas of concern and potential risk. For high school athletes and younger athletes, it is very important that parents or guardians help the athlete with the completion of the history form. This better ensures that all elements of the history are reported accurately (Risser et al 1985).

Surgical history

The past surgical history is important. Athletes and exercise participants who have had previous surgery need the time to heal and to have proper rehabilitation before returning to play.

Medical history

The past medical history uncovers conditions such as asthma, bee sting allergies and diabetes, which require special care to allow safe participation. It is also important to note if the athlete is missing any paired organs in order to discuss protective equipment needs and counseling on the risk to the remaining organ. The presence of sickle cell trait or disease is important as these athletes will be more likely to have heat-related problems and may be at risk for sudden death from sickling of red blood cells with strenuous activity (AAFP, AAP, ACSM, AMSSM, AOSSM, AOASM 2004). A recent history of infectious mononucleosis is important due to the risk of splenomegaly and fragility during the illness that may place the athlete at risk of splenic rupture with activity. These athletes should not participate in physical activity for 21–28 days from the onset of the illness to prevent this complication. It is often helpful to ask participants what is the sickest they have ever been. For most young athletes the answer is usually a viral illness, which is reassuring. Occasionally, this question will help uncover important but forgotten history.

Allergies should be noted on emergency cards that are carried with the team. Athletes often travel and may not be treated by medical personnel who are familiar with their history. Allergies to insects are important, especially in outdoor sports. If a serious allergy is known, such as respiratory distress or tongue swelling after an insect sting, an adrenaline (epinephrine) pen should be available at all times for the athlete. Food and environmental allergies should be noted since athletes may travel and be exposed to different environments. A small number of athletes will even experience urticaria or anaphylaxis related to exercise itself.

Medication history should include current prescription medications as well as any over-the-counter medications. Certain medications have side effects that can affect athletic performance (see Chapter 29). For example, beta-blockers used to control hypertension can affect endurance, diuretics can affect hydration status and the antibiotic tetracycline can increase risk of sunburn. Over-the-counter medications that may seem innocuous can also have unwanted side effects that adversely affect athletic performance. For example, certain cold and cough medications containing sympathetomimetics may cause tachycardia.

It is also helpful to get an accurate history of any vitamin, herbal remedies or supplements. It is useful to ask about these, specifically, as many athletes do not consider these preparations as medications. Often it will be necessary to actually look at the label to determine the components of the supplement as many contain several substances. Athletes are especially prone to taking these preparations if they believe it will improve athletic performance. Often, however, the efficacy and/or safety of these supplements are unknown. Some athletes take ergogenic substances to gain an advantage in athletic competition. It is advisable to inquire about such substances as anabolic steroids and growth hormone.

Some sports governing organizations, including the International Olympic Committee and the National Collegiate Athletic Association (in the USA), have lists of medications that are banned to their athletes (see Chapter 29 for further details). Failure to comply with these restrictions can have serious consequences. Of note is that some of the banned substances are over-the-counter medications. This point was highlighted during the Sydney Olympic Games in 2000 when a gymnast was stripped of their medal for taking a cold medication that was banned.

Cardiac history

The cardiac history is extremely important, as this is the best tool available at this time to detect medical conditions that would place an athlete or exercise participant at risk for sudden cardiac death (Mac 1998) (see Chapter 31). Sudden death in athletes is fortunately an uncommon occurrence, affecting about 0.2 to 0.5 young athletes per 100 000 per year (Maron et al 1996b). Unfortunately, many athletes with cardiac defects that lead to sudden death are asymptomatic until the fatal event occurs, which is usually a ventricular arrhythmia. Warning symptoms during exercise include syncope or near syncope, chest pain, irregular heart rhythms and tachycardia. Athletes may also fatigue earlier than their peers. These symptoms need to be distinguished from deconditioning that usually occurs in the beginning of the season and resolves as the fitness level improves. Previous history of heart murmurs and diagnostic testing, high cholesterol and hypertension should be obtained (Mac 1998).

In the under-35-year-old age group, congenital cardiac abnormalities are the most common cause of sudden cardiac death. A family history of cardiac problems that have led to death before the age of 50 years will give clues toward familial heart disease. Maron et al (1996b) found the following breakdown of causes in 158 athletes in the USA from 1985 to 1995: hypertrophic cardiomyopathy in 36%, anomalous coronary arteries in 19%, increased cardiac mass in 10%, ruptured aorta in 5%, tunneled left anterior descending coronary artery in 5%, aortic stenosis in 4%, myocarditis in 3%, dilated cardiomyopathy in 3%, arrhythomogenic right ventricular dysplasia in 3%, mitral valve prolapse in 2%, coronary artery disease in 2% and other causes in 5%.

The most common cause of sudden death in young athletes, hypertrophic cardiomyopathy, is an asymmetrical hypertrophy of the left ventricle that can lead to outflow obstruction and fatal arrhythmias. Symptoms may include syncope, chest pain, palpitations or dyspnea with exertion or a heart murmur. Often, however, the athlete is asymptomatic. Although it appears more common in males and African Americans, a study from the Centers for Disease Control and Prevention showed a higher incidence in females than previously suspected. The rates of sudden cardiac death increased 30% in females from 1989 to 1996 (Zheng et al 2001).

Marfan's syndrome

Marfan's syndrome, a connective tissue disorder due to lack of fibrillin, should be asked about specifically. Marfan's syndrome diagnosis is made on the presence of at least two of four major features of the disease. These are positive family history, and ocular, cardiac and skeletal abnormalities. These athletes are at risk of sudden death from aortic rupture. If an athlete has any significant positive history responses, further evaluation should be pursued before clearance is given to participate (Cantwell 1986).

Coronary artery disease

In athletes older than 35 years, coronary artery disease is the most common cause of exercise-related sudden death (Maron et al 1996b). Younger athletes with a personal or family history of coronary artery disease should also be assessed. Risk factors include age, family history of coronary artery disease in a first-degree relative, male gender, cigarette smoking, hypercholesterolemia, diabetes, hypertension, obesity and sedentary lifestyle. Males over the age of 40 years and females over the age of 50 years with two or more risk factors should be considered for exercise stress testing prior to the start of an exercise program. Screening questions of symptoms such as those on the Physical Activity Readiness Questionnaire (PAR-Q) (Thomas et al 1992) are helpful in screening at risk athletes (Kenney 1995).

Heat-related illness

Heat illness is important to note as previous heat-related problems would increase risk of recurrent problems. Athletes at the extremes of age, obesity, poor physical fitness, not being acclimatized to the heat and those taking certain medications such as diuretics will be at increased risk of heat related problems. Athletes should be educated during the preparticipation exam about proper hydration and encouraged to monitor their fluid status and take measures to acclimatize to the heat before the season starts. This type of education is also important for athletes traveling to competitions in hotter and more humid climates than they are used to. Fluid status can be monitored by observing the color of the athlete's urine. A well-hydrated athlete will have clear to light yellow urine whereas the dehydrated athlete will have dark yellow, concentrated urine. Another way to monitor hydration status is to weigh the athlete before and after a practice session. Most weight loss will be due to fluid losses and should be replaced before the athlete returns to play. This method allows for the determination of the individual athlete's sweat rate, which allows for accurate fluid replacement (Murray 1994).

Acclimatization is a process inducing physiological adaptations in response to the stress of exercising in the heat. The process takes 7 to 14 days to complete. This will help protect the athlete from heat illness by starting to sweat sooner, decreasing salt loss in sweat, increasing time to exhaustion and improving cardiovascular responses to heat stress. Athletes should exercise in the heat for 60 to 90 min and increase the intensity of the workouts over a 2-week period to achieve these protective changes (Maughan & Shirreffs 1997).

Appropriate guidelines should be given to the athlete about hydration. Athletes should be advised to prehydrate about 2 h before an event with at least 17 ounces (0.5 L) of fluids. During the event, they should drink 4–8 ounces (0.12–0.25 L) of fluids every 20 min and after the event it is best to rehydrate within 2 h. Twenty-four ounces (0.7 L) of fluids should be consumed for every 1 pound (0.45 kg) of weight loss. Fluid breaks should be scheduled into the activity rather than taken as needed. Athletes have been found to replace only two-thirds of their fluid loss by voluntary drinking alone (Coyle 1994). Also, by the time the athlete is thirsty, dehydration has already occurred. Sports drinks that contain 6–8% carbohydrates, sodium and other electrolytes should be favored over water as the taste will encourage increased consumption, and it has been shown that athletes who drink these substances can perform longer with less fatigue (Coyle 1994).

Neurological history

Neurological history includes seizure disorders, history of burners or stingers, previous concussions and loss of consciousness. Level of control of any seizure disorders should be determined. Burners or stingers are transient traction injuries of the brachial plexus of nerves. The history should include frequency of symptoms, residual weakness and any lasting neurological deficits.

A detailed concussion history should be done to assess the number, severity and symptoms and recovery from previous injuries. There have been a lot of changes in the management of concussions over the past several years based on evidence from the use of neuropsychological testing. In 2004 there was an international symposium on concussion in sport which set forth recommendations to improve safety and health of athletes with concussions. These recommendations divide concussions into simple and complex categories. Simple concussions are the most common form of injury and typically resolve progressively over 7–10 days. This type of concussion resolves with rest and there are no complications for return to sport. Complex concussions are characterized with persistent symptoms, especially with exertion, and prolonged cognitive impairment. These athletes often have multiple concussions and repeated concussions occur with less force. Formal neuropsychological and other testing is needed, as well as a multidisciplinary medical treatment team approach. It is recommended that combined measures of recovery from concussion along with a graded exertion protocol for return to play be used to manage concussions. During the acute management phase, an athlete with any symptoms of concussion should not return to play the same day of the injury. The athlete should then have physical and cognitive rest until asymptomatic. The next phase is light aerobic physical activity. If the athlete remains asymptomatic, the third phase is exercise-specific to the sport along with light resistance training. The fourth phase is noncontact training drills and continued resistance training. When the athlete completes this phase, there is medical clearance to perform full contact training, and then progress to game play. It is recommended that a baseline cognitive assessment test and a symptom score or neuropsychological screening be completed on athletes during the preparticipation exam (McCrory et al 2005).

Respiratory history

Respiratory history focuses on detection of exercise-induced bronchospasm (EIB). This condition involves airway obstruction that only occurs related to exercise. The usual symptoms are coughing, wheezing, chest tightness or shortness of breath that occur during or after exercise. At times, the symptoms of EIB are mistaken for deconditioning. A previous history of asthma or allergic rhinitis is a risk factor for the development of EIB. EIB is also more pronounced during exercise in cold, low-humidity environments, and in the presence of environmental allergens (Storms 1999). Most athletes respond well to treatment with short acting bronchodilators, such as albuterol, taken 20–30 min before the start of exercise. Athletes can also induce a refractory period of reduced symptoms by warming up with an intense workout to invoke bronchospasm prior to the start of exercise. This refractory period can last 30–90 min. Athletes with underlying asthma or allergic rhinitis should be treated for these conditions (Storms 1999). Athletes who are identified with asthma or EIB should have baseline peak flow readings or spirometry. Athletes should modify their vigorous exercise routine when the peak flow measurement is less than 80% of their personal best. A written management plan should also be in place to guide medical treatment of athletes and medications should be readily available at all practices and events (AAFP, AAP, ACSM, AMSSM, AOSSM, AOASM 2004).

Vision history

Vision history should determine if the athlete requires correction of visual acuity and whether glasses or contact lenses are used. Glasses should have lenses made of polycarbonate material that will not shatter if they are hit, to avoid eye injury. Previous eye injury or surgery should be noted. The risk of eye injury in sports is often overlooked. The American Academy of Ophthalmology recommends protective eyewear with polycarbonate lenses for all sports that are at high risk for eye injury. These sports include those that use a small ball or sticks (e.g. baseball, tennis, lacrosse), those with close contact (e.g. basketball) and those that cause intentional injury (e.g. boxing) (Vinger 2000).

Skin conditions

Skin conditions should be noted in the history to detect those that may be contagious, such as herpes, molluscum contagiosum and tinea corporis. These are especially important in contact sports, such as wrestling. In the USA, there has been an increase in the incidence of community acquired methicillin resistant *Staphylococcus aureus* infections in otherwise healthy athletes. These infections, which can be very serious, leading to lung and systemic infections, can also be challenging to treat due to the antibiotic resistance. Careful attention and education must be placed on prevention of such infections with proper cleansing and hygiene techniques and early detection through frequent skin inspections. Infectious skin conditions should provoke isolation of the athlete until treatment occurs and the risk of transmission to others is decreased, and appropriate barrier protection (AAFP, AAP, ACSM, AMSSM, AOSSM, AOASM 2004).

Musculoskeletal history

Musculoskeletal history should focus on previous injuries and type of treatment given. Many athletes, especially at school level and younger, have not received adequate rehabilitation of previous injuries. The most important risk factor for a repeat injury is having a previous injury that was not completely rehabilitated (Bar-Or et al 1988). Previous surgery should be cleared for return to play by the surgeon who performed the procedure. Inquiry should also be made about the use of protective equipment such as knee or ankle braces.

Immunization

The preparticipation exam is an opportune time to review immunizations to make sure that they are up to date. This is especially important in team sports where communicable diseases are easily spread. Tetanus immunization booster is given in adolescence and updated every 5–10 years. Two measles, mumps and rubella vaccines are needed. Adolescents who have not had chicken pox need immunization, and meningococcal vaccine should be considered especially for those living in dormitory settings. Hepatitis A and B vaccines should be given to athletes who have not received the series and should be recommended to coaches. Influenza A immunization should be considered especially for team sports where the infection can spread easily and for athletes with asthma and other chronic disease conditions. As discussed in Chapter 31, athletes involved in international travel should receive appropriate immunizations for the area (Centers for Disease Control and Prevention 1999).

Nutrition

Proper nutrition is extremely important for optimum sports performance. It is important to screen athletes for how well they manage their nutritional needs. Questions should focus on their nutritional habits, whether they are trying to lose or gain weight and how they are planning to do so. Calculation of the body mass index (BMI) can help to determine if the athlete is underweight, normal weight, overweight or obese. Underweight athletes are concerning for the risks of eating disorders. There is also an increasing prevalence of overweight and obese athletes. The world is experiencing an epidemic of obesity, especially for children. Obesity leads to the increased risk of comorbidities such as diabetes, hypertension, dyslipidemia and many other conditions that can affect athletic performance. The risk of these comorbid conditions should be screened for and further testing done as appropriate. Nutritional counseling should be provided for all athletes (AAFP, AAP, ACSM, AMSSM, AOSSM, AOASM 2004).

Female athletes

Female athletes deserve special consideration during their examination to evaluate those at risk for the female athlete triad (see Chapter 27). The triad includes amenorrhea, which is the loss of menstruation in a female who previously had menstrual cycles, eating disorders and osteoporosis. This triad of disorders has significant health consequences, which may affect the athlete for the rest of her life, especially with premature osteoporosis. Age at menarche and date of the first day of the last menstrual period should be noted.

Menarche

Menarche is the onset of menses and is often delayed in young athletes who are participating in strenuous activities. Menarche may be delayed by 5 months for every year of intense prepubertal training (Frisch et al 1981). The average age of menarche for non-athletic females has decreased over the years. The mean age for menarche has been reported as 12.88 years in Caucasians and 12.16 years in African Americans (Herman-Giddens et al 1997). The number of normal menstrual periods that occur yearly should be assessed. Secondary amenorrhea is defined as missing at least three consecutive menstrual cycles in a woman who has established menstrual cycles. The most common cause of secondary amenorrhea, even in athletes, is pregnancy and this should be ruled out before concluding that the amenorrhea is related to exercise. Prolonged amenorrhea can have negative effects on bone health, as estrogen is a necessary component to make adequate bone. If the amenorrhea persists for more than 3 years and occurs during the time of peak bone accretion, the effects are usually irreversible (Hobart & Smucker 2000). Athletes should be made aware that amenorrhea is not a normal occurrence and that it should be investigated if it persists. Often, unfortunately, athletes and coaches feel that amenorrhea is a good sign of hard training.

Eating disorders

Eating disorders (see Chapter 27) include a spectrum from disordered eating which does not meet the energy requirements of the athlete, to frank eating disorders such as anorexia nervosa and bulimia nervosa. Anorexia nervosa has the following diagnostic criteria: weight less than 85% of ideal body weight, amenorrhea, distorted body image and intense fear of gaining weight. There are restricting anorexics that decrease intake of food to achieve weight loss and bulimic anorexics that regularly purge or binge eat (American Psychiatric Association 1994).

Bulimia nervosa is characterized by recurrent episodes of binge eating, which involve eating large amounts of food in 2-hour time periods, and using a pathological method to get rid of the food to prevent weight gain. By definition, the binge eating and compensatory behaviors must occur at least twice a week for 3 months (American Psychiatric Association 1994). Bulimics have a distorted self-evaluation based on body shape and weight. There are two types of bulimics: the purging type who use methods such as vomiting, laxatives, diuretics and diet pills to lose the weight; and the non-purging type who use other methods such as excessive exercise to lose weight (American Psychiatric Association 1994).

One approach to begin a discussion on eating behaviors is to inquire how the athlete feels about their current weight. The hallmark of eating disorders is a distorted self-image about weight; athletes with an eating disorder will feel that they are overweight even when they are not. Also ask about pathological weight control behaviors, which include vomiting, taking diet pills and laxatives, using saunas or wearing heavy clothing to sweat and lose weight. Exercise to excess is often used as a way to purge calories, especially in adolescents with eating disorders. At times, it may be difficult to determine when this behavior is pathological as it may be perceived as a sign of being a good athlete. Inquire how much exercise is done in addition to that needed to meet the requirements of the sport. Eating disorder patients often fit in well in an athletic environment because they are typically compulsive in their behaviors and are perfectionists (Thompson & Sherman 1993). Certain sports are more at risk than others. These include sports that have weight classes (e.g. weightlifting, rowing, boxing), those in which appearance is important for judging (e.g. gymnastics, ballet, figure-skating) and endurance sports (Thompson & Sherman 1993).

Osteoporosis

Osteoporosis occurs in the triad due to the lack of the necessary substrates to keep bone formation above bone resorption. The dietary deficits in calcium and vitamin D as well as the low estrogen hormonal status can lead to premature osteoporosis. This usually manifests clinically as stress fractures and other fractures, and recurrent musculoskeletal injuries. Osteoporosis that occurs before menopause is very difficult to treat, and may be largely irreversible (Hobart & Smucker 2000). Hormonal replacement is controversial in its ability to reverse the problem (Taitel & Lippman 1995).

Adolescents

The preparticipation examination is also an opportune time to inquire about the general health of the athlete, especially adolescents. Adolescents are often an under-served population as they may not be evaluated by medical providers on a regular basis. It is also the time when risk-taking behaviors that will have adverse health consequences can begin. Talking to adolescent and young adults about high-risk behaviors requires some preliminary discussion about confidentiality and its limits. If adolescents reveal that they are engaging in high-risk behaviors, they need some reassurance as to what will be done with that information. If there is not an agreement about confidentiality, this information will most likely not be revealed by the athlete. It is also useful to determine the social support systems available to the adolescent to deal with stressful situations. Teenagers who do not have social supports, have poor coping mechanisms to deal with stress, and who feel socially isolated, are more likely to develop high risk behaviors such as smoking, substance abuse, sexual activity and suicide (Goldenring & Cohen 1988). It is often useful to discuss less personal topics first and lead up to more sensitive issues. One mnemonic for this discussion is HEADSS (Goldenring & Cohen 1988). 'H' is for home environment: questions should focus on who lives in the home, who is a support person for the adolescent, and what type of environment is present in the home. 'E' is for education, vocational goals, and employment: adolescents who are failing in

school or who are having behavior problems in school deserve further evaluation. 'A' is for activities in and out of school: this includes peer activities, hobbies, and religious involvement. 'D' is for drug, tobacco and alcohol use by the teenager, peers and family members. 'S' is for sexual activity, sexual orientation, contraception use and sexually transmitted infection history. The other 'S' is for suicidal ideation and depression. Athletes engaging in high-risk behaviors should be counseled for risk factor reduction by appropriate health care personnel and referred as necessary.

Preparticipation physical

The physical examination is a screening examination to rule out pathology that will make athletic participation unsafe. Athletes should be dressed in clothes that will make it possible to visualize the anatomy (AAFP, AAP, AMSSM, AOSSM, AOASM 2004). It is important to be sensitive to exposure of the body in athletes during the examination. Young adolescents are particularly sensitive to the changes in their bodies so it is best to expose only the area that needs to be examined, to cover that area when finished and then to expose the next area.

Vital signs

Vital signs include blood pressure, pulse, height, weight and visual acuity. Blood pressure should be measured in the right arm in the sitting position and the athlete should be sitting with the back and arm supported. If the blood pressure is found to be elevated, it is necessary to repeat the measurement again during the examination. Three consecutive elevated blood pressure measures on three different occasions are needed to diagnose hypertension. It is important to note in adolescent athletes and children that normal blood pressure levels are lower than in adult athletes (National High Blood Pressure Education Program 1996) (Table 12.1). Height and weight should be compared to standard charts. Body mass index or body fat measurements may also be included. This is especially important in sports that have weight limits. Athletes who are over- or underweight should have a dietary evaluation and underweight athletes should be screened for eating disorders, regardless of gender. Visual acuity should be tested using Snellen eye charts. Athletes should have vision that is correctable to 20/40 or better (AAFP, AAP, AMSSM, AOSSM, AOASM 2004, Vinger 2000).

The head, ears, eyes, nose and throat

Examinations of the head, ears, eyes, nose and throat should document the lack or presence of infection. The eyes should be checked for equal pupils. Any asymmetry such as anisocoria should be noted so that if the athlete should receive a head injury, the pupil asymmetry will not be attributed to the trauma. Nasal passages should be checked for symmetry and patent airflow. The pharynx should be checked for signs of infection. The condition of the teeth should be noted, especially for any loose

Table 12.1 Blood pressure measurements in male and female children and adolescents. If systolic or diastolic blood pressure is at or above the 95th percentile, the child may be hypertensive and warrant further observation and consideration of other risk. (Modified from the National High Blood Pressure Education Program 1996.)

Age (years)	5th percentile height	50th percentile height	95th percentile height
Male 95th percentile blood pressure measurements by percentage of height for age			
6	109/72	114/74	117/76
7	110/74	115/76	119/78
8	111/75	116/77	120/80
9	113/76	117/79	121/81
10	114/77	119/80	123/82
11	116/78	121/80	125/83
12	119/79	123/81	127/83
13	121/79	126/82	130/84
14	124/80	128/82	132/85
15	127/81	131/83	135/86
16	129/83	134/85	138/87
17	132/85	136/87	140/89
Female 95th percentile blood pressure measurements by percentage of height for age			
6	108/71	111/73	114/73
7	110/73	113/74	116/76
8	112/74	115/75	118/78
9	114/75	117/77	120/79
10	116/77	119/78	122/80
11	118/78	121/79	124/81
12	120/79	123/80	126/82
13	121/80	125/82	128/84
14	123/81	126/83	130/85
15	124/82	128/83	131/86
16	125/83	128/84	132/86
17	126/83	129/84	132/86

or damaged teeth and dental erosions that may be the result of vomiting in eating disorder patients.

Lungs

Lung examination should assess for equal breath sounds and the presence of wheezing and other abnormal sounds. Athletes with exercise-induced bronchospasm should have normal lung examinations at rest. The presence of wheezing during the screening examination indicates baseline asthma or underlying respiratory infection (Storms 1999). These conditions should be treated appropriately.

Abdomen

Abdominal examination should check for hepatosplenomegaly, which may be the result of infections such as mononucleosis. One should also check for other abdominal masses or tenderness that may require further evaluation.

Skin

Skin examination should check for infectious conditions as well as acne, abnormal lesions and signs of sun exposure. Acne may be exacerbated by helmets and sweating. Any evidence of a communicable skin disease should be treated prior to beginning team training in close contact sports. During the treatment phase, an individualized training schedule should be established for the affected athlete.

Genitourinary tract

Genitourinary examination and level of sexual development should be assessed in male athletes. This examination is not currently recommended in female athletes (AAFP, AAP, AMSSM, AOSSM, AOASM 1996). Testicular examination should check for abnormal lumps, varicocoeles and bilateral descended testicles. Athletes should be given education in how to perform testicular self-examinations, as this form of cancer is more common in young males aged 20 to 35 years (Chan 2001). The presence of hernias should be ruled out. Sexual maturity rating may be done based on development of pubic hair, penis and testicular size. Traditionally, this information was used to help group males according to maturity rather than age in contact sports. It has not been shown, however, that such grouping will prevent injuries to less mature and smaller athletes (AAFP, AAP, AMSSM, AOSSM, AOASM 1996, 2004).

Cardiology

Cardiac examination is important in an attempt to detect cardiac abnormalities that could lead to sudden death. The American Heart Association recommendations include a minimum of auscultation of the heart for murmurs in at least the supine and standing positions, palpation of femoral artery pulses, and evaluation for physical examination findings of Marfan's syndrome. Heart size should be assessed clinically by palpating the point of maximal impulse on the precordium. Heart rate and rhythm should be assessed on auscultation.

The murmur of hypertrophic cardiomyopathy is louder when there is less blood in the heart, which increases outflow tract obstruction. It is therefore important to listen to the heart in different positions to accentuate this murmur. Getting the athlete to perform a Valsalva maneuver or to stand from a squatting position will increase the murmur of hypertrophic cardiomyopathy, as these positions decrease the amount of blood in the left ventricle (Allen et al 1994).

Functional murmurs are a common finding on examination particularly in young athletes. These murmurs are typically louder in the supine position and the change in intensity of sound is reversed in comparison to the above maneuvers for hypertrophic cardiomyopathy.

Palpation of pulses in the upper and lower extremity is important to rule out coarctation of the aorta, which will result in diminished femoral pulses compared to upper extremity pulses (Allen et al 1994).

Marfan's syndrome

The physical examination findings of Marfan's syndrome include cardiac, ocular, musculoskeletal and skin conditions. Cardiac abnormalities include mitral or aortic valve regurgitation murmurs, dilated aortic root, aortic dissection and dysrhythmias. Ocular findings include myopia, lens subluxations and retinal detachment. Musculoskeletal findings include arm span longer than height, tall stature, pectus excavatum deformity of the anterior chest wall, scoliosis, flat feet and hyperextensible joints. Skin findings include stria distensae. Inguinal hernias are more frequent. Athletes with a family history and physical examination findings suggestive of Marfan's syndrome should undergo further evaluation to confirm the diagnosis (Cantwell 1986).

Musculoskeletal

The musculoskeletal examination should be a screening for asymptomatic, at risk athletes and should include a joint-specific examination for previously injured athletes. The objectives are to compare symmetry, side-to-side laxity and assess range of motion, gross strength and neurological function. Any areas of abnormality should be further evaluated with a joint-specific examination. The *Preparticipation Monograph* recommends the following 14-point screening examination (AAFP, AAP, AMSSM, AOSSM, AOASM 1996) (Fig. 12.1): there is a general inspection of body habitus, neck range of motion, trapezius strength, deltoid strength, shoulder range of motion, elbow range of motion, and hand and finger range of motion. Spine assessment begins with inspection with the back towards the examiner, back extension to assess for spondylolysis or spondylolisthesis and back flexion for scoliosis. Lower extremity examination focuses on the range of motion and laxity of the hips, knees and ankles, hamstring flexibility and quadriceps contraction. Functional testing includes squat and duck walk for four steps. To successfully perform these tests, a functional range of motion, adequate strength of the hips, knees and ankles, and balance are required. The lower extremity functional testing is completed by standing on the toes and heels to assess calf symmetry and strength (AAFP, AAP, AMSSM, AOSSM, AOASM 1996).

The joint-specific examination should be performed if there are abnormalities in the above screening examination or if there is a past history of musculoskeletal injury. This should also focus on joints relevant to participation in sports and exercise activities. The shoulder examination should consist of range of motion (particularly internal rotation) and strength testing of the rotator cuff. Instability and impingement testing should be performed. Assessment of neck range of motion, winging of the scapula and evaluation of pulses with the arm in the high five position to assess for thoracic outlet syndrome complete the shoulder examination. Hip evaluation should rule out referred knee pain especially in the adolescent population. The knee examination consists of range of motion, strength testing, ligamentous, patellofemoral and meniscus evaluations and testing for the presence of a painful plica. The ankle examination also consists of range

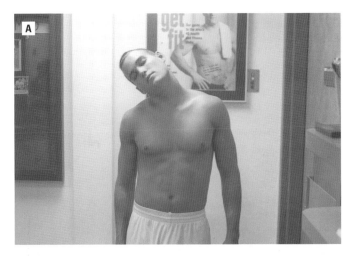

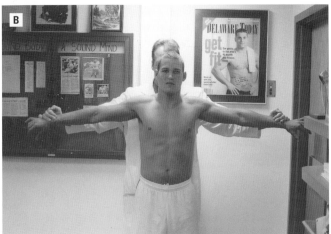

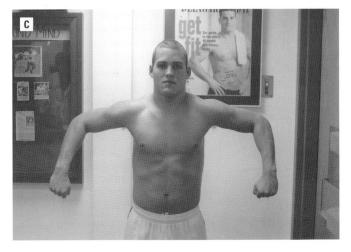

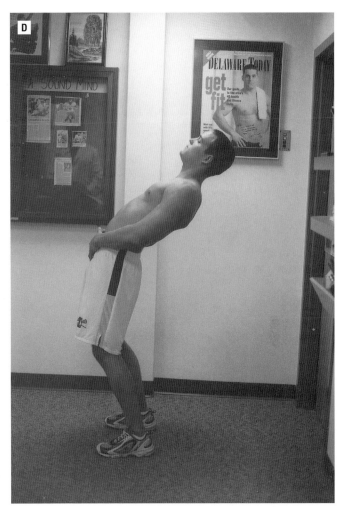

Figure 12.1 • The preparticipation screening musculoskeletal exam. **A:** Inspection, neck range of motion. **B:** Resisted shoulder shrug and deltoid strength. **C:** Range of motion of shoulders, elbows, wrists, fingers. **D:** Inspection of back, hyperextention of back. **E:** Scoliosis check. **F:** Tighten quadriceps, stand on toes and heels, squat and duck walk four steps.

of motion and strength testing. Anterior drawer and talar tilt testing evaluate for lateral ankle laxity. The squeeze test and external rotation stress tests assess syndesmosis injuries and the Thompson's test is used to assess Achilles tendon continuity (AAFP, AAP, AMSSM, AOSSM, AOASM 1996).

Sport-specific considerations

During the preparticipation examination, it is important to consider the demands of the particular sport in which the athlete will be participating. This will help focus the examiner to

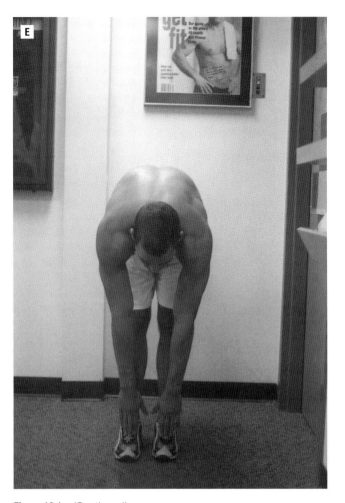

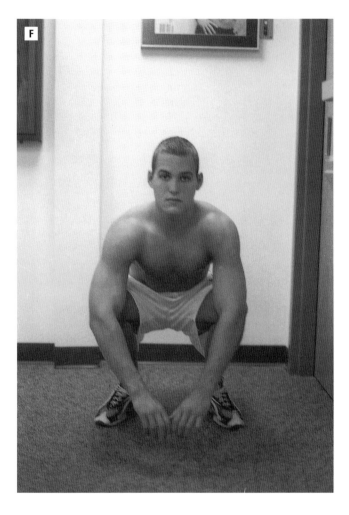

Figure 12.1 • (Continued)

look for physical findings that may correlate to specific injuries in playing that sport.

American football favors athletes who have power, speed and explosive movements. Those athletes who have increased tightness with lateral cervical flexion may be at increased risk of developing stingers or burners (Michael et al 1996).

Basketball involves running, jumping, cutting, pivoting and explosive movements. Injuries to the ankle, knee and foot are the most common in this sport. Athletes who have decreased calf flexibility and decreased ankle eversion strength may be at increased risk of ankle sprains (Dombroski 1995).

Wrestling is an anaerobic sport that involves muscle endurance, strength and flexibility. Injuries most often involve the knee, shoulder, ribs, elbow and back. Athletes with lower abdominal weakness may be at risk for lumbar strain injuries (see Chapter 16).

Overhead sports, such as tennis and volleyball, involve flexibility, strength and muscular endurance. Athletes with scapular dyskinesis and loss of internal rotation may be at risk for ipsilateral shoulder impingement (Nicola 1997).

Swimming involves aerobic endurance, strength and flexibility. Athletes with weak hip flexors may be at risk for contralateral

shoulder impingement. Also, those with tight pectoralis minor muscles may be at risk for ipsilateral shoulder impingement (Hammer 1997).

Soccer involves running, cutting, pivoting and explosive movements. Athletes with rectus femoris tightness may be at risk for quadriceps strains (Barkley 1997).

Fitness and performance testing is an optional component of preparticipation evaluations that can supply valuable extra information for the athlete and the coaching staff but it is often sacrificed due to time constraints and lack of personnel capable of performing the tests. These evaluations by athletic trainers, strength coaches and rehabilitation specialists can be extensive and involve expensive equipment or can be performed in a more basic fashion. There are many options for taking measurements that can be adapted to the evaluation site and level of play. The areas of concern are usually flexibility, strength, endurance, power, speed and agility (Bar-Or et al 1998).

Screening tests are not routinely recommended for asymptomatic athletes during the preparticipation examination. Urinalysis for protein and glucose has been recommended in the past but has not been shown to be cost effective in detecting renal abnormalities and diabetes (Peggs et al 1986). Much attention has been focused on screening large populations of athletes with echocardiogram or electrocardiogram to detect cardiac abnormalities that may lead to sudden death. These methods of evaluation as a screening tool again are not cost effective and the problem of detecting falsely positive abnormalities causes significant delay in clearance to play for asymptomatic athletes (Maron et al 1996a). Hemoglobin and hematocrit levels, especially in female athletes who are more prone to iron deficiency anemia from menstrual blood losses, should be considered in at risk athletes, but not routinely ordered (AAFP, AAP, AMSSM, AOSSM, AOASM 1996).

Determining clearance

The vast majority of preparticipation examinations will result in clearance of the person to participate in the desired sport or exercise activity. Smith & Laskowski (1998) found that only 1.9% of 2739 athletes were disqualified from participation as a result of their examinations. When determining if a condition should disqualify an athlete from participating, the following questions should be considered (AAFP, AAP, AMSSM, AOSSM, AOASM 1996):

1. Will the problem place the athlete at increased risk of sudden death?
2. Will other athletes be placed at higher risk of injury?
3. Can this athlete safely play, with treatment (i.e. medication, protective equipment, rehabilitation)?

The level of competition and the age of the athlete are critical in making these decisions. If the increased risk of injury will have a long-lasting effect on the athlete's future health, the athlete should not be cleared for return to play. If clearance is denied for the chosen sport or exercise activity, it is very important to identify activities in which the person can safely participate. The importance of participating in sport or exercise should not be underestimated. Rifat et al (1995) found that adolescents rated not making the team as more devastating than their parents separating, the death of a close friend or academic failure. It is also important to discuss these decisions with the athletes and their families to determine what they want to be communicated to the coaches and athletic staff. The medical provider has primary responsibility to abide by the athlete's wishes for disclosure of information, and proper permission should be obtained before sharing medical information with others. In the USA there are additional regulations such as the Health Insurance Portability and Accountability Act (HIPPA) and the Family Education Rights and Privacy Act (FERPA) that medical providers may be required to follow (AAFP, AAP, ACSM, AMSSM, AOSSM, AOASM 2004). This, however, may be problematic as coaches and athletic staff expect to be part of the communication process when problems are identified and evaluation is being performed (Mitten 1996).

Table 12.2 Classification of sports by contact (reproduced with permission from the Preparticipation Physical Evaluation [monograph] Leawood, Kansas: American Academy of Family Physicians, American Academy of Pediatrics, American Medical Society for Sports Medicine, American Orthopaedic Society for Sports Medicine, American Osteopathic Academy of Sports Medicine 1996)

Contact/collision sport	Limited contact sport	Non-contact sport
Basketball	Baseball	Archery
Boxing	Bicycling	Badminton
Diving	Cheerleading	Body building
Field hockey	Canoeing/kayaking (whitewater)	Canoeing/kayaking (flat water)
Football	Fencing	Crew/rowing
(flag and tackle)	Field (high jump and pole vault)	Curling
Ice hockey		Dancing
Lacrosse	Floor hockey	Field (discus, javelin, shot put)
Martial arts	Gymnastics	
Rodeo	Handball	Golf
Rugby	Horseback riding	Orienteering
Ski jumping	Racquetball	Power lifting
Soccer	Skating (ice, inline and roller)	Race walking
Team handball		Riflery
Water polo	Skiing (cross-country, downhill and water)	Rope jumping
Wrestling		Running
	Softball	Sailing
	Squash	Scuba diving
	Ultimate frisbee	Strength training
	Volleyball	Swimming
	Windsurfing/surfing	Table tennis
		Tennis
		Track
		Weightlifting

Decisions about participation in a specific sport are made easier by classification of sports according to their physical requirements (Table 12.2).

There are only a few conditions in which participation is contraindicated. These are fever, carditis and diarrhea that is more than mild (AAFP, AAP, AMSSM, AOSSM, AOASM 1996). Fever is generally defined as an oral temperature greater than 100.4°F (38°C). Fever increases heart rate and cardiovascular workload, which can lead to orthostatic hypotension, heat illness and diminished performance. Carditis is an inflammation of the heart muscle or the surrounding myocardium, and is usually the result of a viral illness. This condition places the athlete at risk for sudden death with exertion; therefore, athletes should not participate for at least 6 months after the

Table 12.3 Medical conditions and sports participation

This table is designed to be understood by medical and non-medical personnel. In the 'Explanation' column, the words 'needs evaluation' mean that a physician with appropriate knowledge and experience should assess the safety of a given sport for an athlete with the listed medical condition. Unless otherwise noted, this is because of the variability of the severity of the disease or of the risk of injury among the specific sports, or both. (Reproduced with permission from the Preparticipation Physical Evaluation [monograph] Leawood, Kansas: American Academy of Family Physicians, American Academy of Pediatrics, American Medical Society for Sports Medicine, American Orthopaedic Society for Sports Medicine, American Osteopathic Academy of Sports Medicine 1997.)

Condition	May participate	Explanation
Atlantoaxial instability (instability of the joint between cervical vertebrae 1 and 2)	Qualified yes	Athlete needs evaluation to assess risk of spinal cord injury during sports participation
Bleeding disorder	Qualified yes	Athlete needs evaluation
Carditis (inflammation of heart)	No	May result in sudden death with exertion
Hypertension (high blood pressure)	Qualified yes	Those with significant essential (unexplained) hypertension should avoid weight and power lifting, bodybuilding and strength training. Those with secondary hypertension (caused by a previously identified disease) or severe essential hypertension need evaluation
Congenital heart disease (structural heart defects present at birth) Mild, moderate and severe congenital heart disease are defined in 26th Bethesda Conference: Recommendations for eligibility for competition in athletes with cardiovascular abnormalities. January 6–7, 1994. Med Sci Sports Exerc 1994; 26 (10 suppl):S246–253	Qualified yes	Those with mild forms may participate fully; those with moderate or severe forms, or who have undergone surgery, need evaluation
Dysrhythmia (irregular heart rhythm)	Qualified yes	Athlete needs evaluation because some types require therapy or make certain sports dangerous or both
Mitral valve prolapse (abnormal heart valve)	Qualified yes	Those with symptoms (chest pain, symptoms of possible dysrhythmia) or evidence of mitral regurgitation (leaking) on physical exam need evaluation. All others may participate fully
Heart murmur	Qualified yes	If murmur is innocent (does not indicate heart disease), full participation is permitted. Otherwise, the athlete needs evaluation
Cerebral palsy	Qualified yes	Athlete needs evaluation
Diabetes mellitus (well controlled)	Yes	All sports can be played with proper attention to diet, hydration, and insulin therapy. Particular attention is needed for activities that last 30 min or more
Diarrhea (American Academy of Pediatrics recommendation)	Qualified no	Unless disease is mild, no participation is permitted, because diarrhea may increase the risk of dehydration and heat illness (see Fever below)
Eating disorders (anorexia nervosa, bulimia nervosa)	Qualified yes	These patients need both medical and psychiatric assessment before participation
Functionally one-eyed athlete, loss of an eye, detached retina, previous eye surgery or serious eye injury	Qualified yes	A functionally one-eyed athlete has a best corrected visual acuity of <20/40 in the worse eye. These athletes would suffer significant disability if the better eye was seriously injured as would those with loss of an eye. Some athletes who have previously undergone eye surgery or had a serious eye injury may have an increased risk of injury because of weakened eye tissue. Availability of eye guards approved by the American Society for Testing Materials (ASTM) and other protective equipment may allow participation in most sports, but this must be judged on an individual basis

(Continued)

Table 12.3 (Continued)

Condition	May participate	Explanation
Fever	No	Fever can increase cardiopulmonary effort, reduce maximum exercise capacity, make heat illness more likely, and increase orthostatic hypotension during exercise. Fever may rarely accompany myocarditis or other infections that may make exercise dangerous
Heat illness (history of)	Qualified yes	Because of the increased likelihood of recurrence, the athlete needs individual assessment to determine the presence of predisposing conditions and to arrange a prevention strategy
Human immunodeficiency virus (HIV) infection	Yes	Because of the apparent minimal risk to others, all sports may be played that the state of health allows. In all athletes, skin lesions should be properly covered, and athletic personnel should use universal precautions when handling blood or body fluids with visible blood
Kidney (absence of one)	Qualified yes	Athlete needs individual assessment for contact/collision and limited contact sports
Liver (enlarged)	Qualified yes	If the liver is acutely enlarged, participation should be avoided because of risk of rupture. If the liver is chronically enlarged, individual assessment is needed before contact/collision or limited contact sports are played
Malignancy	Qualified yes	Athlete needs individual assessment
Musculoskeletal disorders	Qualified yes	Athlete needs individual assessment
History of serious head or spine trauma, severe or repeated concussions, or craniotomy	Qualified yes	Athlete needs individual assessment for contact/collision or limited contact sports, and also for non-contact sports if there are deficits in judgment or cognition. Recent research supports a conservative approach to management of concussions
Convulsive disorder (well controlled)	Yes	Risk of convulsion during participation is minimal
Convulsive disorder (poorly controlled)	Qualified yes	Athlete needs individual assessment for contact/collision or limited contact sports. Avoid the following non-contact sports: archery, riflery, swimming, weight or power lifting, strength training or sports involving heights. In these sports, occurrence of a convulsion may be a risk to self or others
Obesity	Qualified yes	Because of the risk of heat illness, obese persons need careful acclimatization and hydration
Organ transplant recipient	Qualified yes	Athlete needs individual assessment
Ovary (absence of one)	Yes	Risk of severe injury to the remaining ovary is minimal
Pulmonary compromise including cystic fibrosis	Qualified yes	Athlete needs individual assessment, but generally all sports may be played if oxygenation remains satisfactory during a graded exercise test. Patients with cystic fibrosis need acclimatization and good hydration to reduce the risk of heat illness
Asthma	Yes	With proper medication and education, only athletes with the most severe asthma will have to modify their participation
Acute upper respiratory infection	Qualified yes	Upper respiratory obstruction may affect pulmonary function. Athlete needs individual assessment for all but mild disease (see Fever above)

(Continued)

Table 12.3 (Continued)

Condition	May participate	Explanation
Sickle cell disease	Qualified yes	It is unlikely that individuals with sickle cell trait (AS) have an increased risk of sudden death or other medical problems during athletic participation except under the most extreme conditions of heat, humidity and possibly increased altitude. These individuals, like all athletes, should be carefully conditioned, acclimatized and hydrated to reduce any possible risk
Skin (boils, herpes simplex, impetigo, scabies, molluscum contagiosum)	Qualified yes	While the patient is contagious, participation in gymnastics with mats, martial arts, wrestling or other contact/collision or limited contact sports is not allowed. Herpes simplex virus probably is not transmitted via mats
Spleen (enlarged)	Qualified yes	Patients with acutely enlarged spleens should avoid all sports because of risk of rupture. Those with chronically enlarged spleens need individual assessment before playing contact/collision or limited contact sports
Testicle (absent or undescended)	Yes	Certain sports may require a protective cup

onset of the illness, and should have cardiac function evaluated before return to play. Moderate to severe diarrhea results in fluid loss that can lead to dehydration and heat illness in exercising individuals. Diarrhea is defined as the frequent passage of watery bowel movements. Participation should be postponed until the diarrhea resolves. There are several cardiac conditions that disallow competitive play. These are detailed in the 26th Bethesda Conference recommendations for determining eligibility in athletes with cardiovascular abnormalities (Bethesda Conference 1994). Hypertrophic cardiomyopathy is a condition that will disqualify most athletes from all but the lowest intensity sport activities. Athletes with congenital coronary artery anomalies should generally not participate in competitive sports. Prolonged Q-T syndrome is also an electrical condition that will disallow athletic participation since these athletes are at risk for sudden death from ventricular arrthymias. Athletes with severe aortic regurgitation or stenosis, multivalvular disease, arrhythomogenic right ventricular dysplasia, pulmonary hypertension or significant ventricular dysfunction should not participate in competitive sports. Individual assessment is needed by a cardiologist of all of these conditions.

For all other medical conditions listed in Table 12.3, participation is allowable based on individual circumstances and ability to use protective gear.

Summary

The preparticipation evaluation is an important intervention for athletic populations. Although it involves many components, the examination can be performed efficiently and in a timely manner. Individual examinations allow for relationship building and education of athletes, whereas coordinated medical team examinations allow for screeners with specific areas of expertise. The medical history can be preprinted and reviewed with the athlete during the visit. Most information that will be of concern will be revealed in the history. The physical examination is a screening that includes all the major body systems with the exception of the genital area in females. The focus in the examination is on finding pathology that may affect athletic performance. Health education and assessment of high-risk behaviors is especially important in adolescents who may not undergo any other health maintenance examination. The information gained from the history and physical examination is utilized to make clearance decisions. Communication with all involved participants is necessary when abnormalities are discovered. Although little evidence exists as to the effectiveness of this evaluation, identification of cardiac abnormalities, medical conditions that can affect long-term health and musculoskeletal injuries that can be rehabilitated are very important health outcomes for athletes. Medical and health care personnel who care for athletes should be well versed in the components of this evaluation.

References

Allen H D, Golinko R J, Williams R G 1994 Heart murmurs in children: when is a workup needed? Patient Care 28:123–151

American Academy of Family Physicians, American Academy of Pediatrics, American Medical Society for Sports Medicine, American Orthopaedic Society for Sports Medicine, American Osteopathic Academy of Sports Medicine (AAFP, AAP, AMSSM, AOSSM, AOASM) 1996 Preparticipation physical evaluation, 2nd edn. McGraw-Hill Healthcare, Minneapolis, MN

American Academy of Family Physicians, American Academy of Pediatrics, American Medical Society for Sports Medicine, American Orthopaedic Society for Sports Medicine, American Osteopathic Academy of Sports Medicine (AAFP, AAP, AMSSM, AOSSM, AOASM) 2004 Preparticipation physical evaluation, 3rd edn. McGraw-Hill Healthcare, Minneapolis, MN

American Psychiatric Association 1994 Diagnostic and statistical manual of mental disorders 4th edn. American Psychiatric Association, Washington, DC, p 539–550

Barkley K L 1997 Soccer. In: Mellion M B, Walsh W M, Shelton G L (eds) The team physician's handbook 2nd edn. Hanley and Belfus, Philadelphia, PA, p 672–684

Bar-Or O, Lombardo J A, Rowland T W 1988 The preparticipation sports exam. Patient Care 22:75–102

Batt M E, Jaques R, Stone M 2004 Preparticipation examination (screening): practical issues as determined by sport: a United Kingdom perspective. Clinical Journal of Sport Medicine 14:178–182

Bethesda Conference 1994 26th Bethesda Conference. Recommendations for determining eligibility for competition in athletes with cardiovascular abnormalities. Journal of the American College of Cardiology 24:845–899

Bratton R L, Agerter D C 1995 Preparticipation sports examinations efficient risk assessment in children and adolescents. Postgraduate Medicine 98:123–132

Brukner P, White S, Shawdon A et al 2004 Screening of athletes: Australian experience. Clinical Journal of Sport Medicine 14:169–177

Cantwell J D 1986 Marfan's syndrome: detection and management. Physician and Sportsmedicine 14(7):51–55

Carek P J, Futrell M 1999 Athlete's view of the preparticipation physical examination attitudes toward certain health screening questions. Archives of Family Medicine 8:307–312

Centers for Disease Control and Prevention 1999 Vaccine-preventable diseases: improving vaccination coverage in children, adolescents, and adults. A report on recommendations from the Task Force on Community Preventive Services. Morbidity and Mortality Weekly Report 48(RR-8):1–15

Chan D 2001 Testicular cancer: an update on recognition and management. Family Practice Recertification 23:27–34

Coyle E E 1994 Fluid and carbohydrate replacement during exercise: how much and what? Sports Science Exchange 7:1–10

Dombroski R T 1995 Wrestling. In: Baker C L (ed) The Hughston Clinic sports medicine book. Williams and Wilkins, Media, PA, p 677–670

Esquivel M T, McCormick D P 1987 Preparticipation sports evaluation: 1. The station-method examination. Family Practice Recertification 9:41–58

Frisch R E, Gotz-Welbergen A V, McArthur J W et al 1981 Delayed menarche and amenorrhea of college athletes in relation to age of onset of training. Journal of the American Medical Association 246:1559–1563

Goldenring J M, Cohen E 1988 Getting into adolescent HEADS. Contemporary Pediatrics 5:75

Hammer R W 1997 Swimming and diving. In: Mellion M B, Walsh W M, Shelton G L (eds) The team physician's handbook, 2nd edn. Hanley and Belfus, Philadelphia, PA, p 718–728.

Herman-Giddens M E, Slora E J, Wasserman R C et al 1997 Secondary sexual characteristics and menses in young girls seen in office practice: a study from the Pediatric Research in Office Settings Network. Pediatrics 99:505–512

Hobart J A, Smucker D R 2000 The female athlete triad. American Family Physician 61:3357–3364

Kenney W L (ed) 1995 Health screening and risk stratification. American College of Sports Medicine's guidelines for exercise testing and prescription, 5th edn. Williams and Wilkins, Media, PA

Mac M 1998 Managing the risks of school sports. School Administrator 55:42–46

McCrory P, Johnston K, Meeuwisse W et al 2005 Summary and agreement statement of the Second International Conference on Concussion in Sport, Prague 2004. Physician and Sportsmedicine 33(4):1–13

Maron B J, Thompson P D, Puffer J C et al 1996a Cardiovascular preparticipation screening of competitive athletes: a statement for health professionals from the sudden death committee and congenital cardiac defects committee, American Heart Association. Circulation 94:850–856

Maron B J, Shirani J, Poliac L C et al 1996b Sudden death in young competitive athletes: clinical, demographic, and pathological profiles. Journal of the American Medical Association 276:199–204

Maron B J, Thompson P D, Puffer J C et al 1998 Cardiovascular preparticipation screening of competitive athletes: addendum. Circulation 97:2294

Maughan R J, Shirreffs S M 1997 Preparing athletes for competition in the heat: developing an effective acclimatization strategy. Sports Science Exchange 10:1–8

Michael D J, Moeller J L, Hough D O 1996 Basketball injuries. In: Sallis R E, Massimino F (eds) Essentials of sports medicine. American College of Sports Medicine, St Louis, MO, p 558–570

Mitten M J 1996 When is disqualification from sports justified? Medical judgment vs patient's rights. Physician and Sportsmedicine 24(10):75–78

Murray B 1994 Fluid replacement: the American College of Sports Medicine position stand. Sports Science Exchange 7:1–10

National High Blood Pressure Education Program 1996 Update on the 1987 Task Force Report on High Blood Pressure in Children and Adolescents. Pediatrics 98:649–658

Nicola T L 1997 Tennis. In: Mellion M B, Walsh W M, Shelton G L (eds) The team physician's handbook, 2nd edn. Hanley and Belfus, Philadelphia, PA, p 816–827

Peggs J F, Reinhardt R W, O'Brien J M 1986 Proteinuria in adolescent sports physical examinations. Journal of Family Practice 22:80–81

Pigozzi F, Spataro A, Faganani F et al 2003 Preparticipation screening for the detection of cardiovascular abnormalities that may cause sudden death in competitive athletes. British Journal of Sports Medicine 37:4–5

Rifat S F, Ruffin M T 4th, Gorenflo D W 1995 Disqualifying criteria in a preparticipation sports evaluation. Journal of Family Practice 41:42–50

Risser W L, Hoffman H M, Bellah G G Jr 1985 Frequency of preparticipation sports examinations in secondary school athletes: are the University Interscholastic League guidelines appropriate? Texas Medicine 81:35–39

Smith J, Laskowski E R 1998 The preparticipation physical examination: Mayo Clinic experience with 2739 examinations. Mayo Clinic Proceedings 73:419–429

Storms W 1999 Exercise induced asthma: diagnosis and treatment for the recreational athlete. Medicine and Science in Sports and Exercise 31 (suppl 1):S33–S38

Taitel H F, Lippman J S 1995 Effects of oral contraceptives on bone mass: a review of the literature. Female Patient 20:30–47

Thomas S, Reading J, Shepard R J 1992 Revision of the Physical Activity Readiness Questionnaire (PAR-Q). Canadian Journal of Sport Science 17:338–345

Thompson R A, Sherman R T 1993 Helping athletes with eating disorders. Human Kinetics, Bloomington, p 45–65

Vinger P F 2000 A practical guide to sports eye protection. Physician and Sportsmedicine 28(6):49–67

Wingfield K, Matheson G O, Meeuwisse W H 2004 Preparticipation evaluation: an evidence-based review. Clinical Journal of Sport Medicine 14:109–122

Zheng Z, Menash G A, Croft J 2001 Sudden cardiac death in young people. Paper presented at American Heart Association's 41st Annual Conference on Cardiovascular Disease Epidemiology and Prevention 2001. Available online at: http//www.cdc.gov/od/oc/media/pressrel/r010301.htm (29 June 2006)

Clinical outcomes in sport and exercise physical therapies

James J. Irrgang and Robert G. Marx

13

CHAPTER CONTENTS

Introduction 206
Framework for identifying clinical outcomes 207
Selection of clinical outcome measures 211
Collecting, analyzing and interpreting clinical
outcome measures 215
Summary 218

Introduction

Outcomes management is the process of data collection, analysis and interpretation of the efficiency and effectiveness of patient treatment, with the intent of improving quality of care and lowering health care costs (Dobrzykowski 1997), and is an integral component of the process of care provided by physical therapists (American Physical Therapy Association 2001). Outcomes data can be used to make patient management decisions, assess clinician and organizational performance and to provide evidence for the effectiveness of interventions provided by physical therapists and other rehabilitation specialists. The validity of the inferences made from outcomes data is dependent on the outcome measures themselves and the circumstances under which the data were collected.

A framework for assessing outcomes of sports physical therapy is presented in Fig. 13.1. Important outcomes of sports physical therapy include clinical outcomes, process outcomes, patient satisfaction and costs (Irrgang 1996). Clinical outcomes are usually the primary interest when attempting to demonstrate effectiveness of rehabilitation and reflect the clinical status of the patient. Disablement schemes, such as the Nagi Disablement Model (Nagi 1991) and the recent International Classification of Impairment, Disability and Health (ICIDH-2) proposed by the World Health Organization (2001) provide a useful framework for identifying relevant clinical outcome measures and will be discussed in greater detail below.

Process outcomes represent the utilization of resources and include measures such as the duration of care, number of visits and number and type of interventions provided to the patient. Evaluation of process outcomes can be used to answer the question 'Did the intervention provided to the patient match the patient's diagnosis (classification) based upon the findings of the examination?' Selection of the most appropriate intervention for a particular patient requires the ability of the clinician to examine, evaluate and diagnose the condition in order to select the most appropriate form of intervention. Achieving optimal process outcomes requires application of the principles of evidence-based practice (see Chapter 1). Evaluation of process outcomes can be used to assess clinician and organizational performance. Expert clinicians would be expected to choose the most optimal interventions given a patient's diagnosis. Sources of process outcomes data may include scheduling and billing databases and patient records.

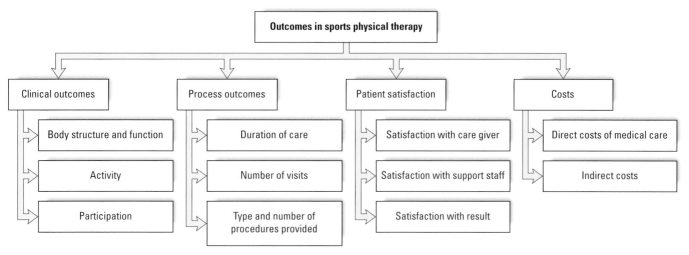

Figure 13.1 • Framework for assessing outcomes of sport physical therapy.

Patient satisfaction may also be an important outcome for sports physical therapy. Aspects of patient satisfaction include satisfaction with the caregiver, support staff and the clinical result. Patient satisfaction is usually measured anonymously using a written survey. Domains of patient satisfaction that are commonly measured in rehabilitation include satisfaction with access to care, physical environment, patient care, billing issues and overall satisfaction with the experience during the episode of care. Patient satisfaction instruments commonly use Likert-type rating scales that reflect the degree of satisfaction or dissatisfaction on a 5 to 7 point scale. Most patient satisfaction instruments have been developed by the user and have not undergone psychometric testing; however, Goldstein et al (2000) developed and tested a 26-item patient satisfaction survey to measure the outcome of physical therapy intervention. Patient satisfaction data can be aggregated to compare the levels of patient satisfaction achieved by individual clinicians or facilities, and may be useful for quality improvement initiatives to identify opportunities for improvement. Development and use of a standardized patient satisfaction instrument to measure the outcomes of sports physical therapy would be valuable to permit benchmarking between providers and organizations.

The costs of care may also be an important outcome of sports physical therapy. The total costs to an individual due to an injury include the direct costs for medical care as well as indirect costs. The direct costs for medical care for an injury go beyond the costs for rehabilitation and include the costs for diagnosis, medical/surgical management and any equipment that may be necessary to facilitate recovery. The indirect costs of an injury may be related to work time lost, decreased productivity or cost related to assistance required to perform activities of daily living or household activities. When discussing costs, one must be careful to distinguish costs from charges. From the perspective of the provider of sports rehabilitation, costs are the costs of providing a service including costs related to manpower, space, equipment and supplies. From the perspective of the patient or payer, costs are the charges for the

services that are rendered. Charges are closely related to the services (i.e. the process outcomes) that are provided during the episode of care. Costs can be used to calculate the value of sports physical therapy, which is defined as the ratio of the benefit of care divided by the costs of providing that care. The aim of sports physical therapy should be to provide high value, which is of large benefit at a relatively low cost. An important question that needs to be answered is 'Does sports physical therapy reduce the total costs associated with an injury?' The answer to this question requires detailed analyses and the expertise of a medical economist.

While process outcomes, patient satisfaction and costs are important outcomes of sports physical therapy to consider, the remainder of this chapter will focus on clinical outcomes. This will include a discussion of a framework for identifying important clinical outcomes, considerations for selecting outcome measures and collecting, analyzing and interpreting outcomes data.

Framework for identifying clinical outcomes

Disablement models provide a useful framework for identifying relevant clinical outcomes of sports physical therapy. Disablement models have been proposed by Nagi (1965, 1991), the World Health Organization (1980, 2001), and the National Center for Medical Rehabilitation Research (National Institutes of Health 1992). Disablement is the impact of injury or illness on the function of specific body systems, on basic human performance, and on an individual's role in society (Jette 1994, Verbrugge & Jette 1994). While the terminology used by the models differs somewhat, each of the models defines disablement at the tissue/cellular level, organ/ body system level, personal level and societal level (Table 13.1).

The Nagi scheme is the model of disablement accepted in the Guide to Physical Therapist Practice (American Physical

Table 13.1 Comparison of disablement schemes

System	Tissue/cellular level	Organ/system level	Personal level	Societal level
Nagi	Active pathology	Impairment	Functional limitation	Disability
ICIDH	Disease	Impairment	Disability	Handicap
NCRMM	Pathophysiology	Impairment	Disability	Societal limitation
ICIDH-2	Impairment of body structure and function	Impairment of body structure and function	Active restriction	Participation restriction

Therapy Association 2001). The Nagi disablement model includes active pathology, impairment, functional limitations and disability. Active pathology may result from infection, trauma, metabolic imbalance and/or degenerative disease conditions, and may interrupt or interfere with normal cellular processes. Active pathology includes the simultaneous efforts by the organism to regain homeostasis. Impairment is a loss or abnormality of an anatomical, mental or emotional nature that results in loss or abnormal function at the organ or body system level. Functional limitations refer to the manifestations of pathology and impairment on the function of the individual as a whole and may include limitation in physical or psychological function. Disability refers to the function of the individual within society and is defined as 'the inability or limitation experienced by the individual in performing socially defined roles and tasks within the context of a socio-cultural and physical environment' (Nagi 1991). Disability may affect family and other interpersonal interactions, work and other economic pursuits, education, recreation and/or self-care.

Recently, the World Health Organization (WHO) introduced a revision of the International Classification of Impairments, Disabilities and Handicaps (ICIDH), called the International Classification of Functioning and Disability (ICF) (World Health Organization 2001). The ICF provides a unified and standard language and framework for the description of health and health-related states that can be used as a framework to measure health outcomes.

In the ICF, health domains are described from the body, individual and societal perspectives in terms of (1) impairment (i.e., to body structure and function), (2) activity and (3) participation. In the ICF, functioning is an umbrella term that refers to all body functions, activities and participation, while disability is the umbrella term for impairments, activity limitations and participation restrictions. Body structures are the anatomical parts of the body, such as organs, limbs and their components. Body function refers to the physiological functions of the body systems including psychological function. Impairments are problems in body structure or function. Activity is the execution of a task or action by an individual, while participation is involvement in life situations. Activity limitations are difficulties an individual may have in executing activities, and participation restrictions are problems an individual may experience in involvement in life situations. The ICF model of functioning and disability provides a detailed description of body structure and function, activity and participation. For example, the activity and participation domain includes learning and applying knowledge, general tasks and demands, communication, mobility, self-care, domestic life, interpersonal interactions and relationships, major life areas and community, social and civic life.

The descriptions of body structure and function, activity and participation provided by the ICF can be used to identify important clinical outcomes of sports physical therapy. To illustrate this, consider an athlete with an acute knee sprain. Impairment of body structure may include disruption of the anterior cruciate ligament (ACL) or injury to the meniscus, articular cartilage or subchondral bone. Clinical outcome measures to evaluate body structure may include radiographs and magnetic resonance imaging. Impairment of body function may include limited range of motion, weakness or laxity of the knee. Measures of clinical outcome at the level of impairment of body function for this individual may include goniometry to measure the range of knee motion, isometric or isokinetic testing to measure quadriceps performance, or use of the KT-1000 (MedMetric, San Diego, CA) to measure anterior tibial laxity. Activity limitations experienced by this individual may include difficulty walking, climbing stairs, running, jumping and landing or cutting and pivoting. The resulting participation restrictions may include the inability to participate in sports such as football, soccer or basketball. Clinical outcome in terms of activity and participation can be measured by observing and rating the performance of the individual while executing a variety of activities, or by the use of standardized self-reports of activity limitations and participation restrictions. In summary, clinical outcome measures of body structure and function may include the results of diagnostic studies such as laboratory tests and imaging studies, as well as the findings from clinical examination of the involved structure or region. Clinical outcome measures of activity and participation may include observation of the individual or use of standardized self-reports of activity limitations and participation restrictions.

Health-related quality of life

Health-related quality of life is an individual's perception of his or her health. Broadly, health-related quality of life encompasses an individual's perception of his or her physical, emotional and social function. Health-related quality of life deals with what people perceive their health condition to be and the consequences of it; hence, it is the individual's subjective sense of wellbeing (World Health Organization 2001). Because health-related quality of life encompasses an individual's physical, emotional and social function, it overlaps with the activity and participation domains of the ICF model. As such, health-related quality of life measures can be used to measure the individual's perception of his or her activity and participation.

Many health-related quality of life measures have been developed. These can be classified as general or specific measures of health-related quality of life. General measures of health-related quality of life are designed to be applicable across a number of disease processes and interventions, and across demographic and cultural subgroups (McSweeney & Creer 1995). General health-related quality of life instruments are designed to give a comprehensive and general overview of health-related quality of life. General health-related quality of life measures are usually multidimensional and scores can be obtained for each dimension, or they can be combined to provide an overall measure. The most widely known and accepted general measure of health-related quality of life is the Medical Outcomes Study Short Form – 36 (McHorney et al 1993, 1994, Ware & Sherbourne 1992).

General measures of health-related quality of life permit comparisons across populations with different health conditions (Guyatt et al 1993, McSweeney & Creer 1995) and are more likely to detect unexpected effects of intervention (Kessler & Mroczek 1995, McSweeney & Creer 1995). An important limitation of general health-related quality of life measures is that they tend to be less responsive than specific measures of health-related quality of life, to changes in health status (Guyatt et al 1993). Therefore, use of general health-related quality of life measures might make it more difficult to detect the effects of an intervention for a specific condition. General measures of health-related quality of life are susceptible to ceiling effects. The presence of ceiling effects limits the ability to detect the effects of intervention, especially when used by young, healthy, high-level functioning individuals such as athletes. Because general measures of health-related quality of life measure a broad range of health including emotional function, the content may appear less relevant to patients and clinicians. Finally, general measures of health-related quality of life tend to be longer and more difficult to score.

Specific health-related quality of life measures are designed to focus on aspects of health that are specific to the primary condition or population of interest, with the intent of creating a more responsive measure (Guyatt et al 1993). Specific measures of health-related quality of life have been developed for specific diseases (e.g. osteoarthritis of the knee), specific populations of patients (e.g. the frail elderly), specific functions (e.g. physical function) or for symptoms (e.g. pain) (Guyatt et al 1993).

Specific measures of health-related quality of life are responsive to small changes in the patient's condition and are easy to administer and interpret (McSweeney & Creer 1995). The increased responsiveness of specific measures of health-related quality of life stems from the fact that they include only those important aspects of health-related quality of life that are relevant to the condition or population being studied (Guyatt et al 1993). Specific health-related quality of life measures usually relate closely to areas commonly assessed by clinicians, therefore they are more likely to be accepted by clinicians for routine use. Since specific health-related quality of life measures relate more closely to a particular condition, they are also more likely to be accepted by patients. Disadvantages of specific measures of health-related quality of life are that they do not measure all aspects of health status and they do not allow for comparisons between different disease states and/or populations.

Specific health-related quality of life measures include disease-specific, region-specific and patient-specific measures. Disease-specific measures of health-related quality of life are developed for a particular injury or illness. The content of disease-specific, health-related quality of life measures includes the symptoms, activity limitations and participation restrictions commonly experienced by individuals with the injury or illness for which the instrument was developed. Examples of disease-specific health-related quality of life measures include the Lysholm Knee Score (Tegner & Lysholm 1985), the Cincinnati Knee Rating System (Noyes et al 1984, Barber-Westin et al 1999) and the Quality of Life Assessment in Anterior Cruciate Ligament Deficiency (Mohtadi 1998) for knee ligament injuries. Also, there is the Western Ontario and McMaster Universities Osteoarthritis Index (WOMAC) (Bellamy et al 1988) for osteoarthritis of the knee and hip, and the Western Ontario Shoulder Instability Index (Kirkley et al 1998) for shoulder instability.

Region-specific, health-related quality of life measures have been developed to determine the effects of a variety of pathologies and impairments affecting a particular region. The content of region-specific measures of health-related quality of life reflects the symptoms, activity limitations and participation restrictions commonly experienced by individuals with impairment of the particular region for which the instrument was developed. Examples of region-specific measures of health-related quality of life include the following:

- Disabilities of the Arm Shoulder and Hand Index (DASH) (Beaton et al 2001a) for the upper extremity
- American Shoulder and Elbow Surgeons Patient Self-Evaluation Form (Richards et al 1994) for the shoulder
- Simple Shoulder Test (Lippitt et al 1993) for the shoulder
- Oswestry Low Back Pain Disability Questionnaire (Fairbank et al 1980) for the lumbar spine
- Quebec Back Pain Disability Scale (Kopec et al 1995) for the lumbar spine
- Lower Extremity Function Scale (Binkley et al 1999) for the lower extremity
- Knee Outcome Survey for the knee (Irrgang et al 1998)
- International Knee Documentation Committee Subjective Knee Form (Irrgang et al 2001) for the knee
- Foot and Ankle Ability Measure (Martin et al 2005) for the foot and ankle.

Patient-specific measures of health-related quality of life are defined by the patient. Patients are requested to provide a list of three to five relevant activities that they are either unable to do or have difficulty doing as a result of their problem, and then provide a rating of the difficulty they have doing each activity on an 11-point scale that ranges from 'unable to do' to 'able to do at preinjury level' (Stratford et al 1994, Westaway et al 1998). Patient-specific measures have been tested for the low back (Stratford et al 1994), knee (Chatman et al 1997) and cervical spine (Westaway et al 1998). Patient-specific measures of health-related quality of life are applicable to a large number of clinical conditions, efficient and easy to administer and record and have been found to have adequate psychometric properties. While patient-specific measures of health-related quality of life are responsive to within-subject change, between-subject comparisons are not possible because the content of each is determined by each patient.

Clinical outcomes that should be measured

The most important clinical outcome of rehabilitation for athletes is whether they can return to their prior level of activity and participation with the same intensity, frequency, duration and skill without symptoms and risk of reinjury. Furthermore, this outcome should be achieved in the shortest period of time possible. While on the surface this outcome appears easy to determine, it is difficult to quantify due to the varying demands of sports and levels of participation. Thus, function (i.e. the activity and participation) of the athlete is an important clinical outcome of sports physical therapy.

In addition to being an important outcome of treatment, sports activity is also an important prognostic factor in the sports medicine population because people who are very active have different expectations and demands than those who are active. In terms of outcome, it is important to know if a patient has returned to his or her preinjury level of sports activity in terms of the frequency, intensity and duration of participation as well as the length of time needed to return to this level. Defining outcome only in terms of absence of symptoms may be misleading if the level of sports activity is not considered. For example, the outcome would be considered suboptimal if prior to injury, an athlete could participate in very strenuous sports that require sprinting, cutting, pivoting, jumping and landing with no symptoms, but after surgery and rehabilitation can only return to moderate sports that involve running and turning without symptoms.

Because the frequency, intensity and duration of sports participation vary widely among patients, it is important for studies evaluating such individuals to clearly describe the patient's activity profile. For example, a study describing a new surgical technique for a knee disorder should document the patients' activity level to ensure that the results can be applied to the appropriate patient population. For studies comparing two groups of patients, it is important for the activity levels of the two groups to be similar in order to avoid a biased comparison.

In a systematic review (Marx et al 2001), five activity level rating scales that are potentially applicable to outcomes studies for knee injuries in sports medicine were identified (Daniel et al 1994, Noyes et al 1989, Seto et al 1988, Straub & Hunter 1988, Tegner & Lysholm 1985). There were inherent problems with each of the available instruments, which led to the construction of a new rating scale for this purpose (Marx et al 2001). This activity rating scale consists of four questions relating to the frequency with which the patient runs, cuts, pivots and decelerates. It has been demonstrated to be reliable and valid (Marx et al 2001). This scale is recommended in addition to a knee-specific health-related quality of life instrument for the evaluation of athletic patients with disorders of the knee. An activity rating scale for the upper extremity has recently been developed and has demonstrated acceptable levels of test retest reliability and validity (Brophy et al 2005).

Using the ICF model of functioning and disability, the range of clinical outcome measures should include measures of body structure and function, activity, and participation. Whyte (1994) suggested that the level of outcome measurement should be at or higher than the level of intervention. For example, the aim of ACL reconstruction is to restore stability of the ACL deficient knee. Thus an appropriate clinical outcome measure of ACL reconstruction is anterior and rotational laxity of the knee. One would expect that if surgery were successful, it would reduce anterior tibial translation as measured with the KT-1000 and eliminate the pivot shift. Also, restoring stability of the knee should allow the athlete to return to running, jumping and landing, cutting and pivoting, and ultimately to sports such as football, soccer or basketball. Thus, potential clinical outcome measures following ACL reconstruction include measurement at the levels of body structure and function, activity, and participation.

As another example, consider an athlete with a grade II posterior cruciate ligament injury with 6 to 10 mm of increased posterior tibial translation compared to the non-involved knee. Non-operative management for this individual may include quadriceps strengthening and a functional exercise progression. In this case, measurement of laxity would not be an appropriate outcome measure for this intervention because the intervention would not be expected to reduce posterior tibial translation. Appropriate clinical outcome measures for this case include strength testing of the quadriceps as well as the ability of the athlete to return to sports activities and participation. Therefore, clinical outcome measures should be thoughtfully selected and be appropriate for the intervention that was provided.

In the past it was believed that there was a direct link between impairment of body structure and function, activity limitations and participation restrictions; however, there is a growing body of literature to the contrary. For example, Snyder-Mackler et al (1997) found no relationship between laxity measured with the KT-1000 and activity and participation measured with the Knee Outcome Survey in ACL deficient copers and non-copers. Pantano et al (2001) obtained similar results 3–5 years after ACL reconstruction. Laxity, range of motion and isokinetic quadriceps and hamstring strength were not significantly related to function and disability as measured with the Knee Outcome Survey. Thus, at least for the knee, there does not appear to be a direct relationship between impairment of body structure and function and the resulting activity limitations and participation restrictions.

This lack of a direct relationship between impairment of body structure and function and activity and participation limitations is inherent in the ICF model (Fig. 13.2). In this model, disability is the outcome of a complex interaction between the

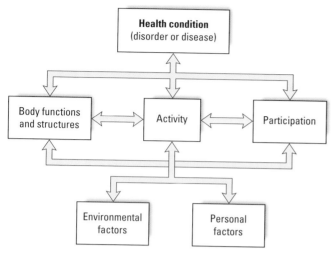

Figure 13.2 • Model of functioning and disability proposed by the World Health Organization in the International Classification of Functioning Disability and Health. (Reproduced with permission from ICF – International Classification of Functioning and Disability, World Health Organization, 2001.)

individual's health condition and contextual factors (World Health Organization 2001). Contextual factors include environmental and personal factors. Environmental factors are the make up of the physical, social and attitudinal environment in which individuals live and conduct their lives. Personal factors include gender, race, age, other health conditions, fitness, lifestyle, habits, upbringing, coping styles, social background, education, profession, past and current experiences, overall behavior pattern and character style, individual psychological assets and other characteristics, all or any of which may play a role in disability (World Health Organization 2001). Research is needed to explore these complex interactions between health conditions and contextual factors and the resulting disability.

The lack of a direct relationship between impairment of body structure and function and the resulting activity limitations and participation restrictions implies that measures of impairment should not be combined with measures of activity limitations and participation restrictions into a single composite score. Rather, reports of clinical outcome should include separate summaries of relevant measures of impairment of body structure and function that are appropriate for the interventions that were provided and valid measures of activity limitations and participation restrictions. Furthermore, because the relationship between impairment and the resulting activity limitations and participation restrictions is not direct, and because activity limitations and participation restrictions are of the utmost concern to the athlete, the primary clinical outcome should be measures of activity limitations and participation restrictions. Activity limitations and participation restrictions may be measured either through direct observation of performance or by general or specific measures of health-related quality of life.

Selection of clinical outcome measures

When selecting clinical outcome measures, one must consider the purpose for which the information will be used as well as practical and psychometric considerations of the instrument. Kirshner & Guyatt (1985) classified health indices according to their purpose as discriminative, predictive or evaluative measures of health. Discriminative health measures are those that distinguish individuals or groups of individuals on an underlying dimension when no external criterion is available for validating the measure. Predictive health indices are those which attempt to classify individuals into a set of predefined categories when an external criterion measure exists concurrently or in the future to determine if the individual has been correctly classified. Evaluative health indices are those that have been developed to measure change within an individual or of a group over time on the dimension of interest. To demonstrate the effects of sports physical therapy, one is interested in measuring change in body structure and function, activity and participation over time. Thus, demonstration of clinical outcomes requires the use of evaluative health indices.

Practical considerations for selection of clinical outcome measures include ease of use, acceptance and costs (McSweeney & Creer 1995). Self-administered health-related quality of life measures are attractive clinical outcome measures because they require minimal resources for administration; however, the reading level must be appropriate for the intended audience. Ease of use of self-administered health-related quality of life measures is determined by the time required for administration and scoring, as well as the effort required to interpret and use the data. Costs for administrating and scoring a measure of health-related quality of life will greatly influence its acceptance in clinical practice and research. Clinical outcome measures that require special expertise or equipment for administration, scoring and interpretation are likely to be more costly and less readily accepted than self-administered health-related quality of life measures that can be scored manually (McSweeney & Creer 1995).

Psychometric considerations for selection of a clinical outcome measure

A number of authors have discussed psychometric considerations for selecting a clinical outcome measure (Guyatt et al 1993, Hoffman et al 1995, Kessler & Mroczek 1995, Kirshner & Guyatt 1985, Lohr et al 1996, McSweeney & Creer 1995, Testa & Nackley 1994, Testa & Simonson 1996). Important psychometric considerations when selecting an evaluative clinical outcome measure include reliability, validity and responsiveness. According to contemporary validity theory, in which validity is defined as 'the degree to which empirical evidence and theoretical rationales support the adequacy and appropriateness of the inferences and actions based on the tests scores' (Messick 1989), these psychometric considerations all fall within the realm of validity. Knowledge of the psychometric characteristics of a clinical outcome measure allows one to interpret the appropriateness and usefulness of the inferences and actions that are based on the scores from the measure. Furthermore, the nature of the evidence that is required to interpret the appropriateness and usefulness of scores from a particular clinical outcome measure is dependent on the intended purpose and/or use of the measure (Kirshner & Guyatt 1985). When selecting a clinical outcome measure, one must consider the psychometric evidence to support the validity of the inferences that will be made and the actions that will be taken based upon the clinical outcome measure.

Validity evidence to support use and interpretation of a clinical outcome instrument to measure change should include evidence that: the items are all related to the construct being measured (i.e. the items are unidimensional), the score is related to other measures of the construct and not unduly related to other constructs (i.e. the score demonstrates convergent and divergent evidence of validity), the score remains stable when the underlying condition measured by the outcome instrument remains stable (i.e. the score demonstrates test re-test reliability) and the score changes with improvement or deterioration of the condition measured by the instrument (i.e. the score is responsive). Among these, evidence for reliability and responsiveness is most important and will be discussed in greater detail below.

Reliability

Reliability of a clinical outcome measure implies consistency of measurement. Measures of reliability include internal consistency and test re-test reliability. Internal consistency is applicable to outcome measures such as measures of health-related quality of life that consist of multiple items. Internal consistency is the degree to which all items on the scale consistently measure the underlying condition and is concerned with measurement errors related to sampling of items that are included on the instrument (Crocker & Algina 1986). Internal consistency is most commonly estimated with coefficient alpha.

Test re-test reliability is the degree to which scores remain stable when there is no change in the underlying construct that is being measured. Test re-test reliability for a clinical outcome measure is estimated by measuring individuals two or more times over a period of time when the individual's condition is expected to remain stable. The amount of time between repeat measurements is an important issue when determining test re-test reliability (Marx et al 2003). The length of time should not be so short that memory or recall artificially inflates the test re-test reliability estimate. Conversely, the length of time between repeat administrations of the clinical outcome measure should not be too long to avoid change in the condition that is being measured. In general, the length of time between repeat administrations of the clinical outcome measure should be relatively short (e.g. 1–3 days) when the condition being measured is expected to change rapidly (e.g. patients within the first 4 weeks after ACL reconstruction). The time between

repeat administrations of the clinical outcome measure should be longer (e.g. 4 weeks or more) when the condition is not expected to change (e.g. individuals who are 3 to 5 years status post-ACL reconstruction). Given this, it is evident that test re-test reliability should not be considered a property of the instrument itself, but rather the degree of consistency of measurement when applied to certain populations under particular measurement conditions (Streiner & Norman 1995).

The type of reliability coefficient used to estimate test re-test reliability is dependent on the nature of the data. Percent agreement and Cohen's kappa statistic, which is the agreement above chance agreement, are recommended for nominal or ordinal level data, while the intraclass correlation coefficient (Shrout & Fleiss 1979) is recommended for interval or ratio level data. Because test re-test reliability is concerned not only with the relative standing of individuals on repeated measurement, but also the degree to which the repeated measurement yields the same score, the intraclass correlation coefficient is recommended over the Pearson correlation coefficient when estimating test re-test reliability for continuous data.

The standard error of measurement can be used to interpret estimates of internal consistency and test re-test reliability. The standard error of measurement (SEM) is defined as:

$$\textbf{SEM} = \sigma\sqrt{1 - r}$$

where σ is the standard deviation of the scores and r is the reliability coefficient. When coefficient alpha is used to determine the standard error of measurement, the interpretation should be limited to the error associated with a measure at a single point in time. If one is concerned with error over repeated measurements, the intraclass correlation coefficient should be used to determine the standard error of measurement. The standard error of measurement can be used to determine a confidence interval that can facilitate interpretation of a score. For example, coefficient alpha for the Activities of Daily Living Scale of the Knee Outcome Survey was found to be 0.92 in a sample of 397 patients presenting for outpatient physical therapy with a variety of knee impairments and the corresponding standard error of measurement was approximately 6 points on the Activities of Daily Living Scale (Irrgang et al 1998). Thus, the 95% confidence interval (i.e. ± 1.96 SEM) for an observed score of 70 ranges from 58 to 82. This means that if an individual has a true score of 70, 95 out of 100 times that the individual is measured the individual would have an observed score between 58 and 82.

When one is concerned about the magnitude of the expected difference between scores on repeat testing, the intraclass correlation coefficient should be used to calculate the SEM. Furthermore, the standard error of measurement should be multiplied by $\sqrt{2}$ to take into account that there is error associated with both the first and second scores (Streiner & Norman 1995). To illustrate this, consider test re-test reliability of the International Knee Documentation Committee Subjective Knee Score, which was found to be 0.94 when estimated over an average interval of 50 days in 33 individuals who were participating in long-term outcome studies following ACL reconstruction, meniscal replacement or proximal and distal realignment of the knee extensor mechanism (Irrgang et al 2001). The standard deviation of the scores for this data was 18. Given this, the 95% confidence interval of the expected difference between the scores was ±12.2 points. Thus, a change in the score over a 7-week interval greater than 12.2 points represents a true change beyond measurement error, while a change less than 12.2 points may occur due to chance alone because of the measurement error at each point in time. The expected difference between scores due to error associated with repeated testing is called the minimal detectable change and is interpreted as the amount of change that needs to be observed before it can be considered beyond the bounds of measurement error for an instrument in a particular application (Beaton 2000).

Responsiveness

Responsiveness is the degree to which a clinical outcome score changes as the underlying condition that is measured by the scale changes. A clinical outcome measure that is responsive will reflect improvement as an individual's condition improves and deterioration as the individual's condition worsens. Demonstration of responsiveness for a clinical outcome measure requires evidence that the measure accurately detects change when change has occurred. Studies to demonstrate responsiveness of a clinical outcome measure should link the amount of change in the outcome score to a construct of change. The construct of change is the way that was used to demonstrate that change has in fact occurred (Beaton 2000). Examples of a construct for change include change from before to after treatment of a known efficacy or change in those deemed to be better or worse, based on an external marker of change (Beaton 2000, Stratford et al 1996).

Factors that will affect the magnitude of change for a given instrument include the patient group under study, the type of treatment being studied, timing of the data collection and the construct for change (Beaton 2000). For example, one would expect greater change over a similar time frame for those with an acute condition compared to those that have a chronic condition. The patient group, type of treatment and timing of data collection must be comparable before the results of a responsiveness study can be applied to a particular clinical setting or used to judge the meaningfulness of a change score (Beaton 2000). The construct for change must also be considered when interpreting the results of a responsiveness study. The construct of change is defined by the answers to: (1) Who is the focus of the analysis? (2) Which scores are being compared? and (3) What kind of change or difference is being examined? (Beaton 2000, Beaton et al 2001b).

The focus of the analysis can be at the group or individual level. When the focus of the analysis is at the group level, summary statistics, such as the mean, standard deviation, median and range or combinations of these statistics in the form of an effect size, standardized response mean or Guyatt's responsiveness index are reported for the entire group or the subgroup of individuals who improved (Beaton 2000). While these group statistics provide useful information about what should be expected for a group of individuals, they do not provide meaningful information that can be used to interpret change of a particular individual.

When the focus of analysis is at the individual level, receiver operating characteristic curves are used to determine the cut-off value for the change score that has the highest sensitivity and specificity for change (Beaton 2000). Sensitivity of change is the proportion of subjects that have improved according to a criterion of change that have a change score above the cutoff point. Specificity of change is the proportion of subjects that have not improved according to a criterion measure of change that have a change score below the cutoff point (Deyo & Centor 1986). When the focus of the analysis is at the individual level, the challenge is to select the cutoff point in the change score that best discriminates between those that have improved and those that have not improved. The results of a responsiveness study, where the focus of analysis has been at the individual level, can be used to determine if a particular individual has improved or not, given the similarities of other aspects of the responsiveness study (e.g. patient group, type of treatment and timing of data collection) (Beaton 2000).

The construct of change for a responsiveness study is also defined by the scores that are being compared (Beaton 2000). Possibilities include comparison of scores within subjects, between subjects or between group differences of within-subject change. A within-subjects comparison of scores is made over time by comparing before and after scores within an individual or group of individuals. A between-subjects comparison entails a comparison of health states between persons at a single point in time. Differences in the scores between pairs of subjects, one of whom states he or she is healthier than the other, can be used to determine minimally clinically important differences; however, it is doubtful that this construct for change is comparable to constructs that link responsiveness to longitudinal change over time (Beaton et al 2001b). A between-groups difference of within-subject change compares the within-group change over time between two or more groups. This comparison is concerned with the amount of change in one group over time compared to the amount of change over the same period of time in another group. An example of this is a clinical trial, in which the within-subject change in the experimental group is compared to the within-subject change in the control group. Demonstration of responsiveness would entail demonstrating that the within-subject change is greater in the experimental group than in the control group. In essence, this comparison is a combination of a within-subjects and between-subjects comparison.

The third determinant of the construct for change is what kind of change is being quantified in the study to provide evidence for responsiveness. The change that is being quantified can include: (1) change that is considered greater than measurement error; (2) change that is observed over time before and after a treatment; (3) change in those that have improved according to a criterion measure of change; or (4) change in those that have had a major improvement according to a criterion measure of change (Beaton 2000, Beaton et al 2001b).

The minimal detectable change is the amount of change that is considered to be greater than measurement error (Christensen & Mendoza 1986). It is calculated as the confidence interval for the standard error of measurement for the expected difference between before and after scores (see Reliability section above). Calculation of the standard error of measurement to determine the minimum detectable change requires the use of the test re-test reliability coefficient and multiplication by $\sqrt{2}$ to correct for error associated with measurements made at two points in time. The minimum detectable change can be considered to be the lowest change score that can be confidently considered to be beyond measurement error. It provides an anchor for interpretation of a change score because only when a change score exceeds the minimum detectable change can the clinician be confident that the change score represents true change of the individual and not measurement error (Beaton 2000).

Observed change is the change that occurs in an individual before and after a treatment or over a period of time that is expected to result in improvement for most individuals (Beaton 2000, Beaton et al 2001b). No criterion measure of change is used to determine if individuals have truly changed. This type of change assumes that with treatment or the passage of time, most subjects will improve and the analysis is performed on all subjects being studied. The observed change provides information on how much change should be expected for individuals receiving a particular treatment or being observed for a similar period of time.

Estimated change utilizes a criterion measure of change to determine whether a change has occurred (Beaton 2000, Beaton et al 2001b). The criterion measure of change is used to separate a group of individuals into those that have improved and those that have not improved. Many different criterion measures of change have been proposed from different perspectives including the patient, clinician, payer or society (Beaton 2000). The analysis involves contrasting the change score between those that have improved and those that have not improved. The estimated change provides an estimate of the magnitude of the change score in individuals who improve, and because a criterion measure of change is used, it provides an opportunity to determine the best change score to use as a threshold for improvement in similar individuals.

Important change is similar to estimated change; however, it implies that not only has change occurred, but the change that has occurred is important to the patient, clinician, payer or society (Beaton 2000, Beaton et al 2001b). Important change is often referred to as the minimum clinically important change. It is determined by using a criterion measure that determines that important change has occurred.

The above taxonomy developed by Beaton (Beaton 2000, Beaton et al 2001b) can be used when judging the usefulness of a clinical outcome measure to evaluate change over time. When selecting an outcome instrument to measure change, one should review the evidence to support its reliability and validity for a particular application. Ideally, the evidence to support use of a clinical outcome measure should be determined under conditions that are similar to those under which the measure will be utilized. This requires careful analysis to determine if the patient group, type of treatment, timing of data collection and construct of change that were used in the study to provide evidence for the usefulness of the clinical outcome measure matches the patient group, type of treatment, timing of data collection and construct for change of the application for which the instrument will be used. To facilitate this, Beaton (2000) has provided guidelines for evaluating evidence to support the use and interpretation of a clinical outcome instrument to measure change (see Box 13.1).

Box 13.1 Guidelines for evaluating evidence to support use and interpretation of a clinical outcome instrument to measure change (reproduced with permission from Beaton D E 2000 Understanding the relevance of measured change through studies of responsiveness. Spine 25:3192–3199)

First, be clear about the type of information you need to know about. Define your patient group and type of change you need to understand. Second, appraise whether this study offers you the right kind of information by asking these questions:

1. Are the patients similar enough to my own?
   Yes
   No
2. Are they looking at a similar type of treatment?
   Yes
   No
   Time between treatment _____
3. What category of responsiveness is being studied?
   A. Who is the focus of the analysis and the results presented? Individuals or groups of patients?
      group level
      individual level
   B. Which data are being contrasted?
      over time (same patients, over time)
      one point in time (between persons)
      hybrid (between group differences of within person change)
   C. What type of change is being quantified?
      minimum change detectable given measurement error
      observed change in a given population
      observed change in those deemed to have changed (estimated change) – according to:
         patient
         clinician/researcher
         payer
         society
      observed change in those deemed to have had an important change – according to:
         patient
         clinician/researcher
         payer
         society

Collecting, analyzing and interpreting clinical outcome measures

Outcomes management requires collection, analysis and interpretation of data to improve the quality of care that is provided and to reduce health care costs. The ultimate aim of an outcomes management system should be to increase value, which is defined as the ratio of quality to costs. High value is achieved by maximizing improvements in quality while minimizing costs. Outcomes data can be used to make patient management decisions, and to provide evidence for the effectiveness of interventions provided by physical therapists and other rehabilitation specialists. When utilized as part of a quality improvement initiative, outcomes data can be used to assess performance of individual clinicians as well as of organizations as a whole. In addition to the quality of the outcome measures, validity of the inferences made from outcomes data is dependent on the circumstances under which the data were collected and interpreted.

Collection of outcomes data

To minimize selection bias, outcomes data should be collected from all individuals with the condition of interest. If this is not possible, then outcomes data should be collected from a representative random sample of individuals. Selection bias in outcomes data can arise when the sample is not representative of the population of individuals that are of interest to the clinician. For example, excluding individuals from the analysis with incomplete follow-up data due to individuals terminating treatment before the course of care is complete may result in an overly favorable outcome. While it is acknowledged that collection of outcomes data from all individuals with the condition of interest or collection of data from a truly random sample may not be possible, attempts should be made to detect bias by determining if the sample of individuals for whom outcomes data is complete is different at the start of care from the sample of individuals with incomplete outcomes data. This requires consistent collection of outcomes data from all individuals at the start of care.

An important concept in the ICF classification system is that contextual factors interact with an individual's health condition to determine the individual's level of functioning (i.e. the individual's activity and participation) (World Health Organization 2001). Contextual factors include both personal and environmental factors. Personal factors include features of the individual that are not part of a health condition such as gender, race, other health conditions, fitness, lifestyle, habits, upbringing, coping styles, social background, education, profession, past and current life experiences, character and psychological status (World Health Organization 2001). Environmental factors include the individual's immediate environment, such as the home, workplace or school, as well as services and systems in the community that can have an impact on the functioning of the individual. Because an individual's level of function and disability are the result of an interaction between the individual's

health condition with personal and environmental contextual factors, attempts to describe the clinical outcome of care provided by the physical therapist should include collection of information that may mediate or modify clinical outcome. Thus, an outcomes data collection system should attempt to capture personal and environmental factors that may impact on clinical outcome.

To make valid inferences, the outcomes data collection system should make use of valid (as broadly defined above) clinical outcome measures. When selecting an outcome measure, use of a 'common currency' will facilitate the ability to compare results between organizations as well as to data in the literature for benchmarking purposes. Linking the outcomes data collection system to scheduling and billing systems will facilitate incorporation of process and cost outcomes. Procedures should be established to facilitate systematic collection of outcomes data to allow for assessment of the individual over time. These procedures should minimize burden on staff and patients required to collect the outcomes data. The use of computer technology can greatly facilitate this process.

Components of a comprehensive outcomes data collection system should include relevant clinical outcome measures. This should include both general and specific health-related quality of life measures to quantify disability in terms of activity limitations and participation restrictions. A general measure of health-related quality of life, such as the SF-36, should be included to provide a comprehensive assessment of health, including physical, emotional and social functioning. Additionally, a general measure of health-related quality of life permits comparisons across populations with different health conditions (Guyatt et al 1993, McSweeney & Creer 1995) and is more likely to detect unexpected effects of intervention (Kessler & Mroczek 1995, McSweeney & Creer 1995). A specific measure of health status, such as the DASH for conditions affecting the upper extremity or the Oswestry Low Back Disability Questionnaire for conditions affecting the low back, should be included to enhance detecting the effects of intervention on an individual's level of function and disability.

As interventions provided by physical therapists are often directed at impaired body structure and function, a comprehensive outcomes data collection system may also include relevant measures of impairment. Inclusion of impairment measures will enable clinicians to determine if interventions directed at impairments were effective at alleviating the impairment and will allow for exploration of relationships between impairment, activity limitations and participation restrictions. However, as noted above, because the relationship between impairment and disability is not direct, and because function and disability are of the utmost concern to the athlete, measures of impairment should not be the only clinical outcome measure included in the outcomes database.

To account for factors that may mediate or modify clinical outcome, contextual factors including characteristics of the individual as well as characteristics of the environment in which the individual must function should be included in a comprehensive outcomes data collection system. Examples of personal factors that may be included are gender, age, level of education and comorbidities. Environmental factors that may be included in an outcomes data collection system are the nature and demands imposed by work or the type of sports activities in which the individual is able to participate. To describe process outcomes, the outcomes data collection system should include information regarding the duration of care, number of visits and type of procedures provided to the individual. This information may be obtained from the scheduling and/or billing systems.

Systematic collection of outcomes data requires the development of forms that are either completed by the patient or clinician. These forms should be user-friendly and utilize a type font size that is easy to read. The forms should include clear instructions to facilitate accurate completion and to minimize the burden of administration. To minimize the burden of completing the form, the form should maximize the use of check boxes. The form should be organized to facilitate scoring and entry of data into a computerized database. Development of forms that can be scanned or faxed into a computerized database can facilitate data entry. Once in a database, routines can be written to automatically score the data and to store it for analysis at a later time.

An alternative to the use of paper forms to collect outcomes data is the use of computers with user-friendly interfaces. Advances in computer technology including the use of touch screens, wireless networks and the internet have opened new avenues for collection of outcomes data.

In the future, it is envisioned that computerized data collection systems that are internet compatible will be available to collect patient-reported outcomes data during an office visit or from the patient's home. In the clinic, the system will make use of touch screen tablet computers that are wirelessly connected to a local server to efficiently and effectively collect clinical outcomes data. Using a computerized system to collect patient-reported outcomes data while the patient is in the clinic takes advantage of unutilized patient time, helps to increase operational efficiency, and provides the clinician and patient with an instantaneous summary of the patient's status. Providing a summary of the patient-oriented data to the clinician at the time of the encounter should facilitate the encounter and should improve the clinician's efficiency. At home, patients could log-on to a secure website to provide patient-reported outcomes data. Being able to collect patient-reported outcomes data from home simplifies data collection and enhances patient follow-up. Clinical data could be input directly into the system using computers located throughout the clinic. This allows for efficient recording of findings from the physical examination as well as the treatment that was provided.

To facilitate efficient longitudinal data collection, the system should make use of condition-, time- and/or protocol-specific algorithms to determine the data that needs to be collected and/or updated at any given encounter. The system should also be able to accommodate algorithms to administer unique questions based upon responses to prior questions. This will allow the data collection process to be tailored to the unique responses from the patient or clinician, which improves efficiency of data capture. These algorithms should be easily adjustable to tailor the data collection process to unique clinical populations. Finally, the system should be designed to meet all HIPAA regulations. As such, each patient should be assigned a unique identification number that allows linking of data from multiple encounters and all data should be encrypted when transmitted over the internet.

Outcomes data should be collected at the initiation of care, at regular intervals during the course of care and at the conclusion of care. Data that should be collected at the initiation of care include general and specific measures of health-related quality of life, as well as personal and environmental factors that may mediate or moderate the outcome of care. To measure the response to intervention during the course of care, specific measures of health-related quality of life should be collected on a regular basis (e.g. every 1–2 weeks) during the course of care. Collection of specific measures of health-related quality of life at regular intervals during the course of care will also ensure that some follow-up outcomes data is available for analysis should an individual terminate care before the episode of care is completed. At the conclusion of care, general and specific measures of health-related quality of life, as well as a measure of patient satisfaction, should be collected. To assess the lasting effects of intervention after the course of care is completed, efforts should be made to collect follow-up data, including general and specific measures of health-related quality of life. Alternatives to having an individual return to the clinic to collect this data include the use of telephone or mailed surveys that may include the use of electronic mail and the world wide web.

Analyzing and interpreting clinical outcomes data

Clinical outcomes data can be analyzed and interpreted at either the individual or group level. At the individual level, clinical outcomes data can be used to determine if a particular individual is better, worse or unchanged as a result of intervention. This entails calculation of a change score, which is the difference in the clinical outcome measure from initiation of care to follow-up. To determine if the individual is better, worse or unchanged, the change score can be compared to either the minimum detectable change or minimal clinically important difference. If the change score exceeds the minimal detectable change, then one can be confident that the amount of change as measured by the clinical outcome instrument exceeds the bounds of measurement error for the instrument in a particular application. If the change score exceeds the minimal clinically important difference, then we can be confident that the change, as measured by the clinical outcome instrument, exceeds the amount of change described by other similar individuals as being an important amount of change. The validity of the decisions made at the individual level is dependent on how well the evidence for interpretation of the change score matches the condition under which the decision is applied. As discussed in the above section on responsiveness, application of evidence supporting responsiveness of a clinical outcome measure should consider the degree to which the patient group, type of treatment, timing of data collection and construct for change used to provide evidence of responsiveness for the clinical outcome measure matches the patient group, type of treatment, timing of data collection and construct for change under which the evidence will be applied.

Measures of central tendency and dispersion are used to summarize data at the group level. Measures of central tendency include the mean, median and mode. The mean is the average score for the group. The median is the middle score or the score at the 50th percentile. The most frequent score is the mode. When data are skewed, such as when there are a few extreme scores, the median will provide a better representation of the entire group than will the mean. This is because the few extreme scores affect the mean, while the median will not be affected as much.

Measures of dispersion include the range, standard deviation and variance. The range is the distance between the highest and lowest score for the entire group. The standard deviation is the square root of the variance. The variance is equal to the average squared distance between each individual score and the group average as given by the following formula:

$$\sigma^2 = \frac{\sum_{i=1}^{n}(x_i - \bar{x})^2}{n}$$

In this formula σ^2 is the variance, x_i is the score of the i-th individual from 1 to n, $\bar{x}$ is the group average and n is the number of individuals in the sample. Scores that are spread over a larger range will have a larger variance and standard deviation, while scores that are very closely distributed to the group mean will have a smaller variance and standard deviation.

A number of indices have been developed to summarize change in the clinical outcome measure over time. These include a change score, effect size, standardized response mean and Guyatt's responsiveness index. A complete description and use of these statistics can be found in Stratford et al (1996); however, the effect size and standardized response mean deserve additional comment. The effect size (ES) is calculated as:

$$ES = \frac{\text{Average change}}{\text{Standard deviation of initial scores}}$$

and the standardized response mean (SRM) is calculated as:

$$SRM = \frac{\text{Average change}}{\text{Standard deviation of change scores}}$$

Both the ES and SRM relate the average change in the clinical outcome score from the initial to follow-up measure to the variability of the scores. The ES relates the average change to the variability of the initial measures, while the SRM relates the average change to the variability of the change scores. The resulting statistics interpret the magnitude of change in terms of the variability of the scores. For example, an ES of 0.5 is

interpreted to mean that the average change from the initial to follow-up measure is equal to one-half of a standard deviation of the initial scores. Cohen (1969) provides guidelines for interpreting the ES: an ES greater than or equal to 0.8 is considered large, 0.5 is considered medium and 0.2 is considered small.

Use of an ES to describe clinical outcomes data is described in Fig. 13.3. This figure is a radar graph that displays the ES over the episode of care for patients with a variety of knee impairments. Each axis of the graph represents the ES for one of the 8 scales of the SF-36. Graphs such as this can be used to benchmark (i.e. compare) the performance of an individual or organization against data from an external organization. For example, in Fig. 13.3, the effect of physical therapy intervention provided by a large outpatient rehabilitation organization in the Pittsburgh, PA, region is compared to data published by Jette & Jette (1996). On average, the improvement in physical function achieved by the outpatient rehabilitation organization in Pittsburgh is approximately 0.1 of a standard deviation larger than that reported by Jette & Jette (1996), and the improvement in social function is approximately 0.3 of a standard deviation larger. While this implies that individuals with knee impairments treated in Pittsburgh may experience slightly better

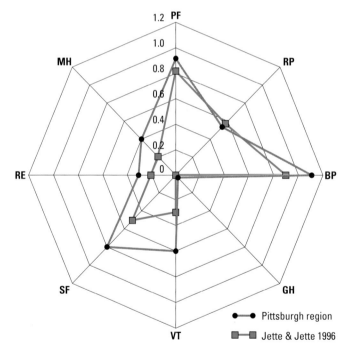

Figure 13.3 • Radar graph of the effect size of each of the 8 scales of the SF-36 following a course of physical therapy in patients with a variety of knee impairments. Data from patients receiving physical therapy from a large multicenter nonprofit outpatient physical therapy organization in the Pittsburgh, PA, region are benchmarked against data reported by Jette & Jette (1996). Each of the axes represents a scale of the SF-36. PF = Physical Function Scale. RP = Role Limitations Due to Physical Function. BP = Bodily Pain. GH = General Health. VT = Vitality. SF = Social Function. RE = Role Limitations Due to Emotional Health. MH = Mental Health.

improvement from a course of physical therapy in health-related quality of life as measured by the SF-36, the results must be interpreted carefully because the validity of this inference is dependent on a number of factors including differences in patient and therapist characteristics, medical diagnosis and length of care between the two samples.

Several statistics can be calculated to determine if the change over time, either within or between groups of individuals, is statistically different from zero. The paired t-test can be used to answer the question 'Is the magnitude of change within a group over time significantly different from 0?', while the independent t-test of change scores can be used to answer the question 'Is the magnitude of change over time in one group larger than the magnitude of change for another group?' The statistical significance of these comparisons is largely dependent on the sample size. A large change may not be significant if the sample size is too small, and a small change may be statistically significant but not clinically meaningful if the sample size is large. Therefore, the significance of any statistical results must be interpreted clinically.

Summary

Clinical outcomes data can be used to facilitate patient management decisions, to assess clinician and organizational performance and to provide evidence for the effectiveness of interventions provided by physical therapists and other rehabilitation specialists. The validity of the inferences made from outcomes data is dependent on the validity of the outcome measures themselves and the circumstances under which the data were collected, analyzed and interpreted. Clinical outcomes may include measures of impairment of body structure and function, activity limitation and participation restriction. However, because the relationship between impairment and the resulting activity limitation and participation restriction is not direct, and because activity limitations and participation restrictions are of the utmost concern to the athlete, the primary clinical outcome should be measures of activity limitation and participation restriction. Activity limitation and participation restriction may be measured either through direct observation of performance or by general or specific measures of health-related quality of life. Clinical outcomes data must be collected systematically to ensure valid inferences from the data.

References

American Physical Therapy Association 2001 Guide to physical therapist practice: 2nd edition. Physical Therapy 81:9–744

Barber-Westin S D, Noyes F R, McCloskey J W 1999 Rigorous statistical reliability, validity, and responsiveness testing of the Cincinnati Knee Rating System in 350 subjects with uninjured, injured, or anterior cruciate ligament-reconstructed knees. American Journal of Sports Medicine 27:402–416

Beaton D E 2000 Understanding the relevance of measured change through studies of responsiveness. Spine 25:3192–3199

Beaton D E, Katz J N, Fossel A H et al 2001a Measuring the whole or the parts? Validity, reliability, and responsiveness of the Disabilities of the Arm, Shoulder and Hand outcome measure in different regions of the upper extremity. Journal of Hand Therapy 14:128–146

Beaton D E, Bombardier C, Katz J N et al 2001b Looking for important change/differences in studies of responsiveness. Journal of Rheumatology 28:400–405

Bellamy N, Buchanan W W, Goldsmith C H et al 1988 Validation study of WOMAC: a health status instrument for measuring clinically important patient relevant outcomes to antirheumatic drug therapy in patients with osteoarthritis of the hip or knee. Journal of Rheumatology 15:1833–1840

Binkley J M, Stratford P W, Lott S A et al 1999 The lower extremity functional scale (LEFS): scale development, measurement properties, and clinical application. Physical Therapy 79:371–383

Brophy R H, Beauvais R L, Jones E C et al 2005 Measurement of shoulder activity level. Clinical Orthopaedics 439:101–108

Chatman A B, Hyams S P, Neel J M et al 1997 The patient-specific functional scale: measurement properties in patients with knee dysfunction. Physical Therapy 77:820–829

Christensen L, Mendoza J L 1986 A method of assessing change in a single subject: an alteration of the RC Index. Behavior Therapy 17:305–308

Cohen J 1969 Statistical power analysis for the behavioral sciences. Academic Press, New York

Crocker L, Algina J 1986 Introduction to classical and modern test theory. Harcourt Brace Jovanovich College Publishers, Fort Worth, TX

Daniel D M, Stone M L, Dobson B E et al 1994 Fate of the ACL-injured patient: a prospective outcome study. American Journal of Sports Medicine 22:632–644

Deyo R A, Centor R M 1986 Assessing the responsiveness of functional scales to clinical change: an analogy to diagnostic test performance. Journal of Chronic Diseases 39:897–906

Dobrzykowski E A 1997 The methodology of outcomes measurement. Journal of Rehabilitation Outcomes Measurement 1:8–17

Fairbank J C T, Couper J, Davies J B et al 1980 The Oswestry Low Back Pain Disability Questionnaire. Physiotherapy 66:271–273

Goldstein M S, Elliott S D, Guccione A A 2000 The development of an instrument to measure satisfaction with physical therapy. Physical Therapy 80:853–863

Guyatt G H, Feeny D H, Patrick D L 1993 Measuring health-related quality of life. Annals of Internal Medicine 118:622–629

Hoffman L G, Rouse M W, Brin B N 1995 Quality of life: a review. Journal of the American Optometric Association 66:281–289

Irrgang J J 1996 Outcomes in sports medicine: classification schemes for physical impairments, functional limitations, and disability. Project Focus 96. Conference on Sports Related Injury. Presented by the Foundation for Physical Therapy. American Physical Therapy Association, Alexandria, VA

Irrgang J J, Synder-Mackler L, Wainner R S et al 1998 Development of a patient-reported measure of function of the knee. Journal of Bone and Joint Surgery (Am) 80A:1132–1145

Irrgang J J, Anderson A F, Boland A L 2001 Development and validation of the International Knee Documentation Committee Subjective Knee Form. American Journal of Sports Medicine 29:600–613

Jette A M 1994 Physical disablement concepts for physical therapy research and practice. Physical Therapy 74:380–386

Jette D U, Jette A M 1996 Physical therapy and health outcomes in patients with knee impairments. Physical Therapy 76:1178–1187

Kessler R C, Mroczek D K 1995 Measuring the effects of medical interventions. Medical Care 33:AS109–AS119

Kirkley A, Griffin S, McLintock H et al 1998 The development and evaluation of a disease-specific quality of life measurement tool for shoulder instability. The Western Ontario Shoulder Instability Index (WOSI). American Journal of Sports Medicine 26:764–772

Kirshner B, Guyatt G 1985 A methodological framework for assessing health indices. Journal of Chronic Diseases 38:27–36

Kopec J A, Esdaile J M, Abrahamowicz M et al 1995 The Quebec Back Pain Disability Scale: measurement properties. Spine 20:341–352

Lippitt S B, Harryman D T II, Matsen F A III 1993 A practical tool for evaluating function: the Simple Shoulder Test. In: Matsen III FA, Fu FH, Hawkins RJ (eds) The shoulder: a balance of mobility and stability. American Academy of Orthopaedic Surgeons, Rosemont, IL, p 501–518

Lohr K N, Aaronson N K, Alonso J et al 1996 Evaluating quality-of-life and health status instruments: development of scientific review criteria. Clinical Therapeutics 18:979–992

McHorney C A, Ware J E Jr, Raczek A E 1993 The MOS 36-Item Short-Form Health Survey (SF-36): II. Psychometric and clinical tests of validity in measuring physical and mental health constructs. Medical Care 31:247–263

McHorney C A, Ware J E Jr, Lu J F R et al 1994 The MOS 36-item short-form health survey (SF-36): III. Tests of data quality, scaling assumptions, and reliability across diverse patient groups. Medical Care 32:40–66

McSweeney A J, Creer T L 1995 Health related quality-of-life assessment in medical care. Disease of the Month 41:6–71

Martin R L, Irrgang J J, Burdett R G et al 2005 Evidence of validity for the Foot and Ankle Ability Measure (FAAM). Foot and Ankle International 26:968–983

Marx R G, Stump T J, Jones E C et al 2001 Development and evaluation of an activity rating scale for disorders of the knee. American Journal of Sports Medicine 29:213–218

Marx R G, Menezes A, Horovitz L et al 2003 A comparison of two time intervals for test-retest reliability of health status instruments. Journal of Clinical Epidemiology 56:730–735

Messick S 1989 Validity. In: Linn R L (ed) Educational measurement, 3rd edn. American Council on Education/Macmillan Series on Higher Education, New York, p 13–103

Mohtadi N 1998 Development and validation of the quality of life outcome measure (questionnaire) for chronic anterior cruciate ligament deficiency. American Journal of Sports Medicine 26:350–359

Nagi S Z 1965 Some conceptual issues in disability and rehabilitation. In: Sussman M B (ed) Sociology and rehabilitation. American Sociological Association, Washington, DC, p 100–113

Nagi S Z 1991 Disability concepts revisited: implication for prevention. In: Pope A M, Tarlov A R (eds) Disability in America: toward a national agenda for prevention. National Academy Press, Washington, DC, p 309–327219

National Institutes of Health 1992 National Advisory Board on Medical Rehabilitation Research. Draft V: report and plan for medical rehabilitation research. National Institutes of Health, Bethesda, MD

Noyes F R, McGinniss G H, Mooar L A 1984 Functional disability in the anterior cruciate insufficient knee syndrome: review of knee rating systems and projected risk factors in determine treatment. Sports Medicine 1:278–302

Noyes F R, Barber S D, Mooar L A 1989 A rationale for assessing sports activity levels and limitations in knee disorders. Clinical Orthopaedics 246:238–249

Pantano K J, Irrgang J J, Burdett R et al 2001 A pilot study on the relationship between physical impairment and activity restriction in persons with anterior cruciate ligament reconstruction at long-term follow-up. Knee Surgery, Sports Traumatology, Arthroscopy 9:369–378

Richards R R, An K-N, Bigliani L U et al 1994 A standardized method for the assessment of shoulder function. Journal of Shoulder and Elbow Surgery 3:347–352

Seto J L, Orofino A S, Morrissey M C et al 1988 Assessment of quadriceps/hamstrings strength, knee ligament stability, functional and sports activity levels five years after anterior cruciate ligament reconstruction. American Journal of Sports Medicine 16:170–180

Shrout P E, Fleiss L 1979 Intraclass correlation: uses in assessing rater reliability. Psychological Bulletin 86:420–428

Snyder-Mackler L, Fitzgerald G Bartolozzi III A R et al 1997 The relationship between passive joint laxity and functional outcome after anterior cruciate ligament injury. American Journal of Sports Medicine 25:191–195

Stratford P W, Binkley J, Solomon P et al 1994 Assessing change over time in patients with low back pain. Physical Therapy 74:528–533

Stratford P W, Binkley J M, Riddle D L 1996 Health status measures: strategies and analytic methods for assessing change scores. Physical Therapy 76:1109–1123

Straub T, Hunter R E 1988 Acute anterior cruciate ligament repair. Clinical Orthopaedics 227:238–250

Streiner D L, Norman G R 1995 Health measurement scales: a practical guide to their development and use. Oxford University Press, New York, p 1–231

Tegner Y, Lysholm J 1985 Rating systems in the evaluation of knee ligament injuries. Clinical Orthopaedics 198:43–49

Testa M A, Nackley J F 1994 Methods for quality of life studies. Annual Review of Public Health 15:535–559

Testa M A, Simonson D C 1996 Assessment of quality-of-life outcomes. New England Journal of Medicine 334:835–840

Verbrugge L M, Jette A M 1994 The disablement process. Social Science and Medicine 38:1–14

Ware J E Jr, Sherbourne C D 1992 The MOS 36-item short-form health survey (SF-36): I. Conceptual framework and item selection. Medical Care 30:473–483

Westaway M D, Stratford P W, Binkley J M 1998 The patient-specific functional scale: validation of its use in persons with neck dysfunction. Journal of Orthopaedic and Sports Physical Therapy 27:331–338

Whyte J 1994 Toward a methodology for rehabilitation research. American Journal of Physical Medicine and Rehabilitation 73:428–435

World Health Organization 1980 International classification of impairments, disabilities and handicaps: a manual of classification relating to the consequences of disease. World Health Organization, Geneva

World Health Organization 2001 International classification of functioning disability and health. World Health Organization, Geneva

Electrophysical agents in sport and exercise injury management

Lynn Snyder-Mackler, Laura A. Schmitt,

Katherine Rudolph and Sara Farquhar

14

CHAPTER CONTENTS

Introduction 220

Treatment of inflammation and edema 220

Treatment of pain 224

Treatment of impaired muscle function 226

Reduced tissue extensibility 228

Treatment of tissue damage 229

Summary 232

Introduction

Rehabilitation of the injured athlete can be particularly challenging as return to a high level of function is expected. The clinician must make prudent decisions to achieve a speedy return-to-play without jeopardizing the wellbeing of the athlete. Athletic injury can be associated with tissue damage that can range from localized cellular damage to ruptured tendon or fracture. Injury is accompanied by inflammation, edema and pain and can result in the loss of muscle strength and function due to disuse or immobilization. The use of electrophysical agents may help to facilitate more rapid healing of damaged tissues. This chapter presents the principles of electrophysical agents that are common in sports medicine and that clinicians may use in conjunction with other rehabilitation interventions.

Treatment of inflammation and edema

Cryotherapy

Cryotherapy is the use of ice and other cold modalities to reduce the harmful effects of tissue injury – hemorrhage, edema, muscle spasm and pain – all of which can lead to loss of function. The application of the RICE principle (rest, ice, compression and elevation) immediately after injury has been successful in minimizing tissue inflammation and edema (Green et al 2001) through a mechanism that involves blood vessel constriction and decreased cellular metabolism (Karunakara et al 1999, Thorsson et al 1985). Reduced circulation and cellular metabolism result in the release of fewer metabolic byproducts, thereby minimizing further tissue injury (Knight 1995). Commonly used application techniques are commercial cold packs, ice bags, ice massage, Cryo/Cuff (AirCast, Summit, NJ) and cold baths.

Temperature of the cold modality, duration of application, area of targeted tissues and the physical makeup of the athlete all affect the depth of tissue cooling. Skin temperatures cool rapidly but may not be a good indicator of the intensity of cooling that occurs in deeper tissues. Palmer & Knight (1996) found greater than 20°C temperature reduction in human skin after the application of an ice pack for 20 min; however, Zemke et al (1998) found only a 4°C reduction at a depth of 1.7 cm in the human calf. Levy & Lintner (1997) found no significant temperature difference in the glenohumeral joint or subacromial space before and after a 90 min application of cold via a Cryo/Cuff (AirCast, Summit, NJ). During treatment, it is unlikely that cryotherapy will produce changes in tissue temperatures at depths greater than 2 cm.

Athletes will typically feel three phases before reaching analgesia: intense cold leading to burning followed by aching. The choice of cold application is dependent on the target tissue depth and size. Smaller target areas, such as the patellar tendon, can be treated with ice massage while larger areas should be treated with a cold whirlpool (Zemke et al 1998). Ice massage is the application of ice directly to the skin for 5–7 min while a cold bath involves immersion of the affected body part in water, typically 15°C (Eston & Peters 1999, Michlovitz 1996). Zemke et al (1998) demonstrated that while both ice massage and ice bags were effective in reducing intramuscular temperature, ice massage was more time efficient. In a busy physical therapy or athletic training facility, ice massage would be an effective and efficient way to reduce pain and inflammation if the area of the target tissue is small.

Cryotherapy is used postsurgically to reduce pain and swelling and improve range of motion. Ohkoshi et al (1999) investigated the effects of prolonged cooling with circulating cold water at 5 and 10°C after anterior cruciate ligament (ACL) reconstruction. The use of cryotherapy at 10°C decreased scores on an analog pain scale and the amount of pain medication administered. The study group treated with the 5°C cooling demonstrated decreased blood loss, but had no decrease in pain ratings (Ohkoshi et al 1999). It must be noted that the applicability of this study may be limited due to the feasibility of applying extreme cold water continuously at such low temperatures for 48 h, but it demonstrates that the use of ice after surgery may be beneficial if the tissues can be cooled adequately.

Many athletes receive ice before or during a sporting event due to previous muscular trauma. Some clinicians may have concerns that the application of cold during athletic activity will decrease sensory perception; however, evidence to the contrary exists. Ingersoll et al (1992) found that a 20-min immersion in 1°C water did not affect the athlete's sensory perception of the ankle or foot. Evans et al (1995) demonstrated no significant difference in agility after immersion of the ankle in 1°C water for 20 min. These studies demonstrate that the application of ice does not significantly affect agility or perception; therefore the fear of returning an athlete to participation after icing does not seem warranted.

A treatment utilizing an ice bag or cold pack typically lasts 10–15 min. In contrast, an ice massage will only last 5–7 min. The goal of the treatment is to cool the affected area and ultimately produce the sensation of analgesia. Contraindications to the use of cold involve hypersensitivity, decreased sensation and poor blood flow. The use of ice to treat athletic injuries is routine but it is not without risk. Application of ice can cause nerve injury to superficial nerves, particularly over the ulnar, peroneal and femoral cutaneous nerves (Bassett et al 1992). When treating tissues over these areas, the athlete's sensation

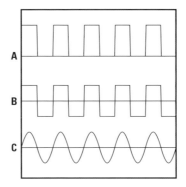

Figure 14.1 • Illustrations of different waveforms. **A:** Interrupted direct current. **B:** Alternating current with a square wave configuration. **C:** Alternating current with a sine wave configuration.

should be monitored closely to determine if treatment should be discontinued.

Electrical stimulation

General principles

Several forms of electrical stimulation are used to affect tissue edema but through very different mechanisms. Before discussing the specific electrical stimulation modalities, a brief overview of electrical stimulation principles will be presented. Electrical stimulation involves the use of electrical current for therapeutic purposes and may result in the activation of excitable tissues, changes in cellular function or the transcutaneous delivery of medications to target tissues.

Two types of current are used, alternating current (AC) and direct current (DC) (Fig. 14.1). Alternating current involves the bidirectional flow of charged particles and can be applied continuously, in pulses or in bursts of current. Direct current is unidirectional and can be applied continuously or in the form of interrupted pulses. Continuous DC is used in applications including wound care and iontophoresis and has chemical effects that warrant special considerations, which will be discussed later. Interrupted DC and AC that are used therapeutically have no chemical effect because the pulse duration is well below the very long pulse durations of 50–300 ms that would result in electrochemical changes at the cellular level (Alon 1991). AC can be delivered continuously or in bursts. The shape of the waveforms can take many forms and can be modified by adjusting the amplitude and phase duration of each pulse. Physiologically, the most important characteristic of a waveform is the amount of electrical charge delivered to the tissues, called the phase charge, which is expressed in coulombs or microcoulombs (10^{-6} coulombs). Phase charge is the time integral of a single phase of current. In a square wave pulse, the phase charge is the pulse amplitude multiplied by the phase duration. When applying pulsed DC, increasing the pulse duration and/or amplitude of a waveform will recruit more neurons (Crago et al 1980). When using AC, decreasing the stimulation frequency will increase the phase charge.

The recruitment of neurons with electrical stimulation occurs differently than in volitional activation. When neurons are recruited volitionally they are activated according to the size principle whereby smaller diameter fibers are recruited before larger diameter fibers (Kandel et al 1995). When using electrical stimulation, the excitation of neurons follows the reverse order. With electrical stimulation, large diameter neurons, whose membrane resistance is lower, are activated before small diameter fibers, whose membrane resistance is higher. Physiologically, this means that the sensory neurons are recruited first, followed by motor neurons and finally neurons that transmit noxious signals. In general, with clinical stimulators, selective activation of sensory neurons is achieved with short pulse durations, from 2 to 50 μs; activation of motor neurons is achieved with pulse durations of 200–600 μs; and pain fibers are activated with long pulse durations upwards of 1 ms.

Clinically, as stimulation intensity is increased, one will typically experience a tingling sensation, followed by a muscle twitch and then a painful sensation. It is important to understand that when applying current transcutaneously, the location of the neuron beneath the skin is also important. For example, when applying a waveform of a given phase charge, a small-diameter neuron that is located close to the surface of the skin will experience higher current than a large-diameter neuron at a deeper location, so the small-diameter fiber may be activated before the neuron with a larger diameter. This explains why in some applications in which the stimulating electrode is located over the motor point of the muscle whose motor neurons are very close to the skin, a motor response may precede a sensory response.

In addition to changing the phase charge, the frequency at which pulses or bursts are delivered affects the intensity of response. For example, when producing a motor response, increasing the frequency of stimulation will produce more summation of twitch forces and may result in a strong tetanic contraction if the frequency is sufficiently high. When AC is delivered in bursts, the carrier frequency refers to the frequency of stimulation within the burst, and the burst frequency is that which affects the force of the contractions. Size and spacing of electrodes need to be considered in order for a treatment to be more effective in effecting a desired response.

Electrical stimulation and tissue edema

Electrical stimulation has been used to lessen the formation of edema and to reduce existing edema. High-volt pulsed current (HVPC) involves the use of pulsed DC consisting of twin spikes of high amplitude (up to 500 V), small pulse duration (50–200 μs) waveforms that are delivered at 1–120 twin spikes per second (Fig. 14.2).

HVPC is commonly used in wound care but it has also been used to prevent the formation of edema in animal models. Studies have shown that the application of HVPC within the first hour after injury can help prevent the formation of edema (Thornton et al 1998). Electrodes have been placed directly on skin overlying the injury or submerged in a water bath and the intensity of stimulation produces a strong sensory response (10%

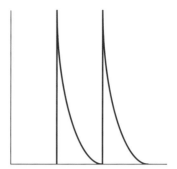

Figure 14.2 • Twin spikes of high-voltage pulsed galvanic electrical stimulation.

below motor threshold) (Taylor et al 1992, 1997, Thornton et al 1998). The evidence suggests that HVPC inhibits microvascular leakage that minimizes further tissue edema (Taylor et al 1992, 1997, Thornton et al 1998). These studies were performed in animal models, so further research is needed to investigate the effects in humans. However, the benefits of early intervention with HVPC appear promising (Mendel & Fish 1993).

The use of electrical stimulation to reduce existing edema has proven less effective. Research has shown that motor level stimulation is no better at reducing tissue edema than compression boots, which mimic the effect of muscle pumping (Griffin et al 1990). Therefore, the added time and expense of using electrical stimulation in this manner appears unfounded. It could be, however, that motor level electrical stimulation might be useful in reducing existing edema when individuals cannot perform volitional contractions.

Iontophoresis

Iontophoresis is the transcutaneous delivery of medication by DC through the mechanism of electrostatic repulsion. Many drugs that are placed in a solution ionize into positively and negatively charged ions that will be affected by an electric field. Negatively charged ions are repelled from the negative electrode, while positively charged ions are repelled from the positive electrode. Electrodes used in iontophoresis include a delivery electrode that is designed to deliver the medication and dispersive electrode to complete the circuit. The delivery electrode is small so it will concentrate the current to deliver medication to a precise area of tissue. The dispersive electrode is larger with a lower density of current so the effect on the skin is minimized.

Due to the continuous nature of direct current, chemical burns at the electrode–skin interface are possible. When the delivery electrode is positive (anode), the chemical reaction on the skin involves the release of hydrogen ions that decreases the pH and results in an acidic reaction. Current density of the positive electrode should be held below 1.0 mA/cm^2. When the delivery electrode is negative (cathode), sodium hydroxide ions are produced that increase the pH in an alkaline reaction. This reaction is more caustic to the skin and current density should not exceed 0.5 mA/cm^2. Most clinical iontophoresis units limit the peak current to 4.0 mA. Commercial electrodes provide even current distribution and typically have buffering systems to help regulate pH minimizing chemical reactions (Schmidt 1993).

When choosing iontophoresis treatment parameters, the clinician must balance time efficiency with patient safety and comfort. Current dosage refers to the total amount of current used to deliver the medication taking into account both peak current and treatment duration. For example, if the treatment consisted of 2 mA delivered over 20 min, the dosage would be 40 mA/min. Dosages used for iontophoresis have ranged from 40 to 80 mA/min. In general, higher peak currents can lead to discomfort in some patients; however, it appears that greater treatment dosages are associated with greater success in treating pain and inflammation (Bertolucci 1982, Braun 1987, Delacerda 1982). Clinicians may choose to alter the treatment dosage by increasing the treatment duration in patients who are less tolerant of high peak currents.

Treatment principles

Prior to beginning the treatment, the skin should be thoroughly inspected. Skin abrasions reduce the resistance to current flow, thereby increasing the potential for skin irritation (Schmidt 1993). Clinicians should be aware that mild to moderate erythema under the delivery or dispersive electrode is a typical response to iontophoresis treatment (Japour et al 1999) and should resolve within several hours after treatment. Skin thickness and skin sensitivity must be considered when deciding on treatment parameters. Tissues that are close to the skin surface are more likely to receive the drug during iontophoresis. Treating areas under thick skin, such as on the palmar surface of the hand and plantar surface of the foot, can be difficult because of increased resistance to ion flow, so an alternative electrode location may be chosen. Electrophysical agents that increase blood flow, such as continuous ultrasound, may drive the drug away from targeted tissue; therefore use of heating agents in conjunction with iontophoresis is not recommended. Three to four treatments should be adequate to determine if iontophoresis is yielding positive results (Braun 1987, Harris 1982, Lark & Gangarosa 1990).

Medications

In sports medicine, the most common medications used for iontophoresis include anti-inflammatories and local anesthetics (Table 14.1) but other medications have been used. Acetic acid has been used to treat calcific tendonitis (Robinson & Snyder-Mackler 1995, Schmidt 1993) and potassium iodide or sodium chloride (2% solution) has been used to treat scar tissue (Schmidt, 1993).

Efficacy of iontophoresis

Heel pain is a common complaint among athletes. Acetic acid (5% solution) has been shown to provide relief of recalcitrant heel pain in 94% of patients who received an average of 5.7 treatments of iontophoresis at an intensity of 30–60 mA/min with the delivery electrode placed over the heel (Japour et al 1999). In a controlled clinical trial, Myerson et al (1986) found

Table 14.1 Medications used in iontophoresis

Drug	Indication	Effect	Delivery electrode
Dexamethasone sodium phosphate (4 mg/mL)	Inflammation	Anti-inflammatory	Negative
Lidocaine (lignocaine) HCL (4% solution with or without adrenaline [epinephrine])	Pain	Local anesthetic	Positive
Acetic acid (2–5% solution)	Calcific tendinitis	May increase solubility of calcium deposits	Negative
Potassium iodide (10% solution)	Scar tissue	Help to break down collagen	Negative
Sodium chloride (2% solution)	Scar tissue	Help to break down collagen	Negative

that 0.4% dexamethasone sodium phosphate reduced heel pain in an average of 6 treatments administered over 2–3 weeks. In this trial, the treatment dose was 80 mA/min and the active electrode was placed on the plantar aspect of the heel. After 6 treatments, the treatment group noted significantly greater improvement based on physical examination and completion of the Maryland Foot Score, which assesses both pain and function of the foot (Myerson et al 1986). Iontophoresis can be an effective modality to decrease inflammation, decrease pain and treat calcifications and scar tissue.

Ultrasound

Ultrasound (US) is the application of high-frequency sound waves, between 1 and 3 MHz, applied continuously or in pulses. Continuous US has thermal effects while pulsed ultrasound does not. The non-thermal effects of pulsed US include cavitation and mechanical and chemical changes that may effect cellular permeability and metabolism (Rivenburgh 1992). Cavitation is the vibrational effect of US on gas bubbles leading to changes in local pressure and improved membrane permeability.

Another manner in which US is used to affect tissue inflammation and edema is through phonophoresis. Phonophoresis is the use of continuous US to enhance the transcutaneous absorption of anti-inflammatory drugs to underlying tissue. Corticosteroid gel, methyl salicate cream and betamethasone in US gel are some commonly used drugs that have demonstrated delivery rates at above 80% (Cameron & Monroe 1992). Because of the high water content of most tissues, an important characteristic of the medication is its affinity to water. The medium in which the drug is delivered must allow transmission by being hydrophilic.

Many creams, such as hydrocortisone, are hydrophobic and do not transmit well (Cameron & Monroe 1992).

Studies have shown beneficial effects of phonophoresis in decreasing pain and inflammation. Ciccone et al (1991) demonstrated the use of trolamine salicylate phonophoresis decreased stiffness and pain greater than US alone. Shin & Choi (1997) applied indomethacin to the temporomandibular joint and evaluated pain relief using a visual analog pain scale and pain threshold. They applied 1% indomethacin cream at 1 MHz, 0.8 to 1.5 w/cm^2 continuous for 15 min to the temporomandibular joint and found decreased pain scale scores and a 14% increase in pain threshold. In contrast, Klaiman et al (1998) showed no significant decrease in tolerance to pressure pain as compared to US alone when using a 0.05% fluocinonide gel on lateral epicondylitis.

Despite the beneficial effect of some phonophoresis applications, the effectiveness of phonophoresis has been questioned in the literature (Bare et al 1996, Benson et al 1989, Byl 1995, Oziomek et al 1991). Bare et al (1996) looked at the delivery of 10% hydrocortisone acetate gel using 1 MHz US at an intensity of 1 w/cm^2 for 5 min and measured its transmission by determining the relative cortisol serum level in the bloodstream. They demonstrated no increase in blood cortisol levels as compared to US alone (Bare et al 1996). Similar studies by Oziomek et al (1991) and Benson et al (1989) on the absorption of salicylate and benzydamine have also found no enhancement of the absorption of the drug with US.

The benefits of phonophoresis appear to be specific to both the drug choice and depth of target tissue. The frequency of the ultrasonic waves is inversely proportional to the depth of tissue penetration. The depth of penetration for 1 MHz US is 2–5 cm while that of 3 MHz US is only 1–2 cm (Michlovitz 1996), so consideration of the depth of the target tissue is important.

Treatment of pain

An important component to successful rehabilitation of the injured athlete is the treatment of pain for which many modalities can be a useful adjunct. As described in Chapter 9, two mechanisms by which pain is relieved are through the gate control mechanism and by the release of endogenous opiates. The gate control theory states that activity of the large diameter sensory fibers can modulate pain impulses from peripheral neurons thereby influencing the experience of pain. The opioid-mediated analgesic system blocks pain transmission through neural and/or hormonal mechanisms whereby endogenous opiates are released in response to painful stimuli. Of note is that the release of endogenous opiates is achieved through exercise as well (Surbey et al 1984).

Heat and cold

Pain reduction has been demonstrated by the application of both heat and cold. Ohkoshi et al (1999) found reduced pain in individuals who received cryotherapy with 10°C circulating water after surgery. Cold can affect pain directly by decreasing nerve conduction velocities of both motor and sensory nerves, thereby interfering with the transmission of nerve signals. Extreme cold has also been found to reduce pain via the release of endogenous opiates (Washington et al 2000).

The application of superficial heat, among other effects, can also produce analgesia (Lehmann et al 1958). Heat should not be used in acute injury since it increases blood flow to the area (Greenberg 1972) and may increase edema. One should wait at least 48 h or until swelling has resolved to allow completion of the inflammatory phase.

Superficial heat is thought to reduce pain following the acute phase of injury by increasing tissue temperature and promoting relaxation, although the exact mechanism is not fully understood. Commonly used forms of heating modalities are hot packs or warm whirlpools. Researchers have speculated that reduction in pain and muscle spasm occurs through the increased blood flow and an elevation of the pain threshold (Lehmann et al 1958, Rivenburgh 1992). The increased blood flow occurs by vasodilatation of blood vessels, while the pain threshold is thought to increase through a thermal effect on free nerve endings (Rivenburgh 1992).

Circulation increases (Abramson et al 1960), muscle relaxes and tissue extensibility increases at 40–45°C (Fountain et al 1960, Gersten 1955). Achieving an elevated tissue temperature is greatly affected by the depth of the target tissue. Superficial heating techniques, such as hot packs and warm whirlpools, warm tissues to a depth of approximately 0.5 cm (Michlovitz 1996), so deeper structures may not benefit from superficial heating methods. Superficial heat is typically applied for 10–15 min.

Continuous US produces thermal effects that result from absorption of sound waves and is often used to heat deeper tissues. Thermal effects include increased soft tissue extensibility, increased blood flow, and decreased muscle spasm (Rivenburgh 1992), all of which can reduce a patient's experience of pain. Klaiman et al (1998) demonstrated decreased pain and increased pressure tolerance in response to an 8-min treatment (1 MHz continuous US at 1.5 w/cm^2) to the elbow. The rise in tissue temperature is typically 2–3°C, which can cause a reduction in muscle spasm and pain relief (Draper & Ricard 1995). Draper & Ricard (1995) demonstrated that a rise of 4°C occurs in 3–4 min when using a 3 MHz US frequency. When a frequency of 1 MHz was used, the rise in temperature took up to 6 min (Draper & Ricard 1995). The composition of the target tissue may influence the heating effect of US. Tissues that are high in collagen content, such as bone, absorb more US energy than tissues with high water content, so caution must be exercised when using continuous US on bony areas. Moving the US applicator more rapidly or reducing the intensity of the US may help improve patient tolerance and prevent tissue damage.

Electroanalgesia

All manners of electrical stimulation (sensory, motor and noxious) are used in reducing pain associated with injury, although the mechanism of pain relief depends on the intensity of stimulation and the patient's subjective experience of the stimulus.

Sensory level stimulation

Two modes of sensory level electrical stimulation that are commonly used for pain relief are conventional transcutaneous electrical nerve stimulation (TENS) and interferential electrical stimulation. Both are thought to reduce pain through the gate control mechanism and are therefore only effective for the duration of the treatment. Although all methods of electrical stimulation used clinically are applied transcutaneously, TENS has become synonymous with a comfortable sensory level of stimulation. The term 'conventional TENS' is used here to differentiate the comfortable sensory sensation from the very intense, often unpleasant sensation associated with high intensity, 'acupuncture-like TENS' that is also used for pain relief.

Jensen et al (1985) studied pain level, amount of pain medication administered and knee range of motion in 90 patients who had undergone arthroscopic knee surgery. The subjects were randomized into three groups: control, sham TENS and TENS. The group that received TENS (pulse duration of 300 μs and pulse rate of 70 Hz) had significantly less pain, needed less pain medication and achieved greater joint range than the sham or control groups (Jensen et al 1985). Conventional TENS is thought to have effects in addition to analgesia including increased blood flow and skin temperature; however, research has yielded conflicting results. Cramp et al (2000) applied conventional TENS for 15 min at 4 Hz and 110 Hz (both at 200 μs) to a healthy population. Skin temperatures as well as blood perfusion levels were measured at 3-min intervals for 30 min. The results showed increased blood flow and skin temperature when 4 Hz TENS as compared to 110 Hz and the control was used (Cramp et al 2000). Neither high- nor low-frequency stimulation demonstrated any changes in skin temperature when compared to the control group, questioning the vasodilatory effects of conventional TENS.

When using conventional TENS, stimulation parameters usually include pulse durations ranging from 2 to 50 μs, stimulation frequency of 50–100 pulses per second (pps) and intensity levels such that a strong but comfortable tingling sensation is experienced. Because of adaptation to the tingling sensation, the intensity is increased throughout the treatment. Analgesic effects of conventional TENS occur only when the stimulation is applied (Johnson et al 1991) for treatment durations ranging from 15–20 min up to hours.

Interferential current involves the application of two unique sinusoidal frequencies that are applied to the tissue simultaneously via two channels. The electrodes of these channels are positioned in the form of an 'X' such that the currents intersect over the painful area. The frequency of the currents typically ranges from 4000 to 4200 Hz, which intersect at deeper tissue layers (Bertoti 2000). Interferential current is purported to provide greater analgesic effects than other forms of electrical stimulation, however, research does not support this assertion. Interferential treatments have been found no better than placebo in decreasing pain (Taylor et al 1987), increasing blood flow (Indergand & Morgan 1995) or decreasing edema (Bertoti 2000, Christie & Willoughby 1990, Nussbaum et al 1990).

Motor and noxious electrical stimulation

Many procedures in rehabilitation are uncomfortable so clinicians often benefit from the opioid-mediated analgesic system. However, the release of endogenous opiates can be initiated intentionally with high intensity electrical stimulation and can be particularly useful in treating subacute and chronic pain. Unlike analgesia produced through the gate control mechanisms, analgesia associated with the release of endogenous opiates lasts several hours. Any stimulation parameters capable of producing a motor or noxious response are adequate to produce analgesia, thus, waveforms with longer pulse durations are usually required.

One type of high-level electrical stimulation used to produce analgesia is sometimes referred to as strong, low-rate TENS or acupuncture-like TENS. With this technique, stimuli are delivered continuously at a low frequency (2–4 pps) with pulse durations over 150 μs to produce a rhythmic muscle contraction. Evidence suggests that stronger contractions are associated with greater pain relief (Picker 1988, 1989). Sometimes the current is delivered at sites remote to the injury corresponding to acupuncture points. Clinical observations indicate that tolerance to intense motor level contractions is limited, so clinicians may have more success when using sites remote to the injury or over areas with no muscle tissue.

High-frequency (>100 pps) stimuli have also been used to produce a noxious sensation that will elicit the release of endogenous opiates. Long pulse durations (1 ms, up to 1 s) are required to activate actual pain fibers (Robinson & Snyder-Mackler 1995); however, clinical stimulators rarely provide such long pulse durations. To compensate for the shorter than desired pulse durations, clinicians should use very small electrodes in order to produce high current density and deliver a stimulus producing a painful sensation. When using waveforms with large phase charges, sensory, motor and possibly pain fibers will be activated. Therefore, it is important to choose electrode placements that avoid areas of muscle tissue if motor level contractions are not desired.

Manal & Snyder-Mackler (1997) described a treatment that produces electroanalgesia with high-intensity electrical stimulation using a current that is sometimes referred to as 'Russian current'. The stimulus characteristics are similar to those used by the Soviet researcher Yakov Kots to strengthen Soviet Olympic athletes (Kots et al 1977). Manal and Snyder-Mackler's protocol involves identifying a specific point of pain and surrounding it by small electrodes through which the current is delivered (Fig. 14.3). The current is a burst-modulated AC sine wave configuration and a 2500 Hz carrier frequency that is applied at 50 bursts per second. Within the burst, the 2500 Hz current is delivered with a duty cycle of 50% (10 ms on, 10 ms off) and the electrical stimulation is provided for 12 s on and 8 s off for a total of 12–15 min (Manal & Snyder-Mackler 1997). The amplitude of the current is increased to maximal tolerance.

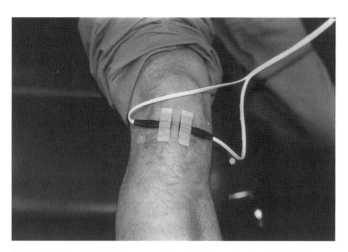

Figure 14.3 • Electrode placement for electroanalgesia with high-intensity electrical stimulation.

The intensity is increased throughout the treatment as tolerance allows. Securing the electrodes with tape and replacing the electrodes frequently helps to maintain good electrode contact. This is important when delivering high current density to minimize the chance of electrical burns, which can sometimes occur with high-intensity AC. Manal & Snyder-Mackler (1997) stated that this protocol often produces long lasting analgesia, well over the several hours that one would expect from an opioid-mediated response. The exact mechanism of its success is not fully understood; however, it appears to be an effective modality to treat palpable, painful, soft tissue structures.

When using any treatment for analgesia, objective documentation of pain relief is essential. Techniques to provoke the patient's signs of pain, as well as pain and functional status questionnaires, should be used to determine the effectiveness of treatment. If significant improvement in symptoms is not noted, another modality may be more appropriate (Manal & Snyder-Mackler 1997).

Treatment of impaired muscle function

Neuromuscular electrical stimulation for muscle strengthening

As discussed previously, motor level electrical stimulation can be used for pain relief and for edema reduction in persons who are unable to activate their muscles volitionally. When using electrical stimulation for treating muscle weakness, some unique issues must be addressed. Rapid restoration of muscle strength, power and endurance are vitally important in the rehabilitation of athletes. Training should target the specific muscles that are impaired and training should be sport-specific. The overload principle states that strength increases in proportion to the amount of overload that the muscle experiences during exercise (Hillebrandt & Houtz 1956). Overload

can be applied to specific weakened muscles through the use of electrical stimulation providing that the peripheral nerve and the muscle are intact.

When using neuromuscular electrical stimulation (NMES), the clinician must balance the need for high force production with the presence of rapid muscle fatigue. Stimulating muscle electrically differs from volitional activity in ways that lead to rapid fatigue. Because of the reversal of the order of motor unit recruitment with electrical stimulation, larger diameter motor neurons, associated with large fast fatigable motor units are stimulated before smaller, slow twitch, fatigue-resistant motor units. In contrast to volitional contractions, when stimulating muscle electrically, motor units are activated synchronously and recover from fatigue only during the times when the stimulation is absent. During the application of NMES, muscle fatigue must be monitored and can be addressed by increasing the rest time between contractions.

Research into the benefits of NMES to strengthen muscle has produced conflicting results. For example, Delitto et al (1988) and Snyder-Mackler et al (1995) found that NMES is superior to volitional exercise in regaining strength after ACL reconstruction, while Paternostro-Sluga et al (1999) found no difference in the same population. Several methodological factors may account for the discrepancy in results. Delitto et al (1988) studied 20 patients who had undergone ACL reconstruction within 6 weeks of participation, half of whom received NMES with burst-modulated AC (2500 Hz, triangle wave form, 50 bursts per second (bps), 15 s on, 50 s off). The other half of the sample performed volitional exercise. Patients in both groups contracted their quadriceps femoris and hamstring muscles simultaneously during rehabilitation, 5 days a week for a 3-week period. Stimulation amplitude was increased to maximal tolerance but no net extension torque was generated due to the activity of the antagonist hamstrings. The voluntary exercise group also performed 15 co-contractions of their quadriceps and hamstrings at a maximal level with no net extension torque, holding for 15 s and resting for 50 s. The NMES group demonstrated greater isometric strength gains than the volitional exercise group, 6 weeks after surgery (Delitto et al 1988). Snyder-Mackler et al (1991) reported similar results in a group of patients following ACL reconstruction that received NMES and volitional exercise or performed volitional exercise alone. Following 4 weeks of treatment, the NMES with volitional exercise group demonstrated significant strength gains in the quadriceps (Snyder-Mackler et al 1991).

In contrast to the previous findings, Paternostro-Sluga et al (1999) studied the effect of NMES on quadriceps strength in persons who had undergone surgery for ACL deficiency. Three groups were evaluated: group 1 – NMES and exercise; group 2 – TENS and exercise; group 3 – control group (exercise alone). NMES was supplied by a battery-powered, portable muscle stimulator with rectangular, monophasic, square wave pulses, daily for 6 weeks. The regimen included two different sets of parameters: set 1 (30 Hz, 5 s on with a 1 s ramp, 15 s off time) was repeated four times and set 2 (50 Hz, 10 s on with a 2 s ramp, 50 s off) was repeated twice. The pulse duration was 200 μs and the amplitude was set to perform a 'strong muscle contraction'. Subjects performed 12 repetitions in each set. The TENS group received analgesic stimulation (biphasic rectangular wave form at 220 μs and 100 Hz, sensory perception, treatment time was 30 min). The results indicated no statistically significant difference between the three groups (Paternostro-Sluga et al 1999). Because a battery-operated portable stimulator was used, it is likely that an appropriate dose of electrical stimulation was not provided. Studies have shown that NMES induced contractions that are below 50% of the volitional force are inadequate to produce strength gains (Snyder-Mackler et al 1994) and portable muscle stimulators may be unable to produce muscle contractions in the quadriceps femoris muscles that are in a therapeutic range.

Recent advances in technology, however, have resulted in improved results and performance using battery-powered stimulators. Laufer et al (2001), using two portable stimulators and one clinical stimulator, investigated force generation production with the use of different waveforms. Muscle fatigue was caused by repeated contractions with these waveforms, and differences in fatigue and muscle force production between genders were examined. The fatiguing test had a 7 s on, 2 s off duty cycle until 48 contractions were produced, or until zero torque was generated. They found that the maximum tolerated muscle contraction produced by the line-powered stimulator was weaker than the portable stimulators with the biphasic or monophasic waveforms. The 2500 Hz AC waveform produced the greatest fatigue and between genders there was no difference in the rate of fatigue. Battery-operated stimulators may prove effective tools with client rehabilitation at home and in the clinic providing that the unit has the capability to generate force.

In a more recent study, Lyons et al (2005) investigated the force generation produced through a portable stimulator and a clinical stimulator, as well as self-reported pain during NMES. They found no differences in peak torque or pain ratings between the clinical and portable stimulator, but the portable stimulator produced a greater average torque integral compared to the clinical stimulator during the course of testing. Testing of the current capacity of each instrument revealed that the portable stimulator used a greater percentage of its capacity as compared to the clinical stimulator, indicating that while the two are comparable at producing torque, the portable stimulator may not have the reserve current capacity to maintain adequate torque as muscle torque increases with training. While improved technology makes use of battery-powered stimulators a feasible option, battery drainage must be monitored, as it will affect the capacity of the stimulator (Lyons et al 2005).

Clinically, NMES for quadriceps strengthening is performed with an isometric contraction of the leg. The parameters used to achieve maximal results include pulse duration of 400–600 μs, stimulation frequency of 50–100 Hz intensity and at least 50% of the maximal volitional isometric contraction. Electrodes are placed over the vastus medialis oblique (VMO) and just distal to the anterior superior iliac spine (ASIS) on the rectus femoris and 10 contractions are elicited for 15 s on and with a 50 s rest period to achieve desired strength gains (Fig. 14.4).

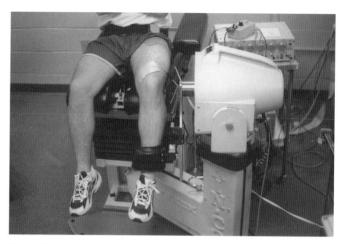

Figure 14.4 • Electrode placement for neuromuscular electrical stimulation for strengthening the quadriceps femoris muscles.

When using burst-modulated current, 400–600 μs pulse durations are achieved with a carrier frequency of approximately 1600–2500 Hz and the frequency is set to 50–100 bps.

While an intensity of at least 50% of the maximal volitional isometric contraction is recommended for strength gains with NMES, strength gains with lesser intensities have been demonstrated (Fitzgerald et al 2003). The strength gains reported by Fitzgerald et al (2003), however, were modest compared to other studies (Snyder-Mackler et al 1991, 1994).

Many investigations of NMES have involved the quadriceps femoris muscles; however, other muscles can benefit from NMES for strengthening. Starring (1991) showed subjective improvement in L5/S1 stability after 2 weeks of NMES with burst-modulated AC. The stimulation parameters were 2500 Hz AC with a burst frequency of 75 bps, 15 s on and 50 s off, and with the electrodes placed over the erector spinae. Kahanovitz et al (1987) performed a randomized controlled clinical trial to investigate strength gains of the low back musculature with electrical stimulation. One hundred and seventeen healthy women were randomly assigned to one of four groups: group 1 – low-frequency electrical stimulation and exercise; group 2 – medium-frequency electrical stimulation and exercise; group 3 – exercise only; group 4 – control. Low-frequency electrical stimulation included the following parameters: amplitude 0–100 mA; voltage 45 V; frequency 35 Hz; duration 300 μs; interpulse width 25 μs; and waveform biphasic symmetrical balanced rectangular pulse. Medium-frequency electrical stimulation included: amplitude 25 mA; voltage 0–105 V; frequency 300 Hz; duration 400–600 μs; and waveform monophasic modified spike wave. Both forms of electrical stimulation were found to significantly influence back muscle endurance compared to the control group. Low-frequency electrical stimulation and exercises were shown to significantly increase isokinetic back muscle strength compared to the control and medium-frequency groups (Kahanovitz et al 1987).

Electrical stimulation parameters for NMES include pulsed DC or burst-modulated AC current with a pulse duration of

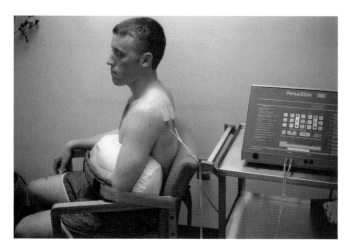

Figure 14.5 • Electrode placement for neuromuscular electrical stimulation for strengthening the rotator cuff muscles.

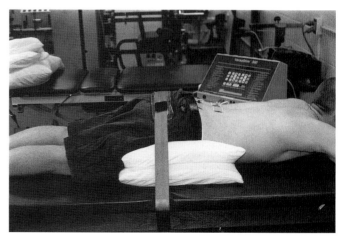

Figure 14.6 • Electrode placement for neuromuscular electrical stimulation for strengthening the lumbar paraspinal muscles.

200–1000 µs, and a frequency of 30–75 pulses or bursts per second (Nalty 2001). Isometric contractions are typically generated for 10–15 s followed by 50–120 s of rest to minimize fatigue (Selkowitz 1989) for a total of 10 contractions. The stimulus intensity is gradually increased to the therapeutic level over several seconds to help patient tolerance; however, the ramp time should be added to the total contraction time to ensure appropriate duration of the contraction at an appropriate level. Electrodes are typically placed over the motor point of the muscle and the intensity of stimulation is increased until the force reaches at least 50% of the force generated volitionally. Patients should receive the NMES treatment at least three times per week to maximize strength gains (Robinson & Snyder-Mackler 1995). Patient positioning depends on the muscle group to be treated. For example, once precautions following surgery have been removed, NMES can be used to restore rotator cuff strength by stabilizing the arm against the side of the body using a belt or sheet. In the case of stimulating the supraspinatus, placing the electrodes near the spine of the scapula helps minimize upper trapezius recruitment (Fig. 14.5). Amplitude is increased to maximum tolerance until a strong contraction is elicited.

When strengthening lumbar paraspinal muscles with NMES, the pelvis must be stabilized to the table and the spine placed in slight flexion to avoid lumbar hyperextension when the stimulation is applied (Fig. 14.6).

The success of NMES treatments depends on correct preparation of the patient by the clinician. It is essential to help patients tolerate very high force contractions in order to produce strength gains because the intensity of the NMES elicited contractions correlates positively with strength gains (Snyder-Mackler et al 1994). Patients rarely refuse the treatment due to discomfort if they realize its benefits. Strategies to improve patient tolerance include increasing the rest time between contractions, reducing the frequency of stimulation, increasing the ramp-up time and, if available, changing the shape of the waveform. Delitto & Rose (1986) found that although no consistent differences in level of comfort were found between NMES with triangular, sine or square wave pulses, individual preferences did exist. Clinicians may use this information as evidence to the patient that use of a different waveform may make the NMES treatment more tolerable.

Reduced tissue extensibility

Another aspect of sport and exercise injury that affects the progress in rehabilitation is that of reduced tissue extensibility that may impair joint range of motion. Superficial heat and the thermal effects of continuous US are commonly thought to affect tissue extensibility and improve range of motion.

Although superficial heat is used prior to range of motion activities, research has shown no effect in improving range of motion when used in an athletic population. Henricson et al (1984) studied the use of an electric heating pad for 20 min at 43°C on the posterior-lateral thigh. The use of heat and stretch did not significantly increase hip flexion, abduction or external rotation. Similarly, Taylor et al (1995) looked at the effect of heat on hamstring length. A 77°C hot pack surrounded by seven dry terry cloth towels for 20 min was used. No significant increase in hamstring flexibility was noted. These studies provide evidence that disputes the use of superficial heat prior to stretching as a way to increase range of motion in an athletic population (Henricson et al 1984, Taylor et al 1995).

In contrast, the thermal effects of continuous US is used to improve collagen extensibility by affecting the viscoelastic properties of collagen tissue (Enwemeka 1989, Jackson et al 1991). The 'heat and stretch' technique is often used to improve muscular flexibility (Reed et al 2000). Muscle tissue typically needs to be heated to between 39 and 47°C to increase extensibility (Gersten 1955). Several investigations have demonstrated increased tissue extensibility of the human calf after application of continuous US (Draper & Ricard 1995, Wessling et al 1987). Draper & Ricard (1995) suggested that the stretch must be applied within 3 min of the application of US to achieve the maximum benefits.

Treatment of tissue damage

Electrical stimulation for fracture repair

Bone has piezoelectric properties in which tension creates positive charge and compression creates negative charge. Therefore, electrical stimulation can be beneficial in promoting fracture repair (Evans et al 2001, Uhl 1989).

DC and pulsed electromagnetic fields (PEMF) have been used in promoting fracture repair. Three types of electrical stimulation applications are used for bone healing: invasive, percutaneous (semi-invasive) and noninvasive (Evans et al 2001). Each has advantages and disadvantages and are chosen based on fracture location, complication factors and patient compliance (Evans et al 2001).

Both DC (Kahanovitz & Arnoczky 1990, Meril 1994) and PEMF (de Hass et al 1980, Marks 2000) have been shown to assist bony healing. Application of PEMF is noninvasive and involves a coil worn over the fracture site for at least 10 hours a day for maximum benefit. The restriction on daily activities affects compliance with the treatment and may be an important factor in choosing this modality (Patterson 2000, Uhl 1989). PEMF can be effective when displacement is less than 1 mm, no signs of synovial pseudoarthrosis are evident and no signs of intracarpal collapse in the case of scaphoid non-union are present (Uhl 1989).

The semi-invasive electrical stimulation units are used to deliver DC. The cathode is anchored to the bone and a self-adherent anode electrode is secured to the skin, which also houses the power source. The anodal electrode is replaced daily and a non-weightbearing cast is applied to prevent motion at the fracture site as well as to reduce tension on the electrode cables. This system requires monitoring of the power source, wire connections and for the possibility of chemical effects associated with DC on the skin under the anode (Evans et al 2001).

Fully invasive units have been utilized in conjunction with spinal fusions to enhance bone formation (Kahanovitz & Arnoczky 1990, Marks 2000, Meril 1994) or when compliance is a concern (Uhl 1989). The electrodes are implanted at the fracture/fusion site and a battery pack is located subcutaneously. Once fusion is achieved, the battery pack may be removed under local anesthesia. The electrodes can remain in the healed fracture site (Uhl 1989).

Laser

Laser is electromagnetic energy found in the visible or infrared spectrums and is used to promote tissue healing. Three properties differentiate laser from other light sources: monochromaticity, coherence and collimated beam. Monochromatic laser contains a single wavelength. Coherent means single wavelengths oscillate in phase. Collimated beams indicate a minimal scattering of photons. Lasers that are used clinically have a frequency of less than 60 milliwatts so the effects are non-thermal. Rather, the effects of laser are due to its ability to alter cellular mechanisms, such as increased phagocytosis or facilitation of collagen synthesis (Basford 1995). Two typical lasers that are used are the helium–neon (HeNe) and the gallium–arsenide (GaAs). Wavelengths typically range from 820 to 904 nm and the dose of the treatment is usually between 1 and 4 J/cm^2 (Basford 1995).

There are two uses of laser in sports medicine: promotion of tissue healing and pain management. However, much of the literature published on laser treatments is anecdotal. There have been few randomized clinical controlled studies on laser (Basford 1995); therefore, the use of laser in sports medicine has not gained acceptance and the US Food and Drug Administration has not approved its use in the USA (Basford 1995).

Possible benefits of laser on wound healing may be due to the lasers' effect on stimulation of capillary growth and the formation of granulation tissue (Basford 1995). Mester et al (1985) cited multiple studies of the use of laser in the healing of ulcers and non-healing wounds, but the limitations of the research involve poor randomization, lack of measurements by blinded observers and lack of control groups. Studies in which blinded researchers were used, found no significant difference in the healing of venous stasis ulcers in response to treatment with HeNe lasers (Lundeberg & Malm 1991, Santoianni et al 1984).

The use of laser in the athletic population has focused predominantly on pain relief. Basford et al (1998) attempted to determine the effectiveness of low-intensity laser therapy on the treatment of pain control for plantar fasciitis. They used a 30 milliwatt continuous wave 0.83 nm GaAlAs diode laser three times a week for 4 weeks and found no statistical difference in pain level and duration of painful walking upon awakening, a common symptom with plantar fasciitis (Basford et al 1998). Similarly, Vecchio et al (1993) investigated the effect of 3-J laser treatments using a 30 milliwatt 830 nm GaAlAs diode twice a week for 8 weeks on rotator cuff tendonitis. No significant differences in pain, range of motion or strength were found between the group treated with laser and that treated with the sham laser. Bingol et al (2005) demonstrated improved palpation sensitivity and passive range of motion of the shoulder following 10 sessions of laser (GaAs 904 nm diode, at 2.98 J/cm^2), but found no significant differences in pain or active range of motion (Bingol et al 2005). Vasseljen et al (1992) showed improvement of pain and strength of lateral epicondylitis with eight treatments of 3.5 J/cm^2 laser using an 18 milliwatt pulsed 904 nm diode. However, the authors stated that the benefits of laser alone would not be as great without other forms of therapy (Vasseljen et al 1992). Lowe et al (1997) investigated the effects of low-level laser on ischemic pain at Erb's point, the junction of the midclavicle and sternocleidomastoid muscle. This area is easily irradiated because nerve trunks from the brachial plexus are most superficial at this point. They found no significant decrease in pain using a GaAlAs 830 nm diode for either 5 or 30 s (Lowe et al 1997). Naeser et al (2002) compared red-beam laser (continuous 15 mW, 632.8 nm HeNe laser) to the affected hand, infrared laser (pulsed, 9.4 W, 904 nm GaAs laser) to deep points of the upper extremity and cervical region, and sham treatment (TENS to the affected wrist) in treating pain associated with carpal tunnel syndrome. There were decreases in McGill Pain

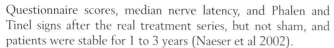

Questionnaire scores, median nerve latency, and Phalen and Tinel signs after the real treatment series, but not sham, and patients were stable for 1 to 3 years (Naeser et al 2002).

Some possible precautions to the use of laser are pregnancy, cancer, acute hemorrhages, placement over growth plates and photosensitive skin. Other risks of laser center on the ability of laser to destroy tissue (Basford 1995).

All lasers used in laser therapy are not the same. The possible benefits of one type of diode laser may not yield the same benefits of another diode (Basford 1995). Having many types of lasers available makes comparisons of the study's results difficult. Depth of target tissue can affect the results. The use of laser currently needs more research to support its use in sports medicine when compared to other widely used modalities in sports medicine. The results found in the literature are conflicting, due to the differing methods of application and other features of the treatment application. The effectiveness of the treatment depends on wavelength, treatment duration, dosage and site of application over nerves, rather than joints. When evaluating the literature, characteristics of the device and application techniques used are helpful in evaluating the results (Brosseau et al 2004).

Hyperbaric oxygen

Hyperbaric oxygen (HBO) involves the application of 100% oxygenated air at high pressures (2–3 times atmospheric pressure) to patients who are enclosed in special tanks. The principle behind HBO is that by delivering oxygen under high pressure, alveolar oxygen pressure is increased, thus producing a rise in plasma oxygen content, which results in enhanced tissue oxygen delivery. Studies have shown that when pressures are twice that of atmospheric pressure, blood oxygen content can increase by 2.5% and the oxygenation of local tissue can increase 10-fold (Bassett & Bennett 1977, Jain 1995).

HBO has been useful in decreasing edema, which should facilitate healing by improving oxygenation to the damaged tissues. HBO has been shown to promote granulation tissue formation, revascularization and epithelialization (Jain 1995, Lavan & Hunt 1990). However, a study by Fabian et al (2000) on full-thickness wound healing in rabbits found that HBO therapy did not significantly improve the rate of healing. Some research has focused on the use of HBO in sports medicine (Best et al 1998, Borromeo et al 1997, Staples et al 1999). The use of HBO early after injury (i.e. in the first 4–6h) has shown the best results for improving the effects of tissue injury (Hunt & Pai 1972, Jain 1995).

Borromeo et al (1997) looked at the effect of HBO on the time to recovery and ankle range of motion after acute ankle sprains. HBO had no effect on decreasing the recovery time or increasing the range of motion of the ankle. The time taken to administer HBO may limit its use in sports medicine because typical treatment duration is approximately 90 min. HBO treatment is contraindicated in patients who have a fever, upper respiratory infection or predisposition to a tension pneumothorax (Staples & Clement 1996). The continued use of HBO needs further prospective randomized trials to demonstrate and elucidate its positive effects on the sports population.

Extracorporeal shock wave therapy

General principles

Extracorporeal shock-wave therapy (ESWT) is an emerging treatment modality for managing pain from musculoskeletal disorders. ESWT is starting to show promise with tendinopathies, such as epicondylitis of the elbow, calcific tendonitis of the shoulder and plantar fasciitis of the foot. As of 2006, the US Food and Drug Administration had only approved the use of electrohydraulic ESWT for treatment of plantar fasciitis. Previously, ESWT has been successfully used in urology to disintegrate kidney and ureteric stones, and was first used for musculoskeletal conditions in the early 1990s (Valchanou & Michailov 1991) to treat fractures that were demonstrating nonunion or delayed union with healing.

The extracorporeal shock wave is an acoustic wave with single-pressure pulses of microsecond (3–5 µs) duration that has a very short rise time followed by a low-pressure phase with peak pressures of 35 to 120 MPa (Ogden et al 2001). Because the pulse duration is short and generated at low frequencies, it is minimally absorbed by body tissues, and no thermal effects are generated. Many of the physical effects are considered to depend on the energy involved, and are affected by pulse pressure, density of propagation medium and the area of the shock wave. For medical use, shock waves are concentrated into very small focal areas of 2–8 mm diameter, in order to optimize the therapeutic effects and minimize the effects on other tissues (Auge & Preminger 2002).

The characteristics of shock waves are determined by the type of device used. They are generated by an electric storage capacitor, which is charged and then rapidly discharged by electroacoustic transducers (Coleman & Saunders 1993). The generators can be electrohydraulic, electromagnetic or piezoelectric, and the source type determines the shape of the pulse (Ogden et al 2001). For all types, the shock wave is focused based upon the geometric arrangement of the head and focal length of the lens. Table 14.2 describes each type briefly, and identifies benefits and disadvantages of the different methods. Electromagnetic and piezoelectric machines generate lower energy shock waves than the electrohydraulic devices. Multiple treatments are often required, and there is no need for a local anesthetic with electromagnetic or piezoelectric devices. High-energy devices require fewer treatment sessions than low-energy devices to produce similar levels of pain relief. At the present time in the USA, high-energy machines require anesthesia, and can therefore only be used by physicians (Cheing & Chang, 2003).

The mechanism of the action of ESWT is unknown, but in soft tissue it is hypothesized to directly stimulate the healing processes, neovascularization and disintegration of calcium deposits. It may also alter cell membrane permeability and act as a nociceptive input. These hypothesized effects, while they remain speculative, have been shown to help reduce pain

Table 14.2 Mechanisms of ESWT and a brief description of each type, along with benefits and disadvantages of each

Mechanism	Description	Benefits	Disadvantages
Piezoelectric	Piezocrystals are mounted on the inner surface of a sphere and receive rapid electric discharge. A pressure pulse in the surrounding water produces a shock wave	Good focusing accuracy Low acoustic power treatment can be performed without analgesia	Low acoustic power may result in inefficiency of treatments or may require repeated treatments
Electrohydraulic	High voltages from a charged capacitor are applied across an electrode, generating a gas bubble filled with vapor. The expansion of the bubble produces a sonic pulse and subsequent implosion that produces a shock wave	Can generate a range of pressures	Pressure fluctuations
Electromagnetic	Strong electric current is passed through a flat coil, inducing a magnetic field. At the same time, another magnetic field is induced over a metal membrane located over the coil. As magnetic poles repel, the magnetic fields repel creating a shock wave	Can generate a range of peak pressures Deep penetration of waves is possible Good focusing accuracy Large distribution area may potentially reduce adverse effects	Cost

Table 14.3 Different responses produced in the body with the use of ESWT, and their potential benefits and adverse reactions (reproduced with permission from Speed C A 2004 Extracorporeal shock-wave therapy in the management of chronic soft-tissue conditions. Journal of Bone and Joint Surgery (Br) 86B:165–171)

Biological response	Potential benefits	Potential adverse effects
Direct tissue trauma or cavitation	Bleeding Mechanical shearing Ultrastructural damage	Stimulation of tissue healing Disintegration of calcium Transient inflammatory response
Altered cell membrane permeability	Cell death	Nociceptive: suppression of pain transmission
Direct effect on nociceptors		Denervation: antinociceptive effect
Peripheral nerve stimulation	Arrhythmias, paresthesias	Hyperstimulation, blocking the gate control mechanism

associated with plantar fasciitis, heel pain, lateral epicondylitis and calcific shoulder tendonitis (Haake et al 2003, Rompe et al 2002, Schmitt et al 2001, Speed et al 2003, Wang 2003). Shock waves may have beneficial or adverse effects on soft tissues (Table 14.3). The passage of shock waves can result in damage to the tissues along the axis of the field of the shock wave that can result in localized bleeding. Cavitation, the movement of gas bubbles in a fluid, is thought to play a role in the development of tissue changes resulting from a shock wave–gas bubble interaction. The bubbles expand within microseconds of the shock wave, and then collapse, generating a second shock wave. Cavitation can have mechanical and chemical effects that may be therapeutic or detrimental. Contraindications for use of ESWT include direct exposure to internal organs and major vascular structures, as well as in the area of the clavicle or first rib. Hemophilia is also a contraindication secondary to the tissue damage that occurs with ESWT.

Treatment parameters

Pulse duration for ESWT is usually fixed at 3–5 μs and the calculation of dose depends on the choice of energy level and the total number of shock wave impulses delivered. Energy flux density (EFD, reported in mJ/mm^2) within the focal region refers to the shock wave flow through an area perpendicular to the direction of propagation, but the total amount of acoustic energy (pulses × energy per pulse) is what determines therapeutic effects. Treatments are usually described according to the number of shocks administered, generator frequency and energy level setting. EFD in the focal region can be adjusted within a range between 0.04 and 0.5 mJ/mm^2. The frequency of the shock impulses can be adjusted between 1 and 4 Hz. A total dose for the duration of treatment may be reported. For example, a total dose of 270 mJ/mm^2 equals 1000 pulses delivered over three treatment sessions, at an EFD of 0.09 mJ/mm^2.

Patient preparation and positioning

Most patients report a sharp pain sensation during the application of ESWT, but require no anesthetic agent. A pinprick test is performed prior to treatment to ensure that the patient has normal sensation. The patient should be positioned comfortably, with the body part stabilized to prevent movement during administration of the treatment. The device should be positioned over the most tender point of palpation for the patient. Ultrasound gel should always be used as a contact medium between the cylinder head and the skin. Care should be taken to focus the ESWT on the same localized spot during each treatment session.

Clinical evidence

Plantar fasciitis

Recent studies assessing the effectiveness of ESWT at decreasing pain in patients with plantar fasciitis have produced conflicting results (Haake et al 2003, Rompe et al 2002, Speed et al 2003). Rompe et al (2002), in a prospective, randomized, controlled clinical trial, investigated three applications of 1000 impulses of low-energy shock waves compared to three applications of 10 impulses of low-energy shock waves, both delivered at $0.08 \, mJ/mm^2$. The dose of 1000 impulses reduced pain significantly compared to 10 impulses with walking, night pain and resting pain. At 5 years follow-up, 5 of 38 people in the 1000 impulse group had surgery while none were receiving other treatment; conversely, in the 10 impulse group, 32 of 40 had surgery or were still receiving other treatments (Rompe et al 2002). Speed et al (2003) randomized subjects to receive either electromagnetic ESWT (1500 pulses at $0.12 \, mJ/mm^2$) or sham treatment. Both groups showed improvement over the course of the study; however, there were no statistically significant differences between groups. The authors concluded that there was no treatment effect of moderate dose of ESWT in these subjects. Efficacy may be dependent upon the type of ESWT and the treatment protocol used. Haake (2003) randomized subjects into two groups, one receiving placebo and one receiving ESWT (4000 pulses of $0.08 \, mJ/mm^2$ with local anesthesia), for 3 treatment sessions spaced 2 weeks apart. Patients were followed for a 1-year period. The authors found no meaningful improvement in clinical outcomes between the two groups; while three-quarters of the subjects in the ESWT group reported good outcomes at 1 year, reasons for the improvement cannot be directly attributed to the treatment.

Rompe et al (2005) demonstrated that anesthetic should not be used with electromagnetic ESWT. The study found that in a group of patients receiving local anesthetic with ESWT for plantar fasciitis, less of an increase in pain was reported compared to those who did not receive a local anesthetic. The authors explained that basic science investigations have demonstrated that high-energy shock waves may lead to selective dysfunction of peripheral sensory unmyelinated nerve fibers without affecting nerve fibers responsible for motor function. This selective destruction of unmyelinated sensory nerve fibers within the focal zone of the ESWT may contribute to analgesic effects. Low-energy shock waves may induce neuropeptide release resulting in a local neurogenic inflammation within the focal area that prevents sensory nerve reinnervation.

Epicondylitis

Haake et al (2002) conducted a multicenter randomized trial investigating the effects of ESWT on the treatment of lateral epicondylitis. Patients received 200 pulses of $0.07–0.09 \, mJ/mm^2$ or placebo therapy; both groups had a success rate of 25%. ESWT was found not effective in this study. Different protocols may affect the results. The authors hypothesized that the difference between their study and previous studies demonstrating the effectiveness of ESWT could be lack of a placebo group for comparison. Rompe et al (2004) investigated the effects of low-energy ESWT on 78 subjects who were randomized into either a control or ESWT group ($0.09 \, mJ/mm^2$ for 3 treatments of 2000 impulses). They reported at 3 months a significant decrease in pain with resisted wrist extension.

Tendonitis and calcific tendonitis

In addition to musculoskeletal conditions found in an athletic population, ESWT has been shown to be effective at breaking down calcium deposits, and has shown promise with calcific tendonitis conditions (Wang et al 2003). In tendonitis of the supraspinatus without calcification (Schmitt et al 2001), it has been shown to be no different than control.

Summary

Tissue damage is associated with most athletic injury. The damage can range from localized cellular damage to ruptured tendon or fracture. The use of electrophysical agents may help to facilitate healing of damaged tissues by addressing inflammation, edema, pain and loss of muscle strength and function due to disuse or immobilization. This chapter presents the principles of electrophysical agents that are common in sports medicine. The benefits and uses of each electrophysical agent must be carefully evaluated when deciding appropriate intervention strategies.

References

Abramson D I, Bell Y, Rejal H et al 1960 Changes in blood flow, oxygen uptake, and tissue temperatures produced by therapeutic physical agents. American Journal of Physical Medicine 39: 87–95.

Alon G 1991 Principles of electrical stimulation. In: Nelson R L, Currier D P (eds) Clinical electrotherapy. Appleton and Lange, Norwalk, CT, p 35–101

Auge B K, Preminger G M 2002 Update on shock wave lithotripsy technology. Current Opinion in Urology 12:87–90

Bare A C, McAnaw M B, Pritchard A E et al 1996 Phonophoretic delivery of 10% hydrocortisone through the epidermis of humans as determined by serum cortisol concentrations. Physical Therapy 76:738–745

Basford B R 1995 Low intensity laser: still not an established clinical tool. Lasers in Surgery and Medicine 16:331–342

Basford B R, Malanga G A, Krause D A et al 1998 A randomized controlled evaluation of low-intensity laser therapy: plantar fasciitis. Archives of Physical Medicine 79:249–253

Bassett B E, Bennett P B 1977 Introduction to the physical and physiological bases of hyperbaric therapy. In: Davis J C, Hunt T K (eds) Hyperbaric oxygen therapy. Undersea Medical Society, Bethesda, MD, p 11–24

Bassett F H 3rd, Kirkpatrick J S, Engelhardt D L et al 1992 Cryotherapy-induced nerve injury. American Journal of Sports Medicine 20:516–518

Benson H A, McElnay J C, Harland R 1989 Use of ultrasound to enhance percutaneous absorption of benzydamine. Physical Therapy 69:113–118

Bertolucci L E 1982 Introduction of antiinflammatory drugs by iontophoresis. Double blind study. Journal of Orthopaedic and Sports Physical Therapy 4:103–108

Bertoti D B 2000 Electrical stimulation: a reflection on current clinical practices. Assistive Technology 12:21–32

Best T M, Loitz-Ramage B, Corr D T et al 1998 Hyperbaric oxygen in the treatment of acute muscle stretch injuries. American Journal of Sports Medicine 26:367–371

Bingol U, Altan L, Yurkturan M 2005 Low-power laser treatment for shoulder pain. Photomedicine and Laser Surgery 23:459–464

Borromeo C N, Ryan J L, Marchetto P A et al 1997 Hyperbaric oxygen therapy for acute ankle sprains. American Journal of Sports Medicine 25:619–624

Braun B L 1987 Treatment of acute anterior disk displacement in the temporomandibular joint: a case study. Physical Therapy 67:1234–1236

Brosseau L, Welch V, Wells G et al 2004 Low level laser therapy (Classes I, II, and III) for treating osteoarthritis. Cochrane Database of Systematic Reviews 3:CD002046

Byl N 1995 The use of ultrasound as an enhancer for transcutaneous drug delivery: phonophoresis. Physical Therapy 75:539–553

Cameron M H, Monroe L G 1992 Relative transmission of ultrasound by media customarily used for phonophoresis. Physical Therapy 72:142–148

Cheing G L Y, Chang H 2003 Extracorporeal shock wave therapy. Journal of Orthopaedic and Sports Physical Therapy 33:337–343

Christie A D, Willoughby G L 1990 The effect of interferential therapy on swelling following open reduction and internal fixation of ankle fractures. Physiotherapy Theory and Practice 6:3–7

Ciccone C D, Leggin B G, Callamaro J J 1991 Effects of ultrasound and trolamine salicylate phonophoresis on delayed-onset muscle soreness. Physical Therapy 71:666–678

Coleman A J, Saunders J E 1993 A review of the physical properties and biological effects of the high amplitude acoustic fields used in extracorporeal lithotripsy. Ultrasonics 31:75–89

Crago P E, Peckham P H, Thrope G B 1980 Modulation of muscle force by recruitment during intramuscular stimulation. IEEE Transactions on Biomedical Engineering 27:679–684

Cramp A F, Gilsen C, Lowe A S et al 2000 The effect of high- and low-frequency transcutaneous electrical nerve stimulation upon cutaneous blood flow and skin temperature in healthy subjects. Clinical Physiology 20:150–157

de Hass W G, Watson J, Morrison D M 1980 Non-invasive treatment of ununited fractures of the tibia using electrical stimulation. Journal of Bone and Joint Surgery (Br) 62B:465–470

Delacerda F G 1982 A comparative study of three methods of treatment for shoulder girdle myofascial syndrome. Journal of Orthopaedic and Sports Physical Therapy 4:51–54

Delitto A, Rose S J 1986 Comparative comfort of three waveforms used in electrically elicited quadriceps femoris contractions. Physical Therapy 66:1704–1707

Delitto A, Rose S J, McKowen J M et al 1988 Electrical stimulation versus voluntary exercise in strengthening thigh musculature after anterior cruciate ligament surgery. Physical Therapy 68:660–663

Draper D O, Ricard M D 1995 Muscle following 3 MHz ultrasound: the stretching window revealed. Journal of Athletic Training 30:304–307

Enwemeka C S 1989 The effects of therapeutic ultrasound on tendon healing. A biomechanical study. American Journal of Physical Medicine and Rehabilitation 68:283–287

Eston R, Peters D 1999 Effects of cold water immersion on the symptoms of exercise induced muscle damage. Journal of Sports Sciences 17:231–238

Evans R, Foltz D, Foltz K 2001 Electrical stimulation with bone and wound healing. Clinics in Podiatric Medicine and Surgery 18:79–95

Evans T A, Ingersoll C, Knight K et al 1995 Agility following the application of cold therapy. Journal of Athletic Training 30:231–234

Fabian T S, Kauffman H J, Lett E D et al 2000 The evaluation of sub-atmospheric pressure and hyperbaric oxygen in ischemic full-thickness wound healing. American Surgeon 66:1136–1143

Fitzgerald G K, Piva S R, Irrgang J J 2003 A modified neuromuscular electrical stimulation protocol for quadriceps strength training following anterior cruciate ligament reconstruction. Journal of Orthopaedic and Sports Physical Therapy 33:492–501

Fountain F P, Gersten J W, Sengir O 1960 Decrease in muscle spasm produced by ultrasound, hot packs, and infrared radiation. Archives of Physical Medicine and Rehabilitation 41:293–298.

Gersten J 1955 Effect of ultrasound on tendon extensibility. American Journal of Physical Medicine 34:362–369

Green T, Refshauge K, Crosbie J et al 2001 A randomized controlled trial of a passive accessory joint mobilization on acute ankle inversion sprains. Physical Therapy 81:984–994

Greenberg R S 1972 The effects of hot packs and exercise on local blood flow. Physical Therapy 52:273–278

Griffin J W, Newsome L S, Stralka S W et al 1990 Reduction of chronic posttraumatic hand edema: a comparison of high voltage pulsed current, intermittent pneumatic compression, and placebo treatments. Physical Therapy 70:279–86

Haake M, Konig I R, Decker T et al 2002 Extracorporeal shock wave therapy in the treatment of lateral epicondylitis: a randomized multi-center trial. Journal of Bone and Joint Surgery (Am) 84A:1982–1991.

Haake M, Buch M, SChoellner C et al 2003 Extracorporeal shock wave therapy for plantar fasciitis: randomised controlled multicentre trial. British Medical Journal 327:75–79

Harris P R 1982 Iontophoresis: clinical research in musculoskeletal inflammatory conditions. Journal of Orthopaedic and Sports Physical Therapy 4:109–112

Henricson A S, Fredrikson K, Persson I et al 1984 The effect of heat and stretching on the range of hip motion. Journal of Orthopaedic and Sports Physical Therapy 6:110–115

Hillebrandt F A, Houtz S J 1956 Mechanisms of muscle training in man: experimental demonstration of the overload principle. Physical Therapy Review 38:319–322

Hunt T K, Pai M P 1972 The effect of varying ambient oxygen tensions on wound metabolism and collagen synthesis. Surgery Gynecology Obstetrics 135:561–567

Indergand H J, Morgan B J 1995 Effect of interference current on forearm vascular resistance in asymptomatic humans. Physical Therapy 75:306–312

Ingersoll C D, Knight K L, Merrick M A 1992 Sensory perception of the foot and ankle following therapeutic applications of heat and cold. Journal of Athletic Training 27:231–234

Jackson B A, Schwane J A, Starcher B C 1991 Effect of ultrasound therapy on the repair of Achilles tendon injuries in rats. Medicine and Science in Sports and Exercise 23:171–176

Jain K K 1995 Textbook of hyperbaric medicine, 2nd edn. Hogrefe and Huber, Toronto

Japour C, Vohra R, Vohra P et al 1999 Management of heel pain syndrome with acetic acid iontophoresis. Journal of the American Podiatric Medical Association 89:251–257

Jensen J E, Conn R R, Hazelrigg G et al 1985 The use of transcutaneous neural stimulation and isokinetic testing in arthroscopic knee surgery. American Journal of Sports Medicine 13:27–33

Johnson M I, Ashton C H, Thompson J W 1991 An in-depth study of long-term users of transcutaneous electrical nerve stimulation: implications for clinical use of TENS. Pain 44:221–229

Kahanovitz N, Arnoczky S P 1990 The efficacy of direct current electrical stimulation to enhance canine spinal fusions. Clinical Orthopaedics and Related Research 251:295–299

Kahanovitz N, Nordin M, Verderame R et al 1987 Normal trunk muscle strength and endurance in women and the effect of exercises and electrical stimulation: 2. Comparative analysis of electrical stimulation and exercises to increase trunk muscle strength and endurance. Spine 12:112–118

Kandel E R, Schwartz J H, Jessell T M 1995 Essentials of neural science and behavior. Appleton and Lange, Stamford, CT

Karunakara R G, Lephart S M, Pincivero D M 1999 Changes in forearm blood flow during single and intermittent cold application. Journal of Orthopaedic and Sports Physical Therapy 29:177–180

Klaiman M D, Shrader J A, Danoff J V et al 1998 Phonophoresis versus ultrasound in the treatment of common musculoskeletal conditions. Medicine and Science in Sports and Exercise 30:1349–1355

Knight K L 1995 Cryotherapy in sports injury management. Human Kinetics, Champaign, IL

Kots Y M, Babkin D, Timtsenko N 1977 Canadian–Soviet Exchange Symposium on Electrostimulation of Skeletal Muscles. Concordia University, Montreal, p 6–15

Lark M R, Gangarosa L P 1990 Iontophoresis: an effective modality for the treatment of inflammatory disorders of the temporomandibular joint and myofascial pain. Cranio 8:108–119

Laufer Y, Ries J D, Leininger P M et al 2001 Quadriceps femoris muscle torques and fatigue generated by neuromuscular electrical stimulation with three different waveforms. Physical Therapy 81:1307–1316

Lavan F B, Hunt T K 1990 Oxygen and wound healing. Clinical Plastic Surgery 17:463–472

Lehmann J D, Brunner G D, Stow R W 1958 Pain threshold measurements after therapeutic application of ultrasound, microwaves, and infrared. Archives of Physical Medicine 39:560–565

Levy A S, Lintner S 1997 Penetration of cryotherapy in treatment after shoulder arthroscopy. Arthroscopy 13:461–464

Lowe A S, McDowell B C, Walsh D M et al 1997 Failure to demonstrate any hypoalgesic effect of low intensity laser irradiation (830 nm) of Erb's point upon experimental ischemic pain in humans. Lasers in Surgery and Medicine 20:69–76

Lundeberg T, Malm M 1991 Low-power HeNe laser treatment of venous leg ulcers. Annals of Plastic Surgery 27:537–539

Lyons C L, Robb J B, Irrgang J J et al 2005 Differences in quadriceps femoris muscle torque when using a clinical electrical stimulator versus a portable electrical stimulator. Physical Therapy 85:44–51

Manal T J, Snyder-Mackler L 1997 Electrotherapy for pain management: high intensity stimulation shows promising results. Rehabilitation Management 65:56–57

Marks R A 2000 Spine fusion for discogenic low back pain: outcomes in patients treated with or without pulsed electromagnetic field stimulation. Advances in Therapy 17:57–67

Mendel F, Fish D 1993 New perspectives in edema control via electrical stimulation. Journal of Athletic Training 28:63–74

Meril A J 1994 Direct current stimulation of allograft in anterior and posterior lumbar interbody fusions. Spine 19:2393–2398

Mester E, Mester A F, Mester A 1985 The biomedical effects of laser application. Lasers in Surgery and Medicine 5:31–39

Michlovitz S L 1996 Thermal agents in rehabilitation, 3rd edn. FA Davis Company, Philadelphia, PA

Myerson M S, Fisher R T, Burgess A R et al 1986 Fracture dislocations of the tarsometatarsal joints. End results correlated with pathology and treatment. Foot and Ankle 6:225–242

Naeser M A, Hahn L A, Lieberman B E et al 2002 Carpal tunnel syndrome pain treated with low-level laser and microamperes transcutaneous electrical nerve stimulation: a controlled study. Archives of Physical Medicine and Rehabilitation 83:177–180

Nalty T 2001 Electrotherapy: clinical procedures manual. McGraw Hill, New York

Nussbaum E, Rush P, Disenhaus L 1990 The effects of interferential therapy on swelling following open reduction internal fixation of ankle fractures. Physiotherapy Canada 76:803–807

Ogden J A, Toth-Kischkat A, Schultheiss R 2001 Principles of shock wave therapy. Clinical Orthopaedics 387:8–17

Ohkoshi Y, Ohkoshi M, Nagasaki S et al 1999 The effect of cryotherapy on intraarticular temperature and postoperative care after anterior cruciate ligament reconstruction. American Journal of Sports Medicine 27:357–362

Oziomek R S, Perrin D H, Herold D A et al 1991 Effects of phonophoresis on serum salicylate levels. Medicine and Science in Sports and Exercise 23:397–401

Palmer J E, Knight K L 1996 Ankle and thigh skin surface temperature changes with repeated ice pack application. Journal of Athletic Training 31:319–323

Paternostro-Sluga T, Fialka C, Alacamliogliu Y et al 1999 Neuromuscular electrical stimulation after anterior cruciate ligament surgery. Clinical Orthopaedics and Related Research 368:166–175

Patterson M 2000 What's the buzz on external bone growth stimulators? Nursing 30:44–45

Picker R I 1988 Current trends: low-volt pulsed microamp stimulation, Part I. Clinical Management in Physical Therapy 9:10–14

Picker R I 1989 Current trends: low-volt pulsed microamp stimulation, Part II. Clinical Management in Physical Therapy 9:28–33

Reed B, Ashikaga T, Fleming B et al 2000 Effects of ultrasound and stretch on knee ligament extensibility. Journal of Orthopaedic and Sports Physical Therapy 30:341–347

Rivenburgh D W 1992 Physical modalities in the treatment of tendon injuries. Clinics in Sports Medicine 11:645–659

Robinson A J, Snyder-Mackler L (eds) 1995 Clinical electrophysiology: electrotherapy and electrophysiologic testing, 2nd edn. Williams and Wilkins, Baltimore, MD

Rompe J D, Schoellner C, Nafe B 2002 Evaluation of low-energy extracorporeal shock-wave application for treatment of chronic plantar fasciitis. Journal of Bone and Joint Surgery (Am) 84A:335–341

Rompe J D, Decking J, Schoellner C et al 2004 Repetitive low-energy shock wave treatment for chronic lateral epicondylitis in tennis players. American Journal of Sports Medicine 32:734–743

Rompe J D, Meurer A, Nafe B et al 2005 Repetitive low-energy shock wave application without local anesthesia is more efficient than repetitive low-energy shock wave application with local anesthesia in the treatment of chronic plantar fasciitis. Journal of Orthopaedic Research 23:931–941

Santoianni P, Monfrecola G, Martellotta D et al 1984 Inadequate effect of helium-neon laser on venous leg ulcers. Photodermatology 1:245–249

Schmidt W 1993 Iontophoresis. Is it drug delivery or electrotherapy? Rehabilitation and Therapy Products Review Sept/Oct:15–20

Selkowitz D 1989 High frequency electrical stimulation in muscle strengthening. American Journal of Sports Medicine 17:103–111

Shin S M, Choi J K 1997 Effect of indomethacin phonophoresis on the relief of temporomandibular joint pain. Journal of Craniomandibular Practice 15:345–348

Snyder-Mackler L, Ladin Z, Schepsis A et al 1991 Electrical stimulation of the thigh muscles after reconstruction of the anterior cruciate ligament. Effects of electrically elicited contractions of the quadriceps femoris and hamstring muscles on gait and strength of the thigh muscles. Journal of Bone and Joint Surgery (Am) 73A:1025–1036

Snyder-Mackler L, Delitto A, Stralka S et al 1994 Use of electrical stimulation to enhance recovery of quadriceps femoris muscle force production in patients following anterior cruciate ligament reconstruction. Physical Therapy 74:901–907

Snyder-Mackler L, Delitto A, Bailey S et al 1995 Strength of the quadriceps femoris muscle and functional recovery after reconstruction of the anterior cruciate ligament. Journal of Bone and Joint Surgery (Am) 77A:1166–1173

Speed C A 2004 Extracorporeal shock-wave therapy in the management of chronic soft-tissue conditions. Journal of Bone and Joint Surgery (Br) 86B:165–171

Speed C A, Nichols D, Wies J et al 2003 Extracorporeal shock wave therapy for plantar fasciitis. A double blind randomized control trial. Journal of Othopaedic Research 21:937–940

Staples J R, Clement D B 1996 Hyperbaric oxygen chambers and the treatment of sports injuries. Sports Medicine 22:219–227

Staples J R, Clement D B, Taunton J E et al 1999 Effects of hyperbaric oxygen on a human model of injury. American Journal of Sports Medicine 27:600–605

Starring D 1991 The use of electrical stimulation and exercise for strengthening lumbar musculature: a case study. Journal of Orthopaedic and Sports Physical Therapy 14:61–64

Surbey G D, Andrew G M, Cervenko F W et al 1984 Effects of naloxone on exercise performance. Journal of Applied Physiology 57:674–679

Taylor B F, Warning C A, Brashear T A 1995 The effects of therapeutic application of heat or cold followed by static stretch on hamstring muscle length. Journal of Orthopaedic and Sports Physical Therapy 21:283–286

Taylor K, Newton R A, Personius W J et al 1987 Effects of interferential current stimulation for treatment of subjects with recurrent jaw pain. Physical Therapy 67:346–350

Taylor K, Fish D, Mendel F et al 1992 Effect of electrically induced muscle contractions on posttraumatic edema formation in frog hind limbs. Physical Therapy 72:127–132

Taylor K, Mendel F, Fish D et al 1997 Effect of high-voltage pulsed current and alternating current on macromolecular leakage in hamster cheek pouch microcirculation. Physical Therapy 77:1729–1740

Thornton R, Mendel F, Fish D 1998 Effects of electrical stimulation on edema formation in different strains of rats. Physical Therapy 78:386–394

Thorsson O, Lilja B, Ahlgren L et al 1985 The effect of local cold application on intramuscular blood flow at rest and after running. Medicine and Science in Sports and Exercise 17:710–713

Uhl R 1989 The use of electricity in bone healing. Orthopaedic Review 18:1045–1050

Valchanou V D, Michailov P 1991 High energy shock waves in the treatment of delayed and nonunion of fractures. International Orthopaedics 15:181–184

Vasseljen O, Hoeg N, Kjeldstad B et al 1992 Low level laser versus placebo in the treatment of tennis elbow. Scandinavian Journal of Rehabilitation Medicine 24:37–42

Vecchio P, Cave M, King V et al 1993 Doubleblind study of the effectiveness of low level laser treatment of rotator cuff tendonitis. British Journal of Rheumatology 32:740–742

Wang C J, Yang K D, Wang F S et al 2003 Shock wave therapy for calcific tendonitis of the shoulder. A prospective clinical study with two year follow up. American Journal of Sports Medicine 31:425–430

Washington L L, Gibson S J, Helme R D 2000 Age-related differences in the endogenous analgesic response to repeated cold water immersion in human volunteers. Pain 89:89–96

Wessling K C, DeVane D A, Hylton C R 1987 Effects of static stretch versus static stretch and ultrasound combined on triceps surae muscle extensibility in healthy women. Physical Therapy 67:674–679

Zemke J E, Anderson J C, Guion W K et al 1998 Intramuscular temperature responses in the human leg to two forms of cryotherapy: ice massage and ice bag. Journal of Orthopaedic and Sports Physical Therapy 27:301–307

Prevention of injury

15

Timothy E. Hewett, Kristin Briem and Roald Bahr

CHAPTER CONTENTS

Introduction 236

Sequence of prevention 237

Methodology in research 242

Example paradigm: ACL injuries in female
athletes 243

Summary 248

Introduction

A physically active lifestyle and participation in sports is undoubtedly important for all age groups. Motives for choosing to participate in sports are many, such as pleasure and relaxation, competition, socialization and a desire to maintain and improve fitness and health. However, sports participation also entails a risk for overuse injuries as well as acute injuries which, although rarely, may even lead to death or permanent disability. It appears that early osteoarthrosis, which frequently results from the more serious knee joint injuries, cannot be prevented with our current treatment methods (Myklebust & Bahr 2005). In addition, long-term absences from work and sports as a result of injury constitute a significant problem for sports, society and for the affected individuals.

Reports indicate that the health benefits from regular physical activity exceed the risks connected with injuries. Sarna et al (1993) conducted a study on male members of a number of Finnish international sports teams during 1920 to 1965. They were subsequently evaluated for incidence of chronic disease and life expectancy. After adjusting for occupation, marital status and age at entry to the cohort of the study, former elite athletes, particularly those in aerobic sports, were found to live longer than less active controls. The increased mean life expectancies were mainly explained by decreased cardiovascular mortality. Kujala et al (1996) looked at the same groups and investigated the men's post-career use of hospital care from all causes, based on national hospital discharge registry data. They found that the athletes needed less overall hospital care, largely explained by lower rates of hospitalization for heart disease, respiratory disease and cancer. However, all groups of athletes were hospitalized for musculoskeletal problems more frequently than men in the control group. At least in part, this may be explained by the increased prevalence of osteoarthritis in former elite athletes (Imwalle et al 2005, L'Hermette et al 2006).

The overall health benefits experienced by the Finnish athletes cannot solely be attributed to their athletic career, but may also result from a physically active lifestyle in later life. The intensity of training and competition in sports has increased several-fold over the last two decades, which undoubtedly has led to more prevalent and more severe acute injuries as well as long-term musculoskeletal problems. However, the relative benefits in terms of increased longevity and reduced morbidity due to reduced risk of lifestyle diseases in athletes may be even greater today due to the ever more sedentary lifestyle in the general population.

This chapter describes some current concepts regarding sports injury epidemiology, as well as the general principles for injury prevention research. However, since potential injury prevention strategies differ considerably between sports, it is not possible to describe practical preventive measures for specific sports within the confines of the present chapter. However, some models will be presented and examples will be given from randomized controlled trails (RCTs) to illustrate the principles involved when trying to prevent injuries. These models may, in turn, be applied to any specific sport. The final section of the chapter will be dedicated to a discussion about the etiology and prevention of the detrimental and costly injury to the anterior cruciate ligament (ACL) in the knee.

As promoters of sports and physical activity from a health perspective, we have a professional obligation to make sports participation as safe as possible. In order to reduce the risk of injury associated with sports, it is necessary to use advances in the epidemiology of sports injuries as a basis for sports policy. In order to set out effective prevention programs, epidemiological studies need to be done on incidence, severity and etiology of sports injuries. In addition, the effect of preventive measures needs to be evaluated as they are introduced.

Sequence of prevention

Measures to prevent sports injuries do not stand by themselves. They form part of what might be called a sequence of prevention (van Mechelen et al 1992) (Fig. 15.1).

First, the magnitude of the problem must be identified and described in terms of incidence and severity of sports injuries. Second, the causes of injury, risk factors and injury mechanisms that play a part in the occurrence of injuries must be identified. Based on that information, the third step is to introduce

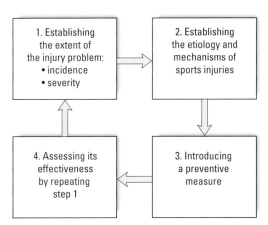

Figure 15.1 • Four-step sequence of injury prevention research. (Reproduced from van Mechelen et al 1992 with permission of Adis International.)

measures that are likely to reduce the future risk and/or severity of sports injuries. Finally, the effect of the measures must be evaluated by repeating the first step, which will determine if they are effective in reducing injury incidence and severity.

Magnitude of the problem

One way of getting an impression of the magnitude of the sports injury problem is by counting the absolute number of injuries. In Scandinavian studies, between 6.3 and 18.1% of all acute injuries seen in an emergency room, casualty department or outpatient clinic setting are sports-induced (de Loes 1990, Lindqvist et al 1996, Maehlum & Daljord 1984, Sandelin et al 1985, Ytterstad 1996). When these absolute numbers are compared with the number of work-related injuries or those resulting from traffic accidents in a particular community, for instance, the relative extent of the sports injury problem for that population can be revealed.

The numbers with regard to injury frequency per type of sport or gender will reflect the number of actual participants and the types of sports in which the population of that community predominantly participates. If the total number of athletes and the total time of participation in the different sports are not known, the numbers give no information on the risks across sports or gender. For instance, if we were to find that half of all sports injuries in South America were sustained while playing soccer and less than one percent in ice hockey, it would not be fair to conclude that soccer is a more dangerous activity than playing ice hockey. Obviously, soccer is much more popular and widely played in that population.

Incidence of sports injuries

Incidence of sports injuries can be defined as the number of new injuries during a particular period, in a given population at risk, which also gives an estimate of risk. In terms of risk assessment, however, allowance needs to be made for actual time of exposure to injury (i.e. the number of hours of active play during which the individual runs the risk of being injured). Expressing injuries as the number of injuries per 1000 or 10 000 hours of exposure time allows for a meaningful comparison across studies, sports or populations, whether looking at absolute number of injuries or particular types of injuries. For example, a soccer team with 16 players who train 8 hours a week during a 40-week season will have a combined exposure time of 5120 practice hours. If the team sustains a combined total of 46 injuries during the same period, the incidence during training is 9 injuries per 1000 hours of exposure ($46/5120 \times 1000$). Methods used to calculate injury incidence need to be adjusted to particular research settings. For instance, the incidence of skiing injuries can be expressed as the number of injuries per 1000 skier days or per 1000 runs or as the number of injuries per 100 000 km skied (Ronning et al 2000).

Prevalence is the best way of describing the occurrence of overuse injuries. It can be defined as the percentage of athletes in a given population with an injury at a given time. For example, the prevalence is 30% if 3 out of 10 javelin throwers state that they have elbow pain at a given time.

Sports injury incidence can only be assessed properly if clear definitions of the sports injury and of the population-at-risk are present. When interpreting and comparing results of different studies it is important to know what definition for 'sports injury' was used, how the injuries were counted and whether the studies were retrospective or prospective. It is also important to know the comparability of the populations-at-risk and the methods used to count the population and record exposure time.

Table 15.1 shows incidence rates found in a number of prospective studies conducted in Scandinavia at the senior level for male teams (Aagaard et al 1997, Arnason et al 1996, Bahr & Bahr 1997, Drogset 1990, Ekstrand & Gillquist 1983, Lorentzon et al 1986, 1988a, 1988b, Luthje et al 1996, Molsa et al 1997, 2000, Nielsen & Yde 1988, 1989, Pettersson & Lorentzon 1993, Poulsen et al 1991, Tegner & Lorentzon 1991, Yde & Nielsen 1988). Although there is a limitation to the number of studies available in some sports, the trend seems relatively clear: Ice hockey is the game with the highest rate of injuries by far: in most studies 50–80 injuries per 1000 player hours during games. Ice hockey is followed by soccer with a match injury incidence of 18–35 per 1000 player hours. Comparable studies from other European countries and the USA show similar numbers for elite men's and women's soccer (Faude et al 2005, Giza et al 2005, Hawkins & Fuller 1999, Morgan & Oberlander 2001, Walden et al 2005), or slightly lower (Giza et al 2005). Although the injury rate for ice hockey is certainly high, the Rugby World Cup 2003 surveillance project had 97.9 injuries per 1000 player hours reported to the tournament medical officer (Best et al 2005). There is only one study available from European team handball, showing an incidence slightly lower than soccer, and volleyball appears to have the lowest injury rate of the most popular Scandinavian team sports. There is no prospective study available from Scandinavian basketball, but other studies have shown rates just slightly higher than volleyball (Arendt & Dick 1995, Colliander et al 1986, Yde & Nielsen 1990, Zelisko et al 1982).

More injuries appear to be sustained during competition than during training. This is primarily due to the higher intensity during matches and most likely also because athletes do not take the same risks when training with their teammates as they do against their opponents during games. The extremely high difference in injury rates between games and training seen in elite ice hockey can be explained by the fact that the teams have an intense match schedule and mainly use their training sessions during the season for recovery and basic skill training purposes.

Severity of sports injuries

To fully understand the risk related to participation in sport, one must consider not only the incidence of injuries but also their severity. A description of the severity of sports injuries is important in making decisions about preventive measures, since the incidence of serious injuries in a given sport does not necessarily coincide with the overall incidence of injuries in that sport. The vast majority of sports injuries heal without permanent disability. Serious injuries such as fractures, ligament, tendon and intra-articular injuries, concussions, spinal injuries and eye injuries can leave permanent damage (residual symptoms). Serious physical damage can cause permanent disability, or even death. Thus, priority should be given to preventive measures in sports where serious injuries are common and to these injury types, even though the particular sport itself may be characterized by a low incidence of sports injuries and/or a low absolute number of participants.

As an example, studies from European team handball show that there is a high incidence of ACL injuries, especially among female players. Myklebust et al (1998) and Strand et al (1990) have found an incidence of 0.91 and 0.82 per 1000 player hours for women during competition in Norwegian team handball, which almost equals the rate of ankle sprains in volleyball (Bahr & Bahr 1997, Bahr et al 1994). An ACL injury is a much greater source of concern than an ankle sprain as the severity of an ACL injury will be reflected in more comprehensive medical treatment, longer absence from sport and work, a greater degree of future disability and functional impairment and higher direct and indirect treatment costs. Ice hockey represents a sport where the total incidence of injury is high, and where a high frequency of concussions and spinal cord injuries is seen (Molsa et al 1999, Tegner & Lorentzon 1996).

According to the literature (van Mechelen 1997) the severity of sports injuries can be described on the basis of the following six criteria: the nature of the sports injury in terms of medical diagnosis, the duration and nature of treatment, loss of sporting time, the length of working or school time lost, permanent disability and the direct and indirect economic cost of the injury, which essentially involves the expression of these criteria in economic terms. The economic costs can be divided into: (1) direct costs, i.e. the cost of medical treatment (diagnostic expenses such as X-rays, doctor's fee, and costs of medicines, hospital admission and rehabilitation) and (2) indirect costs, i.e. expenditure incurred in connection with the loss of productivity due to increased morbidity and mortality levels (loss of school or working time and loss of expertise due to death or handicap).

Table 15.1 Incidence of acute injuries during competition and training in selected team sports, based on studies of Scandinavian elite sports

Sport	Incidence (no. of injuries per 1000 practice hours)	
	In competition	In training
Basketball	2–3	5–6
Soccer	11–35	2–8
Team handball	14	1–2
Ice hockey	29–79	1–3
Volleyball	3–6	1–4

Etiology of sports injuries

Although we have a fair number of studies available documenting the incidence, severity and injury profile of most major sports, very little information available is on risk factors and injury mechanisms.

Risk indicators for sports injuries can be divided into two main categories: intrinsic, personal risk indicators and external, environmental risk indicators (van Mechelen et al 1992). This division is based on partly proven and partly supposed causal relationships between risk factors and sports injuries. The mere presence of these intrinsic and extrinsic indicators is usually not sufficient to produce injury, but the sum of them and the interaction between them may make the athlete vulnerable to injury at a given place, in a given sports situation. Merely to establish these risk factors for sports injuries is not enough; the mechanisms by which the injuries occur must be identified as well.

Studies on the etiology of sports injuries require a dynamic model that accounts for the multifactorial nature of sports injuries. A dynamic model by Meeuwisse (1994), later modified by Bahr & Krosshaug (2005), describes how multiple factors interact to produce injury (Fig. 15.2).

Intrinsic risk indicators

According to the model, the intrinsic or athlete-related factors are classified as predisposing factors that are necessary, but seldom sufficient, to produce injury. Examples include age, aberrant quality or quantity of joint motion, reduced neuromuscular function, e.g. as a result of previous injuries, and osteoporosis. In addition, there may be psychological precursors to injury as outlined in Chapter 11.

Extrinsic risk indicators

In this theoretical model, extrinsic risk factors are classified as enabling factors in that they facilitate the manifestation of injury in the presence of intrinsic risk factors. Examples include floors where the friction is very high or low, an uneven grassy playing field, training or competing in severe weather conditions, running on hard asphalt, on crowded streets or in traffic or wearing inappropriate footwear.

Inciting events

Meeuwisse's (1994) model further describes an inciting event as the final link in the chain of causation to sports injury and suggests that such an inciting event is usually directly associated with the onset of injury. Such events are regarded as necessary causes. The term injury mechanism is often used to describe the inciting event in biomechanical terms. Studies on the etiology of sports injuries tend to focus on the inciting events and neglect the intrinsic and extrinsic risk factors, thereby revealing only a small fraction of the factors and events that lead to sports injury. Although understandable, focusing on inciting events may lead to overweighing the importance of such events in the etiology and prevention of acute and chronic sports injuries.

Bahr & Krosshaug (2005) emphasized the need to use a comprehensive model to describe the inciting event, which accounts for the events leading to the injury situation (playing situation, player and opponent behavior), as well as to include a description of whole body and joint biomechanics at the time of injury. Examples of factors that may be important to understand and describe the injury mechanisms are shown in Table 15.2.

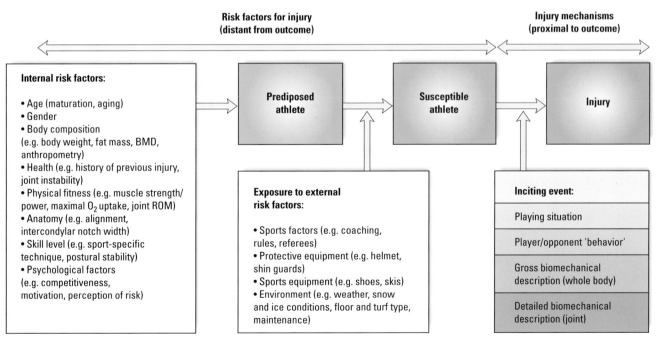

Figure 15.2 • Comprehensive model for injury causation. (Reproduced from Bahr & Krosshaug 2005 with permission from BMJ Publishing Group.)

Table 15.2 Categories of injury mechanism descriptions with examples of elements and descriptions (reproduced from Bahr & Krosshaug 2005 with permission from BMJ Publishing Group)

Category	Elements	Examples of factors describing the injury mechanism			
		Noncontact ACL injury in basketball	ACL injury in a mogul skiing jump landing	Knock-out in boxing	Lower leg stress fracture in football
Playing (sports) situation	Team action Skill performed prior to, and at, the point of injury Court position Player position Ball handling	Fast break Zone defense Charging Cutting Setting up for a shot Defensive rebound Player-to-player defense	Course steepness Jump elements (e.g. twist, helicopter) Jump height and length	Uppercut, hook Counterattack Foot work Forced into the corner/to the ropes Ring-side referee decision Inter-boxer distance	Exposure to matches and training (total load) Midfielder with defensive and offensive tasks (i.e. many runs in matches/training) Hard working team Frequency of duels
Athlete/opponent behavior	Player performance Opponent interaction Player attention	Effort Disturbance by opponent Intention Foot firmly fixed to the floor Intention Technical foul	Rhythm and balance prior to the jump Concentration Balance Boot-binding release Visual control Jumping technique Over-rotation Falling technique	Awareness Aggressiveness Punching power Punching speed Balance	Effort Toe/heel runner Jumping technique Duel technique
Whole body biomechanics	Coarse description – often static – of whole body kinematics and kinetics	Sideways translation Rotation of the body around the fixed foot Speed at impact Foot in front of center of mass	Linear and angular momentum Energy absorption Center of mass to the rear	Center of mass velocity Punching force Punching direction Weight distribution on the legs	Stride length Stride frequency Vertical excursion Ground reaction forces Knee flexion angle
Joint/tissue biomechanics	Detailed description of joint/tissue kinematics and kinetics	Valgus moment Pivot shift of the tibia relative to the femur Notch impingement	Shear forces Anterior drawer Intercondylar lift-off Loading rate	Energy transfer Head acceleration Pressure distribution and localization	Bending moment Shear forces Surface/shoe dynamics

ACL = anterior cruciate ligament

Application of sport science methods may provide a better understanding of the chain of events preceding an injury. Injury mechanisms can be described using different research approaches with a focus on different elements of the inciting event, and suggestions for preventive measures may originate from each category. It is therefore important to investigate all aspects of the injury mechanism. Krosshaug et al (2005) reviewed eight different research approaches to study the mechanisms of injuries in sport, each with its possibilities and limitations. These include interviews of injured athletes, analysis of video recordings of actual injuries, clinical studies (where the clinical joint damage findings are studied to understand the injury mechanism, mainly through plain radiography, MRI, arthroscopy or CT scans), in vivo studies (measuring ligament strain or forces to understand ligament loading patterns), cadaver studies, mathematical modeling and simulation of injury situations, or measurements/estimation from 'close to injury' situations. For most injury types, one research approach alone will not be sufficient to describe all aspects of the injury situation. A broader and more precise understanding could be attained by combining such research approaches as athlete interviews, video analysis and clinical studies, or by combining video analysis and studies using cadavers, dummies or mathematical simulations.

A multifactorial model like the model of Meeuwisse (1994) should be used to study the etiology of sports injuries, and at the same time take intrinsic and extrinsic risk factors into account. However, one limitation of the model is that it does not take the team's training routine and competitive schedule into consideration as potential causes, and the model may therefore be more relevant to describe acute injuries than overuse injuries.

Introducing preventative measures

Haddon's matrix

Ideally, as discussed earlier in relation to the sequence of prevention (Fig. 15.1), injury prevention measures are developed on the basis of research information about the risk factors and the injury mechanisms in various sports. Few studies are available on injury prevention. Strategies for injury control, however, have been developed from other research areas, particularly from research on motor vehicle accidents. One such model, the so-called Haddon's matrix (Haddon 1980), has two dimensions (Table 15.3). Although it was developed primarily for motor vehicle accidents, it can be applied to sports and exemplifies a few measures that may be effective in injury prevention.

Pre-crash measures

Measures related to the pre-crash stage have been developed to counteract potential injury-causing situations, by preventing accidents altogether. In sports, examples of *athlete*-related pre-crash measures include ensuring adequate, sport-specific, physical conditioning of athletes, increasing their skill level and improving neuromuscular control and agility to avoid situations where they might get injured. Psychosocial variables may be addressed in an effort to influence the athletes' resiliency and

Table 15.3 Haddon's matrix applied to sport injury prevention: measures effective in preventing sport injuries

	Pre-crash	Crash	Post-crash
Athlete	Technique Neuromuscular function	Training status Falling techniques	Rehabilitation
Surroundings	Floor friction Playing rules	Safety nets	Emergency medical coverage
Equipment	Shoe friction	Tape or brace Ski bindings Leg padding	First aid equipment Ambulance

injury vulnerability. In addition, sport-specific screens may help identify athletes at risk for injury, as outlined in Chapter 12. Examples of *environmental* pre-crash measures include modifying the friction of the playing surface (too high may lead to twisting injuries to the lower extremity, too low may lead to slipping and falling injuries) or changing regulations to avoid dangerous plays. *Equipment*-related pre-crash measures include modifying shoe friction and choosing cleat length according to the playing surface and weather conditions.

Several RCTs have applied pre-crash measures or actions to examine the efficacy of the intervention on occurrence of sports injuries (Ekstrand 1982, Heidt et al 2000, Jakobsen et al 1994, Pope et al 2000, van Mechelen et al 1993, Wedderkopp et al 1999) and although some showed effectiveness, others did not. Since a lot of the studies included multifactorial prevention programs, effectiveness (or ineffectiveness) of any single action in the programs remain unclear.

Crash measures

Measures related to the second stage, the crash stage, have been developed to protect the athlete against injuries if a potentially harmful situation arises. These measures mainly focus on assisting athletes to withstand the forces involved when a collision or a fall occurs. *Athlete*-related crash measures could involve e.g. a general strength-training program, flexibility program or falling techniques. *Environmental* crash measures include safety nets to avoid falling alpine skiers from flying into the crowd or soft mats protect gymnasts failing a dismount or falling down from an apparatus. There are many examples of *equipment*-related crash measures in sports, such as release-bindings for alpine skiing, helmets and pads for various sports, taping and braces for joints, shin guards and eye protection.

RCTs have shown effectiveness of prophylactic knee braces (Sitler et al 1990), balance-board training (Tropp et al 1985) and semi-rigid ankle stabilizers (Sitler et al 1994, Surve et al 1994).

Post-crash measures

Post-crash measures are designed to minimize the damage resulting from an injury and the risk of reinjury (which is a strong risk factor for sports injuries), and mainly relates to the chain of medical treatment provided after an injury. Post-crash measures in sports may include providing adequate medical services during sports events (personnel and equipment), training athletes and coaches to provide adequate on-field first aid, including quick evacuation procedures to a hospital in the case of severe injuries, and adequate rehabilitation programs for injured athletes before they return to competition. Unfortunately, in sports medicine there are no examples known of effective post-crash measures that have been tested in RCTs.

Assessing effectiveness of preventive measures

The fourth and last step in van Mechelen's sequence of prevention is to evaluate the effectiveness of the intervention that was introduced. From an epidemiological standpoint it is preferable to evaluate the effect of specific preventive measures by means of a RCT in order to see whether the intervention was indeed effective in reducing the risk and/or severity of a specific sports injury. Unfortunately, relatively few RCTs have been conducted in sports injury prevention studies (Ekstrand & Gillquist 1983, Gilchrist et al 2004, Jakobsen et al 1994, Petersen et al 2005, Pope et al 2000, Sitler et al 1990, 1994, Surve et al 1994, Tropp et al 1985, van Mechelen et al 1993, Wedderkopp et al 1999).

When conducting (and also when interpreting the outcomes of) epidemiological sports injury studies one is confronted with a number of methodological issues. The first issue of importance here is the definition of sports injury. Another has to do with the setting in which the study is conducted. The results of various sports injury incidence surveys are not necessarily comparable, if the study setting differs. Thirdly, the extent to which sports injury incidence and sports injury risk can be assessed not only depends on the definition of sports injury or the study setting, but also the methods used to count injuries, to establish the population at risk, and to verify that the sample is representative. It is here that proper research design comes into play.

Methodology in research

Definition of sports injuries

In general, sports injury is a collective name for all types of damage that can occur in relation to sporting activities. Studies define the term sports injury in a number of different ways (Meeuwisse & Love 1997). Some define a sports injury as any injury sustained during sporting activities for which an insurance claim is submitted; in other studies the definition is confined to injuries treated at a hospital casualty or other medical departments (van Mechelen et al 1992); still others rely on reports from athletes or trainers.

Different injury definitions can be grouped in three categories: (1) time loss injuries, where the definition usually is that the player is unable to participate in next match or training session because of injury; (2) game interruption injuries, where the player has to interrupt the game or training session because of an injury; or (3) medical attention injuries, where the player has to seek medical attention for evaluation and/or treatment because of an injury.

To make sports injury surveys as comparable as possible, an unambiguous, universally applicable definition of sports injury is the first prerequisite. This definition should be based on a concept of health different than that customary in standard medicine, and should, for instance, take incapacitation for sports or school into account.

A consensus group met after the First World Congress on Sports Injury Prevention in Oslo in 2005 under the auspices of Fédération Internationale de Football Association (FIFA) Medical Assessment and Research Centre (Fuller et al 2006). The objective was to establish definitions and methodology, implementation and reporting standards that should be adopted for studies of injuries in football (soccer), but which may also be applicable in other sports. This group defined an injury as: 'Any physical complaint sustained by a player that results from a match or training, irrespective of the need for medical attention or time-loss from team activities. An injury that results in a player receiving medical attention is referred to as a "medical-attention" injury and an injury that results in a player being unable to take a full part in future training or match play as a "time-loss" injury.' 'Medical attention' refers to an assessment of a player's medical condition by a qualified medical practitioner. 'A player being unable to take a full part in future football [soccer] training or match play' is independent of whether a training session actually takes place on the day following the injury or whether a player is selected to play in the next match. The term 'future' refers to any time after the onset of injury, including the day of injury. It is important to recognize that variations in medical support and practice and in individuals' tolerances to pain may create differences in the incidence of injury reported in studies.

Study setting

Differences in the injury definition used may partly explain the differing injury rates observed, but the study setting also plays a role. One should bear in mind that if a study is conducted in a setting where courtside medical support is readily available, using a 'Medical attention' injury definition is likely to result in a higher injury incidence rate than a 'Time loss' definition; in such a situation players are likely to seek medical attention for minor injuries not involving time loss. This may be the case in ice hockey, where medical staff is required to be present at all times during training and matches. Conversely, if a study is done in a setting where professional medical support is not as readily available, a 'Time loss' definition is likely to result in a higher injury rate than a 'Medical attention' definition. Players do not always seek medical attention for injuries, not even for time loss injuries.

If sports injuries are recorded through medical channels (for instance through hospital emergency rooms or insurance records), a fairly large percentage of serious, predominantly acute injuries will be observed and less serious and/or overuse injuries will not be recorded. If such a 'limited' definition is used, only part of the total sports injury problem is revealed. This 'tip-of-the-iceberg' phenomenon is commonly described in epidemiological research (Walter et al 1985). This problem is to a large extent found in sport injury epidemiology in youth where many overuse injuries are thought to be found, as well as 'minor' acute injuries.

Research design

Depending on the methods used the researcher will be confronted to a greater or lesser extent with phenomena such as recall bias, overestimation of the hours of sport participation (Klesges et al 1990), incomplete responses, nonresponse, dropout, invalid injury description and problems related to the duration and cost of research. These factors will clearly affect the internal validity of a study.

Study design

Injuries as well as time-at-risk can be assessed retrospectively or prospectively, using questionnaires or person-to-person interviews. However, prospective studies can, by closely monitoring exposure time and injury outcome, more accurately estimate the risk and incidence of sports injury according to the level of sports participation and type of exposure of an athlete. They are therefore superior to retrospective studies. One of the main problems of retrospective studies is the inherent recall bias of the subjects participating in such a study.

A word should be said here about case studies. In sports medical journals clinical case series are commonly described. Conclusions are drawn from these case series regarding the incidence and the risk to sustain sports injuries. However, case studies have the drawback that no information on the population-at-risk is available. Consequently, no valid conclusions can be drawn from case studies; neither with respect to sports injury incidence nor with respect to injury risks (Walter et al 1985).

Sample selection

Special attention has to be paid to the method of assessing the population-at-risk and to ascertain that the sample is representative. If the population-at-risk is not clearly identified it is not possible to calculate reliable incidence data. With regard to representative samples, consideration has to be taken that the performance of athletes in sports, and therefore the incidence of sports injuries, is highly determined by selection. Bol et al (1991) recognized four different kinds of selection: (1) self-selection (personal preferences) and/or selection by social environment (parents, friends, school, etc.), (2) selection by the sports environment (trainer, coach, etc.), (3) selection by sports organizations (organization of competition by age and gender, the setting of participation standards, etc.) and (4) selection by social, medical and biological factors (socioeconomic background, mortality, age, ageing, gender, etc.).

All these issues should be taken into account in the study design, or, if this is not possible, limitations must be readily acknowledged when interpreting the results.

Example paradigm: ACL injuries in female athletes

As described earlier, and shown in Fig. 15.1, measures to prevent sports injuries form part of what might be called a sequence of prevention. First, the magnitude of the problem must be identified and described in terms of incidence and severity of sports injuries.

Establishing the extent of the ACL injury problem

Since the passage of Title IX of the Educational Assistance Act, enacted in 1972, male participation at the high school level has not changed (3.7 to 3.8 million), while female participation has increased approximately 10-fold (National Federation of State High School Associations 2002), roughly doubling every 10 years (from <0.3 million to 3.2 million). The National Federation of State High School Associations reports approximately 3.2 million female participants in high school sports programs (National Federation of State High School Associations 2002). As approximately one in 50 to 70 female athletes at the high school level sustains a serious knee injury during any given year of varsity sports (Chandy & Grana 1985, Hewett et al 1999), high school athletics likely contributes to greater than 40 000 serious knee injuries to female athletes annually. Adolescent females who participate in pivoting and jumping sports suffer ACL injuries at a 3- to 6-fold greater rate than adolescent males participating in the same sports (Arendt & Dick 1995, Chandy & Grana 1985, Hewett et al 1999, Malone et al 1993), so their increased sport participation has led to a parallel rise in knee and ACL injuries.

A fivefold increase in female collegiate (National Collegiate Athletic Association 2002) sport participation has been seen in the last 30 years. The National Collegiate Athletic Association reports approximately 150 000 women participating in varsity sports each year (Hutchinson & Ireland 1995). In a survey of member institutions, an average knee injury incidence of approximately one in every 10 female athletes was reported (Hutchinson & Ireland 1995). Based on these figures, over 15 000 debilitating knee injuries are expected to occur in female athletes at the varsity intercollegiate level during any given year.

Incidence of ACL injury in female athletes

A prospective study of the first two seasons of the Women's United Soccer Association in the USA reported the knee to be by far the most common injury location (30.7%) (Giza et al 2005). Of the 55 knee injuries reported, 8 were ACL injuries. Over the two seasons, the incidence of ACL tear during games and practice was 0.9 and 0.04, respectively, per 1000 player hours, or an overall incidence of 0.09 per 1000 player hours. A prospective study of Norwegian men's and women's team-handball players was conducted during three consecutive seasons (Myklebust et al 1998). They found 28 ACL injuries, of which 23 occurred among women. The incidence of ACL injury during women's competition was 1.60 ± 0.35 per 1000 hours and an overall incidence of 0.31 ± 0.06 injuries per 1000 player hours.

Severity of injury – associated cost

The cost of reconstructing and rehabilitating the ACL injuries in these athletes, at a conservative cost of US$17 000 per athlete (Hewett et al 1999), may approach a billion dollars annually. Aside from direct financial costs, the potential loss of entire seasons of sports participation, scholarship funding, lowered academic performance (Freedman et al 1998), time taken off work and restricted work capacity, long-term disability (Ruiz et al 2002) and significantly greater risk of radiographically diagnosed osteoarthritis must also be considered (Myklebust & Bahr 2005).

A high prevalence of radiographic knee osteoarthritis as well as knee-related symptoms and functional limitations has been found in female soccer players 12 years after an ACL injury (Lohmander et al 2004). The long-term costs of ACL injury, including those related to the near certain risk of osteoarthritis, may be significantly greater than the short-term costs of surgery and rehabilitation. Thus, interventions for ACL injury prevention may provide a reasonable time and financial investment for the coach, athlete and sports medicine staff and society.

Establishing etiology and mechanism of ACL injury

The second step, according to van Mechelen's sequence of prevention, is to identify the risk factors and injury mechanisms that play a part in the occurrence of ACL injuries – specifically in women for the purpose of our paradigm. As outlined earlier, the nature of sports injuries is multifactorial and a dynamic model proposed by Meeuwisse (1991) shows how multiple factors interact to produce injury (Fig. 15.2).

Most ACL injuries in female sports occur during a noncontact episode, typically during deceleration, lateral pivoting or landing tasks that are often associated with high loads on the knee joint (Boden et al 2000, Olsen et al 2004). Sports maneuvers may lead to high external loads in both genders. Why these tasks result in greater incidence of ACL injury in females has, until recently, remained unclear. The following sections will focus on identifying intrinsic factors and inciting events (Olsen et al 2003) which may lead to ACL injury, specifically those that may be modifiable, in hopes of decreasing the incidence of this type of injury in females.

Potential risk factors – modifiable versus non-modifiable

Three major etiological theories have been proposed to explain the gender disparity observed in ACL injury rates: anatomic, hormonal and neuromuscular (Hewett 2000). A number of studies of ACL injury risk factors have focused on *anatomic* or anthropometric measures such as thigh length (Beynnon et al 2001), height and femoral notch width (Scoville et al 2001).

However, static anatomic measures such as Q-angle often do not appear to correlate to dynamic injury mechanism (Endsley et al 2003, Myer et al 2005a). In addition, they are non-modifiable by nature. *Hormonal* factors, particularly those associated with the follicular and ovulatory phases of the menstrual cycle, have also been linked to ACL injury risk (Arendt et al 2002, Hewett 2000, Slauterbeck & Hardy 2001, Wojtys et al 1998, 2002). However, the precise means by which they may contribute to ACL injury risk and the extent to which these hormonal factors can be modified remains unclear. The study of modifiable risk factors has focused on the working hypothesis that ACL injury risks are related to measurable deficits in *neuromuscular* control in female athletes (Ford et al 2003b, 2005a, Hewett et al 2006a). Neuromuscular control deficits are defined as muscle strength, power or activation patterns that lead to increased knee joint and ACL loads.

Hewett et al (2001) hypothesized that female athletes demonstrate neuromuscular control deficits that increase lower extremity joint loads during sports activities. One neuromuscular deficit, which was operationally termed 'ligament dominance', can be defined as an imbalance between the neuromuscular and ligamentous control of dynamic knee joint stability, demonstrated by an inability to control lower extremity coronal plane motion during landing and cutting (Hewett et al 2001). A second neuromuscular control deficit often observed in female athletes can be termed 'quadriceps dominance' and may be defined as an imbalance between knee extensor and flexor strength, recruitment and coordination (Hewett et al 2001). A third neuromuscular control deficit often observed in female athletes is 'leg dominance' which may be defined as an imbalance between the two lower extremities in strength and coordination (Hewett et al 2001).

The three potential neuromuscular control deficits operationally defined above are postulated to be important contributors to knee and ACL injury incidence in female athletes. ACL injury likely occurs under conditions of high dynamic loading of the knee joint, when active muscular restraints do not adequately compensate for and adequately dampen joint loads (Beynnon & Fleming 1998). Neuromuscular control of high load movements is required to maintain dynamic knee stability during landing and pivoting (Besier et al 2001, Li et al 1999). Decreased neuromuscular control of the joint may cause excessive stress to be placed on the passive ligament structures, exceeding the failure strength of the ligament (Li et al 1999, Markolf et al 1978). Methods to identify neuromuscular control deficits during tasks related to ACL injury mechanisms, such as landing, cutting and decelerating, may offer the greatest potential for the development and application of neuromuscular screening interventions targeted to high-risk populations (Boden et al 2000, Olsen et al 2004).

Potential modifiable mechanisms and landing techniques

Hewett et al (1996) tested the hypothesis that insufficient neuromuscular control of lower limb biomechanics, particularly the dynamic biomechanics of the knee joint, lead to high-risk biomechanical patterns in female athletes during execution of common albeit potentially hazardous movements. The results of this study demonstrated that peak landing forces were significantly predicted by valgus torques at the knee in females, that females developed decreased relative knee flexor torque during landing compared to males, and that females had greater side to side differences, or leg dominance, in normalized hamstrings peak torque and power. Ford et al (2003b) demonstrated similar gender differences during the performance of a drop vertical jump. This study determined that female athletes landed with a greater maximum valgus knee angle and greater total valgus knee motion than male athletes. Female athletes also had significant differences between their dominant and nondominant side in maximum valgus knee angle. These differences in valgus measures (ligament dominance) and limb-to-limb asymmetries (leg dominance) reflect neuromuscular deficits that may be indicative of decreased dynamic knee joint control in female athletes (Ford et al 2003b).

Subsequent studies systematically evaluated neuromuscular control at the hip in female athletes (Hewett et al 2006b). The evidence from multiple, potentially high-risk movements indicated that variables at the hip contributed to dynamic valgus while electromyographic (EMG) data demonstrated female to male differences in firing patterns of the hip musculature. The results demonstrated that female athletes had greater hip adduction angles and torques than males during multidirectional single-leg landing. These differences were limited to the frontal plane and were not observed in the sagittal plane. EMG patterns showed increased quadriceps and decreased gluteus firing in females. Another study examined gender differences during single leg landings from either a medial or lateral direction (Ford et al 2006). In addition to greater knee valgus, female athletes had increased hip coronal plane excursion compared to males during both types of landings (Ford et al 2006). The increased hip adduction (hip varus) motion seen in the coronal plane during athletic activities likely contributes to the dynamic valgus knee position that may place the athlete at increased risk of ACL injury (Ford et al 2006, Hewett et al 2005a).

Potential modifiable mechanisms and cutting techniques

In follow-up to the gender assessment of high risk landing positions, subsequent work by Ford et al (2005b) focused on the analysis of unanticipated, high velocity, high load cutting movements. The hypotheses were that female athletes would display increased lower extremity coronal plane motions and similar sagittal plane mechanics during the unanticipated cutting maneuver compared to males. The results showed that female athletes exhibited greater knee abduction (valgus) angles compared to males. McLean et al. (2004) also found increased coronal plane measures at the knee when evaluating a similar side cut task. Imwalle et al (2005) compared unanticipated cutting techniques at different angles to determine the effects of transverse plane rotations on coronal plane motion

related to ACL injury. The results indicated that the mechanisms underlying knee abduction measures, demonstrated by female athletes during cutting tasks, are not dictated by lower extremity transverse plane rotations. Rather, coronal plane motions at the hip may correlate to knee abduction (valgus) motion. Thus, the cutting data corroborate the findings of the landing studies that females demonstrate increased lower extremity valgus alignments and that coronal plane motions at the hip control dangerous dynamic knee alignments during high risk activities (Ford et al 2003a, 2005b, Hewett et al 1996, 2006b, Imwalle et al 2005). These data further explain the gender differences in neuromuscular control during high force, high torque, and high-risk sports maneuvers (Ford et al 2005b, Imwalle et al 2005).

Determining the underlying factors to high-risk mechanisms

Neuromuscular control deficits may lead to the valgus collapse and ACL rupture in females during the performance of high-risk maneuvers (Boden et al 2000, Hewett et al 2005b, Olsen et al 2004, Teitz 2001). Muscle activation strategies underlying the altered biomechanics in females have been examined, specifically those in which neuromuscular control deficits might induce injury during sports maneuvers. Video analyses of ACL injuries during competitive sports play have indicated a common body position associated with ACL injury: the knee is close to full extension, most or all of the weight is shifted to the planted foot and as the limb is decelerated as it collapses into valgus. In addition, the foot is externally rotated.

Gender differences in muscle activation strategies during maneuvers that mimic high ACL injury risk positions have been evaluated. Myer et al (2005a) hypothesized that the ratio of medial quadriceps activation to lateral quadriceps ratio would be decreased in female athletes. Females demonstrated imbalanced quadriceps muscular activation compared to males during a maneuver that mimicked the ACL injury mechanism. This imbalanced firing pattern, specifically a low ratio of medial to lateral quadriceps recruitment, may combine with increased lateral hamstring firing to compress the lateral joint, open the medial joint and increase anterior shear force (Rozzi et al 1999, Sell et al 2004). Repeated performance of high-risk maneuvers with inappropriate muscle activation likely contributes to the dynamic valgus knee motion that may lead to the valgus collapse and ACL rupture during these activities (Boden et al 2000, Hewett et al 2005b, Olsen et al 2004, Teitz 2001).

Relationship of high-risk mechanism to ACL injury

In order to determine if measurable neuromuscular control deficits were actually predictors of ACL injury risk, Hewett et al (2005b) undertook a large scale prospective study in order to determine if prescreened females who demonstrated decreased neuromuscular control and increased valgus joint loading would subsequently sustain an ACL injury. A coupled biomechanical–epidemiological study design was used to accomplish this goal. Prior to their competitive seasons 205 female athletes in the high-risk sports of soccer, basketball and volleyball were prospectively measured for neuromuscular control using three-dimensional kinematics (joint angles) and joint loads using kinetics (joint moments) during a jump landing task. ANOVA, linear and logistic regression isolated predictors of risk in athletes who subsequently ruptured their ACL.

Nine athletes sustained a confirmed ACL rupture during the competitive season. They had demonstrated significantly different knee kinematics and kinetics in the prescreening measurements compared to the 196 who did not go on to an ACL rupture. The mean knee abduction valgus angle at landing was 8° greater in the ACL-injured group than uninjured athletes. ACL injured athletes had a 2.5-times greater knee abduction moment and 20% higher ground reaction force, while stance time was 16% shorter, hence increased motion, force and moments occurred more quickly. Knee abduction moment predicted ACL injury status with 73% specificity and 78% sensitivity. The results of this study clearly demonstrated that female athletes that have increased dynamic valgus and high abduction loads are at increased risk of ACL injury.

Introducing a preventive measure for ACL injury

Haddon's matrix was introduced earlier (Table 15.2) and shows examples of measures that aim at ensuring adequate, sport-specific, physical conditioning of athletes. By increasing skill level and improving neuromuscular control and agility, the athletes may be able to avoid situations where they might get injured. As outlined above, gender differences in neuromuscular control and muscle activation strategies during various sports maneuvers have been identified. Neuromuscular control deficits may be targeted and modified by specific training protocols.

Effects of neuromuscular training on high-risk mechanisms

Training protocols have been developed in order to improve neuromuscular control and decrease the risk of ACL injuries in female athletes. Tables 15.4, 15.5 and 15.6 show an example of a comprehensive neuromuscular training protocol of plyometrics, core stability and strength training developed by Myer et al (2005b) in an attempt to reduce ACL injury risk in female athletes and improve sports-related performance measures. Their protocol resulted in significantly reduced coronal plane measures that increase risk of injury and also improved vertical jump, sprint speed, single leg hop distance and total body (squat) strength. While protocols that incorporate similar techniques may decrease knee injury risk and lower the incidence of injury (Myklebust et al 2003), coaches and athletes will likely find the additional potential to improve physical performance appealing (Hewett et al 2005a, Myer et al 2005b).

Hewett et al (1996) have also evaluated the effects of neuromuscular training on measures of lower extremity neuromuscular control. Females significantly reduced peak landing forces and valgus torques at the knee after six weeks of neuromuscular

Table 15.4 Example of neuromuscular training protocol consisting of plyometrics

	Time (s)	Reps
Plyometric Training (Week 1)		
Wall Jumps	15	5
Squat Jumps	10	
Tuck Jump (with thighs parallel)	10	
Line Jumps (Side to Side)	10	
Line Jump Lateral Max Vertical		5
Lunge Jump	10	
180° Jumps (Height)	15	
Broad Jump Vertical+Step*		8
Bounding in Place	20	
Forward Jumps Over Barriers+Step*		6
Forward Barrier Jumps W/Middle Box+Step*		6
Box Drop Max Vertical+Step*		10
Box Drop+Step*		10
Plyometric Training (Week 3)		
Wall Jumps	15	
Squat Jumps	15	
Tuck Jump (with Abdominal Crunch)	15	
Tuck Jump (with Butt Kick)	15	
Barrier Jumps (Front to Back)	15	
Barrier Jumps (Side to Side)	15	
Hop, Hop, Hop-Athletic Position+Step*		6
180° Jumps (Height)	15	
Broad Jump, Jump, Jump Vertical+Step*		6
Bounding For Distance		6
Lateral Barrier Hops W/Staggered Box Reaction*		6
Back Drop-Box Touch Max Vertical+Step*		10
Lateral Box Drop Max Vertical		5
Power Steps		8
Plyometric Training (Week 6)		
Squat-Tuck Jumps	12	
Barrier Hops Flat (Front to Back)	12	
Barrier Hops Flat (Side to Side)	12	
Crossover Hop, Hop, Hop Athletic Position+Step*		10
180° Jumps (Height)	15	
Broad Jump, Jump, Jump Vertical+Step*		6
3 Barrier Hop-Reaction (3-Way)		3
Forward/Backward Hops Over Barriers+Step*		6
Box Drop-180°-Box Drop-Max Vertical+Step*		8
Box Drop-180°+Step*		8
Lateral Box Drop-Broad Jump+Step*		6
Box Drop Max Vertical-Broad Jump+Step*		6
Approach Max Vertical		4
Crossover Step-Ski Stop Max Vertical		4

* Exercise ends with a quick unanticipated reaction cut/step

Table 15.5 Example of neuromuscular training protocol for core stability

	Time (s)	Reps
Core Stability Training (Week 1)		
Deep Hold Position		5
Box Butt Touch		8
Line Jump (Forward)-Deep Hold		8
Line Jump (Lateral)-Deep Hold		4
Box Drop-Deep Hold		10
Single Leg Squat-Deep Hold		6
BOSU(F) [a] Deep Hold	5	8
BOSU(F) [a] Drop Squats		8
BOSU(R) [b] Jump Stick Landing-Deep Hold		10
BOSE(R) [b] Both Knees Deep Hold	20	
BOSU(R) [b] Crunches		35
BOSU(R) [b] Swivel Crunch (Feet Planted)		40
BOSU(R) [b] Single Leg Pelvic Bridges		12
BOSU(R) [b] Supermans		12
Core Stability Training (Week 3)		
BOSU(F) [a] Drop Stick Deep Hold		10
BOSU(F) [a] Deep Hold Partner Perturbations	20	
Box Drop (Lateral)-Deep Hold		4
Single Leg Line Hop (Front/Back)-Deep Hold		8
Single Leg Line Hop (Side/Side)-Deep Hold		8
Single Leg Squat-Heel Touches		10
Swiss Ball Both Knees Deep Hold	20	
BOSU(R) [b] Single Leg Step-Stick Deep Hold		6
Double Crunch		25
Table Double Crunch		15
Table Double Swivel Crunch		8
Table Reverse Hyperextensions		12
BOSU(R) [b] Lateral Crunch		10
BOSU(R) [b] Swimmers		10
Core Stability Training (Week 6)		
Double BOSU (F) [a] Deep Hold (Partner Perturbations)	10	5
BOSU(F) [a] Drop Single Leg Airex Stick Deep Hold		5
BOSU(R) [b] Single Leg Deep Hold Partner Ball Toss	25	
Swiss Ball Both Knees Deep Hold (Partner Perturbations)	20	
BOSU(R) [b] Single Leg (4 + way) Hop Stick Deep Hold		8
BOSU(F) [a] Single Leg Ball Pick Up		8
Airex Walking Lunges		5
BOSU(F) [a] Single Legs Squats		8
BOSU(F) [a] Single Leg Deep Hold (Partner Perturbations)	30	
Straight Leg Lifts with Toe Punch		15
Straight Leg Lateral Double Crunch		12
BOSU(R) [b] Double Crunch		15
BOSU(R) [b] Opposite Swivel Crunch (Feet Up)		12
Swiss Ball Reverse Back Hyperextensions		12

[a] BOSU flat side up; [b] BOSU round side up

Table 15.6 Example of neuromuscular training protocol for strength

	Sets	Reps
Strength Training (Week 1)		
Dumbbell Hang Snatch	2	12
Bench Butt Touch	1	10
Barbell Squat	2	12
Bench Press	2	12
Lying Leg Curl	2	10
Lat Pulldowns	1	15
Ball Squat Dumbbell Floor Touches	1	10
Dumbbell Shoulder Press	1	15
Russian Hamstring Curl	1	10
Seated Cable Row	1	15
Hip Ab/Abd at 60° and 120°/sec	1	10
Double Crunch	2	20
Strength Training (Week 3)		
Hang Clean	2	8
Leg Press	2	10
Dumbbell Incline Press	2	8
Front Lunges + Press	2	10
Inverted Lying Pull-Ups	1	10
Stretch Dumbbell Dead Lift	1	10
3-Way Dumbbell Shoulder Circuit	1	12
Bench Reverse Hyper Extensions	1	10
Knee Flex/Ext at 120° and 300°/sec	1	12
Band Good Mornings	1	10
Back Extensions	1	20
Ankle Circuit	1	12
Strength Training (Week 6)		
Dumbbell Hang Snatch	3	5
Barbell Squat	2	5
Single Leg Band Assisted Squat	1	8
Bench Press	2	5
Lying Leg Curl	2	8
Lat Pulldowns	1	8
Dumbbell Shoulder Press	1	8
Band Shoulder Press	1	8
Russian Hamstring Curl	1	15
Standing Cable Row	1	8
Hip Ab/Abd at 60° and 120°/sec	1	8
Double Crunch	2	30

*Actual weight and reps used

training. In addition, relative hamstring recruitment increased and side-to-side differences in strength and power measures were normalized. The study demonstrated the potential for neuromuscular control deficits to be modified through neuromuscular training.

Assessing the effectiveness of ACL interventions: repeating step 1

The last step in the sequence of prevention is to evaluate whether the intervention which was introduced was indeed effective in reducing the risk and/or severity of a specific sports injury.

Effects of intervention: neuromuscular training and ACL injury rate

The effects of neuromuscular training on knee and ACL injury in the high-risk female sports population was evaluated by Hewett et al (1999) in a cohort study, in which high school-aged female soccer, basketball and volleyball players were monitored. Fifteen teams with 366 female athletes were included in the neuromuscular training intervention and an additional 15 teams with 463 female athletes were used as a positive control group (no training). Thirteen teams with 434 untrained male athletes were utilized as a negative control group. The intervention consisted of a six-week neuromuscular training intervention performed three times per week prior to the competitive season (Hewett et al 1996). The training intervention focused on plyometrics (jump training) and strength training.

The trained female athletes had statistically fewer serious knee, noncontact knee and noncontact ACL injuries. The rate of serious knee injury was 0.43 in untrained females, 0.12 in trained females and 0.09 in males (injuries per 1000 exposures). Statistical analysis indicated a significant effect of training on group injury rates. Untrained females had a significantly higher incidence of serious knee injury than trained females and males, whereas trained females were not different than untrained males. Training resulted in even greater differences in noncontact injuries between the female groups. This prospective study was the first to demonstrate a decreased incidence of ACL injury following neuromuscular training in the high-risk female sports population.

Hewett et al (2006a) performed a systematic review of the published literature, yielding six publications on the effects of interventions targeted towards ACL injury prevention in female athletes (Heidt et al 2000, Hewett et al 1999, Mandelbaum et al 2005, Myklebust & Bahr 2005, Powell & Barber-Foss 2000, Teitz 2001). A meta-analysis of these six studies demonstrates a significant effect of neuromuscular training programs on ACL injury incidence in female athletes (test for overall effect $Z = 4.31$, $P < 0.0001$). Examination of the similarities and differences between the training regimes gives insight into the development of more effective and efficient interventions (Hewett et al 2006a).

Gilchrist et al (2004) performed a large scale study to determine the incidence of ACL injury rate in a cohort of National Collegiate Athletic Association (NCAA) collegiate female athletes. This RCT studied interventional training as part of the practice and game warm-up. They demonstrated a significant reduction of non-contact ACL injuries in their study group during one competitive season of soccer. The evidence demonstrates that positive steps have been made toward prevention of ACL injuries in female athletes. Further research is needed to determine high-risk athletes, the most effective training methods and the most effective means to increase the implementation of these interventions.

Effects of preventive measures on overall ACL injury incidence

With the positive effect of interventions targeted to reduce ACL injuries in female athletes established, it is necessary to reevaluate the problem to determine if the incidence and severity of the problem has changed (van Mechelen et al 1992). Agel et al (2005) performed a 13-year (1989–2002) retrospective epidemiological study to determine the trends in ACL injury rates of NCAA soccer and basketball athletes. They reported that in male soccer players there was a significant decrease in ACL injuries whereas female soccer athletes showed no change over the same time period. Both female basketball and soccer players showed no change in the rates of noncontact ACL injuries over the study period and the magnitude of difference in rates (3.6 times) between their male counterparts remain unchanged. However, this study was retrospective and it did not examine injury rates in the most recent 3-year period (2002–2005). Neuromuscular training programs have only come into widespread use during these recent years (2000–2005) and, in addition, appropriate preventive measures were not likely applied across the board during the study period. Hewett and colleagues are currently conducting large-scale epidemiological studies at the county and state levels in order to define the current incidence rates in high school basketball and soccer.

Summary

The outcome of research on the extent of the sports injury problem is highly dependent on the definitions of 'sports injury', 'sports injury incidence' and 'sports participation'. The outcome of sports epidemiological research also depends on the research design and methodology, the representativeness of the sample and on whether or not exposure time was considered when calculating incidence. The severity of sports injuries can be expressed by taking six indices into consideration. The etiology of sports injuries is highly multicausal. This fact, as well as the sequence of events leading to a sports injury, should be accounted for when studying the etiology of sports injuries and when trying to prevent them. Finally, one should take determinants of sports and preventive behavior into account in attempts to solve the sports injury problem.

References

Aagaard H, Scavenius M, Jorgensen U 1997 An epidemiological analysis of the injury pattern in indoor and in beach volleyball. International Journal of Sports Medicine 18:217–221

Agel J, Arendt E A, Bershadsky B 2005 Anterior cruciate ligament injury in national collegiate athletic association basketball and soccer: a 13-year review. American Journal of Sports Medicine 33:524–530

Arendt E, Dick R 1995 Knee injury patterns among men and women in collegiate basketball and soccer. NCAA data and review of literature. American Journal of Sports Medicine 23:694–701

Arendt E A, Bershadsky B, Agel J 2002 Periodicity of noncontact anterior cruciate ligament injuries during the menstrual cycle. Journal of Gender-Specific Medicine 5:19–26

Arnason A, Gudmundsson A, Dahl H A et al 1996 Soccer injuries in Iceland. Scandinavian Journal of Medicine and Science in Sports 6:40–45

Bahr R, Bahr I A 1997 Incidence of acute volleyball injuries: a prospective cohort study of injury mechanisms and risk factors. Scandinavian Journal of Medicine and Science in Sports 7:166–171

Bahr R, Krosshaug T 2005 Understanding injury mechanisms: a key component of preventing injuries in sport. British Journal of Sports Medicine 39:324–329

Bahr R, Karlsen R, Lian O et al 1994 Incidence and mechanisms of acute ankle inversion injuries in volleyball. A retrospective cohort study. American Journal of Sports Medicine 22:595–600

Besier T F, Lloyd D G, Cochrane J L et al 2001 External loading of the knee joint during running and cutting maneuvers. Medicine and Science in Sports and Exercise 33:1168–1175

Best J P, McIntosh A S, Savage T N 2005 Rugby World Cup 2003 injury surveillance project. British Journal of Sports Medicine 39:812–817

Beynnon B D, Fleming B C 1998 Anterior cruciate ligament strain in-vivo: a review of previous work. Journal of Biomechanics 31:519–525

Beynnon B D, Slauterbeck J R, Padua D et al 2001 Update on ACL risk factors and prevention strategies in the female athlete. Presented at National Athletic Trainers' Association 52nd Annual Meeting and Clinical Symposia, Los Angeles, CA

Boden B P, Dean G S, Feagin J A et al 2000 Mechanisms of anterior cruciate ligament injury. Orthopedics 23:573–578

Bol E, Schmickli S L, Backx F J G et al 1991 Sportblessures onder de knie. Papendal. NISGZ publication 38

Chandy T A, Grana W A 1985 Secondary school athletic injury in boys and girls: a three-year comparison. Physician and Sportsmedicine 13:106–111

Colliander E, Eriksson E, Herkel M et al 1986 Injuries in Swedish elite basketball. Orthopedics 9:225–227

de Loes M 1990 Medical treatment and costs of sports-related injuries in a total population. International Journal of Sports Medicine 11:66–72

Drogset J O 1990 [Injuries among soccer players in lower division clubs]. Tidsskrift for den Norske Laegeforening 110:385–389

Ekstrand J 1982 Soccer injuries and their prevention. Linköping University, Linköping

Ekstrand J, Gillquist J 1983 Soccer injuries and their mechanisms: a prospective study. Medicine and Science in Sports and Exercise 15:267–270

Endsley M L, Ford K R, Myer G D et al 2003 The effects of gender on dynamic knee stability and Q-angle in young athletes. Presented at Ohio Physical Therapy Association Fall Conference, Columbus, OH

Faude O, Junge A, Kindermann W et al 2005 Injuries in female soccer players: a prospective study in the German National League. American Journal of Sports Medicine 33:1694–1700

Ford K R, Myer G D, Hewett T E 2003a Reliability of dynamic knee motion in female athletes. Presented at American Society of Biomechanics 2003 Annual Meeting, Toledo, OH

Ford K R, Myer G D, Hewett T E 2003b Valgus knee motion during landing in high school female and male basketball players. Medicine and Science in Sports and Exercise 35:1745–1750

Ford K R, Myer G D, Smith R L et al 2005a Use of an overhead goal alters vertical jump performance and biomechanics. Journal of Strength and Conditioning Research 19:394–399

Ford K R, Myer G D, Toms H E et al 2005b Gender differences in the kinematics of unanticipated cutting in young athletes. Medicine and Science in Sports and Exercise 37:124–129

Ford K R, Myer G D, Smith R L et al 2006 A comparison of dynamic coronal plane excursion between matched male and female athletes when performing single leg landings. Clinical Biomechanics (Bristol, Avon) 21:33–40

Freedman K B, Glasgow M T, Glasgow S G et al 1998 Anterior cruciate ligament injury and reconstruction among university students. Clinical Orthopaedics and Related Research 356:208–212

Fuller C W, Ekstrand J, Junge A et al 2006 Consensus agreement on injury definitions and data collection procedures in studies of football (soccer) injuries. British Journal of Sports Medicine 40:193–201

Gilchrist J R, Mandelbaum B R, Melancon H et al 2004 A randomized controlled trial to prevent non-contact ACL injury in female collegiate soccer players. Presented at the American Orthopaedic Society for Sports Medicine, San Francisco, CA

Giza E, Mithofer K, Farrell L et al 2005 Injuries in women's professional soccer. British Journal of Sports Medicine 39:212–216, discussion 212–216

Haddon W Jr 1980 Advances in the epidemiology of injuries as a basis for public policy. Public Health Report 95:411–421

Hawkins R, Fuller C 1999 A prospective epidemiological study of injuries in four English professional football clubs. British Journal of Sports Medicine 33:196–203

Heidt R S Jr, Sweeterman L M, Carlonas R L et al 2000 Avoidance of soccer injuries with preseason conditioning. American Journal of Sports Medicine 28:659–662

Hewett T E 2000 Neuromuscular and hormonal factors associated with knee injuries in female athletes: strategies for intervention. Sports Medicine 29:313–327

Hewett T E, Stroupe A L, Nance T A et al 1996 Plyometric training in female athletes. Decreased impact forces and increased hamstring torques. American Journal of Sports Medicine 24:765–773

Hewett T E, Lindenfeld T N, Riccobene J V et al 1999 The effect of neuromuscular training on the incidence of knee injury in female athletes. A prospective study. American Journal of Sports Medicine 27:699–706

Hewett T E, Myer G D, Ford K R 2001 Prevention of anterior cruciate ligament injuries. Current Women's Health Reports 1:218–224

Hewett T E, Myer G D, Ford K R 2005a Reducing knee and anterior cruciate ligament injuries among female athletes: a systematic review of neuromuscular training interventions. Journal of Knee Surgery 18:82–88

Hewett T E, Myer G D, Ford K R et al 2005b Biomechanical measures of neuromuscular control and valgus loading of the knee predict anterior cruciate ligament injury risk in female athletes: a prospective study. American Journal of Sports Medicine 33:492–501

Hewett T E, Ford K R, Myer G D 2006a Anterior cruciate ligament injuries in female athletes: 2. A meta-analysis of neuromuscular interventions aimed at injury prevention. American Journal of Sports Medicine 34:490–498

Hewett T E, Ford K R, Myer G D et al 2006b Gender differences in hip adduction and torque in collegiate athletes. Journal of Orthopaedic Research 24:416–421

Hutchinson M R, Ireland M L 1995 Knee injuries in female athletes. Sports Medicine 19:288–302

Imwalle L E, Myer G D, Ford K R et al 2005 Hip adduction, not internal rotation, dictates knee motion related to ACL injury during cutting maneuvers. Paper presented at the Medical Student Summer Research Program Conference, Cincinnati, OH

Jakobsen B W, Kroner K, Schmidt S A et al 1994 Prevention of injuries in long-distance runners. Knee Surgery, Sports Traumatology, Arthroscopy 2:245–249

Klesges R C, Eck L H, Mellon M W et al 1990 The accuracy of self-reports of physical activity. Medicine and Science in Sports and Exercise 22:690–697

Krosshaug T, Andersen T E, Olsen O E et al 2005 Research approaches to describe the mechanisms of injuries in sport: limitations and possibilities. British Journal of Sports Medicine 39:330–339

Kujala U M, Sarna S, Kaprio J et al 1996 Hospital care in later life among former world-class Finnish athletes. Journal of the American Medical Association 276:216–220

L'Hermette M, Polle G, Tourny-Chollet C et al 2006 Hip passive range of motion and frequency of radiographic hip osteoarthritis in former elite handball players. British Journal of Sports Medicine 40:45–49

Li G, Rudy T W, Sakane M et al 1999 The importance of quadriceps and hamstring muscle loading on knee kinematics and in-situ forces in the ACL. Journal of Biomechanics 32:395–400

Lindqvist K S, Timpka T, Bjurulf P 1996 Injuries during leisure physical activity in a Swedish municipality. Scandinavian Journal of Social Medicine 24:282–292

Lohmander L S, Ostenberg A, Englund M et al 2004 High prevalence of knee osteoarthritis, pain, and functional limitations in female soccer players twelve years after anterior cruciate ligament injury. Arthritis and Rheumatism 50:3145–3152

Lorentzon R, Wedren H, Pietila T 1986 [The occurrence of injuries in first class ice hockey]. Lakartidningen 83:3432–3433, 3435

Lorentzon R, Wedren H, Pietila T 1988a Incidence, nature, and causes of ice hockey injuries. A three-year prospective study of a Swedish elite ice hockey team. American Journal of Sports Medicine 16:392–396

Lorentzon R, Wedren H, Pietila T et al 1988b Injuries in international ice hockey. A prospective, comparative study of injury incidence and injury types in international and Swedish elite ice hockey. American Journal of Sports Medicine 16:389–391

Luthje P, Nurmi I, Kataja M et al 1996 Epidemiology and traumatology of injuries in elite soccer: a prospective study in Finland. Scandinavian Journal of Medicine and Science in Sports 6:180–185

McLean S G, Lipfert S W, van den Bogert A J 2004 Effect of gender and defensive opponent on the biomechanics of sidestep cutting. Medicine and Science in Sports and Exercise 36:1008–1016

Maehlum S, Daljord O A 1984 Acute sports injuries in Oslo: a one-year study. British Journal of Sports Medicine 18:181–185

Malone T R, Hardaker W T, Garrett W E et al 1993 Relationship of gender to anterior cruciate ligament injuries in intercollegiate basketball players. Journal of the Southern Orthopaedic Association 2:36–39

Mandelbaum B R, Silvers H J, Watanabe D et al 2005 Effectiveness of a neuromuscular and proprioceptive training program in preventing the incidence of ACL injuries in female athletes: two-year follow up. American Journal of Sports Medicine 33:1003–1010

Markolf K L, Graff-Redford A, Amstutz H C 1978 In vivo knee stability: a quantitative assessment using an instrumented clinical testing apparatus. Journal of Bone and Joint Surgery (Am) 60A:664–674

Meeuwisse W H 1991 Predictability of sports injuries. What is the epidemiological evidence? Sports Medicine 12:8–15

Meeuwisse W 1994 Assessing causation in sport injury: a multifactorial model. Clinical Journal of Sport Medicine 4:166–170

Meeuwisse W H, Love E J 1997 Athletic injury reporting. Development of universal systems. Sports Medicine 24:184–204

Molsa J, Airaksinen O, Nasman O et al 1997 Ice hockey injuries in Finland. A prospective epidemiologic study. American Journal of Sports Medicine 25:495–499

Molsa J J, Tegner Y, Alaranta H et al 1999 Spinal cord injuries in ice hockey in Finland and Sweden from 1980 to 1996. International Journal of Sports Medicine 20:64–67

Molsa J, Kujala U, Nasman O et al 2000 Injury profile in ice hockey from the 1970s through the 1990s in Finland. American Journal of Sports Medicine 28:322–327

Morgan B E, Oberlander M A 2001 An examination of injuries in major league soccer: the inaugural season. American Journal of Sports Medicine 29:426–430

Myer G D, Ford K R, Hewett T E 2005a The effects of gender on quadriceps muscle activation strategies during a maneuver that mimics a high ACL injury risk position. Journal of Electromyography and Kinesiology 15:181–189

Myer G D, Ford K R, Palumbo J P et al 2005b Neuromuscular training improves performance and lower-extremity biomechanics in female athletes. Journal of Strength and Conditioning Research 19:51–60

Myklebust G, Bahr R 2005 Return to play guidelines after anterior cruciate ligament surgery. British Journal of Sports Medicine 39:127–131

Myklebust G, Maehlum S, Holm I et al 1998 A prospective cohort study of anterior cruciate ligament injuries in elite Norwegian team handball. Scandinavian Journal of Medicine and Science in Sports 8:149–153

Myklebust G, Engebretsen L, Braekken I H et al 2003 Prevention of anterior cruciate ligament injuries in female team handball players: a prospective intervention study over three seasons. Clinical Journal of Sport Medicine 13:71–78

National Collegiate Athletic Association 2002 NCAA injury surveillance system summary. National Collegiate Athletic Association, Indianapolis, IN

National Federation of State High School Associations 2002 High School Participation Survey. National Federation of State High School Associations, Indianapolis, IN

Nielsen A B, Yde J 1988 An epidemiologic and traumatologic study of injuries in handball. International Journal of Sports Medicine 9:341–344

Nielsen A B, Yde J 1989 Epidemiology and traumatology of injuries in soccer. American Journal of Sports Medicine 17:803–807

Olsen O E, Myklebust G, Engebretsen L et al 2003 Relationship between floor type and risk of ACL injury in team handball. Scandinavian Journal of Medicine and Science in Sports 13:299–304

Olsen O E, Myklebust G, Engebretsen L et al 2004 Injury mechanisms for anterior cruciate ligament injuries in team handball: a systematic video analysis. American Journal of Sports Medicine 32:1002–1012

Petersen W, Braun C, Bock W et al 2005 A controlled prospective case control study of a prevention training program in female team handball players: the German experience. Archives of Orthopaedic and Trauma Surgery 125:614–621

Pettersson M, Lorentzon R 1993 Ice hockey injuries: a 4-year prospective study of a Swedish elite ice hockey team. British Journal of Sports Medicine 27:251–254

Pope R P, Herbert R D, Kirwan J D et al 2000 A randomized trial of preexercise stretching for prevention of lower-limb injury. Medicine and Science in Sports and Exercise 32:271–277

Poulsen T D, Freund K G, Madsen F et al 1991 Injuries in high-skilled and low-skilled soccer: a prospective study. British Journal of Sports Medicine 25:151–153

Powell J W, Barber-Foss K D 2000 Sex-related injury patterns among selected high school sports. American Journal of Sports Medicine 28:385–391

Ronning R, Gerner T, Engebretsen L 2000 Risk of injury during alpine and telemark skiing and snowboarding. The equipment-specific distance-correlated injury index. American Journal of Sports Medicine 28:506–508

Rozzi S L, Lephart S M, Gear W S et al 1999 Knee joint laxity and neuromuscular characteristics of male and female soccer and basketball players. American Journal of Sports Medicine 27:312–319

Ruiz A L, Kelly M, Nutton R W 2002 Arthroscopic ACL reconstruction: a 5–9 year follow-up. Knee 9:197–200

Sandelin J, Kiviluoto O, Santavirta S et al 1985 Outcome of sports injuries treated in a casualty department. British Journal of Sports Medicine 19:103–106

Sarna S, Sahi T, Koskenvuo M et al 1993 Increased life expectancy of world class male athletes. Medicine and Science in Sports and Exercise 25:237–244

Scoville C R, Williams G N, Uhorchak J M et al 2001 Risk factors associated with anterior cruciate ligament injury. Proceedings of the 68th Annual Meeting of the American Academy of Orthopaedic Surgeons. American Academy of Orthopaedic Surgeons, Rosemont, IL, p 564

Sell T, Ferris C M, Abt J P et al 2004 Predictors of anterior tibia shear force during a vertical stop-jump. Journal of Orthopaedic and Sports Physical Therapy 34:A56

Sitler M, Ryan J, Hopkinson W et al 1990 The efficacy of a prophylactic knee brace to reduce knee injuries in football. A prospective, randomized study at West Point. American Journal of Sports Medicine 18:310–315

Sitler M, Ryan J, Wheeler B et al 1994 The efficacy of a semirigid ankle stabilizer to reduce acute ankle injuries in basketball. A randomized clinical study at West Point. American Journal of Sports Medicine 22:454–461

Slauterbeck J R, Hardy D M 2001 Sex hormones and knee ligament injuries in female athletes. American Journal of the Medical Sciences 322:196–199

Strand T, Tvedte R, Engebretsen L et al 1990 [Anterior cruciate ligament injuries in handball playing. Mechanisms and incidence of injuries]. Tidsskrift for den Norske Laegeforening 110:2222–2225

Surve I, Schwellnus M P, Noakes T et al 1994 A fivefold reduction in the incidence of recurrent ankle sprains in soccer players using the Sport-Stirrup orthosis. American Journal of Sports Medicine 22:601–606

Tegner Y, Lorentzon R 1991 Ice hockey injuries: incidence, nature and causes. British Journal of Sports Medicine 25:87–89

Tegner Y, Lorentzon R 1996 Concussion among Swedish elite ice hockey players. British Journal of Sports Medicine 30:251–255

Teitz C C 2001 Video analysis of ACL injuries. In: Griffin L Y(ed) Prevention of noncontact ACL injuries. American Academy of Orthopaedic Surgeons, Rosemont, IL, p 93–96

Tropp H, Askling C, Gillquist J 1985 Prevention of ankle sprains. American Journal of Sports Medicine 13:259–262

van Mechelen W 1997 The severity of sports injuries. Sports Medicine 24:176–180

van Mechelen W, Hlobil H, Kemper H C 1992 Incidence, severity, aetiology and prevention of sports injuries. A review of concepts. Sports Medicine 14:82–99

van Mechelen W, Hlobil H, Kemper H C et al 1993 Prevention of running injuries by warm-up, cool-down, and stretching exercises. American Journal of Sports Medicine 21:711–719

Walden M, Hagglund M, Ekstrand J 2005 UEFA Champions League study: a prospective study of injuries in professional football during the 2001–2002 season. British Journal of Sports Medicine 39:542–546

Walter S D, Sutton J R, McIntosh J M et al 1985 The aetiology of sport injuries. A review of methodologies. Sports Medicine 2:47–58

Wedderkopp N, Kaltoft M, Lundgaard B et al 1999 Prevention of injuries in young female players in European team handball. A prospective intervention study. Scandinavian Journal of Medicine and Science in Sports 9:41–47

Wojtys E M, Huston L J, Lindenfeld T N et al 1998 Association between the menstrual cycle and anterior cruciate ligament injuries in female athletes. American Journal of Sports Medicine 26:614–619

Wojtys E M, Ashton-Miller J A, Huston L J 2002 A gender-related difference in the contribution of the knee musculature to sagittal-plane shear stiffness in subjects with similar knee laxity. Journal of Bone and Joint Surgery (Am) 84A:10–16

Yde J, Nielsen A B 1988 [Epidemiological and traumatological analysis of injuries in a Danish volleyball club]. Ugeskrift for Laeger 150:1022–1023

Yde J, Nielsen A B 1990 Sports injuries in adolescents' ball games: soccer, handball and basketball. British Journal of Sports Medicine 24:51–54

Ytterstad B 1996 The Harstad injury prevention study: the epidemiology of sports injuries. An 8 year study. British Journal of Sports Medicine 30:64–68

Zelisko J A, Noble H B, Porter M 1982 A comparison of men's and women's professional basketball injuries. American Journal of Sports Medicine 10:297–299

Section Three

Regional sport and exercise injury management

16 Spine 255
17 Shoulder 283
18 Elbow 308
19 Wrist and hand 338
20 Pelvis, hip and groin 365
21 Knee 382
22 Patellofemoral joint 402
23 Foot, ankle and lower leg 420
24 Rehabilitation of lower limb muscle and tendon injuries 440

Spine

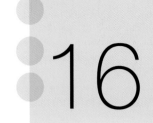

Tara Jo Manal and Anthony Delitto

CHAPTER CONTENTS

Introduction 255

Spinal anatomy and biomechanics 255

Emergency care of spinal injury 256

Examination of the patient. 258

Special cervical spine topics. 271

Special thoracic topics 272

Special lumbar topics 273

Spinal treatments 274

Return to play 277

Summary 278

Introduction

Management of spine injury in an athlete reflects a continuum of care. Some injuries can be severe and require immediate on-field immobilization and transport while others are only symptomatic in situations requiring extreme positions and activity. In order to be effective, sports medicine practitioners are involved in screening, primary rehabilitation and activities that lead up to return to play. The therapist must work effectively with the coach, trainer, physician, athlete and other interested parties (parents, agents, choreographers, technique instructors, etc.) in order to collectively develop and implement a comprehensive rehabilitation program that leads to return to play in a safe and efficient manner.

Spinal anatomy and biomechanics

Anatomical structures of the spine can be a source of concern in the injured athlete. An understanding of the anatomy and function of the spine can assist a therapist in ruling in or out specific structures in spinal dysfunction. The disconnect between patient presentation and pathology in spinal evaluation and treatment challenges the treating therapist to combine tests and measures of movement combined with provocation and easing of symptoms to best direct subsequent physical therapy interventions. The patterns of movement that exist in spinal function can help identify areas that require treatment.

Bony anatomy

The typical vertebra is comprised of an anterior body and a posterior vertebral or neural arch. The body is load bearing with a cortical shell. Injury to the body should be suspected in high-energy axial loading (e.g. falls from height) (White & Panjabi 1990). The strength of the body is related to its size and diminishes with age. The pedicle is the component of the vertebral arch that connects the arch to the vertebral body. The laminae of the neural arch attach the spinous process to the pedicle. The pars interarticularis is located between the superior and inferior articular process (facet contributions). Fracture here can occur in athletes due to repetitive strain or acute injury. This 'isthmic spondylolyis' or spinal stress fracture can be present in 47% of adolescents with low back pain (Micheli & Wood 1995).

The superior and inferior articular processes, when connected to the vertebrae above and below, create the spinal facet (zygapophyseal) joint. The orientation of synovial facet joints dictates movement in the spinal region. In the cervical region, the motion of the facet is upward, opening or distraction with cervical flexion. Due to the anatomy of the cervical spine facets, lateral flexion (sidebending) of the neck occurs in conjunction with rotation to the same side. Extension (closing, compression) of the cervical facet is a combination of posterior gliding and tilting of the spinal segment. Maximal opening of the cervical facet would include the combination of flexion and contralateral rotation while maximal closing includes extension and ipsilateral rotation (Bogduk & Mercer 2000, Panjabi et al 2001). The thoracic spine behaves as a transition region with the upper thoracic spine following motion descriptions similar to the cervical spine and the lower thoracic functions more in-line with the lumbar spine. In the lumbar spine, flexion and extension creates motion very similar to that of the cervical region except that the motion of lateral flexion and rotation are in the opposite direction. Since the superior contribution of the facet joint in the lumbar spine is medial to the inferior contribution, rotation of the spine creates ipsilateral opening of the facet as does contralateral lateral flexion or sidebending. A summary of the mechanics of specific spinal movement is described in Table 16.1.

Disc mechanics

A region of cartilage, the endplate, covers the superior and inferior surface of the vertebral body. This endplate articulates with the intervertebral disc and is attached to the disc and the body. Diffusion through the endplate provides nutrients to the disc and disruption of this plate can allow disc material to invaginate the cancellous cavity of the vertebral body. This protrusion is called a Schmrol's node (Bogduk & Mercer 2000) and can be related to juvenile kyphosis or degenerative disc disease, however, is generally not a source of pain or dysfunction in athletes.

The disc is interposed between two spinal segments and provides support and height to the motion segment (two adjacent vertebrae, disc and soft tissue interposed). The nucleus of the disc has high water content and resists compressive loads (Lundon & Bolton 2001). The annulus of the disc comprises supportive concentric rings of primarily type I collagen to handle tensile forces (Lundon & Bolton 2001). Herniation of a disc is not directly correlated with pain and dysfunction in athletes. Thirty percent of the population has MRI findings of lumbar disc herniation and 10% with cervical herniation, with no discernible signs or symptoms (Boden et al 1990). Therapist must be very careful to use thorough evaluation techniques to determine an effective patient treatment plan rather than relying solely on imaging studies for diagnosis. Corroboration between imaging and signs and symptoms is an essential component to the value of imaging in the diagnostic process (see Chapter 30). In a treatment based classification system, in which evaluation findings and response to evaluation techniques guide the intervention, imaging is used to add insight into 'why' the patient

may be responding to a specific treatment plan rather than guiding the therapist's decision making on 'which' treatment approach should be utilized.

Ligaments of the spine

The ligamentous system of the spine is extensive and contributes to stability of the spine. The anterior longitudinal ligament is stretched with spinal extension and slackened with spinal flexion while the posterior longitudinal, interspinous and supraspinous ligaments are slackened with extension and stretched with flexion. The ligamentum flavum is also stretched with flexion, and hypertrophy of this ligament can encroach on nerve space and in some cases can contribute to nerve impingement. Such encroachment may be a contributing factor to radiculopathy (Kim et al 2004).

Trunk muscles

The muscular anatomy of the trunk becomes of primary importance when dealing with suspected lumbar instability. A thorough review of the trunk muscles is beyond the scope of this chapter; however, in dealing with suspected lumbar instability, therapists should have an accurate knowledge of the key muscles, as these muscles become the targets of exercise interventions whose goal is to improve the lumbar spine's neuromuscular (or 'dynamic') stability. These muscles include: (1) the internal, external oblique and transversus abdominus muscles; (2) the quadratus lumborum; and (3) the erector spinae muscles (e.g. multifidus). Studies have shown that exercises designed to activate and progressively challenge these muscles result in long-term improvement in people with suspected lumbar instability. It is believed that the improvement is a result of greater neuromuscular control of the trunk (Fritz et al 2000, Hayden et al 2005a, 2005b, Hides et al 1996, Koumantakis et al 2005, McGill 1998, 2001, Richardson & Jull 1995, Richardson et al 2002).

Emergency care of spinal injury

Injuries of the head, neck and spine can occur during athletic participation. It is the responsibility of the covering therapist to determine the severity of the injury and make transport or return to play decisions. A three-year study of injuries in 10 popular American high school sports revealed an 11% injury rate in the head, neck and spine regions (Powell & Barber-Foss 1999). Of the sports studied, basketball, American football, and wrestling generated the greatest spinal injuries including neurological compromise from head injury or spinal nerve injury. Using the head as a weapon in some sports can lead to catastrophe. In American football, 'spearing' is a term to describe the use of the top of the head to impact another player and the energy created can result in lower cervical fracture dislocation, paralysis and death (Torg 1990). The sports physical therapist is responsible for proficient on-field examination for spinal injury.

Table 16.1 Specific patterns of motion of the spine

Joint	Flexion	Extension	Lateral flexion (sidebending)	Rotation	Maximal opening (facet distraction)	Maximal closing (facet compression)
Cervical C2–C7	Facet glides upward and open	Facet glides downward and closed	Upward motion and opening on contralateral side	Upward motion and opening on contralateral side	Flexion with contralateral lateral flexion and rotation	Extension with ipsilateral lateral flexion and rotation
Clinical comments	During flexion as unilateral opening is restricted, may see deviation of the trunk to that side as the contralateral side continues its opening activity	During extension if one side is limited in closing, see deviation to the opposite side as the joint continues to close on the uninvolved side	If right lateral flexion is limited, it can be a result of right closing restriction or left opening restriction. Restrictions in flexion or extension or deviations with these movements can assist in the determination. Max. closing or opening can confirm	If right rotation is limited it can be a result of right closing restriction or left opening restriction. Restrictions in flexion or extension or deviations with these movements can assist in the determination. Max. closing or opening can confirm	Maximal testing can confirm suspected limitation in facet opening	Maximal testing can confirm suspected limitation in facet closing
Thoracic			Upper thoracic behave like cervical, lower thoracic behave more like lumbar	Upper thoracic behave like cervical, lower thoracic behave more like lumbar		
Lumbar	Facet glides upward and open	Facet glides downward and closed	Open contralateral and close ipsilateral	Open ipsilateral and close contralateral	Flexion with contralateral sidebending	Extension with ipsilateral sidebending
Clinical comments	Same as cervical above	Same as cervical above	Same as cervical above	If right rotation is limited, it may be the result of right opening or left closing. Restrictions in flexion or extension or deviations with these movements can assist in the determination. Max. closing or opening can confirm	Maximal testing can confirm suspected limitation in facet opening	Maximal testing can confirm suspected limitation in facet closing

Observation of the injury mechanism can provide some insight into possible injured structures. Peripheral nerve traction can occur from stretching of the head and shoulder region, fracture suspicion results from a direct blow by an object or opponent and the most serious events are suspected from significant axial loading or extreme postures.

In order to protect the athlete, those with suspected spinal injuries are immobilized prior to evaluation. As many as 50% of neurological injuries that occur are not created by the initial trauma, but by subsequent movement or activity (Wiesenfarth & Briner 1996). An unconscious athlete is a sign of serious injury and head and spinal injuries should be suspected. The removal of sporting equipment (e.g. helmets, pads) can be sport-specific depending on the impact the removal will have on head and neck positions; however, any component of the equipment blocking access to the airway is removed immediately (Waninger 1998). If airway and breathing are impaired, an airway is established using a chin lift maneuver in which the angle of the mandible is thrust forward to open the airway without hyperextending the cervical spine (American National Red Cross 2001). Such athletes require assessment for bleeding and emergency transport and care.

Conscious athletes with suspected spine injuries may be able to assist in their own assessment. Severe pain with movement, weakness, numbness or paresthesia in the arms or legs are all symptoms of serious spinal injury. Palpable deformity of the spine, abnormal posturing or firm bony end feels with diminished range of motion are signs that require immobilization and further evaluation (Haight & Shiple 2001). Screenings of motor and sensory distributions may also provide greater insight into the areas of spinal injury; however, the absence of positive signs should not be considered indicative of the absence of severe pathology. Patients with cervical fractures may have no neurological signs or symptoms (Davis et al 1993, Gerrelts et al 1991, Kreipke et al 1989, McKee et al 1990). After trauma, adequate cervical X-rays including a lateral view (including the C7–T1 junction), an anteroposterior view and an open-mouth odontoid view are indicated. If all on-field screening examinations are negative, an athlete can be moved to the sidelines and examined further. It is common to delay a second evaluation for a period of time, to allow for the continued development of symptoms. If any worsening of symptoms occurs, or any of the signs and symptoms noted develop, the athlete should be stabilized and transported for further evaluation. In order to successfully manage spinal injuries in athletes a comprehensive emergency plan should be developed, rehearsed and followed by the medical team onsite.

Questionnaires to assist assessment

Region-specific questionnaires can be used to classify the severity of a spinal complaint, clarify the impact of the problem on the athlete's functional level and, with subsequent administration, document progress. The Neck Disability Index (Fig. 16.1) is a questionnaire that describes the impact of the athlete's neck pain on activities of daily living in 10 domains: pain intensity, personal care, lifting, reading, headache, concentration, work, driving, sleeping and recreation (Vernon & Mior 1991). A grading scale of 0–5 is used where 0 indicates no impact on the specific activity and higher numbers indicate greater disability, and an overall disability rating is generated from summing the scores on the 10 domains and multiplying by two. The score on this questionnaire reflects varying degrees of impaired function and results can be grouped into mild, moderate and severe disability categories (Hains et al 1998). The Oswestry Low Back Pain Disability Questionnaire (Fairbank et al 1980), or its modified version (Fritz & Irrgang 2001) utilize the same grading and scoring techniques to describe the intensity of the low back pain and the impact on functional activities including personal care, lifting, walking, sitting, standing, sleeping, social life, traveling and sex life (Fig. 16.2). Disability questionnaires can be helpful in determining the severity of the athlete's pain at initial evaluation and can also be used repeatedly to monitor change resulting from treatment intervention (Fritz & George 2002). This information can be invaluable to a therapist in making decisions regarding treatment progression and overall intervention success. Readers are encouraged to source these questionnaires for use in clinical practice.

Examination of the patient

The examination of the patient begins with history and proceeds to the physical examination. The purpose of the history is threefold: (1) to complete the screening process that will lead to a decision for the patient to be referred for further workup for suspected serious injury or disease; (2) to assess the presence of conditions that may cause the clinician to seek consultation with another health professional to co-manage the case with the rehabilitation professional; and (3) to begin collecting information that will guide the specific treatment intervention.

Treatment-based classification schemes

Classification schemes can be useful in determining how to interpret the information collected throughout the evaluation process. Although many classification systems exist, using one that is based on the success of direct treatment interventions can assist a sports therapist in management of acute low back pain. The Delitto classification scheme has been developed and validated as a classification for the management of patients with acute low back pain (Childs et al 2004, Delitto et al 1995, Fritz 1998, Fritz et al 2000, George & Delitto 2005, Hicks et al 2005). The classification, many aspects of which are described below, uses the athlete's signs and symptoms gathered during motion testing to determine a treatment approach.

Initial screening

Prior to treatment, a sports therapist must decide if an athlete can be managed independently or must be referred for

This questionnaire has been designed to give your therapist information as to how your neck pain has affected your ability to manage in everyday life. Please answer every section by checking the **one choice** that best describes your condition **today**. We realize you may feel that 2 of the statements may describe your condition, but **please mark only the box that most closely describes your current condition.**

Pain Intensity
- I have no pain at the moment.
- The pain is very mild at the moment.
- The pain is moderate at the moment.
- The pain is fairly severe at the moment.
- The pain is very severe at the moment.
- The pain is the worst imaginable at the moment.

Personal Care (washing, dressing, etc.)
- I can look after myself normally without causing extra pain.
- I can look after myself normally but it causes me extra pain.
- It is painful to look after myself and I am slow and careful.
- I need some help but manage most of my personal care.
- I need help everyday in most aspects of self-care.
- I do not get dressed, wash with difficulty and stay in bed.

Lifting
- I can lift heavy weights without extra pain.
- I can lift heavy weights but it causes extra pain.
- Pain prevents me from lifting heavy objects off the floor, but I can manage if they are conveniently position, e.g. on a table.
- Pain prevents me from lifting heavy weights but I can manage light to medium weights if they are conveniently placed.
- I can only lift very light weights.
- I cannot lift or carry anything at all.

Reading
- I can read as much as I want with no pain in my neck.
- I can read as much as I want with slight pain in my neck.
- I can read as much as I want with moderate pain in my neck.
- I can't read as much as I want because of moderate pain in my neck.
- I can hardly read at all because of severe pain in my neck.
- I cannot read at all.

Headache
- I have no headache at all.
- I have slight headaches that come infrequently.
- I have moderate headaches that come infrequently.
- I have moderate headaches that come frequently.
- I have severe headaches that come frequently.
- I have headaches almost all the time.

Concentration
- I can concentrate fully when I want to with no difficulty.
- I can concentrate fully when I want to with slight difficulty.
- I have a fair degree of difficulty in concentrating when I want to.
- I have a lot of difficulty in concentrating when I want to.
- I have a great deal of difficulty in concentrating when I want to.
- I cannot concentrate at all.

Work
- I can do as much as I want to.
- I can only do my usual work, but no more.
- I can do most of my usual work, but no more.
- I cannot do my usual work.
- I can hardly do any work at all.
- I can't do any work at all.

Driving
- I can drive my car without any neck pain.
- I can drive my car as long as I want with slight pain in my neck.
- I can drive my car as long as I want with moderate pain in my neck.
- I can't drive my car as long as I want because of moderate pain in my neck.
- I can hardly drive at all because of severe pain in my neck.
- I can't drive at all.

Sleeping
- I have no trouble sleeping.
- My sleep is slightly disturbed (less than 1 hour sleep loss).
- My sleep is mildly disturbed (1–2 hours sleep loss).
- My sleep is moderately disturbed (2–3 hours sleep loss).
- My sleep is greatly disturbed (3–5 hours sleep loss).
- My sleep is completely disturbed (5–7 hours sleep loss).

Recreation
- I am able to engage in all my recreational activities with no neck pain at all.
- I am able to engage in all my recreational activities with some pain in my neck.
- I am able to engage in most but not all of my usual recreational activities because of pain in my neck.
- I am able to engage in a few of my usual activities because of pain in my neck.
- I can hardly do any recreational activities because of pain in my neck.
- I can't do any recreational activities at all.

Disability Score (x2): _____ %

Figure 16.1 • The neck disability index. (Reproduced from Vernon & Mior 1991 with permission from Elsevier.)

This questionnaire is designed to give us information as to how your back (or leg) trouble affects your ability of manage in everyday life Please answer every section. Mark one box only in each section that most closely describes you today.

Section 1 – Pain intensity
- I have no pain at the moment.
- The pain is very mild at the moment.
- The pain is moderate at the moment.
- The pain is fairly severe at the moment.
- The pain is very severe at the moment.
- The pain is the worst imaginable at the moment.

Section 2 – Personal care (washing, dressing, etc.)
- I can look after myself normally without causing extra pain.
- I can look after myself normally but it is very painful.
- It is painful to look after myself and I am slow and careful.
- I need some help but manage most of my personal care.
- I need help everyday in most aspects of self care.
- I do not get dressed, wash with difficulty and stay in bed.

Section 3 – Lifting
- I can lift heavy weights without extra pain.
- I can lift heavy weight but it gives extra pain.
- Pain prevents me from lifting heavy weights off the floor but I can manage if they are conveniently positioned, e.g. on a table.
- Pain prevents me from lifting heavy weights but I can manage light to medium weights if they are conveniently positioned.
- I can lift only very light weights.
- I cannot lift or carry anything at all.

Section 4 – Walking
- Pain does not prevent me walking any distance.
- Pain prevents me walking more than one mile.
- Pain prevents me walking more than a quarter of a mile.
- Pain prevents me walking more than 100 yards.
- I can only walk using a stick or crutches.
- I am in bed most of the time and have to crawl to the toilet.

Section 5 – Sitting
- I can sit in any chair as long as I like.
- I can sit in my favourite chair as long as I like.
- Pain prevents me from sitting for more than 1 hour.
- Pain prevents me from sitting for more than half an hour.
- Pain prevents me from sitting for more than 10 minutes.
- Pain prevents me from sitting at all.

Section 6 – Standing
- I can stand as long as I want without extra pain.
- I can stand as long as I want but it gives me extra pain.
- Pain prevents me from standing for more than 1 hour.
- Pain prevents me from standing for more than half an hour.
- Pain prevents me from standing for more than 10 minutes.
- Pain prevents me from standing at all.

Section 7 – Sleeping
- My sleep is never disturbed by pain.
- My sleep is occasionally disturbed by pain.
- Because of pain I have less than 6 hours sleep.
- Because of pain I have less than 4 hours sleep.
- Because of pain I have less than 2 hours sleep.
- Pain prevents me from sleeping at all.

Section 8 – Sex life (if applicable)
- My sex life is normal and causes no extra pain.
- My sex life is normal but causes some extra pain.
- My sex life is nearly normal but is very painful.
- My sex life is severely restricted by pain.
- My sex life is nearly absent because of pain.
- Pain prevents any sex life at all.

Section 9 – Social life
- My social life is normal and causes me no extra pain.
- My social life is normal but increases the degree of pain.
- Pain has no significant effect on my social life apart from limiting my more energetic interests, e.g. sport, etc.
- Pain has restricted my social life and I do not go out as often.
- Pain has restricted social life to my home.
- I have no social life because of pain.

Section 10 – Travelling
- I can travel anywhere without pain.
- I can travel anywhere but it gives extra pain.
- Pain is bad but I manage journeys over two hours.
- Pain restricts me to journeys of less than one hour.
- Pain restricts me to short necessary journeys under 30 minutes.
- Pain restricts me from traveling except to receive treatment.

Result

Your ODI = [ ] %

Figure 16.2 • The Oswestry disability index (Version 2.1a). (Reproduced from www.orthosurg.org.uk/odi with permission from J. C. T. Fairbank, P. B. Pynsent and S. Disney.)

further medical evaluation. Major trauma during an athletic injury is a high suspicion for spinal fracture, head injury or neurological compromise. Medical concerns of fever, chills, unexplained weight loss, recent bacterial infection or intravenous drug use require a more extensive evaluation for infection or illness. Cancer can be suspected if the athlete is over 50 or under 20 years old, has a prior cancer history, has unexplained weight loss, has no improvement in symptoms after one month of treatment, has constant pain that is unaffected by posture, position or bed rest, or complains of pain at night (Deyo & Diehl 1988). In general, any athlete with fever and back pain should be referred for more extensive medical evaluation (Wipf & Deyo 1995). Cauda equina compromise from disc herniation is relatively rare and occurs in less than 1 or 2% of disc protrusions; however, it requires immediate referral to an emergency room (Hackley & Wiesel 1993, Wipf & Deyo 1995). Signs of cauda equina syndrome are bladder or bowel dysfunction, paresthesia of the fourth sacral dermatome (saddle region) and severe or progressive lower extremity weakness or clumsiness (Hackley & Wiesal 1993, Wipf & Deyo 1995). Even when combined, the risk factors for cancer, infection and cauda equina syndrome are less than 3.5% of patients with low back pain; however, screening athletes with these questions can identify cases in need of referral for necessary medical care.

Referral for a psychological consultation may also be necessary in the management of spinal dysfunction. In most cases, athletes are very motivated to recover from spinal injury and return to previous levels of activities. However, this is not universal. There are athletes who are fearful of returning to a sport that resulted in an injury and still others who remain concerned that continued athletic participation may compromise future health. Evidence suggests that people with spinal injury, specifically low back injury, demonstrating a high level of fear of activity are less likely to return to the preinjury activity level (Fritz & George 2002, Fritz et al 2004, George et al 2001). The Fear Avoidance Beliefs Questionnaire (Waddell et al 1993) is one way of measuring the impact of fear on the athlete's perception of returning to 'work activity', which in this case represents their sport (Fig. 16.3). Although this has not been studied in the athletic population specifically, an emphasis on reducing fear and encouraging return to activities is a strategy regularly utilized in this population instinctively by the medical staff. It is important to follow basic principles that educate the athlete to focus on success and not concerns with injury and failure. The Back Book is an example of a resource designed to educate the injured person that the spine is strong and recovers, that imaging findings are common even in people with no pain so pain does not mean your back has serious damage, that

Here are some of the things which *other* patients have told us about their pain. For each statement please circle any number from 0 to 6 to say how much physical activities such as bending, lifting, walking or driving affect or would affect *your* back pain.

	COMPLETELY DISAGREE			UNSURE		COMPLETELY AGREE	
1. My pain was caused by physical activity	0	1	2	3	4	5	6
2. Physical activity makes my pain worse	0	1	2	3	4	5	6
3. Physical activity might harm my back	0	1	2	3	4	5	6
4. I should not do physical activities which (might) make my pain worse	0	1	2	3	4	5	6
5. I cannot do physical activities which (might) make my pain worse	0	1	2	3	4	5	6

The following statements are about how your normal work affects or would affect your back pain.

	COMPLETELY DISAGREE			UNSURE		COMPLETELY AGREE	
6. My pain was caused by my work or by an accident at work	0	1	2	3	4	5	6
7. My work aggravated my pain	0	1	2	3	4	5	6
8. I have a claim for compensation for my pain	0	1	2	3	4	5	6
9. My work is too heavy for me	0	1	2	3	4	5	6
10. My work makes or would make my pain worse	0	1	2	3	4	5	6
11. My work might harm my back	0	1	2	3	4	5	6
12. I should not do my normal work with my present pain	0	1	2	3	4	5	6
13. I cannot do my normal work with my present pain	0	1	2	3	4	5	6
14. I cannot do my normal work until my pain is treated	0	1	2	3	4	5	6
15. I do not think that I will be back to my normal work within 3 months	0	1	2	3	4	5	6
16. I do not think that I will ever be able to go back to that work	0	1	2	3	4	5	6

Figure 16.3 • The Fear Avoidance Beliefs Questionnaire. (Reproduced from Waddell et al 1993 with permission from Elsevier.)

there are treatments available to help but participation level is the greatest critical factor and that they will be successful by doing more each day than the day before (Burton et al 1999, Kvist et al 2005). In more severe cases, sport psychologists may be utilized to work with athlete's fears and concerns when they manifest themselves in performance anxiety or an inability to return to sport (Taylor & Taylor 1997, Vlaeyen et al 1995).

There are also athletes who are less motivated for the return to sport than the 'team' around them. Injury can be an opportunity to break from a very hectic schedule of practice and performance. After significant investment in time and money, it is often difficult for athletes who may want a hiatus to express these desires to the support system comprised of those directly involved in the athletic activity (coaches, teammates, parents, etc.) (Mechanic 1980). When the athlete's signs and symptoms do not match expected patterns or behaviors, the therapist may need to consider that the pain is an unconscious strategy to manage emotional conflict and a waning desire for continued sports participation. Referral to a sport psychologist may be required in these situations for resolution of the athlete's physical complaints.

Injury history

History taking in the athlete begins with questions related to the mechanism of injury. An athlete can provide insight into the impact of position or movement on their complaints. If symptoms radiate below the knee, a lower quarter screen, or more inclusive neurological screen, is indicated (Box 16.1). The goal of the screen is to identify patterns of sensory, reflex and muscular changes indicating specific neural involvement. These signs can be monitored to demonstrate treatment success, or in cases of failure to progress, be used to determine appropriate injection strategies (Table 16.2).

Evaluation

The lumbar classification scheme assumes that the pelvic region has been evaluated and cleared as a potential source of dysfunction (see Chapter 20). There are three possible responses to movement testing of acute lumbar pain: the symptoms can worsen, improve or stay status quo. The symptoms are considered to worsen if they move distal from the spine during

---

Box 16.1 Neurological screening for the injured athlete

Level	Reflex	Myotome	Dermatome	Level	Reflex	Myotome	Dermatome
C5	Biceps reflex	Deltoid Biceps	Lateral arm Axillary nerve	L4	Patellar reflex	Knee extension Ankle dorsiflexion	Inner buttock Outer thigh Inside of leg Dorsum of foot
C6	Biceps reflex	Biceps Wrist extension	Lateral forearm Musculocutaneous nerve	L5	None	Extensor hallucis longus Extensor digitorum longus and brevis Tibialis posterior	Buttock Back and side of thigh Lateral aspect of leg Dorsum of foot Inner half of sole First, second and third toes Ankle
C7	Triceps reflex	Triceps Wrist flexors Finger extension Forearm extension at elbow	Middle finger				
C8	Triceps reflex	Finger flexion Hand intrinsics	Medial forearm Medial anterior branch Cutaneous nerve	S1	Achilles reflex	Peroneus longus and brevis Gastrocnemius/ soleus Ankle plantarflexion and knee flexion	Lateral foot and sole Fifth toe Buttock Back of thigh Posterior lower leg
T1	None	Hand intrinsics	Medial forearm Medial anterior branch Cutaneous nerve	S2	Achilles reflex	Ankle plantarflexion and knee flexion	Buttock Back of thigh Lower leg
L1	None	Hip flexion	Back Greater trochanter Groin	S3	None	Intrinsic foot muscles	Groin Inner thigh to knee
L2	Patellar reflex	Hip flexion Hip adductors Quadriceps	Back Front of thigh and knee	S4	None	None	Perineum Genital Lower sacrum
L3	Patellar reflex	Knee extension Hip adductors	Back Upper buttock Front of thigh and knee Medial lower leg				

Table 16.2 Spinal injections

Type	Location	Rationale	Athlete profile	Variation on the procedure	Expected response
Sacroiliac joint blocks	Sacroiliac joint	Diagnosis of sacroiliac joint dysfunction	Athletes with buttock pain below the PSIS, who have been unsuccessful with conservative treatment measures	N/A	If sacroiliac joint is the cause of pain, patient's pain will be reduced and the physician will inject steroids into the region to decrease inflammation, relieving the patient's pain
Epidural block	The epidural area of the spine, outside of the dura of the spinal cord; in the general area of the nerve root level believed to be causing pain	To decrease pain and inflammation causing axial and/or radicular pain	Athletes with moderate to severe back or neck pain with or without arm/leg pain, numbness or tingling; athletes with suspected protruded/herniated discs as the cause of their pain; athletes who have not responded to any other treatment	(1) Caudal block – through sacral gap for lumbosacral nerves (2) Translaminar block – through ligamentum flavum into epidural space (3) Transforaminal block – through neural foramen into epidural space for specific nerve root	Relief of pain if medication reaches source. Generally performed in a series of three every 2–3 weeks, but no consensus has been reached as to the effectiveness of this method
Selective nerve root block	At the specific nerve root believed to be causing pain	To determine whether specific nerve root is generator of pain and decrease pain and inflammation	Athletes with predominantly upper or lower extremity radicular symptoms and a nerve root suspected to be effected by mechanical or chemical irritant	(1) Intercostal (2) Great occipital (3) Lateral femoral cutaneous	Patient's pain is decreased after the injection, confirming that nerve root is pain generator; steroids injected decrease inflammation around the nerve root, decreasing patient's pain
Intra-articular facet joint injection	In general area of facet joint believed to be causing pain	To determine whether a specific facet join is the generator of pain and decrease pain and inflammation	Athletes where facet joint syndrome is suspected	Facet joint injection with local anesthetic to assess response	Patient's pain is decreased after injected confirming that facet joint is pain generator; steroids injected decrease inflammation around the facet joint decreasing patient's pain
Facet joint nerve blocks	At the specific facet joint, the medial branch or nerves that connect with the joint, believed to be causing pain	To confirm that a facet joint(s) is the source of pain and decrease pain and inflammation	Athletes who have failed to see improvement with a directed non-operative treatment program for 4–6 weeks and have a typical pattern of facet involvement: pain with extension, ext and rotation, asymmetrical sidebending	(1) Facet joint nerve ablation – placed parallel to medial branch with radiofrequency to burn area (2) General injection – intra-articular facet joint injection	Decrease in or relief of patient's back or neck pain
Hardware blocks	In area where metal hardware was placed	To determine whether metal hardware used during surgery is contributing to patient discomfort	An athlete having pain post surgery to determine if hardware is causing pain	N/A	If pain is abolished temporarily, hardware implanted is source. If pain remains, hardware is not the source

motion testing (peripheralize). An increase of the athlete's pain level from a 4 on a 10-point pain scale to a 6 on the same scale reflects more pain, that change is defined as 'increased' not 'worsened' in this classification. For 'worsening' to occur, radicular symptoms must exist and they must move in a direction away from the spine.

An alternative symptom response is 'improving' or movement of the symptom from the periphery to the center of the spine (centralization). This symptom response is also called 'directional preference' and reflects a movement of symptoms toward the midline of the body. An athlete's symptoms are considered improved if the symptoms move from the lateral leg and thigh into the buttocks following movement in a specific direction.

Status quo describes the response of increased or decreased pain on a pain scale (e.g. from 3/10 to 5/10 or 8/10 to 2/10) as a result of movement testing; however, with no peripheralization or centralization of symptoms. Most athletes have no associated radiculopathy with their injuries and therefore will end up in this category.

Evaluation of acute lumbar pain

During the evaluation component of the Delitto classification scheme spinal motions are performed to determine if the pain worsens (peripheralizes), improves (centralizes) or remains status quo (increases or decreases in intensity but not direction). Sidebending is assessed to determine if it is symmetrical or asymmetrical. Asymmetrical sidebending will often couple with a specific loss of range of motion or combined motion (Table 16.1) or with centralization or peripheralization with other movements. This information is combined with the rest of the movement responses. Movements assessed are flexion, extension and pelvic translocation. The motions are performed as a single motion, a sustained motion, and then repeated motions with symptom responses being recorded. The examination can be performed in standing in most cases. In more extreme cases, if a patient cannot move through these motions in standing, alternative positions can be adopted. In place of standing flexion, side lying or supine knees to chest can be performed and standing extensions can be replaced with the prone press up position. The therapist can passively move the cervical and lumbar spine to assess for motion in absence of muscular contraction. This information can be helpful in identifying if the activity is limited only by stiffness (cannot be performed actively or passively) or by pain (cannot be performed actively but range is available passively), or a combination of the two. The separation of the passive joint restraint to motion from the active neuromuscular contribution may assist the therapist in determining relevant components of a successful treatment program. The movements are examined for symptom provocation and change, as well as issues of motion quality and quantity.

Testing of the spine motion provides information about the ability and willingness of an athlete to move. Single plane motions are often tested first in order to observe any significant increases or limitation in range. If an athlete's complaint is brought on quickly, with little range or stress, and remains for a protracted period of time, the patient's symptoms are considered irritable. Symptom irritability is often a clustering of the pain severity, ease of onset, intensity and duration. During the history taking, the therapist gathers information about activities that tend to aggravate the athlete's pain. Using information about irritability level and positions of symptom provocation, a therapist can plan an order of data collection that will yield the most clinically useful results, while not aggravating the symptoms. Routinely, if an activity such as sitting is painful, motion testing that reproduces that position (e.g. flexion) would be chosen as the last single plane motion to avoid irritating the athlete's complaint. If the athlete has a high irritability level and performs flexion first in the sequence of range testing, the resulting persistent pain may confound the results of the other planes of motion tested. In the case of an athlete who has pain only after playing for over several hours (i.e. low irritability), the therapist may find symptom reproduction to be challenging. Although range restrictions may still be present, the lack of symptom provocation with moving may make correlation between the sign and symptom difficult. In difficult cases, it may be prudent to perform the evaluation on the athlete after a practice or competition in order to increase the likelihood of successful symptom provocation.

Movement response interpretation

If the patient presents with asymmetry in sidebending and peripheral symptoms, the therapist should assess for a lumbar shift in the coronal plane. In the presence of a lumbar shift, the trunk will be deviated to one side and the space between the arm and the trunk will appear greater on the side to which the trunk is shifted (Fig. 16.4). Active pelvic translocation is performed; the athlete shifts their upper body on a stable pelvis from the right to the left. If the symptoms improve, the patient is treated with pelvic translocation until symptoms resolve or reassessment determines another category of successful treatment intervention. If symptoms peripheralize or worsen, the response to flexion and extension is assessed. Depending on the response to other motions, a category of worsen or improve is ultimately assigned (see below).

Symptoms worsen (peripheralize)

In the athlete's symptoms move distally away from the spine and remain in that location with all movement testing, Delitto et al (1995), Fritz (1998), Fritz et al (2000) and George & Delitto (2005) recommend lumbar traction as the treatment of choice. In this case, no successful motion is identified to help move the symptoms to the center of the spine, so traction is used until a repeat movement assessment yields a new intervention strategy. Other treatment interventions aimed at calming muscle spasm and controlling pain (e.g. transcutaneous electrical nerve stimulation, cryotherapy) may be helpful in conjunction with traction until reassessment identifies a new treatment category.

Symptoms improve (centralize)

If an athlete's symptoms centralize with any single motion in pelvic translocation, flexion or extension, the improving motion

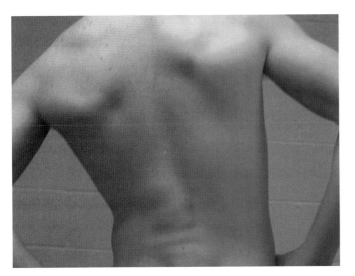

Figure 16.4 • Left lumbar shift. The athlete's spine is shifted to the left as indicated by the direction of the shoulder on the side to which he is shifted. His sidebending would be asymmetrical and his response to movement testing will determine his treatment category.

is repeated to assess the benefit of 8 or 10 repetitions on the symptom centralization. Once an athlete's radiculopathy centralizes, the therapist is directed to do whichever motions created the 'improved' response. Positions that peripheralize the symptoms are avoided and positions that centralize the symptoms are repeated often. In the extension syndrome treatment category, symptoms are centralized with spinal extension; therefore, extension activities are prescribed. These can include walking, prone positioning, prone press-ups, standing lumbar extension, hip extension, skiing machine, etc. Flexion positions would be avoided in this athlete if they contribute to a worsening of these symptoms, including sleeping in a curled position. The opposite would be true for an athlete who improves with flexion and worsens with extension. Athletes in the flexion syndrome category would be encouraged to sit, ride a recumbent bike, perform knee to chest activities, flex in standing and avoid extension postures. Stomach sleepers in the flexion syndrome category should lie over a mound of pillows to avoid irritation while they sleep. In all cases of 'centralization', activities that contribute to centralization of the radicular complaints should be repeated multiple times each day. Athlete's can change categories as a result of treatment and require constant re-evaluation of the motion testing (e.g. flexion and extension) to determine if their response has changed and a new category is indicated.

In the management of spinal radiculopathy, the behavior of pain can clearly provide insight into activities that are likely to irritate the condition and those that may be beneficial in treatment. The patient can usually list things that increase their local spinal pain or cause the pain to travel into the extremities (peripheralize). In the case of a flexion problem, athletes will relate that repetitive or sustained postures in forward bending aggravates their back pain, but symptoms are absent with standing, walking or running. This scenario suggests encouraging extension type postures while avoiding flexion postures until the condition has improved. Motion testing findings should correlate with those activities noted by the athlete in the injury history. The principles learned here can be applied to developing aerobic and lifting guidelines so the athlete can maintain their fitness level while the underlying spinal disability is treated.

Status quo (no radiculopathy – symptoms may increase or decrease)

Most athletes have no radiculopathy and therefore have no ability for their symptoms to worsen or improve. These athletes fall automatically into the status quo category. Their pain complaints may increase or decrease in intensity in response to movement testing. Single plane motion in sidebending or lateral flexion can provide insight into the presence or absence of unilateral dysfunction. When sidebending is equal and undisturbed and the limitation is in the sagittal plane, a cyriax capsular pattern of the motion segment (vertebrae above, intervertebral disc, vertebrae below) is present (Magee 1997). When sidebending is equal, the interpretation is that the restriction is related to a motion segment (e.g. L3/L4). The capsular pattern indicates a limitation of a more general area that would benefit from general mobilizations and stretching depending on the greatest direction of limitation, flexion or extension. Motion testing in flexion and extension can reveal limitation is only one direction or both. The classification is 'general mobilization' indicating that more general mobilization techniques to increase range in one or both directions are indicated. The classification scheme does not dictate which mobilizations should be performed, only that in the status quo category when hypomobility is noted, that some form of general mobilizations are included in the treatment plan.

If sidebending is asymmetrical (i.e. limited more to one side than another), the pattern is considered non-capsular. The involvement may extend to areas beyond the central motion segment, such as to a facet. When sidebending is asymmetrical, motion testing is expected to reveal a pattern that can be used for determination of the best treatment. A description of the coupled motions is included in Table 16.1. Treatment interventions for joint restrictions demonstrating a pattern (e.g. right opening restriction or right closing restriction) should include specific mobilizations aimed at resolving the deficit. There are a myriad of mobilizations purported to resolve specific motion restriction that can be employed. Joint manipulation may be indicated in this general and specific mobilization category as well.

In the described classification scheme, the results of the motion testing can identify specific areas of hypermobility, stiffness or pain. When stiffness is present, mobilization and stretching can be considered, and when hypermobility is present, stabilization may be the treatment of choice (Childs et al 2004, Fritz 1998, Fritz et al 2000, George & Delitto 2005, Hicks et al 2005, Manal & Claytor 2005).

Instability

Evaluation of range can identify excessive range of motion (hypermobility), which is often necessary for specific athletic activities (e.g. gymnastics, figure skating, diving). In these cases, although joint stiffness is unlikely present, the athlete's range may be limited by pain. Identifying instability in an athlete with excessive range can be a clinical challenge. There is much debate about the techniques used to diagnose lumbar instability. The presence of excessive motion may be a requirement for successful sport participation and therefore in no way inherently dysfunctional. As has been demonstrated in the ACL deficient athlete, clinical diagnosis of instability must combine inherent laxity with a corresponding decrease in function (Rudolph et al 2001). The 'non-coper' is an athlete with excessive range and corresponding painful sport participation. Signs of clinical instability often manifest themselves when the patient is required to control laxity with motion testing. Hicks et al (2005) demonstrated that the

presence of aberrant motion during testing of lumbar spine range (e.g. an instability catch, a painful arc of motion, 'thigh climbing' or Gower's sign, or a reversal of lumbopelvic motion) may be a predictor of those who benefited from a stabilization training program. Using the absence or presence of a sign of aberrant movement rather than focusing on the interpretation of a single test, improves the reliability of classification (Hicks et al 2003). In addition, Hicks et al (2005) have published a phase I clinical prediction rule for predicting success after an eight-week lumbar stabilization exercise program. These predictors include at least 3 of the following 4 variables: (1) age <40 years; (2) aberrant movements during active lumbar motion; (3) average straight leg raise of greater than 91°; and (4) a positive prone instability test (Fig. 16.5). Aberrant movements were defined as follows: while

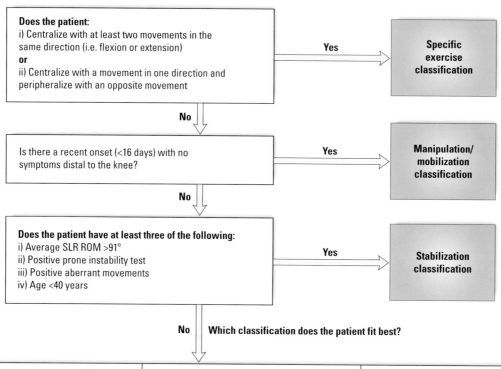

Figure 16.5 • Phase I clinical prediction rule for predicting success after an eight-week lumbar stabilization exercise program. (Reproduced from Hicks et al 2005 with permission of Elsevier.)

standing, the subject flexes the trunk forward as far as possible while the examiner attempts to identify any of the following abnormalities: (1) painful arc in flexion or on return from flexion; (2) Gower's sign; (3) instability catch; (4) reversal of lumbopelvic rhythm. Patients who had at least three of the four variables present during the initial evaluation were four times more likely to be a positive responder (have at least a 50% decrease in their Oswestry score) after an eight-week lumbar stabilization exercise program. The details of the exercise program and the criteria for progression are included in Box 16.2.

The Delitto classification scheme has been developed, refined and tested on patients with low back pain; however, the principle of allowing evaluation findings to inform treatment planning is a universal theme that can apply to all spinal care (Childs et al 2004, Delitto et al 1995, Fritz 1998, Fritz et al 2000, George & Delitto 2005, Hicks et al 2005). The classification scheme provides a framework under which the summary information in the chapter can be understood.

Problem complaint

Screening for dermatomal, myotomal and reflex changes can assist in identifying the likely source of the problem (Box 16.1). Provocative tests can also assist in recreating radicular complaints relating to the lumbar spine (Table 16.3) and cervical spine (Table 16.4). Pain level can also be useful to provide information to the therapist of pain severity and response of the pain to stresses placed on the system during the evaluation and treatment procedures. There is strong evidence for the validity of various measures of pain intensity (Banos et al 1989). The Visual Analog Scale (VAS) is a 10 cm line labeled from 0 (no pain) to 10 (worst possible pain) and the athlete marks a position reflecting their pain level which is converted to a measurement. The verbal and numerical rating scales describe pain with descriptors or numbers from 0 (no pain) to 10 (worst possible pain). Evidence suggests that all of these pain scales are responsive and are helpful clinical methods for recording pain (Banos et al 1989). See Chapter 9 for further details on the assessment of pain.

Symptom behavior

One focus of the physical therapist during an initial evaluation is to identify the offending motion causing the athlete to seek treatment. If the pain cannot be replicated during the examination, it is unlikely that a successful treatment plan will be established. The therapist will ask 'Is this recreating your symptoms?' repeatedly during the evaluation process. Once the therapist can reliably reproduce the complaint, this 'comparable sign' can be re-tested to assess the effectiveness of the intervention and assure the therapist of treatment effectiveness.

The comparable sign can be re-tested after individual interventions to indicate success. For example, if an athlete has complaints of left sided cervical pain with right rotation, the therapist will evaluate the range of motion to observe if a pattern of restriction is present. If the athlete indicates pain and is limited with end-range cervical flexion, right lateral flexion and right rotation, the therapist may suspect an opening restriction of the left side. If the combined motion of maximal opening of the left side confirms the hypotheses, the therapist has many treatment options. The therapist may provide joint mobilizations, a cervical manipulation or independent stretching to gain range. The therapist can use one of the provoking motions (cervical flexion, right sidebending or rotation) to reassess the benefit of each of these interventions on the range restriction and pain levels. This provides immediate and reliable data on the success of each intervention and the benefits of the intervention strategy as a whole.

Box 16.2 Stabilization exercises with criteria for progression of each exercise

Primary Muscle Group*	Exercises	Criteria for Progression
Transversus abdominus	Abdominal bracing	30 repetitions with 8-s hold
	Bracing with heel slides	20 repetitions per leg with 4-s hold
	Bracing with leg lifts	20 repetitions per leg with 4-s hold
	Bracing with bridging	30 repetitions with 8-s hold, then progress to 1 leg
	Bracing in standing	30 repetitions with 8-s hold
	Bracing with standing row exercise	20 repetitions per side with 6-s hold
	Bracing with walking	
Erector spinae/multifidus	Quadruped arm lifts with bracing	30 repetitions with 8-s hold on each side
	Quadruped leg lifts with bracing	30 repetitions with 8-s hold on each side
	Quadruped alternate arm and leg lifts with bracing	30 repetitions with 8-s hold on each side
Quadratus lumborum	Side support with knees flexed	30 repetitions with 8-s hold on each side
	Side support with knees extended	30 repetitions with 8-s hold on each side
Oblique abdominals	Side support with knees flexed	30 repetitions with 8-s hold on each side
	Side support with knees extended	30 repetitions with 8-s hold on each side

*Although certain muscle groups are preferentially activated with each exercise sequence, each exercise progression will promote stability by producing motor patterns of cocontraction among all spinal stabilizing muscles.

Table 16.3 Special tests of the lumbar spine of the injured athlete

Test	Purpose	Position	Expected response	Rationale
L'hermitte's sign	To assess dural irritation	Athlete is long sitting. Examiner flexes the head and hips of the athlete	Sharp pain down the spine or into the upper or lower extremities is considered positive	Hyperflexion of the spine in the presence of compression or inflammation would reproduce radicular complaints
Straight leg raise	To assess the effect of stretching on the neural system	The athlete is lying supine and the leg is passively raised, the angle at which back and or leg symptoms are reproduced is recorded. The peripheral nerve can be further stretched with ankle dorsiflexion, hip internal rotation and adduction, and cervical flexion	Reproduction of the athlete's radicular symptoms is considered a positive test. If stretching modifications are added (ankle dorsiflexion, hip or cervical motion) the symptoms would be expected to come on earlier in the range of motion	Implications of pathology based on straight leg raise angle of symptom onset have been suggested; validity is unclear
Slump test	Provocative test to stress the neural system throughout the spine and periphery simultaneously	The athlete is sitting and slouches through the thoracic and lumbar spine. The knee is then extended and the ankle is dorsiflexed. The cervical spine is then passively flexed. In some descriptions the hip is also adducted	Once the athlete's symptoms are recreated, the test is terminated. Symptoms other than those that are the complaint of the athlete are considered inconsequential. These often included hamstring pulling or muscular complaints	Stretching of the nerve throughout the system is suggested to recreate radicular complaints
Reverse Lasegue test or prone knee flexion test	Described as stretch of L3, or L4 nerve root	Patient is prone or side-lying. Knee is flexed avoiding spinal extension	Reproduction of referred anterior thigh pain is considered positive of L3 or L4 radiculopathy. Stretching of the quadriceps muscle is considered negative	Stretching of the nerve throughout the system is suggested to recreate radicular complaints
Prone instability test	Provocative test to determine lumbar spinal levels generating pain that may benefit from spinal stabilization	Athlete is prone lying with legs off the bed. The examiner performs a posterior-to-anterior (PA) glide for pain. Athlete lifts their feet off the floor, PA glide is reproduced and symptoms recorded	If the pain produced in the first spring test is alleviated or diminished on the re-test, the test is considered positive	If self stabilization during the feet up phase reduce pain, the segment is considered unstable

Table 16.4 Special tests for the cervical spine of an injured athlete

Test	Purpose	Position	Expected response	Rationale
Vertebrobasilar artery test cervical	To assess for compromise of the vertebral artery	Athlete's head is held in extension for 10 seconds, progressed to end range rotation for 10 seconds, finally combined extension and rotation is performed	If the athlete complains of dizziness, difficulty swallowing, speaking, or eye nystagmus is noted, test is considered positive and stopped. If no symptoms are elicited, proceed to next position until complete	Creation of symptoms may indicate compromise of the vertebral artery and medical clearance is needed before performing of end range cervical stretches or return to sport with excessive cervical motion
Alar ligament test	To test the ligaments from the odontoid process to the condyles of the occipital bone	The therapist palpates on one side of C2 and C3 spinous processes with their hand, patient's head is passively moved into sidebending away from the palpating hand.	The sidebending produces immediate and simultaneous rotation of C2 if the alar ligament is intact. Lack of rotation of C2 with sidebending is considered positive and would warrant referral for medical follow-up	If the alar ligament is stabilizing C2, motion will occur at the same time as motion of the head occurs
Atlantoaxial motion	To assess the contribution of the atlantoaxial joint to overall cervical rotation	The athlete's head can be placed in full flexion and the rotation right and left is observed and compared. Alternative position: full cervical extension combined with sidebending, the head is then rotated to the opposite side. This is repeated in the opposite direction	The rotation available at the atlantoaxial joint is expected to be symmetrical bilaterally	When the cervical spine is fully flexed or fully extended and sidebent, there is little contribution to rotation by the cervical levels, therefore, remaining motion in rotation is attributed to the atlantoaxial joint preferentially
Spurling's test	To assess for cervical radiculopathy	Patient is seated and the head is sidebent and rotated to the same side. 7 K of force is produced as an axial load	Complaints of radicular pain or paresthesia are assessed	Compression of the neural foramen coupled with the axial load would produce radiculopathy if the area is compromised
Shoulder abduction sign	To assess for alleviation of pain caused by C5–C6 nerve root compression (these levels are often involved in sports 'burners' or stingers')	Involved arm is abducted and forearm rests on top of the athlete's head	If complaints of arm pain or paresthesia are reduced, C5–C6 is suspected	Position unloads brachial plexus and symptoms are reduced
Median nerve testing	Assessment to determine if the pain complaint is related to stress of the median nerve	Shoulder is depressed and retracted, extended and externally rotated. Elbow is extended, forearm supinated, wrist and fingers are extended. Neck is laterally flexed and rotated away	Athlete's symptoms are reproduced in the distribution of the median nerve	This position has been theorized to preferentially stress the median nerve
Radial nerve testing	Assessment to determine if the pain complaint is related to stress of the radial nerve	Shoulder is retracted and depressed and internally rotated. Forearm is pronated and wrist is flexed and deviated to the ulnar side. Fingers are flexed. Neck is laterally flexed and rotated away	Athlete's symptoms are reproduced in the distribution of the radial nerve	This position has been theorized to preferentially stress the radial nerve
Ulnar nerve testing	Assessment to determine if the pain complaint is related to stress of the ulnar nerve	Shoulder is retracted, depressed, extended and externally rotated. The elbow is flexed and the forearm is supinated. The wrist is extended and radially deviated. Fingers are extended. Neck is laterally flexed and rotated away	Athlete's symptoms are reproduced in the distribution of the ulnar nerve	This position has been theorized to preferentially stress the ulnar nerve

Consider a golfer who complains of pain with hitting down on the ball in high grass; motion-testing reveals decreased right lumbar sidebending and extension. Maximal closing is combined to assess the overall motion loss and level of pain provoked. The therapist discovers that right low lumbar closing is restricted and performs specific mobilizations to the region. Reassessment of the golf swing comparable sign increases the range by 20% with no subsequent change in pain. The therapist returns to data gathering and finds that palpation of the quadratus lumborum is painful and recreates a familiar complaint to the athlete. Following deep tissue work and stretching of the quadratus, the golfer was immediately able to fully swing their imaginary club in the clinic pain-free. Although joint mobilizations had a role in the patient's condition, the role was small in comparison to another likely pain generator. Utilizing a 'comparable sign' assists clinicians in assessing the success of the components of their interventions within and between treatment sessions.

Neurological screening/radiculopathy

The involvement of neural tissue in spinal injury or disability can produce reliable and reproducible responses. Symptoms from irritation of central nerve roots or peripheral nerves follow specific dermatomal distributions and have been mapped. These distributions are 'common' findings from the summation of many subjects and therefore different anatomy and reference texts will have slightly different drawings of the dermatomal distribution patterns of pain, paresthesia or numbness. A summary of relevant distributions for the cervical and lumbar regions is given in Box 16.1. When pain extends down the arm or below the knee, a complete neurological screen is indicated. This procedure may reveal patterns of nerve compromise related to a specific level or levels. These data can be helpful in implicating nerve dysfunction and also can be used to monitor improvement with interventions.

Patterns of weakness in the upper or lower extremity that reflect injury to the innervating nerve can also guide the diagnostic procedure. Weaknesses in the muscles listed in Box 16.1 are considered as spinal level myotomes, and indicate nerve root compromise. Monosynaptic stretch reflexes can also be impaired in nerve compromise and are tested to provide further evidence of nerve injury. Some special tests are designed specifically to stress the nervous system, in general the tests are intended to provoke or alleviate radicular complaints. Examples of those tests are included in Tables 16.3 and 16.4. In general, an athlete is considered to have neurological compromise when they have more than one of the following signs: weakness of a myotomal distribution, sensory changes or pain in a dermatomal distribution, or a positive provocative test such as Spurling's in the cervical region or a Straight Leg Raise in the lumbar region. Treatments that restore reflexes result in a migration of symptoms out of the distal extremity, or restore muscle function are all considered to have a positive impact on the athlete's radiculopathy and should be continued.

Neural tension is a term that has been proposed to characterize the reactivity of a peripheral nerve to stretch. Positions have been described that are purported to selectively stress the ulnar, median, radial and common sciatic peripheral nerves (Tables 16.3 and 16.4).

The lumbar classification scheme indicates nonresponsive radiculopathy receives traction, while activities promoting centralization are encouraged. A similar principle can be followed in the cervical spine, although thoracic manipulation has also been indicated to assist with cervical complaints (Figs 16.6 and 16.7) (Browder et al 2004).

Referred pain

It is not uncommon for referred pain in the upper or lower extremity of an athlete to be present. When a pattern of pain is identified but no other neurological signs or symptoms are present, joint referral or trigger points should be considered (Travell & Rinzler 1952, Simons et al 1998, Travell & Simons 1983, 1983b). This pain caused from a muscular trigger point or joint referral can be significant and limit pain-free sport participation. Trigger points in the quadratus lumborum and hip have been identified to relate to instances of persistent unresolved low back pain and trigger points in the cervical and shoulder

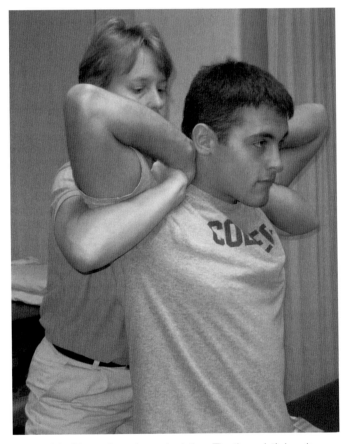

Figure 16.6 • Upper thoracic manipulation. The therapist's hands are looped through the athlete's arms and the therapist's hands are placed at the target joint level. Spinal extension is introduced by shoulder extension and the therapist produces an upward traction through the legs.

region can mimic cervical radiculopathy. Palpation is sufficient to identify a trigger point, and direct pressure, dry needling, saline or steroid injections, aggressive stretching and electrical stimulation have all been suggested as treatment options for trigger points (Hubbard 1998, Johnson 1998, Sjolund et al 1977). The pain distribution patterns outlined by Simons et al (1998) and Travell & Simons (1983) for all regions of the body can help provide a map for sources of pain that are not associated with other neurological signs (Travell & Rinzler, 1952, Simons et al 1998, Travell & Simons 1983). Specific pain referral patterns have been mapped stemming from cervical, thoracic, and lumbar facet joints as well (Aprill et al 1990, Dwyer et al 1990, Manchikanti et al 2004). Not unlike the trigger point patterns, pain is present often in an area remote from the source but it is characterized by the absence of neurological findings. More information about facet joints will follow.

Joint mobility testing

Pain originating from spinal joints can generally be reproduced with joint mobility testing although the results of the mobility assessment can vary (Abbott et al 2005). There are many proposed methods of joint assessment: unilateral and central posterior anterior glides, passive physiological joint motions in sidebending and rotation, and a multitude of other assessments aimed at identifying position and mobility response. Segmental

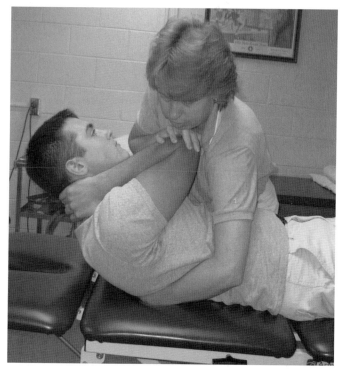

Figure 16.7 • Supine thoracic manipulation. The therapist's hand is placed on the inferior vertebra of the hypomoblie segment. The athlete is supine with hands behind the neck. The therapist applies a downward pressure through the elbows of the athlete in an anterior–posterior direction.

motion testing for sagittal plane flexion and extension is tested with posterior-to-anterior glides (Kulig et al 2004). Although reliability coefficients for posterior-to-anterior glide assessments are fair, the agreement among raters is high and it may be best used to determine those that may benefit from specific interventions such as manipulation (Binkley et al 1995, Childs et al 2004, Hicks et al 2003, Maher & Adams 1994, Maher et al 1998a). Overall, the reliability on individual joint assessment is best when limited to discrete categories of 'hypermobile' or 'hypomobile'. The results from pain provocation testing of spinal segments routinely outperform mobility testing (Maher et al 1998b). Joints that are hypomobile can become painful when loads or positions of the joint exceed its range and ability. These joints would display a pattern of limitation during range of motion testing (Table 16.1), and joint pain provocation testing would likely reproduce the patient's complaints.

In some cases, the overstressed hypermobile joint is the source of pain, and in other cases the stiff joint is painful because it cannot move into positions that are needed for the athlete to perform specific activities. In either case, activities that stress the irritated joint are usually painful. The aggravating activities derived from the patient's history can often lead the therapist to surmise what spinal mechanics are contributing to the problem. Fritz et al (2005) used spinal segmental mobility testing to categorize patients. They determined that subjects with lumbar stiffness benefited more from a manipulation intervention while those deemed hypermobile experienced a greater benefit from stabilization. When stiffness and looseness are juxtaposed, treatments aimed at calming the irritated segments are coupled with mobilization of the hypomobile areas and stabilization of the overworked hypermobile region.

Special cervical spine topics

Burners/stingers

Cervical radiculopathy can occur from traction injuries to nerves or a plexus, called burners or stingers (Cantu et al 1998, Speer & Bassett 1990, Weinstein 1998). This transient neurapraxia is characterized by paresthesia and/or weakness in one arm. Stretching from a combined movement of the shoulder and head in opposite directions or a direct contusion to the neurovascular region can occur in many sports such as martial arts or wrestling. Traction injuries generally improve quickly on their own and may require protected rest and treatment for resulting protective muscle spasms of the neck and shoulder. The 'electric shock' or weakness of the upper extremity resolves quickly, and often this injury is not even reported due to the spontaneous nature of the recovery; however, in some instances the condition is considered more serious when symptoms persist (Cantu et al 1998, Weinstein 1998). Further evaluation is required if the symptoms do not recover within hours or days. Other spinal conditions that compromise neural space, such as facet degeneration and ligamentum flavum hypertrophy, disc herniation and a congenitally small central spinal canal or neural foramen, can contribute to the incidence of burners (Kim et al 2004).

Wry neck or facet syndrome

The term wry neck is used interchangeably with the term torticollis and the etiology ranges from acute articular dislocation to muscle pain and stiffness (Amevo et al 1991, 1992). In the rare case of wryneck developing after a significant trauma, articular process subluxation or even unilateral dislocation may need to be considered. Resultant muscle tone guarding the injured area may be severe enough to prevent reduction. In this case medical intervention is required and the neurological status will be assessed before and after reduction, and the neck will be protected for 6–8 weeks or until healing is complete (McGrory et al 1993).

In some definitions wry neck is linked directly to a shortening of the sternocleidomastoid either actively or passively. The resultant position is sidebending toward the affected side and rotating to the opposite side. This condition can be congenital; however, in the athlete it is more likely the resultant posturing to protect muscle strain or injury. A similar head position can also occur after strenuous sport participation or an insidious onset. In this case, the position relieves the pain, and the pain is posterior in location. The offending position is extension and sidebending and rotation to the opposite side. This has also been called torticollis; however, it is more likely an attempt to avoid closing the contralateral facet joint. The facet joints have been identified as a possible source of neck pain, and the diagnosis of cervical facet syndrome is often one of exclusion (Fukui et al 1996, Johnson 1991). Since a definitive diagnosis of etiology of the pain and dysfunction is unclear in either case, a universal term may be the most appropriate choice.

Clinical features associated with an acute stiff neck include tenderness to palpation over the facet joints or paraspinal muscles, pain with cervical extension or rotation and the absence of neurological signs. Identified components through motion testing, symptom provocation and palpation may lead the therapist to develop a comprehensive intervention addressing all contributing factors, regardless of the label used to describe the condition.

Special thoracic topics

Rib mobility and dysfunction

Thoracic strain and injury can occur during sport and exercise participation. The injury can result from a direct blow to the ribs, or thoracic spine, or excessive stretching into a thoracic end range position such as flexion, extension, sidebending or rotation (Serina & Lieu 1991). Injury can occur to the ribs and surrounding musculature from violent or sustained muscular contractions, or an extreme stretch to the supporting joints and ligaments. Often signs of limited swelling and ecchymosis are present in the case of direct contusions. Pain and protective muscle guarding are also common to immobilize the area. This can be significant in the first few weeks after the injury and severe sprains can require four weeks or more for healing. Thoracic binding has been used with a variety of materials including ace wraps, elastic supports and athletic taping. When a contused area needs to be protected, padding can be applied over the injured area prior to wrapping. Treatments to the area include ultrasound, ice, anti-inflammatory medications, supports and activity modification.

Costal subluxations can also occur and can be palpated and subsequently reduced with direct pressure to the joint (Thomas 1988). Manipulation to the thoracic region is often performed to overcome a motion restriction (Figs 16.6 and 16.7). In the case of rib or thoracic vertebral dysfunction and decreased motion, thoracic/rib joint manipulations can often restore pain free function. In these cases, a significant traumatic injury has been ruled out and the athlete instead complains of pain at the posterior costotransverse junction (between the thoracic vertebrae and the corresponding rib) or central thoracic region. The complaint is often noted on full inhalation or exhalation. The pain may also be produced with thoracic extension (Browder et al 2004, Cleland et al 2005, Pho & Godges 2004). There are many manipulation procedures utilized to restore motion to this area (Browder et al 2004, Cleland 2005, Cleland et al 2005, Pho & Godges 2004). The majority of techniques create distraction or space to allow for motion restrictions to resolve either through traction or anterior/posterior gapping at the vertebral rib interface. Figures 16.6 and 16.7 provide examples of these techniques. The techniques are also utilized in the thoracic area to assist in the resolution of cervical complaints either alone or in conjunction with direct cervical treatment (Browder et al 2004, Cleland et al 2005).

The thoracic vertebrae are well protected by the ribs; therefore, fractures are more likely to occur in the thoracolumbar junction than the thoracic spine itself. Apophysitis or inflammation of the vertebral growth plate is more likely to occur in adolescent athletes with large compressive loads (e.g. weightlifting, wrestling) or in sports that generate smaller but highly repetitive loads such as gymnastics, wrestling and skiing (Rachbauer et al 2001, Sward et al 1993). The apophysitis can eventually result in loss of anterior vertebral body height and is theorized to result from trauma and compressive forces (Sward et al 1993). The presence of Scheuermann's disease or degeneration of the epiphyseal endplate and resultant anterior body height loss may precede or complicate this condition. Scheuermann's kyphosis is twice as prevalent in girls as in boys, and the onset is generally in the early teen years (Bradford 1981, Bradford et al 1980). The incidence of apophysitis is likely sport dependent and may account for less than 20% of back pain complaints (Rachbauer et al 2001); however, since most strains and contusions resolve with modified activity, an athlete with persistent complaints in the thoracic region may require a referral and evaluation by a physician for imaging and diagnosis.

Thoracic outlet

The thoracic outlet space is bounded by the clavicle, the first rib (present in 1% of the population), the costoclavicular ligament and the subclavius and anterior scalene muscle. When the space is compromised, compression of the first rib or between the anterior and middle scalene into the subclavian or axillary artery, vein or lower trunk of the brachial plexus (C8 and T1) can occur. The athlete's complaints can vary from shoulder pain to more distinct vascular and neurological symptoms. There are three types of thoracic outlet syndrome and the athlete may have only one or a combination of areas of compression. In the costoclavicular syndrome, the space between the clavicle and the first rib is compromised. The cervical rib syndrome involves the presence of a cervical rib from C7 or a band of fibrous tissue that traverses the space between C7 and the first rib. Cervical ribs occur in less than 1% of the population so this condition is uncommon. The anterior scalene syndrome describes the compression of the neurovascular bundle between the anterior and medial scalene muscles. The athlete will often complain of numbness or tingling in the ring finger (fourth digit) and little finger (fifth digit), and intrinsic muscle weakness via the ulnar and median nerves. If the vein is involved, arm or hand edema may occur. The athletes may also complain of severe arm and hand fatigue or finger and hand ischemia with vascular involvement (McCarthy et al 1989). Provocative testing can be used to assess the involvement of the structures in the athlete's symptoms. A test for thoracic outlet should be considered positive if it replicates the athlete's complaint, the presence or change in pulse strength alone is insufficient to determine vascular involvement.

The involvement of the artery is tested by determining if pulse obliteration occurs with alternative positioning. The athlete's arm is placed on the thigh in supination, the head is rotated to the affected side and then extended. The athlete holds their breath and any change in pulse from the resting position combined with symptom changes are noted. Hyperabduction of the arm can also stress the brachial plexus across the coracoid, humeral head and pectoralis minor tendon. Shoulder external rotation, inhaling and shrugging shoulders have been added to this test by some authors (Jamieson & Chinnick 1996). A loss of pulse itself is not a positive finding, but coupled with reproduction of the athlete's complaints should be considered significant (Novak et al 1993). Radiographs can determine the presence of a cervical rib. Doppler ultrasonography and cold immersion testing may assist in the diagnosis of vascular compromise. The contribution of nerve conduction testing, electromyography testing and sensory testing is often limited due to the transient nature of the symptoms (Novak et al 1993). In some cases thoracic outlet syndrome can be exacerbated by recurrent anterior shoulder dislocation and the conditions can combine to result in the 'dead arm' complaint (Leffert & Gumley 1987).

Treatment for thoracic outlet syndrome in the athlete should be directed at the cause of the compromise. First rib mobility testing and subsequent mobilizations may be helpful in cases of hypomobility. Stretching of scalene musculature and compromising soft tissue can be attempted to resolve tightness. Concurrent treatment of the shoulder for laxity or pectoralis minor tightness may improve the available range of motion. Surgery may be considered for vascular compromise and cervical rib restriction; however, the surgical outcome data suggest that surgical complications can and do occur; surgery is the treatment of last resort (Cherington et al 1986, Wilbourn 1988).

Special lumbar topics

Spondylolysis/spondylolithesis

Acute fracture of the thoracolumbar and lumbar regions can occur in any sport when the force is sufficient. The same is true for the sacral and coccygeal region. More obscure but possible fractures can occur to the spinous process, transverse process, iliac crest or vertebral endplate apophyseal (as discussed in the special thoracic topics section above). These injuries often result from forceful muscle contractions coupled with extreme motion ranges in sports such as gymnastics, ice-skating and wrestling. Referral to a physician for imaging and diagnosis may be necessary, although treatment of these conditions often involve immobilization and activity modification for symptom management, and progressive return to activity as the athlete tolerates.

It can be difficult to determine if a spinal element injury is an acute traumatic injury or the final blow to a developing isthmic spondylolysis (Sward 1990). Fracture of the pars interarticularis, especially in adolescents, represents a continuum from prespondylolytic stress reaction to spondylolysis, and is likely the result of overuse (Wier & Smith 1989). A single photon emission computerized tomography (SPECT) bone scan (see Chapter 30) is necessary to identify all prespondylolytic lesions and many spondylolytic lesions of the pars (Bellah et al 1991, Rosen et al 1982). Stress fracture may be considered a more incidental finding in adults (5% of back pain); however, in adolescent athletes with back pain spondylolysis was found in 47% of the cases and may be as high as 60% (Micheli & Wood 1995, Rossi 1988). Pars stress reaction is often associated with overuse and hyperextension loading, and early treatment of bracing for immobilization is recommended and may prevent progression to a frank fracture (Micheli et al 1980, Steiner & Micheli 1985). The period of immobilization can persist for 3 to 9 months or greater until healing is complete on SPECT or CT scan (Bellah et al 1991, Congeni et al 1997, Rosen et al 1982). Some authors advocate SPECT scans on any adolescent athlete with back pain of over 3 weeks' duration (Congeni et al 1997, Gerbino & Micheli 1995). If a spondylolysis is present but the SPECT scan is negative, although the defect is present, it is not undergoing active repair. This may be a case of a developmental defect or even an old fracture line that has undergone pseudoarthrosis where the defect fills with scar tissue. In this case, the athlete is managed only for symptom control as bracing for immobilization is not warranted; healing in this case is not expected.

Spondylolisthesis refers to the anterior migration of one vertebra in relation to another as a result of separation of the pars interarticularis. This anterior subluxation occurs primarily at the lumbosacral junction and can result from trauma or repetitive strain. The slippage is graded from Grade 1 (least migration) to Grade 4 (most migration). These patients are managed with an immobilization brace to reduce motion and allow for the area to calm. The goal with these athletes is not to attain bony union but instead to return to activity without pain (Muschik et al 1996). In cases where the slippage is progressing to a high level, neurological symptoms are present or attempts at returning the athlete to play have failed, fusion surgery can be considered (Hardcastle 1993). Prevention of stress fractures and their subsequent complications remains a priority. Consideration of the hours of practice an athlete is involved in, the frequency and force of hyperextension positioning and a family history of spondylolysis or spondylolisthesis are all risk factors that need to be considered in developing and implementing prevention strategies.

Spinal treatments

Joint manipulation and mobilizations

Hypomobility of the spine can be addressed with combinations of joint mobilizations and stretching. Descriptions of joint mobility testing can be found in a myriad of publications (e.g. Boyling & Palastanga 1994, Cleland 2005, Edmond 1993, Greenman 1996, Kaltenborn 1993). Although many books describe spinal joint mobilization techniques, no one technique has been demonstrated to outperform another. Joint mobilization techniques are indicated when accessory joint motion restriction is identified and relates to pain or abnormal movement. Grade 1 or 2 mobilizations are oscillatory techniques in the middle of arthrokinematic range and can be used to reduce pain complaints. Mobilizations that engage the joint-restriction barrier are called Grade 3 or 4 depending on the amplitude of the oscillation, and increase accessory joint mobility. Generally mobilizations of painful limited joints are performed in mid-range joint positions; however, improvements in joint mobility may require more aggressive mobilizations. Mobilizations done at the end ranges of available motion can increase joint capsule stress and allow stretching to occur.

Cervical manipulation

Cervical manipulation has been demonstrated to increase range of motion, although it is less successful in treating pain without motion restriction. Hurwitz et al (1996) estimated the complication rate of cervical manipulation to be 10 in 10 million. Although the risk is minimal compared to other more common risk factors in medicine, using manipulation for any cervical problem may expose the athlete to unnecessary risk. Since manipulation is intended to overcome motion restriction it is most efficacious in increasing range of motion (Childs et al 2004, Cleland 2005, Hurwitz et al 1996). In a situation in which the athlete recently lost previously available range of motion upon waking or after prolonged positioning, in the absence of bony resistance with cervical motion or neurological compromise,

manipulation can be successful in regaining lost motion. In situations where athletes have areas of long-standing hypomobility, the short-term effects of manipulation are unlikely beneficial over a program of mobilizations and stretching. Some authors have demonstrated that in the cervical region, manipulation and mobilizations have equivocal results (Bronfort et al 2004).

Lumbar manipulation

Lumbar manipulation has become one of the most studied interventions in low back pain. There is emerging evidence supporting the efficacy of lumbar manipulation, particularly in a subgroup of patients. Flynn et al (2002) developed a clinical prediction rule for success with manipulation, which has since been validated by Childs et al (2004). The prediction rule consists of at least 4 of 5 of the following variables: (1) duration of back pain <15 days; (2) Fear Avoidance Behavior Questionnaire (work scale) (Waddell et al 1993) of <19; (3) no pain distal to the knee; (4) presence of lumbar hypomobility; and (5) hip internal rotation of >35°. If a patient is positive in at least 4 of the 5 variables in the clinical prediction rule, they are 13 times more likely to have a 50% decline in their Oswestry score within one week. The strongest predictor of nonsuccess included the presence of pain distal to the knee, which had a negative likelihood ratio of 0.16.

The manipulation used in this study is one that has been purported to be directed towards the sacroiliac joint (SIJ) (Fig. 16.8). Interestingly, however, none of the traditional SIJ tests (e.g. pelvic signs related to inominate rotations) were as predictive as the variables outlined in the prediction rule. In fact, the strongest predictors of success with manipulation were from

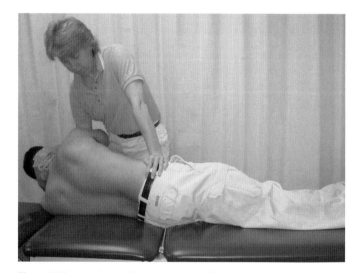

Figure 16.8 • Lumbopelvic manipulation. The athlete is supine with fingers interlocked behind their head. The therapist rotates the patient to end range and thrusts the anterior superior iliac spine in a posterior/inferior direction. The manipulation is performed two times and if symptom improvement is absent or incomplete, it is repeated for two attempts on the opposite side.

history and included duration of <15 days and no pain distal to the knee, which had a positive likelihood ratio of 12.6. This particular manipulation is safe and relatively easy to perform.

Stretching

When treating an area of injury, consideration must be made to evaluate the joints above and below the areas of focus. That is especially true in the management of spinal pain. Tightness in the shoulder range of motion can put abnormal stress on the cervical and thoracic regions. Hip and knee flexibility can place undue burden on the lumbar spine in activities involving excessive ranges of motion. For example, in the case of a rower, flexibility loss in the ankle and hip would require more flexion of the back to place the oar in the water with a full reaching stroke. Soccer (football) goalkeepers require significant hip and low back range of motion to enable them to cover the outer lower corners of the net. Each athlete must be evaluated in context of their sport and the impact the surrounding joints and muscle range can have on sport performance.

Stretching programs should be initiated when impairments are identified and some authors believe that hamstring flexibility is especially detrimental to low back injury and progression (Gerbinao 1995, Herbert & Gabriel 2002, Micheli & Wood 1995).

Electrophysical agents and other modalities

In general, electrophysical agents and other modalities used in spinal care are implemented for pain management (see Chapter 14). In most cases, the target tissue in spinal dysfunction is deep within the body and superficial modalities cannot penetrate the overlying tissue to reach target tissue. Modalities successful in reducing pain may allow the athlete a more rapid return to daily activities and prevent secondary complications of fear avoidance resulting from pain with activity. Ultrasound is indicated for deep heating and increasing blood flow in tissue (Draper et al 1995). Hot packs may be indicated for superficial heating especially combined with painful stretching and stiffness. Cold therapy is often utilized following acute contusion or strain. Use of ice acutely after injury is associated with reductions in pain although the effect on tissue healing is unclear (Bleakley et al 2004, Hubbard & Denegar 2004). Electrical stimulation is used over areas of local pain and may result in decreased oral analgesic use and increased pain relief (Berkman et al 1999). See Chapter 14 for a further discussion of the use of electrophysical agents.

Traction

Traction is hypothesized to affect spinal segments in a myriad of ways. Evidence for the reduction of disc protrusion and altered intradiscal pressure is weak (Mathews 1968); however, beneficial effects on patients with radiculopathy have been found (Moeti & Marchetti 2001, Zylbergold & Piper 1985). There is strong in vivo and in vitro evidence of transitory vertebral

separation although the clinical implications of this impact are unclear (Colachis & Strohm 1969, Wong et al 1992). The evidence does suggest that for intervertebral separation to occur the lumbar traction is targeted at 50% bodyweight or greater plus 4% bodyweight to overcome table friction (Judovich 1955). A study by Wong et al (1992) showed that in the cervical spine, 20 lb of traction was necessary to reverse the cervical lordosis and 50 lb of traction had greater effects than 30 lb. It does not appear that one type of cervical traction is more successful than another. In a study of 25 lb of cervical traction on patients with or without radiculopathy, positive responses were found equally among three different types of traction: manual, intermittent and static (Zylbergold & Piper 1985).

Traction is often considered in patients with radiculopathy who do not centralize with active motions. When no centralization occurs with motion testing during the evaluation, traction may help reduce the acute radiculopathy until a directional preference is identified (Fritz 1998, Fritz et al 2000, George & Delitto 2005, Manal & Claytor 2005). Traction parameters are most often successfully determined by patient response. Increases in the minimal poundage of 20 lb for the cervical spine in neutral and greater than 50% body weight for lumbar traction coupled with increases in treatment duration can both be adjusted to effect treatment dosage. Changes in patient symptom complaints during traction or immediately following traction can assist the therapist in determining the usefulness of this intervention.

Stabilization training

The concept of spinal stabilization and support goes in and out of fashion every few years. This is currently a time of upswing in the concept of the 'core' and the need for 'core strengthening'. The idea that stability in the center of the body will promote more fluid, controlled and forceful motions from the extremities is in a revival. Very often the challenges are in the meaning of 'stabilization'. The role of muscle strengthening or control has not been directly linked with a decrease in passive joint laxity; however, the concept of dynamic control compensating for inherent laxity is an area of interest to explain functional outcomes in the presence of laxity in the knee, shoulder and spine (Tierney et al 2005, Swanik et al 1997, 2002).

The goal in lumbar stabilization is to educate the athlete to maintain a pelvic neutral position while performing muscular contractions of the trunk and extremities. McGill (1998, 2001) has evaluated exercises to promote the greatest EMG of the stabilizing musculature while minimizing disc pressures. The side plank or side bridge exercise promotes high-level muscular contractions in a controlled position (Figs 16.9–16.12). The instructions to the athlete are to pull the trunk to the ceiling while maintaining a pelvic neutral position. The athlete is advised to avoid flexing the hips, a 'pike' position, or using the shoulder to push the body up. The athlete first attempts to raise the trunk with flexed knees and, if successful, progresses to attempting the trunk side lift on fully extended legs. In the most advanced stage of this exercise, the athlete maintains

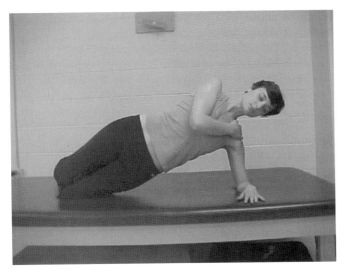

Figure 16.9 • Side support with knees flexed. Patient lies on their side with knees bent and upper body supported on the lower elbow. Then they lift their body from the table with all weight borne on the lower knee and elbow. Hold for 8 seconds. Relax and repeat.

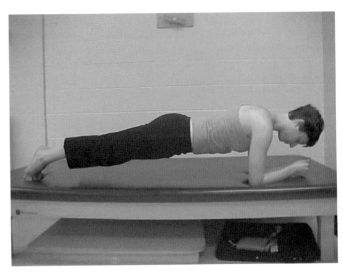

Figure 16.11 • Advanced side bridge (prone). Perform the side support as described in Fig. 16.10. Roll from one elbow to the prone position while abdominally bracing to attain a prone position.

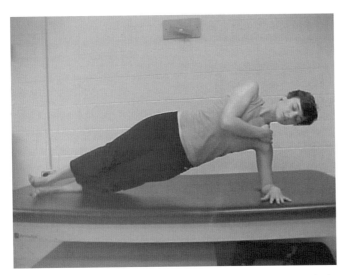

Figure 16.10 • Side support with knees extended. Patient lies on their side with knees straight and upper body supported on the lower elbow. Then they lift their body from the table with all weight borne on the lower foot and elbow. Hold for 8 seconds. Relax and repeat.

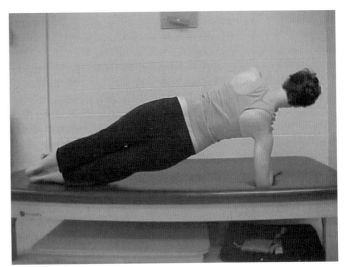

Figure 16.12 • Advanced side bridge (complete). Roll from the prone position illustrated in Fig. 16.11 to the opposite elbow. Then, lower yourself from side support position on the opposite elbow down to the floor.

their stabilized spine while rotating from the elevated lift position to the prone position and then continuing the rotation to the opposite side. The key in designing stabilization programs for athletes is to educate them that a loss of control at the lumbar/pelvic region is a failure of the exercise. Athletes will often sacrifice form to complete the exercise requested. In stabilization training, the purpose of the activity is to stabilize the spine so that any motion from the original lumbopelvic neutral position is a failure. A comprehensive example of a progressive lumbar stabilization program has been developed specifically for figure skaters (Schneider et al 1999).

Strength

Weak muscles are unlikely able to 'control' motion that occurs with high-level activity. Evidence suggests that specificity of exercise is one of the best ways to ensure muscle hypertrophy. Direct training with weights, machines and rubber tubing has demonstrated strength gains in the spinal musculature (Conley et al 1997, Leggett et al 1991, Mansell et al 2005, Rezasoltani et al 2005, Ylinen et al 2003). Resistance training has been demonstrated to increase muscular strength and, more importantly, training may also impact on neuromuscular control (Tierney 1996, Franco & Herzog 1987).

Electrical stimulation has been demonstrated to have success in improving strength of the quadriceps muscles in athletes following injury and surgery (Babkin et al 1977, Delitto & Synder-Mackler 1990, Fitzgerald et al 2003, Snyder-Mackler et al 1991, 1995). Use of high-intensity electrical stimulation to lumbar paraspinals may be a logical extension of this success and has been used with figure skaters with failed lumbar fusions (Manal 2002a). It has also been used on skaters during the period of immobilization while healing from lumbar stress fracture (Goodstadt & Manal 2003, Manal 2002b). An electrical stimulator with power sufficient to generate strong muscular contractions (i.e. 80% of the maximal force output of a quadriceps contraction) is the most effective. The parameters used are: $400\,\mu s$ pulse duration, 50–75 pulses per second, ramp on and off to tolerance, 15 second on time, 50 second off time for 10–15 contractions. The pelvis is stabilized and a single channel is placed on the right side and a second on the left side of the paraspinals at the target spinal level. The pelvis is placed over pillows and strapped down to create a posterior pelvic tilt. When the stimulation intensity is increased to the maximal tolerable level, the belt prevents lumbar extension ensuring an isometric contraction (minimal spinal extension with contraction). Figures 16.13 and 16.14 demonstrate electrical stimulation setup.

Dynamic stability/neuromuscular control

In order to successfully stabilize, the muscles must prepare for and react to movement and load. The dual concept of feed forward and feedback encompasses the duality of preparation and constant readjustment to changing conditions (Swanik et al 1997, 2002). In an often unpredictable athletic environment, players must anticipate muscular power and control needed for execution of their desired action and concurrently respond to externally imposed forces from terrain, individuals and equipment (Mansell et al 2005). Training programs must consider progression to ensure that lessons learned in the clinical setting are translated to the playing field to assist the athlete in return to sport.

Return to play

Management of the injured athlete requires a full understanding of their sport and participation level. Knowledge of the biomechanics and demands of a specific sport position or sport repertoire provide the evaluating therapist with an understanding of positions and stresses occurring during aggravating activities. Baseline knowledge of the sport specific demands of the athlete will also become critical to decisions regarding drills or types of activities an injured athlete can resume. For example, the demands on a singles figure skater versus an ice dancer are as unique as those placed on a soccer goalkeeper versus a striker. Athletes can frequently reliably reproduce the sport

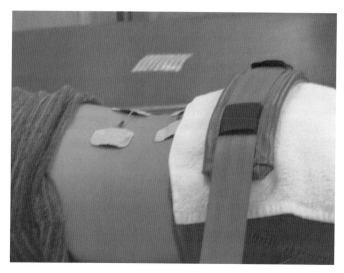

Figure 16.13 • Patient positioning for isometric lumbar electrical stimulation. The athlete is prone over pillows, the pelvis strapped to the table in posterior pelvic tilt. The athlete attempts to perform an anterior tilt to assure the pelvis is stable and immobile.

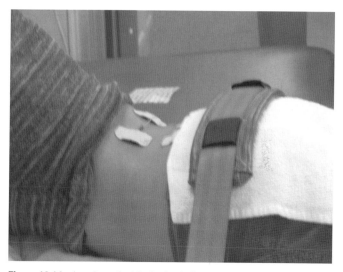

Figure 16.14 • Lumbar electrical stimulation providing a paraspinal contraction. A single channel is placed on the right side of the spine and a second on the left. The stimulus amplitude is increased until a strong visible contraction is seen and the intensity level is the maximal tolerated by the athlete. The treatment is stopped if the athlete complains of any increase in the problem that caused them to seek treatment.

position creating pain and therapists can modify those positions to determine if they can alter pain with participation. The interaction between positional changes and symptom change is important to assist the therapist in confirming hypotheses related to biomechanical stresses in sport specific activities and in developing novel and unique approaches to symptom management.

Safe return to play is allowed after the appropriate sport-specific rehabilitation program is completed and the athlete demonstrates full ROM and proper neutral spine posture with sport-specific activities. In most cases of spinal injury, if the athlete can perform activities of daily living without exacerbating the condition, sport-specific drills are introduced. As long as the athlete can perform progressively increasing sport specific activities return to play is often determined by athlete tolerance. Cases of injury to bone or ligamentous structures can delay the initiation of return to sport progressions by 6–8 weeks or longer.

Medical consultation

Any athlete who has a red flag during history collection should be referred to a physician for follow-up testing. Any athlete with loss of bowel or bladder function or suspected spinal cord injury or fracture requires an immediate referral. In other cases, a referral to a specialist can be requested to confirm a new diagnosis (i.e. lumbar stress fracture) or in the most extreme cases, surgical consultation.

The physician plays a vital role in the successful team management of an athlete and when the relationship between the therapist and physician is strong, the athlete benefits. Nonsurgical spine management reflects a full spectrum of intervention strategies. The use of non-steroidal anti-inflammatory medications (NSAIDs) and steroidal medications (e.g. Prendisone) are prevalent in athletic spine management (Bronfort et al 1996, Harmon & Hawley 2003, Herskovitz et al 1995, Leadbetter 1995).

Corticosteroids are cortisone-like medications that can be used for inflammation. They can be given orally or injected. They mimic cortisol hormones produced by the adrenyl gland and regulated by the pituitary. Glucocorticoids like cortisol control carbohydrate, fat and protein metabolism, and control inflammation via prevention of phospholipid release and a decrease in white blood cells. This contributes to an impaired immune response and potential for delayed healing. The mineralcorticoids like aldosterone control electrolyte and water levels via retention of sodium in the kidneys. This can relate to hypertension, high sodium levels and low potassium levels in the blood. Some drugs mimic the glucocorticiods (dexamethasone) while others combine the actions of gluco- and mineralcorticoids (prendisone) (Cardone & Tallia 2002, Gotzsche & Johansen 2005).

Oral steroid dose is commonly characterized into low dose (<10 mg/day of prednisone), medium (10–20 mg/day) and high dose (>20 mg/day) (Cardone & Tallia 2002, Gotzsche & Johansen 2005, Herskovitz et al 1995). Treatment continuing for more than three months is regarded as long-term use and for most orthopedic conditions the steroid dose packs are short (5, 8 or 11 days). Steroidal dose packs are prescribed in cases of acute radiculopathy (or acute aggravation of a chronic condition) and may reduce the athlete's complaints quickly. In many cases, time is a critical factor in the management of an athlete and although many problems can resolve without a myriad of interventions, speed can be a factor impacting the decision making process.

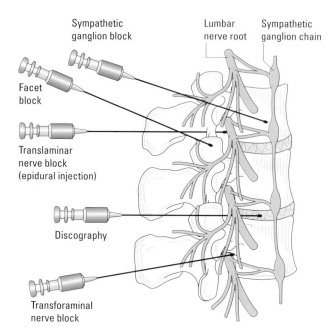

Figure 16.15 • Spinal segment with injection locations identified (Cameron 2000). (Reprinted with permission, copyright the Hughston Foundation, Inc.)

It is not uncommon to offer an athlete one course of treatment during the season and a less aggressive treatment plan in the off-season. Chapter 29 provides a more comprehensive account of the use of pharmacological agents in sport.

Injections are utilized in the nonoperative spine management arsenal with conflicting results (Anderberg et al 2006, Bogduk 1997, Carette et al 1991, Delport et al 2004, Derby 1993). Table 16.2 describes injections available and the correlation of the injection site with the symptoms of the athlete. Figure 16.15 provides an anatomical representation of the injection locations (Cameron 2000). Glucocorticoid steroids are prohibited by the World Anti-Doping Agency (WADA) and any use of this substance (orally or intramuscularly) is prohibited and if necessary requires a Therapuetic Use Exemption Approval (http://www.wada-ama.org/en/exemptions.ch2). This form must be approved prior to participation in international sanctioned competition.

Summary

The purpose of the physical therapy guided history described in this chapter is to rule out significant red flags of more serious pathology, learn about the behavior of the patient's spinal problem and add focus to the evaluation. A systematic approach through a treatment-based classification system can assure the therapist that if multiple components are present, each will be identified and a comprehensive treatment plan can be developed. Special considerations in the management of athletes with spinal pain and dysfunction are considered by a sports physical therapist in their differential diagnosis and subsequent treatment strategy. The physical therapist managing the athlete with spine pain uses information about movement testing, symptom behavior, the biomechanics of the athlete's sport, provocative testing and evidence-based interventions to rapidly return the athlete to the sporting arena.

References

Abbott J, McCane B, Herbison P et al 2005 Lumbar segmental instability: a criterion-related validity study of manual therapy assessment. BMC Musculoskeletal Disorders 6:56

American National Red Cross 2001 American National Red Cross Emergency Response. Staywell, Boston, MA, p 144–145

Amevo B, Worth D, Bogduk N 1991 Instantaneous axes of rotation of the typical cervical motion segments: a study in normal volunteers. Clinical Biomechanics 6:111–117

Amevo B, Aprill C, Bogduk N 1992 Abnormal instantaneous axes of rotation in patients with neck pain. Spine 17:748–756

Anderberg L, Annertz M, Rydholm U et al 2006 Selective diagnostic nerve root block for the evaluation of radicular pain in the multilevel degenerated cervical spine. European Spine Journal 15:794–801

Aprill C, Dwyer A, Bogduk N 1990 Cervical zygapophyseal joint pain patterns: II. A clinical evaluation. Spine 15:458–461

Babkin D, Timtsenko N, Kots Y M 1977 Lectures and laboratory periods. Canadian–Soviet exchange symposium on electrostimulation of skeletal muscles. Concordia University, Montreal

Banos J E, Bosch F, Canellas M et al 1989 Acceptability of visual analogue scales in the clinical setting: a comparison with verbal rating scales in postoperative pain. Methods and Findings in Experimental and Clinical Pharmacology 11:123–127

Bellah R D, Summerville D A, Treves S T 1991 Low back pain in adolescent athletes: detection of stress injury to the pars interarticularis with SPECT. Radiology 180:509–512

Berkman R, Hyman M H, Kaplan E A et al 1999 Percutaneous electrical nerve stimulation for treatment of low back pain. Journal of the American Medical Association 282:941–942

Binkley J, Stratford P, Gill C 1995 Interrater reliability of lumbar accessory motion mobility testing. Physical Therapy 75:786–795

Bleakley C, McDonough S, MacAuley D 2004 The use of ice in the treatment of acute soft-tissue injury: a systematic review of randomized controlled trials. American Journal of Sports Medicine 32:251–261

Bogduk N 1997 International Spinal Injection Society guidelines for the performance of spinal injection procedures: 1. Zygapophysial joint blocks. Clinical Journal of Pain 13:285–302

Bogduk N, Mercer S 2000 Biomechanics of the cervical spine: I. Normal kinematics. Clinical Biomechanics 15:633–648

Boden S D, McCowin P R, Davis D O et al 1990 Abnormal magnetic resonance scans of the cervical spine in asymptomatic subjects: a prospective investigation. Journal of Bone and Joint Surgery (Am) 72A:1178–1184

Boyling J, Palastanga N 1994 Grieve's modern manual therapy: the vertebral column, 2nd edn. Longman, New York

Bradford D S 1981 Vertebral osteochondrosis (Scheuermann's kyphosis). Clinical Orthopaedics and Related Research 158:83–90

Bradford D S, Ahmed K B, Moe J H 1980 The surgical management of patients with Scheuermann's disease. Journal of Bone and Joint Surgery (Am) 62A:705–712

Bronfort G, Goldsmith C H, Nelson C F et al 1996 Trunk exercise combined with spinal manipulative or NSAID therapy for chronic low back pain: a randomized, observer-blinded clinical trial. Journal of Manipulative and Physiological Therapeutics 19:570–582

Bronfort G, Haas M, Evans R L et al 2004 Efficacy of spinal manipulation and mobilization for low back pain and neck pain: a systematic review and best evidence synthesis. Spine Journal 4:335–356

Browder D A, Erhard R E, Piva S R 2004 Intermittent cervical traction and thoracic manipulation for management of mild cervical compressive myelopathy attributed to cervical herniated disc: a case series. Journal of Orthopaedics and Sports Physical Therapy 34:701–712

Burton A K, Waddell G, Tillotson K M et al 1999 Information and advice to patients with back pain can have a positive effect. A randomized controlled trial of a novel educational booklet in primary care. Spine 24:2484–2491

Cameron D T 2000 Spinal injections: getting to the source of your pain. Hughston Health Alert 12(1):www.hughston.com/hha/a_12_1_4.htm

Cantu R C, Bailes J E, Wilberger J E 1998 Guidelines for return to contact or collision sport after a cervical spine injury. Clinics in Sports Medicine 17:137–146

Cardone D, Tallia A 2002 Joint and soft tissue injection. American Family Physician 66:283–288, 290

Carette S, Marcoux S, Truchon R et al 1991 A controlled trial of corticosteroid injections into facet joints for chronic low back pain. New England Journal of Medicine 325:1002–1007

Cherington M, Happer I, Machanic B et al 1986 Surgery for thoracic outlet syndrome may be hazardous to your health. Muscle and Nerve 9:632–634

Childs J D, Fritz J, Flynn T et al 2004 A clinical prediction rule to identify patients with low back pain most likely to benefit from spinal manipulation: a validation study. Annals of Internal Medicine 141:920–928

Cleland J 2005 Orthopaedic clinical examination: an evidence-based approach for physical therapists. WB Saunders, Philadelphia, PA

Cleland J, Childs J, McRae M et al 2005 Immediate effects of thoracic manipulation in patients with neck pain: a randomized clinical trial. Manual Therapy 10:127–135

Colachis S C, Strohm B R 1969 Effects of intermittent traction on separations of lumbar vertebrae. Archives of Physical Medicine and Rehabilitation 50:251–258

Congeni J, McCulloch J, Swanson K 1997 Lumbar spondylolysis. A study of natural progression in athletes. American Journal of Sports Medicine 25:248–253

Conley, M S, Stone M H, Nimmons M et al 1997 Specificity of resistance training responses in neck muscle size and strength. European Journal of Applied Physiology 75:443–448

Davis J W, Phreaner D L, Hoyt D B et al 1993 The etiology of missed cervical spine injuries. Journal of Trauma 34:342–346

Delitto A, Snyder-Mackler L 1990 Two theories of muscle strength augmentation using percutaneous electrical stimulation. Physical Therapy 70:158–164

Delitto A, Earhard R E, Bowling R W 1995 A treatment based classification approach to low back syndrome: identifying and staging patients for conservative treatment. Physical Therapy 6:470–489

Delport E G, Cucuzzella A R, Marley J K et al 2004 Treatment of lumbar spinal stenosis with epidural steroid injections: a retrospective outcome study. Physical Medicine and Rehabilitation 85:479–484

Derby R 1993 Precision percutaneous blocking procedures for localizing spinal pain: 1. The posterior lumbar compartment. Pain 3:89–100

Deyo R A, Diehl A K 1988 Cancer as a cause of back pain. Journal of General Internal Medicine 3:230–238

Draper D, Castel J, Castel D 1995 Rate of temperature increase in human muscle during 1 MHz and 3 MHz continuous ultrasound. Journal of Orthopaedic and Sports Physical Therapy 22:142–150

Dwyer A, Aprill C, Bogduk N 1990 Cervical zygapophyseal joint pain patterns: I. A study in normal volunteers. Spine 15:453–457

Edmond S 1993 Manipulation and mobilization extremity and spinal techniques. Mosby, St Louis, MO

Fairbank J, Couper J, Davies J et al 1980 The Oswestry Low Back Pain Disability Questionnaire. Physiotherapy 66:271–273

Fitzgerald G K, Piva S R, Irrgang J 2003 A modified NMES protocol for quad strengthening following ACL reconstruction. Journal of Orthopaedic and Sports Physical Therapy 33:492–501

Flynn T, Fritz J M, Whitman J et al 2002 A clinical prediction for classifying patients with low back pain who demonstrate short-term improvement with spinal manipulation. Spine 27:2835–2843

Franco L, Herzog A 1987 A comparative assessment of neck muscle strength and vertebral stability. Journal of Orthopaedic and Sports Physical Therapy 8:351–356.

Fritz J M 1998 Use of a classification approach to the treatment of 3 patients with low back syndrome. Physical Therapy 78:766–777

Fritz J, George S 2002 Identifying psychosocial variables in patients with acute work related low back pain: the importance of fear avoidance beliefs. Physical Therapy 82:973–983

Fritz J, Irrgang J A 2001 Comparison of a modified Oswestry Low Back Pain Disability Questionnaire and the Quebec Back Pain Disability Scale. Physical Therapy 81:776–788

Fritz J M, Hicks G E, Mishock J 2000 The role of muscle strength in low back pain. Orthopaedic Physical Therapy Clinics of North America 9:1059–1151

Fritz J M, Whitman J M, Flynn T W et al 2004 Factors related to the inability of individuals with low back pain to improve with a spinal manipulation. Physical Therapy 84:173–190

Fritz J M, Whitman J, Childs J 2005 Lumbar spine segmental mobility assessment: an examination of validity for determining intervention strategies in patients with low back pain. Archives of Physical Medicine and Rehabilitation 86:1745–1752

Fukui S, Ohseto K, Shiotani M et al 1996 Referred pain distribution of the cervical zygapophyseal joints and cervical dorsal rami. Pain 68:79–83

George S Z, Delitto A 2005 Clinical examination variables discriminate among treatment-based classification groups: a study of construct validity in patients with acute low back pain. Physical Therapy 85:306–331

George S, Fritz J, Earhard R 2001 A comparison of fear avoidance beliefs in patients with lumbar spine pain and cervical spine pain. Spine 26:2139–2145

Gerbino P, Micheli L 1995 Back injuries in the young athlete. Clinics in Sports Medicine 14:571–590

Gerrelts B D, Petersen E U, Mabry J et al 1991 Delayed diagnosis of cervical spine injuries. Journal of Trauma 31:1622–1626

Goodstadt N, Manal T 2003 High intensity electrical stimulation of the lumbar paraspinal musculature on an elite junior figure skater with chronic back pain. Paper presented at the Annual Meeting of the American Physical Therapy Association, Tampa, FL

Gotzsche P C, Johansen H K 2004 Short term low-dose corticosteroids vs placebo and nonsteroidal anti-inflammatory drugs in rheumatoid arthritis. Cochrane Database of Systematic Reviews 3:CD000189

Greenman P E 1996 Principles of manual medicine, 2nd edn. Williams and Wilkins, Baltimore, MD

Hackley D R, Wiesel S W 1993 The lumbar spin in the aging athlete. Clinics in Sports Medicine 2:191–215

Haight R, Shiple B 2001 Sideline evaluation of neck pain: when is it time for transport. Physician and Sports Medicine 29:1–15

Hains F, Waalen J, Mior S 1998 Psychometric properties of the neck disability index. Journal of Manipulative Physiological Therapeutics 21:75–80

Hardcastle P H 1993 Repair of spondylolysis in young fast bowlers. Journal of Bone and Joint Surgery (Br) 75B:398–402

Harmon K G, Hawley C 2003 Physician prescribing patterns of oral corticosteroids for musculoskeletal injuries. Journal of the American Board of Family Practice 16:209–212

Hayden J A, van Tulder M W, Tomlinson G 2005a Systematic review: strategies for using exercise therapy to improve outcomes in chronic low back pain. Annals of Internal Medicine 142:776–785

Hayden J A, van Tulder M W, Malmivaara A V et al 2005b Meta-analysis: exercise therapy for nonspecific low back pain. Annals of Internal Medicine 142:765–775

Herbert R D, Gabriel M 2002 Effects of stretching before and after exercise on muscle soreness and risk of injury: systematic review. British Medical Journal 325:468

Herskovitz S, Berger A R, Lipton R B 1995 Low-dose, short-term oral prednisone in the treatment of carpal tunnel syndrome. Neurology 45:1923–1925

Hicks G E, Fritz J M, Delitto A et al 2003 Interrater reliability of clinical examination measures for identification of lumbar segmental instability. Archives of Physical Medicine and Rehabilitation 84:1858–1864

Hicks G E, Fritz J M, Delitto A et al 2005 Preliminary development of a clinical prediction rule for determining which patients with low back pain will respond to a stabilization exercise program. Archives of Physical Medicine and Rehabilitation 86:1753–1762

Hides J A, Richardson C A, Jull G A 1996 Multifidus muscle recovery is not automatic after resolution of acute, first-episode low back pain. Spine 21:2763–2769

Hubbard D 1998 Persistent muscular pain: approaches to relieving trigger points. Journal of Musculoskeletal Medicine 15:16–26

Hubbard T J, Denegar T J 2004 Does cryotherapy improve outcomes with soft tissue injury? Journal of Athletic Training 39:278–279

Hurwitz E, Aker P, Adams A et al 1996 Manipulation and mobilization of the cervical spine: a systematic review of the literature. Spine 21:1746–1760

Jamieson W G, Chinnick B 1996 Thoracic outlet syndrome: fact or fancy? A review of 409 consecutive patients who underwent operation. Canadian Journal of Surgery 39:321–326

Johnson R 1991 Anatomy of the cervical spine and its related structures. In: Torg J S (ed) Athletic injuries to the head, neck, and face, 2nd edn. Mosby-Year Book, St Louis, MO, p 371–383

Johnson R 1998 The analgesic effects and clinical use of acupuncture-like TENS. Physical Therapy Reviews 3:73–93

Judovich B D 1955 Lumbar traction therapy – elimination of physical factors that prevent lumbar stretch. Journal of the American Medical Association 159:549–550

Kaltenborn F M 1993 The spine basic evaluation and mobilization techniques. Olaf Norlis Bokhandel, Minneapolis, MN

Keene J S, Drummond D S 1985 Mechanical back pain in the athlete. Comprehensive Therapy 11:7–14

Kim D Y, Paik N J, Han T R 2004 L5 radiculopathy caused by ossification of the ligamentum flavum: a case report. Electromyography and Clinical Neurophysiology 44:217–221

Koumantakis G A, Watson P J, Oldham J A 2005 Trunk muscle stabilization training plus general exercise versus general exercise only: randomized controlled trial of patients with recurrent low back pain. Physical Therapy 85:209–225

Kreipke D L, Gillespie K R, McCarthy M C et al 1989 Reliability of indications for cervical spine films in trauma patients. Journal of Trauma 29:1438–1439

Kulig K, Landel R, Powers C 2004 Assessment of lumbar spine kinematics using dynamic MRI: a proposed mechanism of sagittal plane motion induced by manual posterior-to-anterior mobilization. Journal of Orthopaedic and Sports Physical Therapy 34:57–64

Kvist J, Ek A, Sporrstedt K et al 2005 Fear of re-injury: a hindrance of returning to sports after ACL reconstruction. Knee Surgery, Sports Traumatology, Arthroscopy 13:393–397

Leadbetter W B 1995 Anti-inflammatory therapy in sports injury. The role of nonsteroidal drugs and corticosteroid injection. Clinics in Sports Medicine 14:353–410

Leffert R D, Gumley G 1987 The relationship between the dead arm syndrome and thoracic outlet syndrome. Clinical Orthopaedics and Related Research 223:20–31

Leggett S H, Graves J E, Pollock M L et al 1991 Quantitative assessment and training of isometric cervical extension strength. American Journal of Sports Medicine 19:653–659

Lundon K, Bolton K 2001 Structure and function of the lumbar intervetebral disk in health, aging, and pathologic conditions. Journal of Orthopaedic and Sports Physical Therapy 31:291–303

McCarthy W J, Yao J S, Schafer M F et al 1989 Upper extremity arterial injury in athletes. Journal of Vascular Surgery 9:317–327

McGill S M 1998 Low back exercises: evidence for improving exercise regimens. Physical Therapy 78:754–765

McGill S M 2001 Low back stability: from formal description to issues for performance and rehabilitation. Exercise and Sport Sciences Review 29:26–31

McGrory B J, Klassen R A, Chao E Y et al 1993 Acute fractures and dislocations of the cervical spine in children and adolescents. Journal of Bone and Joint Surgery (Am) 75A:988–995

McKee T R, Tinkoff G, Rhodes M 1990 Asymptomatic occult cervical spine fracture: case report and review of the literature. Journal of Trauma 30:623–626

Magee D J 1997 The spine in orthopedic physical assessment, 3rd edn. WB Saunders, Philadelphia, PA

Maher C, Adams R 1994 Reliability of pain and stiffness assessments in clinical manual lumbar spine examination. Physical Therapy 74:801–811

Maher C G, Latimer J, Adams R 1998a An investigation of the reliability and validity of posterioranterior spinal stiffness judgements made using a reference based protocol. Physical Therapy 78:829–837

Maher C G, Simmonds M, Adams R 1998b Therapists' conceptualization and characterization of the clinical concept of spinal stiffness. Physical Therapy 78:298–300

Manal T J 2002a Use of electrical stimulation to supplement lumbar stabilization for a figure skater following lumbar fusion. Orthopaedic Practice 14:30–32

Manal, T 2002b Electrical stimulation and lumbar strengthening with performing artists. Paper presented at the Annual Meeting of the American Physical Therapy Association

Manal T J, Claytor R 2005 The Delitto Classification Scheme and the management of lumbar-spine dysfunction. Human Kinetics 10:6–12

Manchikanti L, Boswell M, Singh V et al 2004 Prevalence of facet joint pain in chronic spinal pain of cervical, thoracic, and lumbar regions. BMC Musculoskeletal Disorders 5:1–7

Mansell J, Tierney R T, Sitler M R et al 2005 Resistance training and head–neck segment dynamic stabilization in male and female collegiate soccer players. Journal of Athletic Training 40:310–319

Mathews J A 1968 Dynamic discography: a study of lumbar traction. Annals of Physical Medicine 9:275–279

Mechanic D 1980 The experience and reporting of common physical complaints. Journal of Health and Social Behavior 21:146–155

Micheli L J, Hall J E, Miller M E 1980 Use of modified Boston brace for back injuries in athletes. American Journal of Sports Medicine 8:351–356

Micheli L Y, Wood R 1995 Back pain in young athletes. Archives of Pediatrics and Adolescent Medicine 149:15–18

Moeti P, Marchetti G 2001 Clinical outcome from mechanical intermittent cervical traction for the treatment of cervical radiculopathy: a case series. Journal of Orthopaedic and Sports Physical Therapy 31:207–213

Muschik M, Hahnel H, Robinson P N et al 1996 Competitive sports and the progression of spondylolisthesis. Journal of Pediatric Orthopedics 16:364–369

Novak C B, Mackinnon S E, Patterson G A 1993 Evaluation of patients with thoracic outlet syndrome. Journal of Hand Surgery (Am) 18A:292–299

Panjabi M, Crisco J J, Vasavada A et al 2001 Mechanical properties of the human cervical spine as shown by three dimensional load displacement curves. Spine 26:2692–2700

Pho C, Godges J 2004 Management of whiplash-associated disorder addressing thoracic and cervical spine impairments: a case report. Journal of Orthopaedic and Sports Physical Therapy 34:511–519, 520–523

Powell J, Barber-Foss K 1999 Injury patterns in selected high school sports: a review of the 1995–1997 seasons. Journal of Athletic Training 34:277–284

Rachbauer F, Sterzinger W, Eibl G 2001 Radiographic abnormalities in the thoracolumbar spine of young elite skiers. American Journal of Sports Medicine 29:446–449

Rezasoltani A, Ahmadi A, Nehzate-Khoshroh M et al 2005 Cervical muscle strength measurement in two groups of elite Greco-Roman and free style wrestlers and a group of non-athletic subjects. British Journal of Sports Medicine 39:440–443

Richardson C A, Jull G A 1995 Muscle control – pain control. What exercises would you prescribe? Manual Therapy 1:2–10

Richardson C A, Snijders C J, Hides J A et al 2002 The relation between the transversus abdominis muscles, sacroiliac joint mechanics, and low back pain. Spine 27:399–405

Rosen P R, Micheli L J, Treves S 1982 Early scintigraphic diagnosis of bone stress and fractures in athletic adolescents. Pediatrics 70:11–15

Rossi F 1988 Spondylolysis, spondylolisthesis in sports. Journal of Sports Medicine and Physical Fitness 18:317–340

Rudolph K, Axe M, Buchanan T et al 2001 Dynamic stability in the anterior cruciate ligament deficient knee. Knee Surgery, Sports Traumatology, Arthroscopy 9:62–71

Serina E R, Lieu D K 1991 Thoracic injury potential of basic competition taekwondo kicks. Journal of Biomechanics 24:951–960

Schneider J, Schmitt L, Manal T 1999 Lumbar stabilization progression for figure skaters. University of Delaware Physical Therapy Clinic and Ice Skating Science Development Center Publication, Newark, DE

Simons D G, Travell, J G, Simons L S, Cumings B D 1998 Myofascial pain and dysfunction. The trigger point manual, vol 1. Upper half of body. Lippincott Williams & Wilkins, Baltimore, MD

Sjolund B, Ternis L, Eriksson M 1977 Increased CSF of endorphins after electro-acupuncture. Acta Physiologica Scandinavica 100:382–384

Snyder-Mackler L, Ladin Z, Schepsis A A et al 1991 Electrical stimulation of the thigh muscles after reconstruction of the anterior cruciate ligament. Journal of Bone and Joint Surgery (Am) 73A:1025–1036

Snyder-Mackler L, Delitto A, Bailey S L et al 1995 Strength of the quadriceps femoris muscle and functional recovery after reconstruction of the anterior cruciate ligament. Journal of Bone and Joint Surgery (Am) 77A:1166–1173

Speer K P, Bassett F H 1990 The prolonged burner syndrome. American Journal of Sports Medicine 18:591–594

Steiner M E, Micheli L J 1985 Treatment of symptomatic spondylolysis and spondylolisthesis with the modified Boston brace. Spine 10:937–943

Sward L, Hellstrom M, Jacobsson B et al 1990 Acute injury of the vertebral ring apophysis and intervertebral disc in adolescent gymnasts. Spine 15:144–148

Sward L, Hellstrom M, Jacobsson B et al 1993 Vertebral ring apophysis injury in athletes. Is the etiology different in the thoracic and lumbar spine? American Journal of Sports Medicine 21:841–845

Swanik K A, Lephart S M, Giannantionio F P 1997 Reestablishing proprioception and neuromuscular control in the ACL-injured athlete. Journal of Sports Rehabilitation 6:182–206

Swanik K A, Lephart S M, Swanik C B et al 2002 The effects of shoulder plyometric training on proprioception and muscle performance characteristics. Journal of Shoulder and Elbow Surgery 11:579–586

Taylor J, Taylor S 1997 Psychological approaches to sports injury rehabilitation. Lippincott Williams and Wilkins, Baltimore, MD

Thomas P L 1988 Thoracic back pain in rowers and butterfly swimmers – costovertebral subluxations. British Journal of Sports Medicine 22:81

Tierney R T, Sitler M R, Swanik CB et al 2005 Gender difference in head–neck dynamic stabilization during head acceleration. Medicine and Science in Sports and Exercise 37:272–279

Torg J 1990 The epidemiologic, biomechanical, and cinematographic analysis of football induced cervical spine trauma. Journal of Athletic Training 25:147–155

Travell J, Rinzler S 1952 The myofascial genesis of pain. Postgraduate Medicine 11:425–434

Travell J G, Simons D G 1983 Myofascial pain and dysfunction. The trigger point manual. The lower extremities (vol 2). Williams and Wilkins, Baltimore, MD

Vernon H, Mior S 1991 The neck disability index: a study of reliability and validity. Journal of Manipulative and Physiological Therapeutics 14:409–415

Vlaeyen J W, Kole-Snijders A M, Boeren R G et al 1995 Fear of movement/(re)injury in chronic low back pain and its relation to behavioral performance. Pain 62:363–372

Waddell G, Newton M, Henderson I et al 1993 A Fear-Avoidance Beliefs Questionnaire (FABQ) and the role of fear-avoidance beliefs in chronic low back pain and disability. Pain 52:157–168

Waninger K 1998 On field management of potential cervical spine injury in helmeted football players: leave the helmet on! Clinical Journal of Sports Medicine 8:124–129

Weinstein S M 1998 Assessment and rehabilitation of the athlete with a 'stinger': a model for the management of noncatastrophic athletic cervical spine injury. Clinical Sports Medicine 17:127–135

White A, Panjabi M 1990 Clinical biomechanics of the spine, 2nd edn. Lippincott Williams and Wilkins, Baltimore, MD

Wier M R, Smith D S 1989 Stress reaction of the pars interarticularis leading to spondylolysis. A cause of adolescent low back pain. Journal of Adolescent Health Care 10:573–577

Wiesenfarth J, Briner W 1996 Neck injuries: urgent decisions and actions. Journal of Sports Medicine and Physical Fitness 24:78–83

Wilbourn A J 1988 Thoracic outlet syndrome surgery causing severe brachial plexopathy. Muscle and Nerve 11:66–74

Wipf J E, Deyo R A 1995 Low back pain. Medical Clinics of North America 79:231–246

Wong A, Leong C, Chen C 1992 The traction angle and cervical intervertebral separation. Spine 17:136–138

Ylinen J J, Julin M, Rezasoltani A et al 2003 Effect of training in Greco-Roman wrestling on neck strength at the elite level. Journal of Strength and Conditioning Research 17:755–759

Zylbergold R, Piper R 1985 Cervical spine disorders: a comparison of three types of traction. Spine 10:867–874

Shoulder

17

Brian J. Tovin and Jason P. Reiss

CHAPTER CONTENTS

Introduction 283
Applied anatomy and biomechanics. 283
Clinical examination 285
Principles of treatment. 290
Common sports-related injuries and management . . 296
Summary 305

Introduction

The shoulder complex is designed to achieve the greatest range of motion (ROM) with the most degrees of freedom of any joint system in the body. The excessive mobility of the shoulder at the glenohumeral and scapulothoracic joints is balanced by the stability of the acromioclavicular and sternoclavicular joints. At the glenohumeral joint, a complex ligamentous system contributes to primary stability and an elaborate musculotendinous system serves as secondary stabilizers. This support mechanism allows the shoulder to withstand large external forces, while providing enough mobility for the upper extremity to accomplish complex movement patterns. Perhaps the greatest illustration of the balance between shoulder mobility and stability occurs during sports activities, particularly during activities that require overhead movements.

This chapter will provide a general overview of the anatomy and biomechanics of the shoulder girdle, review common tests and measures performed during a physical assessment, discuss the common shoulder impairments that present to the physical therapist and provide treatment strategies for sport-specific conditions. Although specific tissue pathologies will be presented, this chapter will focus on the surrounding impairments that need to be addressed for return to function. More specifically, the emphasis will be to present general guidelines of shoulder treatment and apply them to sport-specific treatment.

Applied anatomy and biomechanics

Joint anatomy and biomechanics

The shoulder complex consists of four interdependent joints: the sternoclavicular joint (SCJ), the acromioclavicular joint (ACJ), the scapulothoracic (STJ) joint and the glenohumeral joint (GHJ). These joints work in a synergistic pattern allowing the shoulder to function through multiple planes of motion under varying degrees of stress. The shoulder girdle functions with relative stability using a complex interaction of both passive and active stabilization components. An understanding of the anatomy and biomechanics is important for accurate diagnosis of impairments contributing to patient dysfunction and disability.

Sternoclavicular joint

The SCJ is the only bony attachment between the shoulder complex and the axial skeleton. The SCJ is the articulation between the enlarged medial end of the clavicle and the superolateral portion of the manubrium of the sternum and the medial aspect of the first costal cartilage. The joint has two synovial cavities separated by a thick fibrocartilage disc, which functions as a shock absorber to forces transmitted along the clavicle and inhibits medial displacement of the clavicle against medially directed forces.

The SCJ is stabilized through the joint capsule and ligaments. The capsule completely surrounds the joint and is reinforced by the anterior and posterior sternoclavicular ligaments and by the superior interclavicular ligament. Further support is given by the extracapsular costoclavicular ligament which extends from the first rib to the medial/inferior aspect of the clavicle. The joint is rarely dislocated due to the strength of the SCJ supporting structures and sufficient stress would more likely result in fracture.

Movement at this sellar joint includes rotation in the sagittal plane, elevation and depression in the frontal plane and protraction/retraction in the transverse plane. This joint is commonly placed under compressive force through upper extremity weight bearing.

Acromioclavicular joint

The ACJ connects the clavicle to the scapula and is comprised of the anterior aspect of the acromion process and the lateral end of the clavicle. The two joint surfaces both project inferomedially, leaving the lateral clavicle superior in relation to anterior acromion process. A wedge shaped articular disc separates the superior aspect of this joint into halves, improving the congruency between the two joint surfaces.

The passive stabilizing structures of the ACJ include the acromioclavicular ligament and a weak fibrous capsule with secondary support by fibers of the upper trapezius. The ACJ is indirectly supported by two coracoclavicular ligaments, anchoring the lateral clavicle to the coracoid process of the scapula. These ligaments prevent superior displacement of the clavicle (dropping of the scapula) and also play a role in scapulohumoral rhythm by rotating the clavicle as the scapula upwardly rotates. Motion at the ACJ can be described as rotation around three axes; anterior–posterior (scapular upward/ownward rotation), transverse (scapular tipping) and vertical (scapular winging).

Scapulothoracic joint

The STJ is not a true joint because no joint capsule or articular cartilage exists on the surfaces. This articulation is comprised of the scapula and the posterior/lateral aspect of the thoracic cage and is an important dynamic component of the shoulder girdle. This joint has no ligamentous support system, relying on the muscular attachments for stability. Scapular position during a functional activity determines the orientation of the glenoid fossa to the humeral head as well as the length–tension relationship of the rotator cuff (RTC) muscles. Scapular position can be described along three axes. Tilting takes place along an axis parallel to the scapular plane, elevation and depression, and upward and downward rotation takes place along an axis perpendicular to the plane of the scapula; winging occurs along a vertical axis.

Glenohumeral joint

The GHJ is comprised of the shallow glenoid cavity of the scapula and the large humeral head which is 2–3 times the size of the glenoid cavity. The GHJ is supported through dynamic and passive restraints. Passively, the glenoid labrum forms a ring around the periphery of the glenoid and provides anchorage for the capsuloligamentous structures. The labrum contributes to stability by increasing the depth and concavity of the glenoid, and providing proprioceptive feedback contributing to dynamic control of the GHJ. The labrum also provides the concave space necessary to maintain negative pressure, preventing distraction of the joint surfaces and decreasing available translation. Damage to the labrum breaks this negative pressure seal and allows more humeral head translation (Habermeyer et al 1992, Lippitt et al 1993).

The GHJ capsule primarily contains thin and loose fibrous tissue reinforced by intrinsic ligaments, which are thickenings of the capsule and named according to their location. Anteriorly, the glenohumeral ligament (GHL) is separated into three parts: superior (SGHL), middle (MGHL) and inferior (IGHL). The IGHL is part of the inferior glenohumeral ligament complex (IGHLC) that also includes the axillary pouch and posterior glenohumeral ligament (PGHL).

An understanding of anatomical motion restraints within the shoulder in various shoulder positions is important when assessing overuse or traumatic injuries of the GHJ. The SGHL provides humeral suspension and resists inferior humeral translation and humeral external rotation (ER) below 60° of abduction. The MGHL provides restraint against ER from 0 to 90° with the greatest restraint at 45°. The IGHLC is the primary passive restraint to accessory GH movement in all positions besides full adduction. In full adduction, the SGHL and the corocohumeral ligament, found in the rotator interval, provide the primary stabilizing role. At 90° of abduction, the anterior IGHL provides resistance to anterior humeral head translation and the PGHL provides resistance to posterior translation that occurs with internal rotation (IR). Injury to the anterior IGHL at its attachment to the glenoid rim and labrum (common in sports injuries) is called a Bankhart lesion.

The site and nature of damage associated with trauma depends on the age of the subject, the direction and amount of force applied, position of the shoulder during the injury, and the rate and frequency of application of that force. The force needed to rupture the glenohumeral capsule and RTC decreases with age (Kaltsas 1983). Older subjects tend to rupture these structures, whereas younger subjects were more likely to fail at the labral osseous junction or within the labrum itself. Rupture of the RTC concurrent with dislocation of the shoulder is common in subjects over 40 years of age (Gonzalez & Lopez 1991, Neviaser et al 1988).

Muscular anatomy

Rotator cuff

The RTC consists of the tendinous portions of supraspinatus, infraspinatus, teres minor and subscapularis and is the primary dynamic restraint of the GHJ. The RTC muscles originate from the scapula and the tendons converge in a sheath of tissue surrounding the GHJ. The tendons form a nearly continuous sleeve that maintains the humeral head in the glenoid fossa.

The supraspinatus arises from the supraspinatus fossa, the infraspinatus from the infraspinatus fossa, the teres minor from the middle of the lateral border of the scapula and the infraspinatus fascia and the subscapularis from the anterior subscapularis fossa. In addition to the tendinous insertion, the infraspinatus has muscular fibers attaching directly to the posterior surgical neck of the humerus and extending inferiorly for up to 2 cm below the greater tuberosity. The subscapularis has two compartments: the upper 60% forms a collagen-rich tendon that blends MGHL and has a passive stabilizing role against anterior humeral translation; the lower 40% inserts on the humerus, just inferior to the lesser tuberosity.

A structural link exists between the RTC and the capsule, which influences stability. Muscular contraction on one side of the joint will tighten the capsular structures on the other side, providing joint compression and limiting humeral head translation. For example, contraction of the subscapularis pulls the humeral head anteriorly and creates medial rotation of the humerus. This motion results in passive lengthening and therefore tightening the posterior capsule and infraspinatus, restricting posterior translation. Conversely, active contraction of infraspinatus pulls the humeral head posteriorly and causes external rotation of the humerus. This motion prevents anterior humeral head translation by pulling the humeral head posteriorly and tightening the passive anterior stabilizing structures. If this relationship is compromised by a RTC tear, glenohumeral instability may result (Hsu et al 1997).

Long head of the biceps

The long head of biceps (LHB) also contributes to humeral head stability in addition to flexing the elbow. The LHB is intra-articular but extrasynovial, and arises from the superior labrum and supraglenoid tubercle. The tendon passes over the humeral head and leaves the GHJ via the intertubercular (bicipital) groove, between the tendons of supraspinatus and subscapularis.

The LHB is an important dynamic stabilizer of the GHJ, restricting superior migration and anteroposterior translation (Kumar et al 1989). The LHB tendon functions as a 'monorail', guiding humeral rotation, while depressing the humeral head through the rotator interval suspensory system. External rotation tightens the tendon in the floor of the groove, where stabilizing efficiency is enhanced. Both the LHB and the short head of biceps (SHB) contribute to anterior stability in lateral rotation, reducing the load on the passive inferior stabilizing structures. In extreme ranges of external rotation, the stabilizing effect becomes significant only when the inferior stabilizing mechanisms are disrupted.

Scapular stabilizers

The angle of inclination of the scapula has a significant effect on inferior stability of the GHJ, particularly with the arm adducted. An increase in scapular inclination tightens the superior capsule, with the increased upward slope of the glenoid fossa acting as a bony cam, further tightening the rotator interval structures. Altered neuromuscular control may affect the scapular position and decrease the RTC stabilizing mechanism, such that the humeral head is not maintained in the glenoid fossa.

The serratus anterior and trapezius are the primary muscles involved in scapular elevation, although their specific contribution changes as the axis of rotation moves from the root of the scapular spine to the ACJ. Alterations in function found in painful shoulders of athletes (as described below) indicate that the serratus anterior and probably the lower trapezius are the primary stabilizers of the scapulothoracic region.

The subacromial space

Common injuries of the athletic shoulder involve structures lying in the subacromial space. The subacromial space is the area between the coracoacromial arch, consisting of the anterior undersurface of the acromion and the coracoacromial ligament (CAL), and the humeral head. Located in this 9–10 mm space are the subacromial bursa, RTC tendon and the LHB. The coracoacromial arch provides a strong ceiling for the GHJ and is where the RTC tendons glide during shoulder movements. The gliding mechanism of the tendons in this space is facilitated by the subacromial bursa. These structures are vulnerable to compression with any altered mechanics caused by intrinsic or extrinsic factors. Intrinsic factors include swelling of the bursa or muscle tendons, bone spurs at the ACJ or abnormal acromial morphology. Extrinsic factors include abnormal posture, weakness of the RTC, scapular instability, impaired scapulohumoral rhythm or capsular tightness or laxity.

Clinical examination

Overview

The purpose of the clinical examination is to collect enough information in the subjective and objective assessment to guide treatment. Because different healthcare professionals focus on different aspects of treatment, the goals of the clinical examination may vary. For example, physicians may focus more on diagnosis of specific tissue pathology, while rehabilitation specialists may focus more on the relationship between tissue pathology and impairments.

Nagi (1965) presents a model that represents a continuum from tissue pathology to disability. In this model, tissue pathology may lead to impairments which may lead to dysfunction and eventually disability. When applied to the shoulder, the clinician may better understand the disablement process. For example, a RTC tear (tissue pathology) may lead to loss of ROM and strength (impairments). These impairments may limit the patient's ability to throw a baseball (dysfunction). If the patient is a professional baseball player, they may be limited in their ability to perform in his occupation (disability).

The disablement model influences both clinical examination and treatment. In medicine, a detailed history and various tests and measures are used to identify the tissue pathology or disease process associated with the presenting signs and symptoms (Guccione 1991). The first objective is to determine if a patient has a musculoskeletal condition, or suggest additional tests or referral to another health care practitioner if the findings are inconclusive. The second objective is deciding between conservative management with pharmacological therapy or rehabilitation, and surgical intervention. This decision is often based on the age of the patient, the activity level and goals of the patient and the extent of tissue injury.

Conversely, rehabilitation specialists use the clinical examination to identify the specific impairments associated with the tissue pathology or disease process (Guccione 1991). If a thorough history and review of systems indicates that the presenting condition is appropriate for conservative management, the focus of the examination for the rehabilitation specialist is assessing the cause and effect relationship between the tissue pathology and presenting impairments. Establishing this relationship will help the clinician formulate an appropriate treatment plan.

Components of the clinical examination include both a subjective and objective assessment. During the subjective assessment, the clinician will perform a review of systems and take a thorough history. The objective assessment consists of appropriate tests and measures used to confirm or rule out a diagnosis.

Subjective assessment

History and onset

A shoulder evaluation begins with a thorough history and review of systems which guides the physical examination. Because not all tests and measures are appropriate for all patients with complaints of shoulder pain and dysfunction, the physical examination should be based on the information obtained in the history. After a review of systems confirms the condition is musculoskeletal in nature, the clinician can begin to categorize information. A patient is first categorized into a macrotrauma, microtrauma or postoperative group based on the onset. A condition with sudden onset that occurs due to one specific incident usually is referred to as macrotrauma. A condition with a slow, gradual onset or an onset that occurs after an activity, such as painting or playing a sport, is classified as microtrauma.

When macrotrauma is reported in the history, the rehabilitation specialist should determine the exact mechanism,

which may help differentiate which tissue structures may be involved. For example, a patient who reports a glenohumeral dislocation should have had the appropriate tests and measures done by the physician to rule out capsular or labral pathology. If these tests were not previously done, the physical examination by the rehabilitation specialist will need to focus on ruling out significant tissue pathology. In a case where the history and physical examination suggests considerable tissue pathology, a referral back to the physician may be needed for additional imaging studies or for a surgical consultation.

The relationship between tissue pathology and impairments in patients with macrotrauma is clear. The condition usually results from external forces and not primarily from preexisting impairments. In these cases, the patient can usually describe during the subjective examination the impairments that have *resulted* from the tissue pathology or injury. Assuming that the patient is appropriate for conservative management, the rehabilitation specialist must determine a course of treatment that resolves these impairments in a manner that does not overstress the healing tissues.

When microtrauma is reported in the history, the subjective assessment may be considerably longer and more complex than patients involved in macrotrauma. The clinician must determine if the microtrauma is due to overuse, misuse, abuse, or disuse. **Overuse** in sports is performing a task with a frequency that does not allow the tissues to recover and symptoms may be due to lack of muscle strength or endurance. An example of overuse would be a tennis player practicing 3 hours a day, 5 days a week when they had been used to practicing 1 hour, 3 days a week. **Misuse** is using improper form or equipment, which may put abnormal stress on the tissue structures. An example of misuse is a tennis player having faulty mechanics when hitting a backhand or having their racquet strung too tightly. **Abuse** is having excessive force going though normal tissues. An example of abuse is running with ankle weights or swimming with hand paddles. In all of these cases, the tissues cannot accommodate the repetitiveness, force, or stress that is encountered with a specific activity. Pain in these cases can lead to disuse, which may cause associated conditions such as capsulitis.

The relationship between tissue pathology and impairments in patients with microtrauma is less clear than with macrotrauma because the patient can usually not single out a specific event. With microtrauma, the rehabilitation specialist has to discern which impairments may have *contributed* to the condition or injury. By the time patients with microtrauma present to the clinic, the primary complaint is usually pain associated with an inflammatory condition such as tendonitis, bursitis, capsulitis or arthritis. In some cases, repetitive microtrauma can lead to a tissue pathology such as RTC tear.

Often patients with microtrauma present with several impairments which may not be related to the presenting condition. For example, impingement syndrome is a condition that involves encroachment of the soft tissue structures between the acromion and greater tuberosity. Patients with impingement syndrome may have a diagnosis of specific tissue pathology that guides medical treatment, consisting of either pharmacological intervention with oral medication or injections or surgical intervention. However, this diagnosis does not guide conservative treatment because patients with impingement syndrome may present with impaired posture, impaired RTC strength, impaired neuromuscular control, instability or a tight posterior capsule. During the history, the clinician can ask specific questions that may help determine which impairments are contributing most to the impingement syndrome. The objective assessment can focus on specific tests and measures to confirm this relationship.

Description and behavior of symptoms

The subjective examination also provides information about the area, symptom description and behavior of the symptoms in patients with macrotrauma and microtrauma. This information may help the clinician identify potential sources of the symptoms. For example, a patient who points with one finger to the anterior lateral aspect of the shoulder and describes a sharp pain with overhead movements may have involvement of the subacromial region or ACJ. The physical examination would need to focus on these areas. Conversely, a patient who presents with diffuse pain throughout the shoulder and upper extremity and describes burning shooting pains may need to have a detailed evaluation of the cervical spine to rule out spinal pathology.

Other subjective information may help the rehabilitation specialist determine the appropriate amount of testing to be performed during the physical examination. The clinician should determine the level of irritability of a condition during the subjective examination. Irritability is characterized by three parameters: pain level, what it takes to provoke the symptoms and the latency or time it takes the symptoms to resolve after provocation. A highly irritable condition is determined by all three factors. For example, a patient who reports symptoms with a 7/10 pain level that are brought on with lifting the arm above 90° without a load and last for several hours, has a highly irritable condition. Conversely, a patient who reports symptoms with a 9/10 pain level that comes on with lifting 200 lb on a bench press, and last only for a few seconds, has low irritability. The rehabilitation specialist must be cautious during the physical examination of a patient with high irritability because once the symptoms are provoked results from the remaining tests and measures may be unclear.

The subjective examination for a patient who presents with an acute postoperative condition will be focused on collecting information on the history of events that led to the surgery. Important information in these cases includes specifics about the surgical procedure and contraindications.

Objective examination

The objective portion of the examination should not be a laundry list of tests and measures performed in a predetermined order. This chapter will provide the components of an objective assessment, but the clinician must determine which specific assessment tools are appropriate for each patient. As previously described, the subjective examination provides the framework of the objective examination.

The objective examination may vary for patients presenting with microtrauma, macrotrauma or postoperative conditions. The focus of tests and measures for a patient who presents with macrotrauma will be assessing the extent of tissue damage and establishing a prioritized list of impairments that have occurred as a *result* of the trauma. Conversely, the focus of tests and measures for a patient presenting with a history of microtrauma will be on determining which impairments *led* to the tissue pathology or condition. A patient who presents with an acute postoperative condition will have a limited physical examination to ensure that the healing tissues are not overstressed. Additionally, referral of pain from other sources must be ruled out if the mechanism of injury includes involvement of the cervical spine, thoracic spine or thoracic outlet.

In addition to standard tests and measures, knowledge of the biomechanical and physiological demands of a specific sport is valuable in assessment of the overhead athlete, particularly in patients with microtraumatic injuries. Many textbooks and articles have provided summaries of the biomechanics of different sports and how they relate to shoulder injuries (e.g. Andrews & Wilk 1994, Ciullo 1996). Although physical examination of the shoulder complex must include detailed evaluation of the ACJ and SCJ, the focus of this chapter will be on the scapulothoracic articulation, the subacromial space and the GHJ.

Key features in the objective assessment of the athletic shoulder are:

- Upper quarter posture
- Upper quarter screening
- Quality, control and awareness of movement patterns during active range of motion (AROM)
- Assessment of the RTC and scapular stabilizers during strength assessment
- Integrity of the passive stabilizing structures during passive range of motion (PROM)
- Integrity of the subacromial space, capsule and glenoid labrum.

Posture

In an athlete, full body postural assessment is important because of the inter-relationships between the lower quarter, trunk and core musculature, and upper quarter. Abnormal postures in these areas can influence upper quarter muscle function. However, the primary focus is on upper quarter posture including the head and neck, upper trunk and thorax, and shoulder girdle. The relationship between postural impairments in these areas and shoulder function is well documented (Ayub et al 1984, Janda 1978, Rocabado 1983). Cervicothoracic posture influences scapular position and mobility and glenohumeral mobility (Crawford & Jull 1991, Solem-Bertoff et al 1993). Patients who present with a 'forward head posture' usually have rounded shoulders, increased thoracic kyphosis, increased cervical lordosis or back bending, increased scapular protraction, and a humeral head that sits anteriorly in the glenoid fossa. Patients with these postural impairments usually have tight suboccipital and anterior chest musculature and weakness of the interscapular musculature (Janda 1978). All of these impairments can lead to altered position and mechanics in the subacromial region, contributing to impingement.

Upper quarter screening

An upper quarter screening exam is designed to assess myotomes and rule out nerve damage, muscle damage or referred symptoms from another area. The first portion of the screening is performing a break test or resisted isometric contraction to each of the myotomes. During this assessment, the examiner asks the patient to hold the arm in a specific position while resistance is applied to determine if the muscle will 'break' under a given load. The movements typically include resisted shoulder shrug, shoulder abduction/flexion, shoulder internal/external rotation, elbow flexion/extension, wrist flexion/extension and finger abduction/adduction for the hand intrinsics. The examiner should determine if the contraction is strong and painless, indicating no dysfunction. If weakness is detected along with pain, the clinician should rule out pathology of the contractile structures. Weakness detected without pain suggests either a complete tear of a contractile structure or damage to a nerve root or peripheral nerve.

During an upper quarter screen, other structures that could refer pain to the shoulder should be assessed. To rule out referral of symptoms from the cervical spine, the examiner should assess all cardinal plane motions with overpressure added to the end range. In addition, combined movement patterns should be examined, particularly in an extension quadrant where the neural foramen can encroach on a nerve root. If a patient is reporting diffuse pain over a large area of the upper extremity, thoracic outlet testing should also be administered.

Active range of motion

When observing AROM, the rehabilitation specialist should note the willingness of the patient to move into a specific pattern, as well as the quality and control of the movement pattern. Normal motor control allows a patient to dissociate movement of one body segment from another. Careful evaluation for substitution strategies and control of concentric and eccentric movements should be assessed during cardinal plane movements and at speeds and under loads that simulate a specific sports movement. When symptoms are present during active motion, the clinician should determine the relationship between impaired motor control and pain provocation. For example, a clinician may observe excessive anterior humeral head translation and poor upward scapular rotation, accompanied by pain, during active abduction. To determine the association between these two impairments and pain, the rehabilitation specialist can apply manual forces. If a posterior manual force applied to the humeral head to decrease anterior translation during this movement reduces the pain, the symptoms may be due to impaired humeral head translation. However, if this procedure fails to change the symptoms, and manually assisting upward scapular rotation during elevation helps to reduce the pain, the symptoms may be due to impaired scapulohumeral rhythm.

Passive range of motion

Passive ROM is useful for assessing noncontractile structures including the capsule, labrum and ligaments. In addition, the examiner assesses the end-feel or the resistance to movement at the end of motion. If resistance is encountered early in the range of motion, the examiner must determine if the resistance is due to active guarding or a mechanical blockage. A mechanical blockage can be from a severe capsulitis or something inside the joint that is limiting motion such as a bone fragment or torn cartilage. Descriptions of end-feels have been presented in the literature (Maitland 1991). These classifications present normal end-feels for specific joints and abnormal end-feels that suggest specific tissue pathologies.

Strength assessment

Dynamic control of the shoulder girdle is essential for high performance during sports, and strength assessment should include the glenohumeral, scapular and trunk musculature. Individuals involved in sports, particularly with overhead movements, should have a balance between the proximal stabilizing muscles and peripheral mobilizing muscles.

Muscle performance can be assessed with a manual muscle test, but subtle differences in strength may be difficult to assess. Hand held dynamometers and isokinetic dynamometers can quantify the amount of force generated by a specific muscle group. Regardless of the method, the rehabilitation specialist should assess the core and trunk musculature in addition to focusing on the shoulder girdle. Although strength for all muscles of the shoulder girdle should be examined, the primary muscle groups affecting sports performance are the RTC and scapular stabilizing muscles. In addition to rotating the humerus, the RTC stabilizes the humeral head in the glenoid fossa. More specifically, the external rotators play a key role in preventing anterior migration of the humeral head and decelerating the humerus during overhead activities. The scapular stabilizers are a key component for normal scapulohumeral rhythm, which is important for maintaining the proper length–tension relationship of the RTC muscles.

RTC strength should be assessed through resisted internal and external rotation, with the humerus in varying positions of abduction. To assess RTC integrity, the focus is on resisted abduction and external rotation. Marked weakness on both resisted abduction and lateral rotation is a strong predictor of a full thickness RTC tear (Matsen et al 1998a).

The scapular stabilizers can be evaluated in a weight-bearing or non-weight-bearing position. Weight-bearing assessment helps the clinician determine if scapular protractors, such as the serratus anterior, can stabilize the scapula against the thoracic wall. A standard progression from more easy to more difficult positions includes leaning against a wall, leaning on a table, quadruped, prone on elbows and a pushup position. Scapular protraction and retraction is assessed in each of these positions and the ability to hold the scapulae in neutral protraction is then evaluated through different stages and types of loading. If loading in a position fails to demonstrate any impairment, the assessment can be progressed to more challenging positions or demands. Failure to maintain these positions may indicate weakness of the scapular protractors and depressors.

Special tests

Subacromial space

The anatomy of the subacromial space, described earlier in this chapter, illustrates how soft tissue impingement can occur. Impingement is the common term used to describe the compression of soft tissue structures between the greater tuberosity and anterior aspect of the acromion. The most commonly involved tissues include the subacromial bursa, the supraspinatus and the LHB. The traditional impingement tests, the Neer (Neer & Welsh 1977) and Hawkins (Hawkins & Kennedy 1980) tests, use combined movements of elevation with internal rotation, but they are not designed to isolate specific structures or determine why impingement exists.

After determining that subacromial impingement is present, the rehabilitation specialist can perform additional tests to determine which structures may be involved. If a tissue is being compressed, inflammation may result and a subsequent tendonitis can be detected with resisted tests. These include:

- The supraspinatus or 'empty can test' described by Jobe & Moynes (1982) as the position in which electromyographic (EMG) activity is maximal in supraspinatus may be useful to identify specific involvement of this muscle.

- The 'reverse empty can test' loads the shoulder elevation component of LHB function. This test is predicated on the biceps' contribution to glenohumeral abduction and flexion irrespective of elbow activity (Burkhead 1990).

- Shoulder flexion added to the isometric test of elbow flexion/supination selectively loads LHB (Itoi et al 1994).

- Resisted elbow flexion through a full range, and with the shoulder in extension beyond the plane of the body, will stress the LHB. Additionally, tenderness, soft tissue changes and crepitus may be felt in the groove during the movement.

- The 'lift off test': an inability to maintain the hand off the back in the hand behind back position may indicate a tear of supscapularis (Gerber & Krushell 1991, Gerber et al 1996).

Determining why impingement is occurring, particularly for an overhead athlete, is more important to the rehabilitation specialist than determining which tissues are involved. The clinician should assess the following to determine the relationship between impairments and tissue pathology:

- Posture: to determine if the scapulohumeral relationship is altering normal arthrokinematics.

- RTC strength: to determine if the head of the humerus is being centered in the glenoid fossa.

- Motor control: to determine if normal scapulohumeral rhythm exists.

- Glenohumeral accessory motion: to determine if a tight posterior capsule is preventing posterior translation.

- Instability: to determine if impingement is secondary to instability.

Instability

Clinicians sometimes confuse hypermobility with instability. Hypermobility is excessive laxity of the primary stabilizers including the capsule and ligaments, while instability is a clinical syndrome associated with specific signs and symptoms. Individuals with hypermobility can achieve ROM beyond standard limits, without being unstable. For example, baseball pitchers can usually achieve up to 130° of external rotation, or 40° beyond normal. This feat is accomplished because of the loosening of the joint capsule and ligaments which occurs from the repetitive forces of throwing. The musculotendinous unit of the RTC acts as a secondary restraint, inhibiting excessive anterior humeral head translation and preventing a hypermobile joint from being unstable.

The onset of instability can be sudden or acquired. A sudden onset usually involves a history of trauma and dislocation. Studies indicate that the incidence of chronic instability increases with each episode of dislocation (Dines & Levinson 1995, Kvitne & Jobe 1993). The incidence of instability also rises if labral pathology, such as a Bankhart lesion, is present following a dislocation because the vacuum seal between the head of the humerus and glenoid is disrupted. Acquired instability usually occurs with overuse or misuse. The capsuloligamentous structures stretch out due to repetition combined with improper mechanics.

Several tests exist to assess shoulder hypermobility and are used in conjunction with subjective examination to infer instability. The anterior drawer test measures the range of anterior translation in different ranges of scapular plane abduction, with the arm in neutral rotation. Hypermobility is graded by the degree of humeral head translation on the glenoid. For grade I translation, the humeral head stays on the glenoid, and with grade II translation the humeral head translates on to the glenoid rim with immediate relocation. Grade III translation includes humeral head migration over the glenoid rim. Apprehension during translation may cause muscle guarding and limit the value of manual laxity tests for the shoulder (Glousman & Jobe 1996, Levy 1999, Mohtadi 1991).

The posterior drawer test more closely evaluates the primary passive restraints to posterior translation. The test involves horizontal flexion and slight medial rotation combined with a posterior translation. An alternative posterior drawer test can be undertaken in sitting, with the arm in neutral (Allingham 1996), particularly if relaxation is difficult in the supine position. The examiner may palpate a subluxation over the posterior glenoid rim if hypermobility is present.

The inferior glide or sulcus test is performed in sitting or supine (Gerber & Ganz 1984). During this test, the arm is at the side while a distraction force is applied inferiorly. The distance between the superior portion of the humeral head and the inferior aspect of the acromion is assessed. In extreme cases of multidirectional hypermobility, a large sulcus is noted in this area. However, subtle instabilities associated with overhead athletes often do not demonstrate a visible sulcus, but increased translation can be detected with palpation of the gap between the bony surfaces. Distraction can be applied to the arm in a variety of positions to determine maximum inferior translation.

An anteroinferior test provides an assessment of translation in the direction in which instability is most common (Glousman & Jobe 1996, Matsen et al 1991, 1998b, Mohtadi 1991). This test appears less prone to provocation of apprehension or muscle guarding, allowing a more consistent evaluation of range of movement and end feel. Traditional assessment of instability includes an apprehension test, where the humerus is passively abducted, externally rotated and brought into slight horizontal abduction. During this passive motion, the examiner notes the degree of apprehension, including muscle guarding and reluctance or refusal to allow the motion to continue. Apprehension can be due to pain or a feeling that the joint will sublux or dislocate so the clinician should question the patient during this maneuver to determine the difference. Patients with atraumatic instability associated with athletic overuse may not demonstrate the same apprehensive response as patients who have had a dislocation (Glousman & Jobe 1996). Pain provocation on the apprehension without true apprehension may indicate internal impingement.

Internal impingement is the compression of the supraspinatus or infraspinatus tendon into the posterosuperior labrum and a relocation test is used to make a diagnosis (Davidson et al 1995, Jobe et al 1996). During this test, the arm is placed in the same position as a supine apprehension test. During the apprehension test, the examiner places a hand on the posterior aspect of the humeral head and lifts anteriorly to provoke pain. If the pain is relieved when the examiner moves the hand to the anterior aspect of the joint and pushes posteriorly to relocate the humeral head, the test is considered positive.

Glenoid labrum

Both macrotraumatic injuries, such as dislocation, and microtraumatic injuries, such as overuse, can involve disruption to the superior portion of the labrum. Clinical diagnosis of superior labral lesions is challenging upon physical examination and is usually made with the adjunct of an MRI. Most physical examination procedures involve loading of the LHB in different positions, particularly emphasizing shoulder flexion. Because of the insertion at the superior labrum, loading the LHB will indirectly load the superior labrum, and may provoke pain in the presence of labral damage. Recently, a number of tests have been reported to assess superior labral anterior posterior (SLAP) lesions (Liu et al 1996, Mimori et al 1999, O'Brien et al 1998, Zaslav 2001):

- The 'SLAP prehension test' involves sudden medial rotation of the shoulder in 90° of forward flexion and 30° adduction. Clicking in the shoulder and/or pain radiating down the biceps tendon or in the posterior joint constitutes a positive test (Berg & Ciullo 1998). No research verification of this test was provided.

- The 'crank test' consists of medial and lateral rotation performed in maximal forward flexion with axial compression down the humeral shaft. Reproduction of a click and/or pain is considered positive (Liu et al 1996).

- 'O'Brien's active compression test' is performed in the standing position, with the humerus placed in 90° of flexion, 10–15° of horizontal adduction and medial rotation with full elbow extension (O'Brien et al 1998). The examiner applies downward resistance to the arm while the patient attempts to meet the resistance. Resistance is first applied with the forearm pronated and then with the forearm supinated while pain is assessed. In this test position, the tension on the biceps tendon is altered without altering any other load on the shoulder. Pain can indicate dysfunction of the ACJ or labral pathology, depending on location of the symptoms. Pain in the superficial aspect of the anterior lateral shoulder suggests ACJ dysfunction while pain and/or clicking deep in the GHJ suggests labral pathology.

- Mimori et al (1999) advocate a 'pain provocation test' for superior labral tears, performed in a sitting position with the arm in 90–100° of abduction and the elbow flexed to 90°. The examiner resists a biceps contraction in this position with the arm either maximally pronated or supinated. A subjective report of increased symptoms with resisted elbow flexion while the forearm is pronated is considered a positive test for labral pathology. The authors emphasized that this test was useful for SLAP lesions involving the biceps anchor, not those involving superficial fraying of the labrum.

- The 'internal rotation resistance strength test' (IRRST) consists of resisted medial and lateral rotation in a position of 90° abduction in the coronal plane and approximately 80° of lateral rotation (Zaslav 2001). Weakness with or without increased pain on medial rotation, compared with lateral rotation, is positive for intra-articular pathology with the reverse being the case for subacromial pathology.

Principles of treatment

Introduction

The foundation of establishing a treatment plan for the shoulder is having a clear understanding of the impairments, underlying tissue pathologies and resultant functional limitations. Achieving functional goals also requires knowledge of the demands placed on the shoulder during specific sports activities including the specific position, level of competition and frequency of play and practice. This knowledge will guide the rehabilitation specialist to choose exercises that place demands on the shoulder similar to those encountered with a specific sport or position. Prior to initiating a functional exercise progression, the rehabilitation specialist may first need to address soft tissue healing constraints and advance the athlete through a standard exercise program that emphasizes key principles that are similar for any overhead athlete. These exercises will establish a solid foundation to progress to a sport specific rehabilitation program.

Soft tissue healing

The soft tissue healing process which occurs following injury or surgery will guide the development of a safe and effective rehabilitation program. Knowledge of the healing process is used to create a timeline for exercise progression based on the amount of stress imposed on the injured tissues during a specific exercise (Table 17.1). While injured tissues must be protected during the early stages of healing, completely shielding injured tissues from stress can also have deleterious effects. The amount of protection is different for microtraumatic injuries with little to no tissue damage versus macrotraumatic injuries with considerable tissue damage. Additionally, the time frames for the phases of soft tissue healing may be affected by patient age, tissue condition and comorbidities. Therefore, the soft tissue healing process provides general guidelines and should be used in conjunction with a criterion-based progression. A criterion-based progression may advance or slow the rehab process based on signs, symptoms and achievement of predetermined milestones.

Most patients start in a maximum protective phase following macrotrauma or postoperative procedure to avoid overstressing healing tissues. During this phase, the patient may be splinted depending on the degree of soft tissue injury and the type of surgical procedure. The clinician should understand which movements impose the most stress on specific tissue structures. The goal during the maximum protection phase is to provide protection to the healing tissue while minimizing detrimental effects of immobilization so most patients are advanced through a program that involves controlled movements that impart minimal stress to the involved tissue. The most common shoulder pathologies that warrant protection during the healing phase include anterior capsule injuries and related stabilization procedures, posterior capsule injuries and related stabilization procedures, labral pathologies and RTC tears.

During the maximum protection phase following an anterior stabilization procedure or traumatic dislocation, rehabilitation will avoid motions that overstress the anterior capsule such as passive external rotation and any extension past the frontal plane. If surgery was performed, the clinician must know the type of surgical approach. In the case of an anterior stabilization surgery, the subscapularis is often removed and reattached to allow exposure to the joint, so resisted internal rotation is usually omitted in the early stages of rehabilitation. Conversely, resisted external rotation in the available ROM is used in the early stages because this muscle group helps maintain the humeral head centered in the glenoid fossa and when activated correctly, will reduce the stress on the anterior capsule. The period of maximum protection may vary by sport and position. For example, ROM for a baseball pitcher may be advanced more quickly because they need to have the same amount of external rotation as they did prior to surgery or they will not be able to return to their prior functional level.

During the maximum protection phase following a posterior stabilization procedure or posterior dislocation, rehabilitation will avoid motions that stress the posterior capsule. These motions include excessive internal rotation, horizontal adduction and weight-bearing through the upper extremity. The maximum protection phase for patients with labral pathology will vary according to the size and location of the tear. Patients with a Bankhart lesion or tears of the anterior labrum will follow similar restrictions as patients with anterior stabilization procedures, ensuring that the anterior capsule is protected. Patients with a posterior labral tear will follow similar restrictions as patients with posterior stabilization procedures. The one difference in patients with labral pathology occurs when a SLAP lesion is present. Because these tears often involve the attachment of the long head of the biceps, resisted elbow flexion is omitted during the maximum protection phase.

For RTC repairs, the maximum protective stage timeline varies depending on the size, location, tissue condition and operative approach. A repair that is performed arthroscopically will have less soft tissue healing than an open repair, particularly if the deltoid is resected and reattached. Using a deltoid splitting technique may reduce the maximum protection phase for the deltoid, but the same precautions are followed for the RTC repair. The shoulder is often placed in a sling with an abduction pillow to prevent avascularization to the tendon which can occur when the arm is at the side. If a patient has a massive tear or the surgeon was unable to obtain strong fixation of the tissue, active contraction of the RTC may be limited for 4–6 weeks. Patients with smaller, partial tears require less time in the maximum protective phase and may progress to a moderate restriction phase that allows ROM to tolerance, active assisted ROM activities, and submaximal RTC isometrics. In any case, the rehabilitation specialist should be in contact with

Table 17.1 Macrotrauma injury: rehabilitation phases correlated with soft tissue healing stage

Protective phase: Protect healing tissue, maintain uninvolved joint ROM and muscle strength/control	Inflammatory stage: Immediate up to 5 days Proliferation stage: 10 days–6 weeks
Intermediate phase: Impairment resolution	Proliferation stage: 10 days–6 weeks Remodeling stage: 6 weeks–12 months
Functional progression phase: Sport-specific training	Remodeling stage: 6 weeks–12 months

the surgeon to understand the type of repair and any extenuating circumstances that may alter rehabilitation progression.

Criterion-based progression between phases of rehab or within a phase is guided by pain level, achieved ROM, end-feel, quality of ROM, neuromuscular control, proprioception and strength. Although many protocols are available to guide therapists through a rehabilitation of postoperative and nonoperative injuries, understanding soft tissue healing and reason for progression from one stage to the next will enable the therapist to rationalize through individual differences of each athlete.

When planning a rehabilitation program following the protection period, the primary goal is impairment resolution without compromising fixation. Primary impairments include loss of ROM, joint mobility, strength and neuromuscular control. Secondary impairments may impact shoulder function and include postural dysfunction, loss of core strength and lower extremity flexibility restrictions. Addressing primary and secondary impairments is essential for successful return to sport. The following section outlines the essential elements needed for return to overhead sports activities.

Common impairments

In treating the athletic shoulder, common impairments include postural deviations, loss of joint mobility, loss of neuromuscular control and RTC weakness. This section will outline a variety of strategies used in treating some of the most common impairments seen in the athletic population.

Posture

A common postural deviation observed in clinical practice is the forward head, rounded shoulder posture. This posture is typically a combination of several impairments of the upper quarter including increased thoracic kyphosis, decreased cervical lordosis, protracted scapulae and internally rotated/anterior humeral head (Ayub et al 1984). Common soft tissue findings associated with this posture include restricted anterior shoulder musculature, lengthened and weak medial scapular stabilizers, tight GH posterior capsule and weak anterior cervical flexors (Janda 1978).

These postural impairments are treated through joint/soft tissue mobilization, flexibility and strengthening/stabilization exercises of the scapular retractors and deep cervical flexors. Tight anterior shoulder musculature including the pectoralis minor can be self stretched or manually stretched. Care must be taken to avoid overstretching the anterior capsule. One method that allows the anterior chest to be stretched without overstressing the anterior capsule is to apply a low load on the anterior aspects of the shoulder using cuff weights while the patient lies supine over a bolster. This position allows the scapulae to retract over the bolster so the stretch is concentrated on the anterior chest musculature (Fig. 17.1).

Joint mobility

In the overhead athlete, posterior capsule tightness often accompanies anterior shoulder laxity and should be addressed

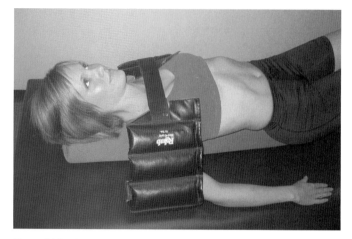

Figure 17.1 • Anterior chest stretch on bolster.

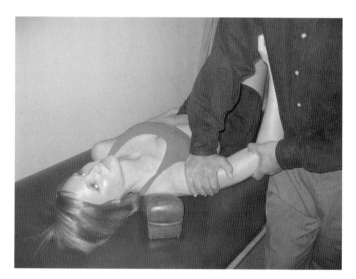

Figure 17.2 • Posterior capsule mobilization.

by the rehabilitation specialist. Posterior capsule mobilizations can be performed with the patient in supine and the shoulder blade supported in the scapular plane using a mobilization wedge or folded towel (Fig. 17.2). The clinician holds the arm in mid range abduction, applies a gentle GH distraction while placing a posterior glide to the proximal humerus. A self-stretch to the posterior capsule can also be applied by lying on the involved side with the shoulder flexed to 90°. The patient applies a self-stretch by applying a downward force to the distal forearm towards the plinth (Fig. 17.3).

Sufficient joint mobility of the SCJ and ACJ is needed for proper scapulohumeral rhythm. Hypomobility of these joints is treated with joint mobilization with the patient in a sitting or supine position. The ACJ is mobilized using a cupping grip of the shoulder with the patient in a sitting position (Fig. 17.4). The physical therapist uses one hand to stabilize the acromion and the other mobilizing the clavicle. The SCJ is mobilized either in

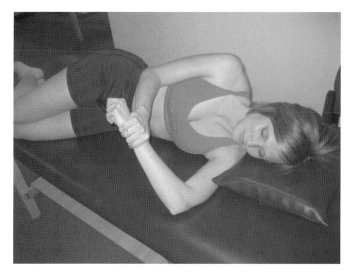

Figure 17.3 • Self-stretch to posterior capsule.

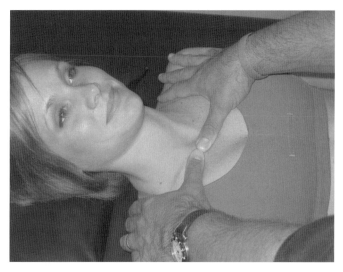

Figure 17.5 • Sternoclavicular mobilization.

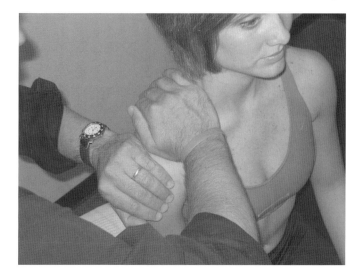

Figure 17.4 • Acromioclavicular mobilization.

an inferior medial direction or superior lateral direction using a thumb or hypothenar contact over the clavicle (Fig. 17.5).

Neuromuscular control

Scapular stability and proper scapulohumoral rhythm is essential in shoulder rehabilitation. Scapular position directly affects humeral head position and determines the length–tension relationship for the RTC as these muscles originate on the scapula (Kibler 1991). An unstable scapula or faulty movement patterns can change the demands on the RTC muscles, potentially leading to microtrauma injuries (Kibler 1998). The rehabilitation specialist should assess the muscles essential to scapular stability such as the middle and lower trapezius, serratus anterior and rhomboids. Scapular position and improper movement patterns are treated with a combination of soft tissue release and neuromuscular re-education to inhibit overactive, dominant muscle and facilitate weak or inhibited muscles.

Numerous studies have identified ideal methods of strengthening the scapular muscles (Ballantyne et al 1993, Moseley et al 1992, Townsend et al 1991). This research demonstrates that the highest activity of the middle trapezius occurs with prone rowing and horizontal abduction with ER while the greatest activity in the rhomboids occurs with prone horizontal abduction in neutral rotation and scaption in ER (Moseley 1992). Prone scapular stability exercises are assessed by the ability to recruit targeted muscles and control the movement without compensation. For prone exercises, the clinician should instruct the patient to maintain the scapula in retraction/depression while palpating the upper trapezius to ensure no compensation is occurring.

Figures 17.6–17.9 illustrate some common prone table exercises used for shoulder strengthening and scapular stabilization. The rowing motion is accomplished with humeral extension with elbow flexion (Fig. 17.6). For prone extension, the patient extends the shoulder with the elbow extended and thumb facing away from the body (Fig. 17.7). For prone horizontal abduction, the patient horizontally abducts the arm with the elbow extended and either neutral rotation or external humeral rotation (Fig. 17.8). During these exercises, the clinician should instruct the patient to retract the scapula prior to and during the humeral motion. The patient should also know not to advance the humerus beyond the plane of the body, particularly if an injury or postoperative condition warrants protection of the anterior capsule. Scapular protraction and stabilization in the protracted position are trained through a series of exercises, starting with a supine punch. The patient is positioned supine with the arm held in 90° flexion with full elbow extension and maintained in the scapular plane. During the movement, the patient is told to move the hand towards the ceiling, by protracting the scapula (Fig. 17.9). Manual resistance or weights can be added to this motion as the patient advances. These exercises may also be used in conjunction with weight-bearing exercises.

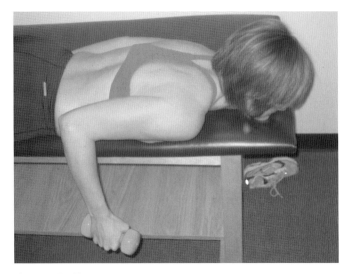

Figure 17.6 • Prone row.

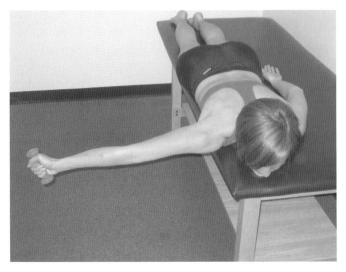

Figure 17.8 • Prone horizontal abduction with external rotation.

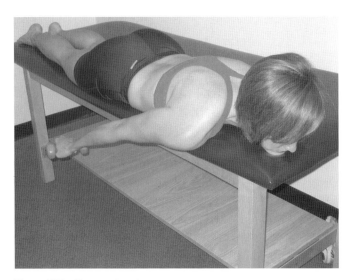

Figure 17.7 • Prone extension.

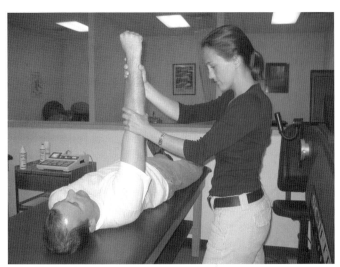

Figure 17.9 • Manually resisted scapular protraction.

Weight-bearing exercises for scapular stabilization are illustrated in Figs 17.10–17.16. Patients are advanced from prone on elbows (Fig. 17.10) to quadruped (Fig. 17.11) to a push up position (Fig. 17.12). As the patient improves, the lower extremities can be elevated to increase resistance (Fig. 17.13). A dynamic component can be added to higher level athletes who demonstrate good control with the preceding exercises. These patients can perform these exercises with the upper extremities on a wobble board (Fig. 17.14), 'walk-outs' with their upper extremities with the lower quarter on a gym ball (Fig. 17.15), or 'step-overs' using the upper extremities to 'walk' up and down over a foot stool (Fig. 17.16). A slide board is also an excellent device to use for dynamic upper extremity stabilization. Patients can be progressed from performing horizontal abduction and adduction on their knees and eventually on their toes. For these exercises, patients are instructed to maintain scapular protraction during the activity to strengthen the serratus anterior.

RTC strength

Strengthening exercises for the RTC are progressed based on the presenting condition and the ability of the patient. The range of RTC strengthening exercises may include isometric, concentric, eccentric and plyometric activities. As healing allows, shoulder strengthening is initiated with isometrics including rhythmic stabilization drills, which are exercises to challenge a patient to maintain the upper extremity in a variety of positions while the rehabilitation specialist challenges the position with manual resistance. The exercise selection should be based on positions that do not overstress the healing tissues. This activity helps restore proprioceptive feedback to the central nervous system through mechanoreceptors of the shoulder girdle and prepares the shoulder for isotonic strengthening.

Isotonic strengthening of the RTC can be accomplished with different types of resistance in different positions. Resistance

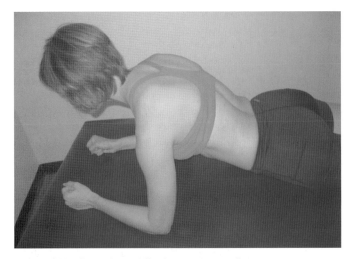

Figure 17.10 • Scapular stabilization: prone on elbows.

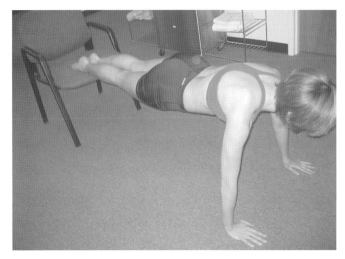

Figure 17.13 • Scapular stabilization: push-up position with elevated lower extremities.

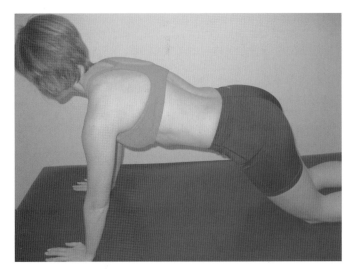

Figure 17.11 • Scapular stabilization: quadruped.

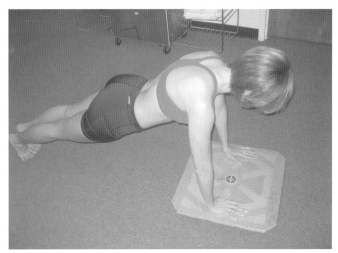

Figure 17.14 • Scapular stabilization: upper extremities on wobble board.

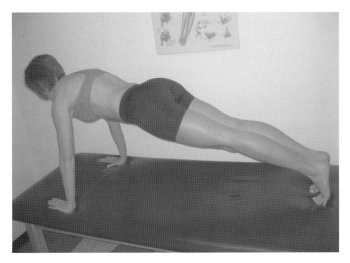

Figure 17.12 • Scapular stabilization: push-up position.

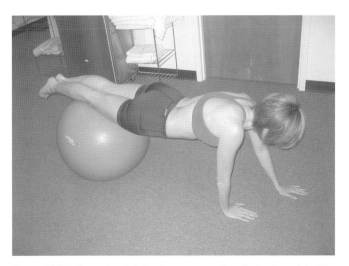

Figure 17.15 • Scapular stabilization: upper extremity 'walk-outs' with Swiss ball.

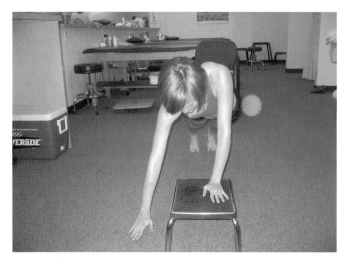

Figure 17.16 • Scapular stabilization: upper extremity 'walk-overs' using a stool.

can be applied manually, with resistive bands or with weights. The advantage of using manual resistance is that the therapist can vary the resistance to accommodate the output from the patient. The advantage of using resistive bands is that the patient can perform functional movement patterns against resistance. However, this form of resistance does not allow a clinician to quantify the amount of resistance, which is the advantage of using weights. When choosing a position for RTC strengthening, the rehabilitation specialist should have a goal for the exercise. If the goal is to fix the scapula, exercising in supine may be the best position because the scapula is stabilized against the table. Patients can be progressed to a side lying position to work against gravity or in standing position to simulate functional movement patterns. Patients should be encouraged to exercise in the scapular plane and the position of humeral abduction can advance to reproduce the position the arm is in during a specific sport.

RTC exercises are performed and advanced based on the available ROM. Due to the importance of the eccentric component of the RTC in overhead sports, this mode of exercise should be integrated into the rehabilitation program, particularly for external rotation. The infraspinatus and teres minor contract to stabilize the humeral head by maintaining a posterior pull to counter any anterior translatory forces. Devices such as 'inertia' pulleys that emphasize eccentric strengthening are incorporated into the rehabilitation program.

Common sports-related injuries and management

The shoulder is commonly injured during participation sports, particularly with overhead activities. Most injuries are attributed to microtauma rather than macrotrauma. Microtrauma is usually attributed to a combination of impairments and training errors. These training errors can be classified into overuse, misuse or abuse as described earlier in this chapter. Clinicians can usually assess the impairments based on a thorough history and physical examination. However, to gain insight into possible training errors, the rehabilitation specialist should have an understanding of the mechanics of the individual sports and training techniques. This section will review common injuries in various sports, present possible reasons for occurrence and provide treatment strategies for return to sports. These specific sports have been chosen because each presents a set of unique challenges for the rehabilitation specialist based on unique shoulder mechanics and forces at the shoulder during the activity.

Swimming

Biomechanics

Shoulder pain is the most common musculoskeletal complaint in swimming with reports of incidence of disabling shoulder pain in competitive swimmers ranging from 27 to 87% (Allegrucci et al 1994, Bak 1996, Bak & Faunø 1997, Beach et al 1992, Ciullo 1986, McMaster & Troup 1993, McMaster et al 1998, Richardson et al 1980, Stocker et al 1995). Swimming requires several different motions of the shoulder, most being performed during circumduction in clockwise and counter-clockwise directions. The following section will provide an overview of swimming mechanics related to the shoulder. For more detailed analysis of swimming biomechanics, the reader is referred to other sources (Pink & Jobe 1996, Pink et al 1991, 1992, 1993a).

The *freestyle* stroke requires a combined motion of scapular retraction and elevation, with humeral abduction and external rotation during the recovery. During the pull-through phase, the scapula is protracted while the humerus is adducted and internally rotated. Because the trunk is rotated away from the side that is beginning to pull, the shoulder avoids a true impingement position of forward flexion with internal rotation and horizontal adduction.

The *butterfly* stroke has a similar motion at the shoulder as freestyle, but the stresses are different because both arms are moved through the same motion simultaneously rather than alternating. For this reason, no trunk rotation occurs so the demand of the medial scapular stabilizers and retractors is greater with butterfly than freestyle. In addition, the humeral head moves into an impingement position at the end of recovery.

The motion at the shoulder during the *backstroke* is also similar to freestyle, but the stress at the shoulder is different and movement is in the opposite direction. Due to trunk rotation, the swimmer is rarely flat on the back during the movement, spending more time on the side. The arm position is different with the elbow extended (rather than flexed) during the recovery. During hand entry, the shoulder is in a position of full abduction and external rotation with scapular retraction, placing increased stress on the anterior capsule.

Movement at the shoulder during *breaststroke* can vary, with more motion occurring below the surface of the water than any other stroke. Like the butterfly, the arms are moved simultaneously through a motion that starts in full flexion with internal rotation. However, the elbows remain flexed during the pull-through until the humerus is fully adducted and brought into horizontal adduction with forearms touching each other. Unlike the other strokes, the hands never move below the hips so the tensile forces on the RTC that occur during the other strokes at the end of pull-thorough do not occur.

Etiology of swimmer's shoulder

The etiology of swimmer's shoulder is multifactorial and usually presents as subacromial impingement involving the RTC tendon, bicipital tendon or subacromial bursa (Bak & Faunø 1997). Primary subacromial impingement may occur in swimmers due to a tight posterior capsule, causing the humeral head to migrate anteriorly, or due to abnormal acromial morphology. The more common cause of impingement in swimmers is due to the prevalence of glenohumeral hyperlaxity that can lead to instability. Secondary impingement due to instability develops through a series of events.

The mechanism of secondary impingement usually starts with a swimmer that has increased anterior glenohumeral laxity. Shoulder ROM in swimmers is similar to that of overhead athletes, with excessive external rotation and limited internal rotation. This shift in ROM towards greater external rotation ROM is adjustment to the demands on the GHJ which goes through approximately 4000 strokes daily (Allegrucci et al 1994). The acquired anterior laxity permits excessive external rotation, but places greater demand on the RTC and the LHB to reduce humeral head elevation and anterior translation. Loss of the ability of these muscle groups and the scapular stabilizers to maintain the humeral head in the glenoid fossa, can lead to instability and secondary impingement.

Another proposed impingement mechanism involves the microvasculature of the RTC. Studies indicate that when the shoulder is abducted, the vessels of the supraspinatus and LHB are filled. Conversely, when the arm is adducted and at the side, the vascular system to these tendons is compromised (Rathbun & McNab 1970). This phenomenon is referred to as a 'wringing out' of the tendon, causing a temporary avascular zone 1 cm proximal to the insertion on the humeral head. This response also occurs when the humerus is adducted and flexed, a position that occurs with faulty mechanics or muscle fatigue.

Research has documented changes in muscle activity that occurs in swimmers with painful shoulders compared with swimmers with healthy shoulders (Bak & Magnusson 1997, Perry et al 1992, Pink et al 1993b). The proposed sequence of events for the development of swimmer's shoulder initiates with the onset of muscle fatigue. For example, the serratus anterior in the healthy shoulder stabilizes the scapula in upward rotation and protraction, creating adequate subacromial space for the biceps tendon and RTC and maintaining good approximation between the humeral head and the glenoid fossa. During the pulling motion of swimming, the serratus anterior effectively reverses origin and insertion to propel the body over the arm, while maintaining the subacromial space and joint GHJ congruency. When the serratus anterior becomes fatigued, the scapula fails to protract and upwardly rotate and the subacromial space is compromised. Additionally, the space between the humeral head and glenoid increases, contributing to more laxity.

Symptoms that develop as a result of fatigue can also affect stroke mechanics (Perry et al 1992, Pink et al 1993b, Scovazzo et al 1991). Many swimmers will inherently adjust their stroke to avoid painful movement patterns. For example, during early pull-through, the hand usually enters the water close to the midline with the elbow above the surface of the water. The upper extremity then continues to 'reach' forward below the surface of the water towards the midline of the body. In swimmers with painful shoulders, the hand enters further away from the midline with the elbow dropped closer to the surface of the water. This change is usually made to avoid an impingement position of full elevation with internal rotation and horizontal adduction. Another adjustment occurs at the end of the pull-through phase, when the hand should be close to the thigh with internal rotation of the shoulder but instead externally rotated and the pull-through phase shortened to avoid impingement.

Treatment strategies

Resolve impairments

The first step in addressing swimmers shoulders is to address any impairment. Because the clinical presentation usually involves pain related to inflammation, initial treatments may use modalities and manual techniques, such as grade I or II mobilizations, to address pain (Maitland 1991). As pain resolves, the rehabilitation specialist should prioritize the problem list related to the symptoms. Potential common impairments that need to be addressed are a tight posterior capsule, tight anterior chest musculature, hypomobility of the thoracic spine and impaired strength and endurance of the RTC and scapular stabilizers.

Address training errors

Overuse is a classic training error that occurs in swimming as athletes typically train 10–12 hours per week in the water in addition to dry-land training (Shapiro 2001). Swimmers can average 10 000 yards per day of training. The high level of repetitions, estimated at 4000 strokes per side, that occur during training sessions can cause fatigue, leading to the conditions discussed earlier. Modification of swim yardage may need to be emphasized if the swimmer wants to prevent an injury from getting worse.

Abuse is another training error that can occur in swimming, causing increased external stress on the shoulder. The use of hand paddles increases stress on the upper extremity by increasing surface area and resistance to movement. Kickboards put the arm in a position of full elevation and internal rotation, leading to subacromial joint compression. Use of these devices should be omitted or limited for a swimmer returning from a shoulder injury.

Misuse in swimming occurs if an individual has faulty stroke mechanics. An example of improper technique is when the hand crosses the mid-line during the pull-through phases of the freestyle stroke. This motion is common in swimmers who have excessive body roll and can predispose them to impingement. Optimal body roll allows the arm to stay close to the plane of the scapula, thus reducing the stress of soft tissue structures in the anterior shoulder region. Optimal body roll also allows greater lengthening of the oblique abdominal muscles, shoulder adductors/medial rotators and scapular retractors so that at the beginning of the pull-through, these muscles have a mechanical advantage. Conversely, a lack of adequate body roll forces the recovering arm into a greater range of shoulder extension, hori-zontal abduction, and medial rotation in order to clear the hand from the water, causing encroachment of the subacromial space.

An important issue to consider when working with swimmers is their reluctance to stay out of the water. Although swimmers are involved in dry-land training, no suitable substitute exists for swimming. Modification of training schedules and techniques allow the patient to continue swimming, enabling the physical therapist to establish or maintain credibility with the swimmer. In extreme cases, the swimmer may need a short dry-land period to allow for adequate soft tissue healing. In these cases, the rehabilitation specialist should educate the swimmer so that the reason for the lay-off is understood. Time spent out of the water should be kept as short as possible, even if the swimmer is doing primarily kicking activities. Although returning to the water may not be ideal for rehabilitation, keeping a swimmer out of the water for a lengthy period may result in a rehabilitation program that is ignored. Activity modification in swimming may consist of the following tasks:

- Temporarily reduce training distance and frequency
- Alter training patterns so that different strokes are used more frequently throughout the practice. This alteration will reduce the repetitive pattern at the glenohumeral and allow the muscles to function differently
- Avoid the use of hand paddles, kickboards, and surgical tubing.
- Use swim fins to enhance the propulsion from the legs and reduce the stress on the shoulder
- Technique modification to eliminate inappropriate stresses to the tissues.

Throwing

Biomechanics

To understand the specific etiology of these microtraumatic conditions, the rehabilitation specialist should understand the basic biomechanics of throwing. For a more detailed analysis of throwing biomechanics, the reader is referred to other sources (Andrews & Wilk 1994, DiGiovine et al 1992, Fleisig et al 1995, Jobe et al 1983, 1984). Throwing has six components: windup, stride, arm cocking, arm acceleration, arm deceleration and follow-through (Dillman et al 1993). The windup is the initial movement used to prepare the body for energy transfer from the lower extremity and trunk to the upper thorax and upper extremity. The stride is the movement of the contralateral lower extremity towards home plate and finishes when the foot is planted on the ground. At the end of this phase, the arm is in a cocked position prepared for acceleration. After arm cocking, the upper extremity accelerates through ball release, and than decelerates rapidly before follow-through. The shoulder is vulnerable to injury when the foot hits the ground in the cocking phase. The deceleration phase is another point in the pitching cycle where injuries occur due to the eccentric demand on the RTC and biceps musculature.

The foot position at the end of the stride should be almost in line with the rearfoot and the foot should be pointed slightly in. If the stride leg lands across the midline of the body, the hips will not have full rotation and the pitcher will not have optimal energy transfer from the lower extremity. As a result, the pitcher 'throws across the body' which can lead to subcoracoid impingement during follow-through (Gerber & Sebesta 2000, Gerber et al 1987). Conversely, if the stride leg lands away from the midline, the hips will rotate too early and lack the proper energy transfer from the lower extremities. In this case, where the pitcher is too 'open', the humerus is left behind the plane of the scapula and excessive stress is placed on the anterior capsule. In addition to normal mechanics, the throwing athlete should have excellent dynamic stabilizers to avoid injury.

Etiology of common throwing injuries

Microtraumatic injuries related to throwing occur due to the combination of excessive ROM, high compressive and translatory forces, rapid acceleration/deceleration and ballistic movement patterns. Jobe & Pink (1993) proposed a continuum of shoulder injuries in the overhead athlete to provide insight to the relationship between impairments, throwing biomechanics and tissue pathology. This classification scheme consists of four groups, with the first three being microtraumatic. Group I consists of older patients with isolated impingement and no instability, but no reason for the impingement is presented. Underlying impairments in this group may be a tight posterior capsule, poor neuromuscular control including RTC weakness or abnormal acromial morphology. Group II includes young patients with impingement secondary to instability. This group has acquired laxity and may also have poor neuromuscular control. Group III is also young patients who have generalized ligamentous laxity in various joints, which is most likely congenital. Group IV is instability attributed to macrotrauma, such as a dislocation. The criticism of this classification system is that the groups do not represent all injuries with the overhead athlete so others have elaborated on this classification system (Meister 2000, Meister & Andrews 1993).

As with swimming, microtrauma usually initiates with fatigue of the dynamic stabilizers of the shoulder girdle. If dynamic stabilizers are not functioning properly, increased stress is placed on the glenoid labrum and anterior capsule at the end of the cocking phase and beginning of the acceleration phase, while increased stress is placed on the posterior capsule and labrum during deceleration of follow through. As a result of poor stabilization at the GHJ, various tensile and compressive injuries may result.

Tensile injuries occur as a result of failure of the muscles to stabilize the GHJ in the presence of increased laxity. The initial injuries may be inflammation of the biceps tendon, RTC and joint capsule. Repetitive tensile stress may eventually lead to tendon failure or labral pathology. Increased tensile stresses on the posterior band of the inferior glenohumeral ligament that occurs during deceleration can lead to exostosis of posterior inferior border of the glenoid labrum, referred to as a Bennett's lesion (Meister et al 1999). This lesion can also lead to tearing of the posterior labrum and posterior RTC.

Tensile stress on the biceps tendon can lead to tendonitis and excessive pulling at the insertion on the labrum. Excessive stress from the biceps tendon and humeral head translation can lead to a SLAP lesion of the labrum. A deceleration mechanism has been proposed for biceps anchor tears, associated with the large forces transmitted via the biceps tendon to the superior labrum as the muscle contracts eccentrically to decelerate the elbow (Andrews et al 1985, 1991, McLeod & Andrews 1986). However, other research suggests that posterior SLAP lesion is more likely to occur during late cocking rather than during deceleration (Kuhn et al 2000).

The biceps tendon plays a key role in preventing excessive superior humeral head migration (Kumar et al 1989). The biceps tendon provides compression of the humeral head in the glenoid fossa when the shoulder is in an abducted externally rotated position, limiting torsional forces (Meister 2000). Loss of the biceps anchor mechanism may result in increased strain on the IGHLC. Increased activity in the biceps reported in unstable shoulders is hypothesized to be an attempt to compensate for the loss of passive restraints (Glousman 1993).

RTC pathology usually develops from compressive forces caused by primary impingement or secondary impingement from instability (Glousman & Jobe 1996). Primary impingement is compression of the structures in the subacromial space and occurs from a tight posterior capsule or abnormal acromial morphology. Throwing athletes usually have hyperlaxity of the GHJ so impingement often has a component of instability. Inflammation from impingement may lead to fraying of the tendon and eventually RTC tears. Internal impingement is compression of the undersurface of the RTC on the posterosuperior glenoid, which occurs when excessive anterior translation of the humeral head occurs at the end of external rotation.

A different mechanism of internal impingement has been proposed, based on the loss of internal rotation in throwing athletes, leading to labral pathology (Burkhart et al 2000). In this model, associated tightness in the posterior capsule causes a shift of the axis of humeral rotation. External rotation results in increased contact between the RTC and labrum and increased forces at the posterosuperior biceps–labral attachment. Although the authors are adamant that the primary lesion is loss of medial rotation and that evidence of antero-inferior laxity is 'pseudolaxity' associated with disruption of the superior labrum rather than capsular laxity, each mechanism may occur in different patients.

The clinical presentation of the thrower's shoulder may vary. The thrower with internal impingement may complain of posterior shoulder pain with loss of control associated with early ball release secondary to painful loss of external rotation (Meister 2000). Episodes of clicking or clunking may be reported related to labral pathology (Andrews et al 1991) and a sensation of 'looseness' associated with instability (Allen & Warner 1995). The term 'dead arm' syndrome is used to describe the symptoms associated with recurrent transient anterior subluxation during throwing (Burkhart et al 2000, Rowe 1987, Rowe & Zarins 1981). Burkhart et al (2000, p. 126) redefined the 'dead arm' as a 'pathologic shoulder condition in which the thrower is unable to throw with his preinjury velocity and control because of a combination of pain and subjective unease in the shoulder'. Transient neurological symptoms may also be a component of the problem (Allen & Warner 1995, Rowe & Zarins 1981).

Treatment strategies

Resolve impairments

The throwing athlete may present with impaired joint mobility, muscle performance or motor control. When assessing these impairments, the clinician should consider the entire kinetic chain as throwing is a complex motion that involves mobility and muscle performance at the lower extremities, pelvic girdle, trunk and thorax, as well as the shoulder girdle. Common impairments that may be missed beyond the shoulder girdle include impaired joint mobility of the thoracolumbar spine, pelvic girdle and hips. Impaired muscle flexibility may be detected in the anterior chest musculature, hamstrings, hip flexors and adductors. Tightness of these muscle groups may affect throwing mechanics. When assessing strength and motor control beyond the shoulder girdle, the rehabilitation specialist should evaluate the lower extremities, pelvic girdle and core stabilizers. Once these potential impairments are addressed, the clinician can focus on the shoulder girdle and the common impairments that directly influence throwing mechanics.

Common impairments at the shoulder girdle include anterior chest tightness, posterior capsule restriction, decreased thoracic spine mobility and weakness or poor motor control of the RTC and scapular stabilizers. Treating soft tissue restriction of the anterior chest may be challenging if the clinician is also trying to protect the anterior GHJ capsule. Many stretches for the anterior chest musculature consist of pulling the arms back into retraction and horizontal abduction, causing stress to the anterior shoulder. One solution is to use the technique described earlier in this chapter, where the athlete lies supine over a bolster with weights applied to the anterior shoulder, pushing posteriorly (Fig. 17.1). Treating thoracic spine hypomobility is accomplished through joint mobilization procedures. To obtain full scapular retraction, the thoracic spine has to extend or backward bend. Figures 17.17 and 17.18

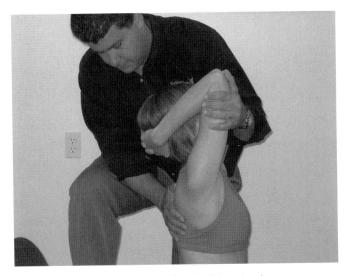

Figure 17.17 • Thoracic spine mobilization into extension.

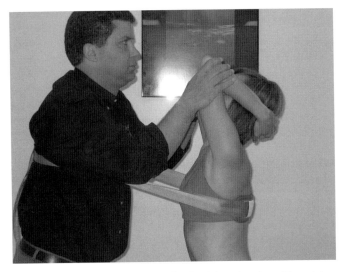

Figure 17.18 • Thoracic spine mobilization into extension with assistance of a belt.

show two different methods of mobilizing the thoracic spine into extension. Treatment for posterior capsule tightness may involve stretching or mobilization techniques presented earlier in the chapter.

Once the secondary impairments are addressed, the key for successful rehabilitation of the throwing athlete is strengthening and motor control of the shoulder girdle muscles. The primary emphasis is on the muscle groups that control the arm during throwing. Most stress on the shoulder occurs at the end range of cocking and during the follow-through phases, when muscles have to work eccentrically. The dynamic stabilizers of the GHJ during these phases are the RTC, scapular stabilizers, LHB and latissimus dorsi. During the later stages of rehabilitation, the goal is to incorporate exercises that simulate the forces encountered during a throwing motion. Exercises that incorporate stretch-shortening drills that rely on eccentric muscle control are the key element for functional strengthening of

the throwing athlete (Wilk & Voight 1994, Wilk et al 1993). These exercises combine strength, proprioception and neuromuscular control. Some examples include throwing and catching medicine balls with the physical therapist, throwing against a rebounding device or dribbling a ball against a wall.

Many training errors in the throwing athlete can be addressed through proper mechanics and activity modification. *Overuse* in baseball can be carefully controlled by tracking the pitch-count of the athlete. Although some youth organizations may limit the number of innings pitched per week, the number of pitches thrown during those innings can vary a great deal. The recommended pitch count for athletes under 15 years old is 75 per game and 600 per season. Various throwing programs have been presented to adequately develop the shoulder musculature in young pitchers and prevent injuries (Axe et al 1996).

Abuse can occur in the throwing athlete in different ways. Although a pitch count may be controlled, the type of pitches may have deleterious effects on the shoulder particularly in younger athletes. Some experts suggest that a limit should be placed on the number of curve balls thrown during a game because of increased stress to the upper extremity during this motion. Throwing at high speeds without an adequate warm-up period or with lack of eccentric stabilization can also lead to injury.

Misuse in throwing may be hard to detect without a trained eye or understanding of throwing biomechanics. Altered mechanics in stride length, foot placement, hip/trunk rotation and upper extremity position can lead to increased stress on the shoulder and potential injury. Upon return to throwing activities, the rehabilitation specialist should observe throwing mechanics.

Diving injuries

Biomechanics of diving

Competitive diving consists of 1 m and 3 m springboard events and a 10 m platform event (O'Brien 1992). When learning a new dive or warming up for the 10 m platform, divers perform 'lead-ups' at lower heights of 1, 3, 5 and 7 m. Six different types of dive groups are used in competition. The first four groups are classified based on the position the diver is in when leaving the board or platform. In a *forward* dive, the diver is facing the front of the board or platform and dives or spins towards the water. In a *backward* dive, the diver stands at the end of the board or platform and faces inward towards the back of the board and dives or spins with the back towards the water. A *reverse* or *gainer* dive begins the same way as a forward dive, but after the diver leaves the board or platform, the rotation of the dive is back towards the board. An *inward* dive starts the same way as a backward dive, but after the diver leaves the board or platform the dive rotates toward the board. The fifth group is comprised of dives that include a *twisting* component. The sixth group is only used for platform diving and includes dives beginning in an *armstand* position.

Diving components include the approach/hurdle, press/take-off, flight and entry (O'Brien 1992). Diving injuries can occur from a variety of factors, but the predominant cause is the high forces encountered when hitting the water during entry. Because divers can reach speeds of 35 mph before hitting the water (Kimball et al 1985), diving can be classified as a contact sport. The shoulder is the most commonly injured joint in competitive diving (Kimball et al 1985). One reason is the balance of shoulder mobility and stability needed for the sport. Divers need to achieve full humeral and scapular elevation at entry while maintaining stability to withstand external forces at entry. The development of a diver's shoulder is mutifactorial.

Etiology of common diving injuries

Shoulder injuries occur in diving usually as a result of fatigue of the stabilizing muscles around the shoulder girdle (Tovin & Neyer 2001). The primary stabilizing muscles include the scapular upward rotators, RTC and triceps. During entry, the scapular elevators and upward rotators stabilize the scapula, the RTC stabilizes the humeral head in the glenoid fossa and the triceps maintains elbow extension needed for proper entry. Failure of these muscle groups can lead to excessive stress on the static stabilizers, resulting in increased laxity of the capsuloligamentous system and possible instability.

Diving can cause excessive compressive forces at the GHJ. These compressive forces can lead to subacromial impingement and labral pathology. If glenohumeral instability is present, excessive humeral head translation can also put sheer forces across the labrum, while increasing tensile stress on the RTC and biceps tendons. Resulting injuries could be a SLAP lesion and tendonopathy, which are common shoulder injuries in divers.

Faulty mechanics can also lead to shoulder injuries in divers. Excessive stress usually occurs when divers 'miss' their hands upon entry and cannot place the upper extremities into the proper position. A similar fault occurs when a diver attempts to 'save' a dive, a technique used in flight to adjust position when a diver knows the dive will be 'short' (under rotated or short of vertical). To prevent appearing short to the judges upon entry, the diver will reach the arms posteriorly to the head and neck (Fig. 17.19). This position places increased stress on the anterior capsule and may result in glenohumeral dislocation.

A training device commonly used in diving, referred to as a 'bubbler', can lead to injury if not operated properly. This equipment is an air sparging system that operates in the water and uses a compressor to produce a combination of air and water creating turbulent bubbles at the surface. Use of this device breaks the surface tension of the water by 80%, providing a 'softer' surface for the divers. The turbulence should be adjusted to the height of the dive and size of diver. The turbulence should be turned off as the diver leaves the board to prevent excessive upward force from the water. The machine is ideal for learning a new dive, but can be detrimental for divers entering the water in a vertical position if not used correctly.

Treatment strategies

Address impairments

In addition to traditional shoulder strengthening methods, divers need to have exercises that emphasize achieving strength

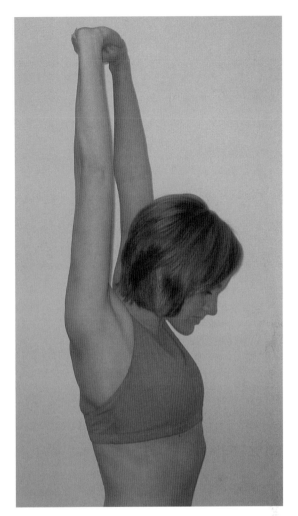

Figure 17.19 • Faulty position of the head and upper extremities when attempting to 'save' a dive.

and ROM in positions that simulate diving. Full upper extremity and scapular elevation with upward rotation is needed at entry to ensure the diver is in a streamline position. To achieve this position, divers also need to have adequate flexibility of the anterior chest musculature, glenohumeral mobility and extension of the thoracic spine. Stretching and joint mobilization techniques can address these potential impairments. Resistive tubing is an ideal way to provide resistance to the upper extremities to simulate elevation of the arms from neutral to full elevation (Fig. 17.20).

Address training errors

Overuse in diving may occur from performing too many dives in a practice or too many practices in a week, particularly from the 10 m platform where impact forces exceed 2.0 g. Age group divers should have their dive count limited depending on their age and ability, and the height of dives. *Abuse* in diving may be defined as excessive forces going through the shoulder in a practice. Forces increase with height and may be affected by the use of training devices such as the 'bubbler'. In these cases, injury may not be due to the number of repetitions (overuse), but the

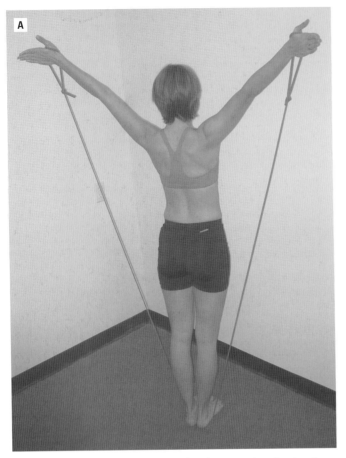 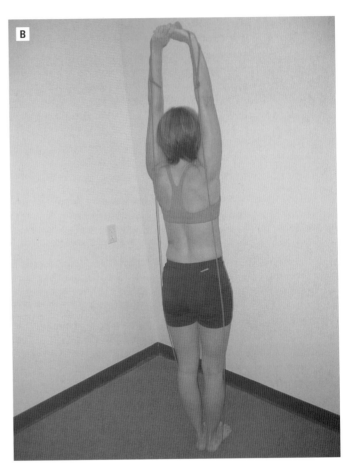

Figure 17.20 • A: Start position for resisted upper extremity elevation reproducing diving movement. **B:** Finish position simulating upper extremity position at entry.

dive height. Divers who are less advanced should be limited to simple dives at heights of 3 m and above. *Misuse* can lead to shoulder injuries when dive mechanics are flawed. The primary mechanical faults are an inability to attain a 'lock out' position (Fig. 17.21) with the upper extremities or failure to keep the head and neck in line with the upper extremities (Fig. 17.19).

Different strategies exist to facilitate a return to diving after shoulder injury. The first is to emphasize dry-land training to avoid impact forces. Divers can train with a bungee cord device attached to a metal ring that allows the divers to spin and rotate. This apparatus is attached to a spotting belt so the coach can control the dive in the air from a trampoline or dry-land diving board. Another strategy is to use feet-first entries when the diver returns to the water. A final strategy is to progress slowly from 1 m boards to higher levels and advance over several days or weeks based on symptoms.

Volleyball

Biomechanics

Volleyball consists of six different movements: serving, digging, passing, setting, spiking and blocking (Drexler et al 2001). Of these motions, only serving and spiking require quick acceleration/deceleration movement patterns at the shoulder and will be the only components reviewed in this section. For additional information on volleyball mechanics, the reader is referred to Drexler et al (2001).

The act of spiking, or hitting the ball downward, is similar to overhead throwing. A spike consists of different phases including the approach, takeoff, cocking, acceleration, contact, follow-through and landing. The shoulder is vulnerable during the middle phases of cocking, acceleration, contact and follow-through. During these phases the shoulder advances in a whipping motion from abduction and external rotation with elbow flexion to extension, adduction and internal rotation with elbow extension. Proper hitting mechanics are dependent upon synchronous movements of other body parts. For example, during the cocking phase the thoracolumbar spine must extend and rotate towards the spiking upper extremity while the contralateral upper extremity is also flexed and abducted with the elbow extended. The acceleration movement is initiated by the non-hitting extremity moving into extension and adduction while the trunk moves into counter-rotation. During contact, the hitting extremity should be in extension at the elbow and shoulder to maximize the moment arm of the limb

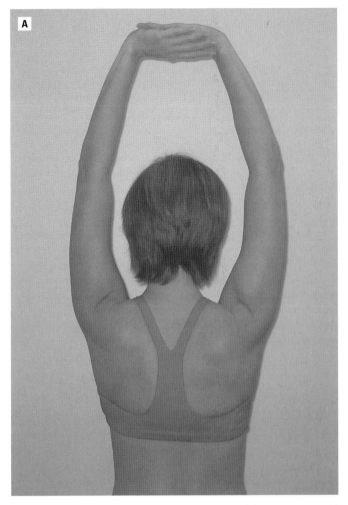 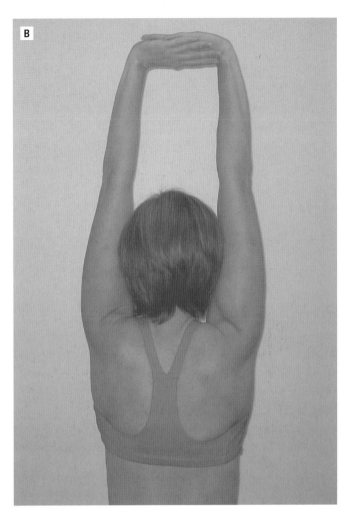

Figure 17.21 • Moving into the 'lockout' position of the upper extremities illustrating full upper extremity elevation and full scapular elevation with upward rotation (note position change from **A** to **B**).

and increase velocity. If contact is made prior to attaining this position, excessive stress may be imparted on the elbow and shoulder.

Serving is another overhead motion that can lead to shoulder dysfunction in volleyball players. This motion is similar to spiking a ball, but the wrist does not rapidly flex or 'snap' the ball and the arm is rapidly decelerated with little to no follow-through. By terminating the follow-through, the player is able to 'float' the ball causing more side-to-side movement in the air and a more difficult return. This serving motion places increased stress on the posterior RTC.

Etiology of volleyball shoulder injuries

Volleyball has progressed into an explosive game where ball speeds can reach 80–90 mph (Drexler et al 2001). Unlike other overhead sports such as baseball, the arm during a volleyball serve makes contact with a ball at the peak of acceleration causing more stress to the shoulder. Much of the success of a volleyball player is determined by the ability to spike and

serve. This emphasis results in increased practice of this overhead activity and it is estimated that an athlete practicing and playing 16–20 hours per week may perform as many as 40 000 spikes per year.

To accommodate this motion, the athlete needs to have excessive external rotation and scapular retraction. Although baseball pitchers are encouraged not to bring the humerus beyond the scapular plane in horizontal abduction, volleyball players often move into excessive horizontal abduction with shoulder abduction and external rotation to generate a forceful hit. This motion puts increased stress on the anterior shoulder capsule. Over time, anterior glenohumeral laxity may result. If the posterior RTC is unable to maintain the head of the humerus posteriorly, instability may result.

Another difference between volleyball and throwing sports is the rapid deceleration that occurs after contacting a ball when serving. This quick deceleration that stops the upper extremity without a follow-through puts great strain on the posterior cuff, particularly the infraspinatus. This mechanism can lead to a traction injury of the suprascapular nerve at the myoneural junction, suprascapular notch or spinoglenoid notch (Ferretti et al 1987, 1998, Holzgraefe et al 1994, Sandow & Ilac 1998). External rotation strength should be assessed during preseason physicals and signs of neuropathy, such as atrophy, should be noted.

Another mechanism of injury may be due to increased stress on the shoulder due to lack of strength or mobility at the trunk. Approximately 85% of the force required to spike a ball is generated from the legs and trunk (Drexler et al 2001). Therefore, optimal shoulder function is dependent on the synchronous movement patterns and strength generated at the lower extremities, hips and trunk. If this system is compromised, excessive forces may be imposed on the shoulder. For example, if a player cannot extend the thoracolumbar spine enough to generate force for spiking, the shoulder may need to compensate by moving further into scapular retraction and external rotation.

Treatment strategies

Address impairments

In addition to traditional shoulder strengthening methods, volleyball players need to have exercises that emphasize achieving strength and ROM in positions that simulate volleyball. The mechanics of overhead activities taking place in volleyball involve several motions directly tied to the shoulder including thoracolumbar extension and rotation, scapular retraction, horizontal abduction of the humerus and external rotation. To achieve this position, players need to have adequate flexibility of the anterior chest musculature, glenohumeral mobility and good mobility of the thoracolumbar spine. Stretching and joint mobilization techniques can address these potential impairments.

Once the secondary impairments are addressed, the key for successful rehabilitation of a volleyball player is strengthening and motor control of the shoulder girdle muscles. The primary emphasis is on the muscle groups that control the arm during spiking and serving. Resistive tubing is an ideal way to provide resistance to the upper extremities to simulate these motions. Most stress on the shoulder occurs at the contact phase and during the follow through phases, when muscles have to work eccentrically. The dynamic stabilizers of the GHJ during these phases are the RTC, scapular stabilizers, LHB and latissimus dorsi. Many of the exercises that are used for the throwing athlete can be used for volleyball players. One component that must be emphasized is eccentric loading of the external rotators, as these simulate the quick deceleration and stop that occurs after making contact with the ball while serving.

Address training errors

Overuse in volleyball may occur from performing too many spikes or serves in a practice or too many practices in a week. Athletes may need to limit these activities to prevent microtrauma injuries to the shoulder. *Abuse* in volleyball is not very common as training devices are not used as widely as with other sports. *Misuse* can lead to shoulder injuries when spiking or serving mechanics are flawed. The primary mechanical faults are moving the humerus beyond the plane of the body during spiking or serving. Different strategies exist to facilitate a return to volleyball after shoulder injury. The primary goal is to decrease spiking and serving, the activities that place the most stress on the shoulder.

Tennis and other racket sports

Biomechanics

Tennis is made up of three primary movement patterns: forehand, backhand and serve. These strokes can vary as some players use a two-handed backhand or forehand. The forehand and backhand are comprised of three phases including the backswing, contact and follow-through. The tennis serve may vary in mechanics, but consists of four primary phases including the windup, cocking, acceleration and follow-through. The reader is referred to other sources for detailed descriptions of tennis biomechanics (Ellenbecker 1994, 1995, Kibler 1995, Lee 1995, Ryu et al 1988).

Etiology of tennis injuries

High injury rates are reported in all levels of tennis, ranging from 10–30% in elite juniors to 74% of world-class players (Ellenbecker 1995, Lehman 1988). The characteristic 'tennis shoulder' is associated with a postural change of shoulder girdle depression associated with an apparent scoliosis (Priest 1988). Anterior pain was reported most frequently, provoked by the serve or overhead smash. Other injury reports indicate that tennis players are likely to experience the same problems as the thrower as a result of the comparable mechanics of the sports (Kibler 1995, Lee 1995, Ryu et al 1988). Most stress and injuries occur during the explosive overhead strokes (Ellenbecker 1994, 1995, Kibler 1995, Lee 1995, McCann & Bigliani 1994, Priest 1988). Chandler et al (1992) reported an imbalance of the external rotators compared to the medial rotators that predisposed the shoulder to injury and recommended strengthening of the external rotators to maintain a more even strength balance to reduce the chance of overload injury.

Faulty mechanics and inadequate racket selection can also lead to injuries (Lehman 1988, Lee 1995). The most common error made in tennis is the breakdown of the kinetic chain, with the player failing to use muscles from the trunk, hips and lower extremity to generate force. In this case, the player uses an 'all-arm' stroke, causing increased stress to upper extremity joints. Another cause of injury may be related to a timing problem. In this case, the player has a momentary 'hitch' and loses momentum needed to hit the ball forcefully so compensation from the upper extremity occurs.

Due to the biomechanics of the forehand, backhand and serve, the shoulder often is in a position of adduction and internal rotation. This position may predispose a tennis player to impingement. This condition usually results from a combination of poor mechanics and impairments such as poor flexibility, poor scapular stability, weak RTC or decreased joint mobility. Studies indicate that a significant loss of internal rotation ROM occurs over time as result of playing tennis (Ellenbecker 1994).

Treatment strategies

Address impairments

The common impairments that need to be addressed in tennis players are posterior capsule mobility, RTC strength, scapular stabilizing strength and anterior chest mobility. The clinician should introduce exercises that emphasize achieving strength and ROM in positions that simulate tennis. The mechanics of overhead tennis strokes involve several motions directly tied to the shoulder including thoracolumbar extension and rotation, scapular retraction, horizontal abduction of the humerus and external rotation. To achieve this position, players need to have adequate flexibility of the anterior chest musculature, glenohumeral mobility and good mobility of the thoracolumbar spine. Stretching and joint mobilization techniques can address these potential impairments.

A key element of successful rehabilitation of a tennis player is strengthening and motor control of the shoulder girdle muscles. The primary emphasis is on the muscle groups that control the arm during overhead strokes and serving. Resistive tubing tied to a racket is an ideal way to provide resistance to the upper extremities to simulate these motions. Most stress on the shoulder occurs at the contact phase and during the follow-through phases, when muscles have to work eccentrically. The dynamic stabilizers of the GHJ during these phases are the RTC, scapular stabilizers, LHB and latissimus dorsi. Eccentric loading of the external rotators in a position that simulates overhead hitting and serving should be emphasized.

Training errors

Overuse in tennis may occur from performing too many overhead strokes in a practice or too many practices in a week. Players may need to limit these activities to prevent microtrauma injuries to the shoulder. Abuse in tennis may occur from a player using the wrong type of racket. One aspect of tennis that is different to other overhead sports is the influence of the tennis racket on upper extremity stress (Ryu et al 1988). Stress on the upper extremity is affected by grip size, grip position and racket string size and tension. These external factors can put excessive stress on the shoulder. Misuse can lead to shoulder injuries when stroke mechanics are flawed, particularly with a serve or overhead smash. The primary mechanical faults are not using the trunk, hips and lower extremities effectively enough to reduce the stress on the upper extremity. Different strategies exist to facilitate a return to tennis playing after shoulder injury. The primary goal is to decrease overhead motions, the activities that place the most stress on the shoulder.

Summary

Understanding the relationship between impairments and tissue pathology is needed for proper diagnosis of shoulder conditions in the overhead athlete. In some cases, impairments such as instability may predispose an athlete to tissue pathology such as a labral tear. Conversely, tissue pathology such as tendonitis can lead to impairments such as altered scapulohumeral rhythm. Clinicians working with these athletes should determine the etiology of the condition and address each impairment, while allowing proper time guidelines for injured tissues to heal. Without resolving all impairments, the healed tissues will remain susceptible to further injury.

After impairments are resolved and tissues have healed, the clinician should facilitate a safe return to sport. In accomplishing this goal, the physical therapist should understand the demands of the athlete's sport and position so that the rehabilitation program incorporates exercises that simulate the movements and forces that will be encountered. Advancement during the return-to-activity phase of rehabilitation should be based on achieving specific milestones that reflect normal ROM, strength, proprioception and motor control during the functional activities. Careful monitoring of throws, strokes, swings or hits will ensure that the athlete is advanced slowly, reducing the likelihood of exacerbations.

References

Allegrucci M, Whitney S L, Irrgang J J 1994 Clinical implications of secondary impingement of the shoulder in freestyle swimmers. Journal of Orthopaedic and Sports Physical Therapy 20:307–318

Allen A A, Warner J J P 1995 Shoulder instability in the athlete. Orthopedic Clinics of North America 26:487–504

Allingham C 1996 The shoulder complex. In: Zuluaga M, Briggs C, Carlisle J et al (eds) Sports physiotherapy: applied science and practice. Churchill Livingstone, Melbourne, p 357–406

Andrews J R, Wilk K E 1994 Shoulder injuries in baseball. In: Andrews J R, Wilk K E (eds) The athlete's shoulder. Churchill Livingstone, New York, p 369–390

Andrews J R, Carson W G, McLeod W D 1985 Glenoid labrum tears related to the long head of biceps. American Journal of Sports Medicine 13:337–341

Andrews J R, Kupferman S P, Dillman C J 1991 Labral tears in throwing and racquet sports. Clinics in Sports Medicine 10:901–911

Axe M J, Snyder-Mackler L, Konin J G et al 1996 Development of a distance-based interval throwing program for Little League-aged athletes. American Journal of Sports Medicine 24:594–602

Ayub E, Glasheen-Wray M, Kraus S 1984 Head posture: a study of the effects on the rest position of the mandible. Journal of Orthopaedic and Sports Physical Therapy 14:179–184

Bak K 1996 Nontraumatic glenohumeral instability and coracoacromial impingement in swimmers. Scandinavian Journal of Medicine and Science in Sports 6:132–144

Bak K, Faunø P 1997 Clinical findings in competitive swimmers with shoulder pain. American Journal of Sports Medicine 25:254–260

Bak K, Magnusson S P 1997 Shoulder strength and range of motion in symptomatic and pain-free elite swimmers. American Journal of Sports Medicine 25:454–460

Ballantyne B T, O'Hare S J, Paschall J L et al 1993 Electromyographic activity of selected shoulder muscles in commonly used therapeutic exercises. Physical Therapy 73:668–681

Beach M L, Whitney S L, Dickoff-Hoffman S A 1992 Relationship of shoulder flexibility, strength and endurance to shoulder pain in competitive swimmers. Journal of Orthopaedic and Sports Physical Therapy 16:262–268

Berg E E, Ciullo J V 1998 A clinical test for superior glenoid labral or 'SLAP' lesions. Clinical Journal of Sports Medicine 8:121–123

Burkhart S S, Morgan C D, Kibler W B 2000 Shoulder injuries in overhead athletes. The 'dead arm' revisited. Clinics in Sports Medicine 19:125–158

Burkhead W Z 1990 The biceps tendon. In: Rockwood C A, Matsen F A (eds) The shoulder. WB Saunders, Philadelphia, PA, p 791–836

Chandler J, Kibler B, Stracener E C et al 1992 Shoulder strength, power and endurance in college tennis players. American Journal of Sports Medicine 20:455–458

Ciullo J V 1986 Swimmer's shoulder. Clinics in Sports Medicine 5:115–137

Ciullo J V 1996 Shoulder injuries in sport. Human Kinetics, Champaign, IL

Crawford H J, Jull G A 1991 The influence of thoracic form and movement on range of shoulder flexion. Physiotherapy, Theory and Practice 9:143–148

Davidson P A, El Attrache N S, Jobe M et al 1995 Rotator cuff and posterior-superior glenoid labrum injury associated with increased glenohumeral motion: a new site of impingement. Journal of Shoulder and Elbow Surgery 4:384–390

DiGiovine N M, Jobe F W, Pink M et al 1992 An eletromyographic analysis of the upper extremity in pitching. Journal of Shoulder and Elbow Surgery 1:15–25

Dillman C J, Fleiseg G S, Andrews J R 1993 Biomechanics of pitching with emphasis upon shoulder kinematics. Journal of Orthopedics and Sports Physical Therapy 18:402

Dines D M, Levinson M 1995 The conservative management of the unstable shoulder including rehabilitation. Clinics in Sports Medicine 14:797–816

Drexler D M, Briner W W, Reeser J C 2001 Volleyball. In: Shamus E, Shamus J (eds) Sports injury: prevention and rehabilitation. McGraw Hill, New York, p 73–102

Ellenbecker T S 1994 Shoulder injuries in tennis. In: Andrews J R, Wilk K E (eds) The athlete's shoulder. Churchill Livingstone, New York, p 399–409

Ellenbecker T S 1995 Rehabilitation of shoulder and elbow injuries in tennis players. Clinics in Sports Medicine 14:107–108

Ferretti A, Cerullo G, Russo G 1987 Suprascapular neuropathy in volleyball players. Journal of Bone and Joint Surgery (Am) 69A:260–263

Ferretti A, DeCarli A, Fontana M 1998 Injury of the suprascapular nerve at the spinoglenoid notch. The natural history of infraspinatus atrophy in volleyball players. American Journal of Sports Medicine 26:759–763

Fleisig G S, Andrews J R, Dillman C J et al 1995 Kinetics of baseball pitching with implications about injury mechanisms. American Journal of Sports Medicine 23:233–239

Gerber C, Ganz R 1984 Clinical assessment of instability of the shoulder, with special reference to anterior and posterior drawer tests. Journal of Bone and Joint Surgery (Br) 66B:551–556

Gerber C, Krushell R J 1991 Isolated rupture of the tendon of the subscapularis muscle: clinical features in 16 cases. Journal of Bone and Joint Surgery (Br) 73B:389–394

Gerber C, Sebesta A 2000 Impingement of the deep surface of the subscapularis tendon and the reflection pulley on the anterosuperior glenoid rim: a preliminary report. Journal of Shoulder and Elbow Surgery 9:483–490

Gerber C, Terrier F, Zehnder R et al 1987 The subcoracoid space: an anatomic study. Clinical Orthopaedics and Related Research 215:132–138

Gerber C, Hersche O, Farron A 1996 Isolated rupture of subscapularis tendon. Journal of Bone and Joint Surgery (Am) 78A:1015–1023

Glousman R E 1993 Instability versus impingement syndrome in the throwing athlete. Orthopedic Clinics of North America 24:89–99

Glousman R, Jobe F W 1996 Anterior shoulder instability, impingement and rotator cuff tear. In: Jobe F W (ed) Operative techniques in upper extremity sports injuries. Mosby, St Louis, MO, p 191–210

Gonzalez D, Lopez R A 1991 Concurrent rotator-cuff tear and brachial plexus palsy associated with anterior dislocation of the shoulder. Journal of Bone and Joint Surgery (Am) 73A(4):620–621

Guccione A A 1991 Physical therapy diagnosis and the relationship between impairments and function. Physical Therapy 71:499

Habermeyer P, Schüller U, Wiedemann E 1992 The intra-articular pressure of the shoulder: an experimental study on the role of the glenoid labrum stabilizing the joint. Arthroscopy 8:166–172

Hawkins R J, Kennedy J C 1980 Impingement syndrome in athletes. American Journal of Sports Medicine 8:151–158

Holzgraefe M, Kukowski B, Eggert S 1994 Prevalence of latent and manifest suprascapular neuropathy in high-performance volleyball players. British Journal of Sports Medicine 28:177–179

Hsu H-C, Luo Z-P, Cofield R H et al 1997 Influence of rotator cuff tearing on glenohumeral stability. Journal of Shoulder and Elbow Surgery 6:413–422

Itoi E, Motzkin N E, Morrey B F et al 1994 Stabilizing function of the long head of the biceps in the hanging position. Journal of Shoulder and Elbow Surgery 3:135–142

Janda V 1978 Muscles, central nervous motor regulation and back problems. In: Korr I M (ed) The neurobiologic mechanisms in manipulative therapy. Plenum, New York, p 27–41

Jobe C M, Pink M, Jobe F W et al 1996 Anterior shoulder instability, impingement and rotator cuff tear. In: Jobe F W (ed) Operative techniques in upper extremity sports injuries. Mosby, St Louis, MO, p 164–176

Jobe F W, Moynes D R 1982 Delineation of diagnostic criteria and a rehabilitation program for rotator cuff injuries. American Journal of Sports Medicine 10:336–339

Jobe F W, Pink M 1993 Classification and treatment of shoulder dysfunction in the overhead athlete. Journal of Orthopaedic and Sports Physical Therapy 18:427–432

Jobe F W, Tibone J E, Perry J et al 1983 An EMG analysis of the shoulder in throwing and pitching. A preliminary report. American Journal of Sports Medicine 11:3–5

Jobe F W, Moynes D R, Tibone J E et al 1984 An EMG analysis of the shoulder in pitching. A second report. American Journal of Sports Medicine 12:218–220

Kaltsas D S 1983 Comparative study of the properties of the shoulder joint capsule with those of other joint capsules. Clinical Orthopaedics and Related Research 173:20–26

Kibler W B 1991 Role of the scapula in the overhead throwing motion. Contemporary Orthopedics 22:525–533

Kibler W B 1995 Biomechanical analysis of the shoulder during tennis activities. Clinics in Sports Medicine 14:79–85

Kibler W B 1998 The role of the scapula in athletic shoulder function. American Journal of Sports Medicine 26:325–339

Kimball R J, Carter R L, Schneider R C 1985 Competitive diving injuries. In: Schneider R C, Kennedy J C, Plant M L (eds) Sports injuries: mechanisms, prevention, and treatment. Lippincott Williams and Wilkins, Baltimore, MD, p 192–211

Kuhn J E, Bey M J, Huston L J et al 2000 Ligamentous restraints to external rotation of the humerus in the late-cocking phase of throwing. A cadaveric biomechanical investigation. American Journal of Sports Medicine 28:200–205

Kumar V P, Satku K, Balasubramaniam P 1989 The role of the long head of biceps brachii in the stabilization of the head of the humerus. Clinical Orthopaedics and Related Research 244:172–175

Kvitne R S, Jobe F W 1993 The diagnosis and treatment of anterior instability in the throwing athlete. Clinical Orthopaedics and Related Research 291:107–123

Lee H W M 1995 Mechanisms of neck and shoulder injuries in tennis players. Journal of Orthopaedics and Sports Physical Therapy 21:28–37

Lehman R C 1988 Shoulder pain in the competitive tennis player. Clinics in Sports Medicine 7:309–327

Levy 1999 Intra- and interobserver reproducibility of the shoulder laxity examination. American Journal of Sports Medicine 27:460–468

Lippitt S B, Vanderhooft E, Harris S L et al 1993 Glenohumeral stability from concavity-compression: a quantitative analysis. Journal of Shoulder and Elbow Surgery 2:27–35

Liu S H, Henry M H, Nuccion S et al 1996 Diagnosis of glenoid labral tears: a comparison between magnetic resonance imaging and clinical examinations. American Journal of Sports Medicine 24:149–154

McCann P D, Bigliani L U 1994 Shoulder pain in tennis players. Sports Medicine 17:53–64

McLeod W D, Andrews J R 1986 Mechanisms of shoulder injuries. Physical Therapy 66:1901

McMaster W C, Troup J 1993 A survey of interfering shoulder pain in United States competitive swimmers. American Journal of Sports Medicine 21:67–70

McMaster W C, Roberts A, Stoddard T 1998 A correlation between shoulder laxity and interfering pain in competitive swimmers. American Journal of Sports Medicine 26:83–87

Maitland G D 1991 Peripheral manipulation. Butterworth Heinemann, London

Matsen F A, Harryman D T, Sidles J A 1991 Mechanics of gleno-humeral stability. Clinics in Sports Medicine 10:783–788

Matsen F A, Arntz C T, Lippitt S B 1998a Rotator cuff. In: Rockwood C A, Matsen F A (eds) The shoulder. 2nd edn. WB Saunders, Philadelphia, PA, p 755–839

Matsen F A, Thomas S C, Rockwood C A et al 1998b Glenohumeral instability. In: Rockwood C A, Matsen F A (eds) The shoulder, 2nd edn, vol 2. WB Saunders, Philadelphia, PA, p 611–754

Meister K 2000 Injuries to the shoulder in the throwing athlete: 1. Biomechanics/pathophysiology/classification of injury. American Journal of Sports Medicine 28:265–274

Meister K, Andrews J R 1993 Classification and treatment of rotator cuff injuries in the overhand athlete. Journal of Orthopaedic and Sports Physical Therapy 18:415–421

Meister K, Andrews J R, Batts J et al 1999 Symptomatic thrower's exostosis. American Journal of Sports Medicine 27:133–142

Mimori K, Muneta T, Nakagawa T et al 1999 A new pain provocation test for superior labral tears of the shoulder. American Journal of Sports Medicine 27:137–146

Mohtadi N G H 1991 Advances in the understanding of anterior instability of the shoulder. Clinics in Sports Medicine 10:863–870

Moseley B, Jobe F W, Pink M et al 1992 Analysis of the scapular muscles during a shoulder rehabilitation program. American Journal of Sports Medicine 19:128–134

Nagi S Z 1965 Some conceptual issues in disability and rehabilitation. In: Sussman M B (ed) Sociology and rehabilitation. American Sociological Association, Washington, DC, p 100

Neer C S, Welsh P 1977 The shoulder in sports. Orthopedic Clinics of North America 8:583–590

Neviaser R J, Neviaser T J, Neviaser J S 1988 Concurrent rupture of the rotator cuff and anterior dislocation of the shoulder in the older patient. Journal of Bone and Joint Surgery (Am) 70A:1308–1311

O'Brien R 1992 Diving for gold. Leisure Press, Champaign, IL

O'Brien S J, Pagnani M J, Fealy S et al 1998 The active compression test: a new and effective test for diagnosing labral tears and acromio-clavicular joint abnormality. American Journal of Sports Medicine 26:610–614

Perry J, Pink M, Jobe F W et al 1992 The painful shoulder during the backstroke: an EMG and cinematographic analysis of 12 muscles. Clinical Journal of Sports Medicine 2:13–20

Pink M M, Jobe F W 1996 Biomechanics of swimming. In: Zachazewski J E, Magee D J, Quillen W S (eds) Athletic injuries and rehabilitation. WB Saunders, Philadelphia, PA, p 317–331

Pink M, Perry J, Browne A et al 1991 The normal shoulder during freestyle swimming. An eletromyographic and cinematographic

analysis of twelve muscles. American Journal of Sports Medicine 19:569–576

Pink M, Jobe FW, Perry J et al 1992 The normal shoulder during the backstroke: an EMG and cinematographic analysis of 12 muscles. Clinical Journal of Sports Medicine 2:6–12

Pink M, Jobe F W, Perry J et al 1993a The normal shoulder during the butterfly swim stroke: an electromyographic and cinematographic analysis of twelve muscles. Clinical Orthopaedics and Related Research 288:48–59

Pink M, Jobe F W, Perry J et al 1993b The painful shoulder during the butterfly stroke: an electromyographic and cinematographic analysis of twelve muscles. Clinical Orthopaedics and Related Research 288:60–72

Priest J D 1988 The shoulder of the tennis player. Clinics in Sports Medicine 7:387–402

Rathbun J B, McNab I 1970 The microvascular pattern of the rotator cuff. Journal of Bone and Joint Surgery (Br) 52B:540–553

Richardson A B, Jobe F W, Collins H R 1980 The shoulder in competitive swimming. American Journal of Sports Medicine 8:159–163

Rocabado M 1983 Biomechanical relationship of the cranial, cervical, and hyoid regions. Journal of Cranio-mandibular Practice 1:61–66

Rowe C R 1987 Recurrent transient anterior subluxation of the shoulder. The 'dead arm' syndrome. Clinical Orthopaedics and Related Research 223:11–19

Rowe C R, Zarins B 1981 Recurrent transient subluxation of the shoulder. Journal of Bone and Joint Surgery (Am) 63A:863–872

Ryu R K N, McCormick J, Jobe F W et al 1988 An electromyographic analysis of shoulder function in tennis players. American Journal of Sports Medicine 16:481–485

Sandow M J, Ilic J 1998 Suprascapular nerve rotator cuff compression syndrome in volleyball players. Journal of Shoulder and Elbow Surgery 7:516–521

Scovazzo M L, Browne A, Pink M et al 1991 The painful shoulder during freestyle swimming. American Journal of Sports Medicine 19:577–582

Shapiro C 2001 Swimming. In: Shamus E, Shamus J (eds) Sports injury prevention and rehabilitation. McGraw-Hill. New York, p 103–154

Solem-Bertoff E, Thuomas K-A, Westerberg C-E 1993 The influence of scapular retraction and protraction on the width of the subacromial space. An MRI study. Clinical Orthopaedics and Related Research 296:99–103

Stocker D, Pink M, Jobe F W 1995 Comparison of shoulder injury in collegiate- and master's-level swimmers. Clinical Journal of Sport Medicine 5:4–8

Tovin B J, Neyer M 2001 Diving. In: Shamus E and Shamus J (eds) Sports injury: prevention and rehabilitation. McGraw Hill, New York, p 155–184

Townsend H, Jobe F W, Pink M et al 1991 Electromyographic analysis of the glenohumeral muscles during a baseball rehabilitation program. American Journal of Sports Medicine 19:264–272

Wilk K E, Voight M L 1994 Plyometrics for the shoulder complex. In: Andrews J R, Wilk K E (eds) The athlete's shoulder. Churchill Livingstone, New York, p 543–566

Wilk K E, Voight M L, Keirns M A et al 1993 Stretch-shortening drills for upper extremities: theory and clinical application. Journal of Orthopedic and Sports Physical Therapy 17:225–239

Zaslav K R 2001 Internal rotation resistance strength test: a new diagnostic test to differentiate intra-articular pathology from outlet (Neer) impingement syndrome in the shoulder. Journal of Shoulder and Elbow Surgery 10:23–27

Elbow

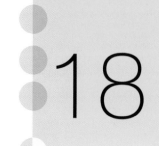

Michael M. Reinold and Kevin E. Wilk

CHAPTER CONTENTS

Introduction 308

Anatomy 308

Elbow biomechanics in sport 312

Clinical examination 314

Overview of elbow rehabilitation 315

Common sport-related injuries 324

Less common sport-related injuries 334

Summary 336

Introduction

Injuries to the elbow joint complex occur frequently in the athletic population. Rehabilitation following these injuries is often challenging to the clinician due to the significant amount of stress applied to the unique anatomy of the elbow joint during sport-specific movements. Mechanisms of injuries include repetitive microtraumatic forces from overuse, as well as macrotraumatic overload of excessive forces (Wilk & Levinson 2001, Wilk et al 1993a). Athletes experience sport-specific injury patterns based on the unique demands involved with each particular sport. Overhead athletes such as throwers and tennis players typically present with injuries caused by chronic stress overload or repetitive traumatic stress (Fleisig & Barrentine 1995). Conversely, athletes participating in contact sports such as football, ice hockey, wrestling, gymnastics and soccer are more susceptible to traumatic injuries including fractures and dislocations due to the aggressive nature of each sport.

Rehabilitation of the elbow joint requires a thorough knowledge of the anatomical, biomechanical and pathomechanical factors associated with athletic participation. The purpose of this chapter is to overview the anatomy and biomechanics of the elbow joint during sports, followed by a detailed description of common clinical examination techniques for the injured athlete. Several nonoperative and postoperative rehabilitation programs will be discussed for specific sport injuries utilizing a multiphased, progressive rehabilitation approach based on current scientific research and clinical experience. The ultimate goal of rehabilitation is to gradually restore function and return the athlete to competition as quickly and safely as possible.

Anatomy

Sport-specific applied anatomy of the elbow joint complex can be broken down into osseous, capsuloligamentous, musculotendinous and neurological structures.

Osseous Structures

The elbow joint complex includes the humerus, radius and ulna, articulating to form the humeroulnar, humeroradial, proximal radioulnar and distal radioulnar joints.

The humeroulnar joint is generally considered a uniaxial, diarthrodial joint with one degree of freedom allowing flexion and extension in the sagittal plane around a coronal axis. Morrey (1985) described the humeroulnar joint as a modified hinge joint due to the small amounts of internal and external rotation that occur at extreme ranges of flexion and extension. The anterior aspect of the distal humerus contains the convex trochlea, an hourglass-shaped surface covered with articular cartilage. The trochlear groove is located centrally within the trochlea and runs obliquely in the anterior–posterior direction. The distal end of the humerus exhibits 30° of anterior rotation with respect to the long axis of the humerus. A corresponding version is seen at the proximal ulna with 30° of posterior rotation in respect to the shaft of the ulna. This anatomical rotation of the humerus and ulna allows for excessive elbow flexion from 145° to 150° and enhances static stability when the elbow is in full extension (Lehmkuhl & Smith 1983).

The proximal ulna contains a centrally located ridge that runs between two bony prominences, the coronoid process anteriorly and the olecranon posteriorly. Two fossae are located on each side of the corresponding articular surfaces of the humerus. Anteriorly, the coronoid fossa articulates with the coronoid process of the ulna during flexion. Posteriorly, the olecranon fossa receives the olecranon process of the ulna, serving to limit extension. The congruency achieved by these articulations makes the humeroulnar joint one of the most stable joints in the human body (Morrey & An 1983).

Also of significance to the humeroulnar joint is the medial epicondyle of the humerus. Located proximal and medial to the trochlea, the medial epicondyle serves as the attachment site of the flexor-pronator muscle group and the ulnar collateral ligament (UCL). Hoppenfeld (1976) states that the size and prominence of the medial epicondyle provides an important mechanical advantage for the medial stabilizing structures of the elbow joint. The cubital tunnel is located posterior to the medial epicondyle and serves to protect the ulnar nerve as it transverses distally.

The humeroradial joint is similarly a diarthrodial, uniaxial joint allowing elbow flexion and extension with the humeroulnar joint. In addition, the humeroradial joint pivots around a longitudinal axis to allow rotation movements in association with the proximal radioulnar joint, thus making the joint a combination hinge and pivot joint (Norkin & Levangie 1985).

The articular surfaces of the humeroradial joint include the concave radial head and the spherical convex capitulum on the distal aspect of the humerus (Kapandji 1970). The capitulum and trochlea are separated by a groove within the humerus, the capitulotrochlear groove. This groove guides the radial head as the elbow moves in flexion and extension.

Immediately proximal to the capitellum on the anterior aspect of the humerus is the radial fossa. The radial fossa receives the anterior aspect of the radial head in the maximally flexed elbow position. The lateral epicondyle lies laterally to the radial fossa and serves as an attachment site of the wrist extensor muscle group. The radial tuberosity is located on the radius just distally to the radial head. This area serves as the attachment site for the biceps brachii tendon.

The proximal and distal radioulnar joints are intricately related, together allowing for one degree of freedom in the transverse plane around a longitudinal axis. These two joints allow forearm supination and pronation. During supination and pronation, the head of the radius rotates within a ring formed by the annular ligament and radial notch of the ulna. Little motion occurs in the ulna. The radius and ulna lie parallel to each other while in the supinated position. As the forearm rotates into pronation, the radius crosses over the ulna. The radius and ulna are also connected midway between the two bony shafts by an interosseous membrane, which serves as an additional attachment site for the forearm musculature.

The bony articulation of the elbow joint forms the carrying angle of the elbow. This is defined as the angle formed by the long axis of the humerus and the ulna and results in the abducted position of the forearm in relation to the humerus. This angle is measured in the frontal plane with the elbow extended and averages 11–14° in males and 13–16° in females (Atkinson & Elftman 1945, Keats et al 1966). The carrying angle changes linearly as the elbow joint is flexed and extended, diminishing in flexion and increasing with extension (Morrey 1985).

Capsuloligamentous structures

The joint capsule is a relatively thin but significantly strong structure. The anterior capsule is normally a thin transparent structure that allows visualization of the bony prominence when the elbow is fully extended. The anterior capsule inserts proximally above the coronoid and radial fossa. Distally, the capsule attaches to the anterior margin of the coronoid medially and into the annular ligament laterally. Posteriorly, the capsule attaches just above the olecranon fossa and distally along the medial and lateral margins of the trochlea. The capsule exhibits significant strength from the transverse and obliquely directed fibrous bands. The anterior capsule is taut into extension and lax with elbow flexion. The greatest capacity occurs at approximately 80° of flexion (Johansson 1962). The synovial membrane lines the joint capsule and is attached anteriorly above the radial and coronoid fossa to the medial and lateral margins of the articular surface, and posteriorly to the superior margin of the olecranon fossa.

The ligaments of the elbow consist of thickened parts of the medial and lateral capsules. The UCL is located on the medial aspect of the elbow. This ligamentous complex can be divided into three distinct portions, the anterior, posterior and transverse bundles. The anterior bundle originates from the inferior surface of the medial epicondyle and inserts at the medial aspect of the coronoid process. Due to the posterior orientation of the ligament in relation to the center of rotation, the anterior bundle is taut throughout the range of motion. The anterior bundle can be further divided into two bands: the anterior band, which is taut in extension, and the posterior band, which tightens in flexion (Morrey et al 1985, Schwab et al 1980). The anterior bundle of the UCL is the main ligamentous support to valgus strain at the elbow.

The transverse bundle of the UCL originates from the medial olecranon and inserts into the coronoid process. The posterior bundle originates from the medial epicondyle posteroinferiorly and fans out to attach onto the posteromedial aspect of the olecranon. Several authors report that these two bundles provide minimal amounts of medial elbow stability (Morrey & An 1983, Morrey et al 1985, Schwab et al 1980).

Laterally, the ligamentous complex helps stabilize against varus stress and is made up of several components including the radial collateral ligament, the annular ligament, the accessory lateral collateral ligament and the lateral ulnar collateral ligament (Morrey & An 1983).

The radial collateral ligament (RCL) is not as well defined as the UCL. Originating from the lateral epicondyle, the RCL fans out and inserts into the annular ligament. The RCL origin is in line with the axis of joint rotation, allowing little change in length as the elbow moves through full range of motion.

The annular ligament is a strong fibro-osseous ring that encircles and stabilizes the radial head in the radial notch of the ulna. Its origin and insertion occur along the anterior and posterior radial notch of the ulna. The anterior portion of this ligament becomes taut with supination while the posterior portion becomes taut with pronation (Spinner & Kaplan 1970).

The accessory lateral collateral ligament (ALCL) originates from the inferior margin of the annular ligament and inserts discretely into the tubercle of the supinator crest of the ulna. The ALCL further assists the annular ligament in varus stabilization (Martin 1958).

The lateral ulnar collateral ligament (LUCL) originates from the lateral epicondyle and inserts into the tubercle of the crest of the supinator. This ligament provides posterolateral stability of the humeroulnar joint (O'Driscoll et al 1991).

The elbow joint is one of the most congruent joints in the human body and is thus one of the most stable (Morrey & An 1983). Stability is provided by the interaction of soft tissue and articular constraints. The static soft tissue stabilizers include the capsular and ligamentous structures. Table 18.1 summarizes the influence of the ligamentous and articular components of the elbow joint (Morrey & An 1983). When the elbow is in full extension, the anterior capsule provides approximately 70% of the restraint to distraction, whereas the UCL provides approximately 78% of the distraction at 90° of elbow flexion. The restraint to valgus displacement varies significantly depending on the elbow flexion angle. When the elbow is in full extension, the capsule provides 38% of the restraint, the UCL provides 31% and the articulation provides the remaining 31%. Conversely, at 90° of flexion, the primary restraint is the UCL, which provides 54% of the restraint, followed by the osseous articulation, which provides 33%, and the capsule, which provides 13%. Varus stress is controlled in extensions by the joint articulation (54%), RCL (14%) and joint capsule (32%). As the elbow flexes, the RCL and capsule contribute 9 and 13%, respectively, while the joint articulation provides 75% of the stabilizing force (Morrey & An 1983).

Table 18.1 Contributing forces to displacement of the elbow (modified from Morrey & An 1983)

Elbow position	Stabilizing structure	Distraction (%)	Varus (%)	Valgus (%)
Elbow extended (0°)	UCL	6	–	31
	LCL	5	14	–
	Capsule	85	32	38
	Articulation	–	55	31
Elbow flexed (90°)	UCL	78	–	54
	LCL	10	9	–
	Capsule	8	13	10
	Articulation	–	75	33

Musculotendinous structures

The elbow joint musculature can be divided into six groups based on the functions of each muscle. These groups include the elbow flexors, extensors, flexor pronators, extensor supinators, primary pronators and primary supinators.

The three primary flexor muscles of the elbow include the biceps brachii, the brachioradialis and the brachialis. The biceps brachii typically consists of a long head and a short head. The long head of the biceps brachii originates on the superior glenoid and attaches directly to the glenoid labrum. The long head passes directly through the glenohumeral joint capsule and through the intertubercular groove of the humerus until it joins with the short head of the biceps brachii. The short head of the biceps originates from the coracoid process of the scapula. The two heads of the biceps brachii join to form a common attachment onto the posterior portion of the radial tuberosity and via the bicipital aponeurosis, which attaches to the anterior capsule of the elbow joint. The biceps is responsible for the vast majority of elbow flexion strength when the forearm is supinated and generates its highest torque values when the elbow is flexed between 80–100° (Norkin & Levangie 1985). The biceps also acts secondarily as a supinator of the forearm, principally when the elbow is in a flexed position.

The brachialis muscle originates from the lower half of the anterior surface of the humerus. The brachialis muscle extends distally to cross the anterior aspect of the elbow joint and inserts into the ulnar tuberosity and coronoid process. The brachialis muscle is active in flexing the elbow in all positions of the forearm (Basmajian & DeLuca 1985).

The brachioradialis muscle originates from the proximal two-thirds of the lateral supracondylar ridge of the humerus and along the lateral intermuscular septum distal to the spiral groove. The brachioradialis muscles insert into the lateral aspect of the base of the styloid process of the radius. The brachioradialis muscle inserts distant from the joint axis; therefore, exhibiting a significant mechanical advantage as an elbow flexor (Norkin & Levangie 1985).

The triceps brachii and the anconeus muscles serve as the primary extensors of the elbow. The triceps brachii is a large three-headed (long, lateral and medial) muscle that comprises almost the entire posterior brachium. The long head of the triceps originates from the infraglenoid tubercle, crossing the shoulder joint. The other two heads, the lateral and medial heads, originate from the posterior and lateral aspects of the humerus. At the distal portion of the humerus, the three heads converge to form a common muscle that inserts into the posterior surface of the olecranon.

The small anconeus muscle originates from a broad area on the posterior aspect of the lateral epicondyle and inserts into the olecranon. The anconeus muscle covers the lateral portion of the annular ligament, the radial head, and the posterior surface of the proximal ulna. Electromyographic (EMG) activity of the anconeus muscle during the early phases of elbow extension has been noted, and this muscle appears to have a stabilizing role during pronation and supination movements (Pavly et al 1967).

The flexor pronator muscles include the pronator teres, flexor carpi radialis, palmaris longus, flexor carpi ulnaris and flexor digitorum superficialis. All these muscles originate completely or in part from the medial epicondyle, and all serve secondary roles as elbow flexors. Their primary roles are associated with the wrist and hand. This muscle group may provide a limited amount of dynamic stability to the medial aspect of the elbow against valgus stress (Jobe et al 1984).

The extensor supinator muscles include the brachioradialis, extensor carpi radialis brevis and longus, supinator, extensor digitorum, extensor carpi ulnaris and extensor digiti minimi muscles. Each muscle originates near or directly from the lateral epicondyle of the humerus. The primary functions of the extensor supinator muscles involve the wrist and hand and provide dynamic support over the lateral aspect of the elbow. This muscle group, as well as the flexor pronator musculature, is susceptible to various overuse muscle strains.

The pronator quadratus and pronator teres muscles act on the radioulnar joints to produce pronation. The pronator quadratus originates from the anterior surface of the lower ulna. Insertion occurs at the distal and lateral border of the radius. The pronator quadratus acts as a significant pronator in all positions of the elbow and forearm.

The pronator teres, which possesses humeral and ulnar heads, originates from the medial epicondyle and coronoid process of the ulna. The two heads join together and insert along the middle of the lateral surface of the radius. The pronator teres is a strong pronator muscle that generates its highest contractile force during rapid or resisted pronation (Soderberg 1981). However, the pronator teres' contribution to pronation strength diminishes when the elbow is positioned in full extension (Norkin & Levangie 1985). The flexor carpi radialis and brachioradialis also act as secondary pronators.

The biceps brachii and the supinator muscles are the primary supinators of the forearm, while the brachioradialis also acts as an accessory supinator. The supinator muscle originates from three separate locations: the lateral epicondyle, the proximal anterior crest and depression of the ulnar distal to the radial notch, and the radial collateral and annular ligaments. The supinator muscle then winds around the radius to insert into the dorsal and lateral surfaces of the proximal radius. The supinator is the primary supinator of the forearm but appears to be generally weaker than the biceps (Morrey 1985). The supinator acts alone with unresisted slow supination in all elbow and forearm positions and with unresisted fast supination with the elbow extended (Kapandji 1970). The effectiveness of the supinator is not altered by elbow position; however, elbow position does significantly affect the biceps. The supinator originates at the radial collateral and annular ligaments, suggesting that the muscle may also act as a supportive or stabilizing muscle to the lateral aspect of the elbow.

Neurological structures

The four nerves that play significant roles in normal elbow function and pathologies are the median, ulnar, radial and musculocutaneous nerves. Box 18.1 shows the effect of injury to specific peripheral nerves.

The median nerve arises from branches of the lateral and medial cords of the brachial plexus. Nerve root levels include C5 to C8 and T1. This nerve proceeds distally over the anterior brachium, continuing to the medial aspect of the antecubital fossa. From the fossa, the nerve continues its course under the bicipital aponeurosis and passes most often between the two heads of the pronator teres. The median nerve can be compressed between the two heads of the pronator teres or by the bicipital aponeurosis, resulting in either pronator syndrome or anterior interosseous syndrome. Although relatively uncommon, highly repetitive and strenuous pronation movements of the forearm can also lead to entrapment of the median nerve (Magee 1987).

The ulnar nerve emanates from the C8 and T1 levels and descends into the proximal aspect of the upper extremity from the medial cord of the brachial plexus. The ulnar nerve passes from the anterior to posterior compartments of the brachium through the arcade of Struthers. This arcade represents a fascial bridging between the medial head of the triceps and medial intermuscular septum. The nerve continues distally, passing behind the medial epicondyle and through the cubital tunnel. At the cubital tunnel, bony anatomy provides little protection for the nerve. Ulnar nerve injury, which can occur by compression or stretching, takes place most frequently in the cubital tunnel. The cubital tunnel retinaculum flattens with elbow flexion, thus decreasing the capacity of the cubital tunnel. This can be noted clinically as stimulating nerve symptoms when osteophytes are present on the ulna or medial epicondyle (St John & Palmaz 1986). Injury to the medial capsular ligaments can result in increased traction forces against the medial elbow, resulting in a change in length of the ulnar nerve. This change in length may result in neuropathy or ulnar nerve subluxation. The nerve enters the forearm by passing between the two heads of the flexor carpi ulnaris and continues distally between the flexor digitorum profundus and the flexor carpi ulnaris.

The radial nerve originates from the posterior cord of the brachial plexus and derives its nerve supply from the C6, C7

Musculocutaneous nerve (C5, C6, C7)

Sensory supply

Lateral half of the anterior surface of the forearm from the elbow to the thenar eminence

Effect of injury

- Severe weakness of elbow flexion
- Weakness of supination
- Loss of biceps deep tendon reflex
- Loss of sensation, cutaneous distribution

Radial nerve (C5, C6, C7, C8, T1)

Sensory supply

Back of arm, forearm, wrist, radial half of the dorsum of the hand, back of thumb, index finger, and part of the middle finger

Effect of injury

- Loss of triceps deep tendon reflex
- Weakness of elbow flexion
- Loss of supination (when elbow is extended)
- Loss of wrist extension
- Weakness of ulnar and radial deviation
- Loss of extension at the MCP joints
- Loss of extension and abduction of the thumb

Median nerve (C5, C6, C7, C8, T1)

Sensory supply

Radial half of the palm, palmar surface of the thumb, index, middle, and radial half of the ring finger, and dorsal surface of the same fingers

Effect of injury

- Loss of complete pronation (brachioradialis can bring the forearm to midpronation but not beyond)
- Weakness with flexion and radial deviation (ulnar deviation with wrist flexion)
- Loss of flexion at MCP joints
- Loss of thumb opposition or abduction, loss of flexion at IP and MCP joints

Ulnar nerve (C7, C8, T1)

Sensory supply

Dorsal and palmar surfaces of the ulnar side of the hand, including the little finger, and ulnar half of the ring finger

Effect of injury

- Weakness of wrist flexion and ulnar deviation (radial deviation with wrist flexion)
- Loss of flexion of DIP joints of ring and little fingers
- Inability to abduct or adduct fingers
- Inability to adduct thumb
- Loss of flexion of fingers, especially ring and little fingers at the MCP joints
- Loss of extension of fingers, especially ring and little fingers at the IP joint

IP – interphalangeal; MCP – metacarpophalangeal; DIP – distal interphalangeal

and C8 levels with variable contributions from the C5 and T1 levels. At the midpoint of the brachium, the radial nerve descends laterally through the radial groove of the humerus and continues in a path lateral and distal. The nerve descends anteriorly behind the brachioradialis and brachialis muscles, and at the level of the joint, the nerve divides into the posterior interosseous and superficial radial branches.

The musculocutaneous nerve originates from the lateral cord of the brachial plexus at nerve root levels C5 to C7. The nerve passes between the biceps and brachialis muscles to pierce the brachial fascia lateral to the biceps tendon. The nerve continues distally and terminates as the lateral antebrachial cutaneous nerve, which provides sensation over the anterolateral aspect of the forearm. Compression between the biceps tendon and the brachialis fascia can cause entrapment of the musculocutaneous nerve.

Sensory nerves innervate the elbow cutaneously and are derived from specific nerve root levels. The lateral arm is innervated by branches of the axillary nerve of the C5 root level while the lateral forearm is innervated by the musculocutaneous nerve of the C6 root level (Andrews et al 1993). The medial arm is innervated by the brachial cutaneous nerve from the T1 nerve root level. The medial forearm is innervated by branches of the antebrachial cutaneous nerve from the C8 root level (Andrews et al 1993). The T2 dermatome extends from the axilla to the posteromedial elbow (Magee 1987). Variability exists regarding the extent of each nerve root innervation; overlap between dermatome distribution occurs.

Elbow biomechanics in sport

Injuries to the elbow may occur in many different sports. The repetitive motions required for competition in many athletic events result in several common elbow injuries. These injuries are most often related to the tremendous amounts of force applied to the elbow joint during these sport-specific motions. The following section discusses the biomechanics and pathomechanics of the elbow during three sports that commonly produce elbow injuries: baseball pitching, tennis, and golf.

Biomechanics of baseball pitching

The biomechanics of the elbow during overhead baseball pitching can be broken down into six phases: windup, stride, arm cocking, arm acceleration, arm deceleration and follow through.

During the windup and stride, minimal elbow kinetics and muscle activity are present. As the foot contacts the ground, the elbow is flexed to approximately 85° (Werner et al 1993).

The arm-cocking phase begins as the foot comes into contact with the ground and continues until the point of maximum shoulder external rotation. As the arm moves into external rotation, a varus torque is produced at the elbow to prevent valgus stress (Werner et al 1993). Shortly before maximum external rotation, the elbow is flexed to 95° and a varus torque of approximately 64 Nm is produced (Fleisig & Barrentine 1995).

At this critical instant, excessive valgus strain may cause injury to the medial stabilizing structures of the elbow, particularly the UCL. As previously discussed, Morrey & An (1983) report that at this moment, the UCL is contributing approximately 54% of the valgus strain. Assuming that the UCL produces 54% of the 64 Nm of valgus strain observed during the arm cocking phase, 35 Nm would be applied to the UCL approaching the maximum capacity of load before failure in the UCL (Fleisig & Barrentine 1995, Fleisig et al 1995).

Also, as the elbow joint sustains a valgus strain, lateral compression is applied, possibly leading to compressive injuries of the lateral compartment of the elbow as the radial head and humeral capitellum are approximated. This compression may lead to avascular necrosis, osteochondritis dissecans or osteochondral chip fractures.

As the arm accelerates from maximal external rotation to ball release, the elbow extends at approximately 2500°/s (Fleisig & Barrentine 1995). As the elbow extends and resists valgus strain simultaneously, the olecranon can impinge against the medial aspect of the trochlear groove and olecranon fossa (Fleisig & Barrentine 1995). This impingement may lead to posteromedial osteophyte formation and loose body formations. This has been described by Wilson et al (1983) as valgus extension overload.

As the arm decelerates and continues into the follow-through phase, eccentric contraction of the elbow flexors must control the distractive forces at the elbow joint. Moderate activity of the biceps brachii and brachioradialis has been reported (Werner et al 1993). Muscular activity of the elbow flexors may assist in the prevention of olecranon impingement as the elbow is rapidly extended. The elbow remains in a flexed position of approximately 20° as the arm continues into follow through. Minimal kinetic and muscular activity is present during this final phase.

Biomechanics of the elbow during tennis

The kinematic and kinetic data during tennis varies dependent on the type of stroke, and the biomechanics of the serve and groundstrokes will be discussed separately. The overhead serve has been compared to the mechanics of overhead throwing (Fleisig & Barrentine 1995). The elbow has been reported to extend at 982°/s and pronate at 347°/s during acceleration and deceleration phases of the tennis serve (Kibler 1994). Morris et al (1989) report high activity of the triceps and pronator teres during the tennis serve in order to produce significant racket velocity. Because of this excessive angular velocity, the eccentric contraction of the elbow flexors and supinators is critical for the prevention of injuries to the elbow.

During groundstrokes, in both the forehand and the backhand, the wrist extensors are predominantly active as the athlete prepares the racket for impact (Morris et al 1989). The extensor carpi radialis longus, brevis and extensor communis musculature are active during both strokes, with the forehand showing additional muscle activity of the biceps brachii and brachioradialis (Kelley et al 1994, Morris et al 1989, Rhu et al

1988). As the racket comes into contact with the ball and begins the follow through, continued activity of the extensor carpi radialis brevis is noted, while the backhand produces additional activity of the biceps brachii as the elbow decelerates into extension (Kelley et al 1994, Morris et al 1989, Rhu et al 1988).

Kelley et al (1994) compared the muscular activity of the elbow during the backhand stroke in subjects with and without lateral epicondylitis. Results indicated that the group of subjects exhibiting lateral epicondylitis showed a significant increase in EMG activity of the extensor carpi radialis longus and brevis, pronator teres and flexor carpi radialis. These retrospective findings may have an impact in explaining the etiology of lateral epicondylitis.

Biomechanics of the golf swing

The biomechanics of the golf swing pertaining to elbow and wrist injuries can be broken down into five phases: the backswing, transition, downswing, impact and follow through. As the athlete swings the club, the lead arm and back arm are susceptible to injuries at various moments of the swing.

The backswing phase produces few injuries to the elbow. As the backswing progresses, the lead wrist pronates, flexes and radially deviates. The back arm flexes at the elbow and the wrist supinates, extends and radially deviates. The wrist flexors exhibit minimal EMG activity, whereas the wrist extensors exhibit 33% of a maximum voluntary isometric contraction (MVIC) (Glazebrook et al 1994). As the clubhead approaches the top of the backswing, the musculature of the elbow must eccentrically contract to control the clubhead and transition from the backswing to the downswing. This motion places a great deal of stress on the stretched flexor pronator mass of the back arm (Stanish et al 1994).

As the downswing progresses, the wrists must uncoil to produce clubhead speed. The wrist and elbow uncoil to return to the neutral position initially observed at setup to prepare for impact. The downswing is characterized by increased muscle activity of both the wrist extensors, which exhibit 45% MVIC, and the wrist flexors, which exhibit 35% MVIC. During impact, the wrist and hands decelerate due to the force of impact (Glazebrook et al 1994). McCarroll & Gioe (1982) report that more than twice as many injuries occur during the downswing compared to the backswing, as the elbow and wrist move approximately three times as fast during this phase. This deceleration of force places a great deal of strain on the forearm musculature as it attempts to maintain control of the club (Stanish et al 1994). The majority of elbow injuries take place during impact as the lateral epicondyle of the lead arm and the medial epicondyle of the backarm are placed under significant strain. The lead elbow extensor mass has been reported to be under even greater stress at impact due to the compressive force from ball impact and divots (McCarroll 1985) At ball contact, the wrist flexor activity significantly increases to 91% MVIC. Additionally, the wrist extensors exhibit EMG activity of approximately 58% MVIC (Glazebrook et al 1994).

Following impact, the arm continues into the follow through. Minimal injuries occur during this phase. The wrist and hands follow the pattern of the backswing in reverse; the lead arm flexes at the elbow, supinates, extends and radially deviates while the back arm pronates, flexes and radially deviates at the wrist. During the follow through, the wrist extensors EMG activity is approximately 60 to 70% MVIC. The repetitive nature of elbow and wrist motion observed may be responsible for overuse injuries to the forearm musculature.

When comparing the muscular activity patterns of golfers with medial epicondylitis and golfers without injuries, the golfers with medial epicondylitis exhibit significantly greater wrist flexor muscle activity during the backswing, transition, and downswing (Glazebrook et al 1994).

Clinical examination

The clinical examination of the athletic elbow relies on a complete and thorough history, extensive knowledge of the anatomy and biomechanics of the joint and a well-organized physical examination. The goal of the examination is to identify the areas of dysfunction and determine an appropriate course of rehabilitation.

History

Before the examination begins, a complete and thorough history is imperative. The location, intensity and duration of pain should be clearly identified. The date and mechanism of injury should be explained thoroughly, as this will assist in determining involved structures and the chronicity of the injury. Other subjective reports such as aggravating factors, previous injuries and primary complaints should be recorded to assist in the assessment and development of patient specific treatment and goals.

Observation

For a thorough inspection, the patient should completely expose the trunk and arms to provide a full view of the neck, shoulder and elbow. The skin should be evaluated for areas of contusion, ecchymosis, swelling, burns, surgical scars, redness, blanching, petechiae and venous congestion. The carrying angle should also be assessed during this portion of the examination.

Palpation

The palpation of the elbow begins with the identification of specific bony landmarks. The clinician should palpate each to determine if tenderness or deformity exists.

The medial epicondyle may exhibit tenderness for various reasons including epicondylitis, muscle strains and UCL injury. The medial supracondylar ridge should be examined for osteophytes, which may be entrapping the median nerve. The olecranon is easily palpated and is covered by the insertion of the triceps and the olecranon bursa, both of which may be tender if pathological. Osseous changes on the posteromedial olecranon may be associated with valgus extension overload in overhead athletes. The ulnar border should also be palpated for stress fractures, which are sometimes present in the throwing population. The lateral epicondyle is often irritable when palpated in the presence of epicondylitis. Lastly, the radial nerve lies approximately 2 cm distally from the lateral epicondyle and should be palpated during passive supination and pronation.

When palpating the soft tissues of the elbow, it is helpful to divide the elbow into four distinct regions: the medial, posterior, lateral and anterior aspects. The major structures of the medial aspect of the elbow include the ulnar nerve, flexor pronator muscle group, the UCL and the supracondylar lymph nodes. The clinician should determine if the ulnar nerve is capable of dislocating from the bony sulcus. This is done by abduction, externally rotating the shoulder with the patient supine, while the elbow is flexed to 20–70° (Andrews et al 1993). The medial epicondyle is palpated to determine tenderness to the flexor pronator muscle mass or the UCL. The UCL is exposed and can be easily palpated with the arm at 90° of abduction and full external rotation.

The posterior elbow contains the olecranon, which should be palpated for inflammation of a swollen bursa. The triceps insertion points should also be palpated for tenderness.

Laterally, the wrist extensor group is palpated. The brachioradialis is made prominent by having the patient close their fist, place the forearm in a neutral position and resist elbow flexion. Resisted wrist flexion allows for easy palpation of the extensor carpi radialis longus and brevis.

The anterior structures of the elbow pass through the cubital fossa. These structures from medial to lateral are the median nerve, brachial artery and the biceps tendon. The biceps can be made prominent by resistance in elbow flexion.

Range of motion

The normal range of motion (ROM) of the elbow is 0° of extension, 140–150° of flexion, 80° of pronation and 80° of supination (Norkin & White 1995). Passive ROM is assessed in each direction and compared to the contralateral elbow. Although full extension (0°) is considered normal, osseous adaptations from sport activities are common. For example, overhead athletes, such as baseball pitchers, often exhibit loss of full extension. This is often asymptomatic and should be considered chronic adaptations of the anterior soft tissue and the posterior osseous structures.

In addition, the end feel of movement should be assessed. Normal end feels of the elbow are different for each movement; elbow extension exhibits a hard, bony end feel, flexion a soft tissue approximation and forearm pronation and supination a capsular end feel (Cyriax 1982).

Muscle testing

Muscle testing of the elbow musculature begins with the patient seated (Kendall & McCreary 1983). The brachialis is tested with the elbow flexed and forearm pronated. The biceps is tested with the forearm supinated and shoulder flexed to 45–50°. The brachioradialis is tested with the elbow flexed with neutral wrist rotation. Triceps extension is performed with the shoulder flexed to 90° and elbow flexed 45–90°. Pronation and supination of the elbow is performed with the arm by the side and elbow flexed to 90° and neutral wrist rotation. Resistance is applied at the distal forearm as the patient attempts to rotate in either direction. Wrist extension and flexion are performed with the elbow flexed to 30° and with the elbow fully extended. Isokinetic testing may also be applied to determine specific objective data of muscular strength.

Special tests

Special tests for the elbow joint are used to elicit specific signs or symptoms of pathologies. Laxity assessment is used to evaluate the integrity of the medial and lateral stabilizing structures. Varus and valgus testing may be performed by stabilizing the arm with one hand and applying a fulcrum at the elbow joint with the other. The examiner imparts a varus or valgus stress and notes the amount of gapping and the end-feel motion. The tests are compared bilaterally and may be performed at 0° of extension and at 30° of flexion. Pain, excessive gapping or a soft end feel may all indicate pathology to the stabilizing structures.

The clinical test for valgus extension overload involves the examiner grasping the elbow in a flexed position. As the examiner forces the elbow into extension, a valgus stress is simultaneously applied to the elbow. The examiner palpates the posteromedial joint for tenderness and/or crepitation. Pain over the posteromedial olecranon process signifies a positive test (Wilson et al 1983).

A lateral pivot shift test is used to assess posterolateral rotatory instability (O'Driscoll et al 1991). Patients that have sustained an elbow dislocation often report a posterolateral rotatory mechanism of injury that is replicated during this test. The patient is supine and the examiner holds the arm over the head with 90° of shoulder flexion and maximal external rotation. The examiner applies a valgus and supination moment while flexing the elbow, resulting in the semilunar notch of the ulna displacing from the trochlea of the humerus; maximal displacement occurs at approximately 40° (O'Driscoll et al 1991). This test is often not tolerated by the patient without general anesthesia; however, signs of apprehension during testing indicate a positive clinical test in the awake patient (Kelly & Weiland 2001).

Neurological testing

The deep tendon reflexes that are significant in examination of the elbow are the biceps reflex, brachioradialis reflex and the triceps reflex, which are controlled by spinal levels C5, C6 and C7, respectively. A slight response is normal whereas an increased response could signify an upper motor neuron lesion, and a decreased response may indicate the presence of a lower motor neuron lesion.

The biceps tendon reflex can be elicited with the elbow relaxed and in a flexed position; the examiner places their thumb over the biceps tendon in the cubital fossa and gently taps the thumb with a reflex hammer. The brachioradialis reflex is elicited by tapping the tendon at the lateral distal end of the radius with the flat edge of a reflex hammer. The triceps tendon reflex is elicited by tapping over the triceps tendon with a reflex hammer.

Sensory perception is assessed by using a pinprick or light touch to the skin and noting the patient's response. The contralateral extremity is used for comparison. The lateral arm is innervated by the axillary nerve (C5) and the lateral forearm is innervated by branches of the musculocutaneous (C6). The medial arm is innervated by the brachial cutaneous (C8) and the medial forearm is innervated by the antebrachial cutaneous (T1) nerve.

Diagnostic images

Plane view radiographs, computed tomography (CT) arthrogram and magnetic resonance imaging (MRI) may be useful adjuncts to the clinical examination. Radiographs will allow the clinician to identify the presence of fractures, loose bodies and posterior olecranon osteophytes.

A diagnostic CT arthrogram is extremely useful when a UCL tear is suspected. Contrast dye is injected into the elbow, and X-rays are taken to determine if the dye has escaped the capsule through a tear. Complete UCL tears will provide a positive arthrogram. A CT scan, performed immediately following the arthrogram, can enhance visualization of a capsuloligamentous injury.

MRI of the elbow is also helpful in diagnosing complete UCL tears, particularly when the elbow is injected with saline prior to testing. A UCL tear is indicated by a leakage of dye along the medial side of the elbow proximally and distally along the medial olecranon. Timmerman & Andrews (1994) referred to this as a 'T-sign'.

Overview of elbow rehabilitation

Rehabilitation following elbow injury or elbow surgery follows a sequential and progressive multiphased approach. The ultimate goal of elbow rehabilitation is to return the athlete to their previous functional level as quickly and safely as possible. Several key principles must be addressed when rehabilitating the athlete's elbow: (1) the effects of immobilization must be minimized, (2) healing tissue must not be overstressed, (3) the patient must fulfill certain criteria throughout the phases of rehabilitation, (4) the program must be based on current scientific and clinical research, (5) the process must be adaptable to each patient and their specific goals and (6) the rehabilitation program must be a team effort between the physician, physical therapist, athletic trainer and patient. Communication between each team member is essential to successful outcomes. The following section will provide an overview of the rehabilitation process following elbow injury (Box 18.2) and surgery (Box 18.3); rehabilitation protocols for specific pathologies will follow.

Box 18.2 Nonoperative rehabilitation program for elbow injuries

PHASE I. Acute (week 1)

Goals

- Improve motion
- Diminish pain and inflammation
- Retard muscle atrophy

Exercises

1. Stretching for wrist and elbow joint, stretches for shoulder joint
2. Strengthening exercises, isometrics for wrist, elbow and shoulder musculature
3. Pain and inflammation control cryotherapy, high-voltage stimulation, ultrasound and whirlpool

PHASE II. Subacute (weeks 2–4)

Goals

- Normalize motion
- Improve muscular strength, power, and endurance

Week 2

1. Initiate isotonic strengthening for wrist and elbow muscles
2. Initiate exercise, tubing exercises for shoulder
3. Continue use of cryotherapy, etc.

Week 3

1. Initiate rhythmic stabilization drills for elbow and shoulder joint
2. Progress isotonic strengthening for entire upper extremity
3. Initiate isokinetic strengthening exercises for elbow flexion/extension

Week 4

1. Initiate Thrower's Ten program
2. Emphasize eccentric biceps work, concentric triceps and wrist flexor work
3. Program endurance training

4. Initiate light plyometric drills
5. Initiate swinging drills

PHASE III. Advanced strengthening (weeks 4–8)

Goals

- Preparation of athlete for return to functional activities

Criteria to progress to advanced phase:

1. Full nonpainful range of motion
2. No pain or tenderness
3. Satisfactory isokinetic test
4. Satisfactory clinical examination

Weeks 4–5

1. Continue strengthening exercises, endurance drills, and flexibility exercises daily
2. Thrower's Ten program
3. Progress plyometric drills
4. Emphasize maintenance program based on pathology
5. Progress swinging drills (i.e. hitting)

Weeks 6–8

1. Initiate interval sport program once determined by physician Phase I program

PHASE IV. Return to activity (weeks 6–9)

Weeks 6 through 9

When you return to play depends on your condition and progress, your physician will determine when it is safe

1. Continue strengthening program, Thrower's Ten program
2. Continue flexibility program
3. Progress functional drills to unrestricted play

Phase I – immediate motion phase

The first phase of elbow rehabilitation is the immediate motion phase. The goals of this phase are to minimize the effects of immobilization, re-establish nonpainful range of motion, decrease pain and inflammation and to retard muscular atrophy. The rehabilitation specialist must not overstress healing tissues during this phase.

Early ranges of motion activities are performed to nourish the articular cartilage and assist in the synthesis, alignment and organization of collagen tissue (Coutts et al 1981, Dehne & Tory 1971, Haggmark & Eriksson 1979, Noyes et al 1987, Perkins 1954, Salter et al 1980, 1984, Tipton et al 1978, Wilk et al 1993a). Range of motion (ROM) activities are performed for all planes of elbow and wrist motions to prevent the formation of scar tissue and adhesions. Re-establishing full elbow extension is the primary goal of early ROM activities to minimize the occurrence of elbow flexion contractures (Akeson et al 1980, Green & McCoy 1979, Nirschl & Morrey 1985). The elbow is predisposed to flexion contractures due to the

intimate congruency of the joint articulations, the tightness of the joint capsule, and the tendency of the anterior capsule to develop adhesions following injury. The brachialis muscle also attaches to the capsule and crosses the elbow joint before becoming a tendinous structure. Injury to the elbow may cause excessive scar tissue formation of the brachialis muscle as well as functional splinting of the elbow.

Grade I and II joint mobilizations may be performed during this early phase of rehabilitation as tolerated (Maitland 1977). Posterior glides with oscillations are performed in the midrange of motion to assist in regaining full elbow extension. Aggressive mobilization techniques are not utilized until later stages of rehabilitation when pain has subsided. Grade I and II mobilization techniques are also utilized to neuromodulate pain by stimulating type I and type II articular receptors (Maitland 1977, Wyke 1966).

If the patient continues to have difficulty achieving full extension using ROM and mobilization techniques, a low load, long duration (LLLD) stretch may be performed to produce a creep of the collagen tissue, which will result in tissue elongation

Box 18.3 Postoperative rehabilitation protocol for elbow arthroscopy

PHASE I. Initial (week 1)

Goal

Full wrist and elbow range of motion, decrease swelling, decrease pain, retardation of muscle atrophy

A. Day of surgery

Begin gently moving elbow in bulky dressing

B. Post-op day 1 and 2

1. Remove bulky dressing and replace with elastic bandages
2. Immediate post-op hand, wrist and elbow exercise
   a. Putty/grip strengthening
   b. Wrist flexor stretching
   c. Wrist extensor stretching
   d. Wrist curls
   e. Reverse wrist curls
   f. Neutral wrist curls
   g. Pronation/supination
   h. Active/active-assisted range of motion elbow ext/flex

C. Post-op day 3 through 7

1. Passive range of motion elbow ext/flex (motion to tolerance)
2. Begin progressive resistance exercises with 1 lb weight
   a. Wrist curls
   b. Reverse wrist curls
   c. Neutral wrist curls
   d. Pronation/supination
   e. Broomstick roll-up

PHASE II. Intermediate (Weeks 2–4)

Goal

Improve muscular strength and endurance; normalize joint arthrokinematics

A. Week 2 ROM exercises (overpressure into extension)

1. Addition of biceps curl and triceps extension
2. Continue to progress progressive resistance exercise weight and repetitions as tolerable

B. Week 3

1. Initiate biceps and triceps eccentric exercise program
2. Initiate rotator cuff exercises program
   a. External rotators
   b. Internal rotators
   c. Deltoid
   d. Supraspinatus
   e. Scapulothoracic strengthening

PHASE III. Advanced (weeks 4–8)

Goals

Preparation of athlete for return to functional activities

Criteria to progress to advanced phase:

1. Full non-painful range of motion
2. No pain or tenderness
3. Isokinetic test that fulfills criteria to throw
4. Satisfactory clinical exam

A. 3 through 6 weeks

1. Continue maintenance program, emphasizing muscular strength, endurance, and flexibility
2. Initiate interval throwing program phase I

(Kottke et al 1966, Sapega et al 1976, Warren et al 1971, 1976). We have found this exercise to be extremely beneficial for regaining full elbow extension (Wilk & Levinson 2001, Wilk et al 1993a). The patient lies supine with a towel roll placed under the brachium to act as a cushion and fulcrum. Light resistance exercise tubing is applied to the wrist of the patient and secured to the table or a dumbbell on the ground (Fig. 18.1). The patient is instructed to relax as much as possible for 10–12 min. The amount of resistance applied should be of low magnitude to enable the patient to perform the stretch for the entire duration without pain or muscle spasm.

The aggressiveness of stretching and mobilization techniques is dictated based on healing constraints of involved tissues as well as the amount of motion and end feel. If the patient presents with a decrease in motion and hard end feel without pain, aggressive stretching and mobilization technique may be used. Conversely, a patient exhibiting pain before resistance and/or empty end feel will be progressed slowly with gentle stretching.

Cryotherapy and high-voltage stimulation may be performed as required to assist in reducing pain and inflammation. Once the acute inflammatory phase has passed, moist heat, warm whirlpool and ultrasound may be used at the onset of treatment

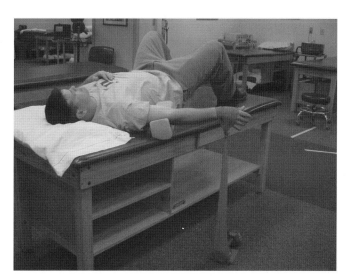

Figure 18.1 • Low load, long duration stretch into elbow extension.

to prepare the tissue for stretching and to improve the extensibility of the capsule and musculotendinous structures.

The early phases of rehabilitation must also focus on retarding muscular atrophy. Subpainful and submaximal isometrics are performed initially for the elbow flexor and extensor, as well as the wrist flexor, extensor, pronator and supinator muscle groups. Isometrics should be performed at multiple angles for 2–3 sets of 10 repetitions, holding each contraction for 6–8 s. Shoulder isometrics may also be performed during this phase with caution against internal and external rotation exercises if painful. Alternating rhythmic stabilization drills for shoulder flexion/extension/horizontal abduction/adduction and shoulder internal/external rotation are performed to begin reestablishing proprioception and neuromuscular control of the upper extremity.

Phase II – intermediate phase

Phase II, the intermediate phase, is initiated when the patient exhibits full ROM, minimal pain and tenderness and a good (4/5) manual muscle test of the elbow flexor and extensor musculature. The emphasis of this phase includes enhancing elbow and upper extremity mobility, improving muscular strength and endurance and reestablishing neuromuscular control of the elbow complex.

Stretching exercises are continued to maintain full elbow flexion and extension. Mobilization techniques may be progressed to more aggressive grade III techniques, as needed, to apply a stretch to the capsular tissue and end range. Flexibility is progressed during this phase to focus on wrist flexion, extension, pronation and supination. Shoulder flexibility is also maintained in athletes with emphasis on flexion, external and internal rotation, and horizontal adduction.

Strengthening exercises are progressed during this phase to include isotonic contractions. Emphasis is placed on elbow flexion and extension, wrist flexion and extension and forearm pronation and supination. The weight of the arm is initially used before progressing to a 1 lb dumbbell. Resistance is then progressed by 1 lb per week to gradually stress the involved tissues. The shoulder and scapular muscles are also placed on a progressive resistance program during the later stages of this phase. Emphasis is placed on strengthening the shoulder external rotators and scapular muscles, and training eccentric control of the elbow flexors. Shoulder internal and external rotation are performed with exercise tubing at 0° of abduction; standing scaption with external rotation (full can), standing abduction, prone horizontal abduction and prone rowing are all included in this phase.

Muscular endurance activities are also performed during this phase. High repetition, low resistance dumbbell exercises, as previously described, and the upper body ergometer may be used.

Neuromuscular control exercises are initiated in this phase to enhance the muscles' ability to control the elbow joint during athletic activities. These exercises include proprioceptive neuromuscular facilitation exercises with rhythmic stabilizations

(Wilk et al 2001b) and slow reversal manual resistance elbow/wrist flexion drills (Fig. 18.2).

Phase III – advanced strengthening phase

The third phase involves a progression of activities to prepare the athlete for sport participation. The goals of this phase are to gradually increase strength, power, endurance and neuromuscular control, to prepare for a gradual return to sport. Specific criteria that must be met before entering this phase include full nonpainful ROM, no pain or tenderness and strength that is 70% of the contralateral extremity.

Advanced strengthening activities during this phase include aggressive strengthening exercises emphasizing high speed and eccentric contraction and plyometric activities. Strengthening exercises are progressed to include the Thrower's Ten program (Fig. 18.3). The design of these exercises is based on numerous EMG studies (Blackburn et al 1990, Fleisig & Escamilla 1996, Moseley et al 1992, Reinold et al 2004, Townsend et al 1991) and they are designed to strengthen all of the shoulder, scapular, elbow and wrist muscles that are utilized during upper extremity athletic activities. Internal and external rotation exercises with exercise tubing are progressed to a function position of 90°

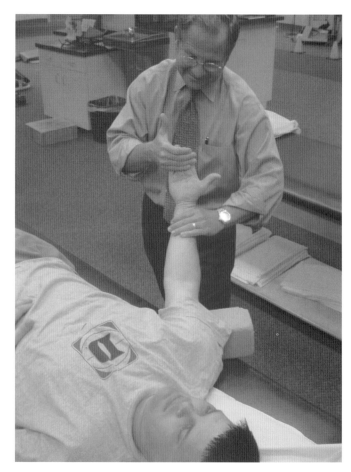

Figure 18.2 • Manual resisted elbow and wrist flexion using both concentric and eccentric contractions of the elbow flexors.

The Thrower's Ten Program is designed to exercise the major muscles necessary for throwing. The Program's goal is to be an organized and concise exercise program. In addition, all exercises included are specific to the thrower and are designed to improve strength, power and endurance of the shoulder complex musculature.

1A Diagonal Pattern D2 Extension:
Involved hand will grip tubing handle overhead and out to the side. Pull tubing down and across your body to the opposite side of leg. During the motion, lead with your thumb.
Perform _____ sets of _____ repetitions _____ times daily.

1B Diagonal Pattern D2 Flexion:
Gripping tubing handle in hand of involved arm, begin with arm out from side 45° and palm facing backward. After turning palm forward, proceed to flex elbow and bring arm up and over involved shoulder. Turn palm down and reverse to take arm to starting position.
Perform _____ sets of _____ repetitions _____ times daily.

2A External Rotation at 0° Abduction:
Stand with involved elbow fixed at side, elbow at 90° and involved arm across front of body. Grip tubing handle while the other end of tubing is fixed. Pull out arm, keeping elbow at side. Return tubing slowly and controlled.
Perform _____ sets of _____ repetitions _____ times daily.

2B Internal Rotation at 0° Abduction:
Standing with elbow at side fixed at 90° and shoulder rotated out. Grip tubing handle while other end of tubing is fixed. Pull arm across body keeping elbow at side. Return tubing slowly and controlled.
Perform _____ sets of _____ repetitions _____ times daily.

2C (Optional) External Rotation at 90° Abduction:
Stand with shoulder abducted 90°. Grip tubing handle while the other end is fixed straight ahead, slightly lower than the shoulder. Keeping shoulder abducted, rotate shoulder back keeping elbow at 90°. Return tubing and hand to start position.
I Slow Speed Sets: (slow and controlled)
Perform _____ sets of _____ repetitions _____ times daily.
II Fast Speed Sets:
Perform _____ sets of _____ repetitions _____ times daily.

2D (Optional) Internal Rotation at 90° Abduction:
Stand with shoulder abducted to 90°, externally rotated 90° and elbow bent to 90°. Keeping shoulder abducted, rotate shoulder forward, keeping elbow bent at 90°. Return tubing and hand to start position.
I Slow Speed Sets: (slow and controlled)
Perform _____ sets of _____ repetitions _____ times daily.
II Fast Speed Sets:
Perform _____ sets of _____ repetitions _____ times daily.

Figure 18.3 • The Thrower's Ten program.

3 Shoulder Abduction to 90°:
Stand with arm at side, elbow straight, and palm against side. Raise arm to the side, palm down, until arm reaches 90° (shoulder level). Perform _____ sets of _____ repetitions _____ times daily.

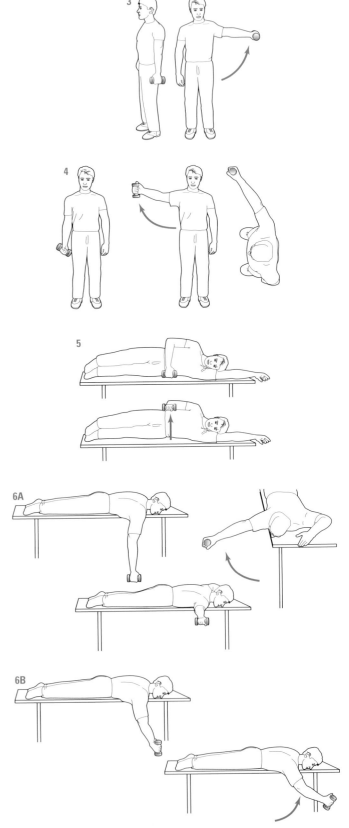

4 Scaption, External Rotation:
Stand with elbow straight and thumb up. Raise arm to shoulder level at 30° angle in front of body. Do not go above shoulder height. Hold 2 seconds and lower slowly.
Perform _____ sets of _____ repetitions _____ times daily.

5 Sidelying External Rotation:
Lie on uninvolved side, with involved arm at side of body and elbow bent to 90°. Keeping the elbow of involved arm fixed to side, raise arm. Hold 2 seconds and lower slowly.
Perform _____ sets of _____ repetitions _____ times daily.

6A Prone Horizontal Abduction (Neutral):
Lie on table, face down, with involved arm hanging straight to the floor, and palm facing down. Raise arm out to the side, parallel to the floor. Hold 2 seconds and lower slowly.
Perform _____ sets of _____ repetitions _____ times daily.

6B Prone Horizontal Abduction (Full ER, 100° ABD):
Lie on table face down, with involved arm hanging straight to the floor and thumb rotated up (hitchhiker). Raise arm out to the side with arm slightly in front of shoulder, parallel to the floor. Hold 2 seconds and lower slowly.
Perform _____ sets of _____ repetitions _____ times daily.

Figure 18.3 • (Continued)

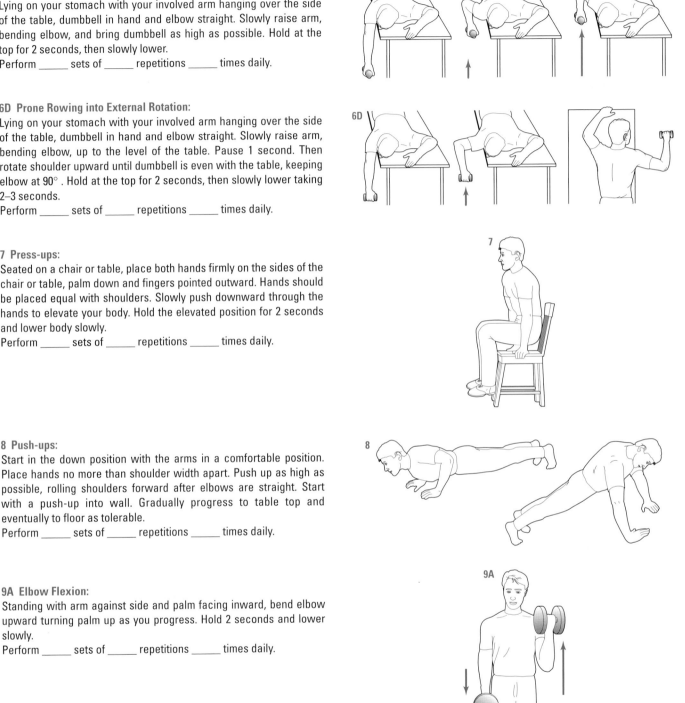

6C Prone Rowing:
Lying on your stomach with your involved arm hanging over the side of the table, dumbbell in hand and elbow straight. Slowly raise arm, bending elbow, and bring dumbbell as high as possible. Hold at the top for 2 seconds, then slowly lower.
Perform _____ sets of _____ repetitions _____ times daily.

6D Prone Rowing into External Rotation:
Lying on your stomach with your involved arm hanging over the side of the table, dumbbell in hand and elbow straight. Slowly raise arm, bending elbow, up to the level of the table. Pause 1 second. Then rotate shoulder upward until dumbbell is even with the table, keeping elbow at 90°. Hold at the top for 2 seconds, then slowly lower taking 2–3 seconds.
Perform _____ sets of _____ repetitions _____ times daily.

7 Press-ups:
Seated on a chair or table, place both hands firmly on the sides of the chair or table, palm down and fingers pointed outward. Hands should be placed equal with shoulders. Slowly push downward through the hands to elevate your body. Hold the elevated position for 2 seconds and lower body slowly.
Perform _____ sets of _____ repetitions _____ times daily.

8 Push-ups:
Start in the down position with the arms in a comfortable position. Place hands no more than shoulder width apart. Push up as high as possible, rolling shoulders forward after elbows are straight. Start with a push-up into wall. Gradually progress to table top and eventually to floor as tolerable.
Perform _____ sets of _____ repetitions _____ times daily.

9A Elbow Flexion:
Standing with arm against side and palm facing inward, bend elbow upward turning palm up as you progress. Hold 2 seconds and lower slowly.
Perform _____ sets of _____ repetitions _____ times daily.

Figure 18.3 • (Continued)

9B Elbow Extension (Abduction):
Raise involved arm overhead. Provide support at elbow from uninvolved hand. Straighten arm overhead. Hold 2 seconds and lower slowly.
Perform _____ sets of _____ repetitions _____ times daily.

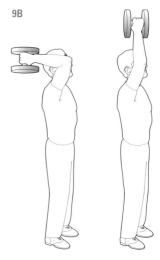

10A Wrist Extension:
Supporting the forearm and with palm facing downward, raise weight in hand as far as possible. Hold 2 seconds and lower slowly.
Perform _____ sets of _____ repetitions _____ times daily.

10B Wrist Flexion:
Supporting the forearm and with palm facing upward, lower a weight in hand as far as possible and then curl it up as high as possible. Hold for 2 seconds and lower slowly.
Perform _____ sets of _____ repetitions _____ times daily.

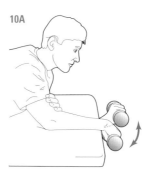
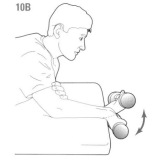

10C Supination:
Forearm supported on table with wrist in neutral position. Using a weight or hammer, roll wrist taking palm up. Hold 2 seconds and return to starting position.
Perform _____ sets of _____ repetitions _____ times daily.

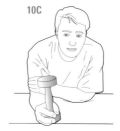
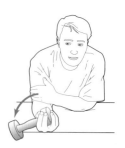

10D Pronation:
Forearm should be supported on a table with wrist in neutral position. Using a weight or hammer, roll wrist taking palm down. Hold 2 seconds and return to starting position.
Perform _____ sets of _____ repetitions _____ times daily.

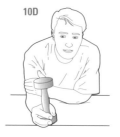
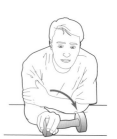

Figure 18.3 • (Continued)

abduction with 90° elbow flexion. Exercises may be performed at slow and fast speeds. Scapulothoracic exercises are progressed to include prone horizontal abduction at 100° and full external rotation as well as prone rows into external rotation.

Elbow flexion exercises are progressed to emphasize eccentric control. The biceps muscle is an important stabilizer during the follow-through phase of overhead throwing to eccentrically control the deceleration of the elbow, preventing pathological abutting of the olecranon within the fossa (Andrews & Frank 1985, Fleisig & Escamilla 1996). Elbow flexion can be performed with elastic tubing to emphasize slow and fast speed concentric and eccentric contractions.

Aggressive strengthening exercises with weight machines are also incorporated during this phase. These most commonly begin with bench press, seated rowing and front latissimus dorsi pull-downs.

Neuromuscular control exercises are progressed to include side-lying external rotation with manual resistance. Concentric and eccentric external rotation is performed against the clinician's resistance with the addition of rhythmic stabilizations (Wilk et al 2001b). This manual resistance exercise may be progressed to standing external rotation with exercise tubing at 0° and finally at 90° (Fig. 18.4).

Plyometric drills are an extremely beneficial form of exercise for training the upper extremity musculature (Wilk et al 1993b). The physiological principles of plyometric exercise utilize an eccentric prestretch of the muscle tissue, thereby stimulating the muscle spindle to produce a more forceful concentric contraction. Plyometric exercises are performed using a weighted medicine ball during the later stages of this phase to train the upper extremity musculature to develop and withstand high levels of stress. Plyometric exercises are initially performed with two hands performing a chest pass, side-to-side throw and overhead soccer throw. These may be progressed to include one hand activities such as 90/90 throws (Fig. 18.5),

external and internal rotation throws at 0° of abduction and wall dribbles (Wilk et al 1993b, 2001b). Specific plyometric drills for the forearm musculature include wrist flexion flips (Fig. 18.6) and extension grips.

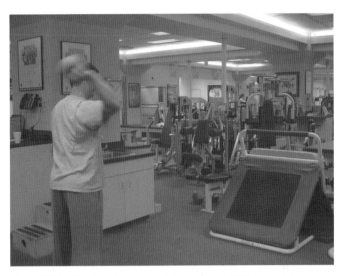

Figure 18.5 • One-handed plyometric throws at 90° of shoulder abduction and 90° of elbow flexion using a 2 lb weighted ball.

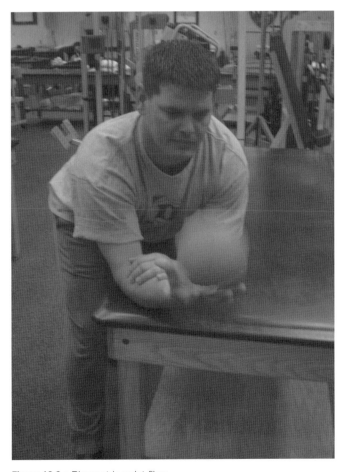

Figure 18.6 • Plyometric wrist flips.

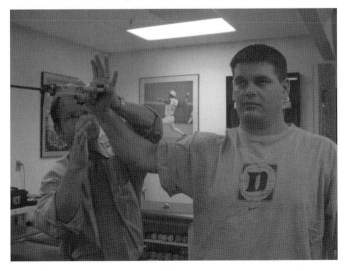

Figure 18.4 • External rotation at 90° of shoulder abduction with tubing and manual resistance.

Phase IV – return-to-activity phase

The final phase of elbow rehabilitation, the return-to-activity phase, allows the athlete to return progressively to full competition using an interval return to sport program (Wilk et al 2001a). Sport-specific functional drills are performed to prepare the athlete for the stresses involved with each particular sport.

Before an athlete is allowed to begin the return-to-activity phase of rehabilitation, the athlete must exhibit full ROM, no pain or tenderness, a satisfactory isokinetic test and a satisfactory clinical examination. Isokinetic testing is commonly utilized to determine the readiness of the athlete to begin an interval sport program. Athletes are routinely tested at 180 and 300°/s. Successful results of isokinetic testing are listed in Table 18.2.

Upon achieving the previously mentioned criteria to return to sport, we begin a formal interval sport program (Reinold et al 2002). For the overhead thrower, we initiate a long-toss interval throwing program (Box 18.4). The athlete throws three times per week with a day off from throwing in between each session. Each step is performed at least twice on separate days before we allow the athlete to progress to the next step. Throwing should be performed without pain or significant increase in symptoms. If the athlete experiences symptoms at a particular step within the program, the athlete is instructed to regress to the prior step until symptoms subside. We believe it is important for the overhead athlete to perform stretching and an abbreviated strengthening program prior to and after performing the interval sport program. Typically, our overhead throwers warm-up, stretch and perform one set of their exercise program before throwing, followed by two additional sets of exercises after throwing. This provides an adequate warm-up but also ensures maintenance of necessary range of motion and flexibility of the shoulder joint.

Following the completion of a long-toss program, pitchers will progress to phase II of the throwing program – throwing off a mound (Box 18.5). In phase II, the number of throws, intensity and type of pitch are progressed to gradually increase stress on the shoulder joint.

Interval sport programs for tennis and golf follow the same guidelines as the baseball program. A specific interval program for tennis is outlined in Box 18.6. As the athlete progresses, the number of forehand and backhand shots are gradually increased. Overhead serving is typically initiated during the third week of the program and games are allowed during the fourth week if symptoms have not exacerbated.

Box 18.7 outlines an interval golf program. The program begins with simple putting and chipping and progresses to include short iron swings by the end of week 1, medium irons by week 2 and long irons by week 3. Medium and long iron shots are hit using a tee, to minimize the forces at the elbow observed while taking a divot. Woods are initiated at the end of week 3 and progressed to include drives by the fourth week. The athlete can play 9 holes during the end of the fourth week if asymptomatic.

The following sections will briefly overview the clinical presentations, findings and rehabilitation programs of numerous elbow joint disorders commonly seen in athletes, followed by several non-common sport-related pathologies. Nonoperative injuries will be presented first, followed by postoperative procedures.

Common sport-related injuries

Medial and lateral epicondylitis

Medial and lateral epicondylitis may result from numerous factors, many of which have been previously discussed. The majority of causes are related to repetitive microtrauma and poor biomechanics, which are sport specific. Medially, overhead throwers most often exhibit pronator tendonitis, and golfers present with wrist flexor tendonitis, whereas lateral epicondylitis is most often seen in tennis players. Patients most often present with tenderness near the epicondyle and along the flexor pronator and extensor supinator muscle masses, which may be exacerbated by contraction or stretching of the musculature.

Clinical examination should attempt to distinguish the structures involved. For medial epicondylitis, manual resistance of wrist flexion should be performed as well as pronation to determine if a pronation strain has occurred. For lateral epicondylitis, testing the extensor carpi radialis longus is performed with

Table 18.2 Satisfactory isokinetic test results

Bilateral comparisons				
Velocity °/s	Elbow Flex	Elbow Ext		
180	110–120%	105–115%		
300	105–115%	100–110%		
Velocity °/s	Shoulder ER	Shoulder IR	Shoulder Abd	Shoulder Add
180	98–105%	110–120%	98–105%	110–128%
300	85–95%	105–115%	96–102%	111–129%

Unilateral muscle ratios				
Velocity °/s	Elbow Flex/Ext	Shoulder ER/IR	Shoulder Abd/Add	Shoulder ER/Abd
180	70–80%	66–76%	78–84%	67–75%
300	63–69%	61–71%	88–94%	60–70%

Peak torque to body weight ratios				
Velocity °/s	Shoulder ER	Shoulder IR	Shoulder Abd	Shoulder Add
180	18–23%	28–33%	26–33%	32–38%
300	12–20%	25–30%	20–25%	28–34%

Abd – abduction; Add – adduction; ER – external rotation; Ext – extension; Flex – flexion; IR – internal rotation

Box 18.4 Interval throwing program for baseball players – phase I

The interval throwing program (ITP) is designed to gradually return motion, strength and confidence in the throwing arm after injury or surgery by slowly progressing through graduated throwing distances. The ITP is initiated upon clearance by the athlete's physician to resume throwing, and performed under the supervision of the rehabilitation team (physician, physical therapist and athletic trainer).

The program is set up to minimize the chance of reinjury and emphasize prethrowing warm-up and stretching. In the development of the ITP, the following factors are considered most important:

1. The act of throwing the baseball involves the transfer of energy from the feet through the legs, pelvis, trunk, and out of the shoulder through the elbow and hand. Therefore, any return to throwing after injury must include attention to the entire body.
2. The chance for reinjury is lessened by a graduated progression of interval throwing.
3. Proper warm-up is essential.
4. Most injuries occur as the result of fatigue.
5. Proper throwing mechanics lessen the incidence of reinjury.
6. Baseline requirements for throwing include:
   - Pain-free range of motion
   - Adequate muscle power
   - Adequate muscle resistance to fatigue

Because there is an individual variability in all throwing athletes, there is no set timetable for completion of the program. Most athletes, by nature, are highly competitive individuals and wish to return to competition at the earliest possible moment. While this is a necessary quality of all athletes, the proper channeling of the athlete's energies into a rigidly controlled throwing program is essential to lessen the chance of reinjury during the rehabilitation period. The athlete may have the tendency to want to increase the intensity of the throwing program. This will increase the incidence of reinjury and may greatly retard the rehabilitation process. It is recommended to follow the program rigidly as this will be the safest route for return to competition.

During the recovery process the athlete will probably experience soreness and a dull, diffuse aching sensation in the muscles and tendons. If the athlete experiences sharp pain, particularly in the joint, stop all throwing activity until this pain ceases. If pain continues, the physician should be contacted.

Weight-training. The athlete should supplement the ITP with a high repetition, low weight exercise program. Strengthening should address a good balance between anterior and posterior musculature so that the shoulder will not be predisposed to injury. Special emphasis must be given to posterior rotator cuff musculature for any strengthening program. Weight-training will not increase throwing velocity, but will increase the resistance of the arm to fatigue and injury. Weight-training should be done the same day as the athlete throws; however, it should be after throwing is completed, using the day in between for flexibility exercises and a recovery period. It should be stressed at this point that a weight-training pattern or routine is a 'maintenance program.' This pattern can and should accompany the athlete into and throughout the season as a deterrent to further injury. It must be stressed that weight-training is of no benefit unless accompanied by a sound flexibility program.

Individual variability. The ITP is designed so that each level is achieved without pain or complications before the next level is started. This sets up a progression that a goal is achieved prior to advancement instead of advancing to a specific timeframe.

Because of this design, the ITP may be used for different levels of skills and abilities, from those in high school to professional levels. The reasons for being in the ITP will vary from person to person. Example: one athlete may wish to use alternate days throwing with or without using weights in between; another athlete may have to throw every third or fourth day due to pain or swelling. 'Listen to your body – it will tell you when to slow down'. Again, completion of the steps of the ITP will vary from person to person. There is no set timetable in terms of days to completion.

Warm-up. Jogging increases blood flow to the muscles and joints, thus increasing their flexibility and decreasing the chance of reinjury. Since the amount of warm-up will vary from person to person, the athlete should jog until developing a light sweat, then progress to the stretching phase.

Stretching. Since throwing involves all muscles in the body, all muscle groups should be stretched prior to throwing. This should be done in a systematic fashion beginning with the legs and including the trunk, back, neck and arms. Continue with capsular stretches and L-bar range of motion exercises.

Throwing mechanics. A critical aspect of the ITP is maintenance of proper throwing mechanics throughout the advancement. The use of the crow-hop method simulates the throwing act, allowing emphasis of the proper body mechanics. This throwing method should be adopted from the set in the ITP. Throwing when flat-footed encourages improper body mechanics, placing increased stress on the throwing arm and, therefore, predisposing the arm to reinjury. The pitching coach and sports biomechanist (if available) may be valuable allies to the rehabilitation team with their knowledge of throwing mechanics.

Components of the crow-hop method are first a hop, then a skip, followed by the throw. The velocity of the throw is determined by the distance, whereas the ball should have only enough momentum to travel each designed distance. Again, emphasis should be placed upon proper throwing mechanics when the athlete begins phase two: 'throwing off the mound' or from the athlete's respective position, to decrease the chance of reinjury.

Throwing. Using the crow-hop method, the athlete should begin warm-up throws at a comfortable distance (approximately 30–45 ft) and then progress to the distance indicated for that phase. The program consists of throwing at each step, 2 to 3 times without pain or symptoms, before progressing to the next step. The object of each phase is for the athlete to be able to throw the ball the specified number of feet without pain (45, 60, 90, 120, 150, 180 ft), 75 times at each distance. After being able to throw at the prescribed distance without pain the athlete will be ready for throwing from flat ground 60 ft 6 in. in the normal pitching mechanics or return to the athlete's respective position (step 14). At this point, full strength and confidence should be restored in the athlete's arm. It is important to stress the crow-hop method and proper mechanics with each throw. Just as the advancement to this point has been gradual and progressive, the return to unrestricted throwing must follow the same principles. A pitcher should first throw only fast balls at 50%, progressing to 75% and 100%. At this time, the pitcher may start more stressful pitches such as breaking balls. The position player should simulate a game situation, again progressing at 50–75 to 100%. Once again, if an athlete has increased pain, particularly at the joint, the throwing program should be backed off and re-advanced as tolerated, under the direction of the rehabilitation team.

Batting. Depending on the type of injury that the athlete has, the time of return to batting should be determined by the physician. It should be noted that stress placed upon the arm in the batting

Box 18.4 (Continued)

motion is very different from the throwing motion. Return to unrestricted use of the bat should also follow the same progression guidelines as seen in the training program. Begin with dry swings progressing to hitting off the tee, then soft toss and finally live pitching.

Summary. In using the ITP in conjunction with a structured rehabilitation program, the athlete should be able to return to full competition status, minimizing any chance of reinjury. The program and its progression should be modified to meet the specific needs of each individual athlete. A comprehensive program consisting of a maintenance strength and flexibility program, appropriate warm-up and cool-down procedures, proper pitching mechanics, and progressive throwing and batting will assist the baseball player in returning safely to competition.

45 ft Phase

Step 1:
A. Warm-up throwing
B. 45 ft (25 throws)
C. Rest 5–10 min
D. Warm-up throwing
E. 45 ft (25 throws)

Step 2:
A. Warm-up throwing
B. 45 ft (25 throws)
C. Rest 5–10 min
D. Warm-up throwing
E. 45 ft (25 throws)
F. Rest 5–10 min
G. Warm-up throwing
H. 45 ft (25 throws)

60 ft Phase

Step 3:
A. Warm-up throwing
B. 60 ft (25 throws)
C. Rest 5–10 min
D. Warm-up throwing
E. 60 ft (25 throws)

Step 4:
A. Warm-up throwing
B. 60 ft (25 throws)
C. Rest 5–10 min
D. Warm-up throwing
E. 60 ft (25 throws)
F. Rest 5–10 min
G. Warm-up throwing
H. 60 ft (25 throws)

90 ft Phase

Step 5:
A. Warm-up throwing
B. 90 ft (25 throws)
C. Rest 5–10 min
D. Warm-up throwing
E. 90 ft (25 throws)

Step 6:
A. Warm-up throwing
B. 90 ft (25 throws)
C. Rest 5–10 min
D. Warm-up throwing
E. 90 ft (25 throws)
F. Rest 5–10 min
G. Warm-up throwing
H. 90 ft (25 throws)

120 ft Phase

Step 7:
A. Warm-up throwing
B. 120 ft (25 throws)
C. Rest 5–10 min
D. Warm-up throwing
E. 120 ft (25 throws)

Step 8:
A. Warm-up throwing
B. 120 ft (25 throws)
C. Rest 5–10 min
D. Warm-up throwing
E. 120 ft (25 throws)
F. Rest 5–10 min
G. Warm-up throwing
H. 120 ft (25 throws)

150 ft Phase

Step 9:
A. Warm-up throwing
B. 150 ft (25 throws)
C. Rest 5–10 min
D. Warm-up throwing
E. 150 ft (25 throws)

Step 10:
A. Warm-up throwing
B. 150 ft (25 throws)
C. Rest 5–10 min
D. Warm-up throwing
E. 150 ft (25 throws)
F. Rest 5–10 min
G. Warm-up throwing
H. 150 ft (25 throws)

Step 11:
A. Warm-up throwing
B. 180 ft (25 throws)
C. Rest 5–10 min
D. Warm-up throwing
E. 180 ft (25 throws)

Step 12:
A. Warm-up throwing
B. 180 ft (25 throws)
C. Rest 5–10 min
D. Warm-up throwing
E. 180 ft (25 throws)
F. Rest 5–10 min
G. Warm-up throwing
H. 180 ft (25 throws)

180 ft Phase

Step 13:
A. Warm-up throwing
B. 180 ft (25 throws)
C. Rest 5–10 min
D. Warm-up throwing
E. 180 ft (25 throws)

Step 14: Begin throwing off the mound or return to respective position

The throwing program should be performed every other day, unless otherwise specified by the physician or rehabilitation specialist.

Perform each step __ times before progressing to next step

Flat ground throwing

A. Warm-up throwing
B. Throw 60 ft (10–15 throws)
C. Throw 90 ft (10 throws)
D. Throw 120 ft (10 throws)
E. Throw 60 ft (flat ground) using pitching mechanics (20–30 throws)

Flat throwing

A. Warm-up throwing
B. Throw 60 ft (10–15 throws)
C. Throw 90 ft (10 throws)
D. Throw 120 ft (10 throws)
E. Throw 60 ft (flat ground) using pitching mechanics (20–30 throws)
F. Throw 60–90 ft (10–15 throws)
G. Throw 60 ft (flat ground) using pitching mechanics (20 throws)

Box 18.5 Interval throwing program for baseball players – throwing off the mound – phase II

After the completion of phase I of the interval throwing program (ITP) and when able to throw to the prescribed distance without pain, the athlete will be ready for throwing off the mound or to return to the athlete's respective position. At this point, full strength and confidence should be restored in the athlete's arm. Just as the advancement to this point has been gradual and progressive, the return to unrestricted throwing must follow the same principles. A pitcher should first throw only fast balls at 50%, progressing to 75 and 100%. At this time, the athlete may start more stressful pitches such as breaking balls. The position player should simulate a game situation, again progressing at 50–75–100%. Once again, if an athlete has increased pain, particularly at the joint, the throwing program should be backed off and re-advanced as tolerated, under the direction of the rehabilitation team.

Summary. In using the ITP in conjunction with a structured rehabilitation program, the athlete should be able to return to full competition status, minimizing any chance of reinjury. The program and its progression should be modified to meet the specific needs of each individual athlete. A comprehensive program consisting of a maintenance strength and flexibility program, appropriate warm-up and cool-down procedures, proper pitching mechanics, and progressive throwing and batting will assist the baseball player in returning safely to competition.

STAGE ONE: FASTBALLS ONLY

Step 1:	Interval throwing 15 throws off mound 50%
Step 2:	Interval throwing 30 throws off mound 50%
Step 3:	Interval throwing 45 throws off mound 50%
Step 4:	Interval throwing 60 throws off mound 50%

Step 5:	Interval throwing 70 throws off mound 50%
Step 6:	45 throws off mound 50% 30 throws off mound 75%
Step 7:	30 throws off mound 50% 45 throws off mound 75%
Step 8:	65 throws off mound 75% 10 throws off mound 50%

STAGE TWO: FASTBALLS ONLY

Step 9:	60 throws off mound 75% 15 throws in batting practice
Step 10:	50–60 throws off mound 75% 30 throws in batting practice
Step 11:	45–50 throws off mound 75% 45 throws in batting practice

STAGE THREE

Step 12:	30 throws off mound 75% warm-up 15 throws off mound 50% BREAKING BALLS 45–60 throws in batting practice (fastball only)
Step 13:	30 throws off mound 75% 30 breaking balls 75% 30 throws in batting practice
Step 14:	30 throws off mound 75% 60–90 throws in batting practice (gradually increase breaking balls)
Step 15:	SIMULATED GAME: PROGRESSING BY 15 THROWS PER WORKOUT (pitch count) (Use interval throwing to 120 ft Phase as warm-up)

ALL THROWING OFF THE MOUND SHOULD BE DONE IN THE PRESENCE OF THE PITCHING COACH TO STRESS PROPER THROWING MECHANICS
(Use speed gun to aid in effort control)

---

the elbow flexed to 30° and resistance given to the second metacarpal bone (Kendall & McCreary 1983). The extensor carpi radialis brevis is tested with the elbow fully flexed and resistance given to the third metacarpal bone (Kendall & McCreary 1983). In addition, the extensor carpi ulnaris can be differentiated by resisting ulnar deviation (Kendall & McCreary 1983).

The nonoperative approach for treatment of epicondylitis varies based on the exact pathology and the chronicity of symptoms. Treatment for acute epicondylitis (Box 18.8) focuses on diminishing pain and gradually improving muscular strength. The primary goals of rehabilitation are to control the applied loads and create an environment for healing. The initial treatment consists of phonophoresis, iontophoresis (Fig. 18.7), stretching exercises and light strengthening exercises to stimulate a healing response. High-voltage stimulation and cryotherapy are used following treatment to decrease pain and postexercise inflammation. The athlete should be cautioned against excessive gripping activities. Once the patient's symptoms have subsided, an aggressive stretching and strengthening program with emphasis on eccentric contractions is initiated. Wrist flexion and extension activities should be performed initially with the elbow flexed 30–45°. Once the athlete can

perform these isotonic exercises with a 3 lb weight, they can be performed with the elbow fully extended. A gradual progression through plyometric and throwing activities precedes the initiation of the interval sport program. Because poor mechanics are often a cause of this condition, an analysis of sport mechanics and proper supervision through the interval sport program are critical.

The treatment for chronic epicondylitis varies greatly from the acute condition. As the chronicity of the pathology progresses, inflammation subsides and tissue degeneration occurs, creating a tendinosis rather than tendonitis. Thus anti-inflammatory treatments are avoided and a healing environment is encouraged by attempting to stimulate blood flow to the area. Treatment includes moist heat or a warm whirlpool, ultrasound (Fig. 18.8), transverse friction massage and eccentric strengthening, which places greater stress on the muscle tendon. The patient is encouraged to exercise in an environment that induces mild microtrauma to the area to create a healing response. Therefore, patients should experience mild discomfort when performing their workouts. We recommend that patients experience a 3–4 (out of a 0–10 pain scale) for the general orthopedic population and 5–6 pain scale for athletes during their exercises.

Box 18.6 Interval tennis program

The same principles should be followed with the interval tennis program as for the interval baseball program. Proper warm-ups, stretching, and strengthening should still be implemented throughout the entire interval tennis rehabilitation program. As you start your program, remember that mechanics play an important role in your recovery. If you have any further questions, please contact your physician or therapist.

OH – overhead shots

FH – forehand shots

BH – backhand shots

	MONDAY	WEDNESDAY	FRIDAY
1st week	12 FH	15 FH	15 FH
	8 BH	8 BH	10 BH
	10 min rest	10 min rest	10 min rest
	13 FH	15 FH	15 FH
	7 BH	7 BH	10 BH
2nd week	25 FH	30 FH	30 FH
	15 BH	20 BH	25 BH
	10 min rest	10 min rest	10 min rest
	25 FH	30 FH	30 FH
	15 BH	20 BH	15 BH
			10 BH
3rd week	30 FH	30 FH	30 FH
	25 BH	25 BH	30 BH
	10 OH	15 OH	15 OH
	10 min rest	10 min rest	10 min rest
	30 FH	30 FH	30 FH
	25 BH	25 BH	15 OH
	10 OH	15 OH	10 min rest
			30 FH
			30 BH
			15 OH
4th week	30 FH	30 FH	30 FH
	30 BH	30 BH	30 BH
	10 OH	10 OH	10 OH
	10 min rest	10 min rest	10 min rest
	Play 3 games	Play set	Play 1½ sets
	10 FH	10 FH	10 FH
	10 BH	10 BH	10 BH
	5 OH	5 OH	3 OH

Ice after each day of play

Ulnar neuropathy

There are several theories regarding the cause of ulnar neuropathy of the elbow in athletes (Glousman 1990). Ulnar nerve changes can result from tensile forces, compressive forces or nerve instability. Any one or a combination of these mechanisms may be responsible for ulnar nerve symptoms (Glousman 1990).

A leading mechanism for tensile force on the ulnar nerve is valgus stress. This may be coupled with an external rotation-supination stress overload mechanism. The traction forces are further magnified when underlying valgus instability from UCL injuries is present (Andrews & Whiteside 1993). Ulnar neuropathy is often a secondary pathology of UCL insufficiency.

Box 18.7 Interval golf program

The same principles should be followed with the interval golf program as for the interval baseball program. Proper warm-up, stretching and strengthening should still be implemented throughout the entire interval golf rehabilitation program. As you start your program, remember that mechanics play an important role in your recovery. If you have any further questions, please contact your physician or rehabilitation specialist.

	MONDAY	WEDNESDAY	FRIDAY
1st week	10 putts	15 putts	20 putts
	10 chips	15 chips	20 chips
	5 min rest	5 min rest	5 min rest
	15 chips	25 chips	20 putts
			20 chips
			5 min rest
			10 chips
			10 short irons
2nd week	20 chips	20 chips	15 short irons
	10 short irons	15 short irons	20 medium irons
	5 min rest	10 min rest	(5 iron/tee)
	10 short irons	15 short irons	10 min rest
	15 medium irons	15 chips	20 short irons
	(5 iron off tee)	Putting	
		15 medium irons	
		(5 iron/tee)	
3rd week	15 short irons	15 short irons	15 short irons
	20 medium irons	15 medium irons	15 medium irons
	10 min rest	10 long irons	10 long irons
	5 long irons	10 min rest	10 min rest
	15 short irons	10 short irons	10 short irons
	15 medium irons	10 medium irons	10 medium irons
	10 min rest	5 long irons	10 long irons
	20 chips	5 wood	10 wood
4th Week	15 short irons		
	15 medium irons		
	10 long irons	Play 9 holes	Play 9 holes
	10 drives		
	15 min rest		
	Repeat		
5th week	9 holes	9 holes	18 holes

Key to golf programs

Flexibility exercises before hitting

Use ice after hitting

Chips – pitching wedge; short irons – W, 9, 8; medium irons – 7, 6, 5; long irons – 4, 3, 2; woods – 3, 5; drives – driver

Compression of the ulnar nerve is often due to hypertrophy of the surrounding soft tissues or the presence of scar tissue. The nerve may also be trapped between the two heads of the flexor carpi ulnaris (Glousman 1990).

Repetitive flexion and extension of the elbow with an unstable nerve can irritate or inflame the nerve. The nerve may sublux or rest on the medial epicondyle, rendering it vulnerable to direct trauma. Complete dislocation of the nerve may occur anteriorly leading to friction neuritis.

Box 18.8 Epicondylitis rehabilitation protocol

PHASE I. ACUTE

Goals

- Decrease inflammation
- Promote tissue healing
- Retard muscular atrophy

Cryotherapy

Whirlpool

Stretching to increase flexibility
   wrist extension/flexion
   elbow extension/flexion
   forearm supination/pronation

Isometrics
   wrist extension/flexion
   elbow extension/flexion
   forearm supination/pronation

High-voltage stimulation

Phonophoresis

Friction massage

Iontophoresis (with anti-inflammatory, e.g. dexamethasone)

Avoid painful movements (e.g. gripping, etc.)

PHASE II. SUBACUTE

Goals

- Improve flexibility
- Increase muscular strength/endurance
- Increase functional activities/return to function

Exercises

Emphasize concentric/eccentric strengthening

Concentration on involved muscle group

Wrist extension/flexion

Forearm pronation/supination

Elbow flexion/extension

Initiate shoulder strengthening (if deficiencies are noted)

Continue flexibility exercises

May use counterforce brace

Continue use of cryotherapy after exercise/function

Gradual return to stressful activities

Gradually re-initiate once painful movements

PHASE III. CHRONIC

Goals

- Improve muscular strength and endurance
- Maintain/enhance flexibility
- Gradual return to sport/high level activities

Exercises

Continue strengthening exercises (emphasize eccentric/concentric)

Continue to emphasize deficiencies in shoulder and elbow strength

Continue flexibility exercises

Gradually decrease use of counterforce brace

Use of cryotherapy as needed

Gradual return-to-sport activity

Equipment modification (grip size, string tension, playing surface)

Emphasize maintenance program

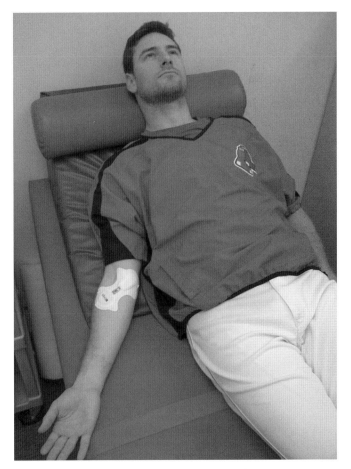

Figure 18.7 • Iontophoresis applied via the Empi Actionpatch (Empi Corp., St Paul, MN). The Actionpatch allows the transmission of anti-inflammatory medication over a longer duration of time (typically 3–5 hours) than traditional iontophoresis applications. This allows the medication to be slowly transmitted into the affected area.

There are three stages of ulnar neuropathy (Alley & Pappas 1995). The first stage includes an acute onset of radicular symptoms. The second stage is manifested by a recurrence of symptoms as the athlete attempts to return to competition. The third stage is associated with persistent motor weakness and sensory changes. Once the athlete presents in the third stage of injury, conservative management may not be effective.

Clinical examination often reveals tenderness along the cubital tunnel. Additionally, the examiner may perform a Tinel test by tapping on the cubital tunnel (Magee 1987). A positive Tinel test results in paresthesia or tingling over the ulnar nerve distribution.

The nonoperative treatment of ulnar neuropathy focuses on diminishing ulnar nerve irritation, enhancing dynamic medial joint stability, and gradually returning the athlete to competition.

Following the diagnosis of ulnar neuropathy, throwing athletes are instructed to discontinue throwing activities for at

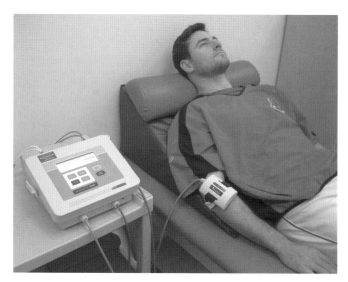

Figure 18.8 • Ultrasound application via the Richmar Autosound (Richmar Corp., Inola, OK). The Autosound contains four crystals that can alternate transmission, allowing the applicator to be applied to a focal point without the risk of overheating the soft tissue structures.

least 4 weeks. The athlete progresses through the immediate motion and intermediate phases over the course of 4 to 6 weeks with emphasis placed on eccentric and dynamic stabilization drills. Plyometric exercises are utilized to facilitate dynamic stabilization of the medial elbow. The athlete is allowed to begin an interval throwing program when the following criteria are fulfilled: (1) full pain-free ROM, (2) a satisfactory clinical examination, (3) no neurological symptoms, (4) adequate medial stability and (5) satisfactory muscular performance. The athlete may gradually return to play if progression through the interval sport program does not reveal neurological symptoms.

Ulnar nerve transposition

Surgical transpositioning of the ulnar nerve involves stabilizing the nerve with fascial slings. Caution is taken so that the soft tissue structures involved in the relocation of the nerve are not overstressed. The rehabilitation following an ulnar nerve transposition is outlined in Box 18.9. A posterior splint at 90° of elbow flexion is used for the first 2 weeks postoperatively to prevent excessive ROM and tension on the nerve. The splint is discharged at week 2 and light ROM activities are initiated. Full ROM is usually restored by weeks 3–4. Gentle isotonic strengthening is begun during week 4 and progressed to the full Thrower's Ten program by 6 weeks following surgery. Aggressive strengthening including eccentric and plyometric training is incorporated by weeks 7 to 8 and an interval sport program at weeks 8 to 9, if all previously outlined criteria are met. A return to competition usually occurs between weeks 12 and 16 postoperatively.

Box 18.9 Postoperative rehabilitation following ulnar nerve transposition

PHASE I. IMMEDIATE POSTOPERATIVE (WEEK 0–2)
Goals

- Allow soft tissue healing of relocated nerve
- Decrease pain and inflammation
- Retard muscular atrophy

A. Week 1

1. Posterior splint at 90° elbow flexion with wrist free for motion (sling for comfort)
2. Compression dressing
3. Exercises such as gripping exercises, wrist range of motion, shoulder isometrics

B. Week 2

1. Remove posterior splint for exercise and bathing
2. Progress elbow range of motion (passive range of motion 15° to 120°)
3. Initiate elbow and wrist isometrics
4. Continue shoulder isometrics

PHASE II. INTERMEDIATE (WEEKS 3–7)
Goals

- Restore full pain-free range of motion
- Improve strength, power and endurance of upper extremity musculature
- Gradually increase functional demands

A. Week 3

1. Discontinue posterior splint
2. Progress elbow range of motion, emphasize full extension
3. Initiate flexibility exercise for wrist extension/flexion, forearm supination/pronation and elbow extension/flexion
4. Initiate strengthening exercises for wrist extension/flexion, forearm supination/pronation, elbow extensors/flexors and a shoulder program

B. Week 6

1. Continue all exercises listed above
2. Initiate light sport activities

PHASE III. ADVANCED STRENGTHENING (WEEKS 8–12)
Goals

- Increase strength, power, endurance
- Gradually initiate sporting activities

A. Week 8

1. Initiate eccentric exercise program
2. Initiate plyometric exercise drills
3. Continue shoulder and elbow strengthening and flexibility exercises
4. Initiate interval throwing program

PHASE IV. RETURN TO ACTIVITY (WEEKS 12–16)
Goals

- Gradually return to sporting activities

A. Week 12

1. Return to competitive throwing
2. Continue Thrower's Ten exercise program

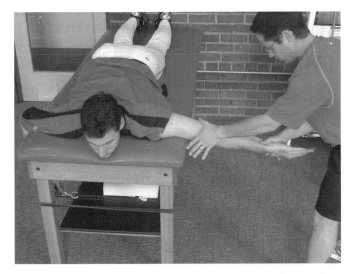

Figure 18.9 • Clinical test for valgus extension overload. The examiner forcefully extends the elbow while applying a valgus stress.

Valgus extension overload

Valgus extension overload occurs in repetitive sport activities such as throwing, tennis serving and swimming. Injury usually occurs during the acceleration or deceleration phase as the olecranon wedges up against the medial olecranon fossa during elbow extension (Wilson et al 1983). This mechanism may result in osteophyte formation and potentially loose bodies. Repetitive extension stress from the triceps may further contribute to this injury. There is often a certain degree of underlying valgus instability in these athletes, further facilitating osteophyte formation through compression of the radiocapitellar joint and the posteromedial elbow (Anderson 2001).

Athletes typically present with pain in the posteromedial aspect of the elbow that is exacerbated with forced extension and valgus stress. The clinical test for valgus extension overload involves the examiner grasping the elbow in a flexed position. As the examiner forces the elbow into extension, a valgus stress is simultaneously applied to the elbow (Fig. 18.9). The examiner palpates the posteromedial joint for tenderness and/or crepitation. Pain over the posteromedial olecranon process signifies a positive test (Wilson et al 1983).

A conservative treatment approach is often attempted before considering surgical intervention. Initial treatment involves relieving the posterior elbow of pain and inflammation. As symptoms subside and ROM normalizes, strengthening exercises are initiated. Emphasis is placed on improving eccentric strength of the elbow flexors in an attempt to control the rapid extension that occurs at the elbow during athletics. Manual resistance exercises of concentric and eccentric elbow flexion are performed, as well as elbow flexion with exercise tubing.

Posterior olecranon osteophyte excision

Surgical excision of posterior olecranon osteophytes is performed using an osteotome or motorized burr. Approximately 5–10 mm of the olecranon tip is removed concomitantly and a motorized burr is used to contour the coronoid, olecranon tip and fossa to prevent further impingement with extreme flexion and extension (Martin & Baumgarten 1996).

The rehabilitation program following arthroscopic posterior olecranon osteophyte excision is slightly more conservative in restoring full elbow extension secondary to postsurgical pain. ROM is progressed within the patient's tolerance; by 10 days postoperatively, the patient should exhibit at least 15–100° of ROM, and 10–110° by day 14. Full ROM is typically restored by day 20 to 25 postsurgery. The rate of ROM progression is most often limited by osseous structure pain and synovial joint inflammation.

The strengthening program is similar to the previously discussed progression. Isometrics are performed for the first 10 to 14 days and isotonic strengthening from weeks 2 to 6. The full Thrower's Ten program is initiated by week 6. An interval sport program is included by weeks 10 to 12. The rehabilitation focus is similar to the non-operative treatment of valgus extension overload. Emphasis is placed on eccentric control of the elbow flexors and dynamic stabilization of the medial elbow.

Andrews & Timmerman (1995) reported on the outcome of elbow surgery in 72 professional baseball players. 65% of these athletes exhibited a posterior olecranon osteophyte and 25% of the athletes who underwent an isolated olecranon excision, later required an ulnar collateral ligament reconstruction (Andrews & Timmerman 1995). This may suggest that subtle medial instability may accelerate osteophyte formation.

Conversely, there is a certain amount of concern related to the effects of excising the posterior olecranon on medial elbow stability; by altering the static stability of the humeroulnar articulation, medial elbow stability may be compromised. Andrews et al (2001) examined the amount of stress applied to the anterior bundle of the UCL with varying amounts of posterior olecranon excisions. UCL strain was measured with intact olecranons and with 2 mm incremental resections of the medial olecranon up to 8 mm. A further resection of 13 mm was also performed. The UCL was then strained to failure during an applied valgus stress at varying degrees of elbow flexion from 50° to 100°. Results indicate no significant differences in strain on the UCL with change in level of osteotomy for a given applied load and angle of flexion. Thus, it appears that UCL strain is not significantly increased with posterior olecranon resection.

Ulnar collateral ligament injury

Injuries to the UCL are becoming increasingly more common in overhead throwing athletes, although the higher incidence of injury may be due to our increased ability to diagnose these injuries. As described briefly in the biomechanics section, the elbow experiences a tremendous amount of valgus stress during overhead throwing. These stresses approach the ultimate failure load of the ligament with each throw. The repetitive nature of overhead sport activities such as baseball pitching, football passing, tennis serving and javelin throwing further

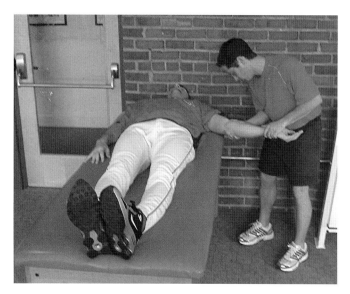

Figure 18.10 • Clinical test for ulnar collateral ligament instability in the supine position.

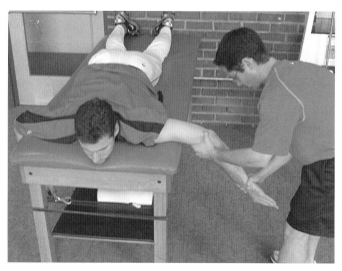

Figure 18.11 • Clinical test for ulnar collateral ligament instability in the prone position.

increase susceptibility to UCL injury by exposing the ligament to repetitive microtraumatic forces.

The athlete with an injury to the UCL usually presents with pain and tenderness to the medial elbow. Generalized joint effusion may also be present. The patient's subjective history typically reveals either recurring medial elbow symptoms or a single traumatic incident of medial elbow pain while throwing, etc. The patient recalls a sudden, sharp, medial elbow pain, often with a popping sensation.

There are several clinical tests that are used to test the integrity of the UCL. We will describe the two most common techniques that we utilize in our clinic. The patient is positioned supine while the examiner holds the elbow and externally rotates the shoulder, blocking the upper extremity from further rotating (Fig. 18.10). The UCL is easily palpated in this position. The elbow is tested at 5° and 25–30° of flexion. A valgus stress is imparted upon the elbow to determine the integrity of the ligament. The amount of opening, or gapping, is assessed as well as the end feel of motion. Excessive gapping, a soft end feel or localized medial pain may all be indicative of UCL injury (Andrews et al 1993).

Next, the patient moves to the prone position with the involved arm hanging over the edge of the table. The examiner internally rotates the shoulder and stabilizes the elbow before placing a valgus stress on the elbow at 5° and 25–30° of flexion (Fig. 18.11). Again the amount of opening and end feel are assessed. We feel that the prone valgus stress test is the most sensitive test for UCL pathology due to the increased ability of the examiner to provide valgus stress without additional movement of surrounding joint.

Furthermore, an MRI enhanced with intra-articular dye injection may be useful in the athlete with a suspected UCL injury. A UCL tear is indicated by a T-sign as previously discussed (Timmerman & Andrews 1994).

Various opinions exist regarding the efficacy of nonoperative treatment for UCL strains or partial tears for the throwing athlete. If an injury to the UCL is suspected, the rehabilitation program outlined in Box 18.10 is initiated. Range of motion is initially permitted in a nonpainful arc of motion, usually 10–100°, to allow for a decrease in inflammation and the alignment of collagen tissue. A brace may be used to restrict motion as well as prevent valgus strain. Isometric exercises are performed for the shoulder, elbow and wrist to prevent muscular atrophy. Ice and anti-inflammatory medications are prescribed to control pain and inflammation.

Range of motion of both flexion and extension is gradually increased during the second phase of treatment as tolerated. Full ROM should be achieved by at least 3–4 weeks. Rhythmic stabilization exercises are initiated to develop dynamic stabilization and neuromuscular control of the upper extremity. As dynamic stability is advanced, isotonic exercises are incorporated for the entire upper extremity.

The advanced strengthening phase is usually initiated at 6 to 7 weeks postinjury. During this phase, the athlete is progressed to the Thrower's Ten isotonic strengthening program and plyometric exercises. An interval return to sport program is initiated once the athlete regains full motion, adequate strength and dynamic stability of the elbow. The athlete is allowed to return to competition following the asymptomatic completion of the interval sport program. If symptoms continue to persist, the athlete is reassessed and possible surgical intervention is considered.

Ulnar collateral ligament reconstruction

Surgical reconstruction of the UCL attempts to restore the stabilizing functions of the anterior bundle of the UCL (Andrews et al 1996). The palmaris longus or gracilis tendon, is taken and

Box 18.10 Conservative treatment following ulnar collateral sprains of the elbow

PHASE I. IMMEDIATE MOTION (WEEKS 0 THROUGH 2)

Goals

- Increase range of motion
- Promote healing of ulnar collateral ligament
- Retard muscular atrophy
- Decrease pain and inflammation

1. *ROM*

 Brace (optional) nonpainful ROM (20–90°)

 AAROM, PROM elbow and wrist (nonpainful range)

2. *Exercises*

 Isometrics – wrist and elbow musculature

 Shoulder strengthening (no ext. rotation strengthening)

3. *Ice and compression*

PHASE II. INTERMEDIATE (WEEKS 3 THROUGH 6)

Goals

- Increase range of motion
- Improve strength/endurance
- Decrease pain and inflammation
- Promote stability

1. *ROM*

 Gradually increase motion 0° to 135° (increase 10° per week)

2. *Exercises*

 Initiate isotonic exercises:

 wrist curls

 wrist extensions

 pronation/supination

 biceps/triceps

 dumbbells: external rotation, deltoid, supraspinatus, rhomboids, internal rotation

3. *Ice and compression*

PHASE III. ADVANCED (WEEKS 6 AND 7 THROUGH 12 AND 14)

Criteria to progress:

1. Full range of motion
2. No pain or tenderness
3. No increase in laxity
4. Strength 4/5 of elbow flexor/extensor

Goals

- Increase strength, power and endurance
- Improve neuromuscular control
- Initiate high-speed exercise drills

Exercises

Initiate exercise tubing, shoulder program:

 Thrower's Ten program

 Biceps/triceps program

 Supination/pronation

 Wrist extension/flexion

 Plyometrics throwing drills

PHASE IV. RETURN TO ACTIVITY (WEEK 12 THROUGH 14)

Criteria to progress to return to throwing:

1. Full nonpainful ROM
2. No increase in laxity
3. Isokinetic test fulfills criteria
4. Satisfactory clinical examination

Exercises

Initiate interval throwing

Continue Thrower's Ten program

Continue plyometrics

AAROM – active-assisted range of motion; PROM – passive range of motion; ROM – range of motion

passed in a figure-of-eight pattern through drill holes in the sublime tubercle of the ulna and the medial epicondyle (Andrews et al 1996). An ulnar nerve transposition is often performed at the time of reconstruction (Andrews et al 1996).

The rehabilitation program following UCL reconstruction varies based on the surgical technique, method of transpositioning of the ulnar nerve and the overall extent of injury to the elbow. The rehabilitation program we currently use following UCL reconstruction is outlined in Box 18.11. The athlete is placed in a posterior splint with the elbow immobilized at 90° of flexion for the first 7 days postoperatively. This allows adequate healing of the UCL graft and soft tissue slings involved in the nerve transposition. The patient is allowed to perform wrist ROM, and gripping and submaximal isometrics, for the wrist and elbow. The patient is progressed from the posterior splint to an elbow ROM brace, which is adjusted to allow ROM from 30 to 100° of flexion. Motion is increased by 5° of extension and 10° of flexion thereafter to restore full ROM by the end of week 5–6 (0–145°). The brace is discontinued by weeks 5 to 6.

Isometric exercises are progressed to include light resistance isotonic exercises at week 4 and the full Thrower's Ten program by week 6. Sport-specific exercises are incorporated at weeks 8 to 9. Focus is again placed on developing dynamic stabilization of the medial elbow. Due to the anatomical orientation of the flexor carpi ulnaris and flexor digitorum superficialis overlaying the UCL, isotonic and stabilization activities for these muscles may assist the UCL in stabilizing valgus stress at the medial elbow.

Aggressive exercises involving eccentric and plyometric contractions are included in the advanced phase, usually weeks 9 through 14. An interval sport program is allowed at week 18 postoperatively. In most cases, throwing from a mound is progressed within 2 months following the initiation of an interval throwing program and a return to competitive throwing at approximately 8 to 12 months following surgery.

Box 18.11 Postoperative rehabilitation following chronic ulnar collateral ligament reconstruction using autogenous graft

PHASE I. IMMEDIATE POSTOPERATIVE (0–3 WEEKS)

Goals

- Protect healing tissue
- Decrease pain/inflammation
- Retard muscular atrophy

A. Postoperative week 1

1. Posterior splint at 90° elbow flexion
2. Wrist AROM extension/flexion
3. Elbow compression dressing (2–3 days)
4. Exercises such as gripping exercises, wrist ROM, shoulder isometrics (except shoulder ER), biceps isometrics
5. Cryotherapy

B. Postoperative week 2

1. Application of functional brace 30° to 100°
2. Initiate wrist isometrics
3. Initiate elbow flex/ext isometrics
4. Continue all exercises listed above

C. Postoperative week 3

Advance brace 15–110° (gradually increase ROM; 5° extension/10° flexion per week)

PHASE II. INTERMEDIATE (WEEKS 4–8)

Goals

- Gradual increase in range of motion
- Promote healing of repaired tissue
- Regain and improve muscular strength

A. Week 4

1. Functional brace set (10–120°)
2. Begin light resistance exercises for arm (1 lb) wrist curls, extensions pronation/supination elbow ext/flexion
3. Progress shoulder program, emphasize rotator cuff strengthening (avoid ER until 6th week)

B. Week 6

1. Functional brace set 0–130°); AROM 0–145° (without brace)
2. Progress elbow strengthening exercises
3. Initiate shoulder external rotation strengthening
4. Progress shoulder program

PHASE III. ADVANCED STRENGTHENING (WEEKS 9–13)

Goals

- Increase strength, power, endurance
- Maintain full elbow ROM
- Gradually initiate sporting activities

A. Week 9

1. Initiate eccentric elbow flexion/extension
2. Continue isotonic program; forearm and wrist
3. Continue shoulder program – Thrower's Ten program
4. Manual resistance diagonal patterns
5. Initiate plyometric exercise program

B. Week 11

1. Continue all exercises listed above
2. May begin light sport activities (i.e. golf, swimming)

PHASE IV. RETURN TO ACTIVITY (WEEKS 14–26)

Goals

- Continue to increase strength, power, and endurance of upper extremity musculature
- Gradual return-to-sport activities

A. Week 14

1. Initiate interval throwing program (phase 1)
2. Continue strengthening program
3. Emphasis on elbow and wrist strengthening and flexibility exercises

B. Weeks 22 through 26

Return to competitive throwing

Less common sport-related injuries

Osteochondritis dissecans

Osteochondritis dissecans of the elbow may develop due to the valgus strain on the elbow joint, which produces not only medial tension but also a lateral compressive force. This is observed as the capitulum of the humerus compresses with the radial head. Patients often complain of lateral elbow pain upon palpation and valgus stress. Morrey (1994) described a three-stage classification of pathological progression. Stage one describes patients without evidence of subchondral displacement or fracture, whereas stage two referred to lesions showing evidence of subchondral detachment or articular cartilage fracture. Stage three lesions involve detached osteochondral fragments, resulting in intra-articular loose bodies. Nonsurgical treatment is attempted for stage one patients only and consists of relative rest and immobilization until elbow symptoms have resolved.

Nonoperative treatment includes 3 to 6 weeks of immobilization at 90° of elbow flexion. ROM activities for the shoulder, elbow, and wrist are performed 3–4 times a day. As symptoms resolve a strengthening program is initiated with isometric exercises. Isotonic exercises are included after approximately 1 week of isometric exercise. Aggressive high speed, eccentric and plyometric exercises are progressively included to prepare the athlete for the start of an interval sport program.

If nonoperative treatment fails, or evidence of loose bodies exists, surgical intervention including arthroscopic abrading and drilling of the lesion with fixation or removal of the loose body is indicated (Roberts & Hughes 1950). Long-term follow-up studies regarding the outcome of patients undergoing surgery to drill or reattach the lesions have not produced favorable results, suggesting that prevention and early detection of symptoms may be the best form of treatment (Baur et al 1992, Woodward & Bianco 1975).

Degenerative joint disease

Degenerative joint disease (DJD) of the elbow may occur prematurely in certain athletes who participate in sport activities that repetitively load the articular surfaces of the elbow joint. Acceleration of joint degeneration and osteophyte formation may occur. Pain and joint effusion may be observed during examination, as well as tenderness to palpation over the joint lines. Although this particular pathology may not restrict normal function and activities of daily living, the pain and motion loss associated with DJD may restrict further participation in sports.

Conservative treatment is thus focused on first diminishing pain and inflammation and secondly, improving ROM and soft tissue flexibility. Warm whirlpool prior to stretching and gentle joint mobilization techniques may be beneficial to enhance soft tissue extensibility. As pain and ROM normalize, an overall enhancement of upper extremity strength and endurance is emphasized. In the event that conservative treatment does not produce favorable results, an open or arthroscopic debridement may be indicated to alleviate symptoms.

Synovitis

Generalized joint synovitis may occur from the repetitive nature of throwing and other overhead sports. Patients often complain of a diffuse joint pain not specific to one area and a flexion contracture is revealed upon examination. Initial treatment includes anti-inflammatory medications and activity modification to allow for a period of rest and recovery.

The rehabilitation program is focused on restoring elbow extension. ROM, stretching and mobilization exercises are performed as necessary to restore and maintain full ROM. The clinician must be cautioned against overaggressive stretching and mobilization during the acute phases of recovery to avoid contributing to the inflammatory synovial reaction. Tepid to warm whirlpool treatment may be used prior to ROM exercises. Contrast treatment (cold to warm) may also be beneficial. Submaximal isometric exercises are performed until the inflammatory response has diminished, followed by the initiation of an isotonic strengthening program. A return to sport-specific drills and an interval sport program are instituted once the patient has achieved proper strength and a satisfactory clinical examination.

Dislocations

Dislocations of the elbow joint most commonly occur in contact sports such as football and wrestling or in noncontact sports as the athlete lands onto an outstretched hand. A hyperextension injury occurs as the olecranon is forced into the olecranon fossa and the trochlea translates posteriorly or posterolaterally over the coronoid process (Andrews & Whiteside 1993). Disruption of the UCL and possibly the RCL may occur. Fractures of the radial head or capitulum may also be seen concomitantly (Andrews & Whiteside 1993).

A lateral pivot shift test may be used to assess posterolateral stability of the elbow (O'Driscoll et al 1991). Initial reduction of the injury may be performed by applying traction to the forearm and humerus with the elbow in 30° of flexion (Andrews & Whiteside 1993). Neurovascular integrity should be assessed immediately and surgical intervention may be necessary to repair concomitant ligament instability and osseous fractures.

Treatment depends greatly on the severity of injury and the associated injuries that are present. An initial period of rest and immobilization may be warranted to allow for soft tissue healing and a decrease in pain and inflammation. Early motion should be initiated within the first week following injury to minimize the chances of motion loss, which is one of the primary complications following elbow dislocation (Richardson & Iglarsh 1994). Progression through rehabilitation follows a progressive sequence similar to the previously described program to regain motion and strength of the elbow and forearm.

Fractures

Various fractures of the elbow may occur in the athletic population, including extra- and intra-articular distal humerus fractures, radial head fractures and olecranon fractures (Richardson & Iglarsh 1994). Stress fractures of the olecranon have been reported in overhead throwers and can occur in any part of the olecranon, especially in the midarticular area (Bennett 1941). The most likely cause of injury involves repetitive stresses applied to the olecranon as the elbow extends from triceps contraction during the acceleration, deceleration and follow-through phases of throwing. Patients often subjectively report an insidious onset of pain in the posterolateral elbow while throwing. Symptoms appear similar to triceps tendonitis; however, tenderness over the involved site of the olecranon is often detected upon palpation. Plane radiographs are typically taken and diagnosis may be further enhanced with the aid of a bone scan and/or an MRI.

Aggressive stretching and strengthening exercises are restricted for the first 6 to 8 weeks to allow adequate healing of the fracture site. The athlete should maintain motion with light ROM exercises. Heavy lifting, plyometrics and sport-specific drills are not allowed until bony healing is seen on radiographic evaluation, typically by 8 to 12 weeks. Once adequate healing has been documented, an interval sport program may be allowed. Complete recovery occurs in approximately 3 to 6 months following injury. An open reduction internal fixation may be indicated if conservative management fails.

Arthrolysis

Many of the previous pathologies that have been discussed have involved motion loss as a primary complication. The elbow joint is one of the most frequent joints to develop motion loss (Green & McCoy 1979, Timmerman & Andrews 1994). Following injury, the elbow flexes in response to pain and hemarthrosis. The periarticular soft tissue and joint capsule become shortened, fibrotic, and loss of motion develops. An arthroscopic arthrolysis may be necessary in patients that do not respond to conservative treatment.

During the first postoperative week, the patient is instructed to perform elbow and wrist range of motion exercises hourly. Treatment to regain ROM at this time is cautiously aggressive (Wilk 1994). Full motion should be obtained quickly; however, a pace that does not cause additional inflammation of the joint capsule is necessary to avoid further pain and reflexive splinting. LLLD stretching has been an extremely beneficial treatment technique for us clinically. Full passive ROM is usually restored by day 10 to 14.

Isometric strengthening is begun during week 2 and progressed to isotonic dumbbell exercises during the third to fourth week. Strengthening exercises are progressed as tolerated by the patient. Emphasis during the later phases of rehabilitation continues to be placed on maintaining motion. Patients are educated to continue a motion maintenance program several times per day and before and after sport activities for at least 2 to 3 months following surgery.

Summary

The elbow joint is a common site of injury in the athletic population. Injuries vary widely from repetitive microtraumatic injuries to gross macrotraumatic dislocations. A thorough understanding of the sport-specific anatomy and biomechanics of the joint are necessary for a successful clinical examination, assessment and rehabilitation prescription. Rehabilitation of the elbow, whether postinjury or postsurgical, must follow a progressive and sequential order to ensure that healing tissues are not overstressed. A rehabilitation program that limits immobilization, achieves full ROM early, progressively restores strength and neuromuscular control and gradually incorporates sport-specific activities is essential to successfully return athletes to their previous level of competition as quickly and safely as possible.

References

Akeson W H, Amiel D, Woo S L Y 1980 Immobilization effects on synovial joints. The pathomechanics of joint contracture. Biorheology 17:95–107

Alley R M, Pappas A M 1995 Acute and performance-related injuries of the elbow. In: Pappas A M (ed) Upper extremity injuries in the athlete. Churchill Livingstone, New York, p 339–364

Anderson K 2001 Elbow arthritis and removal of loose bodies and spurs, and techniques for restoration of motion. In: Altchek D W, Andrews J R (eds) The athlete's elbow. Lippincott Williams and Wilkins, Philadelphia, PA, p 219–230

Andrews J R, Frank W 1985 Valgus extension overload in the pitching elbow. In: Andrews J R, Zarins B, Carson W B (eds) Injuries to the throwing arm. WB Saunders, Philadelphia, PA, p 250–257

Andrews J R, Timmerman L 1995 Outcome of elbow surgery in professional baseball players. American Journal of Sports Medicine 23:245–250

Andrews J R, Whiteside J A 1993 Common elbow problems in the athlete. Journal of Orthopaedic and Sports Physical Therapy 17(6):289–295

Andrews J R, Wilk K E, Satterwhite Y E et al 1993 Physical examination of the thrower's elbow. Journal of Orthopaedic and Sports Physical Therapy 17(6):296–304

Andrews J R, Jelsma R D, Joyse M E et al 1996 Open surgical procedures for injuries to the elbow in throwers. Operative Techniques in Sports Medicine 4(2):109–113

Andrews J R, Heggland E J H, Fleisig G S et al 2001 Relationship of ulnar collateral ligament strain to amount of medial olecranon osteotomy. American Journal of Sports Medicine 29(6):716–721

Atkinson W B, Elftman H 1945 The carrying angle of the human arm as a secondary sex character. Anatomical Record 91:49–54

Basmajian J V, DeLuca C J 1985 Muscles alive: their function revealed by electromyography. Williams and Wilkins, Baltimore, MD, p 279–280

Baur M, Jonsson K, Josefson P O et al 1992 Dissecans of the elbow: a long-term follow-up study. Clinical Orthopaedics and Related Research 284:156–160

Bennett G E 1941 Shoulder and elbow lesions of the professional baseball player. Journal of the American Medical Association 117:510–514

Blackburn T A, McCleod W D, White B 1990 EMG analysis of posterior rotator cuff exercises. Journal of Athletic Training 25:40–45

Coutts R, Rothe C, Kaita J 1981 The role of continuous passive motion in the rehabilitation of the total knee patient. Clinical Orthopaedics and Related Research 159:126–132

Cyriax J 1982 Textbook of orthopedic medicine, vol 1. Diagnosis of soft tissue lesions, 8th edn. Baillière Tindall, London, p 52–54

Dehne E, Tory R 1971 Treatment of joint injuries by immediate mobilization based upon the spiral adaptation concept. Clinical Orthopaedics and Related Research 77:218–232

Fleisig G S, Barrentine S W 1995 Biomechanical aspects of the elbow in sports. Sports Medicine and Arthroscopy Review 3:149–159

Fleisig G S, Escamilla R F 1996 Biomechanics of the elbow in the throwing athlete. Operative Techniques in Sports Medicine 4:62–68

Fleisig G S, Andrews J R, Dillman C J et al 1995 Kinetics of baseball pitching with implications about injury mechanisms. American Journal of Sports Medicine 23:233–239

Glazebrook M A, Curwin S, Islam M N et al 1994 Medial epicondylitis. An electromyographic analysis and an investigation of intervention strategies. American Journal of Sports Medicine 22:674–679

Glousman R E 1990 Ulnar nerve problems in the athlete's elbow. Clinics in Sports Medicine 9:365–377

Green D P, McCoy H 1979 Turnbuckle orthotic correction of elbow flexion contractures. Journal of Bone and Joint Surgery (Am) 61(A):1092

Haggmark T, Eriksson E 1979 Cylinder or mobile cast brace after knee ligament surgery: a clinical analysis and morphologic and enzymatic studies of changes of the quadriceps muscle. American Journal of Sports Medicine 7:48–56

Hoppenfeld S 1976 Physical examination of the spine and extremities. Appleton-Century-Crofts, New York, p 35–55

Jobe F W, Moynes D R, Tibone J E et al 1984 An EMG analysis of the shoulder in pitching. American Journal of Sports Medicine 12:218–220

Johansson O 1962 Capsular and ligament injuries of the elbow joint. Acta Chirurgica Scandinavica 287 (suppl):1–159

Kapandji I A 1970 The physiology of the joints, vol 1. E & S Livingston, London, p 82–83, 112–117

Keats T E, Teeslink R, Diamond A E et al 1966 Normal axial relationships of the major joints. Radiology 87:904

Kelley J D, Lombardo S J, Pink M et al 1994 EMG and cinematographic analysis of elbow function in tennis players with lateral epicondylitis. American Journal of Sports Medicine 22:359–363

Kendall F P, McCreary E K 1983 Muscles, testing, and function 3rd edn. Williams and Wilkins, Baltimore, MD, p 86–87

Kibler W B 1994 Clinical biomechanics of the elbow in tennis: implications for evaluation and diagnosis. Medicine and Science in Sports and Exercise 26:1203–1206

Kottke F J, Pauley D L, Ptak R A 1966 The rationale for prolonged stretching for connective tissue. Archives of Physical Medicine and Rehabilitation 47:345–352

Lehmkuhl D L, Smith L R 1983 Brunnstrom's clinical kinesiology. FA Davis, Philadelphia, PA, p 149–170

McCarroll J R 1985 Golf. In: Schneider R C et al (eds) Sports injuries: mechanisms, prevention, and treatment. Williams and Wilkins, Baltimore, MD, p 290–294

McCarroll J R Gioe T J 1982 Professional golfers and the price they pay. Physician and Sports Medicine 10:64–70

Magee D J 1987 Orthopaedic physical assessment. WB Saunders, Philadelphia, PA

Maitland G D 1977 Peripheral manipulation. Butterworth, Boston, MA

Martin B F 1958 The annular ligament of the superior radioulnar joint. Journal of Anatomy 52:473

Martin S D, Baumgarten T E 1996 Elbow injuries in the throwing athlete: diagnosis and arthroscopic treatment. Operative Techniques in Sports Medicine 4:100–108

Morrey B F 1985 Anatomy of the elbow. In: Morrey B F (ed) The elbow and its disorders. Saunders, Philadelphia, PA, p 7–40

Morrey B F 1994 Osteochondritis dissecans. In: DeLee J C, Drez D (eds) Orthopedic sports medicine. Saunders, Philadelphia, PA, p 908–912

Morrey B F, An K N 1983 Articular and ligamentous contributions to the static stability of the elbow joint. American Journal of Sports Medicine 11:315–319

Morrey B F, An K N, Dobyns J 1985 Functional anatomy of the elbow ligaments. Clinical Orthopaedics and Related Research 201:84

Morris M, Jobe F W, Perry J et al 1989 EMG analysis of elbow function in tennis players. American Journal of Sports Medicine 17:241–247

Moseley V B, Jobe F W, Pink M 1992 EMG analysis of the scapular muscles during a shoulder rehabilitation program. American Journal of Sports Medicine 20:128–134

Nirschl R P, Morrey B F 1985 Rehabilitation. In: Morrey B F (ed) The elbow and its disorders. WB Saunders, Philadelphia, PA, p 147–152

Norkin C, Levangie P 1985 Joint structure and function: a comprehensive analysis. FA Davis, Philadelphia, PA, p 191–210

Norkin C C, White D J 1995 Measurement of joint motion: a guide to goniometry, 2nd edn. FA Davis, Philadelphia, PA

Noyes F R, Mangine R E, Barber S E 1987 Early knee motion after open and arthroscopic anterior cruciate ligament reconstruction. American Journal of Sports Medicine 15:149–160

O'Driscoll S W, Bell D F, Morrey B F 1991 Posterolateral rotatory instability of the elbow. Journal of Bone and Joint Surgery (Am) 73A:440–446

Pavly J E, Rushing J L, Scheving L E 1967 Electromyographic study of some muscles crossing the elbow joint. Journal of Anatomy 159:47–53

Perkins G 1954 Rest and motion. Journal of Bone and Joint Surgery (Br) 35(B):521–539

Rhu K N, McCormick J, Jobe F W et al 1988 An electromyographic analysis of shoulder function in tennis players. American Journal of Sports Medicine 16:481

Reinold M M, Wilk K E, Reed J et al 2002 Interval sport programs: guidelines for baseball, tennis, and golf. Journal of Orthopedic and Sports Physical Therapy 32:293–298

Reinold M M, Wilk K E, Fleisig G S 2004 Electromyographic analysis of the rotator cuff and deltoid musculature during common shoulder external rotation exercises. Journal of Orthopedic and Sports Physical Therapy 34:385–394

Richardson J K, Iglarsh Z A 1994 Clinical orthopaedic physical therapy. WB Saunders, Philadelphia, PA, p 227–230

Roberts W, Hughes R 1950 Osteochondritis dissecans of the elbow joint: a clinical study. Journal of Bone and Joint Surgery (Br) 32B:348–360

St John J N, Palmaz J C 1986 The cubital tunnel in ulnar entrapment neuropathy. Musculoskeletal Radiology 158:119

Salter R B, Simmonds D F, Malcolm B W et al 1980 The effects of continuous passive motion on healing of full thickness defects in articular cartilage. Journal of Bone and Joint Surgery (Am) 62A:1232–1251

Salter R B, Hamilton H W, Wedge J H 1984 Clinical application of basic research on continuous passive motion for disorders and injuries of synovial joints. A preliminary report of a feasibility study. Journal of Orthopedic Research 1:325–342

Sapega A A, Quedenfeld T C, Moyer R A et al 1976 Biophysical factors in range of motion exercise. Archives of Physical Medicine and Rehabilitation 57:122–126

Schwab G H, Bennett J B, Woods G W et al 1980 The biomechanics of elbow stability: the role of the medial collateral ligament. Clinical Orthopaedics and Related Research 146:42

Soderberg G L 1981 Kinesiology application to pathological motion. Williams and Wilkins, Baltimore, MD, p 131–136

Spinner M, Kaplan E B 1970 The quadrate ligament of the elbow: its relationship to the stability of the proximal radioulnar joint. Acta Orthopaedica Scandinavica 41:632

Stanish W D, Loebenberg M I, Kozey J W 1994 The elbow. In: Stover C N, McCarroll J R, Mallon W J (eds) Feeling up to par: medicine from tee to green. FA Davis, Philadelphia, PA, p 143–149

Timmerman L A, Andrews J R 1994 Undersurface tears of the ulnar collateral ligament in baseball players. A newly recognized lesion. American Journal of Sports Medicine 22:33–36

Tipton C M, Mathies R D, Martin R F 1978 Influence of age and sex on strength of bone–ligament junctions in knee joints in rats. Journal of Bone and Joint Surgery (Am) 60A:230–236

Townsend H, Jobe F W, Pink M et al 1991 Electromyographic analysis of the glenohumeral muscles during a baseball rehabilitation program. American Journal of Sports Medicine 19:264–272

Warren C G, Lehmann J F, Koblanski J N 1971 Elongation of rat tail tendon: effect of load and temperature. Archives of Physical Medicine and Rehabilitation 52:465–474

Warren C G, Lehmann J F, Koblanski J N 1976 Heat and stretch procedures: an evaluation using rat tail tendon. Archives of Physical Medicine and Rehabilitation 57:122–126

Werner S, Fleisig G S, Dillman C J et al 1993 Biomechanics of the elbow during baseball pitching. Journal of Orthopaedic and Sports Physical Therapy 17:274–278

Wilk K E 1994 Rehabilitation of the elbow following arthroscopic surgery. In: Andrews J R, Soffer S R (eds) Elbow arthroscopy. Mosby, St Louis, MO, p 109–116

Wilk K E, Levinson M 2001 Rehabilitation of the athlete's elbow. In: Altchek D W, Andrews J R (eds) The athlete's elbow. Lippincott Williams and Wilkins, Philadelphia, PA, p 249–273

Wilk K E, Arrigo C, Andrews J R 1993a Rehabilitation of the elbow in the throwing athlete. Journal of Orthopaedic and Sports Physical Therapy 17:305–317

Wilk K E, Voight M, Keirns M D et al 1993b Plyometrics for the upper extremities: theory and clinical application. Journal of Orthopaedic and Sports Physical Therapy 17:225–239

Wilk K E, Andrews J R, Arrigo C A et al 2001a Preventive and rehabilitative exercises for the shoulder and elbow, 6th edn. American Sports Medicine Institute, Birmingham

Wilk K E, Reinold M M, Andrews J R 2001b Postoperative treatment principles in the throwing athlete. Sports Medicine and Arthroscopy Review 9:69–95

Wilson F D, Andrews J R, Blackburn T A et al 1983 Valgus extension overload in the pitching elbow. American Journal of Sports Medicine 11:83–88

Woodward A H, Bianco A J Jr 1975 Osteochondritis dissecans of the elbow. Clinical Orthopaedics and Related Research 110:35–41

Wyke B D 1966 The neurology of joints. Annals of the Royal College of Surgeons (London) 41:25–29

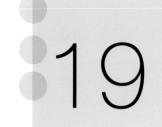

Wrist and hand

Paul LaStayo, Susan Michlovitz and Michael Lee

CHAPTER CONTENTS

Introduction 338

Sport-specific applied anatomy 338

Examination – general concepts related to the
wrist and hand 341

Common sport-related injuries 341

Less common sport-related injuries of the wrist
and hand 361

Summary 362

Introduction

The incidence of all sport-related injuries occurring to the wrist and hand is 3–9% (Arendt 1999). These injuries are more common in the adolescent athlete than in the adult. Wrist injuries typically occur during contact sports or with frequent weight-bearing activities through the upper extremity (e.g. gymnastics where the incidence of wrist problems ranges from 46 to 87% of participants) (Rettig 2003). Athletic finger injuries such as sprains, fractures, dislocations and tendon ruptures occur more often in ball-handling sports (e.g. basketball, baseball and volleyball) (Arendt 1999). Overuse injuries, such as tendonitis, occur most frequently in racquet sports, volleyball, handball and gymnastics (accounting for 25 to 50% of upper extremity injuries) (Rettig 2004). This chapter will focus on wrist and hand sport-related injuries, including the examination and management of these injuries.

Sport-specific applied anatomy

The wrist complex

The distal radius, distal ulna and two rows of carpal bones make up the wrist complex. The distal articular surface of the radius angles palmarly 10–15° and inclines radially 15–25° (Palmer 1993). Restoration of these angles and the bony relationships is imperative after injury (Kaukonen et al 1988, Laseter & Carter 1996, McQueen 1988) because badly united fractures, especially dorsal angulation and shortening of the radius (relative to the ulna), can lead to limited range of motion (ROM) (Kazuki et al 1993), mid-carpal instability (Taliesnik & Watson 1984), ulnar wrist pain (due to alterations in the transmission of axial forces) (Short et al 1987) and reduced grip strength (Villar & Marsh 1987).

Both the radiocarpal and mid-carpal joints contribute to wrist motion. Normally the wrist flexion/extension arc is 160–180° and the radial/ulnar deviation arc is 60°. Functional ROM, however, is 40° for both flexion and extension and a 40° arc of deviation (Ryu et al 1991). The distal radioulnar joint (DRUJ), in concert with the proximal radioulnar joint, is responsible for the 170° arc of forearm rotation (Chidgey 1995). Within the proximal carpal row, two of the most important intrinsic stabilizing ligaments are the scapholunate (SL) and lunotriquetral (LT), while at the DRUJ, the critical soft tissues are encompassed in the triangular

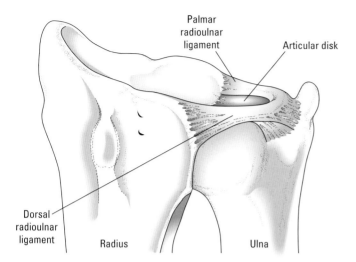

Figure 19.1 • Triangular fibrocartilage complex (TFCC) ligaments and articular disk. The ligaments of the TFCC that provide stability to the distal radioulnar joint (DRUJ) are the dorsal and palmar radioulnar ligaments. The centrally located articular disk is the fibrocartilaginous component of the TFCC which does not provide stability to the DRUJ.

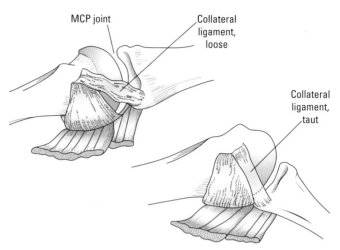

Figure 19.2 • The metacarpophalangeal (MCP) joint collateral ligament is loose in joint extension and taut in joint flexion. If immobilized in extension, the collateral ligaments structurally shorten, thereby preventing MCP flexion.

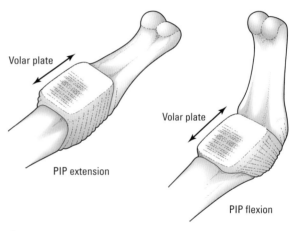

Figure 19.3 • The proximal interphalangeal joint (PIP) volar plate is relatively non-compliant and does not change length with joint motion, hence it is a primary stabilizer to the PIP joint. To allow PIP joint movement the volar plate glides proximally and distally. If the excursion of the volar plate is restricted, particularly the distal excursion, loss of PIP extension occurs.

fibrocartilage complex (TFCC) (Berger & Garcia-Elias 1991, Horii et al 1991, Ruby et al 1987). The radioulnar ligamentous components of the TFCC and the interosseous membrane are the primary stabilizers of the DRUJ. The articular disk (triangular fibrocartilage) of the TFCC, however, does not contribute to joint stability (Chidgey 1995, Kihara et al 1995) (Fig. 19.1).

The finger joints

The finger joints include the metacarpophalangeal (MCP), proximal interphalangeal (PIP) and distal interphalangeal (DIP) joints. A disruption of the surrounding soft tissue structures can cause a characteristic deformity or motion loss. PIP joint dislocations, extensor and flexor tendon ruptures and collateral ligament sprains or tears will be discussed later in this chapter.

The MCP joints of the digits are formed by the cam-shaped distal end of the metacarpal and the biconcave proximal end of the proximal phalanx. This osseous arrangement provides little bony stability. Flexion/extension and radial/ulnar deviation, with a small amount of supination and pronation, occurs at the MCP joints. In extension, the true or band fibers of the MCP collateral ligaments are in their slack position, and in a fully flexed position, these ligaments are lengthened to a taut position (Fig. 19.2). For this reason, there is minimal radial and ulnar deviation at the MCP joint when it is fully flexed. Injury to the true collateral ligament will cause excessive deviation (radial/ulnar) on passive motion when the joint is fully flexed. On the volar joint surface, the main supporting structure is the volar or palmar plate. The volar plate at the MCP joint is less constraining than at the PIP and DIP, thus allowing significant hyperextension (30–45°) at that joint. This motion, coupled

with ulnar deviation, is important for activities requiring palmar push off or ball handling. MCP flexion values greater than 90° occur at the 5th digit for a strong and tight fist (Werner 1996).

The PIP and DIP joints have more inherent bony stability and a stiffer, less compliant volar plate than the MCP joint. Unlike the MCP joint, the true collateral ligaments are taut throughout the range of motion. The injured PIP joint has a propensity for flexion deformity, initially due to joint effusion and ultimately due to limited gliding of the volar plate (Fig. 19.3). Normal flexion ROM at the PIP is 100–110° and at the DIP it can be up to 90° (Freeland & Sennett 1996).

Carpometacarpal joints (including the thumb)

The carpometacarpal (CMC) joints act as a link between the wrist and the digits. The first CMC joint, termed the basal joint of the thumb, has 3° of freedom, permitting flexion/extension, abduction/adduction and opposition/reposition. There is 40° abduction, 50° flexion and 80° opposition (Cooney et al 1981). During pinch, the forces at this joint are 12 times that at the tips of the fingers (Cooney et al 1981). The primary stabilizing structure preventing posterior translation of the metacarpal on the trapezium during pinch is the volar oblique (beak) ligament (Pellegrini 1991). Attenuation of this ligament has been implicated in the commonly occurring instability/osteoarthritis of the basal joint. This arthritis has its highest prevalence in postmenopausal women. The 2nd and 3rd CMC joints are relatively immobile and act to transmit weightbearing loads from the metacarpals through the capitate and trapezoid. A degenerative osteophyte, termed a carpal boss, can occur about these joints. The 4th and 5th CMCs have 20–25° of flexion, motion that is necessary for 'cupping' of the hand around spherical and conical objects as well as making a full fist.

The two distal joints of the thumb, the MCP and interphalangeal (IP), work in concert with the CMC to position the thumb. The thumb is rotated 90° from the plane of the fingers and has the added motion of opposition to position the thumb against the fingers for prehension and precision activities. Because of the position of the thumb, it is vulnerable to lateral stresses, such as that which occur with the so-called 'ski pole' injury (injury to the ulnar collateral ligament of the MCP joint). In addition to the stability provided by the collateral ligaments, stability against lateral stress is provided by the aponeurosis of the adductor pollicis muscle, which inserts on the base of the proximal phalanx and has an intimate relationship with the ulnar collateral ligament (UCL).

Muscle/tendon structures of the wrist and hand

Extensor tendons and compartments of the wrist

The three primary wrist extensors are: the extensor carpi radialis longus (ECRL) and brevis (ECRB) in the second compartment, and the extensor carpi ulnaris (ECU) in the sixth compartment. The ECRL is most effective as a wrist extensor when the elbow is extended and when radial deviation is balanced by the primary ulnar deviator (the ECU) (Brand & Hollister 1993). The ECRB is a more effective wrist extensor due to its insertion on the base of the third metacarpal, its larger moment arm for wrist extension and the fact it is not influenced by elbow position (Brand & Hollister 1993).

The first dorsal compartment contains the abductor pollicis longus (APL) and the extensor pollicis brevis (EPB) tendons. The APL and EPB tendons may be separated by septations (fibrous or osseofibrous divisions), which create separate compartments and potential sites of compression (Kirkpatrick 1990). Septations are commonly found in patients with De Quervain's disease, also known as stenosing tenovaginitis (Kirkpatrick 1990).

Ruptures of tendons that cross the wrist are more commonly seen at the third compartment where the extensor pollicis longus (EPL) tendon turns radially at Lister's tubercle. This is most common in patients with rheumatoid arthritis and/or fractures of the distal radius (Rosenthal 1990). Blending with the dorsal wrist capsule is the floor of the fourth and fifth compartments, which contain the extensor digitorum communis (EDC), extensor indicis proprius and the extensor digiti quinti. They become primary wrist extensors when extension of the wrist follows digital extension in an obligate fashion. This is, however, an unnatural functional sequence as it limits the spatial positioning of the hand and grasping power and is often limited during rehabilitation following wrist fractures (Rosenthal 1990).

Finger extensors and extensor mechanism of the fingers

EDC tendons are maintained in position over the dorsum of MCP joints by sagittal bands, which are components of the dorsal hood. Injury to sagittal bands results in painful subluxation of these tendons during digital flexion and extension. The EDC tendons are also maintained in position through their juncturae tendinae on the dorsum of the hand. The conjoint lateral bands of the lumbricals and interossei travel dorsally to the axis of motion of the PIP and DIP. Injury to the extensor tendon, the central slip component, over the PIP joint and/or the triangular membrane over the middle phalanx can cause volar migration of the lateral bands and a subsequent boutonnière deformity (PIP flexion + DIP hyperextension). Dorsal displacement of the lateral bands can cause a swan neck deformity (PIP hyperextension + DIP flexion). Distally, the terminal tendon inserts onto the distal phalanx for DIP extension. Direct impact to the tip of the finger can tear or avulse the terminal tendon and result in an extension deficit called mallet finger. The mallet finger can also precipitate a swan neck deformity.

Finger flexors of the digits

The tendons which flex the digits stem from the muscle bellies of the flexor digitorum superficialis (FDS) and the flexor digitorum profundus (FDP). Both tendons travel through a synovial sheath in the fingers. Nutrition to the tendons occurs via perfusion extrinsically via vincula, and diffusion intrinsically as the tendons move through synovial fluid within the tendon sheath. The confined structure of the tenosynovial sheath, with its two tendons within, is an area for adhesion formation after phalangeal fractures, crush injuries and flexor tendon injuries and repair. The tendons are reinforced within their tendon sheaths, to maintain their moment arms and mechanical advantage, via fibrous annular (A) pulleys. The A1 pulley is the location where a tendon stenosis can occur resulting in a trigger finger. The A2 and A4 pulleys are the most important as they maintain optimal moment arms and facilitate optimal tendon excursion. All tendons travel in a synovial sheath through the carpal tunnel with the median nerve. In addition to carpal tunnel syndrome (CTS), flexor tenosynovitis can occur at the wrist. The flexor pollicus longus (FPL) tendon also travels through the carpal tunnel with the long finger flexors (FDS and FDP) and has a continuous tendon sheath to its insertion on the distal phalanx of the thumb.

Neurological and vascular structures of the wrist and hand

The median nerve, originating from the nerve roots of C5–7, provides cutaneous innervation to the radial side of the palm, volar thumb, index, middle and radial half of the ring finger, and the dorsum of these digits over the distal phalanx (Pratt 1996). The palmar cutaneous branch of the median nerve branches off proximal to the wrist joint and primarily innervates the skin of the thenar eminence. The remainder of the median nerve has cutaneous and motor branches and travels under the transverse carpal ligament, through the carpal tunnel. The common and proper digital nerves provide cutaneous innervation to the aforementioned digits, with the recurrent branch innervating the muscles of the thenar eminence. Carpal tunnel syndrome involves the median nerve distal to the palmar cutaneous branch.

The radial nerve, originating from the nerve roots of C6–8, only has a cutaneous branch at the level of the hand, supplying the skin to the dorsum of the thumb and hand including digits 2 and 3 and the radial half of the ring finger to the level of the distal phalanx. This superficial branch originates near the elbow, deep to the brachioradialis as the radial nerve splits to the superficial and deep (posterior) interosseous branches. This nerve can become irritated due to a blow to the radial side of the wrist or with surgery (particularly external fixation of distal radius fractures) on that side of the wrist, often producing dysesthesia and hyperesthesia, both of which are difficult to treat.

The ulnar nerve, originating from the nerve roots of C8–T1, splits into two branches before entering the wrist and hand. One branch travels dorsally (dorsal cutaneous branch of the ulnar nerve) to provide sensation to the ulnar dorsum of the hand and the dorsum of the ulnar half of the ring finger and to the little finger. On the volar surface, the other branch of the ulnar nerve travels between the pisiform and hamate to innervate the hypothenar muscles, interossei, 4th and 5th lumbricales, adductor pollicus and 50% of the flexor pollicus brevis. The ulnar nerve also provides sensation to the volar surfaces of the little and ulnar half of the ring fingers.

The blood supply to the hand is via the ulnar and radial arteries, with two major 'arches' formed. The superficial palmar arterial arch is supplied by the ulnar artery, and the superficial palmar branch of the radial artery. This superficial arch forms the digital arteries to all but the thumb and radial aspect of the index finger. These lateral digits are perfused by the radial artery. The deep palmar arterial arch is formed by the radial artery and deep branch of the ulnar artery (Pratt 1996). With arterial occlusion, there will be a spontaneous onset of digital pain. Inadequate blood flow results in pain, cold sensitivity, cyanosis, weakness and may lead to ulceration and tissue necrosis (Coleman & Anson 1961, Smith et al 2004).

Examination – general concepts related to the wrist and hand

Taking a thorough history, performing a meticulous physical examination and corroborating these findings with additional studies (e.g. imaging and electrophysiology) are the hallmark of the assessment of wrist/hand pain and impairment (Beckenbaugh 1984, Cyriax 1982). The tenets of the examination are:

- The patient should describe and perform the task or maneuver that precipitates their symptoms, starting at the least symptomatic region and concluding with the most symptomatic region.
- The exam progression, as suggested by Cyriax (1982), is: active range of motion → passive range of motion → isometric resistive tests → provocative maneuvers → palpation.
- Provocative maneuvers (predicted to be painful) should be the last maneuver performed.
- Assessing the status of cutaneous nerves with sensory testing if a nerve injury is suspected, e.g. reduced or abnormal sensations.
- Grip strength testing is an index of muscle performance and of a joint's ability to withstand a load.
- Electromyography (EMG) and nerve conduction velocity (NCV) can help locate an area of nerve injury/entrapment and can determine the nerve and muscle's status.
- Radiographic images (see Chapter 30) directly reveal the integrity, relationships and contours of the wrist/hand osseous structures and indirectly, the ligamentous status.
- A generic and/or condition-specific outcome measure can assess a patient's perception of disability and should be coupled with physical measures (see Chapter 13).

Common sport-related injuries

Management of wrist and hand pain and impairment

In this section, the following will be presented: (1) an algorithmic approach toward managing radial (Fig. 19.4), central (Fig. 19.5) and ulnar-based (Fig. 19.6) wrist pain and impairment; (2) management principles for sport-specific hand and finger injuries; and (3) treatment concepts, options and caveats (Table 19.1) for major diagnostic categories that affect the hand and wrist.

Radial wrist pain and impairment

Fractures

Scaphoid fractures encompass 70% of all carpal fractures, which are more often noted in young males participating in athletic events (Botte & Gelberman 1987, Zemel & Stark 1986).

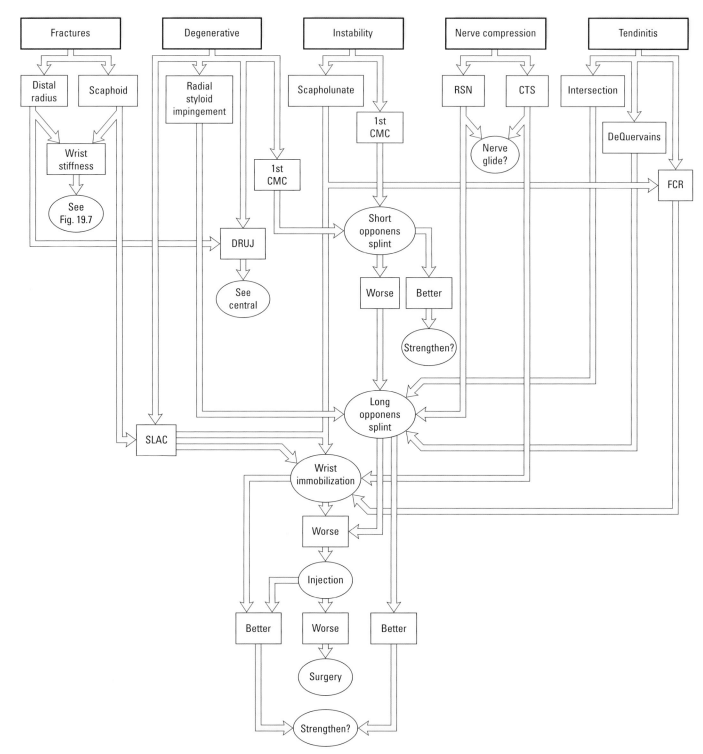

Figure 19.4 • An algorithm to guide the differential diagnosis and treatment concepts of radial wrist pain and impairment. SLAC = scapholunate advanced collapse; DRUJ = distal radioulnar joint; CMC = carpometacarpal joint; RSN = radial sensory neuritis; CTS = carpal tunnel syndrome; FCR = flexor carpi radialis.

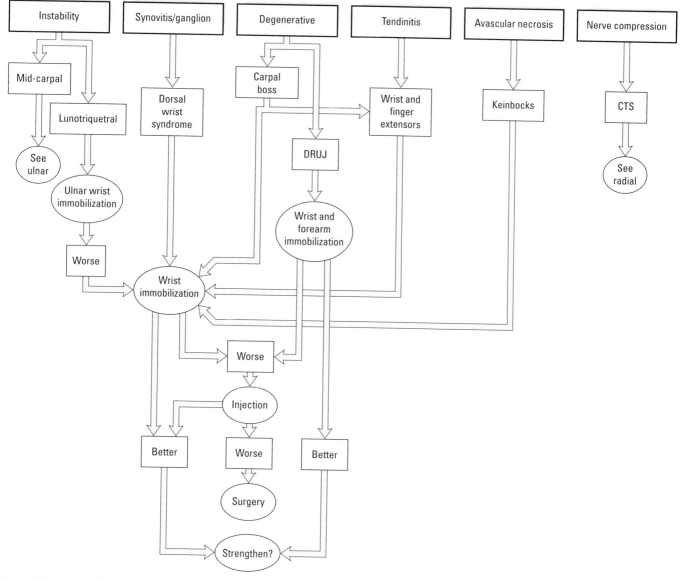

Figure 19.5 • An algorithm to guide the differential diagnosis and treatment concepts of central wrist pain and impairment. DRUJ = distal radioulnar joint.

Unfortunately, scaphoid non-unions are not uncommon due to the scaphoid's dependence on a single interosseous blood supply that is often disrupted after fracture (Gelberman et al 1983, Prosser & Herbert 1996). In particular, the proximal pole of the scaphoid has a worse prognosis for healing and is more prone to non-union due to this vascular anatomy (Rettig 2003). Hyperextension and carpal supination forces, due to a fall on an outstretched hand (FOOSH), are the typical mechanisms of action in distal radius and scaphoid fractures (and/or ligamentous instability) (Mayfield 1981, Weber & Chao 1978). The distal radius osteoporotic fracture in the elderly is common (Laseter & Carter 1996). The higher velocity distal radius fracture, the most common snowboarding injury, tends to have greater soft tissue damage than the typical osteoporotic-type

elderly fracture, hence, problems with swelling and return of ROM are more pronounced in the former than the latter.

Following the immobilization and fracture healing of either the scaphoid or distal radius, there is often a limitation of wrist extension (additionally forearm supination in the latter) and pain at the extremes of motion (Weber 1980). Grip strength is also reduced by more than 50% (Laseter & Carter 1996, Prosser & Herbert 1996). Overcoming wrist stiffness and a return to functional wrist motion is a priority. Treatment options and approaches are presented in Fig. 19.7 and Table 19.1.

After addressing the passive range of motion (PROM) limitations, one must not underestimate the importance of reconstituting active wrist extension via the ECRL and ECRB, rather than the digital extensors prior to strengthening activities. Treatment

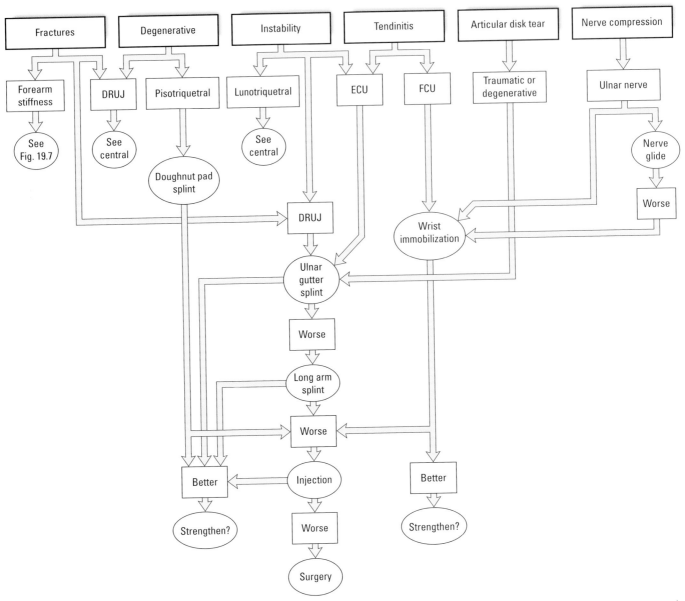

Figure 19.6 • An algorithm to guide the differential diagnosis and treatment concepts of ulnar wrist pain and impairment. ECU = extensor carpi ulnaris; DRUJ = distal radioulnar joint; FCR = flexor carpi radialis.

guidelines for radius and scaphoid fractures are outlined in Table 19.2. In the pediatric wrist patient, especially gymnasts, epiphyseal plate injuries are not uncommon. Radiographic findings are often negative, but the clinical signs of pain (with palpation) and swelling over the physis are indicative of this injury (Sotereanos et al 1994).

Tenderness in the anatomical snuff box following a FOOSH is thought to be pathopneumonic for a scaphoid fracture in younger individuals. This region, however, needs to be explored proximally in the older athlete, at the distal radius where the radial styloid process is located, as symptomatic degenerative changes in the posttraumatic and aged patient are not uncommon.

Tenderness and edema in this region may be present (and accentuated with radial deviation) especially when the radial styloid is fractured and/or a scaphoid irritation is occurring on the radial styloid (radial styloid impingement). If the latter is noted on radiograph and coupled with pain on forced radial deviation, as with decelerating a golf club at the peak of a backswing, rest and protection with a long opponens splint (Fig. 19.8) coupled with an alteration of the task are required. (Watson & Ryu 1986, Whipple 1992). Instability of the scaphoid (via non-union or a ligamentous disruption) can be associated with the scapholunate advanced collapse (SLAC) wrist condition. SLAC wrist pathology is a pattern of degenerative changes that are based on and

Table 19.1 Treatment of wrist and hand pain and impairment: concepts, applications, adjuncts and caveats

	Concept	Treatment application	Caveats	Treatment adjunct(s)
Protection/rest (Shultz-Johnson 1996)	Rigid immobilization Semi-rigid immobilization Incomplete immobilization and/or athletic participation	Casting Pre-fabricated or custom splinting Athletic taping, silicone rubber, neoprene, foam rubber	Too long duration = stiffness Too short duration = non/delayed union, instability	Anti-inflammatories by mouth and/or transdermally (e.g. iontophoresis, phonophoresis; Ch. 14) Electrophysiological agents (Ch. 14)
Strengthening (See Ch. 10)	To overload or not with wrist/hand patients?	Resistance exercises (see Ch. 10)	The potential risks (overstressing structures before they are biologically prepared for such stressors, promoting inflammation and pain) versus benefits (increasing muscle mass, function and overall performance) must be considered before implementing a strengthening program	Consider eccentric loading for high muscle tensions
Joint stiffness (Flowers & LaStayo 1994, Threlkeld 1992)	HLBS (Threlkeld 1992) LLPS (TERT) (Flowers & LaStayo 1994)	Joint mobilization Dynamic splinting, prolonged positioning	Pain, inflammation, increased stiffness See algorithm (Fig. 19.7) (McClure et al 1994)	Manipulation under anesthesia, or surgical joint release
Instability (Wright & Michlovitz 1996)	Protect and rest (complete or partial) 4–8 weeks No pain prior to strengthening/ROM	See protection and rest as above	Transient joint stiffness may not be detrimental Joint pain indicates inadequate protection and/or excessive joint loading	Anti-inflammatories and modalities as above Surgical stabilization
Degenerative joint disease (Eaton & Littler 1969 Jaffe et al 1996, Michlovitz & Kozin 2000)	Avoid provocative activities Protect/rest as above	Behavioral modification See protection and rest as above	Strengthening not always a good option if it aggravates degenerative region	Anti-inflammatories and modalities as above Injections (e.g. anesthetic, corticosteroid)
Tendonitis/synovitis (Mennell 1964, Cyriax 1982)	Avoid provocative activities Protect/rest as above	Behavioral modification See protection and rest as above	Gentle stretching and resistance exercises can be helpful if the dosages are minimal to moderate	Anti-inflammatories and modalities as above Injections (e.g. anesthetic, corticosteroid)
Nerve (Mackinnon & Novak 1997, Sweeney & Harms 1996)	Protection/rest or nerve mobilization	See protection and rest as above Avoid traction to nerve Nerve gliding	If protection increases symptoms add motion If traction/gliding increases symptoms stop nerve mobilization	Anti-inflammatories and modalities as above Surgical decompression

HLBS = high load brief stress; LLPS = low load prolonged stress; ROM = range of motion

caused by articular alignment problems between the scaphoid, lunate, capitate and the radius. Pain and impairments are pronounced and are exacerbated by axial loading (gripping) and radial deviation (Watson & Ballet 1984).

Instability

In addition to fractures, a FOOSH can result in isolated ligamentous damage, with injury to the SL ligament being the most common (Wright & Michlovitz 1996). Ligament injuries in

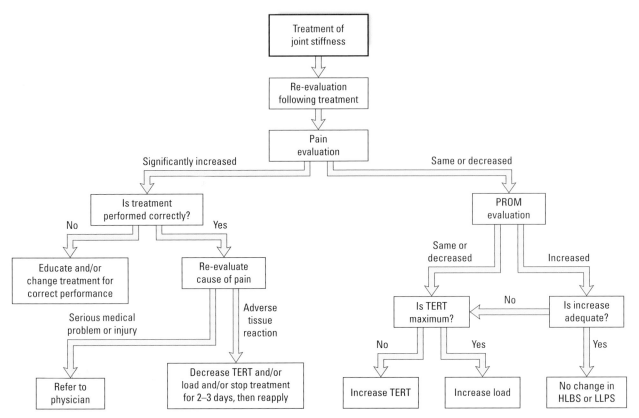

Figure 19.7 • An algorithm to guide the use of treatments for joint stiffness secondary to structural changes to periarticular soft tissues. HLBS = high load brief stress; LLPS = low load prolonged stress; TERT = total end range time (duration × frequency of treatment per treatment session). Load = the amount of force applied during treatment session. Adverse tissue reaction = swelling, heat, pain. (Adapted from McClure P W, Blackburn L G, Dusold C 1994 The use of splints in the treatment of joint stiffness: biologic rationale and an algorithm for making clinical decisions. Physical Therapy: 74:1101–1107, with permission of the American Physical Therapy Association.)

association with fractures occur frequently (>50%) (Richards et al 1997). In SL dissociations (e.g. rotary subluxation of the scaphoid), there is a characteristic dorsal/radial swelling of the wrist, lack of ROM, pain with gripping, a positive scaphoid shift test (Watson's Test) (Watson et al 1988, 1993) (Table 19.3), and a radiographic carpal instability pattern will sometimes be noted (Weber 1984). An intact SL ligament forces the lunate to move with the scaphoid into palmar flexion with radial deviation. With a disrupted SL ligament, however, the lunate is free to assume its natural (and triquetrum-influenced) dorsiflexed position, while the scaphoid continues to palmarflex (hence the rotary subluxation of the scaphoid). This instability pattern, a dorsiflexion intercalated segment instability (DISI), is in reference to the lunate's position (Wright & Michlovitz 1996). In many instances a dynamic instability is present, especially in those with a diagnosis of a 'wrist sprain', whereby an axial load (gripping) must be employed to create the DISI and pain (Wright & Michlovitz 1996). Often a carpal instability radiographic series with the patient making a fist (axially loaded film) is required to pick up dynamic instabilities (Gilula & Yin 1996). The flexor carpi radialis (FCR) can often become inflamed with overuse in racket sports and with throwing. This

tendon's intimate relationship to the scaphoid warrants close assessment of an underlying scaphoid instability.

Vigorous ROM activities are contraindicated in the presence of wrist instabilities. Stability can sometimes be restored with wrist splinting, either a long opponens (Fig. 19.8) or a wrist control (Fig. 19.9) and avoidance of axial loading (resistive fisting), but surgical stabilization is often required. To ensure no fisting activity, a distal block of finger flexion may need to be incorporated into the splint. Treatment options and caveats are outlined in Table 19.1, while Table 19.2 describes management during the phases of recovery from wrist instability.

Degenerative disorders

The 1st CMC joint of the thumb has the greatest amount of ROM in the wrist and hand and experiences relatively high loads (4–5 times the applied external load) with pinching and grasping (Cooney & Chao 1977). Therefore, the impairments related to osteoarthritis of the basal joint of the thumb include a spectrum of disorders ranging from instability (in the young) and degenerative joint disease (DJD)/deformities (in older individuals). Problems with pinching and grasping in tasks such

Table 19.2 Treatment guidelines for wrist fractures (radius and scaphoid) and carpal instabilities

	Protective phase (immobilization)	Motion phase (following immobilization)	Strength and function phase
Time frame	6–12 wks (longer duration typically required for scaphoid fractures) – duration of immobilization will be less with some internal fixation techniques	Starting immediately after immobilization	PROM $\gg$ AROM PROM >25% normal Wrist joint is not painful
Goals	Protect fracture and/or stabilized segment Control swelling, avoid pin site (if present) infections Full finger ROM, no grip strengthening	Active wrist extension, flexion, and forearm supination PROM 1 week later if needed	Increase wrist extension, and grip strength
Techniques	Cast, splint, surgical fixation/ stabilization, external fixator Elevation, retrograde massage compressive wraps, daily pin site cleaning Active and passive gentle fisting	AROM: wrist extension with finger flexion PROM: manual, gravity assisted weight assisted, dynamic splinting	Isometric progressing to isotonic exercises Putty grip exercises
Comments and precautions	Finger ROM should be attained during this phase Nerve symptoms, 'pins and needles', and any CRPS must be monitored closely	Pain, swelling secondary too vigorous ROM exercise Avoid excessive ROM following instability Wrist flexion is a priority following stabilization to the dorsal wrist Any stabilization procedure that fuses one of the carpal rows should result in ~50% return of wrist ROM	Excessive overload, irritated tissues (i.e. tendonitis, joint instability) Any stabilization procedure that fuses one of the carpal rows should result in ~75% return of grip strength

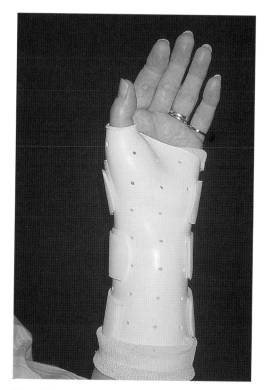

Figure 19.8 • Long opponens splint is used for many of the problems that plague the radial side of the wrist/hand.

as writing or swinging a racket or club are usually coupled with pain and swelling. The axial compression-adduction 'grind test' (Table 19.3) (Eaton & Littler 1969) is used to identify CMC joint arthrosis and to assess the stability of the CMC joint.

Splinting (Figs 19.8 and 19.10) or taping (Fig. 19.11) that will allow both protection and rest of the unstable 1st CMC joint can be fashioned in many ways; however, the principle of providing stability at the joint while pinching is essential. Several splint designs can provide the needed support; however, the short opponens is typically preferred (Fig. 19.10) (Weiss et al 2000).

Tendonitis

De Quervain's tenosynovitis of the EPB and APL in the first dorsal compartment of the wrist is common with repetitive sporting activities or tasks requiring ulnar deviation and thumb movement (Keon-Cohen 1951). De Quervain's is seen in sports such as golf, fly fishing, squash, badminton (Rettig 2004), rowing (Rumball et al 2005) and volleyball (Rossi et al 2005). Palpation of the first extensor compartment proximal to the anatomical snuff box may reveal tenderness, swelling and tendinous nodules (Berger & Dobyns 1996). More proximally, intersection syndrome (see table for provocative test), where the APL and EPB muscles lie across the radial wrist extensors (~3 cm proximal to the radial styloid), is a disorder that mimics de Quervain's and frequently causes crepitus and swelling along the radial forearm

Table 19.3 Provocative tests for radial, central, and ulnar lesions that cause pain and impairment

Radial tests	Technique	Central tests	Technique	Ulnar tests	Technique
Scaphoid shift for scaphoid instability (LaStayo & Howell, 1995, Watson et al 1988)	Stabilize wrist. Thumb pressure on palmar scaphoid. Passive wrist movement into ulnar deviation/ extension, then radial deviation and flexion. Remove thumb pressure. Positive test = relocating 'thunk', reproduction of pain	DRUJ grind and rotate for DJD of DRUJ (Schernberg 1990)	Manual compression of ulnar head into sigmoid notch while rotating forearm. Positive test = reproduction of pain	AD shear for AD tears (LaStayo & Howell 1995)	Dorsal glide of the pisotriquetral complex coupled with a volar glide of ulnar head, thereby shearing the AD. Positive test = reproduction of painful symptoms and/or excessive laxity in TFCC region
1st CMC grind for DJD (Eaton & Littler 1969)	Axial compression and adduction of metacarpal on trapezium. Palpate for instability or crepitus. Positive test = painful crepitus and/or instability	Ballottement for lunotriquetral joint instability (Reagan et al 1984, LaStayo & Howell 1995)	Stabilize lunate and glide pisotriquetral complex volarly and dorsally. Positive test = laxity and/or a reproduction pain	GRIT for ulnar impaction syndrome (LaStayo & Weiss 2001)	Grip strength in 3 forearm positions: first in neutral, then in full supination and finally in pronation. Calculate a ratio (supination:pronation) grip strength. Positive test = GRIT ratio on involved side >1.0 while on the uninvolved side the GRIT ratio is no different than 1.0
Finkelstein for De Quervain's (Finkelstein 1930)	Thumb actively adducted and held tightly in the palm with the other fingers. Wrist actively in ulnar deviation. Positive test = sharp lancinating pain at the first dorsal compartment	Volar/dorsal translation for DRUJ instability (Chidgey 1995)	Volar/dorsal glide of ulna on radius in various positions of forearm rotation (initially in neutral forearm rotation then in extreme positions of supination and pronation). Positive test = ulnar translation at extremes of rotation equals that of the neutral translation	Catch up clunk for CIND instability (Lichtman et al 1981)	Active wrist radial and ulnar deviation. Positive test = clunk or thud and pain at a point just beyond neutral as the wrist moves into ulnar deviation
Traction for radial sensory neuritis (Kenneally et al 1988)	Radial nerve tensioning. Positioning: (1) elbow extension, (2) forearm pronation, (3) wrist flexion, (4) wrist ulnar deviation, (5) digital flexion, (6) sidebending of cervical spine to contralateral side. Positive test = reproduction of pain	Middle finger extension for dorsal wrist syndrome (Watson & Weinzweig 1997)	Resisted middle finger extension (over the PIPJ) with wrist flexed. Positive test = pain in the scapholunate/ dorsal wrist region	Pisotriquetral grind for pisotriquetral DJD (Schernberg 1990)	Compress and translate the pisiform against the triquetrum. Positive test = reproduction of pain
Intersection for intersection syndrome	Active wrist extension with concomitant active thumb circumduction. Positive test = pain, crepitus ± squeaking sound from intersection region			ECU subluxation for instability (Burkhart et al 1982)	Passive supination followed by wrist ulnar deviation ± resistance to ulnar deviation. Positive test = visible and palpable painful subluxation

AD = articular disk; CMC = carpometacarpal joint; CIND = carpal instability nondissociative; DJD = degenerative joint disease; DRUJ = distal radioulnar joint; ECU = extensor carpi ulnaris; PIPJ = proximal interphalangeal joint; TFCC = triangular fibrocartilage complex

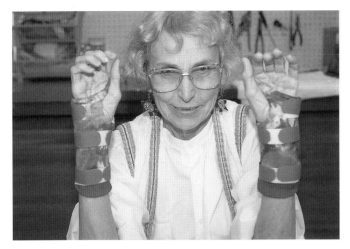

Figure 19.9 • Wrist control splint. The splint most often used to limit wrist motion.

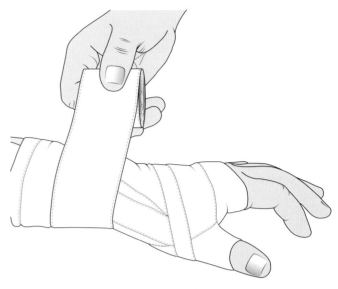

Figure 19.11 • An example of protection and rest with incomplete immobilization using athletic taping. Taping can provide protection and rest of the wrist and thumb as depicted here. Also, taping can be used at the hand and with the fingers.

thumb CMC DJD and/or provoke an established radial sensory neuritis or intersection syndrome.

The primary goal of treatment is to reduce pain and inflammation with splinting (Fig. 19.8) and modalities such as iontophoresis (Table 19.1). Education as to postures and sport-related techniques that both irritate (thumb adduction and wrist radial deviation) and relieve de Quervain's tenosynovitis is essential. Taping (Fig. 19.11) during sport can provide temporary relief. Strengthening of the small thumb tendons should be progressed slowly or omitted. If pain is elicited with strengthening activities, these exercises should be stopped. Factors that affect tendonitis and synovitis (Table 19.1), and specifically the recovery of de Quervain's, are outlined in Table 19.4.

Nerve compression and traction

The radial sensory nerve (RSN) along the radial aspect of the wrist is susceptible to compression and traction injuries. Symptoms can vary from paresthesias to pain or numbness over the dorsoradial aspect of the forearm and wrist. The RSN can get irritated 7–9 cm proximal to the radial styloid, where the nerve becomes superficial from under the distal aspect of the brachioradialis. The RSN can become irritated by traction with repetitive wrist flexion and ulnar deviation (Table 19.3) or may be compressed by a scissoring action between the brachioradialis and the ECRL tendons with repetitive forearm supination and pronation as in racket sports (Dellon & Mackinnon 1986, Kleinert & Mehta 1996). Avoiding these composite postures with educational training and/or a long arm splint (Fig. 19.12), which must cross proximal to the elbow for controlling forearm rotation, is essential for the nerve to recover. Tinel's percussion testing over the nerve can help localize the lesion (Tinel 1915). Light touch perception may be altered over the first dorsal web

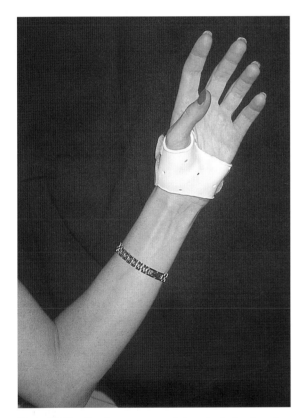

Figure 19.10 • Short opponens splint protects the thumb carpometacarpal joint. The distal margin of the thumb component can be extended distally to also incorporate the metacarpophalangeal joint.

in weightlifters and rowers (Rettig 2004, Wood & Dobyns 1986). A Finkelstein's test (Table 19.3) is the classic evaluative provocative maneuver for de Quervain's and is positive if intense pain is experienced along the styloid process of the radius in the region of the 1st dorsal compartment (Finkelstein 1930). In addition, however, the Finkelstein testing position may irritate

Table 19.4 Factors that affect recovery from de Quervain's stenosing tenovaginitis

	Protective phase (immobilization)	Motion phase (following immobilization)	Strength and function phase
Time frame	Surgical repair: 6–8 weeks Debridement: 1–3 weeks Longer (6 weeks) if ulnar shortening osteotomy with plate fixation is performed	Surgical repair: starting immediately after immobilization Debridement: typically protected intermittent ROM during immobilization phase Followed by unrestricted ROM in motion phase	Surgical repair/debridement PROM $\gg$ AROM PROM >25% normal Wrist complex is not painful
Goals	Surgical repair: protect stabilized DRUJ, no forearm rotation Control swelling, full finger ROM Debridement: avoid painful forearm rotation positions Control swelling, full finger ROM No forceful gripping	Surgical repair/debridement: active forearm rotation PROM 1 week later if needed	Surgical repair/debridement: increase forearm rotation, wrist and grip strength
Techniques	Surgical repair: cast, splint, surgical fixation/stabilization Elevation, retrograde massage, compressive wraps, active gentle fisting Debridement: cast, splint Elevation, retrograde massage, compressive wraps, active gentle fisting	Surgical repair/debridement: AROM forearm rotation PROM manual, gravity assisted eight assisted, dynamic splinting	Surgical repair/debridement: isometric progressing to isotonic exercises Putty grip exercises
Comments and precautions	Surgical repair: must be rigorously protected Debridement alone needs little protection, debridement with ulnar osteotomy/plate fixation requires bone healing Surgical repair/debridement: finger ROM should be attained during this phase Nerve symptoms, 'pins and needles' and any CRPS must be monitored closely	Surgical repair/debridement: pain, swelling secondary to vigorous ROM exercise Functional forearm rotation is 50° supination and 50° pronation. Many sport activities, however, require more ROM	Surgical repair/debridement: excessive overload, irritated tissues (i.e. tendonitis, joint instability)

space distribution of the nerve. In many instances, gentle nerve gliding (using the progressive positioning noted in the RSN traction test (Table 19.3) may be helpful, especially following a nerve release. Other effective interventions may simply involve removing the irritant (watch band, strap, tight jewelry) and changing the hand and wrist posture during activity.

Central wrist pain and impairment

Degenerative

The DRUJ lies in the center of this region. Degenerative changes to the articular surfaces of the DRUJ are not uncommon, especially after distal radius fractures with or without ulnar variance discrepancies. If the normally smooth motion of the sigmoid notch of the radius rotating around the ulnar head, with concomitant ulnar translation, is disrupted, then pain, swelling, crepitus and limitation of forearm rotation are often present. A simple provocative grind and rotate maneuver (Table 19.3) is often helpful in identifying these patients. As with the conservative management of other forms of DJD in the upper extremity, the primary course of treatment is rest with a long arm splint (Fig. 19.12) to prevent forearm rotation, anti-inflammatory medication and patient education (Table 19.1).

In this central region, pain can be due to a carpal boss, which is an osteoarthritic spur that develops at the base of the second and/or third carpometacarpal joints. A carpal boss is often confused with a dorsal wrist ganglion (Watson 1979). A wrist splint, limiting wrist extension (Fig. 19.9), can control symptoms, but often an injection, aspiration or surgical excision is required (Angelides 1999).

Instability

Injury to the LT joint can precipitate central wrist pain, but like DRUJ instability, is often described as a source of ulnar wrist pain. LT injuries are usually the result of a FOOSH where the axial load is applied with the wrist in extension and radial deviation (Rettig 2003). Signs and symptoms of LT injury include: diminished motion, weakness of grip, a sensation of instability

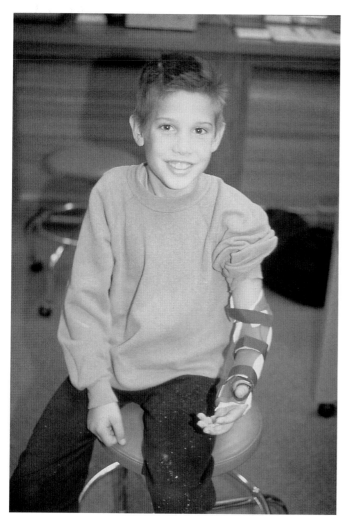

Figure 19.12 • Long arm splint is essential for protecting and restricting the wrist and hand from forearm rotation. The proximal margin must have components that sit medially and laterally over the epicondyles of the elbow, but the volar proximal portion should be flared distally to allow some elbow flexion and extension.

or giving way, ulnar nerve paresthesias and a positive ballottement test (Table 19.3) (Bishop & Reagan 1998). Typically, a simple wrist control resting splint (Fig. 19.9) will suffice in LT strains but conservative and postoperative management principles described in Table 19.1 and 19.2 should be followed. As with any carpal instability, care must be taken when applying axial loads (e.g. fisting and/or FOOSH) to the wrist so as not to compromise the healing of ligamentous/capsular tissue.

Synovitis and ganglion

Dorsal wrist pain postactivity and/or with forced wrist extension, especially in sporting activities that require weightbearing through the wrist, can be the result of a dorsal wrist syndrome. Watson describes dorsal wrist syndrome as localized SL synovitis secondary to overstress to ligaments in this area, or it may

represent an occult ganglia (Watson & Weinzweig 1997, Watson et al 1997). Dorsal wrist ganglia, which comprise 60–70% of all hand and wrist ganglia, can be either palpable or occult and may indicate a dorsal wrist syndrome. Clicks and palpable subluxation from this region should also increase the examiner's suspicion that underlying SL pathology is present (Watson et al 1988, 1997). Tenderness in the SL region coupled with a positive middle finger extension test (Table 19.3) are indicators of a dorsal wrist syndrome (Watson et al 1997). A wrist splint, limiting wrist extension (Fig. 19.9), can control symptoms, but often an injection, aspiration or surgical excision is required.

Avascular necrosis

The lunate, located ulnar to the scaphoid along the proximal margin of the mid-carpal joint, may also cause central wrist pain and impairment. Tenderness over the lunate is suggestive of a fracture and/or Kienbock's disease (idiopathic osteonecrosis) (Skirvin 1996, Watson et al 1997). The latter is often associated with an ulnar negative variance. Ulnar variance is a measure (obtained radiographically) of the distance that the ulnar head extends below (negative) or above (positive) the articular surface of the radius. In all carpal bone or joint lesions causing central wrist pain and impairment, a rigid or semi-rigid block of wrist extension (Fig. 19.9) and diminished axial loading (fisting) is required.

Tendonitis

It is important to differentiate tenderness in this central region as either coming from the lunate or the tendons of the fourth extensor compartment where tenosynovitis can occur. If tendonitis is present at the insertion of the ECRL and ECRB at the base of the 2nd and 3rd metacarpal, one must identify if a carpal boss is the irritant. Also, any systemic cause of inflamed tendons, e.g. rheumatoid arthritis, needs to be ruled out. Using the selective tensioning of tissue approach advocated by Cyriax (1982) is helpful in diagnosing tendonitis. AROM may be painful, while PROM is generally painless; PROM tends to selectively tension inert, non-contractile tissues. Tendonitis should be suspected when pain is elicited with isometric resistance. Wrist motion should be avoided with a protective device (Fig. 19.9) or taping (Fig. 19.11). Modalities should be used as needed and an emphasis on education should be employed in all cases. If strengthening is required after a resolution of pain, an eccentric component to the strengthening exercise is suggested. Guidelines for treatment are described in Table 19.1.

Nerve compression

Carpal tunnel syndrome, the most common entrapment neuropathy, is due to compression/traction injury to the median nerve within the carpal tunnel. Various etiologies including anatomical anomalies, repetitive activity, hormonal changes that occur in pregnancy and systemic diseases such as diabetes mellitus have been implicated in contributing to the occurrence of this disorder. The signs and symptoms of CTS are paresthesias with

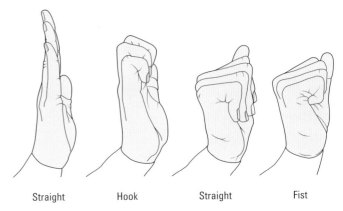

Straight Hook Straight Fist

Figure 19.14 • Tendon gliding exercises: different fist positions accentuating active differential tendon gliding of the extrinsic flexors and active/passive gliding of the extrinsic extensors.

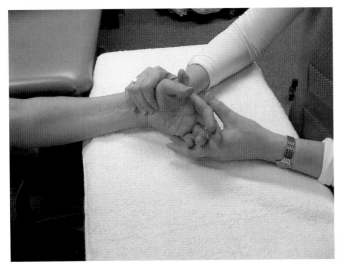

Figure 19.13 • Median nerve compression coupled with wrist flexion is a provocative position used to identify carpal tunnel syndrome as the external compression and flexed position increase pressures on the median nerve.

or without pain in the volar thumb, index, middle and radial half of the ring fingers (paresthesia may only occur in portions of median distribution); paresthesias awaken the individual at night and worsen with repetitive activity. There is a feeling of clumsiness in handling small objects and a weakness of grip and pinch. Provocative maneuvers for carpal tunnel include a positive reproduction of symptoms and a median nerve compression/wrist flexion test (Fig. 19.13) (Massey-Westropp et al 2000, Tetro et al 1998). A sensory evaluation (Breger 1987, Gellman et al 1986), the differential Tinel's percussion test over the nerve, can help isolate the compression site (Tinel 1915). Quantifying symptoms using the symptoms severity scale (Levine et al 1993) is also suggested. The judicious use of nerve and muscle electrodiagnostic studies that can clarify the location and extent of the injury are often helpful. Surgical decompression of the nerve is reserved for cases resistant to conservative care or in instances when nerve compression has led to muscle atrophy.

Conservative treatment (Table 19.1) involves techniques to reduce compression of the median nerve within the carpal tunnel. These interventions include splinting the wrist in neutral (Fig. 19.9) (Burke et al 1994, Kuo et al 2001, Walker et al 2000, Weiss et al 1995) and avoiding sustained pressure on the palm (Cobb et al 1995) and/or sustained grip activities (Seradge et al 1995). Nerve and tendon gliding exercises (Fig. 19.14) have also been suggested (Rozmaryn et al 1998). Additionally, ultrasound has been found to be an effective treatment modality for mild to moderate cases of CTS (Ebenbichler et al 1998). If conservative treatment fails or if there is atrophy of the thenar intrinsic muscles, then surgical release of the transverse carpal ligament is indicated.

Following surgery, grip and pinch strengths will be diminished, sometimes for up to 6 months. There will often be pillar (Ludlow et al 1997) and/or scar tenderness limiting the ability to bear weight on the palm for a number of weeks. Postoperative therapy may assist the individual to return to activity sooner than without therapy (Provinciali et al 2000). General guidelines for postoperative care include: tendon and nerve gliding exercises (Wehbe & Hunter 1985), and strengthening of grip and pinch beginning at about 4 weeks (Maser et al 2001).

Ulnar wrist pain and impairment

Fractures

Any fracture of the distal radius or ulna can compromise the DRUJ, limit ROM and/or produce instability in the distal forearm joint, especially if it is intra-articular in nature and/or has resulted in a malunion. Even what appears to be a benign ulnar styloid fracture can cause instability or wrist/forearm stiffness. An uncommon, yet debilitating sport-related fracture is to the hook of the hamate. Typically, ulnar wrist pain localized to the hook of the hamate after a forceful swing, either with a bat or golf club, is the mechanism of injury.

If stiffness is the primary problem then the clinician must be ensured that a bony abnormality is not blocking motion. This can be done using imaging studies as a primary resource and supplementing that clinically with the type of end feel that is present at the joints end range; which is either soft or hard indicating the absence or presence of an osseous limitation respectively. If soft tissue structural changes are causing stiffness then appropriate treatments for joint stiffness should be used as described in Fig. 19.7 and Table 19.1. A bevy of splints and end-range positioning devices are now available to help restore forearm rotation (Jaffe et al 1996, Lee et al 2003, Schultz-Johnson 1996).

Distal radioulnar joint instability

If DRUJ/TFCC instability and pain are the main concerns, due either to a lack of bony support from the DRUJ (an ulnar styloid non-union with or without a torn TFCC), or an isolated TFCC (dorsal radial ulnar ligament or palmar ulnar ligament

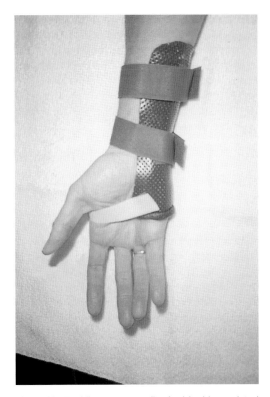

Figure 19.15 • Ulnar gutter splint for blocking wrist ulnar deviation and partially limiting wrist flexion and extension.

Table 19.5 Postoperative management guidelines after TFCC surgery (repair and debridement)

	Factors affecting recovery: de Quervain's
Acute versus chronic	*Acute:* typically resolved with complete rest, avoidance of thumb adduction and wrist ulnar deviation, and judicious use of NSAIDs *Chronic:* often complete rest is not a panacea Gentle (non-painful) wrist ROM, modalities, intermittent splinting/taping, and biomechanical/ergonomic education is required
Concomitant lesions	Irritation to the radial sensory nerve, 1st CMC joint or the intersection region delay recovery. Fortunately, the avoidance of thumb adduction and ulnar deviation will facilitate healing of all of these lesions
Conservative versus operative	The prognosis for conservative treatment is good if symptoms resolve within 1–2 weeks. The surgical prognosis is good if all septations are released, the tendons are painlessly mobilized postoperatively and there are no concomitant lesions.

NSAID = non-steroidal anti-inflammatory drug

specifically) tear, a supportive splint or cast is necessary. DRUJ/TFCC instability can cause central (± ulnar) pain. To test the stability of the DRUJ, and concomitantly the supportive function of the TFCC, one can use a simple volar/dorsal translation provocative maneuver (Table 19.3).

The DRUJ/TFCC stabilizing options can include circumferential taping around the wrist/DRUJ, a simple ulnar gutter (Fig. 19.15) or a long arm splint (Fig. 19.12) (Jaffe et al 1996). The taping and ulnar gutter splint does not prevent forearm rotation, but often provides enough support for palliative relief. If the ulnar gutter is not therapeutic then segueing to a long arm splint is necessary (Jaffe et al 1996). For restricting forearm rotation a long arm splint, which crosses the wrist as well as the elbow joint, can be fashioned to allow flexion and extension of the elbow while preventing supination and pronation. Adequate protection (limited forearm rotation) for 6–8 weeks is necessary. If stability of the DRUJ is not restored with conservative treatment then surgical repair of the torn structures is necessary. Table 19.5 describes the postoperative management.

Degenerative disorders

An ulnar-based site of DJD is between the sesamoid pisiform bone and the triquetrum at the base of the hypothenar eminence. Although most commonly seen in the elderly, any individual can have volar ulnar pain if there is a history of direct injury to the pisiform. Typically, there is a complaint of pain when pressure is exerted on the pisiform, as in resting the hand on a table when writing, or gripping a racket, bat or club handle. A grinding type of provocative maneuver (Table 19.3) is typically positive when this DJD is present.

The splinting options here should include a pad interface between an ulnar gutter splint (Fig. 19.15) and the pisiform. This pad is shaped like a doughnut, so as to prevent compressive forces across the joint when laying the hands on a hard surface.

Articular disk of the triangular fibrocartilage tear

Isolated tears in the articular disk will not typically result in instability of the DRUJ or the ulnar carpal structures of the TFCC. They do, however, often cause clicking, and ulnar-sided wrist pain, which is worsened with gripping and forearm pronation. The articular disk shear test and gripping rotatory impaction test (GRIT) can help identify articular disk lesions (Table 19.3). Ulnar impaction syndrome, secondary to a positive ulnar variance, can precipitate articular disk tears. The pain increases with ulnar deviation, being most profound with gripping and during forearm pronation (due to maximal potential for a positive ulnar variance).

During axial loading (gripping), the radiocarpal joint transmits 80% of the force through the radial aspect of the wrist and forearm while the ulna, through its articulation with the ulnar carpus and the TFCC, carries 20% of the load (Palmer 1993). With malunited distal radius fractures and DRUJ incongruity, loads through the radius and ulna shift, and can exceed physiological limits (Palmer & Werner 1984). Ulnar variance can also affect this force distribution markedly. Ulnar positive variance increases ulnar-sided forces and, conversely, ulnar negative variance increases radial-sided forces (hence it also decreases forces transmitted through the ulnar side) (Palmer & Werner 1984). Ulnar variance changes in a positive direction with forearm pronation and gripping (Epner et al 1982, LaStayo & Weiss 2001, Palmer et al 1982). Gripping and pronating can adversely impact ulnar-sided structures such as the TFCC, lunate and LT ligament, and may be a source of pain during such maneuvers as a tennis serve, swinging a bat or any sports requiring gripping in a pronated position. Athletes with a positive or neutral ulnar variance are therefore more prone to TFCC injury either due to acute injury or attritional changes secondary to chronic repetitive loading (Dailey & Palmer 2000).

Traumatic or degenerative tears within the centrally located avascular articular disk region cause pain which is often recalcitrant, having very minimal to no potential for healing. Radially based tears, however, have some vascularity and are surgically repairable (Cooney 1998). Wrist arthroscopy has been recommended for a variety of TFCC tears and is often a viable choice for athletes as it allows earlier initiation of rehabilitation and return to sports participation (Dailey & Palmer 2000). Table 19.5 outlines the postoperative care following debridement or repair of articular disk tears.

Nonsurgical management options include taping (Fig. 19.11) for sport activities, an ulnar gutter splint (Fig. 19.15) and education which emphasizes avoiding functional activities that require forearm pronation and gripping. This education is most effectively imprinted when one gets patients to reproduce their pain by having them grip with simultaneous movement into forearm pronation. If the patient is having problems modifying this painful behavior, and/or the pain is not improving with the static ulnar gutter splint, then forearm pronation must be limited with a long arm splint (Fig. 19.12). If the clinician feels that strengthening is appropriate, i.e. grip strength, then care must be taken to progress the resistive gripping program from a supinated position, to a neutral forearm position and then finally into pronation if there is no pain.

Instability

Mid-carpal row instability is a non-dissociative type of carpal instability, classified as carpal instability non-dissociative (CIND) and is typically difficult to diagnose, as static imaging studies are often unremarkable. The typical patient has a ligamentous laxity at the wrist and other joints. Typically, this instability is noticed first on clinical examination and then confirmed with cineradiography. If excessive laxity is noted, the tests for dissociative conditions within the proximal row (i.e. the scaphoid shift and ballotement tests for SL and LT tears respectively) may produce false positives. Perhaps the most notable clinical characteristic of mid-carpal instability is the abrupt carpal shift that occurs with ulnar deviation during the catch-up clunk test (Table 19.3) (Lichtman et al 1981). Since gripping and deviation of the wrist are common in sport activities, taping (Fig. 19.11) is essential during training or competition. A special pad addition to the wrist splint, along the pisiform for boosting it dorsally, is helpful in reducing the painful clunk.

The ECU tendon can also be the source of ulnar sided pain as it is apt to move about in its groove in the ulna if the 6th dorsal extensor compartment of the wrist can no longer stabilize it. The ECU subluxation test (Table 19.3) amplifies this instability. Visible or palpable subluxation of the ECU with this maneuver indicates instability. Attempts have been made with wrist cuffs and/or wrist circumferential taping to stabilize the ECU in a conservative manner, but often the tendon still exhibits excessive motion with ulnar deviation. Consequently, preventing ulnar deviation with an ulnar gutter splint (Fig. 19.15) is often effective. If this is unsuccessful then, a surgical procedure for stabilization of the ECU tendon is performed.

Tendonitis

Irritation or inflammation (tendonitis) of the flexor carpi ulnaris (FCU) and ECU tendons is thought to contribute to ulnar wrist pain. ECU tendonitis is particularly common, second to only de Quervain's tendonitis in frequency in the athlete (Rettig 2004). This diagnosis should be based on findings of swelling and crepitus over the tendons and pain with manual isometric resistance of wrist flexion/ ulnar deviation (for FCU) and wrist extension/ ulnar deviation for (ECU). The selective tensioning of musculotendinous tissue via isometric resistance should be accompanied by active and passive ROM testing in the assessment format put forth by Cyriax (1982). These lesions, however, may present themselves only as a result of some other primary lesion. A classic example is an ECU tendonitis resulting from a subtle ECU instability. Unfortunately, if the primary lesion is not addressed, often the secondary tendonitis remains recalcitrant. Splinting or taping (Fig. 19.11), in the form of an ulnar gutter (Fig. 19.15), for the FCU and ECU problems can often be helpful in both classic tendonitis and/or tendon instability. Modalities that address inflammation when present are often helpful, but heat also can be comforting when tenosynovitis is the culprit. Additionally, taping/splinting to rest the tendon and, ultimately, eccentric exercise after the tendon has healed, are appropriate (Table 19.1).

Nerve compression

Compression of the ulnar nerve can cause an aching pain and paresthesias on the ulnar side of the hand; however, it more often occurs when the lesion is at the level of the wrist than the elbow. It is important then to rule out compression of the ulnar nerve in the cubital tunnel at the elbow, which is a commonly occurring entrapment neuropathy. Ulnar nerve compression at the wrist can occur with prolonged weightbearing activities, such as bicycling without adequate palmar padding or when the straps to the bike gloves are fastened too tightly during a long ride. When ulnar nerve compression at the wrist is causing the ulnar wrist pain then the use of a wrist control splint (Fig. 19.9) with a protective pad over the hypothenar eminence is the first option in the conservative care. If the clinician is interested in using any nerve mobilization to treat this lesion, care must be taken to avoid straining the nerve. Unfortunately, compression of the nerve in Guyon's canal may not be detected until there is intrinsic muscle atrophy. The option for intervention then is surgical, with the postoperative course including nerve gliding exercise and avoidance of pressure over the thenar eminence.

Management of finger and thumb joint and skeletal injuries

Joint injuries and fractures of the hand are commonly seen as a result of sports activities. Some supposed 'simple' injuries of the hand, such as PIP joint sprains, may not be taken seriously by the initial treating practitioner, and consequently are not treated accurately or aggressively. This can lead to stiffness, deformity and disability. The care of a fracture of the hand includes fracture reduction, immobilization so the fracture fragment(s) can heal, and subsequent mobilization and strengthening to regain function. The clinician must know when it is safe to mobilize the hand and how to protect the hand, when necessary, during sports activities.

Ulnar collateral ligament injuries – thumb metacarpophalangeal joint

During pinch activities, stability of the MCP joint of the thumb is critical. The UCL, dorsal joint capsule and volar plate, in conjunction with the adductor pollicus aponeurosis, stabilize the ulnar side of that joint (Minami et al 1985). When the thumb is torqued into an abducted or valgus position, such as can occur when falling forward with the hand gripping a 'planted' ski pole, damage can occur to the UCL of the thumb MCP joint. The magnitude of the force will determine the extent of the injury.

A mild valgus force can cause a grade I sprain and a severe force can tear the ligament completely, resulting in a grade III sprain. A grade II is intermediary (Wright & Rettig 1995). When the UCL is completely torn, the proximal ligament stump may get 'stuck' under the adductor pollicus muscle's aponeurosis, creating the so-called Stener's lesion (Stener 1962). In this case, surgical intervention is required to remove the aponeurosis from between the two ends of the UCL.

Grade I and II thumb MCP UCL injuries

The MCP joint is frequently swollen, tender and painful to valgus stress. The initial treatment consists of rest, ice, compression and elevation. Grade I or mild sprains can be treated with early mobilization and a thermoplastic splint (Figs 19.8 and 19.10) for pain control. When a partial tear of the ligament is suspected (grade II) a thumb spica cast, with the interphalangeal joint left free, is worn for 4–5 weeks (Wright & Rettig 1995). Some physicians will manage this injury with a forearm or hand based cast or thermoplastic removable splint (Fig. 19.10), rather than a thumb spica cast that crosses the wrist.

After cast immobilization is concluded, a removable splint is fabricated (Figs 19.8 and 19.10) and gradual mobilization is started. Progression of exercise is from active MCP flexion and extension to active abduction/adduction and opposition. Pain

can be used as a guideline for progressing exercise. High-load brief stressors (HLBS) via joint mobilization, using high-grade (III or IV) volar glide of the proximal phalanx on the metacarpal, followed by passive flexion via a manual stretch, can be used to restore flexion of the MCP joint. With resistant flexion limitations, a low-load prolonged stress (LLPS) program with a progressive static flexion splint may be necessary (Table 19.1). A volar glide mobilization of the distal phalanx on the proximal phalanx can be performed for gaining IP flexion. The goal for flexion is to match the uninjured side. Side-to-side comparison is essential due to the wide variability in thumb MP range of motion, from about 25° to 70° (Bostock & Morrie 1993).

Strengthening activities, such as grip and lateral pinch, are instituted at approximately 4 weeks for grade I injuries and 6 weeks for grade II injuries. Activities that stress the thumb in an abducted and opposed position, for example, tip pinch, should be avoided for up to 8 weeks after injury (Brody 1999). Specialized foam or rubber playing casts are also options that can be explored (Wright & Rettig 1995).

Grade III or complete UCL tears

Complete tears require surgery to repair or reconstruct the ligament and adductor aponeurosis. With a grade III injury, a Stener's lesion may exist (Stener 1962). Following surgery, the MCP joint is immobilized for 4 weeks in a thumb spica cast (Zeiman et al 1998). The principles for management during this phase are the same as with the nonoperative case. Because surgery has been performed, there may be more swelling of the hand and more of a necessity for patient education than in the nonoperative case. A general schema for management guidelines during recovery after a repair or reconstruction of the UCL is outlined in Table 19.6. Losses of ROM of the MCP after surgery can be about 20% (Mitsionis et al 2000) to 30% (Downey et al 1995). Grip and pinch strengths usually are between 90 and 100% of the uninjured side (Downey et al 1995, Melone et al 2000).

Proximal interphalangeal joint sprain and dislocation

Common consequences of 'jamming' or hyperextending the finger during activities like volleyball and basketball include proximal interphalangeal joint dislocations and sprains, or disruption of the digital extensor tendon (the central slip and/or the terminal tendon), leading to a boutonnière or mallet finger deformity respectively. Good emergent care and regular follow-up of these injuries is necessary to prevent flexion contractures, in the case of the proximal interphalangeal (PIP) injury, and loss of active terminal finger extension in the case of an extensor tendon injury. With these injuries, regaining joint extension is more challenging than regaining flexion. Injuries of the PIP joint always result in edema and stiffness of that joint. Therapy is implemented to minimize these problems, maximize motion and protect the healing structures about the joint. Overzealous treatment can contribute to prolonged swelling, a flexion deformity and disability. Edema control should be emphasized and implemented

Table 19.6 General schema of rehabilitation after repair or reconstruction of the thumb metacarpophalangeal (MCP) ulnar collateral ligament (UCL)

	Protective phase	Motion phase	Strength and function phase
Timeframe	Weeks 0–3	Weeks 3–6	Weeks 6–10
Goals	Prevent loss of motion of fingers and thumb IP Control digital swelling	Restore thumb MCP flexion	By discharge should have use of thumb for pinch and torque activities (e.g. using tools, opening jars)
Techniques	Instruction in elevation AROM of thumb IP and all joints of four fingers Prevent adherent and sensitive scar	AROM and PROM of MCP and IP P–A and A–P glides to restore MCP flexion and extension. If regaining flexion is difficult, splinting can be used. Scar massage. Silicone mold over scar. Desensitization techniques if scar hypersensitive	Pinch and grip strengthening activities
Precautions	If a thermoplastic splint is used, education of patient about risks of removing splint Must protect repair/reconstruction	Avoid radially directed torque to the MCP joint (resisted adduction forced abduction, or resisted opposition)	

P–A = posterior to anterior glide (joint mobilization); A–P = anterior to posterior glide (joint mobilization)

by string wrapping and retrograde massage (Flowers 1988) with compression wraps of the digit used between therapy sessions.

The management of PIP joint injuries varies with the diagnosis and the stability of the joint. Dorsal dislocations or subluxations are most common and require anatomical reduction. Most PIP joint dislocations are stable and will not redislocate during active motion. These injuries can be treated by a brief period of splinting (3–5 days) and early motion. In contrast, injuries that are not aligned, and that are unstable after closed reduction, require physical blocks to full PIP extension and longer protection (2–3 weeks).

If the PIP joint is stable (i.e. without evidence of dorsal subluxation or medial or lateral deformity) it may be protected by buddy strapping the injured finger to the adjacent finger, or by immobilization for 3 to 5 days in full extension. The goals of therapy are to maintain gliding of the tendons that cross the PIP joint and prevent a PIP flexion contracture. If the injured finger is 'buddy' strapped to the adjacent finger, active range of motion exercises of the PIP and DIP joints should be implemented to reduce the likelihood of adhering tendons, collateral ligaments and the proximal portion of the volar plate. In addition, exercises should include DIP flexion and extension with the PIP joint blocked in extension (Fig. 19.16). This is done to promote volar and distal glide of the lateral bands and to prevent adherence of the oblique retinacular ligament. If the PIP joint is immobilized in a splint, the DIP joint is left free for range of motion exercises. Full DIP motion should be encouraged to maximize tendon gliding of the FDP and lateral bands of the extensor mechanism. It may be necessary to splint the PIP joint in full available extension at night to reduce the likelihood of a flexion deformity secondary to joint effusion.

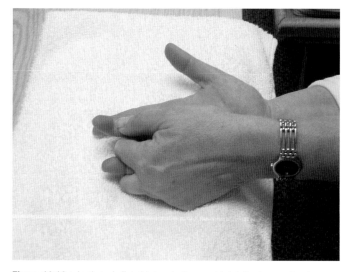

Figure 19.16 • Isolated distal interphalangeal joint flexion and extension with blocking of PIP motion.

A general schema of rehabilitation after a PIP joint injury is outlined in Table 19.7.

If the PIP joint has been immobilized, it is likely to be stiff. Therapy should emphasize regaining flexion while preventing a flexion contracture. PIP flexion contractures which are not fixed (i.e. not resistant to stress) may respond to a period of LLPS. LLPS techniques utilizing progressive static splinting, such as serial casting, can be effective in reducing flexion contractures (Table 19.1) (Flowers & LaStayo 1994). An additional advantage of serial casting is the circumferential pressure

Table 19.7 General schema of rehabilitation after PIP joint injury

	Protective phase	Motion phase	Strength and function phase
Time frame	0 to 2–3 weeks	3 to 6 weeks	6 to 10 weeks
Goals	Control digit edema Promote flexor and extensor tendons excursions	Restore active and passive PIP flexion and extension Prevent or reduce a PIP flexion contracture	Restore functional grip strength
Techniques	Compression wraps Buddy strap injured finger to uninjured Splint PIP joint in full extension at night	AROM, PROM PIP joint PIP flexion contracture should be aggressively managed using a low load prolonged stress (serial cast)	Putty exercise Graded hand held grippers
Precautions	Monitor for extension lag	Increased PIP joint swelling indicates that the vigor of exercise may be excessive; adjust exercise accordingly	

Note: in the case of an unstable injury where surgery is required, the protective phase is extended and limits on motion are more stringent

to control and reduce edema. If this treatment is successful, gains of 5° to 10° per week can be expected. When the flexion contracture is less than 20°, dynamic splinting via spring-wire splints can be used intermittently during the day to promote extension. At that point the patient can also work on regaining PIP flexion through passive flexion strapping and light resisted grip exercises. The balance between regaining full flexion and extension can be challenging. Even though full motion would be ideal, the goal should be at least 90° to 95° of flexion at the PIP joint. An extension deficit of 10° to 15° is an acceptable outcome for most functional activities. Surgical release of a chronic unremitting flexion contracture may be needed to optimize function (Abbiati et al 1995).

Strengthening exercises can begin 4–6 weeks after injury, when swelling and pain are controlled. An additional increase in flexion may occur with grip strengthening exercises due to high forces transmitted through the flexor tendons by the extrinsic flexor muscles, which have a relatively greater cross-sectional area than the extensors. The therapy program during this phase should include sport-specific grip activities to prepare for return to maximum function, e.g. impact activities like hammering nails into wood. If vibration, such as in batting or racket sports is an issue, a support wrap around the digit and buddy strapping can be used during activity until the joint can tolerate vibration and impact. While swelling may persist for months after this injury, return to full function can be expected within 8 to 10 weeks.

With severe disruption of the PIP joint, the joint may be unstable, and emergency care should emphasize restoration of joint stability. If an unstable fracture/dorsal dislocation has adequate joint contact, the goal is to maintain the reduction while allowing a safe ROM. Extension block (approximately 30°) splinting is used in these circumstances (Hamer & Quinton 1992). This technique maintains joint reduction within a safe range by limiting extension. The same principle can be applied to managing volar plate injuries. Immediate active motion (both flexion and extension) to encourage healing of periarticular

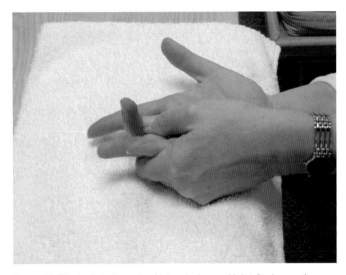

Figure 19.17 • Isolated proximal interphalangeal joint flexion and extension with blocking of MCP motion.

structures and promote good collagen alignment is permitted within the confines of the dorsal blocking splint.

When reduction cannot be maintained with extension block splinting, then a volar plate arthroplasty (Durham-Smith & McCarten 1992) may be indicated to restore the stability of the PIP joint by constructing a volar 'check-rein' to subluxation of the middle phalanx. The repair is protected using a short arm dorsal extension-blocking splint. Flexor tendon gliding exercises (Fig. 19.14) are important as there may be adhesions within the flexor tendon sheath after manipulation of the tendons in surgery. The exercises, performed within the confines of the extension block splint, can include flexion of the PIP with the MCP blocked in extension (Fig. 19.17) and flexion of the DIP with the PIP stabilized in extension (Fig. 19.16). This procedure is continued for 4 weeks, after which the extension block is removed. Therapeutic measures (Table 19.1; Fig. 19.7) for joint stiffness can then be instituted to regain extension. A PIP flexion or extension contracture is inevitable, but an anatomical reduction must be the goal.

Metacarpal fractures

The tendons of the flexors and extensors as well as the intrinsic (interossei and lumbrical) muscles are aligned by the position of the metacarpal bones. This close proximity and dependent relationship between the metacarpals and surrounding musculotendinous structures can produce deforming forces across the fracture site and adversely influence function.

Metacarpal fractures can be caused by a direct blow to the metacarpal or an indirect twisting force through the finger. As with other hand fractures, the soft tissue injury that occurred with the fracture will influence outcome and is often underestimated because the initial focus is often on the fracture. The treatment of the metacarpal fractures must provide a stable bony construct to allow early motion (Kozin et al 2000). Undisplaced and stable fractures are allowed to heal in a hand- or forearm-based splint. After the cast or brace is removed, gradual mobilization and exercise is encouraged. Specific hand motions include: a full fist, a claw fist into the intrinsic minus position (Fig. 19.18), and a table-top posture into the intrinsic plus position (Fig. 19.19); these are used to regain movement.

Irreducible fractures, open fractures, multiple fractures, fractures with bone loss and fractures associated with tendon laceration usually require surgery to restore stability to the metacarpal(s) and hand. Stable fixation, which is usually obtained with screw, or plate and screw, can be treated by early active range of motion as soon as the acute pain from surgery subsides. This is important to prevent contracture, disuse osteopenia and muscle atrophy. A dorsal surgical approach can limit extensor tendon gliding. Active and active assisted motion of the fingers and wrist promotes tendon gliding, primarily of the extensor tendons, and limits adhesion formation. An extension assist splint may be useful in providing resistance during flexion to promote tendon gliding. Selective gliding of the extensor digitorum tendons can be done by actively extending the MCP joints while the PIP and DIP joints are held in flexion: the hook fist. Scar management techniques can include a silicone mold worn over the scar, and vibration, scar massage and gentle suction over the scar.

Passive motion should be limited until bony union is apparent, as aggressive movement can disrupt the fracture fixation. A splint is used between exercise sessions and is necessary to rest the hand, protect the healing fracture and prevent contracture. The therapy goals are to maintain MCP flexion while minimizing PIP flexion contractures. The splint should be made to position the MCP joint in flexion and the interphalangeal joints in extension (Fig. 19.19). When more vigorous attempts to regain flexion are permitted (and this is guided by evidence of fracture consolidation), buddy strapping of the injured digit to the adjacent digit can be used. The uninjured digit, which presumably has more flexion will drag the other finger along with it into flexion.

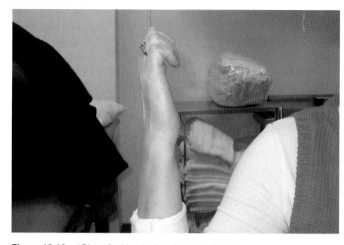

Figure 19.18 • 'Claw fist' intrinsic minus position.

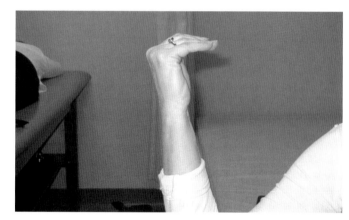

Figure 19.19 • 'Table-top' intrinsic plus position.

Phalangeal fractures

Extra-articular distal phalangeal fractures (i.e. tuft fractures) are usually the result of a crush injury and have a concomitant nail bed laceration. These fractures are treated with splint immobilization until fracture union. Pain and limited function following this injury are seldom from the fracture and more likely to be from the nail bed injury. Therapy is warranted if the magnitude of sensitivity causes the patient to guard the use of the hand. In this case, therapy is done using progressive exercises for functional use of the hand for prehension and precision activities. In contrast, proximal and middle phalangeal fractures are more problematic and can result in hand impairment due to the likelihood of PIP flexion contractures and limited tendon gliding (see Fig. 19.14 for tendon gliding exercises) due to scar.

Stable phalangeal fractures are either not displaced or stable after closed reduction. A nondisplaced fracture can be treated by immobilization for a few days until the swelling subsides and then with protected motion (using buddy taping) until union. The hand is immobilized in the 'safe position' with MCP flexion

Table 19.8 General schema of rehabilitation after unstable hand fractures treated by surgical intervention

	Protective phase	Motion phase	Strength and function phase
Timeframe	A few days for fractures with rigid fixation Up to a few weeks for fracture less rigid fixation (e.g. k-wire) Consult with physician regarding timing of motion	3–5 days to 6 weeks following rigid fixation 3 (or more) to 6 weeks for less rigid fixation	6 weeks and onward May be delayed if complications such as delayed union of fracture
Goals	Edema control Motion of uninvolved joints	Promote maximum joint motion Prevent flexion contractures Promote tendon gliding	Promote maximum grip and pinch strength Sports-specific functional training
Techniques	Elevation String wrap and retrograde massage Compressive wraps Protective padding and/or splinting if physician allows sports participation	Active and active assisted ROM Tendon gliding exercises Joint mobilization if fracture consolidated May need protective padding	Putty and hand held grippers Closed chain grip and torque activities Upper body strengthening and conditioning Functional activities to match sports-specific requirements
Precautions	Avoid undue stresses across fracture site Reduce motion exercises if edema persists for more than 2 h following exercise	Avoid undue passive joint motion or joint loading if articular surfaces are damaged; motion goals will be reduced Monitor for complications	Delay introduction of activities if pain increases

and IP extension (Fig. 19.19) to prevent contracture. Since the interossei muscles traverse volar to the MCP joint, this position also relaxes the interossei, which can act as deforming forces in phalangeal fractures. Protected motion, where the fractured digit is buddy taped to the adjacent digit, should be used continuously for 4–6 weeks until union occurs, to promote tendon gliding. Clinical fracture union is indicated by lack of tenderness at the fracture site and will precede radiographic union (bony bridging across fracture site). This can create confusion as an X-ray report may still indicate a visible fracture line despite clinical union. At this point, strengthening and resistive exercises can be initiated as the strength across the fracture site can withstand these forces.

Unstable, displaced fractures are managed surgically by closed reduction and percutaneous pinning or open reduction and internal fixation using compression screws, interosseous wiring, screws or mini-plate and screws (Oulette & Freeland 1996). There is a greater propensity for adhesions and loss of tendon gliding in phalangeal fractures in comparison to metacarpal fractures due to the intimate proximity of the dorsal extensor hood. Therefore, a fixation that allows early motion is preferred, to diminish the consequences of immobilization.

To plan an exercise program, the therapist must know the status of the fixed fracture. Stable rigid fixation can be treated by early range of motion to encourage tendon gliding and to prevent contracture and atrophy (Oulette & Freeland 1996). Nonrigid fixation, however, must be protected. Static splinting is necessary between exercise sessions to rest the injured digit(s) and to prevent surrounding joint contracture. This early motion regimen, in rigidly fixed fractures, is usually instituted 3–7 days after surgery and requires careful supervision.

Active and active assisted motion exercises are utilized until union. MCP, PIP (Fig. 19.19) and DIP (Fig. 19.16) blocking exercises with appropriate support are used. Passive motion can be started after fracture union, usually at about 4–6 weeks. This should be verified with the patient's physician who performed the fracture reduction. HLBS joint mobilization (Table 19.1) to restore both flexion and extension are then cautiously instituted. LLPS-like activities (Table 19.1; Fig. 19.7) such as strapping of the fractured digit into flexion or the use of a progressive static splint may be needed to regain flexion. Potential complications following hand fractures include: scarring of the soft tissues in the skin, around tendons or in joint capsules leading to stiffness; and malunion, which is typically characterized by malrotation, angulation or shortening (Page & Stern 1998). Nerve or artery injuries can result from the initial trauma or be iatrogenic (from surgery). Sensory nerves along the dorsum of the hand are particularly prone to neuroma formation. Complex regional pain syndrome type I or II (reflex sympathetic dystrophy) may also occur. The general schema of rehabilitation after unstable digit or metacarpal fractures is described in Table 19.8.

Management of finger tendon injuries

Flexor tendons

Active finger flexion is necessary to perform many tasks including manipulation of small objects and grasping around objects. The long flexors of the digits are integral in performing these tasks. Following a laceration of a flexor tendon, the desirable outcome after intervention is to flex the finger to touch the palm. Surgical

Table 19.9 Techniques used during protective phase after flexor tendon repair

	Immobilization	Passive flexion/passive extension[a]	Passive flexion/active extension[b]	Early active (or short arc motion) [c]
Candidates	Children Unreliable adult	Reliable adult	Reliable adult	Minimum: 4-strand epitenon
Splint	Wrist: 30–40° flexion Digit(s): MCP 50–60° flexion IPs extended	Same MCP: same Rubber band traction to flex IPs or straps over IPs removed for exercise	Same MCP: same Rubber band traction to flex IPs	Same MCP: same Rubber band traction to flex MCPs
Exercises	Maintain motion of non-immobilized joints	Passively flex finger joints Passively extend finger joints within confines of splint		

[a] Duran & Houser (1975); [b] Kleinert et al (1973); [c] Silverskold & May (1994)

repair and subsequent postoperative management are designed to restore anatomy as closely as possible and to facilitate healing and maximum gliding of the tendon within its tendon sheath. There must be a balance of sufficient scar at the repair site to maximize tensile strength, yet avoidance of excessive scar within the tendon sheath, to maximize tendon gliding.

Unlike some other areas of rehabilitation, much valuable information on rehabilitation following flexor tendon repair exists (Evans 1989, Pettengill 2005). The quantity of basic science and clinical research addressing flexor tendon management parallels or exceeds that of injuries to the ACL of the knee. Studies have addressed healing in animal models, tensile strengths with various suturing techniques, techniques of protection (i.e. splinting after tendon repair) and methods of exercise, which are outlined in Table 19.9 (Chow et al 1988, Duran & Houser 1975, Kleinert et al 1973, May et al 1992).

Flexor tendon injuries usually occur by a laceration that directly cuts the tendon(s). The treatment of the lacerated flexor tendon(s) is by direct repair. The ultimate goal of the suture method is to allow earlier active motion which will often decrease adhesion formation and optimize functional outcome. Closed rupture of the flexor tendons is less common than open lacerations. The FDP can rupture distally with an extension force against a flexed DIP joint. This occurs often in football as the flexed digit (most commonly in the ring finger) is holding onto the jersey and is quickly extended during an attempted tackle. This injury has been termed the rugger or football jersey injury. The jersey injury involves rupture or avulsion of the FDP tendon from its bony insertion and occurs most commonly in the ring finger (Stamos & Leddy 2000). Often a fragment of the distal phalanx will avulse. A recovery period of 12 weeks is necessary for maximizing the strength of the repair (in the case of ruptured tendon) or good bony consolidation (in the case of avulsion with bony fragment).

Closed ruptures are treated by early repair of the avulsed FDP tendon to its insertion at the base of the distal phalanx. In order to protect the repaired tendon from rupture or attenuation (gapping) at the repair site, the hand and wrist are immobilized in flexion in the operating room. Within 2–5 days after surgery, the surgical dressings and posterior cast shell are removed and replaced by a thermoplastic molded splint. Postoperative splint application and immobilization depends upon the rehabilitation method selected, strength of the suture technique and magnitude of associated injuries.

The general schema of rehabilitation is outlined in Table 19.10. During the first few days after surgery, intervention is directed toward pain and edema control, fabrication and application of a thermoplastic splint and initiating motion. Early postoperative management during the protective phase varies from complete immobilization for 3 weeks to early active motion in flexion and progressing to more vigorous blocked tendon exercises (Figs 19.16 and 19.17) and tendon gliding exercises (Fig. 19.14). The greatest variations in treatment techniques occur during the first 3 weeks following repair.

Extensor tendons

In sports, closed injuries to extensor tendons can commonly occur. A direct blow to the tip of the finger can often cause a tearing/avulsion of the terminal extensor tendon or the central slip. The respective mallet finger (DIP) or boutonnière deformity (PIP) is treated with static extension splinting for 6 weeks, with the uninjured IP joint free. This is followed by motion (active motion initially) exercises to restore finger flexion. A night splint to hold the respective IP joint fully extended is worn for 6 more weeks (Newport 1997). Problems in recovery include an extension lag of the joint. If a lag occurs, further extension splinting, coupled with resistance extensor tendon gliding exercises are indicated.

Overall, extensor tendon injuries in the hand are easier to surgically repair than their synovially bathed flexor antagonists. Hence, longer periods of protection and immobilization are

Table 19.10 General schema of rehabilitation following flexor tendon repair in the digits

	Protective phase	**Motion phase**	**Strength and function phase**
Timeframe	0 to 3 (or 4) weeks	3 weeks (or longer) to 8 weeks	8 weeks through 12 weeks
Goals	Prevent tendon rupture Restore full passive digital flexion Prevent PIP flexion contracture Control edema	Restore active flexion Reduce flexion contractures if present Protect against tendon rupture	Promote tendon glide if active insufficiency of digit flexion is occurring
Techniques	Splint wrist/hand to protect repair Splint PIP in extension at night Digit compression wrap/elevation Protected motion	Use a wristlet with rubber band traction for digits to protect from grabbing and lifting objects	Putty Free weights Progress to functional activities
Precautions	No simultaneous wrist and digit extension	If tendon gliding is freely occurring protect longer If tendon is adhered, motion attempts can be more vigorous	No more than 5 lb grip force until about 10 weeks

needed which can often result in tendon adherence and some residual active extension deficit (Newport 1997).

Less common sport-related injuries of the wrist and hand

Osteochondrosis – Kienbock's

The progressive collapse of the lunate, secondary to avascular necrosis can cause significant wrist impairment and disability. Although no single factor can be attributed to Kienbock's, it is likely that in the athletic population, repetitive compressive forces can cause cancellous fractures. This may be relevant in those with an ulnar minus variant, as axial forces are shifted predominately across the lunate and scaphoid, and those with an osseous vascular compromise (Gelberman et al 1975, 1983). However, other studies have shown that an ulnar minus variant is not a predisposing factor in the development of Kienbock's disease (D'Hoore et al 1994, Tsuge & Nakamura 1993). Immobilization in the early stages can rectify the impairment and disability, but later stages require surgical redistribution of forces across the radiocarpal joint with either an ulnar lengthening or radial shortening. Vascularized pedicle and/or bone grafting procedures may be performed for revascularization of the lunate (Allan et al 2001). A limited carpal fusion or salvage procedure like a proximal row carpectomy is also utilized if collapse of the carpus is advanced (Allan et al 2001, McCue & Bruce 1994). Postoperatively, the emphasis is on return of ROM and strength.

Vascular thrombosis

Thrombosis of the ulnar artery in Guyon's canal (also in a persistent median artery in the carpal tunnel) can occur following blunt and/or repetitive trauma to the palm (Costigan et al 1959). Thrombosis of the ulnar artery in Guyon's canal is termed hypothenar hammer syndrome (Conn et al 1970). Generally, the thrombosis can precipitate an acute neuropathy and a tender mass in the hypothenar area. Allen's test will be abnormal with poor filling through the ulnar artery. Doppler ultrasound and/or an arteriogram can help confirm the diagnosis. Although splinting of the wrist is helpful, the most widely accepted treatment is surgical resection. Vigorous activity is restricted for 6 weeks and the wrist is protected in sport for 3 months after surgery (McCue & Bruce 1994).

Mallet thumb

Disruption of the EPL insertion into the base of the distal phalanx, most often secondary to contact with a ball, can result in flexion deformity similar to that seen in the fingers. Splinting dorsally across the interphalangeal joint only in slight hyperextension for 6 weeks is often helpful, however, operative repair of the extensor tendon is more predictably effective if the tendon is lacerated or avulsed (Miura et al 1986).

Bennet's fracture

A Bennet's fracture is an avulsion of the ulnar volar aspect of the metacarpal base by an intact ulnar oblique ligament (Wilson & Hazen 1995). This injury can occur as the result of an adduction force on a partially flexed thumb such as a quarterback striking a helmet during a follow-through motion (Rettig 2004). Initiation of ROM exercises depends upon the type of fixation used and varies from five to 10 days after surgery with screw fixation, to four weeks with pin fixation (Rettig 2004). Nonthrowers typically return to athletic activities in two to three weeks, while quarterbacks are not able to return for six to 10 weeks (Rettig 2004).

Summary

Although injuries to the wrist and hand are not the most common injury type in sport and exercise, some sporting activities place participants at greater risk. Given the large number of structures in the wrist and hand, injuries can involve several joints and soft tissue structures. The examination of wrist and hand injuries is complex and involves many different joints. Fractures, instability, degenerative disorders, tendonitis and nerve injuries are the most common injuries found in this region.

References

Abbiati G, Delaria G, Saporiti E et al 1995 The treatment of chronic flexion contractures of the proximal interphalangeal joint. Journal of Hand Surgery (Br) 3B:385–389

Allan C H, Atul J, Lichtman D M 2001 Kienbock's disease: diagnosis and treatment. Journal of the American Academy of Orthopaedic Surgeons 9:128–136

Angelides A C 1999 Ganglions of the hand and wrist. In: Green D P, Hotchkiss R N, Pederson W C (eds) Operative hand surgery, 4th edn. Churchill Livingstone, New York, p 2171–2183

Arendt E A 1999 Orthopaedic knowledge update: sports medicine 2. American Academy of Othopaedic Surgeons, Rosemont, IL

Beckenbaugh R D 1984 Accurate evaluation and management of the painful wrist following injury. Orthopedic Clinics of North America 15:289–306

Berger R A, Dobyns J H 1996 Physical examination and provocative maneuvers of the wrist. In: Gilula L A, Yin Y (eds). Imaging of the wrist and hand. WB Saunders, Philadelphia, PA, p 5–22

Berger R A, Garcia-Elias M 1991 General anatomy of the wrist. In: An K N, Berger R A, Cooney W P (eds). Biomechanics of the wrist joint. Springer-Verlag, New York, p 1–22

Bishop A T, Reagan D S 1998 Lunotriquetral sprains. In: Cooney W P, Linscheid R L, Dobyns J H (eds) The wrist: diagnosis and operative treatment. Mosby, St Louis, MO, p 527–549

Bostock S, Morrie M A 1993 The range of motion of the MP joint of the thumb following operative repair of the ulnar collateral ligament. Journal of Hand Surgery (Br) 18B:710–711

Botte M J, Gelberman R H 1987 Fractures of the carpus, excluding the scaphoid. Hand Clinics 3:149–61

Brand P W, Hollister A 1993 Clinical mechanics of the hand. Mosby Year Book, St Louis, MO

Breger D 1987 Correlating Semmes-Weinstein monofilament mappings with sensory nerve conduction parameters in Hansen's disease patients: an update. Journal of Hand Therapy 1:33–37

Brody L T 1999 The elbow, forearm wrist and hand. In: Hall C M, Brody L T (eds). Therapeutic exercise: moving toward function. Lippincott Williams and Wilkins, Philadelphia, PA, p 626–665

Burke D T, McHale-Burke M, Stewart G W 1994 Splinting for carpal tunnel syndrome: in search of the optimal angle. Archives of Physical Medicine and Rehabilitation 75:1241–1244

Chidgey L K 1995 The distal radioulnar joint: problems and solutions. Journal of the American Academy of Orthopaedic Surgeons 3:105–109

Chow J A, Thomes L J, Dovell S 1988 Controlled motion rehabilitation after flexor tendon repair and grafting: a multi-centre study. Journal of Bone and Joint Surgery (Br) 70B:591–595

Cobb T K, An K-N, Cooney W P 1995 Externally applied forces to the palm increase carpal tunnel pressure. Journal of Hand Surgery (Am) 20A:181–185

Coleman S S, Anson B J 1961 Arterial patterns in the hand based upon a study of 650 specimens. Surgery, Gynecology and Obstretrics 113:409–424

Conn J, Bergan J, Bell J 1970 Hypothenar hammer syndrome: posttraumatic digital ischemia. Surgery 68:1122–128

Cooney W P 1998 Tears of the triangular fibrocartilage of the wrist. In: Cooney W P, Linscheid R L, Dobyns J H (eds) The wrist: diagnosis and operative treatment. Mosby, St Louis, MO, p 710–742

Cooney W P, Chao E Y S 1977 Biomechanical analysis of static forces in the thumb during hand function. Journal of Bone and Joint Surgery (Am) 59A:27

Cooney W P, Lucca M J, Chao E Y et al 1981 The kinesiology of the thumb trapeziometacarpal joint. Journal of Bone and Joint Surgery (Am) 63A:1371

Costigan D G, Riley J M, Coy F E 1959 Thrombofibrosis of the ulnar artery in the palm. Journal of Bone and Joint Surgery (Am) 41A:702–704

Cyriax J 1982 Textbook of orthopaedic medicine, vol I. The diagnosis of soft tissue lesions, 8th edn. Baillière-Tindall, London

Dailey S W, Palmer A K 2000 The role of arthroscopy in the evaluation and treatment of triangular fibrocartilage complex injuries in athletes. Hand Clinics 16:461–476

Dellon A L, Mackinnon S E 1986 Radial sensory nerve entrapment. Archives of Neurology 43:833–837

D'Hoore K, DeSmet L, Verellen K et al 1994 Negative ulnar variance is not a risk factor for Kienbock's disease. Journal of Hand Surgery (Am) 19A:229–231

Downey D J, Monheim M S, Omer G E 1995 Acute gamekeepers thumb. Quantitative outcome of surgical repair. American Journal of Sports Medicine 23:222–226

Duran R J, Houser R G 1975 Controlled passive motion following flexor tendon repair in Zones II and III. In: American Academy of Orthopaedic Surgeons symposium on tendon surgery of the hand. CV Mosby, St Louis, MO, p 73–92

Durham-Smith G, McCarten G M 1992 Volar plate arthroplasty for closed proximal interphalangeal joint injuries. Journal of Hand Surgery (Br) 14B:422–428

Eaton R G, Littler J W 1969 A study of the basal joint of the thumb. Treatment of its disabilities by fusion. Journal of Bone and Joint Surgery (Am) 51A:661–668

Ebenbichler G R, Resch K L, Nicolakis P et al 1998 Ultrasound treatment for treating the carpal tunnel syndrome: randomised 'sham' controlled trial. British Medical Journal 316:731–735

Epner R A, Bowers W H, Guilford W B 1982 Ulna variance: the effect of wrist positioning and roentgen filming technique. Journal of Hand Surgery (Br) 7B:298–305

Evans R 1989 Management of the healing tendon: what must we question? Journal of Hand Therapy 2:61–65

Finkelstein H 1930 Stenosing tenovaginitis at the radial styloid process. Journal of Bone and Joint Surgery 12:509–540

Flowers K R 1988 String wrapping versus massage for reducing digital volume. Physical Therapy 68:57–59

Flowers K R, LaStayo P C 1994 Effect of total end range time on improving passive range of motion. Journal of Hand Therapy 7:150–157

Freeland A E, Sennett B J 1996 Phalangeal fractures. In: Peimer C A (ed) Surgery of the hand and upper extremity, vol 1. McGraw Hill, New York, p 149–173

Gelberman R H, Salamon P B, Jurist J M 1975 Ulnar variance in Kienbock's disease. Journal of Bone and Joint Surgery (Am) 57A:674–676

Gelberman R H, Panagis J S, Taleisnik J et al 1983 The arterial anatomy of the human carpus. Journal of Hand Surgery (Am) 8A:367–375

Gellman H, Gelberman R H, Tan A M et al 1986 Carpal tunnel syndrome: an evaluation of the provocative diagnostic tests. Journal of Bone and Joint Surgery (Am) 68A:735–737

Gilula L A, Yin Y 1996 Imaging of the wrist and hand. WB Saunders, Philadelphia, PA

Hamer D W, Quinton D N 1992 Dorsal fracture subluxation of the distal interphalangeal joint of the finger and the interphalangeal joint of the thumb treated by extension block splintage. Journal of Hand Surgery (Br) 17B:591–594

Horii E, Garcia-Elias M, An K N et al 1991 A kinematic study of lunotriquetral dissociations. Journal of Hand Surgery (Am) 16A:355–362

Jaffe R, Chidgey L K, LaStayo P C 1996 The distal radioulnar joint: anatomy and management of disorders. Journal of Hand Therapy 9:129–138

Kaukonen J P, Karaharju E O, Porras M et al 1988 Functional recovery after fractures of the distal forearm. Analysis of radiographic and other factors affecting the outcome. Annales Chirurgiae et Gynaecologiae 77:27–31

Kazuki K, Kusunoki M, Yamada J et al 1993 Cineradiographic study of wrist motion after fracture of the distal radius. Journal of Hand Surgery (Am) 18A:41–46

Keon-Cohen B 1951 De Quervain's disease. Journal of Bone and Joint Surgery (Br) 33B:96–99

Kihara H, Short W H, Werner F W et al 1995 The stabilizing mechanisms of the distal radioulnar joint during supination and pronation. Journal of Hand Surgery (Am) 20A:930–936

Kirkpatrick W H 1990 De Quervain's disease. In: Hunter J M, Schneider L H, Mackin E J et al (eds) Rehabilitation of the hand: surgery and therapy. CV Mosby, St Louis, MO, p 433–478

Kleinert H E, Kutz J E, Atasoy E et al 1973 Primary repair of flexor tendons. Orthopedic Clinics of North America 4:865–876

Kleinert J M, Mehta S 1996 Radial nerve entrapment. Orthopedic Clinics of North America 27:305–315

Kozin S H, Thoder J T, Lieberman G 2000 Operative treatment of metacarpal and phalangeal shaft fractures. Journal of the American Academy of Orthopaedic Surgeons 8:111–121

Kuo M-H, Leong C-P, Cheng Y-F et al 2001 Static wrist position associated with least median nerve compression. American Journal of Physical Medicine and Rehabilitation 80:256–260

Laseter G F, Carter P R 1996 Management of distal radius fractures. Journal of Hand Therapy 9:114–128

LaStayo P C, Weiss S 2001 The GRIT: a quantitative measure of ulnar impaction syndrome. Journal of Hand Therapy 14:173–179

Lee M J, LaStayo P C, vonKersberg A E 2003 A supination splint worn distal to the elbow: a radiologic, electromyographic, and retrospective report. Journal of Hand Therapy 16:190–198

Levine D W, Simmons B P, Koris M J et al 1993 A self-administered questionnaire for the assessment of severity of symptoms and functional status in carpal tunnel syndrome. Journal of Bone and Joint Surgery (Am) 75A:1585–1592

Lichtman D M, Schneider J R, Swafford A R et al 1981 Ulnar midcarpal instability: clinical and laboratory analysis. Journal of Hand Surgery (Am) 6A:515–523

Ludlow K S, Merla J L, Cox J A et al 1997 Pillar pain as a postoperative complication of carpal tunnel release: a review of the literature. Journal of Hand Therapy 10:277–282

McClure P W, Blackburn L G, Dusold C 1994 The use of splints in the treatment of joint stiffness: biologic rationale and an algorithm for making clinical decisions. Physical Therapy 74:1101–1107

McCue F C, Bruce J F 1994 Hand and wrist. In: DeLee J C, Drez D (eds) Orthopaedic sport medicine: principles and practice. WB Saunders, Philadelphia, PA, p 102–147

McQueen M 1988 Colles fracture: does the anatomical result affect the final function? Journal of Bone and Joint Surgery (Br) 70B:649–651

Maser B M, Clark C M, Girard D 2001 Carpal tunnel syndrome: postoperative management. In: Maxey L, Magnusson J (eds) Rehabilitation for the postsurgical orthopedic patient. Mosby, St Louis, MO, p 157–203

Massey-Westropp N, Grimmer K I, Bain G 2000 A systematic review of the clinical diagnostic tests for carpal tunnel syndrome. Journal of Hand Surgery (Am) 25A:120–127

May E J, Silfverskiold K L, Sollerman C J 1992 Controlled mobilization after flexor tendon repair in zone II: a prospective comparison of three methods. Journal of Hand Surgery (Am) 17A:942–952

Mayfield J K 1981 Mechanisms of carpal injuries. Clinical Orthopaedics and Related Research 149:45–54

Melone C P, Beldner S, Basuk R S 2000 Thumb collateral ligament injuries: an anatomic basis for treatment. Hand Clinics 16:345–357

Minami A, An K-N, Cooney W P et al 1985 Ligament stability of the metacarpophalangeal joint: a biomechanical study. Journal of Hand Surger (Am) 10A:255–260

Mitsionis G I, Varitimidis S E, Sotereanos G G 2000 Treatment of chronic injuries of the ulnar collateral ligament of the thumb using a free tendon graft and bone suture anchors. Journal of Hand Surgery (Br) 25B:208–211

Miura T, Nakamura R, Torii S 1986 Conservative treatment for a ruptured extensor tendon on the dorsum of the proximal phalanges of the thumb (mallet thumb). Journal of Hand Surgery (Am) 11A:229–233

Newport M L 1997 Extensor tendon injuries in the hand. Journal of the American Academy of Orthopaedic Surgeons 5:59–66

Oulette E A, Freeland A E 1996 Use of the minicondylar plate in metacarpal and phalangeal fractures. Clinical Orthopaedics and Related Research 327:38–46

Page S M, Stern P J 1998 Complications and range of motion following plate fixation of metacarpal and phalangeal fractures. Journal of Hand Surgery (Am) 23A:827–832

Palmer A K 1993 Fractures of the distal radius. In: Green D P (ed) Operative hand surgery. Churchill Livingstone, New York, p 929–985

Palmer A K, Werner F W 1984 Biomechanics of the distal radioulnar joint. Clinical Orthopaedics and Related Research 187:26–35

Palmer A K, Glisson R R, Werner F W 1982 Ulnar variance determination. Journal of Hand Surgery (Am) 7A:376–379

Pellegrini V D Jr 1991 Osteoarthritis of the thumb trapeziometacarpal joint – a study of the pathophysiology of articular cartilage degeneration: I. Anatomy and pathology of the aging joint. Journal of Hand Surgery (Am) 16A:967–974

Pettengill K M 2005 The evolution of early mobilization of the repaired flexor tendon. Journal of Hand Therapy 18:157–168

Pratt N E 1996 Clinical musculoskeletal anatomy. JB Lippincott, Philadelphia, PA

Prosser R, Herbert T 1996 The management of carpal fractures and dislocations. Journal of Hand Therapy 9:139–147

Provinciali L, Giattini A, Splendiani G et al 2000 Usefulness of hand rehabilitation after carpal tunnel surgery. Muscle and Nerve 23:211–216

Rettig A C 2003 Athletic injuries of the wrist and hand: I. Traumatic injuries of the wrist. American Journal of Sports Medicine 31:1038–1048

Rettig A C 2004 Athletic injuries of the wrist and hand: II. Overuse injuries of the wrist and traumatic injuries to the hand. American Journal of Sports Medicine 32:262–273

Richards R S, Bennett J D, Roth J H et al 1997 Arthroscopic diagnosis of intra-articular soft tissue injuries associated with distal radius fractures. Journal of Hand Surgery (Am) 22A:772

Rosenthal E A 1990 The extensor tendons. In: Hunter J M, Schneider L H, Mackin E J et al (eds) Rehabilitation of the hand: surgery and therapy. CV Mosby, St Louis, MO, p 498–541

Rossi C, Cellocco P, Margaritondo E et al 2005 De Quervain disease in volleyball players. American Journal of Sports Medicine 33:424–427

Rozmaryn L M, Douvelle S, Rothman E R 1998 Nerve and tendon gliding exercises and the conservative management of carpal tunnel syndrome. Journal of Hand Therapy 11:171–179

Ruby L K, An K N, Linscheid R L et al 1987 The effects of scapholunate ligament section on scapholunate motion. Journal of Hand Surgery (Am) 12A:767–771

Rumball J S, Lebrun C M, DiCiacca S R et al 2005 Rowing injuries. Sports Medicine 35:537–555

Ryu J Y, Cooney W P 3rd, Askew L J et al 1991 Functional ranges of motion of the wrist joint. Journal of Hand Surgery (Am) 16A:409–419

Schultz-Johnson K 1996 Splinting the wrist: mobilization and protection. Journal of Hand Therapy 9:165–178

Seradge H, Jia Y-C, Owens W 1995 In vivo measurement of carpal tunnel pressure in the functioning hand. Journal of Hand Surgery (Am) 20A:855–859

Short W H, Palmer A K, Werner F W et al 1987 A biomechanical study of distal radial fractures. Journal of Hand Surgery (Am) 12A:523–534

Skirvin T 1996 Clinical examination of the wrist. Journal of Hand Therapy 9:96–107

Smith H E, Dirks M, Patterson R B 2004 Hypothenar hammer syndrome: distal ulnar artery reconstruction with autologous inferior epigastric artery. Journal of Vascular Surgery 40:1238–1242

Sotereanos D G, Levy J A, Herndon J H 1994 Hand and wrist injuries. In: Fu F H, Stone D A (eds) Sports injuries: mechanisms, prevention and treatment. Williams and Wilkins, Baltimore, MD, p 753–801

Stamos B D, Leddy J P 2000 Closed flexor tendon disruption in athletes. Hand Clinics 16:359–365

Stener B 1962 Displacement of the ruptured ulnar collateral ligament of the metacarpophalangeal joint of the thumb: a clinical and anatomical study. Journal of Bone and Joint Surgery (Br) 44B:869–879

Taliesnik J, Watson H K 1984 Midcarpal instability caused by malunited fractures of the distal radius. Journal of Hand Surgery (Am) 9A:350–357

Tetro A M, Evanoff B A, Hollstien S B et al 1998 A new provocative test for carpal tunnel syndrome. Journal of Bone and Joint Surgery (Br) 80B:493–498

Tinel J 1915 Le Signe du 'Fourmillement' dans les lesions des Nerfs Peripheriques. Press Med 47:388–389

Tsuge S, Nakamura R 1993 Anatomical risk factors for Kienbock's disease. Journal of Hand Surgery (Br) 18(B):70–75

Villar R N, Marsh D 1987 Three years after Colle's fracture: a prospective review. Journal of Bone and Joint Surgery (Br) 69B:635–638

Walker W C, Melzler M, Cifu D X et al 2000 Neutral wrist splinting in carpal tunnel syndrome: a comparison of night-only versus full-time wear instructions. Archives of Physical Medicine and Rehabilitation 81:424–429

Watson H K 1979 The carpal boss: surgical treatment and etiological considerations. Plastic and Reconstructive Surgery 63:88–93

Watson H K, Ballet F L 1984 The SLAC wrist: scapholunate advanced collapse pattern of degenerative arthritis. Journal of Hand Surgery (Am) 9A:358–365

Watson H K, Ryu J 1986 Evolution of arthritis of the wrist. Clinical Orthopaedics and Related Research 202:57–67

Watson H K, Weinzweig J 1997 Physical examination of the wrist. Hand Clinics 13:17–34

Watson H K, Ashmead D, Makhlouf M V 1988 Examination of the scaphoid. Journal of Hand Surgery (Br) 13B:657–660

Watson H K, Ottoni L, Pitts E C et al 1993 Rotary subluxation of the scaphoid: a spectrum of instability. Journal of Hand Surgery (Br) 18B:62–64

Watson H K, Weinzweig J, Zeppieri J 1997 The natural progression of scaphoid instability. Hand Clinics 13:39–49

Weber E R 1980 Biomechanical implications of scaphoid wrist fractures. Clinical Orthopaedics and Related Research 149:83–90

Weber E R 1984 Concepts governing the rotational shift of the intercalated segment of the carpus. Orthopaedic Clinics of North America 15:193–207

Weber E R, Chao E Y 1978 An experimental approach to the mechanism of scaphoid wrist fractures. Journal of Hand Surgery (Am) 3A:142–148

Wehbe M A, Hunter J M 1985 Flexor tendon gliding in the hand: II. Differential gliding. Journal of Hand Surgery (Am) 10A:626–632

Weiss N D, Gordon L, Bloom T et al 1995 Position of the wrist associated with the lowest carpal-tunnel pressure: implications for splint design. Journal of Bone and Joint Surgery (Am) 77A:1695–1699

Weiss S, LaStayo P C, Mills A et al 2000 Prospective analysis of splinting the first carpometacarpal joint: an objective, subjective and radiographic assessment. Journal of Hand Therapy 13:218–226

Werner F W 1996 Principles of musculoskeletal biomechanics – hand. In: Peimer C A (ed) Surgery of the hand and upper extremity, vol 1. McGraw-Hill, New York, p 56–83

Whipple T L 1992 Preoperative evaluation and imaging. In: Whipple T L (ed) Arthroscopic surgery: the wrist. JG Lippincott, Philadelphia, PA, p 89–104

Wilson R L, Hazen J 1995 Management of joint injuries and intraarticular fractures of the hand. In: Hunter J M, Mackin E J, Callahan A D (eds) Rehabilitation of the hand: surgery and therapy, 4th edn. Mosby, St Louis, MO, p 377–394

Wood M, Dobyns J 1986 Sports related extra-articular wrist syndromes. Clinical Orthopaedics and Related Research 202:93–102

Wright H H, Rettig A C 1995 Management of common sports injuries. In: Hunter J M, Mackin D J, Callahan A D (eds) Rehabilitation of the hand: surgery and therapy, 4th edn. CV Mosby, St Louis, MO, p 2076–2104

Wright T W, Michlovitz S L 1996 Management of carpal instabilities. Journal of Hand Therapy 9:148–156

Zeiman C, Hunter R E, Freeman J R et al 1998 Acute skier's thumb repaired with a proximal phalanx suture anchor. American Journal of Sports Medicine 26:644–649

Zemel N, Stark H 1986 Fractures and dislocations of the carpal bones. Clinics in Sports Medicine 5:709–772

Pelvis, hip and groin

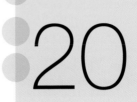

Michael T. Cibulka

CHAPTER CONTENTS

Introduction 365
Sport-specific applied anatomy 365
Clinical considerations when considering
problems with the pelvis 368
Hip joint 372
Hip problems in the athlete 374
Groin injuries in athletes 377
Summary 378

Introduction

The pelvis, hip and groin share one common anatomical component, the innominate bone. The innominate bone comprises three bones, the ilium, pubis and ischium, which are fused together as one. All three bones fuse together at the acetabulum, with each contributing a third to the make up of the acetabulum. The pelvis consists of the paired left and right innominate bones along with the sacrum. The hip joint consists of the acetabulum along with the head of the femur bone. The groin or adductor triangle consists of the hip flexor muscles, the adductor muscles and the femoral nerve, artery and vein. While the pelvis and hip have some of the strongest and thickest ligaments, muscles and bones in the body (Solonen 1957), it is no wonder that it is often the joints in this area that are the frequent sites of problems; for example, many runners, especially in middle and long distance, develop anterior hip joint pain. Unilateral low back pain, from the sacroiliac joint, is common in many athletes. The pelvis is a vital structure; it is where our center of gravity is located and it evenly distributes the weight of our upper extremities and trunk to the lower extremities.

Sport-specific applied anatomy

Kinesiology of the sacroiliac and symphysis pubis joints

Anatomy and arthrology

The sacroiliac joints (SIJ) are two paired joints formed by the connection of the left and right iliac bones to the sacrum. The sacrum consists of five fused vertebrae. The joint capsule differentiates into two structures, an external fibrous capsule and an inner synovial layer (Bernard & Cassidy 1991, Schunke 1938). The cartilage is hyaline, which is thicker on the sacral side (3–4 mm thick) than the iliac side (1–2 mm thick) (Kampen & Tillman 1998, Sasabili et al 1995, Sashin 1930, Schunke 1938). By the third decade after birth, the iliac surface develops a convex ridge that runs centrally along the entire length of the joint surface, limiting motion to anterior/posterior tilting (rotation) (Brunner et al 1991, Wilder et al 1980).

The SIJs are diarthrodial joints with the characteristic features of synovial joints including a joint capsule, synovial fluid, hyaline cartilage, surrounding ligaments and movement between the joint surfaces (Alderink 1991, Bernard & Cassidy 1991, Portefield & DeRosa 1990, 1991, Sashin 1930, Schunke 1938, Solonen 1957). The joint is formed through the connection of the ilium to the sacrum. The joint articular surface has been described as 'C','L' or 'kidney bean' shaped (Fig. 20.1) with its convexity located anteriorly (Alderink 1991, Beal 1982, Bernard & Cassidy 1991, Portefield & DeRosa 1990,1991, Sashin 1930, Schunke 1938, Solonen 1957). The SIJ follows the ventral portion of the bodies of the sacral segments of the S1, S2 and S3 fused vertebrae. The sacrum's articular surfaces are predominantly concave, while the two ilial articular surfaces of the SIJs are convex (Weisl 1955a).

Joint movements of the bicondylar SIJs

Movements at the SIJs are restricted to motion along their curved articular surfaces, and have been described as an oblique sagittal

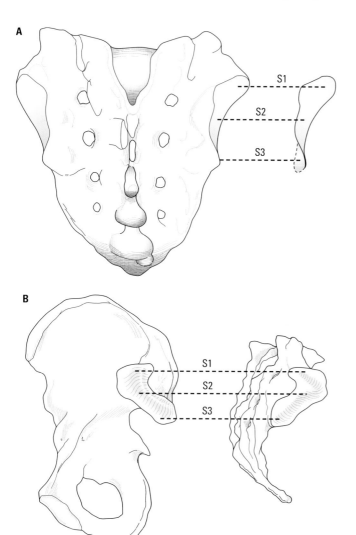

Figure 20.1 • A: Sacrum. **B:** Iliac bone and sacroiliac joint articular surfaces.

plane motion with movement primarily developing in an anterior or posterior direction. Some minor motion also occurs in both the frontal and horizontal planes (Smidt et al 1995, Sturreson et al 1989, 2000, Weisl 1955b, Wilder et al 1980). Smidt et al (1997) confirmed this in a recent cadaveric study where he showed that the innominate bones move in all three planes; however, with most of the motion developing in the sagittal plane. The sellar SIJs are also identified as bicondylar joints (Lavignolle et al 1983, Weisl 1955a). Bicondylar joints, so called because they articulate with two distinct articular condyles, have only two degrees of freedom (MacConaill & Basmajian 1977). The two degrees of freedom consequently limit joint motion around just two axes of motion, each lying perpendicular to each other (MacConaill & Basmajian 1977). As with all bicondylar joints, a movement of one joint must be accompanied by a correlative movement at the other (MacConaill & Basmajian 1977).

A characteristic feature of synovial joints is that the shape and orientation of the articular surfaces determine the type of movement that can occur (MacConnaill & Basmajian 1977). Therefore, the SIJ, being a synovial joint, follows the curvature of its articular surfaces during movement. The characteristic movement of the SIJ is a simultaneous anterior or posterior oblique movement of the left and right innominate bones on the sacrum. This motion develops during symmetrical trunk movements or symmetrical hip motion, for example, trunk forward bending, performing a pelvic tilt or when moving from sitting to standing (Egund et al 1978, Sturesson et al 1989). The second and only other movement possible at the SIJs must therefore be an equal yet opposite (antagonistic) movement where one innominate bone moves anteriorly while the other side moves posteriorly. This occurs in accordance with the rules that govern movement of bicondylar joints where, as outlined previously, movement of one side must be accompanied by a correlative movement of the other side (MacConaill & Basmajian 1977). Sturesson et al (1989) suggest that the two innominate bones rotate as a unit around the sacrum. Presumably innominate bone motion could thus develop as either agonistic (in the same direction) or antagonistic (in opposite directions) motion.

Although agonistic motion has been accepted for years, only recently has evidence for antagonistic motion of the innominate bones been demonstrated. During asymmetrical hip motions, where one hip flexes and the other extends, for example in walking, running or kicking a ball, antagonistic innominate motion has been demonstrated (Barakatt et al 1996, Sturesson et al 2000). However, the first reported description of antagonistic movement of the innominate bones was by Pitkin & Pheasant (1936) who proposed that an unpaired unilateral motion of one innominate bone would rupture the symphysis pubis. Using asymmetrical standing positions and an inclinometer to measure innominate bone tilt, they showed that the left and right innominate bones tilt in opposite (antagonistic) directions. Later, Lavignolle et al (1983) showed antagonistic (dissymmetrical) innominate motion after orthogonally measuring the pelvis while flexing one hip and extending the other. Cibulka et al (1988) observed antagonistic innominate movement after applying a manipulative technique directed at the SIJ in patients who had low back pain with signs of SIJ dysfunction. Cummings et al (1993) repeated Pitkin & Pheasant's (1936) work, using a different type of inclinometer, but still found the same antagonistic motion between the innominate bones when an imposed leg length discrepancy was artificially created. Finally, Barakatt et al (1996), using a Metrecom, showed that with asymmetrical hip positions (one hip maximally flexed and the other maximally extended), the left and right innominate bones move in an equal and opposite direction (antagonistic motion) from each other. So far, there is only anecdotal evidence to show that innominate bone motion can occur independently, except in disruption of the pelvic ring. Conversely, considerable evidence does exist to show antagonistic motion (Barakatt et al 1996, Smidt et al 1997, Sturesson et al 2000), thus supporting the concept that the SIJs are bicondylar joints.

Thus, research studies have shown that the SIJ's rotatory motion ranges from 1° to 19° (Barakatt et al 1996, Colachis et al 1963, Egund et al 1978, Frigerio et al 1974, Lavignolle et al 1983, Smidt et al 1995, 1997, Sturesson et al 1989, 2000). Although all reports agree that motion primarily develops in the sagittal (x) plane, motion also develops in both the frontal and transverse planes (y, z) during different movements. Regardless of how much motion actually takes place at the SIJ, which is probably somewhere in between these ranges, perhaps the most important point is that all studies agree that both agonistic and antagonistic movements of the innominate bones take place at the SIJ.

Joint movement of the amphiarthrodial symphysis pubis

For the SIJs to function as bicondylar joints, motion must be absent or severely limited at the symphysis pubis joint. The symphysis pubis is an amphiarthrodial joint (a fibrous joint with little or no motion available) (Walheim et al 1984). The reported amount of movement measured at the symphysis pubis is no more than 2mm in females and 0.5 mm in males (Chamberlain 1930, Walheim & Selvik 1984, Walheim et al 1984). Sturesson et al (1989) reports that the symphysis pubis allows the two innominate bones to rotate only as a unit around the sacrum, therefore allowing both paired innominate motion and antagonistic innominate motion on the sacrum. Pregnancy, of course, can significantly increase the symphysis pubis mobility (Borrel & Fernestrom 1957, Death et al 1982). In pregnancy, the amount of movement possible at the pubis increases (Borrel & Fernestrom 1957). Therefore, except for pregnancy, the symphysis pubis should probably be regarded functionally as a 'fused' joint.

Ligaments and their role in limiting SIJ movement

The ligaments of the pelvis are among the strongest in the body. In the SIJ, most of the ligaments are short and thick (Walker 1992). Anteriorly, the SIJ ligament is loose and thin, while posteriorly, the dorsal sacroiliac and interosseous ligaments are very thick and strong. The dorsal SIJ ligaments run in two directions, one along the length of the articular surface and the second in a ventral to dorsal direction (Weisl 1954). The primary purpose of the dorsal SIJ ligaments is to prevent the sacrum from falling into the pelvic brim or outlet (Weisl 1954). Since the sacrum is tapered dorsally, the sacrum is limited in moving dorsally by its wedge shape. The majority of the ligaments of the SIJ are short (25mm in length) (Weisl 1954), perhaps explaining why no study has described ligament strain as the cause of SIJ dysfunction.

The sacrotuberous and sacrospinous ligaments are the only long ligaments of the SIJ, and they limit ventral sacral motion (Weisl 1954). The sacrotuberous ligament is continuous with the origin of the hamstring muscles and is thought to play some unexplained role in function. No study has yet shown that either of these two ligaments is a common cause of pain or is commonly strained.

Muscles and their effect on SIJ movement

Any muscle that is attached to the pelvis theoretically has the potential to have an effect on movement of the SIJ. However, not all muscles attached to the pelvis are aligned in such a way that they may produce SIJ motion. For example, since the SIJ moves primarily in the sagittal plane and the abductor and adductor muscles lie in the frontal plane, their line of pull could not theoretically create sagittal plane movement. Thus, the primary muscles that theoretically can create movement of the pelvis are muscles in the sagittal plane, which include the trunk muscles (specifically, the erector spinae and the abdominal muscles), and the hip muscles, which include the hip flexors, extensors, medial and lateral rotators.

From a theoretical perspective the muscles of the spine, except for the iliopsoas muscle, by virtue of attachment have little if any direct affect on SIJ motion. It has been suggested that the transverse abdominis can create a force that compresses the SIJ and gives 'force closure' and restricts SIJ motion, a concept that has been recently advocated by European researchers (Mens et al 2002, Pool-Goudzwaard et al 1998, Vleeming et al 1990a, 1990b). They suggest that since load transfer from spine to pelvis passes through the SIJs, effective stabilization of these joints is essential (Pool-Goudzwaard et al 1998) and can be increased in two ways. First, by interlocking of the ridges and grooves on the joint surfaces (form closure); second, by compressive forces of structures like muscles, ligaments and fascia (force closure) (Pool-Goudzwaard et al 1998, Vleeming et al 1990a, 1990b). Muscle weakness and insufficient tension of SIJ ligaments can lead to diminished compression, influencing load transfer negatively. Continuous strain of pelvic ligaments may create a result leading to low back pain (Pool-Goudzwaard et al 1998). They also suggest that for treatment purposes stabilization techniques and the subsequent specific muscle strengthening procedures are outlined (Pool-Goudzwaard et al 1998).

The seminal theory behind form and force closure relies wholly on the concept that the SIJs are hypermobile. Hypermobility is a plausible hypothesis and an often cited explanation for SIJ recurrence. Although form and force closure makes sense when using a mechanical theory (Vleeming et al 1997), the simple fact remains that no study has yet to show that this theory is true in patients with SIJ pain or whether hyper-mobility of the SIJ actually exists in patients with SIJ pain.

Van Wingerden et al (2004) studied the affect of muscular contribution to force closure of the pelvis in the stabilization of the SIJ in vivo. When looking at the biceps femoris, gluteus maximus, erector spinae and contralateral latissimus dorsi muscles this study showed that SIJ stiffness increased when the erector spinae, biceps femoris and gluteus maximus muscles were individually activated. They contended the increase in SIJ stiffness seen with minimal muscle activity supports the notion that effectiveness of load transfer from spine to legs is improved when muscle forces actively compress the SIJ and prevents shear. Although this study sounds impressive so far it is just a model and thus results cannot be validated.

Neurology of the SIJ

Solonen (1957) describes the innervation of the SIJ ventrally from the spinal nerves of L3 to S2 and the superior gluteal nerve, and dorsally from the first and second spinal sacral nerves (S1–S2). Therefore, the widespread innervation suggests that pain from the SIJ may radiate anywhere in the lower extremity if irritated enough.

Clinical considerations when considering problems with the pelvis

The evidenced-based practice (EBP) approach described by Sackett et al (1985) allows for an unbiased choice when selecting the best tests and intervention for a problem or condition (Sackett et al 1998). Many clinicians currently use the method of differential diagnosis in selecting tests and not EBP. When using the differential diagnosis method, the first step is to develop a list of possible causes that may explain the signs and symptoms. Different strategies often help to refine the examiner's thought processes when making the diagnosis; for example, when using the anatomical method, each specific tissue (e.g. ligament) is tested or stressed to determine its response (Friedland et al 1998). The major problem when using this approach is that tests and interventions may be selected in a biased fashion. Conversely, when using EBP, the best available evidence is assembled in an unbiased fashion to select and interpret the most appropriate diagnostic tests and for guidance in the assessment of potentially useful interventions.

The most common pelvic problem seen by physical therapists is low back pain related to impairment of the SIJs (Broadhurst 1989, DonTigny 1979, 1985, Erhard & Bowling 1977, Goldthwaite & Osgood 1905, Schwarzer et al 1995, Shaw 1992). Symphysis pubis problems are much less common. Muscle pulls of one joint hip flexor, and the extensor muscles, external and internal rotators and abductor muscles are extremely rare. Muscle strains or 'pulls' of two joint hip/thigh muscles, for example, the hamstring and adductor or groin muscles, are much

more frequent, especially in sports. Hamstring muscle pulls will be covered in another chapter, while groin muscle pulls will be covered later in this chapter.

History

When using EBP, the prevalence of the disorder is established before any diagnostic tests are selected (Freidland et al 1998, Sackett et al 1998). It is important to determine the prevalence because if the likelihood of a disorder is low (i.e. it has low prevalence), most diagnostic tests will have limited diagnostic importance (Diamond & Forrester 1979). Moreover, as prevalence of the disorder decreases, the predictive value of a positive test decreases and thus the possibility of finding a false positive test result increases (Diamond & Forrester 1979, Sackett et al 1985). Consequently, it is important to determine the prevalence of the disorder before any specific diagnostic tests are performed (Diamond & Forrester 1979).

If prevalence of a disorder is not known, which is common, the EBP method increases the prediction of the prevalence by estimating its pretest probability (Sackett et al 1985, 1998). Pretest probability, defined, is the prior assessment of diagnostic possibilities before any tests are performed (Sackett et al 1985). Pretest probabilities most often come from the patient's history or presentation (Sackett et al 1998); using clinical experience, an estimate of the probability of the presence of the disorder can be made. Pretest probabilities may also come from published literature or data and can be expressed in rank order as high, medium and low or be given a percentage to reflect relative probability (Sackett et al 1985, 1998).

Pretest probability data on SIJ dysfunction are sparse. Most of the data describing SIJ dysfunction have been obtained from textbooks as few published studies exist. Calvillo et al (2000) suggest that adjacent spinal structures may cause pain to be referred to the SIJ; precise diagnosis can be difficult. However, studies have shown that pain near the posterior superior iliac spine (PSIS) is suggestive of SIJ dysfunction. In one study, Fortin et al (1994) injected the SIJ with an irritant and found unilateral pain around the PSIS. Fortin et al (1994) also showed that pain can refer down the leg in the dermatomal region from L3 to S2. Although often described, no specific or single mechanism of SIJ dysfunction has been shown to create SIJ pain (Dreyfuss et al 1996). SIJ dysfunction usually develops without provocation or incident. Other features of SIJ dysfunction included moderate pain (e.g. Modified Oswestry score around 38%) (Fritz & George 2000). A list of the pretest probabilities that was developed from my own experience is in Box 20.1. Also, a list of pretest probabilities not associated with SIJ dysfunction, and which can help rule out SIJ dysfunction, is listed in Box 20.2.

Examination of the pelvis

Confirmation of SIJ dysfunction has been a continued source of controversy. No doubt this is exacerbated by the fact that, so far, no 'gold standard' of diagnosis has been established for the presence of SIJ dysfunction. Reasons include its deep location, small

Box 20.1 Pretest probability for sacroiliac joint dysfunction in an outpatient physical therapy clinic

1. Unilateral pain in or around the posterior superior iliac spine
2. No mechanism of injury
3. No neurological signs or symptoms
4. Full painless trunk range of motion
5. Minimal to moderate pain (2–4 on a 0–10 pain scale)
   For all five 75%: pretest probability
   For four 50%: pretest probability
   For three or less 40%: pretest probability

Box 20.2 Pretest probability for no sacroiliac joint dysfunction in an outpatient physical therapy clinic

1. Central low back pain or pain radiating below the knee
2. Specific mechanism of injury
3. Neurological signs and symptoms
4. Painful limited trunk range of motion
5. Constant pain
6. Moderate severe or severe low back pain (above 5 on a 0–10 pain scale)

motion, irregular shape and orientation of articular surfaces, all of which make direct examination, visual appraisal of motion and injection difficult (Bernard & Cassidy 1991). Therefore, it is easy to understand that most individual tests used to detect SIJ dysfunction have been shown to be unreliable (Delitto et al 1992, Potter & Rothstein 1985). Clinicians, however, rarely use just one test to detect SIJ dysfunction (Beal 1982, Cibulka & Koldehoff 1999, Delitto et al 1992). Research shows that when SIJ tests are combined, reliability as well as diagnostic specificity improves (Cibulka & Koldehoff 1999, Diamond & Forrester 1979). Cibulka & Koldehoff (1999) and Dreyfuss et al (1996) found high specificity in identifying patients with SIJ dysfunction when combining SIJ tests. Levangie (1999) also found high test specificity when using the Gillet test and sitting flexion test (93%) to detect pelvic asymmetry, an often described feature of SIJ dysfunction. Laslett & Williams (1994) also found good reliability, when using SIJ provocation tests. Freburger & Riddle (2001) recently evaluated the use of pelvic calipers in the clinic and found unacceptable reliability; however, few therapists routinely use pelvic calipers in the clinic to assess pelvic landmarks on patients.

Most SIJ tests can be divided into three different groups. The first group includes tests that attempt to detect limited or abnormal motion of the SIJ, the second group tests for signs of pelvic obliquity and the last group uses tests that provoke the joint to determine irritability. Tests used to detect abnormal SIJ motion usually try to compare motion on one side with the other side. A major problem with using tests to detect abnormal or limited motion is that since bicondylar joint motion is relative (i.e. both sides move together), it is highly unlikely that abnormal or limited motion can be palpated. Also, the few studies that have been performed on patients with SIJ dysfunction have shown no difference in motion between healthy subjects and those identified with SIJ dysfunction (Sturesson et al 1989, 2000). However, admittedly, in these studies, the sample size was small, no control group was used and the roentgen stereophonogrammetric analysis (RSA) setup that was used to make these studies was difficult to interpret. Currently, we do not have any other convincing evidence that motion at the SIJ is increased, decreased or altered in patients with SIJ dysfunction. Nevertheless, since no study has yet to show that movement is altered in SIJ dysfunction, I do not suggest using specific tests to detect movement, at this time, for the SIJ.

The second most common method of testing for SIJ dysfunction is to use four tests for pelvic obliquity (Cibulka & Koldehoff 1999). Pelvic obliquity has long been considered a common element of SIJ dysfunction (Bourdillon & Day 1987, Cibulka et al 1988, Erhard & Bowling 1977, Mennell 1960, Mitchell et al 1979). Detecting the presence of pelvic obliquity, especially when sitting, suggests SIJ dysfunction (Cibulka et al 1986, Mitchell et al 1979). The sitting position eliminates the possible chance that any difference in leg lengths could create pelvic asymmetry. When sitting, the landmarks of the pelvis (e.g. the PSIS) should normally be level. Uneven pelvic landmarks when sitting, suggest innominate bone asymmetry (Fig. 20.2). Innominate bone asymmetry, which is not the result of leg length disparity, can only be produced by an antagonistic innominate bone tilt, where one innominate bone is tilted anteriorly and the other posteriorly. Normally, the innominate bones should remain symmetrical while sitting. It is not known how the innominate bones assume this asymmetrical position; however, some have suggested hip muscle imbalance, although there is presently no evidence available to confirm this (Cibulka 1992, Porterfield & DeRosa 1990,1991). A major caveat in detecting pelvic bone landmarks is that palpation often depends on working with a patient in whom it is possible to reliably and accurately detect uneven pelvic landmarks. Janos (1992) found poor reliability when palpating pelvic landmarks. However, when using a cluster of similar tests (Cibulka & Koldehoff 1999, Delitto et al 1992), the reliability of detecting SIJ dysfunction was found to have improved considerably. The four tests used by Cibulka & Koldehoff (1999) are different methods used to detect pelvic obliquity and include the standing flexion test (Fig. 20.3), the prone knee flexion test (Fig. 20.4), the supine long sitting test and uneven PSIS heights when sitting (Fig. 20.2). It is important when interpreting the results of a cluster of tests that all of the results converge, that is, that they should all suggest the same direction of innominate bone tilt and not contradict each other. Therefore, SIJ dysfunction is defined by the presence of antagonistic innominate bone asymmetry that is present when, normally, the innominate bones should be symmetrical. Thus the two normal antagonistic movements possible, the first where the left innominate bone tilts posteriorly and the right anteriorly, and the second where the right innominate bone tilts posteriorly and the left anteriorly, define the two types of SIJ dysfunctions that can develop. Knowledge of the direction of the innominate bone's tilt is extremely important when planning treatment of SIJ dysfunction.

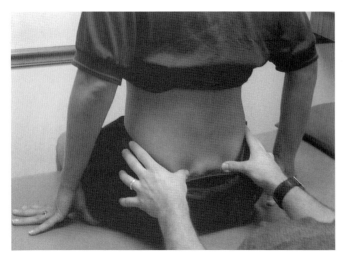

Figure 20.2 • Observation of pelvic landmarks in sitting. The position of the physical therapist's thumbs on the posterior superior iliac spine suggests innominate asymmetry.

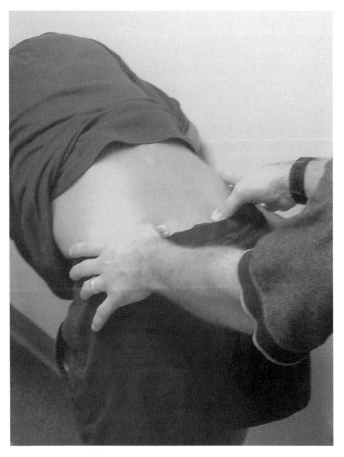

Figure 20.3 • The standing flexion test for examination of the pelvis.

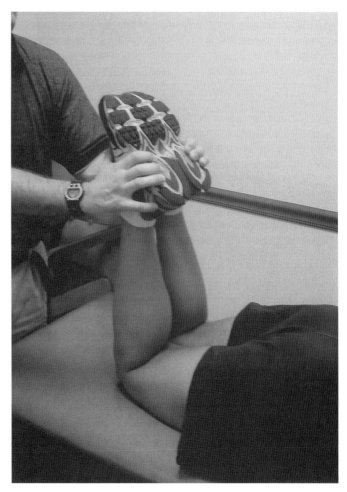

Figure 20.4 • Prone knee flexion test for sacroiliac joint dysfunction.

SIJ dysfunction. Potter & Rothstein (1985) also found good reliability with provocation tests. Other studies, however, have shown poor test specificity with individual provocation tests (Dreyfuss et al 1994, Maigne et al 1996). Broadhurst and Bond (1998) showed that when provocation tests are combined, they have a high predictive value for detecting SIJ dysfunction. Laslett et al (2005) recently examined the measurement properties of SIJ provocation tests using SIJ injection as their reference standard. The tests included sacral thrust, Gaenslen's test, posterior shear, SIJ compression and SIJ gapping. When using a combination of tests (four or more) the measurement properties (sensitivity and specificity) improved. A problem with this study was they used a population that had low back pain for almost 3 years, were off work for nearly 2 years and had very 'high' pain levels. Using an 80% reduction in pain after injection in this sort of population is questionable, such a distorted assembly makes inferences of this study dubious at best. Another major problem with provocation tests is that although they may be useful in identifying the presence of SIJ dysfunction, they have limited clinical usefulness because they have not shown any ability to either guide prognosis or treatment. Also, positive provocation tests have been found in asymptomatic patients (Dreyfuss et al 1994), which

Provocation tests are used to try and recreate a similar painful response by provoking the SIJ through compression or gapping of the SIJs. Laslett & Williams (1994) have shown the reliability of some provocation tests and have suggested their use in identifying can lead to false positive findings. Therefore, provocation tests have limited clinical usefulness.

Doppler method of detecting SIJ dysfunction

Doppler imaging, a noninvasive ultrasound method to detect laxity of the SIJs through vibration, has been used in a number of recent studies (Damen et al 2001, 2002a, 2002b). Subjects usually lie prone while vibrations are applied unilaterally to the anterior superior iliac spine, which are then propagated through the ilium to the SIJ. The imaging unit allows measurements by comparing the vibration amplitude/intensity of the ilium and sacrum (Damen et al 2002a). Differences in threshold levels between the ilium and sacrum (measured in threshold units or TU) are related to the vibration amplitude of the bone (Damen et al 2002b). A minimal difference between threshold levels of the sacrum and ilium is usually an indication of a stiff joint (less than 2 TU), while a large difference is indicative of a loose joint (greater than 5 TU) (Damen et al 2002b). A left to right difference in SIJ laxity ≥3 TU is considered to indicate asymmetric laxity of the SIJs (Damen et al 2002a). Damen et al (2002b) found this method reliable (ICC 0.53 to 0.80) for inter-tester reliability, suggesting that changes can be confidently determined if larger than 1.94 TU to 3.6 TU (Damen et al 2002b). The problem with Doppler imaging is there has been no research on its validity for this measure. We do not know if Doppler imaging actually measures or determines SIJ laxity. Furthermore, as mentioned in an earlier section, we really do not know if joint laxity is an important problem in patients with SIJ pain. Thus the issue of validity must be seriously examined before accepting the Doppler method.

The EBP approach, where pretest probabilities are combined with one or more tests that have good measurement properties (e.g. high likelihood ratios, or high specificity or sensitivity), is the best method of making the diagnosis of SIJ dysfunction. Box 20.1 lists pretest probabilities that are used in my clinic to help increase prediction of the prevalence of SIJ dysfunction. A next step is to go online and via the sites PUBMED (www.ncbi.nlm.nih.gov/pubmed/) to search for those tests that have shown high sensitivity, specificity or likelihood ratios and that are used to determine the post-test probability, and therefore rule in the diagnosis of SIJ dysfunction. The tests used include the four tests for pelvic obliquity mentioned earlier (Cibulka & Koldehoff 1999). Positive results in at least three out of four tests suggest SIJ dysfunction (Cibulka & Koldehoff 1999). Also, all of the SIJ tests must converge or agree suggesting that the exact same problem exists in all of them (e.g. a left posterior innominate bone). The problem with using a cluster of tests is that a gold standard currently does not exist; however, using a cluster as a clinical standard has already shown its usefulness in helping physical therapists guide successful intervention, which is the primary purpose of any examination.

A diagnosis of SIJ dysfunction is made by finding a high post-test probability from the results of the pretest probability for the disorder, and the likelihood ratio generated from the positive test results. For example, one could predict a pretest probability of 75% if the patient had unilateral PSIS pain primarily, had no trauma, had full trunk range of motion and indicated a pain score of around 4/10 on a 1–10 analog pain scale. Then, on examination, if all four SIJ tests were found to be positive (all suggesting a left posterior innominate SIJ dysfunction), the positive likelihood ratio of finding at least three out of four tests positive for SIJ dysfunction is 6.83. Thus, as a result of doing the mathematics, the pretest probability of 0.75 and the likelihood ratio of 6.83 would give a post-test probability of 96%. A post-test probability of 96% strongly suggests that it is likely that the patient has SIJ dysfunction.

Prognosis in SIJ dysfunction

No published data exist on the prognosis of SIJ dysfunction. Numerous reports describe SIJ dysfunction as a recurring problem. The ubiquitous use of SIJ fixation belts is one example of the clinician's quest to reduce the incidence of this problem. Although unilateral low back pain is the most common symptom of SIJ dysfunction, hip pain and hamstring muscle strain have also been shown to be related to SIJ dysfunction (Cibulka & Delitto 1993, Cibulka et al 1992).

Intervention strategies

Much has been written on the treatment of the SIJ; unfortunately most is anecdotal and no randomized clinical trials have been performed so far; therefore, little published evidence is available to guide clinicians. In the only randomized clinical trial (Erhard et al 1994) on SIJ intervention, treatment involved both the SIJ and the lumbar spine, thus making inferences difficult. In another study (Cibulka et al 1988), manipulation, presumably directed at the SIJ, was shown to restore innominate bone symmetry in patients with previous innominate bone asymmetry and with signs and symptoms of SIJ dysfunction; unfortunately no data were collected on symptomatic improvement. Most of the non-peer-reviewed literature on the treatment of the SIJ is extremely confusing. Some treatments aim to restore mobility while others seek to restrict mobility. However, without a reliable or valid measure of motion, these treatments currently appear speculative at best. Since, so far, no data have shown that SIJ mobility is altered in patients with SIJ dysfunction; it may be better to abandon the idea of treating the joint with too much or too little motion until we have some convincing evidence.

Mobilization, although used widely, has not been performed in any randomized control trial so far; therefore, we are left with primarily anecdotal descriptions of mobilizations that were successful in patients with SIJ dysfunction. When using mobilization, unlike manipulation, the direction that the innominate bones tilt must be known for this technique to be effective (Freburger & Riddle 2001). Many textbooks describe these techniques, which primarily include the movement of one or both innominate bones in a direction that would restore innominate bone symmetry (Bourdillon & Day 1987, Lee 1989, Stoddard 1959, Wells 1986, Woerman 1989).

As already mentioned, manipulation has been shown to restore pelvic symmetry in patients with SIJ dysfunction who previously had innominate bone asymmetry (Cibulka et al 1988). Tullberg et al (1998), however, recently questioned the effect manipulation has on the SIJ. Using an RSA technique, where markers were placed only on the dorsal surface of the pelvis of the 'dysfunctional side', they found no change in position between the side of the dysfunctional ilium and the sacrum, before and after a manipulative treatment aimed at the SIJ. The technical setup of this RSA study is questionable primarily because of Tullberg's marker placement. As previously discussed, inadequate marker placement limits the interpretation of movement between the innominate bones and sacrum. The data acquired from the frontal plane markers cannot possibly describe sagittal plane motion between the sacrum and innominate bones. The study by Cibulka et al (1988), in which pelvic calipers were used, showed that in patients who had a cluster of SIJ signs, a manipulative technique aimed at the SIJ restored innominate bone symmetry in all 10 patients who previously had measurable innominate bone asymmetry. A weakness of this study was that reliability of the pelvic calipers was not determined before the study. However, despite this, and with the examiner also being blinded to who was being treated, a significant difference in pelvic tilt was noted in all 10 patients in the experimental group. Also, the cluster of tests not only agreed with the innominate bone measurement of tilt, as to the direction of innominate bone tilt, but also was able to predict that no movement developed in 9 of the 10 patients in the control group. Therefore, in this study, a manipulative technique aimed at the SIJ convincingly restored innominate bone symmetry.

Recently, Childs et al (2004) developed a clinical prediction rule (CPR) that was aimed at improving the accuracy in predicting which patients with low back pain would show a favorable clinical outcome after a physical therapy intervention (manipulation) was applied to the SIJ. Child's criteria included: Fear Avoidance Beliefs Questionnaire score below 19 points, duration of current episode less than 16 days, no symptoms extending distal to the knee, at least one hypomobile lumbar vertebra (judged by spring test) and at least one hip with greater than $35°$ of hip internal rotation. This paper gives future direction at least in the acute patient. The advantage of the CPR is that it helps clinicians determine who is likely to improve with a SIJ manipulation; the disadvantage is that patients with SIJ dysfunction often have recurrences and this rule gives no help or guidance in preventing these relapses.

How does a unilateral manipulative technique restore bilateral innominate bone symmetry? I am not sure; however, since the two SIJs are considered to be one bicondylar joint, manipulating one side must also move the opposite side. More research is needed on this interesting subject.

Prevention of SIJ dysfunction recurrence

Recurrence is considered a problem in patients with low back pain from the SIJ. A significant part of the problem, I believe, is a lack of knowledge of the SIJ. Many clinicians believe that the SIJ moves with three degrees of freedom, describing these motions as unilateral innominate bone movement, sacral flexions, rotations and upslips (Mitchell et al 1979, Oldrieve 1996, 1998). All of these movements are impossible at this bicondylar joint. Furthermore, no data exist to prove that any of these motions exist. Puzzlingly, many of these motions often describe the exact same phenomena. I believe that what is important in the prevention of recurrence is to define the diagnosis of SIJ dysfunction and determine the possible reason for innominate bone symmetry. The movements of the SIJs are related to the motion of the hip and lumbar spinal joints; evaluation of these two areas is mandatory in recalcitrant SIJ problems. Interestingly, a number of studies have shown the importance of the hip in SIJ mechanics; for example, patients with hip joint impairments, including patients with amputations of the thigh (Matanovic & Granic-Husic 1991), and osteoarthritis (OA) of the hip and total hip replacements (Aalam & Hoffman 1975, Hebling 1978, Pap et al 1987), have all demonstrated significant changes in their SIJ. Furthermore, studies have reported that unilateral limited hip rotation is related to low back and SIJ dysfunction (Cibulka et al 1998, LaBan et al 1978). I recommend that with any recurrent SIJ problem, the hip and lumbar spine should be assessed.

Two examples of treatment options for recurrent SIJ dysfunction are arthrodesis (Buchowski et al 2005) and debridement (Haufe & Monk 2005). Buchowski et al (2005) investigated the health-related quality of life outcomes after SIJ arthrodesis for recurrent SIJ disorders and found that significant improvement occurred in the following domains: physical functioning, role physical, bodily pain, vitality, social functioning, role emotional and neurogenic and pain indices. The patient population consisted of 20 patients undergoing SIJ arthrodesis in which previous nonoperative treatment was not successful and the diagnosis was confirmed by pain relief with intraarticular SIJ injections under fluoroscopic guidance. Buchowski recommends arthrodesis for carefully selected patients. In a recent retrospective study, Haufe & Mork (2005) examined 38 patients who underwent SIJ debridement as a treatment for confirmed SIJ pain (via preoperative modified SIJ injection). Assessing the degree of pain relief in patients at 12-month intervals following debridement 61% of the patients had 50–100% reductions of their VAS and 53% had greater than 75% improvement for more than 2 years. This one study, although interesting, is not enough to base any future conclusions.

Hip joint

Joint movements of the hip

The hip joint is the connection between the head of the femur bone and the acetabulum of the innominate bone. The hip joint is an ovoid, or ball and socket, joint and is the largest synovial joint in the body. The joint is very stable and strong because of its ligamentous attachments and its congruent fit. The hip joint's major function is to allow movement for walking and running; however, hip joint motion is important in movement of the trunk.

The two identical synovial joints of the left and right hip are considered to be unmodified ovoid joints with three degrees of freedom allowing motion in the frontal, sagittal and transverse planes. The hip moves primarily in the sagittal plane with 10–15° of extension and 135° of flexion. Movement in the frontal and transverse planes is more varied with measures of: abduction 30–45°, adduction 20–30°, internal rotation 30–75° and external rotation 25–75°. The frontal and transverse plane hip movements have a wider variation of motion. Although the range is quite wide, very little difference is found when comparing left and right sides of the same motion (e.g. left and right medial rotation) in the asymptomatic and young. The head of the femur forms about two-thirds of a sphere with a diameter of 4–5 cm (Kapandji 1970). The head is supported by the femoral neck which runs obliquely from the femoral shaft at an angle of about 125° (within a range of 90–135°). The femoral neck enhances hip motion by placing the femoral shaft away from the pelvis laterally. The concave acetabulum faces in an oblique, anterior, lateral and inferior direction.

The close-pack position of the hip, where the capsule and majority of the ligaments are taut and the joint articular surfaces are congruent, is where the hip is extended, internally rotated and abducted (MacConaill & Basmajian 1977). The loose-pack position, where the capsule and most of the hip ligaments are slackened and the joint articular surfaces are incongruent, is where the hip is flexed, externally rotated and adducted (MacConaill & Basmajian 1977). Walmsley (1928) reports that the hip is in full congruence only when the hip transmits weight and is incongruent in all other positions. The hip joint moves from a loose-pack position at heel-strike to a close-pack position at heel-off and then back again. The loose-pack position at heel-strike is necessary so that the eccentrically contracting muscles of the hip and thigh can absorb the force of ground impact over time; at heel-off, the hip must be in the close-pack position in order to push off a rigid lever to propel the body forward as the hip and thigh muscles contract primarily concentrically.

Ligaments and their role in hip joint motion

The hip joint is surrounded by a strong and dense articular capsule that has a cylindrical shape and that runs from the iliac bone to the upper end of the femur. The hip joint capsule consists of two sets of fibers, one circular and the other longitudinal. The circular fibers are deeper and form a collar around the neck of the femur, while most of the longitudinal fibers are in the anterior aspect of the joint capsule. The capsule is partially blended with the posterior and anterior ligaments.

The hip joint has three very strong ligaments that strengthen the hip anteriorly and posteriorly: the ischiofemoral, pubofemoral and iliofemoral ligaments (Grubel Lee 1983). The ischiofemoral ligament is the only posterior ligament. The pubofemoral ligament runs from the pubis to the trochanteric fossa, while the iliofemoral ligament runs from the lower part of the anterior inferior iliac spine to the trochanter line. All of the three hip ligaments become taut in extension and are relaxed during flexion. During medial hip rotation, the anterior

ligaments are relaxed while the posterior ischiofemoral ligament remains taut, and during external rotation, the iliofemoral and pubofemoral ligaments become taut while the ischiofemoral becomes relaxed (Kapandji 1970). During adduction, the ischiofemoral and pubofemoral ligaments relax, while during abduction, they tighten (Kapandji 1970). The iliofemoral ligament, however, becomes taut during adduction.

The ligamentum teres is a minor supporting ligament with adduction being the only movement where it becomes taut; however, the role of the ligamentum teres in the development of osteophytes is interesting.

Functionally, the transverse ligament of the acetabulum is a portion of the acetabular labrum; however, it is not cartilagenous. It consists of strong fibers which cross the acetabular notch, forming a foramen.

The fibrocartilaginous labrum of the acetabulum is a tough, mobile annulus that attaches to the bony acetabular rim but does not extend over the acetabular notch. The labrum increases the depth of the acetabulum and thus stabilizes the hip joint. The labrum extends beyond the greatest circumference of the head of the femur, thus preventing femoral head dislocation from the acetabulum. The labrum holds the femoral head so effectively that the head can be removed from the acetabulum only if the labrum is stretched or ruptured. The superior margin of the labrum is mobile and may fold into the hip joint cavity of a congenitally dislocated hip, preventing reduction of the dislocated femoral head.

The articular cartilage covers a portion of the acetabulum forming a broad horseshoe-shaped area that opens downward. The upper portion of the acetabulum is the major weight-bearing site of the articulation. The articular cartilage is thickest at this upper area and around the outer periphery of the horseshoe shape as it carries the body weight. Thinning of the cartilage occurs toward the center and lower portion of the acetabulum. The non-articular portion of the acetabulum or acetabular fossa and a fat pad covered with synovial fluid are found within the horseshoe. The subchondral bone and synovial fluid provide nutrition for the articular cartilage. Repair of damaged articular cartilage in the hip joint is limited because blood vessels do not directly supply the cartilage.

Muscle and its role in hip joint movement

Many of the muscles surrounding the hip have hybrid functions: they may be prime movers in one direction and assist in one or more other motions. The muscles that allow flexion of the hip include the iliopsoas, pectineus, sartorious, tensor fascia latae and rectus femoris. The hip extensor muscles include the gluteus maximus and the hamstring muscle group. The hip abductor muscles include the gluteus medius, the gluteus minimus and the tensor fascia latae. The hip adductor muscles include the gracilis, and the three adductor muscles: the longus, magnus and brevis. The hip internal rotator muscles include the gluteus minimus, the anterior fibers of the gluteus medius and the tensor fascia latae. The hip external rotator muscles include the piriformis, quadratus femoris, gemelli superior and inferior and obturator internus and externus. Muscles of the hip may change their role according to the position the hip joint is in, for example, with the hip in 90° of hip flexion, the angle of pull of hip external rotators allows hip abduction instead of hip external rotation.

Neurology of the hip joint

The hip joint is densely supplied with nerves formed from articular nerves that also innervate the surrounding muscles of the hip. The hip joint innervation is supplied primarily by the obturator nerve (Warwick & Williams 1973). Three articular nerves supply the hip joint and they include the posterior branch, the medial articular branch and the nerve to the ligamentum capitus femoris. The posterior articular nerve has the greatest nerve supply to the hip; it supplies the posterior and inferior aspects of the hip joint capsule (Dee 1969). The medial articular nerve arises from the anterior division of the obturator nerve (from the ventral rami of the second, third and fourth lumbar nerves) and divides into two branches (Dee 1969); the medial branch of this nerve supplies the anteromedial and inferior aspects of the joint capsule. The nerve to the ligamentum capitis femoris arises from the muscular branch of the posterior division of the obturator nerve (Warwick & Williams 1973) and it primarily supplies the ligamentum teres. The hip joint may also be supplied by a small number of nerves, coming from accessory articular nerves, which are from surrounding muscle supplied by the femoral nerve (from the dorsal branches of the ventral rami of the second, third and fourth lumbar nerves) (Dee 1969).

Blood supply

The hip joint receives its blood supply from the obturator, gluteal and femoral arteries. These arteries supply the acetabulum, and the femoral head and neck (Warwick & Williams 1973). The blood supply is clinically important in a number of hip disorders. The acetabulum branch of the obturator artery supplies blood to the medial aspect of the acetabulum. A small branch of this artery also supplies the ligamentum teres and therefore a limited portion of the superior aspect of the femoral head (Warwick & Williams 1973). The superior and inferior gluteal artery supplies part of the acetabulum. The femoral artery gives rise to the medial and lateral circumflex arteries (ascending branches) that supply the proximal end of the femur, from the femoral neck to the subcapital sulcus, and give rise to the retinacular arteries which supply the head of the femur (Warwick & Williams 1973). The retinacular arteries that supply the femoral head do not have any anastomoses, thus preventing the femoral head from having access to an alternative blood supply in case of injury.

Hip problems in the athlete

The two most common athletic problems that trouble the hip include hip joint pain from incongruence which creates capsular or labral problems, and hip pointers. Other conditions such as rheumatoidarthritis, ankylosing spondylitis as well as childhood diseases and conditions, such as septic arthritis, Legg–Calvé–Perthes disease, slipped capital femoral epiphysis (SCFE) and congenital hip dislocation, can and do affect the hip; however, these diseases and conditions are rare in the athlete. Hip dislocation, although rare, can occur during contact sports such as American football.

History

In most nontraumatic hip pain, the history of the pain is often unremarkable. Those who have had a childhood disease, such as Legg–Calvé–Perthes disease or SCFE, are often more likely to develop hip pain later in life. The primary complaint is one of either anterior groin pain or lateral greater trochanter region pain (Roberts & Williams 1988). Pain posteriorly, in the buttock region, is more suggestive of a lumbar problem than hip pain (Roberts & Williams 1988). Published data on hip pain (Khan & Woolson 1998) show that hip pain is usually referred to the groin and occasionally to the knee. Acute hip pain in a child of 3–10 years with weightbearing, spasm and fever is suggestive of septic synovitis that should be referred on immediately (Hart 1996). If there is anterior hip pain in the prepubescent child, Legg–Calvé–Perthes disease should be suspected (Adkins & Figler 2000), while in adolescents, SCFE should not be overlooked (Adkins & Figler 2000, O'Kane 1999). Stress fracture of the femoral neck should be suspected if there is a history of anterior hip pain in distance runners (Adkins & Figler 2000, Sterling et al 1993). Pain along the iliac crest is more suggestive of a hip pointer, often with a history of a direct blow, pain on palpation, occasional ecchymosis and frequently pain with a valsalva maneuver (e.g. coughing or sneezing), or abdominal muscle contraction. Hip dislocation during sport is always traumatic and very painful.

Physical examination of the hip

Using the history can be important in problems of the hip in ruling out specific diagnoses, such as in the case of septic arthritis, Legg–Calvé–Perthes disease or SCFE. In septic arthritis the disease is not common, but very serious. It is most common in children less than 2 years old, less common in older children and rare in adults. The pain in septic arthritis is severe and increased with any hip movement. Children or adults receiving prolonged adrenocorticosteroid therapy have a higher than average incidence. In Legg–Calvé–Perthes disease the patient's age is 2–12 years with most around 6 years old. The disease is often found in white children and more often in males than females. In SCFE the age range is generally 10–17 years for boys with the mode about 13–14 years and 8–15 years for girls with the mode about 11 years. The disorder occurs at least twice as often in boys than in girls and about twice as often in black children as white children. About 75% of the cases occur in obese children with delayed maturation. Bilateral involvement occurs about 15% of the time. The evaluation of a hip joint often helps to crystallize the diagnostic process. Thus the history and age, as described above, are important in helping to guide the clinician's thought process.

The examination of the hip starts first with active hip motion during functional movements. Functional movements depend on age and agility, and such activities can include squatting, going from sitting to standing, trunk forward bending, one-legged standing, walking and running. Passive hip range of motion is assessed next, especially hip rotation, since internal rotation is often the first motion lost in OA (Altman et al 1991, Birrell et al 2001). Muscle length (Thomas and Ober tests) and strength are also assessed. Guidance for the examination of these tissues can be found in many textbooks. An examination of the pelvis, including leg lengths, is also performed on all patients with hip pain, since any alteration in innominate bone tilt can result in unequal concentration of pressure on the hip joints. Other tests for the hip include Faber's (Patrick's) test (Fig. 20.5) to determine hip joint irritability, tests for leg length to detect pelvic obliquity and the Trendelenburg test to test the hip abductor muscles functionally for strength. Altman et al (1991) also proposes a test where passive internal rotation of the hip is used to determine hip joint irritability.

In the adult hip, where trauma is not involved, few mechanical disorders develop. The most common hip problem is pain that comes from the hip joint itself. This is usually just called hip pain (Grubel Lee 1983, Reynolds & Freeman 1989). Other diagnoses, like bursitis and tendinitis, around the hip are rare. Ligament strain of the hip joint has not been described in the literature. Muscle injury to the one-joint muscles surrounding the hip is very uncommon, although the two-joint rectus femoris, adductor and hamstring muscles are frequently strained during athletic activity. The most common problem within the hip is joint inflammation that is usually the result of capsular shortening, which leads to incongruence, abnormal joint contact pressures and eventually arthritic changes (Loyd-Roberts 1953, Pauwels 1976, Reynolds & Freeman 1989, Walmsley 1928). Abnormal stress imposed on the hip has also been related to tears of the acetabular labrum (Dorrell & Catterall 1986) which may

also create anterior hip pain. In traumatic conditions, such as hip dislocation, motion is very painful, weightbearing is impossible, and deformity of the hip, such as shortening and angulation, is visually obvious.

The problem of congruence between the head of the femur and acetabulum and the development of abnormal hip joint pressure is important in understanding the development of hip OA (Bullough et al 1973, Pauwels 1976, Walmsley 1928). The reduction or realignment of stress on the hip joint is of major importance in treating hip joint pain (Pauwels 1976). Many potential risk factors can influence joint congruence within the hip joint including joint range of motion, hip joint muscle force (including both muscle length and strength), pelvic obliquity and a history of childhood hip disease. Many of these factors may alter hip joint motion, which in turn can either increase or decrease hip joint pressure by not allowing the hip joint to attain a full close-pack or loose-pack position during gait (Grubel Lee 1983). Articular cartilage is dependent on the repetitive loading and unloading of the hip for nutrition and lubrication, therefore reducing hip joint mobility through either capsular shortening or muscle weakness can diminish the health of the hip joint (Grubel Lee 1983, Loyd-Roberts 1953, Reynolds & Freeman 1989).

During heel-strike, the joints of the hip are primarily in their loose-pack position, allowing the eccentrically contracting muscles of the hip, and not the hip joint, to withstand the impact of ground force. However, if the hip joint cannot attain a full position of loose-pack (flexion, adduction, and external rotation) at the time of heel-strike, excessive compressive forces may develop within the hip. At heel-off, just the opposite problem may develop. At heel-off, the majority of the hip muscles are contracting concentrically to push the limb from the ground; therefore the hip joint must attain a close-pack position to allow the muscle enough momentum to push off. However, if the hip joint cannot attain full close-pack position (the combined movement of internal rotation, extension and abduction), force cannot be equally disseminated across the hip joint and thus excessive pressures can develop leading to hip pain and eventually arthritis.

The presence of anterior or groin pain, pain with weight bearing relieved by rest, limited hip internal rotation (Fig. 20.6) (when comparing the left and right sides), excessive hip external rotation (Fig. 20.7), signs of pelvic obliquity, short hip flexor muscles with the Thomas test and hip muscle weakness also suggest hip joint pain. Birrell et al (2001) or Altman (1987) and Altman et al (1991) criteria and data can be used for those who are unsure in the diagnosis of OA of the hip.

Some have reported a poor relationship between radiological signs of OA of the hip and clinical symptoms (Bierma-Zeinstra et al 2002). This has led some to recommend that in the early and moderate stages of hip OA the diagnosis should be obtained through the clinical examination (Roos 2002). Different studies have been performed to try and help the clinician detect early and moderate OA of the hip. Early detection of hip OA is important in the athlete because it allows for early intervention. Two of the three studies use a composite approach to predict hip joint OA. Age, sex, passive hip range of motion and morning stiffness are the most common variables that are used.

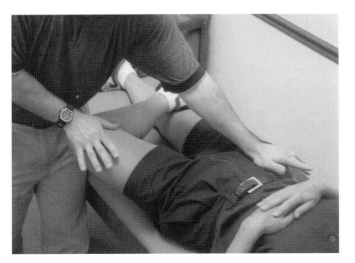

Figure 20.5 • Faber's (Patrick's) test.

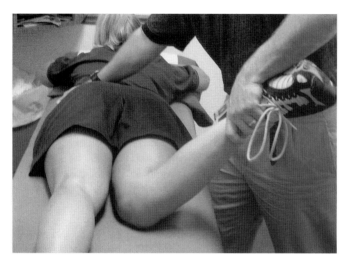

Figure 20.6 • Test for hip internal rotation.

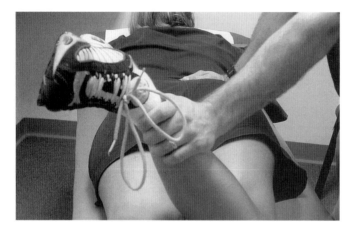

Figure 20.7 • Test for hip external rotation.

There are pros and cons to each of the three different methods used to clinically predict hip joint OA.

Altman et al (1991) developed two clinical criteria for detecting OA of the hip. The first included: hip medial rotation less than 15°, morning stiffness for ⩾60 minutes, age ⩾50 years; the second included: medial rotation less than 15°, an erythrocyte and 45 mm/hour (if no ESR) than hip flexion less than 115°. The reference standard of comparison was radiographic OA including joint space narrowing, presence of osteophytes, cyst formation, subchondral sclerosis, femoral buttressing or remodeling, avascular necrosis and congenital or developmental hip dysplasia. These items were graded as absent, mild, moderate or severe. Osteoarthritis was considered present if each item had a score of 1 or more. The sensitivity for this method was 86%, and specificity was 75%.

More recently Birrell et al (2001) developed a different classification scheme to predict hip joint OA. Using three different passive hip range of motions (flexion, medial and lateral rotation) and a criteria of a minimum joint space of 1.5 mm or less they found that limited hip medial rotation was the best discriminating motion for detecting hip OA and flexion was the least. When one motion was limited the sensitivity was 100%, while the specificity was 69%; when two motions were limited the sensitivity was 81%, and the specificity 69%; with three motions limited the sensitivity was 54%, while the specificity was 88%.

Bierma-Zienstra et al (2002) developed a clinical classification system based on a large number of signs/symptoms determined by history and physical examination and radiological joint space narrowing of ⩽2.5 mm. Signs/symptoms included: age over 60 years, tenderness over the inguinal ligament, decreased lateral rotation, decreased medial rotation, decreased adduction, bony restriction on passive range and muscle weakness of the abductors. On finding five signs/symptoms, the sensitivity was 72% and specificity was 98%; when six signs/symptoms were present the sensitivity was 40% and specificity was 100%; and when finding all seven signs/symptoms present the sensitivity was 8% and specificity was 100%. In the Altman and Bierma-Zienstra studies the use of age as criteria is a major obstacle when trying to diagnose someone who is under the age of 50 with early hip OA. We hope that new criteria will be developed that will be able to overcome this problem. Birrell et al (2001) is clinically useful; however, the confusion comes from trying to interpret guidelines for what is considered the cutoff for limited motion, and this was not clear in the paper. Radiographic measurements especially the measurement of joint space narrowing, especially in more advanced cases, are more accurate as well as specific in making the diagnosis of hip OA (Birrell et al 2001).

Prognosis for hip problems

The prognosis for almost all nonsurgical hip problems in the athlete is very good. Usually hip pain in the young is self-limiting and eventually goes away with or without intervention, especially if activity is restricted. Persistent hip pain in the adult that is related to capsular shortening, diminished range of motion and incongruence, may lead to OA (Grubel Lee 1983, Reynolds & Freeman 1989). Also, those with persistent anteversion of the hip may also be at higher risk for development of hip OA (Halpern et al 1979, Terjesen et al 1982). In nontraumatic conditions, the athlete who develops a femoral head stress fracture is of particular concern. Stress fracture of the femoral head is uncommon but has been described in distance runners who ignore their hip pain (Adkins & Figler 2000, Sterling et al 1993).

Intervention strategies

Strategies for dealing with problems attaining the close-pack position

Problems with the close-pack position include those where the hip cannot achieve the full close-pack position, or congruence, especially during the heel-off portion of the gait when muscles are contracting concentrically. Three major reasons exist for this. First, the joint does not have full range of motion in abduction, extension or medial rotation (in any or all of these movements).

Lack of motion can be due to muscular or capsular problems, or both. The Thomas test can determine if the hip flexor muscles are shortened. Second, muscle strength may not be sufficient to achieve full close-pack, that is, any or all of the hip abductors, hip extensors and hip medial rotator muscles may be weak. Third, the hip may not be able to attain full close-pack range of motion because the pelvis is oblique. Two types of pelvic obliquity can develop, one from a leg length disparity and the second from SIJ dysfunction, as described previously. In all types of pelvic obliquity, the change in acetabular orientation creates a frontal plane shift in the hip joint, on the long leg side, where the hip is adducted; while on the short leg side, the hip is abducted (Gofton 1971, Morscher 1977). In SIJ dysfunction, the hip joint adducts on the posterior tilted side and abducts on the anterior tilted side. Treatment strategies include restoring joint mobility, muscular strength, and eliminating the reason for pelvic obliquity (by leveling leg lengths or treating the SIJ).

Strategies for dealing with problems attaining the loose-pack position

Strategies for achieving a loose-pack position of the hip are just the opposite of those for a close-pack position problem. Problems with loose-pack position include those where the hip cannot achieve the full loose-pack position. The loose-pack position is needed during heel-strike and during the swing phase of the gait. Three major reasons can prevent the hip from gaining the loose-pack position. First, the hip joint has lost some of its range of motion in the direction of adduction, flexion or lateral rotation movements. Lack of motion can be due to muscular or capsular problems, or both. Second, hip muscle strength may not be sufficient to achieve full loose-pack, that is, any or all of the hip abductors, hip flexors and hip lateral rotator muscles may be weak, thus not allowing full loose-pack. Third, the hip may not be able to attain full loose-pack range of motion because the pelvis is oblique. Pelvic obliquity creates hip adduction on the long leg side, while on the short leg side, the hip is abducted (Gofton 1971). In SIJ dysfunction, the hip is adducted on the posterior tilted side and abducted on the anterior tilted side. Treatment strategies are aimed at restoring hip joint mobility, muscular strength and eliminating any pelvic obliquity.

Prevention of recurrent hip pain

The lack of research and data on the recurrence of hip pain helps to explain why the prevention of recurrent hip pain is not very well understood. Some suggest that the persistence of pelvic obliquity is one possible reason for recurrent hip pain (Bjerkreim 1974, Cibulka & Delitto 1993, Halpern et al 1979, Jorring 1980) while Terjesen et al (1982) suggest that increased femoral anteversion is also a predisposing factor in OA of the hip. This factor is similar to unilateral hip rotation asymmetry, which has been shown to be related to anterior and posterior hip pain (Cibulka & Delitto 1993, Cibulka et al 1998). Presumably, anything that does not allow the hip to gain its full close-pack or full loose-pack position may be considered a potential risk factor in the development of recurrent hip pain. Therapists should determine the best course of intervention to insure attainment of full hip range of motion.

Groin injuries in athletes

The groin region, which may also be termed the inguinal area or femoral triangle region, is a common site for athletic injuries. The most common athletic problems in this region include adductor muscle strains (also including gracilis muscle strain), osteitis pubis and, less commonly, hernia. Therapists must be aware of the specific signs and symptoms of each in order to determine a quick referral or an effective treatment for each problem. The groin region consists of the symphysis pubis, described previously, an amphiarthrodial or cartilagenous joint, which has very little movement (2 mm or less normally); the adductor muscles, including the brevis, longus, magnus; the gracilis muscle; and the medial hip flexor muscles, primarily the pectineus, and iliopsoas muscles. The neurology of the groin region is slightly more complex than other regions, owing to the vast amount of different nerves supplying the genitals, as well as the skin, muscles and surrounding joints. The lumbar plexus (L2, L3, L4) gives rise to the iliohypogastric nerve (L1) which supplies a branch (the anterior cutaneous branch) to the skin of the abdomen above the pubis (Warwick & Williams 1973). The ilioinguinal nerve, which also arises from the first lumbar nerve, supplies the skin of the genitals and the skin of the superiomedial area of the thigh (Warwick & Williams 1973), the most common area of groin pain. The genitofemoral nerve supplies the genitals and the area of skin over the upper part of the femoral triangle, just lateral to the groin region.

History

Most of the injuries in and around the groin are traumatic injuries. Muscle strains always have a mechanism of injury. Muscle does not develop fatigue failure like bone, therefore there has to be another reason for the muscle strain. Most commonly, lateral running, skating, jumping or any other quick motion in the frontal plane that requires a forceful contraction of the involved muscle, often while the muscle is also elongating, is the mechanism of muscle injury. As muscle ruptures, it bleeds which results in ecchymosis and, later, the appearance of integumentary contusion. Blood will often migrate distally with the amount of ecchymosis dependent on the degree of muscle injury. Pain from muscle strain is never referred beyond the boundary of the injured muscle; for example, pain from an adductor muscle strain stays within the adductor muscle.

Osteitis pubis is usually characterized by a forceful contraction of the adductor or rectus abdominus muscles (Briggs et al 1992). Adductor muscle strains and osteitis pubis are usually caused by the same adduction motion. The mechanism of injury of osteitis pubis, like adductor muscle strain, includes sudden changes in direction or sprinting (Batt et al 1995). Osteitis pubis is often aggravated by exercise, specifically movements such as running, kicking or pivoting on one leg and is usually relieved by rest (Andrews & Carek 1998). Pain distribution for osteitis pubis can be in several areas including the pubic, groin, lower abdominal, perineal, testicular, suprapubic and inguinal regions (Andrews & Carek 1998). Climbing stairs, coughing or sneezing can create groin symptoms (Andrews & Carek 1998).

Physical examination of the groin region

Examination of the groin includes: examining hip active and passive range of motion, to rule out referred pain from the hip; sacroiliac examination, since Major & Helms (1997) demonstrated that SIJ problems are associated with osteitis pubis; muscle testing (both muscle length and strength) to rule out adductor muscle and abdominal muscle strain; and if no physical impairments are found, examination for possible hernia. Adductor muscle strain (including the gracilis muscle) is tested by examining muscle length and strength. Muscle strains are characterized by reproduction of pain on elongating muscle and on resisted contraction. Thus passive abduction of the hip usually aggravates most adductor muscle strains. Also, resisted muscle contraction of adduction for the adductor muscles, and resisted adduction and knee flexion for the gracilis usually reproduces pain. Lastly palpation is useful as a strained muscle is usually painful when palpated, especially over the anatomical location of the strain (Box 20.3).

Osteitis pubis is characterized by pubic tenderness and pain with active hip abduction. Osteitis pubis is the most common inflammatory condition affecting the symphysis pubis (Andrews & Carek 1998). Adductor muscle strain must be ruled out when osteitis pubis is considered. Williams et al (2001) suggests that radiographic examination (using a flamingo view) that shows more than 2 mm vertical displacement would indicate pubic symphysis instability.

Treatment

Treatment of adductor muscle strains includes restoring adductor muscle length and strength. Initially, like all acute injuries, the area is treated with ice, elevation and compression and avoidance of activities that aggravate the pain. Once symptoms subside, gentle stretching exercises to the involved muscle can begin. As the muscle regains approximately 75% of its length, muscle strengthening exercises follow. The goal in the rehabilitation of injured muscle is to restore the full length and strength of the injured muscle. Additional physical modalities can be used to hasten the rehabilitation process. Later, once muscle length and strength is restored, sport-specific training can begin.

Treatment of osteitis pubis is usually in the form of symptomatic relief, with physical modalities, rest and anti-inflammatory medications; surgery is rarely indicated and reserved only for those whose symptoms are not relieved by conservative therapy (Vincent 1993).

Summary

This chapter demonstrates the complexity of the anatomy around the pelvis, hip and groin area. A thorough knowledge of the anatomical structures and their relationship to each other is necessary to accurately diagnose pain and injuries in this region. When considering treatment options for such injuries, the nature of the sport or exercise activity that the athlete is involved in should be considered, and appropriate biomechanical analysis of movements carried out. In managing injuries in this region both manual and exercise treatment should be combined with biomechanical correction of movement patterns.

References

Aalam M, Hoffman P 1975 Deterioration of the ilio-sacral joints through serious unilateral hip joint disease. Archiv fur Orthopadische und Unfall-Chirurgie 82:257–262

Adkins S B 3rd, Figler R A 2000 Hip pain in athletes. American Family Physician 61:2109–2118

Alderink G J 1991 The sacroiliac joint: review of anatomy, mechanics, and function. Journal of Orthopaedic and Sports Physical Therapy 13:71–84

Altman R D 1987 Criteria for the classification of osteoarthritis of the knee and hip. Scandinavian Journal of Rheumatology 65 (suppl):31–39

Altman R D, Alarcon G, Appelrouth D et al 1991 The American College of Rheumatology criteria for the classification and reporting of osteoarthritis of the hip. Arthritis and Rheumatism 34:505–514

Andrews S K, Carek P J 1998 Osteitis pubis: a diagnosis for the family physician. Journal of the American Board of Family Practice 11:291–295

Barakatt E, Smidt G L, Dawson J D et al 1996 Interinnominate motion and symmetry: comparison between gymnast and nongymnast. Journal of Orthopaedic and Sports Physical Therapy 23:309–319

Batt M E, McShane J M, Dillingham M F 1995 Osteitis pubis in collegiate football players. Medicine and Science in Sports and Exercise 27:629–633

Beal M C 1982 The sacroiliac problem: review of anatomy, mechanics, and diagnosis. Journal of the American Osteopathic Association 81:667–679

Bernard T N, Cassidy J 1991 The sacroiliac joint syndrome: pathophysiology, diagnosis, and management. In: Frymoyer J W (ed) The adult spine: principle and practice. Raven Press, New York

Bierma-Zeinstra S M, Oster J D, Bernsen R M et al 2002 Joint space narrowing and relationship with symptoms and signs in adults consulting for hip pain in primary care. Journal of Rheumatology 29:1713–1718

Birrell F, Croft P, Cooper C et al 2001 Predicting radiographic hip osteoarthritis from range of movement. Rheumatology 40:506–512

Bjerkreim I 1974 Secondary dysplasia and osteoarthrosis of the hip in functional and fixed obliquity of the pelvis. Acta Orthopaedica Scandinavica 45:873–882

Bourdillon J F, Day E A 1987 Spinal manipulation. William Heinemann Medical, London

---

> **Box 20.3** Diagnosis of groin muscle strain
>
> 1. Described mechanism of muscle injury
> 2. Pain localized only to the muscle itself, no radiation of pain
> 3. Pain on palpation of the injured muscle
> 4. Pain on elongation of the injured muscle
> 5. Pain on contraction of the injured muscle

Borrel U, Fernestrom I 1957 The movements of the sacro-iliac joints and their importance to changes on pelvic dimensions during parturition. Acta Obstetrica Gynecologica Scandinavica 36:42–57

Briggs R C, Kolbjornsen P H, Southall R C 1992 Osteitis pubis, Tc-99m MDP, and professional hockey players. Clinical Nuclear Medicine 17:861–863

Broadhurst N A 1989 Sacroiliac joint dysfunction as a cause of low back pain. Australian Family Physician 18:626–627

Broadhurst N A, Bond M J 1998 Pain provocation tests for the assessment of sacroiliac joint dysfunction. Journal of Spinal Disorders 11:341–345

Brunner C, Kissling R, Jacob H 1991 The effects of morphology and histopathology. Spine 16:1111–1117

Buchowski J M, Kebaish K M, Sinkov V et al 2005 Functional and radiographic outcome of sacroiliac arthrodesis for the disorders of the sacroiliac joint. Spine Journal 5:520–528, discussion 529

Bullough P, Goodfellow J, O'Conner J 1973 The relationship between degenerative changes and load bearing in the human hip. Journal of Bone and Joint Surgery (Br) 55B:746–758

Calvillo O, Skaribas I, Turnispeed J 2000 Anatomy and pathophysiology of the sacroiliac joint. Current Reviews in Pain 4:356–361

Chamberlain W E 1930 The symphysis pubis in the roentgen examination of the sacroiliac joint. American Journal of Roentgenology 24:621–624

Childs J D, Fritz J M, Flynn T W et al 2004 A clinical prediction rule to identify patients with low back pain most likely to benefit from spinal manipulation: a validation study. Annals of Internal Medicine 141:920–928

Cibulka M T 1992 The treatment of the sacroiliac joint component to low back pain: a case report. Physical Therapy 72:917–922

Cibulka M T, Delitto A 1993 A comparison of two different methods to treat hip pain in runners. Journal of Orthopaedic and Sports Physical Therapy 17:172–176

Cibulka M T, Koldehoff R M 1999 Clinical usefulness of a cluster of sacroiliac joint tests in patients with and without low back pain. Journal of Orthopaedic and Sports Physical Therapy 29:83–92

Cibulka M T, Rose S J, Delitto A et al 1986 Hamstring muscle strain treated by mobilizing the sacroiliac joint. Physical Therapy 66(8):1220–1223

Cibulka M T, Delitto A, Koldehoff R M 1988 Changes in innominate tilt after manipulation of the sacroiliac joint in patients with low back pain: an experimental study. Physical Therapy 68:1359–1363

Cibulka M T, Erhard R E, Delitto A 1992 Pain patterns in patients with and without sacroiliac joint dysfunction. In: Vleeming A, Mooney V, Snijders C et al (eds) Proceedings of the First Interdisciplinary World Congress on Low Back Pain and its Relation to the Sacroiliac Joint. San Diego, CA

Cibulka M T, Sinacore D R, Cromer G S et al 1998 Unilateral hip rotation range of motion asymmetry in patients with sacroiliac joint regional pain. Spine 23:1009–1015

Colachis S C, Warden R E, Bechtol C O et al 1963 Movement of the sacroiliac joint in the adult male: a preliminary report. Archives of Physical Medicine and Rehabilitation 44:490–498

Cummings G, Scholz J P, Barnes K 1993 The effect of imposed leg length difference on pelvic bone symmetry. Spine 18:368–373

Damen L, Buyruk H M, Guler-Uysal F et al 2001 Pelvic pain during pregnancy is associated with asymmetric laxity of the sacroiliac joints. Acta Obstetricia et Gynecologica Scandinavica 80:1019–1024

Damen L, Buyruk H M, Guler-Uysal F et al 2002a The prognostic value of asymmetric laxity of the sacroiliac joints in pregnancy-related pelvic pain. Spine 27:2820–2824

Damen L, Stijnen T, Roebroeck M E et al 2002b Reliability of sacroiliac joint laxity measurement with Doppler imaging of vibrations. Ultrasound in Medicine and Biology 28:407–414

Death A B, Kirby R I, MacMillan C L 1982 Pelvic ring mobility: assessment by stress radiography. Archives of Physical Medicine and Rehabilitation 63:129–135

Dee R 1969 Structure and function of hip joint innervation. Annals of the College of Surgeons England 45:357–374

Delitto A, Shulman A D, Rose S J 1992 Reliability of a clinical examination to classify patients with low back syndrome. Physical Therapy Practice 1:1–9

Diamond G A, Forrester J S 1979 Analysis of probability as an aid in the clinical diagnosis of coronary artery disease. New England Journal of Medicine 300:1350–1358

DonTigny R L 1979 Dysfunction of the sacroiliac joint and its treatment. Journal of Orthopaedic and Sports Physical Therapy 1:23–35

DonTigny R L 1985 Function and pathomechanics of the sacroiliac joint, a review. Physical Therapy 65:35–44

Dorrell J H, Catterall A 1986 The torn acetabular labrum. Journal of Bone and Joint Surgery (Br) 68B:400–403

Dreyfuss P, Dreyer S, Griffin J 1994 Positive sacroiliac screening tests in the asymptomatic adults. Spine 19:1138–1143

Dreyfuss P, Michaelsen D C, Pauza K et al 1996 The value of medical history and physical examination in diagnosing sacroiliac joint pain. Spine 21:2594–2602

Egund N, Olsson T H, Schmid H et al 1978 Movements in the sacroiliac joints demonstrated with roentgen stereophotogrammetry. Acta Radiologica Diagnostica 19:833–846

Erhard R, Bowling R 1977 The recognition and management of the pelvic component of low back pain and sciatica pain. Bulletin of the Orthopaedic Section, American Physical Therapy Association 2:4–15

Erhard R E, Delitto A, Cibulka M T 1994 Relative effectiveness of an extension program and a combined program of manipulation and flexion and extension exercises in patients with acute low back syndrome. Physical Therapy 74:1093–1100

Fortin J, Aprill C N, Ponthieux R T et al 1994 Sacroiliac joint: pain referral maps upon applying a new injection/arthrography technique: II. Clinical evaluation. Spine 19:1483–1489

Freburger J K, Riddle D L 2001 Using published evidence to guide the examination of the sacroiliac joint region. Physical Therapy 81:1135–1143

Friedland D J, Go S A, Davoren J B et al 1998 Evidence-base medicine. A framework for clinical practice. Appleton and Lange, Stamford, CT

Frigerio N A, Stowe R R, Howe J W 1974 Movement of the sacroiliac joint. Clinical Orthopaedics and Related Research 100:370–377

Fritz J M, George S 2000 The use of a classification approach to identify subgroups of patients with acute low back pain. Spine 25:106–114

Gofton J P 1971 Studies in osteoarthrosis of the hip: II. Osteoarthrosis of the hip and leg length disparity. Canadian Medical Association Journal 104:791–799

Goldthwaite J E, Osgood R B 1905 A consideration of the pelvic articulation from an anatomical, pathological and clinical standpoint. Boston Medical and Surgical Journal 152:593–601

Grubel Lee D M 1983 Disorders of the hip. JB Lippincott, Philadelphia, PA

Halpern A A, Tanner J, Rinsky L 1979 Does persistent fetal femoral anteversion contribute to osteoarthritis. Clinical Orthopaedics and Related Research 145:213–215

Hart J J 1996 Transient synovitis of the hip in children. American Family Physician 54:1587–1591

Haufe S M, Mork A R 2005 Sacroiliac joint debridement: a novel technique for the treatment of sacroiliac joint pain. Photomedicine and Laser Surgery 23:596–598

Hebling R 1978 The sacroiliac joint after hip arthrodesis. Zeitschrift fur Orthopadie 116:113–23

Janos S C 1992 Palpation of selected bony landmarks in the lumbopelvic region. In: Proceedings of the International Federation of Orthopaedic Manipulative Therapists, Fifth International Conference, Vail, CO

Jorring K 1980 Osteoarthritis of the hip, epidemiology and clinical role. Acta Orthopaedica Scandinavica 51:523–530

Kampen W U, Tillmann B 1998 Age-related changes in the articular cartilage of human sacroiliac joints. Anatomy and Embryology (Berlin) 198:505–513

Kapandji I A 1970 Physiology of the Joints, 2nd edn, vol 2. Churchill Livingstone, London

Khan N Q, Woolson S T 1998 Referral patterns of hip pain in patients undergoing total hip replacement. Orthopedics 21(2):123–126

LaBan M M, Meerschaert J R, Taylor R S et al 1978 Symphyseal and sacroiliac joint pain associated with pubic symphysis instability. Archives of Physical Medicine and Rehabilitation 59:470–472

Laslett M, Williams M 1994 The reliability of selected pain provocation tests for sacroiliac joint pathology. Spine 19:1243–1249

Laslett M, Aprill C N, McDonald B et al 2005 Diagnosis of sacroiliac joint pain: validity of individual provocation tests and composites of tests. Manual Therapy 10:207–218

Lavignolle B, Vital J M, Senegas J et al 1983 An approach to the functional anatomy of the sacroiliac joints in vivo. Anatomica Clinica 5:169–176

Lee D 1989 The pelvic girdle. Churchill Livingstone, Edinburgh

Levangie P K 1999 Four clinical tests of sacroiliac joint dysfunction: the association of test results with innominate torsion among patients with and without low back pain. Physical Therapy 79:1043–1057

Loyd-Roberts G C 1953 The role of the capsular changes in osteoarthritis of the hip joint. Journal of Bone and Joint Surgery (Br) 35B:627–642

MacConaill M A, Basmajian J V 1977 Muscles and movements. Robert E. Krieger, Huntington, NY

Maigne J, Aivaliklis A, Pfefer F 1996 Results of sacroiliac joint double block and value of sacroiliac joint pain provocation tests in 54 patients with low back pain. Spine 15:1889–1892

Major N M, Helms C A 1997 Pelvis stress injuries: the relationship between osteitis pubis (symphysis pubis stress injury) and sacroiliac joint abnormalities in athletes. Skeletal Radiology 26:711–717

Matanovic B, Granic-Husic M 1991 Degenerative changes in the sacroiliac joint in persons with amputations of the thigh and biomechanical disorders of gait. Reumatizam 38:9–13

Mennell J M 1960 Back pain: diagnosis and treatment using manipulative techniques. Little, Brown, Boston, MA

Mens J M, Vleeming A, Snijders C J et al 2002 Responsiveness of outcome measurements in rehabilitation of patients with posterior pelvic pain since pregnancy. Spine 27:1110–1115

Mitchell F L, Moran P S, Pruzzo N A 1979 An evaluation and treatment manual of osteopathic muscle energy technique procedures. Mitchell, Moran and Pruzzo, Valley Park, MO

Morscher E 1977 Progress in orthopaedic surgery 1. In: Hungerford DS (ed) Leg length discrepancy: the injured knee. Springer-Verlag, Berlin

O'Kane J W 1999 Anterior hip pain. American Family Physician 60:1687–1696

Oldrieve W L 1996 A critical review of the literature on the anatomy and biomechanics of the sacroiliac joint. Journal of Manual and Manipulative Therapy 4:157–165

Oldrieve W L 1998 A classification of, and a critical review of the literature on, syndromes of the sacroiliac joint. Journal of Manual and Manipulative Therapy 6:24–30

Pap A, Maager M, Kolarz G 1987 Functional impairment of the sacroiliac joint after total hip replacement. International Rehabilitation Medicine 8:145–147

Pauwels F 1976 Biomechanics of the normal and diseased hip. Springer-Verlag, Berlin

Pitkin H C, Pheasant, H C 1936 Sacroarthrogenetic telagia. Journal of Bone and Joint Surgery (Am) 18A:111–133

Pool-Goudzwaard A L, Vleeming A, Stoeckart R et al 1998 Insufficient lumbopelvic stability: a clinical, anatomical and biomechanical approach to 'a-specific' low back pain. Manual Therapy 3:12–20

Porterfield J A, DeRosa C 1990 The sacroiliac joint. In: Gould J A (ed) Orthopaedic and sports physical therapy. CV Mosby, St Louis, MO

Porterfield J A, DeRosa C P 1991 Mechanical low back pain: perspectives in functional anatomy. WB Saunders, Philadelphia, PA

Potter N A, Rothstein J M 1985 Intertester reliability for selected clinical tests of the sacroiliac joint. Physical Therapy 65:1671–1675

Reynolds D, Freeman M 1989 Osteoarthritis of the young adult hip. Churchill Livingstone, Edinburgh

Roberts W N, Williams R B 1988 Hip Pain. Primary Care 15:783–793

Roos E 2002 [Clinical criteria best foundation for diagnosis of mild to moderate arthritis. Symptoms, not radiological results, dictate choice of treatment]. Lakartidningen 99:4362–4364

Sackett D L, Haynes R B, Tugwell P 1985 Clinical epidemiology. A basic science for clinical medicine. Little Brown, Boston, MA

Sackett D L, Richardson W S, Rosenberg W et al 1998 Evidence-based medicine. How to practice and teach EBM. Churchill Livingstone, Edinburgh

Sasabili N, Valojerdy M R, Hogg D A 1995 Variation in thickness of articular cartilage in the human sacroiliac joint. Clinical Anatomy 8:388–390

Sashin D 1930 A critical analysis of the anatomy and the pathological changes of the sacroiliac joint. Journal of Bone and Joint Surgery (Am) 12A:891–910

Schunke G 1938 The anatomy and development of the sacroiliac joint in man. Anatomical Record 72:313–331

Schwarzer A C, Aprill C N, Bogduk M 1995 The sacroiliac joint in chronic low back pain. Spine 20:31–37

Shaw J L 1992 The role of the sacroiliac joint as a cause of low back pain and dysfunction. In: Vleeming A, Mooney V, Snijders C et al (eds) Proceedings of the First Interdisciplinary World Congress on Low Back Pain and its Relation to the Sacroiliac Joint, San Diego, CA

Smidt G L, McQuade K, Wei S H et al 1995 Sacroiliac kinematics for reciprocal straddle positions. Spine 20:1047–1054

Smidt G L, Wei S H, McQuade K et al 1997 Sacroiliac motion for extreme hip positions. A fresh cadaver study. Spine 22:2073–2082

Solonen K A 1957 The sacro-iliac joint in the light of anatomical, roentgenological and clinical studies. Acta Orthopaedica Scandinavica 27 (suppl):1–27

Sterling J C, Webb R F, Meyers M C et al 1993 False negative bone scan in a female runner. Medicine and Science in Sports and Exercise 25:179–185

Stoddard A 1959 Manual of osteopathic technique. Hutchinson, London

Sturesson B, Selvik G, Uden A 1989 Movements of the sacroiliac joint. A roentgen stereophotogrammetric analysis. Spine 14:162–165

Sturesson B, Uden A, Vleeming A 2000 A radiostereometric analysis of the movement of sacroiliac joints in the reciprocal straddle position. Spine 25:214–217

Terjesen T, Benum P, Anda S et al 1982 Increased femoral anteversion and osteoarthritis of the hip joint. Acta Orthopaedica Scandinavica 53:571–575

Tullberg T, Blomberg S, Branth B et al 1998 Manipulation does not alter the position of the sacroiliac joint. A roentgen stereophotogrammetric analysis. Spine 23:1124–1128

Vincent C 1993 Osteitis pubis. Journal of the American Board of Family Practice 6:492–496

van Wingerden J P, Vleeming A, Buyruk H M et al 2004 Stabilization of the sacroiliac joint in vivo: verification of muscular contribution to force closure of the pelvis. European Spine Journal 13:199–205

Vleeming A, Stoeckart R, Volkers A C et al 1990a Relation between form and function in the sacroiliac joint: I. Clinical anatomical aspects. Spine 15:130–132

Vleeming A, Volkers A C, Snijders C J et al 1990b Relation between form and function in the sacroiliac joint: II. Biomechanical aspects. Spine 15:133–136

Vleeming A, Snijders C J, Stoeckart R et al 1997 The role of the sacroiliac joints in coupling between spine, pelvis, legs, and arms. Churchill Livingstone, New York

Walheim G G, Selvik F 1984 Mobility of the pubis symphysis. In vivo measurements with an electromechanic method and a roentgen stereophotogrammetric method. Clinical Orthopaedics and Related Research 191:129–135

Walheim G G, Olerud S, Ribbe T 1984 Mobility of the pubis symphysis. Measurements by an electromechanical method. Acta Orthopaedica Scandinavica 55:203–208

Walker J M 1992 The sacroiliac joint. A critical review. Physical Therapy 72:903–916

Walmsley T 1928 The articular mechanism of the diarthrosis. Journal of Bone and Joint Surgery (Am) 10A:40–45

Warwick R, Williams P 1973 Gray's anatomy, 35th British edn. WB Saunders, Philadelphia, PA

Weisl H 1954 The ligaments of the sacro-iliac joint examined with particular reference to function. Acta Anatomica 20:201–213

Weisl H 1955a The articular surfaces of the sacro-iliac joint and their relation to the movement of the sacrum. Acta Anatomica 23:80–91

Weisl H 1955b The movement of the sacro-iliac joint. Acta Anatomica 23:80–91

Wells P E 1986 The examination of the pelvic joints. In: Grieve G P (ed) Modern manual therapy of the vertebral column. Churchill Livingstone, Edinburgh

Wilder D G, Pope M H, Frymoyer J W 1980 The functional topography of the sacroiliac joint. Spine 5:575–579

Williams P R, Thomas D P, Downes E M 2000 Osteitis pubis and instability of the pubic symphysis. When nonoperative measures fail. American Journal of Sports Medicine 28:350–355

Woerman A L 1989 Evaluation and treatment of dysfunction in the lumbar-pelvic-hip complex In: Donatelli R, Wooden M J (eds) Orthopedic physical therapy. Churchill Livingstone, Edinburgh

Knee

Terese L. Chmielewski, Susan M. Tillman and
Lynn Snyder-Mackler

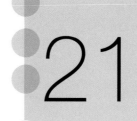

CHAPTER CONTENTS

Introduction 382
Anatomy and biomechanics 382
Knee examination 384
Rehabilitation of common sports-related injuries. . . . 389
Rehabilitation of less common injuries 394
Summary 398

Introduction

The knee joint is a common site for sports injuries, particularly ligamentous injuries, because ligaments contribute a great deal to knee joint stability. A solid knowledge of knee anatomy and biomechanics is necessary to properly assess the injury and devise a rehabilitation program that creates the best environment for healing. Criterion-based rehabilitation protocols are used because they outline milestones that must be met for progression, eliminating subjectivity in clinical decision-making. The rate of progression can differ between athletes and is dependent on the individual rate of healing and the demands of the athlete's activity level. Within each phase of the rehabilitation protocol, clinicians must choose therapeutic exercises that gradually introduce stresses to the healing tissue and that are tailored to preparing the athlete to return to the demands of the sport. Only after completing all phases of rehabilitation and meeting functional testing criteria are athletes allowed to return to sport activities.

Anatomy and biomechanics

Bony structure

The tibiofemoral joint is created by the interface of the distal femur and proximal tibia. The distal femur is characterized by two bony prominences, the medial and lateral condyles, which are separated by an intercondylar notch. Both condyles are rounded inferiorly and project posteriorly, but the medial femoral condylar projection is longer. The longer projection of the medial femoral condyle partially dictates the biomechanics of the knee joint. The greater surface area of the medial condyle requires greater accessory motion in the medial half of the knee in comparison to the lateral half. Thus, when the knee is flexed, the tibiofemoral joint undergoes a small but significant amount of internal rotation to sustain congruency between the condyles. When the knee approaches full extension, the tibiofemoral joint undergoes a subsequent external rotation, as the medial aspect of the knee must exhibit greater motion to maintain joint congruency.

When viewed from above, the proximal tibia appears flattened with a raised central region that divides the surface into medial and lateral components. The central region is known as the intercondylar region, or tibial eminence, and serves as a ligamentous attachment site. The tibial eminence protrudes into the corresponding intercondylar notch of the femur. On either side of the tibial eminence lie the medial and lateral tibial plateaus. The tibial plateaus articulate with their respective femoral condyles.

Surrounding the tibiofemoral joint is a joint capsule, which runs along the femoral condyles proximally and attaches distally around the circumference of the tibia. The joint capsule travels more superiorly on the anterior aspect of the femur and much closer to the joint line as it moves posteriorly. The capsule is deficient posteriorly at the lateral femoral condyle to allow passage of the popliteus tendon. The knee joint capsule is lined with a synovial membrane that surrounds, but does not encompass, the cruciate ligaments. The anterosuperior projection of the synovial membrane is called the suprapatellar pouch. On the posterior aspect of the knee, the synovium projection is not as extensive, as it is dictated by the capsular insertion closer to the joint line.

Slightly distal to the lateral aspect of the tibial plateau is the proximal tibiofibular joint, composed of the fibular head and the fibular notch located on the lateral tibia. This articulation is mentioned here due to its proximity to the tibiofemoral joint. The tibiofibular joint has its own joint capsule and is not continuous with the tibiofemoral joint.

Ligaments

Ligaments of the tibiofemoral joint serve to provide structural stability and to guide knee motion. The ligaments can be subclassified as capsular, intracapsular and extracapsular, based on the relationship of the ligament to the joint capsule. Capsular ligaments are distinct thickenings of the joint capsule, intracapsular ligaments are located within the joint capsule and extracapsular ligaments are located outside of the joint capsule. The medial collateral ligament (MCL), posterior oblique ligament (POL) and arcuate ligament are all capsular ligaments of the tibiofemoral joint. The lateral collateral ligament (LCL) is a capsular ligament at its superior end; however, distally it is extracapsular. The anterior cruciate ligament (ACL), posterior cruciate ligament (PCL) and meniscofemoral ligaments are all intracapsular ligaments.

The MCL is located on the medial aspect of the knee and is composed of both superficial and deep fibers (Fig. 21.1). The superficial fibers of the MCL extend from the medial femoral condyle, anterior to the adductor tubercle, to the anteromedial aspect of the tibial plateau. The deep fibers of the MCL travel from the same origin to insert onto the medial meniscus. On the posteromedial aspect of the knee lies the POL, which originates from the adductor tubercle and inserts onto the posterior aspect of the capsule.

On the lateral side of the knee joint, the LCL courses between the lateral femoral condyle and the fibular head (Fig. 21.1). The arcuate ligament arises from the posterior fibular head and spans the posterolateral aspect of the knee, inserting on the intercondylar region of the tibia and the posterior region of the lateral femoral condyle (Fig. 21.2). The LCL, the arcuate

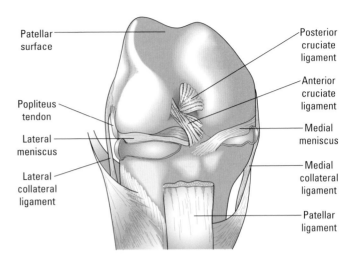

Figure 21.1 • Anterior view of the knee with the patella removed.

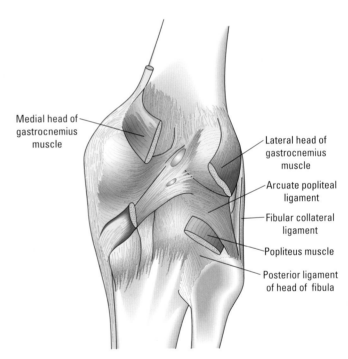

Figure 21.2 • Posterior view of the knee.

ligament, the popliteus tendon and the lateral head of the gastrocnemius are collectively considered the arcuate complex.

The ACL originates on the posteromedial aspect of the lateral femoral condyle and inserts on the tibial ridge of the tibial plateau (Fig. 21.1). The ACL is composed of fascicles that can be divided into two bundles: an anteromedial bundle and a posterolateral bundle. The significance of the bundles is that they each are taut in different portions of the range of motion, allowing tension to be produced in the ACL throughout the entire range. The posterolateral bundle is taut when the knee is extended, whereas the anteromedial bundle becomes tight as the knee is flexed.

The PCL has a more vertical orientation, originating on the medial aspect of the intercondylar notch and inserting on the tibial ridge of the tibial plateau, just posterior to the ACL (Fig. 21.1). The PCL is comprised of two bundles, an anterolateral bundle and a posteromedial bundle. Similar to the ACL, the bundles are tight in reciprocal fashion. The anterolateral bundle becomes tight when the knee is flexed, and the posteromedial bundle is tight with knee extension.

The meniscofemoral ligaments, the ligament of Humphries and the ligament of Wrisberg are accessory ligaments that surround and augment the PCL (Heller & Langman 1964). These ligaments are variably present; however, at least one ligament has been found in 70–100% of knees (Girgis et al 1975, Heller & Langman 1964). When present, these ligaments are located in the intercondylar notch, forming an attachment between the posterior horn of the lateral meniscus and the lateral border of the medial femoral condyle. The ligament of Humphries is located anterior to the PCL, and the ligament of Wrisberg is located posteriorly.

Menisci

The menisci, located on the surface of the tibial plateaus (Fig. 21.1), are vascularized by the genicular arteries at birth; however, this vascularity recedes with increasing age until only the peripheral 10–30% is vascularized (Arnoczky & Warren 1982, Clark & Ogden 1983). The menisci are slightly concave superiorly, increasing the congruity between the tibia and femur interface, and creating a greater contact area for distribution of joint load. The menisci further assist in load transmission during weight bearing through their compression.

Medial and lateral menisci have differing amounts of movement during knee motion. Both menisci are secured to the anterior tibial plateau through attachments called coronary ligaments. The medial meniscus, however, has firm attachments through extensions of the joint capsule, whereas the capsular attachments to the lateral meniscus are less firm. Consequently, the medial meniscus translates about 2–5 mm on the tibial plateau in an anterior–posterior direction during knee motion, and the lateral meniscus about 9–11 mm (Fu & Baratz 1994).

The location of femoral contact on the menisci changes during knee motion. With increasing knee flexion, there is greater contact on the posterior part, or posterior horn, of the mensici. Conversely, as the knee moves into extension, the femur contacts the anterior aspect, or anterior horn (Fu & Baratz 1994).

Knee examination

General guidelines

Every knee examination begins with a patient interview during which information is gathered about the mechanism of injury and the location and severity of pain. The patient interview assists the clinician in generating a hypothesis about which anatomical structure has been injured. This hypothesis guides the examination, helping the examiner avoid superfluous testing and aiding the development of the examination sequence. Tests that may provoke pain in the structure hypothesized to be injured are typically performed near the end of the evaluation because pain can cause muscle guarding which, in turn, can confound the results of subsequent testing procedures.

In most sport injury evaluations, three basic principles can be used to improve the accuracy and validity of the physical examination. First, the patient should be positioned comfortably during the examination. If the patient is not relaxed, muscle contraction may obviate proper technique during testing maneuvers. Second, the knee examination tests should be performed on the contralateral side before testing the injured side. Testing the contralateral side first reveals the amount of inherent laxity to form a baseline against which the injured side can be compared. Also, patients are more likely to be relaxed when they know what to expect during testing. Finally, examination tests must isolate a structure to conclusively test the integrity of the structure. Structures that contribute the majority of the restraint against a force in a given direction are called primary restraints. Secondary restraints are structures that contribute less to counteracting forces in a specific direction or provide significant restraint only after the primary restraint is injured. The most sensitive examination procedure is one in which the tested structure is the primary restraint.

Many knee examination tests are designed to assess the integrity of a ligament. A positive ligamentous test is indicated either by pain in the ligament when force is applied, or an increase in laxity compared to the uninjured side. The examiner may also evaluate ligament integrity by the quality of the end feel in comparison to the other side.

Grading scales are often used to allow clinicians to communicate information about the severity of ligament compromise. A scale that assigns a grade based on the amount of laxity during testing is grade 1+ = 0–5 mm, grade 2+ = 5–10 mm and grade 3+ = 10–15 mm (Hughston & Andrews 1976). The principal consideration concerning grading scales is that clinicians that work together must use a common scale to ensure clear communication.

Ligament testing

Medial collateral ligament

The medial collateral ligament (MCL) is best suited to protect the knee against valgus forces because of its location on the medial side of the knee. When the knee is in full extension, the superficial and deep portions of the MCL share the role of primary restraint against valgus stress (Grood et al 1981, Inoue et al 1987). With the knee in 30° of flexion, the superficial portion of the MCL, the portion most commonly injured, is the primary restraint (Grood et al 1981).

To perform a valgus stress test, the patient is positioned supine with the leg to be tested near the edge of the examining table (Fig. 21.3). The examiner faces the patient, supporting the lateral aspect of the distal femur and the medial aspect

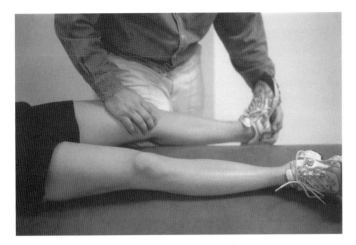

Figure 21.3 • Valgus stress test for the knee.

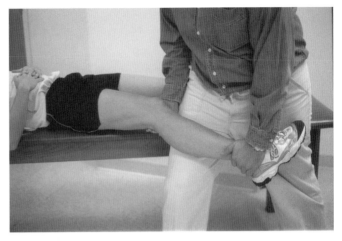

Figure 21.4 • Varus stress test for the knee.

of the distal tibia, with the knee joint in approximately 30° of flexion. The distal femur is held in position while a laterally directed force is applied to the distal tibia, producing a valgus force at the knee joint. Pain with application of the valgus force or increased joint laxity compared to the uninjured side is considered a positive test.

Posterior oblique ligament

The posterior oblique ligament (POL) contributes to resisting valgus stress when the knee is extended, and becomes slack when the knee is in 30° of flexion (Grood et al 1981). External rotation of the tibia moves the POL from a posteromedial position to nearly a pure medial arrangement. Once the POL is in this medial position, applying a valgus stress with the knee in extension can test POL integrity. Similar to the valgus stress test, pain with application of the valgus force or increased joint laxity compared to the uninjured side is considered a positive test.

Lateral collateral ligament

The lateral collateral ligament (LCL) is well suited to resist varus forces at the knee secondary to its lateral location. At full knee extension, the LCL shares the protective role with the arcuate complex (Gollehon et al 1987, Grood et al 1981); however, as the knee becomes more flexed, the LCL becomes a primary restraint (Grood et al 1981).

For varus stress testing, the patient is positioned supine, with the test leg close to the edge of the table (Magee 2002). The examiner faces the patient and abducts the leg to allow the examiner to stand between the edge of the table and the test leg (Fig. 21.4). The distal femur is supported medially, and the distal tibia is supported laterally, with the knee flexed to approximately 30°. While firmly stabilizing the femur, the examiner applies a medially directed force to the distal tibia to produce varus force at the knee joint. An alternate way to perform this test, in order to improve femur stabilization, is to hold the distal femur against the edge of the table while applying the force at the distal tibia, using the edge of the table as a fulcrum to cause a varus stress at the knee joint.

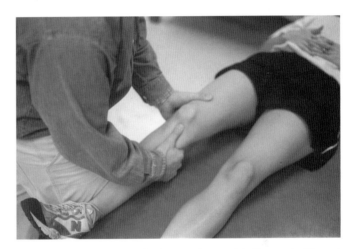

Figure 21.5 • Lachman test for the anterior cruciate ligament of the knee.

Anterior cruciate ligament

The anterior cruciate ligament (ACL) is the primary restraint against anterior displacement of the tibia on the femur. With the knee flexed to 30°, the ACL provides 87% of the restraint against anterior displacement (Butler et al 1980). In addition, the ACL acts as a secondary restraint for valgus stress at full extension (Inoue et al 1987, Markolf et al 1990).

Many tests have been described to test the integrity of the ACL. The Lachman test has been found to have both high sensitivity (80–99%) and specificity (85%) for testing the ACL (Liu et al 1995, Malanga et al 2003). To perform a Lachman test, the patient is positioned supine (Magee 1992). The examiner stands facing the patient, supporting the lateral aspect of the distal femur and grasping the medial aspect of the proximal tibia, keeping the knee flexed to approximately 20° (Fig. 21.5). The examiner then pulls the proximal tibia anteriorly, keeping the femur stabilized. If the femur is adequately stabilized, the applied stress will be localized to the knee. A positive test is indicated by increased anterior tibial translation compared to

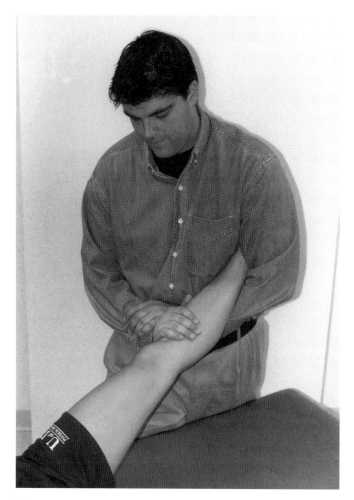

Figure 21.6 • Pivot shift test for the anterior cruciate ligament of the knee.

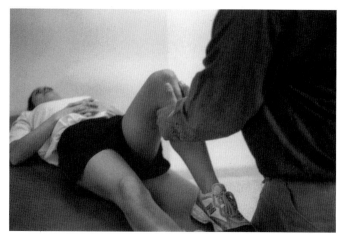

Figure 21.7 • Posterior drawer test for the posterior cruciate ligament of the knee.

caused by the pull of the iliotibial band, which becomes a knee flexor at approximately 20° of flexion.

Posterior cruciate ligament

The posterior cruciate ligament (PCL) is the primary restraint to posterior displacement of the tibia on the femur (Fukubayashi et al 1982, Gollehon et al 1987). The PCL additionally acts as a secondary restraint to varus stress at 0° and 30° knee flexion (Gollehon et al 1987).

Injury to the PCL can be assessed by many tests. One test is called the posterior drawer (Veltri & Warren 1993). To perform the posterior drawer test, the patient is positioned supine with the knee flexed to 90° (Fig. 21.7). The examiner grasps the proximal tibia with both hands, with the thumbs on the anterior aspect of the tibia, and applies a posteriorly directed force. Position of the tibial condyles and the amount of laxity are compared to the uninjured side, and increased laxity on the injured side indicates a positive test. The posterior drawer test is associated with both high sensitivity and specificity (Malanga et al 2003).

Another test with high sensitivity and specificity for diagnosing a PCL tear is the posterior sag test (Malanga et al 2003, Veltri & Warren 1993). For this test, the patient is positioned supine while the examiner passively flexes the hips and knees to 90°. To maintain the 90–90 position, the examiner either cradles the distal tibia or places the patient's foot on a chair of appropriate height. If the tibial tubercle on the injured side is less prominent than the tibial tubercle on the uninvolved side, the test is considered positive. The 'sag', or posterior displacement, of the tibia during this test is a consequence of gravitational pull.

The third test commonly used to assess PCL integrity is the quadriceps active test (Veltri & Warren 1993). The patient is positioned supine with the knee flexed to approximately 90°. The examiner stabilizes the patient's foot on the examining table and instructs the patient to try to extend the knee. This will result in an isometric contraction of the quadriceps. If there is PCL compromise, the posteriorly subluxed tibia will be

the uninjured side and a 'soft' end point. The examiner should also palpate the hamstrings while stabilizing the femur to ensure that the anterior pull is not being impaired by hamstring contraction.

Another test to assess injury to the ACL is the pivot shift test (Galway et al 1972). This test reproduces the 'giving way' sensation of the knee; therefore patient relaxation is problematic. Testing under anesthesia produces a greater percentage of positive results in ACL deficient knees (Donaldson et al 1985) because the tendency for muscle guarding is reduced. To perform a pivot shift test, the examiner holds the patient's lower leg with one hand and applies a valgus stress at the lateral aspect of the knee joint with the other hand while the patient's knee is in a fully extended position (Fig. 21.6). In this position, the valgus force produces a rotational subluxation of the lateral tibia. The examiner then moves the knee into approximately 30° of flexion, maintaining the valgus stress at the knee joint. A positive pivot shift test will be perceived as a 'sliding' motion of the tibia as the knee reaches approximately 20–30° of flexion, which is actually a reduction of the tibia. The tibial reduction is

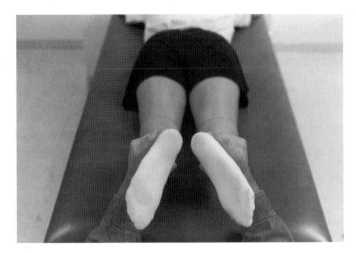

Figure 21.8 • Prone external rotation test for the arcuate complex.

drawn anteriorly by the quadriceps, causing the tibial tubercle to become more prominent.

Arcuate complex

The arcuate complex is the primary restraint to external rotation of the tibia (Gollehon et al 1987). The arcuate complex is tested by the prone external rotation (dial) test with the knee in 30° of flexion (Veltri & Warren 1993). The test is performed with the patient prone (Fig. 21.8). Both knees are flexed to 30° by the examiner and the feet are externally rotated, causing tibial external rotation. External rotation of the foot relative to the thigh is compared between the injured and uninjured legs. An increase in the amount of external rotation by 10° or more compared to the uninjured side is considered a positive test (Veltri & Warren 1993, Wind et al 2004).

Meniscal tests

Meniscal tears are difficult to diagnose by physical examination. McMurray's test is commonly used to diagnose meniscal tears and is performed by fully flexing the patient's injured knee, then grasping the foot and rotating the tibia on the femur while the knee remains flexed (Corea et al 1994). A 'clicking' sensation in the knee indicates a positive test. Although McMurray's test is commonly used to diagnose meniscal tears, the sensitivity of the test is only 59% (Corea et al 1994). McMurray's test, however, has a high specificity, reported to be between 77 and 98%, thus a positive test has favorable predictive value (Malanga et al 2003, Scholten et al 2001). Recently, tests involving standing on the injured leg with the knee in 20° of flexion and performing internal and external rotation of the knee and body (Thessaly test), or standing with both legs in maximal internal or external rotation and performing a squat (Ege's test) have been reported as optional methods for detecting meniscal tears (Akseki 2004, Karachalios et al 2005). Clinicians should have a high index of suspicion for a meniscal tear when symptoms of joint line tenderness, clicking in the knee and knee locking are present

(Anderson & Lipscomb 1986, Eren 2003, Shakespeare & Rigby 1983).

Knee effusion

Assessing knee effusion allows the clinician to monitor the patient's recovery after injury and the patient's response to treatment progression. Girth measurements do not adequately quantify effusion, particularly if the effusion is small. Instead, the stroke test can give more meaningful information about the presence and amount of effusion (Magee 2002). The stroke test is performed with the patient supine and the knee relaxed in full extension. The test starts with the examiner performing several strokes upward from the medial joint line towards the suprapatellar pouch in an attempt to move effusion out of the medial aspect of the knee. The examiner then strokes downward on the lateral side of the knee from the suprapatellar pouch towards the lateral joint line, observing the medial aspect of the knee in an effort to appreciate a fluid wave emanating from the suprapatellar pouch (Magee 2002). At our facility, we use four different grades to describe the amount of effusion. If no wave is produced with the downward stroke, there is no effusion present. If the downward stroke produces a small wave on the medial side of the knee, the effusion is given a 'trace' grade; a larger bulge is given a '1+' grade. If the effusion returns to the medial side of the knee without a downward stroke, the effusion is given a '2+' grade. The inability to move the effusion out of the medial aspect of the knee equates to a '3+' grade.

Special topics related to knee evaluation

Arthometer testing

Arthrometer testing is most often used to quantify knee joint laxity when ACL injury is suspected. Many different knee arthrometers have been developed; however, results obtained with these different systems are not necessarily generalizable to each other (Anderson et al 1992). The KT 1000 arthrometer (Medmetrics, San Diego, CA) is a commonly used arthrometer. Results using KT 1000 with a manual maximum pull have shown a 3 mm difference between sides to be greater than 90% sensitive for an ACL rupture (Liu et al 1995, Rangger et al 1993). In addition, the KT 1000 arthrometer is sometimes used after ACL reconstruction to determine graft status. Although arthrometer testing provides an objective measure of the amount of knee joint laxity, the results do not indicate functional outcome (Snyder-Mackler et al 1997, Tyler et al 1999).

Quadriceps strength testing

Quadriceps weakness is a common sequela after knee injury with important clinical implications. Biomechanical studies have demonstrated that the quadriceps strength deficit is correlated with altered knee kinematics and kinetics during walking, jogging and stair climbing (Lewek et al 2002, Morrissey et al 2004, Patel et al 2003, Snyder-Mackler et al 1995). In addition, the quadriceps strength deficit shows moderate correlations with

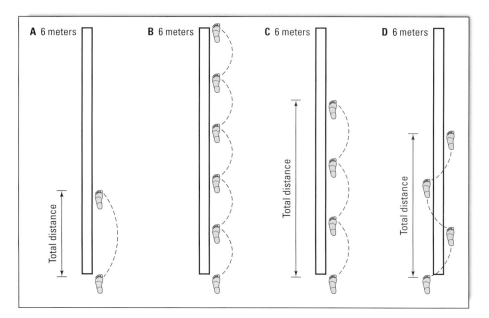

Figure 21.9 • Hop tests for the knee.
A: Single hop for distance. **B:** Timed hop.
C: Triple hop for distance. **D:** Cross-over hop for distance.

hop test scores (Petschnig et al 1998, Pincivero et al 1997, Wilk et al 1994) and subjective ratings of function (Liu-Ambrose et al 2003, Wilk et al 1994). Therefore, measurement of quadriceps strength is important to ensure full resolution of this impairment prior to return to sport.

A variety of methods can be used to test quadriceps strength. The two most common methods used in the clinical setting are manual muscle testing and isokinetic testing. Manual muscle testing is one of the easiest to employ; however, results are less accurate when a patient is able to generate high force or when the strength difference between limbs is minimal. Isokinetic testing offers the benefit of objective measurement through a force transducer, but there is controversy about which is the most clinically significant testing speed. Faster speeds better approximate speed of joint motion during function; however, they tend to underestimate strength deficits (Gapeyeva et al 2000, Keays et al 2000, Morrissey et al 2004).

Neither manual muscle testing nor isokinetic testing measure the patient's effort or offer a method for assessing quadriceps inhibition (i.e. inability to fully activate the quadriceps voluntarily). Quadriceps inhibition can result after knee injury and interfere with the resolution of quadriceps strength deficits (Chmielewski et al 2004, Snyder-Mackler et al 1994a). The burst-superimposition method of testing quadriceps strength is used more commonly in research than a clinical setting; however, this method offers the ability to measure muscle inhibition (Snyder-Mackler et al 1994a). For this type of testing, an electrical stimulus is administered (superimposed) while the patient produces a maximal voluntary isometric contraction. If the patient has fully activated the quadriceps, there will be no force augmentation when the electrical stimulus is delivered. Alternatively, an increase in force when the electrical stimulus is applied signifies the presence of quadriceps inhibition. If the burst-superimposition method of testing is not available to the

clinician, force targets should be set and verbal encouragement given during testing to improve quality of effort.

Hop testing

Hop testing is a commonly used clinical test of function. Many clinics use one or all of the hop tests described by Noyes et al (1991), which include: the single hop test, triple hop test, cross-over triple hop test and timed hop test (Fig. 21.9). Testing in an uninjured population showed that 92–93% had a symmetry index (side-to-side comparison) of at least 85% for the single hop and timed hop tests (Barber et al 1990); thus a score less than 85% on the hop tests can be indicative of disability. Hop testing has been shown to have good reliability, particularly when patients are given more than one practice trial (Bolgla & Keskula 1997). A current limitation of hop testing is that compensatory movements are not regulated. It has been suggested that prohibiting compensatory movements may increase the sensitivity of hop tests for identifying patients with abnormal function (Phillips et al 2000).

Self-report questionnaires

Self-report questionnaires can assist the clinician in measuring disability and monitoring changes in functional status during the course of treatment. Knee-specific (e.g. Lysholm Scale [Lysholm & Gillquist 1982], International Knee Documentation Committee Subjective Form [Irrgang et al 2001]) and general health status questionnaires (e.g. SF-36 [Ware & Shelbourne 1992]) both provide important, but very different information. Knee-specific questionnaires give insight into disability caused by the knee injury, whereas general health status questionnaires reveal mental and emotional states that may impact on rehabilitation. Clinicians should select knee-specific questionnaires that include questions related to high-level activities; otherwise, an athlete may reach the highest score even when some disability remains. Furthermore, clinicians should check the literature to make sure the selected questionnaire has high reliability and is sensitive to changes in functional status.

Rehabilitation of common sports-related injuries

General rehabilitation guidelines

Rehabilitation guidelines are structured to direct the clinician in returning athletes to preinjury activity levels as quickly and safely as possible. Guidelines should be based upon current scientific evidence and have criteria for progression in rehabilitation. Criterion-based protocols eliminate subjectivity in clinical decisions regarding progression through rehabilitation by dictating the milestones that must be reached in order to progress to the next phase. Clinicians should prescribe therapeutic interventions within each phase that are tailored to the patient's particular impairments and anticipated activity level. Prescribing therapeutic interventions in a 'cookbook' fashion for each particular diagnosis is a disservice to the patient.

Phases of rehabilitation

Three phases of rehabilitation will be discussed: the acute phase, advanced phase and return-to-play phase (Box 21.1). It should be noted that many variations on rehabilitation programs for knee injuries are possible and that only some of these approaches are presented in this chapter.

Acute phase

In the acute phase of rehabilitation, strategies are focused on controlling the effects of inflammation (pain, effusion, loss of motion and muscle atrophy). The goal of the acute phase is to restore full range of motion, reduce effusion, retard muscle atrophy and ambulate without an assistive device (Box 21.1). Ice, compression and elevation of the injured limb can assist in counteracting the effects of inflammation. Relative rest is usually indicated to allow for healing to occur without the detrimental effects of strict immobilization, such as articular cartilage degradation, arthrofibrosis and deconditioning.

In the acute stage, ambulation with an assistive device is indicated if the athlete walks with a limp. A knee brace that limits tibiofemoral motion is often used in conjunction with an assistive device to safely allow early weightbearing. Use of an assistive device is maintained until the athlete can walk without a limp, joint effusion is controlled and the quadriceps have recovered sufficiently to provide protection of healing tissues (typically 60% of the uninvolved side).

Range of motion deficits should also be resolved in this phase of rehabilitation. Most often, regaining knee extension is more difficult than regaining knee flexion, so priority should be placed on achieving full passive extension. If knee motion is restricted, the clinician should evaluate the numerous possible contributing

---

Box 21.1 Phases of rehabilitation

Acute phase

Goals
- Decrease pain
- Increase range of movement
- Retard muscle atrophy
- Unassisted ambulation

Common interventions
- Cryotherapy
- Neuromuscular electrical stimulation
- Patellar mobilization
- Soft tissue mobilization at incision site (if surgical intervention)
- Isometric exercise (quadriceps sets)
- Range of motion exercises
- Gait training
- Cardiovascular exercise (stationary bike, swimming)

Advanced phase

Criteria to enter
- Full range of motion and effusion controlled (below 2+)

Goal
- Increase muscle strength and endurance

Common interventions
- Isotonic (both open and closed chain) and isokinetic exercise
- Neuromuscular electrical stimulation
- Proprioception exercise
- Flexibility exercise
- Running program
- Cardiovascular exercise (stationary bike, StairMaster, elliptical machine)

Return-to-play phase

Criteria to enter
- Quadriceps strength ≥80% of the uninjured side

Goal
- Prepare athlete for a return to competition

Common interventions
- Isotonic (both open and closed chain) and isokinetic exercise
- Agility training
- Sport-specific exercise

---

sources including: decreased patella mobility, poor quadriceps recruitment, decreased quadriceps strength, decreased accessory motion of the tibiofemoral joint and muscle guarding and tightness. Interventions should be chosen that address the specific cause of restricted range, for example low-load sustained stretching (often through serial casting), joint mobilizations of the patella and tibiofemoral joints and modalities to control pain and resultant muscle spasm. The development of arthrofibrosis (internal scarring of the joint) is a fairly rare but potentially debilitating complication following knee injury or surgery. Efforts to decrease joint inflammation and early, protected joint motion help to minimize the risk of arthrofibrosis development.

Rapid and significant quadriceps femoris weakness is a common concern following injuries to the tibiofemoral joint (Morrissey 1989, Nyland 1999, Snyder-Mackler et al 1994a). Efforts to retard atrophy and facilitate volitional quadriceps activation form the basis of early progressive strengthening programs (Snyder-Mackler et al 1991). Successful early quadriceps strengthening will facilitate efforts to gain full knee extension, restore normal patellar mobility and correct antalgic gait patterns.

If the athlete is experiencing difficulty producing a strong quadriceps contraction, neuromuscular electrical stimulation (NMES) is indicated (see Chapter 14). Parameters for NMES of athletes include: frequency of 50–75 Hz, wavelength of 200–400 μs, ramp time of 2 s, 10 s of on time, 50 s of off time, and ten contractions during a session, 2–3 sessions a week. The success of NMES depends upon achieving adequate levels of electrical stimulation to provide stimulus to promote strength gains. Patients are counseled to relax while the electrically elicited isometric contractions are increased in an effort to achieve 50% of the injured leg's maximal volitional isometric contraction. Intensity levels that are below 50% of maximal voluntary isometric contraction (MVIC) have limited capacity to assist in strength gain beyond volitional exercise alone (Snyder-Mackler et al 1994b). Use of this high intensity NMES is maintained until the involved limb achieves strength equal to 80% of the uninvolved side.

Advanced phase

The advanced phase of rehabilitation is initiated when range of motion is full and effusion controlled (below grade 2+) (Box 21.1). The goal of this phase is to increase muscle strength and endurance. Higher intensity resistance training can be initiated and should include exercises for all muscles of the lower extremity. If the intensity of therapeutic exercise creates an increase in knee joint effusion, intensity levels are reduced to the previous level. Progression to higher activity is dictated by the presence of soreness after exercise (Box 21.2).

Rehabilitation exercises are commonly categorized as open or closed chain exercises. Open chain exercises are those in which the distal end is free to move (e.g. knee extension), and closed chain exercises are those in which the distal end is fixed (e.g. squat). Optimal strengthening requires a combination of both open and closed chain exercises (Fitzgerald 1997, Mikkelsen et al 2000, Morrissey et al 2000). When athletes perform closed chain exercises, clinicians should be cognizant of the tendency to compensate for weak muscles in the kinetic chain. Reliance on the ankle plantar flexors and hip extensors is a common substitution pattern during closed chain exercises following knee injury.

Box 21.2 Exercise progression guidelines based on soreness

- If no soreness is present from previous exercise, progress exercise by modifying one variable.
- If soreness is present from previous exercise, but recedes with warm-up, stay at same level.
- If soreness is present from previous exercise, but does not recede with warm-up, decrease exercise to the level prior to progression. Consider taking the day off if soreness is still present with the reduced level of exercise. When exercise is resumed, it should be at the reduced level.

Often, exercises designed to improve dynamic joint stability are started in this phase and continue through the final (return-to-play) phase of rehabilitation. Such exercises have been interchangeably called balance, proprioceptive, neuromuscular control or reactive neuromuscular control exercises. Balance exercises using unstable surfaces and perturbation devices are included. The effect of many of these exercises on rehabilitation outcomes is unknown; however, positive changes in muscle activity, corresponding with improved movement patterns and subjective reports of function, have been reported in patients with ACL deficiency that complete a specific program involving progressive postural destabilization exercises (Chmielewski et al 2002, 2005).

Progression of aerobic condition often includes a running program that is usually initiated in this phase of rehabilitation. To start running, the athlete's injured side quadriceps strength must be restored to at least 80% of the uninvolved side, and sufficient healing of the injured structure must have occurred (e.g. ACL reconstruction approximately 8 weeks, grade I MCL injury at 1–2 weeks). Soft tissue healing is usually sufficient at 4–6 weeks. Running progression starts on a treadmill and moves to running on a track. Track workouts are initiated with running the straight-a-ways and walking corners. The intensity is gradually increased until the athlete can run the full length of the track. Road running and finally off-road running represent the least controlled training situations and are instituted as a final stage in running progression. Jogging duration may start with as much as 2 miles and may be progressed on a weekly basis if there is no pain or swelling (Box 21.2). Completing a full running progression can take as long as 2–3 months.

Return-to-play phase

The goal of the return-to-play phase is to prepare the athlete to return to the demands of competition (Box 21.1). The athlete is allowed to enter this phase when intense resistance training and a running program do not increase effusion. Therapeutic exercise interventions should follow the SAID (specific adaptations to imposed demands) principle. This concept is based on the notion that the body will adapt to accommodate the stress and strains applied to it. Therefore, exercises should attempt to mimic the demands of activities required for the athlete to successfully return to sport.

The return-to-play phase is characterized by sport-specific exercise such as plyometric exercise, agility training and interval sport programs. Plyometric exercise (see Chapter 10) is thought to prepare injured athletes for the speeds, forces and planes of movement experienced during sport. Although plyometric exercise is associated with many neuromuscular and performance benefits in uninjured individuals, little is known regarding the benefits of plyometric exercise in a rehabilitation setting (Chmielewski et al 2006). Plyometric exercise should be initiated at a lower intensity and progressed to more difficult, higher intensity levels, with an emphasis on correct technique and symmetrical movement patterns regardless of intensity level. Likewise, less complex agility drills (e.g. shuffle, shuttle run) should be used initially, moving to more complex agility drills (e.g. figure-of-eight, braiding). The volume of plyometric exercise and agility activities should be graded by frequency, duration and intensity. Only one variable should be modified at one time, otherwise it is difficult to determine what factor caused an adverse response (increased pain or effusion) to the treatment, should an adverse response occur. Practice drills are started, leading to competition level activities.

Athletes are cleared to return to sport when they have progressed through all phases of rehabilitation without symptoms and have met the criteria of return-to-play testing. Return-to-play testing involves quadriceps strength testing, hop testing and self-report questionnaires. Athletes must score 90% on all tests before returning to competition (Manal & Snyder-Mackler 1996).

Anterior cruciate ligament

Mechanism of injury

The ACL is injured when the tibia translates too far anterior relative to the femur. The majority of ACL injuries (around 70%) occur by noncontact mechanisms; the remaining injuries involve contact with another person or object (Boden et al 2000). Noncontact injuries typically involve a sharp deceleration with the knee close to extension, with or without a change in direction, or landing from a jump (Boden et al 2000). Injury to the ACL can also occur when the knee is hyperextended, or when contact results in valgus collapse of the knee (Boden et al 2000). Female athletes, compared to male athletes in the same sports, are 4–6 times more likely to rupture their ACL in a noncontact injury (Arendt & Dick 1995). The amount of valgus knee motion and frontal plane moments at the knee have been identified as important predictors of ACL injury in female athletes (Hewett et al 2005).

Nonoperative treatment

Most athletes who tear their ACL experience knee instability during sports that involve cutting or jumping (Shelton et al 1997). Nonoperative treatment has primarily been reserved for those willing to reduce their activity level; however, nonoperative treatment can be a short-term option for athletes if certain conditions are met. A screening examination has been developed to assess an athlete's potential for dynamically stabilizing the injured knee, to determine if an athlete is a good candidate for nonoperative treatment. The screening examination is composed of a variety of clinical tests and is administered when there is no knee effusion present, full knee range of motion has been restored and the patient experiences no pain with unilateral hopping. In order to qualify for nonoperative treatment, the athlete must: (1) have no more than one episode of giving way (i.e. buckling) since the initial injury, (2) score at least 80% on the timed hop test, (3) score at least 80% on the Knee Outcome Survey-Activities of Daily Living Scale (Irrgang et al 1998) and (4) score at least 60% on the Global Rating Scale (Fitzgerald et al 2000a). If the athlete meets the criteria

of the screening examination, then nonoperative treatment can be offered as a viable option, otherwise surgical intervention is recommended. Nonoperative treatment should only be considered when there is no concomitant ligamentous injury greater than grade I, no repairable meniscal tear and no full-thickness articular cartilage defect.

Athletes who pass the criteria of the screening examination are enrolled in a ten-session rehabilitation program that includes lower extremity strengthening exercises, agility training and perturbation training (Fitzgerald et al 2000b). In a randomized controlled trial, perturbation training augmented rehabilitation was compared to a program consisting of only strengthening exercises and agility training, and was found to result in greater success in returning to sport without episodes of giving way (Fitzgerald et al 2000b). Chmielewski et al (2002, 2005) demonstrated changes in muscle activity after completing perturbation training that reflect improved dynamic knee stabilization: the timing and magnitude of quadriceps activity became coordinated with hamstring and soleus activity, and the magnitude of co-contraction between the vastus lateralis and lateral hamstrings or vastus lateralis and medial gastrocnemius was reduced. Perturbation training involves the application of controlled forces to the lower extremity through support surface movement. Rockerboard, rollerboard and rollerboard with a stationary platform are used to apply the perturbations during this type of training (Figs 21.10–21.12). The force, direction and predictability of the perturbations are progressed throughout the ten sessions. Athletes wear a functional brace during agility training and when they return to sport activity. This protocol is given as a short-term option for athletes who wish to complete their competitive season; operative intervention is recommended when the competitive season is finished.

Operative treatment

Operative treatment should be considered for any athlete who wishes to return to sports that require cutting, jumping and lateral movement. Athletes may benefit from preoperative rehabilitation to decrease inflammation and improve knee motion. Surgery less than 1 month from injury was found to be one of the factors related to a loss of motion following surgery (Harner et al 1992). This may be explained by subsequent findings that preoperative effusion and limited motion were factors that correlated with the development of arthrofibrosis after ACL reconstruction (Mayr et al 2004).

ACL reconstructions are performed with a variety of grafts. Typical autogenous graft choices include the middle third of the patellar tendon or doubled semitendinosis-gracilis tendons. Allograft choices include fresh frozen Achilles or patellar tendon.

Advances in surgical fixation allow for full weightbearing and the ability to obtain full knee extension in the immediate postoperative phase without concern for graft failure. Considerable research has been conducted to determine which exercises may impose harmful strain to the ACL graft, thus contributing to graft stretching. Some studies suggest that performing knee

391

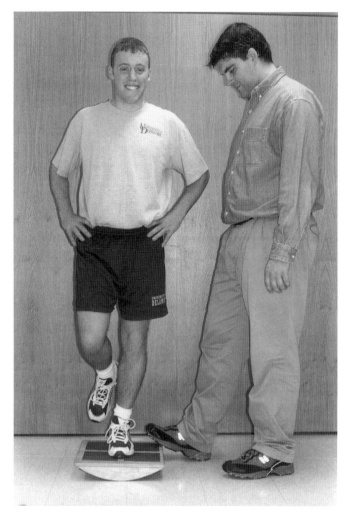

Figure 21.10 • Perturbation training for nonoperative ACL rehabilitation (rockerboard technique).

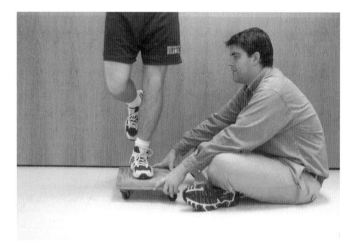

Figure 21.11 • Perturbation training for nonoperative ACL rehabilitation (rollerboard technique).

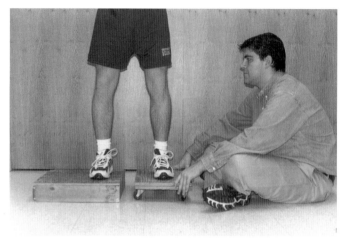

Figure 21.12 • Perturbation training for nonoperative ACL rehabilitation (rollerboard with stationary platform technique).

extension in a range from 0 to 40° may impose high strain on the ACL; however, other studies show that the amount of strain may be comparable to that during weightbearing (Beynnon et al 1997, Escamilla et al 1998, Lutz et al 1993). Clinicians should, therefore, prescribe knee extension exercises in a terminal range judiciously. It is important to remember that absence of strain can also be detrimental, since strain is essential for graft remodeling. Unfortunately, the optimal strain level has not yet been determined.

Postoperative treatment

The primary concerns immediately after surgery are the restoration of quadriceps function and knee motion (particularly knee extension) in addition to reducing knee effusion and pain. Immediately after surgery, patients may experience difficulty producing a quadriceps contraction, particularly if an autogenous patellar tendon graft was used, because of donor site pain associated with quadriceps contraction. An inability to produce a quadriceps contraction, coupled with donor site healing, can lead to a restriction of superior patellar mobility and loss of knee extension. Superior patellar mobilization is therefore essential for these patients. By the second week after surgery, 90° of active knee flexion should be achieved, and by 6–8 weeks after surgery, the patient should achieve full active range of motion (Manal & Snyder-Mackler 1996). If knee extension is not recovered, serial casting may be considered.

In the advanced phase of rehabilitation (6–12 weeks postoperatively), strengthening exercises should be progressed. Approximately 8 weeks after surgery, a running program can be initiated if the patient's involved side quadriceps strength is 80% of the uninvolved side (Manal & Snyder-Mackler 1996).

In the return-to-play phase (12–20 weeks postoperatively), athletes are allowed to gradually increase the complexity and intensity of activities. Athletes are allowed to return to sport approximately 4–6 months after surgery, provided they have met all clinical milestones and progressed through all phases of rehabilitation. The athlete should demonstrate quadriceps strength and hop testing scores that are 90% of the uninjured side before being cleared to return to sport (Manal & Snyder-Mackler 1996). A functional brace may be prescribed for a return to sport and is worn until the patient feels confident in the stability of the knee.

Medial collateral ligament

Mechanism of injury

The majority of isolated MCL injuries involve lateral impact to the lower thigh or upper leg (Indelicato 1995). Injury to the MCL can also occur in combination with an ACL injury, and possibly a POL injury, when the knee is subjected to a large valgus force with external rotation (Indelicato 1995).

Nonoperative treatment

Nonoperative treatment is recommended for most MCL injuries because the MCL has a rich blood supply and associated high healing potential. Nonoperatively managed, incomplete MCL injuries (grade I and II) typically result in an unrestricted return to activity (Derscheid & Garrick 1981, Holden et al 1983). Isolated, complete MCL ruptures can also have good outcomes, although the recovery time will be longer and greater residual laxity will remain (Indelicato et al 1990, Jones et al 1986).

The duration of the acute phase may be as brief as a few days for a grade I MCL sprain and as long as 4 weeks for grade III MCL injuries. In the acute phase of rehabilitation, valgus stress to the knee is avoided to allow initial healing of the MCL. Patients may complain of pain when the knee nears full extension because the MCL is in a lengthened position in extension. For grade II and III MCL sprains, an immobilizer or brace that prohibits knee extension past 30° may be used to reduce pain and to decrease strain of the MCL. Often, an immobilizer is worn initially, and then the athlete is progressed to a brace which restricts range of motion. Total duration of motion restriction is 1–4 weeks, dependent on the severity of the sprain (Holden et al 1983, Indelicato 1983). The location of a grade III injury may also be used in treatment decision-making. Injuries to the proximal attachment of the MCL on the femur tend to lead to stiffness; therefore, they are not treated with strict immobilization. Injuries to the distal attachment of the MCL on the tibia tend to lead to residual laxity and therefore may be treated with cast immobilization for 4–6 weeks. Patients who are limited from full knee extension should initially be encouraged to perform range of motion exercises in a pain-free range, gradually working on increasing range of motion.

In the advanced phase of rehabilitation, valgus stress to the knee can gradually be introduced. Either side-stepping over cones or hip adduction exercises can be used to introduce valgus stress at the knee. Resistance for hip adduction exercises should initially be placed proximally on the tibia and move distally as the patient is able to tolerate and control a longer lever arm. If the patient was limited from full knee extension in the acute phase, resistance in a terminal range should be progressed gradually.

In the return-to-play phase, agility drills should be initiated in the sagittal plane and progressed to the frontal plane. Agility drills in the frontal plane, such as shuffles, braiding or side jumping, all increase valgus stress across the knee and should be progressed with caution. Functional braces may be worn when the athlete returns to sport, but long-term use is discouraged (Indelicato 1995).

Operative treatment

Operative treatment is usually reserved for complete (grade III) ruptures of the MCL, or complete MCL ruptures in combination with other ligamentous ruptures. The operative procedure is usually primary repair. If the primary repair fails, or if the time-frame between injury and surgery is greater than 2 weeks, the MCL reconstruction may be performed with allograft tissue.

Postoperative treatment

Postoperative treatment after MCL repair follows a protocol similar to non-operative treatment of grade III MCL injuries, with the exception that attention must be paid to incision site mobility. An immobilizer is typically worn for 4–6 weeks to protect against valgus forces, and crutches are used for ambulation. Touchdown weight bearing is used for approximately 4 weeks with progression to weight bearing as tolerated at 6 weeks after surgery. Knee motion exercises are gradually progressed over the first 6 weeks after surgery. Patient comfort and ability to meet clinical milestones dictate progression between rehabilitation phases (Indelicato 1995).

Menisci

Mechanism of the injury

Meniscal tears can occur in isolation or in combination with a ligamentous injury. One mechanism for an isolated meniscal injury is pivoting, in which the femur rotates on the meniscus while the meniscus is compressed. Another mechanism for meniscal injury is rising from a squat. This results because weight is transferred to the posterior horns with increasing knee flexion, then as the athlete begins the ascent phase of the squat, the menisci are pushed forward while the posterior horn remains trapped.

Nonoperative treatment

Nonoperative treatment may be recommended for an isolated meniscal tear that is stable and nonsymptomatic. Rehabilitation is directed at resolving knee impairments, and progression is based on symptoms.

Operative treatment

Repair of the meniscus is always preferred to excision or debridement; however, healing potential dictates what procedure is performed. The meniscal rim is vascularized and has been termed the 'red zone'; the central portion of the meniscus is devoid of vascularity and has been termed the 'white zone' (DeHaven & Arnoczky 1994). A tear in the white zone has poor healing potential and is usually treated with debridement. Tears that occur in the red zone or the transition to the white zone (red–white zone) have greater healing potential and may be treated with a repair, if deemed appropriate by the physician. The type of tear can also affect the chosen surgical intervention. Single plane tears, especially in a vertical direction, show greater healing potential than multiple plane or degenerative tears.

Postoperative treatment

Postoperative rehabilitation depends on whether the meniscal tear was debrided or repaired. If the tear was treated with debridement, progression is entirely based on symptoms. There is little tissue morbidity associated with meniscal debridement resulting in a fairly rapid progression in rehabilitation. The clinician should be aware that removal of the meniscus has been associated with increased risk of osteoarthritic changes; therefore, attention should be paid to quadriceps strength deficits, since improving quadriceps strength can provide potential chondroprotective benefits (Slemenda et al 1998). The progression after lateral meniscectomy often lags behind medial meniscectomy by about 10–14 days due to greater amounts of postoperative swelling.

Protocols reported for postoperative meniscal repair rehabilitation vary in the initiation of weight bearing and motion exercises. Some protocols allow motion from 0° to 90° immediately after surgery (Cooper et al 1991); others recommend keeping the knee in full extension for 2 weeks, then beginning a range of motion progression (DeHaven & Arnoczky 1994). Weightbearing to tolerance after surgery has not been associated with any detrimental effects to the repair (Shelbourne et al 1996), although an immobilizer that keeps the knee in full extension may be used for the first 4–6 weeks to protect the repair site. Patients are advised to avoid deep squatting for the first 4 weeks to allow healing of the repair site if it is in the posterior part of the meniscus because of the strain on the posterior horn in moving from knee flexion to extension. Isolated hamstring strengthening is not initiated until 6 weeks after a posterior horn meniscal repair to allow for surgical healing. Because of the attachment of the hamstrings on the posterior horn of the meniscus and joint capsule, there is potential to disrupt the surgical repair if isolated hamstring exercises are initiated prior to adequate healing. Running is usually initiated around 3 months after surgery and a return to sports occurs approximately 4–6 months after surgery. Patient tolerance and ability to meet clinical milestones dictate progression through the phases of rehabilitation.

Rehabilitation of less common injuries

Posterior cruciate ligament and posterolateral corner injuries

Mechanism of the injury

Compared to the ACL and MCL, the PCL is less commonly injured; however, there is suspicion that many injuries go unreported or are misdiagnosed. PCL injuries during sports usually occur as a result of a posteriorly directed blow to the proximal tibia. Often this occurs when the athlete falls onto a flexed knee with the foot plantar-flexed. This injury is common in ice hockey players or figure skaters who slip and fall on the ice. The PCL can also be compromised in a knee hyperextension injury.

Injuries to the PCL classically create long-term impairments and functional limitations due to secondary pathology of degenerative arthritic changes in the medial tibiofemoral and patellofemoral joints (Harner & Höher 1998, Keller et al 1993). Some authors have gone so far as to state that degenerative changes in the tibiofemoral joint following PCL injury 'are inevitable' (Cross & Powell 1984). Concomitant quadriceps weakness found after PCL tears often compounds the disability of these conditions.

The posterolateral corner is described as the LCL, the popliteus complex, the arcuate ligament complex, fabellofibular ligament, biceps femoris tendon and the posterolateral capsular structures (Covey 2001). Injury to these ligamentous and muscular components that surround the posterior aspect of the lateral femoral condyle rarely occurs in isolation; rather, it is usually a concomitant injury with the PCL. The posterolateral corner is typically injured with a posteriorly directed force to the anteromedial tibia with the knee in hyperextension (Baker et al 1985, Covey 2001). Injury to the posterolateral corner can often be missed in an examination of knee ligamentous support, especially with a concomitant PCL injury (Harner & Höher 1998, Noyes & Barber-Westin 1996). Those patients with combined PCL and posterolateral corner injuries have a greater predisposition to degenerative changes than isolated PCL injured patients (Baker et al 1985, Torg et al 1989). Also, the addition of a posterolateral corner to a PCL injury is unlikely to be satisfactorily stabilized with sole reconstruction of the PCL (Harner et al 2000).

Nonoperative treatment

Nonoperative treatment is usually recommended after a grade I or II injury to the PCL. This corresponds with an isolated PCL injury with posterior translation of less than 10 mm (Veltri & Warren 1993). Multiple directional laxity as a result of concomitant ACL, MCL or posterolateral corner injury is usually treated with operative reconstruction (Harner & Höher 1998, Harner et al 2000).

Restoring quadriceps strength is the cornerstone of conservative rehabilitation following PCL injury (Torg et al 1989, Wilk 1994). Early efforts to improve quadriceps strength must be tempered by the potentially detrimental posterior stresses that are generated by some types of strengthening exercises. Several studies have investigated the potential posterior translation with open and closed chain knee extension exercises. Open chain knee extensions beyond 60° can create posterior tibial translation (Jurist & Otis 1985, Kaufman et al 1991, Lutz et al 1993). Closed chain exercise also induces high posterior displacement forces on the tibia relative to the femur, and these forces increase with increased knee flexion (Lutz et al 1993, Stuart et al 1996). Caution should be taken in using open chain knee flexion exercises or closed kinetic chain exercises with deep knee flexion following PCL injury due to the associated posterior forces.

During the first 2 weeks following injury, the athlete typically wears a knee brace that limits motion to near full extension. Range of motion exercises from 0 to 60°, progressing to tolerance, are performed 3–4 times a day along with isometric and short arc (0–30°) open chain quadriceps exercises. Use of isometric NMES usually starts at 30° of knee flexion (Axe et al 2001).

When sufficient range of motion is attained, stationary biking may be used for range of motion efforts (Wilk 1994). The open chain knee extension exercise range is progressed to 0–60° with progressive resistance. General strengthening of the calf musculature can be initiated at this time. Range of motion is typically progressed until the patient achieves 0–110° by their fourth week.

At the start of the fourth week, the patient should have restored gait without a limp. Limited range, closed chain strengthening exercises can be initiated if they are purely sagittal plane exercises of no deeper than 45° of flexion (Wilk 1994). The main emphasis of quadriceps strengthening should continue to be open chain knee extension in limited range. Anterior knee pain is common in this patient population and modifications to open chain exercises to avoid painful strengthening should be employed. Open chain (isolated) hamstring strengthening is not performed in order to avoid the posterior shear of the tibia on the femur associated with this exercise. Full range of motion should be achieved by 4–6 weeks after injury. By approximately 8 weeks after injury, rehabilitation may progress to the return-to-play phase with close monitoring of patellofemoral joint pain and changes in posterior laxity.

Posterolateral corner instability in combination with PCL injury usually slows the speed of progression in nonoperative and operative rehabilitation. There are a number of operative techniques to correct this instability, but currently there is no 'gold standard' for operative measures (Covey 2001). Attempts to improve the dynamic stability of the knee using techniques comparable to nonoperative rehabilitation following ACL injury appear to be the best nonoperative treatment option to correct for knee instability that lacks a viable surgical correction. A combination of perturbation training and completion of a functional progression represent the nonoperative treatment of posterolateral corner injuries (DeLeo et al 2003).

Operative treatment

Reconstruction as operative management of posterior laxity is typically indicated if the patient has functional instability or pain, early degenerative changes in the tibiofemoral joint, or combined ligamentous injuries (Harner et al 2000). PCL reconstructions can be performed using either a single tunnel or two-tunnel technique using two separate grafts. Typical autograft material for reconstruction consists of bone–patellar tendon–bone,

semitendinous and gracilis, and quadriceps tendon–bone (Axe et al 2001). Most allografts are Achilles tendon or bone–patellar tendon–bone (Bullis & Paulos 1994). A surgical repair may be performed if a bone fragment has avulsed with the PCL. Relatively little is known concerning fixation strength and graft incorporation following PCL operative treatment.

Postoperative treatment

Rehabilitation following surgery is governed by the relatively poor strength of the fixation of the reconstructed ligament. Increased posterior laxity is a more frequent complication than arthrofibrosis and subsequent loss of flexion range of motion. Therefore, early rehabilitative efforts are focused on controlling inflammatory processes, and preventing arthrofibrosis and atrophy without excessively stressing the newly reconstructed graft.

Physical therapy following surgery is very similar to conservative treatment for a grade III PCL tear but involves a longer protective phase to ensure that posterior laxity does not develop. Again, open chain knee flexion exercises are avoided, as they will likely cause deleterious posterior stress on the newly reconstructed ligament. Patients are usually braced in full extension for at least 2 weeks and as long as 4 weeks. A knee range of motion of 0–60° is the milestone for 2 weeks after surgery. Quadriceps control should improve to the point that, at 2 weeks, the patient is able to maintain full knee extension without a lag against gravity.

At 3–4 weeks, the athlete can start to be weaned from the brace and gait training should be initiated if there is demonstration of adequate quadriceps control (Wilk 1994). Open chain knee extensions can be performed from 0 to 60° of flexion. Closed chain exercises can be incorporated at this point as the patient moves through the advanced rehabilitation stage. Progression into the return-to-play phase will start at approximately 3 months after surgery if the corresponding criteria are met.

Reconstruction for posterior laxity with a combined posterolateral corner injury requires an even greater protection period. Combined posterolateral corner laxity has been identified as a potential cause of graft failure in PCL reconstruction (Harner et al 2000). There are no clear guidelines to performing a reconstruction or repair of this rotational laxity, even when it is recognized (Harner et al 2000). The athlete must be counseled regarding a diminished likelihood of a rapid return to sport with an injury involving combined posterior and posterolateral instability. Clinical milestones should be delayed by 2 weeks compared to isolated PCL injury, and return to cutting and rotational activities will be implemented in a more gradual fashion.

Combined PCL and posterolateral corner reconstructions involve the greatest amount of restrictions following surgery due to the severity of the injury and the reconstruction (Wilk 1994). Crutches are typically discontinued after about 2 weeks but a knee immobilizer is used to lock the knee in full extension for 6 weeks with no motion allowed during this period. At about 6 weeks, strengthening moves beyond isometric quadriceps activities to active and active assisted motions and is progressed as for PCL reconstruction. Typically, full range of motion is achieved at about 8 weeks postoperatively (Wilk 1994). Return to strenuous activities varies from 18 to 21 weeks following surgery.

Tibial plateau fracture

Mechanism of the injury

A significant varus, valgus or compressive force at the knee can cause a fracture of the tibial plateau. Tibial plateau fractures commonly occur in loaded, twisting injuries or direct blows to the knee causing a direct compressive force through a femoral condyle into the tibial plateau. Due to the natural valgus angulation of the knee, lateral tibial plateau fractures are more common than medial fractures (Kennedy & Bailey 1968). Tibial plateau fractures are categorized as medial, lateral or bicondylar; nondisplaced or displaced; and depressed or nondepressed.

Nonoperative treatment

If a tibial plateau fracture is treated nonoperatively, there is no attempt to restore the anatomical position of the joint surface through surgical reduction. The knee is commonly placed in a cast-brace, with or without traction. Many researchers believe that traction will allow spontaneous reduction via 'ligamentotaxis'; early motion will further contribute to reduction by 'molding' displaced bone fragments (Apley 1979). Allowing at least 2 weeks of immobilization before beginning motion exercises has resulted in greater gains in knee flexion range of motion (Gausewitz & Hohl 1986). Weightbearing can be initiated within the first 7–14 days for all types of tibial plateau fractures, except fractures that are both displaced and depressed, and has positive effects on knee range of motion and avoidance of valgus deformity (Segal et al 1993).

Rehabilitation is dictated first and foremost by the need for physiological healing of the fracture. Weightbearing exercises like squatting are avoided for the first 4–6 weeks in order to allow the fracture sufficient time to heal. Quadriceps strengthening and obtaining passive knee extension should be a focus of treatment in the acute phase. However, given the fact that tibial plateau fractures are placed in a cast-brace, regaining knee flexion will also become a priority once the cast-brace is removed. In the advanced phase, patients are allowed to progress to strenuous weightbearing exercise, such as deep squatting, once callus formation is seen on X-ray. Progression in the return-to-play phase is dictated by patient symptoms.

Operative treatment

Operative management of tibial plateau fractures begins with the decision of whether or not the patient needs internal fixation of the fracture. Open reduction with internal fixation (ORIF) is currently the surgical choice, as most tibial plateau fractures are displaced or display more than 4 mm of tibial plateau depression (Lachiewicz & Funcik 1990, Segal et al 1993). Bone grafting into the fracture site or into the depressed tibial plateau is a common adjunct to surgery. Lachiewicz & Funcik (1990) found that the absence of a bone graft with ORIF was associated with less than excellent results postoperatively. Surgical reduction can also help to prevent arthritic changes to the tibiofemoral joint surfaces by restoring joint congruency and correcting for damaging varus/valgus joint instability.

Postoperative treatment

Postoperatively, tibial plateau fractures are treated similarly to nondisplaced, nonsurgical fractures. Weightbearing, in a cast-brace, is best initiated within 7–14 days for the best range of motion results and least valgus deformity (Segal et al 1993). In surgically treated displaced fractures, allowing knee motion before 2 weeks postinjury has allowed for the most knee flexion range of motion at 6-month follow-ups (Gausewitz & Hohl 1986). Like nonoperative treatment of tibial plateau fractures, rehabilitation must allow for physiological healing of the reduced joint surface. Weightbearing exercises should be avoided for the first 4–6 weeks. Progression in the advanced and return-to-play phases of rehabilitation is similar to the nonoperative treatment protocol.

Arthritis and the athlete

More people are remaining active for longer periods of their life. Decisions regarding treatment of an athlete should be based on their desired activity level and not their biological age. The eventual consequence of sports injuries such as meniscal tears, ligamentous sprains or articular surface damage play a substantial role in developing secondary knee osteoarthritis (Felson et al 2000, Gelber et al 1999, 2000, Kujala et al 1994, Lundberg & Messner 1997, Messner et al 2001). An important factor to remember in treating athletes with these injuries is that there is no cure for osteoarthritis. Once cartilage damage has occurred, it cannot be perfectly repaired with more hyaline cartilage (Buckwalter 1998). Thus, to slow continued deterioration is a goal of rehabilitative interventions.

Nonoperative treatment for osteoarthritis

Counseling is one of the most important aspects in the course of treatment for osteoarthritis. Efforts to reduce weight should be strongly encouraged as obesity is a recognized risk factor in the development of osteoarthritis (Felson et al 1997, Stürmer et al 2000). Loss of body weight can have a pronounced affect on stresses at the knee as the loss of a 1 lb of body weight can correlate to a loss of 3 lb of force at the knee (Schipplein & Andriacchi 1991).

Joint-sparing activities should be used as a mainstay to provide minimal risk to the knee joint while still providing adequate stimulus to maintain strength and conditioning. Non-impact or low-impact aerobic exercises take the place of running type activities. Examples include, but are not limited to, cross-country skiing, swimming, bicycling, roller-blading, elliptical running simulators, walking and water aerobics. Avoidance of aerobic exercise should not be counseled, as increased weight associated with inactivity would be likely to have a detrimental affect on the knee. If the athlete insists on the need to continue impact activities, instruction on improved footwear choices, and encouraging exercise on a more forgiving surface, will help to attenuate stresses on the arthritic knee.

Quadriceps strength can play an important role in preserving activity level and potentially decreasing the risk for progressive osteoarthritis (O'Reilly et al 1998, Slemenda et al 1998). Several studies that have investigated strengthening protocols for knee osteoarthritis have reported modest strength gains, but significant reduction in pain and increased function (Fisher et al 1991, 1997, Hurley & Newham 1993, Hurley & Scott 1998). In general, strengthening programs should include an emphasis on open chain exercise to avoid the additional compressive force present during weighted, closed chain strengthening exercise. Efforts should be taken to prescribe exercises that do not cause pain during their execution and do not stimulate an inflammatory response. A process of trial and error is used to prescribe the best exercises for each patient.

In patients with unicompartmental arthritis, additional mechanical interventions can be attempted to reduce load to the affected compartment. Medial involvement is the most common site of unicompartment joint degeneration. An unloading brace or a lateral heel wedge can potentially decrease the external varus moment at the knee and decrease pain in patients with this form of the disease (Hewett et al 1998, Keating et al 1993, Kerrigan et al 2002, Pollo 1998, Tohyama et al 1991).

Typically, pain management for osteoarthritis can be achieved through the simple use of analgesics such as acetaminophen (Bradley et al 2001, Brandt 2000). Non-steroidal anti-inflammatory drugs (NSAIDs) can be used as well, but have higher risk for gastrointestinal, renal or hepatic side effects from long-term use (see Ch. 29). For arthritic knees that present with continual effusion, NSAIDs may be more effective in controlling symptoms than analgesics. Joint aspiration and intra-articular corticosteroid injections may also provide pain relief for patients who have effused joints (Creamer 1997, Fadale & Wiggins 1994, Livesley et al 1991). In the knee that is painful without the presence of an effusion, injections of hyaluronic acid have been shown to have pain-reducing properties that are similar to NSAIDs. This relief can last for months after treatment (Altman & Moskowitz 1998, Brandt et al 2001). This treatment usually consists of 3–5 injections given over 15 days and presents a relatively high financial risk for the patient due to the high cost of this form of management.

Recent studies have also supported the use of some 'nutraceuticals' in managing symptoms and potentially protecting remaining articular cartilage in knee osteoarthritis. In particular, the oral supplements chondroitin sulphate and glucosamine (sulphate or hydrochloride) have been studied with mixed results. Several studies document efficacy of these supplements in decreasing symptoms of pain in patients with mild osteoarthritis, with few to no known side effects (Bourgeois et al 1998, Lippiello et al 2000, Mazieres et al 2001, Muller-Fassbender et al 1994, Reginster et al 2001). A recent large-scale trial showed that pain reduction was not greater in individuals that received chondroitin sulfate or glucosamine hydrocholoride, alone or in combination, than in individuals receiving placebo (Clegg et al 2006). Hochberg (2006) has recommended, based on current evidence, that patients take glucosamine sulfate if they choose to use supplements to control osteoarthritis symptoms and consider combining with chondroitin sulfate for potential additive effects.

Operative treatment

Several operative treatments are available to reduce the signs and symptoms of an arthritic knee. Arthroscopic lavage has been proven to provide relief, albeit temporary, from the pain associated with osteoarthritis (Kalunian et al 2000, Livesley et al 1991). Little soft tissue injury is involved with this procedure and the majority of rehabilitation is centered on resolving impairments of pain, loss of range of motion and weakness.

Chondral lesions, either chronic degenerative injuries or resulting from traumatic blows such as involved in an ACL tear, have limited potential for repair or reconstruction. Symptoms include pain and clicking, often with a joint effusion. The operative procedure chosen is dependent on the size of the lesion. For lesions less than $1\,cm^2$, arthroscopy is often performed to debride the unstable cartilage flap. Full-thickness lesions that are $1.5\,cm^2$ or less are often treated with operative procedures that evoke a vascular response from the underlying subchondral bone and bone marrow to 'scar' the lesion with fibrocartilage (Buckwalter 1998, Buckwalter & Lohmander 1994), for example microfracture or drilling techniques (Friedman et al 1984). A full thickness lesion that extends up to $2.5\,cm^2$ may be treated with an OATS (osteochondral autogenous transplantation) procedure in which one or more chondral grafts taken from a non-weightbearing portion of the femur are transplanted into the area of chondral defect (Bobic 1996, Matsusue et al 1993). Severe chondral lesions extending beyond $2.5\,cm^2$ are addressed with autologous chondrocyte implantation, in which donor chondrocytes harvested from the knee are cultured in a laboratory and then reintroduced into the chondral defect under a protective, autologous periosteal flap. This procedure may allow the defect to fill with hyaline-like cartilage (Brittberg et al 1994, Gillogly et al 1998).

Postoperative treatment

Rehabilitation following operative procedures for cartilage defects is focused on limiting early weightbearing to allow for fibrocartilage to mature at the site of microfracture or abrasion. Patients are typically restricted to no greater than touch down weightbearing for 4–6 weeks following microfracture or OATS procedures (Irrgang & Pezzullo 1998, Suh et al 1997) and up to 12 weeks after autologous chondrocyte implantation (Axe & Snyder-Mackler 2005). Isometric exercises and NMES at joint angles that do not engage the repaired tissue are used to improve quadriceps femoris muscle function during this period of limited weightbearing (Irrgang & Pezzullo 1998). Range of motion and stretching efforts are encouraged as immobilization has a detrimental effect on chondrocytes, cartilage thickness and proteoglycan concentration (Behrens et al 1989, Palmoski & Brandt 1982). In addition, nutraceuticals and viscosupplementation may also be recommended postoperatively (Axe & Snyder-Mackler 2005).

Weightbearing is slowly progressed from this point. Closed chain exercise is used sparingly in ranges that do not engage the repaired tissue and progression is slow. An unloading brace and/or heel wedge(s) can be used to unweight the repaired chondral defect. Chances for joint effusion are high following these procedures and if patients demonstrate increased effusion, then the activity level is reduced. This may mean they go back to the use of crutches to assist in efforts to control inflammation.

Aquatic rehabilitation can be used to slowly advance impact. Walking in progressively shallow water and instituting aquajogging can assist in facilitating conditioning while providing progressive stress to assist in remodeling the healing cartilage surface. Returning to impact activities such as jogging will be instituted as late as 8 months after the repair (Gillogly et al 1998). Most patients who undergo operative procedures for chondral defects should be counseled in joint-sparing lifestyle changes.

Summary

High loads experienced during sport activity, long lever arms and a considerable reliance on capsular and ligamentous support for joint stability make the knee joint susceptible to traumatic injury. The primary focus of clinicians rehabilitating traumatic knee injuries is resolving impairments that have the greatest potential to decrease functional outcomes, specifically loss of knee extension, quadriceps weakness and insufficient dynamic joint stability. Clinicians should also be cognizant of the increased risk for developing post-traumatic knee osteoarthritis many years after a traumatic knee injury and take measures to protect articular cartilage. As a result of increased specialization and competitiveness in athletics, there is increased pressure and demands on athletes to return to competition as quickly as possible after a knee injury. Physical therapists can use rehabilitation protocols as guidelines for the judicious and progressive application of forces and interventions to maximize healing potential and expedite recovery. These rehabilitation protocols must, however, be individualized to the specific needs of the patient and integrated with current evidence and clinical experience in order to produce the highest level of functional recovery.

References

Altman R D, Moskowitz R 1998 Intraarticular sodium hyaluronate (Hyalgan) in the treatment of patients with osteoarthritis of the knee: a randomized clinical trial. Hyalgan Study Group 25:2203–2212

Anderson A F, Lipscomb A B 1986 Clinical diagnosis of meniscal tears. Description of a new manipulative test. American Journal of Sports Medicine 14:291–293

Anderson A F, Snyder R B, Federspiel C F et al 1992 Instrumented evaluation of knee laxity: a comparison of five athrometers. American Journal of Sports Medicine 20:135–140

Apley A G 1979 Fractures of the tibial plateau. Orthopaedic Clinics of North America 10:61–74

Arnoczky S P, Warren R F 1982 Microvasculature of the human meniscus. American Journal of Sports Medicine 10:90–95

Akseki D, Ozcan O, Boya H et al 2004 A new weight-bearing meniscal test and a comparison with McMurray's test and joint line tenderness. Arthroscopy: Journal of Arthroscopic and Related Surgery 20:951–958

Arendt E, Dick R 1995 Knee injury patterns among men and women in collegiate basketball and soccer: NCAA data and review of literature. American Journal of Sports Medicine 23:694–701.

Axe M J, Snyder-Mackler L 2005 Postoperative management of orthopaedic surgeries. Independent Study Course 15.2.3. Orthopaedic Section, American Physical Therapy Association

Axe M J, Swigart K H, Snyder-Mackler L 2001 Surgical options and procedure-modified rehabilitation for PCL injury. Athletic Therapy Today 6:16–22

Baker C L Jr, Norwood L A, Hughston J C 1985 Acute combined posterior cruciate and posterolateral instability of the knee. American Journal of Sports Medicine 12:204–208

Barber S D, Noyes F R, Mangine R E et al 1990 Quantitative assessment of functional limitations in normal and anterior cruciate ligament-deficient knees. Clinical Orthopaedics and Related Research 255:204–214

Behrens F, Kraft E L, Oegema T R Jr 1989 Biochemical changes in articular cartilage after joint immobilization by casting or external fixation. Journal of Orthopaedic Research 7:335–343

Beynnon B D, Johnson R J, Fleming B C et al 1997 The strain behavior of the anterior cruciate ligament during squatting and active flexion–extension. A comparison of an open and a closed kinetic chain exercise. American Journal of Sports Medicine 25:823–829

Bobic V 1996 Arthroscopic osteochondral autograft transplantation in anterior cruciate ligament reconstruction: a preliminary clinical study. Knee Surgery, Sports Traumatology, Arthroscopy 3:262–264

Boden B P, Dean G S, Feagin J A Jr et al 2000 Mechanisms of anterior cruciate ligament injury. Orthopedics 23:573–578

Bolgla L A, Keskula D R 1997 Reliability of lower extremity functional performance tests. Journal of Orthopaedic and Sports Physical Therapy 26:138–142

Bourgeois P, Chales G, Dehais J et al 1998 Efficacy and tolerability of chondroitin sulfate 1200 mg/day vs chondroitin sulfate 3 × 400 mg/day vs placebo. Osteoarthritis and Cartilage 6 (suppl A):25–30

Bradley J D, Katz B P, Brandt K D 2001 Severity of knee pain does not predict a better response to an anti-inflammatory dose of ibuprofen than to analgesic in patients with osteoarthritis. Journal of Rheumatology 28:1073–1076

Brandt K D 2000 The role of analgesics in the management of osteoarthritis pain. American Journal of Therapeutics 7:75–90

Brandt K D, Block J A, Michalski J P et al 2001 Efficacy and safety of intraarticular sodium hyaluronate in knee osteoarthritis. Clinical Orthopaedics and Related Research 385:130–143

Brittberg M, Lindahl A, Nilsson A et al 1994 Treatment of deep cartilage defects in the knee with autologous chondrocyte transplantation. New England Journal of Medicine 331:889–895

Buckwalter J A 1998 Articular cartilage: injuries and potential for healing. Journal of Orthopaedic and Sports Physical Therapy 28:192–202

Buckwalter J, Lohmander S 1994 Operative treatment of osteoarthrosis. Current practice and future development. Journal of Bone and Joint Surgery (Am) 76A:1405–1418

Bullis D W, Paulos L E 1994 Reconstruction of the posterior cruciate ligament with allograft. Clinics in Sports Medicine 13:581–597

Butler D L, Noyes F R, Grood E S 1980 Ligamentous restraints to anterior-posterior drawer in the human knee. A biomechanical study. Journal of Bone and Joint Surgery (Am) 62A:259–270

Chmielewski T L, Rudolph K S, Snyder-Mackler L 2002 Development of dynamic knee stability after acute ACL injury. Journal of Electromyography and Kinesiology 12:267–274

Chmielewski T L, Stackhouse S, Axe M J et al 2004 A prospective analysis of incidence and severity of quadriceps inhibition in a consecutive sample of 100 patients with complete acute anterior cruciate ligament rupture. Journal of Orthopaedic Research 22:925–930

Chmielewski T L, Hurd W J, Rudolph K S et al 2005 Perturbation training improves knee kinematics and reduces muscle co-contraction after complete unilateral anterior cruciate ligament rupture. Physical Therapy 85:740–749

Chmielewski T L, Myer G D, Kauffman D et al 2006 Plyometric exercise in the rehabilitation of athletes: physiological responses and clinical application. Journal of Orthopaedic and Sports Physical Therapy 36A:308–319

Clark C R, Ogden J A 1983 Development of the menisci of the human knee joint. Morphological changes and their potential role in childhood meniscal injury. Journal of Bone and Joint Surgery (Am) 65:538–547

Clegg D O, Reda D J, Harris C L et al 2006 Glucosamine, chondroitin sulfate, and the two in combination for painful knee osteoarthritis. New England Journal of Medicine 354:795–808

Cooper D E, Arnoczky S P, Warren R F 1991 Meniscal repair. Clinics in Sports Medicine 10:529–548

Corea J R, Moussa M, Al Othman A 1994 McMurray's test tested. Knee Surgery, Sports Traumatology, Arthroscopy 2:70–72

Covey D C 2001 Current concepts review injuries of the posterolateral corner of the knee. Journal of Bone and Joint Surgery (Am) 83A:106–118

Creamer P 1997 Intra-articular corticosteroid injections in osteoarthritis: do they work and if so, how? Annals of Rheumatic Diseases 56:634–636

Cross M J, Powell J F 1984 Long-term followup of posterior cruciate ligament rupture: a study of 116 cases. American Journal of Sports Medicine 12:292–297

DeHaven K E, Arnoczky S P 1994 Meniscus repair: basic science, indications for repair and open repair. Instructional Course Lectures 43:65–76

DeLeo A T, Woodzell W W, Snyder-Mackler L 2003 Resident's case problem: diagnosis and treatment of posterolateral instability in a patient with lateral collateral ligament sprain. Journal of Orthopaedic and Sports Physical Therapy 33:185–195

Derscheid G L, Garrick J G 1981 Medial collateral ligament injuries in football: nonoperative management of grade I and grade II sprains. American Journal of Sports Medicine 9:365–368

Donaldson W F, Warren R F, Wickiewicz T 1985 A comparison of acute anterior cruciate ligament examinations. Initial versus examination under anesthesia. American Journal of Sports Medicine 13:5–9

Escamilla R F, Fleisig G S, Zheng N et al 1998 Biomechanics of the knee during closed kinetic chain and open kinetic chain exercise. Medicine and Science in Sports and Exercise 30:556–569

Eren O T 2003 The accuracy of joint line tenderness by physical examination in the diagnosis of meniscal tears. Arthroscopy: Journal of Arthroscopic and Related Surgery 19: 850–854

Fadale P D, Wiggins M E 1994 Corticosteroid injections: their use and abuse. Journal of the American Academy of Orthopaedic Surgeons 2:133–140

Felson D T, Zhang Y, Hannan M T et al 1997 Risk factors for incident radiographic knee osteoarthritis in the elderly. Arthritis and Rheumatism 40:728–733

Felson D T, Lawrence R C, Dieppe P A et al 2000 Osteoarthritis: new insights: 1. The disease and its risk factors. Annals of Internal Medicine 133:635–646

Fisher N D, Pendergast D R, Gresham G E et al 1991 Muscle rehabilitation: its effect on muscular and functional performance of patients with knee osteoarthritis. Archives of Physical Medicine and Rehabilitation 72:367–374

Fisher N M, White S C, Yack H J et al 1997 Muscle function and gait in patients with knee osteoarthritis before and after muscle rehabilitation. Disability and Rehabilitation 19:47–55

Fitzgerald G K 1997 Open versus closed kinetic chain exercises: issues in rehabilitation after anterior cruciate ligament reconstructive surgery. Journal of Orthopaedic and Sports Physical Therapy 77:1747–1754

Fitzgerald G K, Axe M J, Snyder-Mackler L 2000a A decision-making scheme for returning patients to high-level activity with nonoperative treatment after anterior cruciate ligament rupture. Knee Surgery, Sports Traumatology, Arthroscopy 8:76–82

Fitzgerald G K, Axe M J, Snyder-Mackler 2000b The efficacy of perturbation training in nonoperative anterior cruciate ligament rehabilitation programs for physically active individuals. Physical Therapy 80:128–140

Friedman M, Berasi C, Fox J et al 1984 Preliminary results with abrasion arthroplasty in the osteoarthritic knee. Clinical Orthopaedics and Related Research 82:200–205

Fu F H, Baratz M E 1994 Meniscal injuries. In: DeLee J C, Drez D Jr (eds) Orthopaedic sports medicine. Principles and practice. WB Saunders, Philadelphia, PA, p 1146–1162

Fukubayashi T, Torzilli P A, Sherman M F et al 1982 An in vitro biomechanical evaluation of anterior–posterior motion of the knee. Tibial displacement, rotation, and torque. Journal of Bone and Joint Surgery (Am) 64A:258–264

Galway H R, Beaupre A, MacIntosh D L 1972 Pivot shift: a clinical sign of symptomatic anterior cruciate deficiency. Journal of Bone and Joint Surgery (Br) 54B:763–764

Gapeyeva H, Paasuke M, Ereline J et al 2000 Isokinetic torque deficit of the knee extensor muscles after arthroscopic partial meniscectomy. Knee Surgery, Sports Traumatology, Arthroscopy 8:301–304

Gausewitz S, Hohl M 1986 The significance of early motion in the treatment of tibial plateau fractures. Clinical Orthopaedics 202:135–138

Gelber A C, Hochberg M C, Mead L A et al 1999 Body mass index in young men and the risk of subsequent knee and hip osteoarthritis. American Journal of Medicine 107:542–548

Gelber A C, Hochberg M C, Mead L A et al 2000 Joint injury in young adults and risk for subsequent knee and hip osteoarthritis. Annals of Internal Medicine 133:321–328

Gillogly S D, Voight M, Blackburn T 1998 Treatment of articular cartilage defects of the knee with autologous chondrocyte implantation. Journal of Orthopaedic and Sports Physical Therapy 28:241–251

Girgis F G, Marshall J L, Monajem A R S 1975 The cruciate ligaments of the knee: anatomical, functional and experimental analysis. Clinical Orthopedics 106:216–231

Gollehon D L, Torzilli P A, Warren R F 1987 The role of the posterolateral and cruciate ligaments in the stability of the human knee. A biomechanical study. Journal of Bone and Joint Surgery (Am) 69A:233–242

Grood E S, Noyes F R, Butler D L et al 1981 Ligamentous and capsular restraints preventing straight medial and lateral laxity in intact human cadaver knees. Journal of Bone and Joint Surgery (Am) 63A:1257–1269

Harner C D, Höher J 1998 Evaluation and treatment of posterior cruciate ligament injuries. American Journal of Sports Medicine 26:471–482

Harner C D, Irrgang J J, Paul J et al 1992 Loss of motion after anterior cruciate ligament reconstruction. American Journal of Sports Medicine 20:499–506

Harner C D, Vogrin T M, Höher J et al 2000 Biomechanical analysis of a posterior cruciate ligament reconstruction. Deficiency of the posterolateral structures as a cause of graft failure. American Journal of Sports Medicine 28:32–39

Heller L, Langman J 1964 The menisco-femoral ligaments of the human knee. Journal of Bone and Joint Surgery (Br) 46B:307–313

Hewett T E, Noyes F R, Barber-Westin S D et al 1998 Decrease in knee joint pain and increase in function in patients with medial compartment arthrosis: a prospective analysis of valgus bracing. Orthopedics 21:131–138

Hewett T E, Myer G D, Ford K R et al 2005 Biomechanical measures of neuromuscular control and valgus loading of the knee predict anterior cruciate ligament injury risk in female athletes: a prospective study. American Journal of Sports Medicine 33:492–501

Hochberg M C 2006 Nutritional supplements for osteoarthritis: still no resolution. New England Journal of Medicine 354:858–860

Holden D L, Eggert A W, Butler J E 1983 The nonoperative treatment of Grade I and II medial collateral ligament injuries to the knee. American Journal of Sports Medicine 11:340–343

Hughston J C, Andrews J R 1976 Classification of knee ligament instabilities: I. The medial compartment and cruciate ligaments. Journal of Bone and Joint Surgery (Am) 58A:159–172

Hurley M V, Newham D J 1993 The influence of arthrogenous muscle inhibition on quadriceps rehabilitation of patients with early, unilateral osteoarthritic knees. British Journal of Rheumatology 32:127–131

Hurley M V, Scott D L 1998 Improvements in quadriceps sensorimotor function and disability of patients with knee osteoarthritis following a clinically practicable exercise regime. British Journal of Rheumatology 37:1181–1187

Indelicato P A 1983 Nonoperative treatment of complete tears of the medial collateral ligament of the knee. Journal of Bone and Joint Surgery (Am) 65A:323–329

Indelicato P A 1995 Isolated medial collateral ligament injuries in the knee. Journal of the American Academy of Orthopaedic Surgeons 3:9–14

Indelicato P A, Hermansdorfer J, Huegel M 1990 Nonoperative management of complete tears of the medial collateral ligament of the knee in intercollegiate football players. Clinical Orthopaedics and Related Research 256:174–177

Inoue M, McGurk-Burleson E, Hollis J M et al 1987 Treatment of the medial collateral ligament injury: the importance of anterior cruciate ligament on the valgus-varus knee laxity. American Journal of Sports Medicine 15:15–21

Irrgang J J, Pezzullo D P 1998 Rehabilitation following surgical procedures to address articular cartilage lesions in the knee. Journal of Orthopaedic and Sports Physical Therapy 28:232–240

Irrgang J J, Snyder-Mackler L, Wainner R S et al 1998 Development of a patient-reported measure of function of the knee. Journal of Bone and Joint Surgery (Am) 80A:1132–1145

Irrgang J J, Anderson A F, Boland A L et al 2001 Development and validation of the International Knee Documentation Committee Subjective Knee Form. American Journal of Sports Medicine 29:600–613

Jones R E, Henley M B, Francis P 1986 Nonoperative management of isolated Grade III collateral ligament injury tears in high school football players. Clinical Orthopaedics 213:137–140

Jurist K A, Otis J C 1985 Anteroposterior tibifemoral displacements during isometric extension efforts. The roles of external load and knee flexion angle. American Journal of Sports Medicine 13:254–258

Kalunian K C, Moreland L W, Klashman D J et al 2000 Visually-guided irrigation in patients with early knee osteoarthritis: a multicenter randomized, controlled trial. Osteoarthritis and Cartilage 8:412–418

Karachalios T, Hantes M, Zibis A H et al 2005 Diagnostic accuracy of a new clinical test (the Thessaly test) for early detection of meniscal tears. Journal of Bone and Joint Surgery (Am) 87A:955–962

Kaufman K R, An K N, Litchy W J et al 1991 Dynamic joint forces during knee isokinetic exercise. American Journal of Sports Medicine 19:305–316

Keating E M, Faris P M, Ritter M A et al 1993 Use of lateral heel and sole wedges in the treatment of medial osteoarthritis of the knee. Orthopaedic Review 22:921–924

Keays S L, Bullock-Saxton J, Keays A C 2000 Strength and function before and after anterior cruciate ligament reconstruction. Clinical Orthopaedics and Related Research Apr:174–183

Keller P M, Shelbourne K D, McCarroll J R et al 1993 Nonoperatively treated isolated posterior cruciate ligament injuries. American Journal of Sports Medicine 21:132–136

Kennedy J C, Bailey W H 1968 Experimental tibial plateau fractures: studies of mechanism and a classification. Journal of Bone and Joint Surgery (Am) 50A:1522

Kerrigan D C, Lelas J L, Goggins J et al 2002 Effectiveness of a lateral-wedge insole on knee varus torque in patients with knee osteoarthritis. Archives of Physical Medicine and Rehabilitation 83:889–893

Kujala U M, Kaprio J, Sarno S 1994 Osteoarthritis of weight bearing joints of lower limbs in former elite male athletes. British Medical Journal 308:231–234

Lachiewicz P F, Funcik T 1990 Factors influencing the results of open reduction and internal fixation of tibial plateau fractures. Clinical Orthopaedics 259:210–215

Lewek M, Rudolph K S, Axe M J et al 2002 The effect of insufficient quadriceps strength on gait after anterior cruciate ligament reconstruction. Clinical Biomechanics 17:56–63

Lippiello L, Woodward J, Karpman R et al 2000 In vivo chondroprotection and metabolic synergy of glucosamine and chondroitin sulfate. Clinical Orthopaedics and Related Research 381:229–240

Liu S H, Osti L, Henry M et al 1995 The diagnosis of acute complete tears of the anterior cruciate ligament. Comparison of MRI, arthrometry and clinical examination. Journal of Bone and Joint Surgery (Br) 77B:586–588

Liu-Ambrose T, Taunton J E, MacIntyre D et al 2003 The effects of proprioceptive or strength training on the neuromuscular function of the ACL reconstructed knee: a randomized clinical trial. Scandinavian Journal of Medicine and Science in Sports 13:115–123

Livesley P J, Doherty M, Needoff M et al 1991 Arthroscopic lavage of osteoarthritic knees. Journal of Bone Joint Surgery (Br) 73B:922–926

Lundberg M, Messner K 1997 Ten-year prognosis of isolated and combined medial collateral ligament ruptures: a matched comparison in 40 patients using clinical and radiographic evaluations. American Journal of Sports Medicine 25:2–6

Lutz G E, Palmitier R A, An K N et al 1993 Comparison of tibiofemoral joint forces during open-kinetic-chain and closed-kinetic-chain exercises. Journal of Bone and Joint Surgery (Am) 75A:732–739

Lysholm J, Gillquist J 1982 Evaluation of knee ligament surgery results with special emphasis on use of a scoring scale. American Journal of Sports Medicine 10:150–154

Magee D J 2002 Orthopedic physical assessment, 4th edn. WB Saunders, Philadelphia, PA

Malanga G A, Andrus S, Nadler S F et al 2003 Physical examination of the knee: a review of the original test description and scientific validity of common orthopedic tests. Archives of Physical Medicine and Rehabilitation 84:592–603

Manal T J, Snyder-Mackler L 1996 Practice guidelines for anterior cruciate ligament rehabilitation: a criterion-based rehabilitation progression. Operative Techniques in Orthopaedics 6:190–196

Markolf K L, Gorek J F, Kabo J M et al 1990 Direct measurement of resultant forces in the anterior cruciate ligament. An in vitro study performed with a new experimental technique. Journal of Bone and Joint Surgery (Am) 72A:557–567

Matsusue Y, Yamamuro T, Hama H 1993 Arthroscopic multiple osteochondral transplantation to the chondral defect in the knee associated with anterior cruciate ligament disruption. Arthroscopy 9:318–321

Mazieres B, Combe B, Van A P et al 2001 Chondroitin sulphate in osteoarthritis of the knee: a prospective, double blind, placebo controlled multicenter clinical study. Journal of Rheumatology 28:173–181

Mayr H O, Weig T G, Plitz W 2004 Arthrofibrosis after ACL reconstruction: reasons and outcome. Archives of Orthopaedic and Trauma Surgery 124:518–522

Messner K, Fahlgren A, Persliden J et al 2001 Radiographic joint space narrowing and histologic changes in a rabbit meniscectomy model of early knee osteoarthrosis. American Journal of Sports Medicine 29:151–160

Mikkelsen C, Werner S, Eriksson E 2000 Closed kinetic chain alone compared to combined open and closed kinetic chain exercises for quadriceps strengthening after anterior cruciate ligament reconstruction with respect to return to sports: a prospective matched follow-up study. Knee Surgery, Sports Traumatology, Arthroscopy 8:337–342

Morrissey M C 1989 Reflex inhibition of thigh muscles in knee injury. Causes and treatment. Sports Medicine 7:263–276

Morrissey M C, Hudson Z L, Drechsler W I et al 2000 Effects of open versus closed kinetic chain training on knee laxity in the early period after anterior cruciate ligament reconstruction. Knee Surgery, Sports Traumatology, Arthroscopy 8:343–348

Morrissey M C, Hooper D M, Drechsler W I et al 2004 Relationship of leg muscle strength and knee function in the early period after anterior cruciate ligament reconstruction. Scandinavian Journal of Medicine and Science in Sports 14:360–366

Muller-Fassbender H, Bach G L, Haase W et al 1994 Glucosamine sulfate compared to ibuprofen in osteoarthritis of the knee. Osteoarthritis and Cartilage 2:61–69

Noyes F R, Barber-Westin S D 1996 Surgical restoration to treat chronic deficiency of the posterolateral complex and cruciate ligaments of the knee joint. American Journal of Sports Medicine 24:415–426

Noyes F R, Barber S D, Mangine R E 1991 Abnormal lower limb symmetry determined by function hop tests after anterior cruciate ligament rupture. American Journal of Sports Medicine 19:513–518

Nyland J 1999 Rehabilitation complications following knee surgery. Clinics in Sports Medicine 18:905–925

O'Reilly S C, Jones A, Muir K R et al 1998 Quadriceps weakness in knee osteoarthritis: the effect on pain and disability. Annals of Rheumatic Diseases 57:588–594

Palmoski M, Brandt K 1982 Immobilisation of the knee prevents osteoarthritis after anterior cruciate ligament resection. Arthritis and Rheumatism 25:1201–1208

Patel R R, Hurwitz D E, Bush-Joseph C A et al 2003 Comparison of clinical and dynamic knee function in patients with anterior cruciate ligament deficiency. American Journal of Sports Medicine 31:68–74

Petschnig R, Baron R, Albrecht M 1998 The relationship between isokinetic quadriceps strength test and hop tests for distance and one-legged vertical jump test following anterior cruciate ligament reconstruction. Journal of Orthopaedic and Sports Physical Therapy 28:23–31

Phillips N, Benjamin M, Everett T et al 2000 Outcome and progression measures in rehabilitation following anterior cruciate ligament injury. Physical Therapy in Sport 1:106–118

Pincivero D M, Lephart S M, Karunakara R G 1997 Relation between open and closed kinematic chain assessment of knee strength and functional performance. Clinical Journal of Sports Medicine 7:11–16

Pollo F E 1998 Bracing and heel wedging for unicompartmental osteoarthritis of the knee. American Journal of Knee Surgery 11:47–50

Rangger C, Daniel D M, Stone M L et al 1993 Diagnosis of an ACL disruption with KT-1000 arthrometer measurements. Knee Surgery, Sports Traumatology, Arthroscopy 1:60–66

Reginster J Y, Deroisy R, Rovati L C et al 2001 Long-term effects of glucosamine sulphate on osteoarthritis progression: a randomised, placebo-controlled clinical trial. Lancet 357:247–248

Schipplein O D, Andriacchi T P 1991 Interaction between active and passive knee stabilizers during level walking. Journal of Orthopaedic Research 9:113–119

Scholten R J, Deville W L, Opstelten W et al 2001 The accuracy of physical diagnostic tests for assessing meniscal lesions of the knee: a meta-analysis. Journal of Family Practice 50:938–944

Segal D, Mallik A R, Wetzler M J et al 1993 Early weight bearing of lateral tibial plateau fractures. Clinical Orthopaedics 294:232–237

Shakespeare D T, Rigby H S 1983 The bucket-handle tear of the meniscus. A clinical and arthrographic study. Journal of Bone and Joint Surgery (Br) 65B:383–387

Shelbourne K D, Patel D V, Adsit W S et al 1996 Rehabilitation after meniscal repair. Clinics in Sports Medicine 15:595–612

Shelton W R, Barrett G R, Dukes A 1997 Early season anterior cruciate ligament tears. A treatment dilemma. American Journal of Sports Medicine 25:656–658

Slemenda C, Heilman D K, Brandt K D et al 1998 Reduced quadriceps strength relative to body weight. A risk factor for knee osteoarthritis in women? Arthritis and Rheumatism 41:1951–1959

Snyder-Mackler L, Ladin Z, Schepsis A A et al 1991 Electrical stimulation of the thigh muscles after reconstruction of the anterior cruciate ligament. Effects of electrically elicited contractions of the quadriceps femoris and hamstring muscles on gait and on strength of the thigh muscles. Journal of Bone and Joint Surgery (Am) 73A:1025–1036

Snyder-Mackler L, De Luca P F, Williams P R et al 1994a Reflex inhibition of the quadriceps femoris muscle after injury or reconstruction of the anterior cruciate ligament. Journal of Bone and Joint Surgery (Am) 76A:555–560

Snyder-Mackler L, Delitto A, Stralka S W et al 1994b Use of electrical stimulation to enhance recovery of quadriceps femoris muscle force production in patients following anterior cruciate ligament reconstruction. Physical Therapy 74:901–907

Snyder-Mackler L, Delitto A, Bailey S L et al 1995 Strength of the quadriceps femoris muscle and functional recovery after reconstruction of the anterior cruciate ligament. A prospective, randomized clinical trial of electrical stimulation. Journal of Bone and Joint Surgery (Am) 77A:1166–1173

Snyder-Mackler L, Fitzgerald G K, Bartolozzi A R 3rd et al 1997 The relationship between passive joint laxity and functional outcome after anterior cruciate ligament injury. American Journal of Sports Medicine 25:191–195

Stuart M J, Meglan D A, Lutz G E et al 1996 Comparison of intersegmental tibiofemoral joint forces and muscle activity during various closed kinetic chain exercises. American Journal of Sports Medicine 24:792–799

Stürmer T, Klaus-Peter G, Brenner H 2000 Obesity, overweight and patterns of osteoarthritis: the Ulm Osteoarthritis Study. Journal of Clinical Epidemiology 53:307–313

Suh J, Åroen A, Muzzonigro T et al 1997 Injury and repair of articular cartilage: related scientific issues. Operative Techniques in Orthopaedics 7:270–278

Tohyama H, Yasuda K, Kaneda K 1991 Treatment of osteoarthritis of the knee with heel wedges. International Orthopaedics 15:31–33

Torg J S, Barton T M, Pavlov H et al 1989 Natural history of the posterior cruciate deficient knee. Clinical Orthopaedics and Related Research 246:208–216

Tyler T F, McHugh M P, Gleim G W 1999 Association of KT-1000 measurements with clinical tests of knee stability 1 year after anterior cruciate ligament reconstruction. Journal of Orthopaedic and Sports Physical Therapy 29:540–545

Veltri D M, Warren R F 1993 Isolated and combined posterior cruciate ligament injuries. Journal of the American Academy of Orthopaedic Surgeons 1:67–75

Ware J E Jr, Shelbourne C D 1992 The MOS 36-item short-form health survey (SF-36): I. Conceptual framework and item selection. Medical Care 30:473–483

Wilk K E 1994 Rehabilitation of isolated and combined posterior cruciate ligament injuries. Clinics in Sports Medicine 13:649–677

Wilk K E, Romaniello W T, Soscia S M et al 1994 The relationship between subjective knee scores, isokinetic testing, and functional testing in the ACL-reconstructed knee. Journal of Orthopaedic and Sports Physical Therapy 20:60–73

Wind W M, Bergfeld J A, Parker R D 2004 Evaluation and treatment of posterior cruciate ligament injuries: revisited. American Journal of Sports Medicine 32:1765–1775

Patellofemoral joint

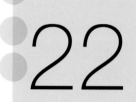

Kay Crossley, Sallie Cowan, Kim Bennell and Jenny McConnell

CHAPTER CONTENTS

Introduction 402

Applied anatomy 402

Examination 405

Management 407

Efficacy of multimodal physical therapy
management 414

Summary 415

Introduction

Patellofemoral pain (PFP) describes anterior or retropatellar pain in the absence of other knee pathology. It occurs commonly, with prospective cohort studies reporting incidence rates of 7–15% in sporting and general populations (Almeida et al 1998, 1999, Heir & Glomsaker 1996, Jones et al 1993, Kowal 1980, Milgrom et al 1991, Schwellnus et al 1990, Shwayhat et al 1994, Witvrouw et al 2000a). In addition, PFP is one of the most common conditions presenting to clinicians involved in the management of sports injuries, accounting for 2–30% of all presentations (Baquie & Brukner 1997, Clement et al 1981, DeHaven & Lintner 1986, Devereaux & Lachmann 1984, James et al 1978, Kannus et al 1987, Macintyre et al 1991, Matheson et al 1989, Pagliano & Jackson 1987).

This chapter will examine the relevant anatomy and biomechanics of the patellofemoral joint, and outline the signs and symptoms of conditions of patellofemoral origin to assist in differential diagnosis and provide assessment procedures and intervention strategies for the clinician.

Applied anatomy

Patellofemoral joint

The patella articulates with the femoral trochlea during knee flexion and extension. The patella is a sesamoid bone located within the patellar ligament. Its posterior surface has five facets, which articulate with the femur: superior, inferior, medial, lateral and odd. The geometry of the articular facets of the patella varies between individuals and may affect patellar tracking (Ahmed et al 1987, Heegard et al 1994, van Kampen & Huiskes 1990). In normal subjects, a static restraint on the natural tendency of the patella to track laterally (Farahmand et al 1998) is provided by the lateral aspect of the femoral trochlea, which extends further anteriorly than the medial aspect (Grelsamer & Klein 1998). Thus, the bony components of the patellofemoral joint provide inherent stability once the patella is within the confines of the trochlea (from 20 to 30° knee flexion). Prior to this point, there is no bony support for the patella, and passive stability is provided by the medial and lateral retinaculum and the joint capsule. The stability of the patella is also affected by the starting position of the femur. Femoral anteversion changes the interrelationship of the patella and the femur (McConnell 2002).

Soft tissue structures

The lateral side of the knee is made up of various fibrous layers, forming the superficial and deep lateral retinaculum. The anterior portion of the superficial layer of the lateral retinaculum consists of the fibrous expansion of the vastus lateralis, running longitudinally along the lateral border and inserting into the patellar tendon (Reider et al 1981a). Fibers from the iliotibial band interdigitate with fibers from the vastus lateralis and the patellar tendon to form the superficial oblique retinaculum. In particular, lateral support is provided by the two distal components of the iliotibial band, the iliopatellar band and the iliotibial tract (Terry et al 1986, Williams & Warrick 1989). Most of the lateral retinaculum arises from the iliotibial band, thus excessive lateral tracking, lateral patellar tilt and compression may arise if the iliotibial band is tight.

The medial retinaculum is thinner than the lateral retinaculum, and is thought to play a lesser role in influencing patellar position or tracking. Three ligaments, the patellofemoral, patellomeniscal and patellotibial, lie beneath the retinaculum and are described as palpable thickenings in the joint capsule (Fulkerson & Shea 1990, Reider et al 1981a). The medial patellofemoral ligament forms the primary restraint to lateral patellar translation, the medial patellomeniscal ligament is less important (Conlan et al 1993, Desio et al 1998, Hautamaa et al 1998), and the patellotibial ligament and superficial fibers of the medial retinaculum are not functionally useful (Desio et al 1998).

Muscular structure

Most of the active stabilization of the patella is provided by the quadriceps muscle, and in particular, the vastus medialis and vastus longus (VL) components. The vastus medialis is commonly divided into the oblique portion, the vastus medialis oblique (VMO), and the more vertical component, the vastus medialis longus (VML) (Bose et al 1980, Lieb & Perry 1968, 1971, Raimondo et al 1998, Scharf et al 1985, Thiranagama 1990). While there is often difficulty accurately distinguishing the VMO and VML as separate entities, most authors agree that they act as two distinct functional units due to their fiber orientation and attachments, and thus angle of force on the patella.

The VMO is more obliquely aligned than the VML or VL, thus providing a mechanical advantage to promote a medial stabilizing force to the patella. This is supported by studies of muscle fiber type, which indicate that the vastus medialis functions more as a stabilizer than the VL. The mechanical advantage gained by the fiber orientation is required to counter the relatively larger cross-sectional area and thus force producing capacity of the VL.

The VML acts with the rest of the quadriceps to extend the knee. Although the VMO does not extend the knee, it is active throughout knee extension to keep the patella centered in the trochlea of the femur, thus enhancing VL efficiency during knee extension (Bull et al 1998, Goh et al 1995, Lieb & Perry 1968).

This synergistic relationship between the medial and lateral vasti, which appears to be important in maintaining the alignment of the patella within the femoral trochlea, is supported by electromyographic (EMG) studies. Consistently, studies have demonstrated that the EMG activity of VMO and VL in the normal population is relatively balanced in terms of activation magnitude and timing in a wide variety of static, dynamic, weightbearing and non-weightbearing activities (Baecke et al 1982, Brownstein et al 1985, Cowan et al 2001b, Gryzlo et al 1994, Isear et al 1997, Karst & Willett 1997, Lange et al 1996, Mariani & Caruso 1979, Morrish & Woledge 1997, Powers et al 1996, Reynolds et al 1983, Signorile et al 1995, Smith et al 1995, Wild et al 1982). These results conflict with a common belief that the VMO needs to activate prior to the VL to counter the larger force producing capacity of the VL and maintain patellar alignment (Grabiner et al 1994). It is possible that the mechanical advantage gained by superior fiber alignment of the VMO may be sufficient to balance the greater force and velocity generating capacities of the VL.

Patellofemoral biomechanics

Kinematics

A number of studies have used cadaveric models to investigate the three-dimensional motion of the patella relative to the femur (Ahmed et al 1983, Chew et al 1997, Heegard et al 1994, Nagamine et al 1995, Reider et al 1981b, van Kampen & Huiskes 1990). In general, the patella moves caudally during knee flexion and is predominantly patellar flexion accompanied initially by a wavy (from medial displacement until 90° followed by lateral) patellar tilt and a lateral displacement. Differences in results may be attributed to the different methodologies, and in particular, the relative fixing of the tibia or femur as a reference point.

Kinetics

The magnitude of the patellofemoral joint (PFJ) reaction force is dependent on the angle of knee flexion, the quadriceps muscle tension and the patellar tendon tension. A greater quadriceps muscle tension is required to resist the flexion moment of body weight as knee flexion increases and the resultant PFJ reaction force increases. Thus, during daily activities, such as stair ascent and descent, the PFJ reaction force can reach 3.3 times body weight (Hungerford & Barry 1979, Reilly & Martens 1972). The increase of PFJ reaction force with flexion offers an explanation for the aggravation of patellofemoral symptoms experienced by individuals during bent knee activities.

Patellar tracking

Patellar tracking describes the patella articulation with the femur and its motion during knee flexion. The normal function of the patellar tracking system is to enhance quadriceps function in various static and dynamic activities. As the PFJ load increases, so too does the surface area of contact between the patella and the femur, thus minimizing the pressure through the joint. Patellar motion can be viewed as an interaction between osseoligamentous structures, muscles and neuromotor control systems (Cowan 2002). These are interdependent components of the patellar tracking system, with one system capable of compensating for deficits in another. Therefore, patellar tracking affects the magnitude and distribution of the forces acting at the PFJ and thus PFJ contact pressures (Grabiner et al 1994).

It is commonly believed that abnormal patellar tracking contributes to the development of patellofemoral pain (Fulkerson & Shea 1990). Altered patellar tracking may lead to an uneven distribution of normal patellofemoral loads, and thus increase the stress or strain on one or more structures around the PFJ.

Sources of pain

There are a number of structures in the PFJ that are susceptible to damage when subjected to loads greater than the load that the structure is able to withstand. There are two important components of patellofemoral load: (1) magnitude of load, which is influenced by the degree of knee flexion during weightbearing and by the quadriceps muscle force; and (2) distribution of load, which is related to patellar tracking (structural alignment and muscle balance).

The pathology of PFP is not clearly understood. Since a variety of pathologies may present with similar signs and symptoms, PFP is an 'umbrella' term used to encompass all anterior or retropatellar pain in the absence of other pathology. It is likely that the cause of the pain is not the same for all patients. The subjective nature of this condition is a major limitation to determining the exact pathology and hence it may be more appropriate to discuss the potential sources of patellofemoral pain (Dye & Vaupel 1994).

Current evidence indirectly indicates that various intra-articular components of the knee generate neurosensory signals that ultimately result in conscious perception. Dye et al (1998) found that palpation of the anterior synovium and fat pad elicited the strongest sensation of pain, followed by the medial and lateral retinacula, tibial and femoral insertions of the anterior cruciate ligament (ACL) and posterior cruciate ligament (PCL), then the mid regions of the ACL and PCL, the capsular margins of the menisci, and the articular cartilage surfaces. This study confirms the findings of Bierdert et al (2000) who described the highest number of afferent nerve fibers in the retinacula and medial/posteromedial capsuloligamentous structures.

Infrapatellar fat pad

The infrapatellar fat pad is a highly potent source of pain due to its rich innervation and relationship with the highly innervated synovium. This was confirmed recently by Dye et al (1998) who observed severe pain during arthroscopic palpation of the fat pad. Since the fat pad innervation is linked to that of the entire knee joint structure, it is possible that this structure may be affected by pathology in various knee joint components (Duri et al 1996). Furthermore, Witonski & Wagrowska-Danielewicz (1999) found that, in subjects with anterior knee pain, nerve fibers were immunoreactive for substance-P in the fat pad retinacula and synovium, but not the articular cartilage. There were more substance-P positive nerve fibers in the medial and lateral retinacula and in the fat pad of patients with PFP, compared with patients undergoing surgery for ACL reconstruction or with knee joint osteoarthritis (OA). A recent study by Bennell et al (2004) where the fat pad of asymptomatic individuals was injected with hypotonic saline, confirmed the finding that the fat pad can be a potent source of knee pain symptoms which are not just confined to the infrapatellar region but can refer to the proximal thigh as far as the groin.

Patellofemoral joint cartilage

While it is accepted that patellofemoral articular cartilage cannot directly be a source of pain, there are a number of mechanisms for patellofemoral chondropathy to evoke patellofemoral pain. Damage to the articular cartilage may originate in the superficial layer, or deeper within the intermediate or deep layers of the cartilage. Superficial cartilage lesion may lead to chemical or mechanical synovial irritation (see later section) or may progress to subchondral bone erosion (Fulkerson & Hungerford 1997, Insall et al 1976, Moller et al 1989, Ohno et al 1988, Outerbridge 1961). Alternatively, matrix degeneration in the intermediate or deep layers of the cartilage may lead to synovial irritation, altered pressure and thus pain perception in subchondral bone (Goodfellow et al 1976, Ohno et al 1988).

Subchondral bone

A number of studies have revealed that increased intraosseous pressure of the patella can result in pain (Arnoldi 1991, Dye & Vaupel 1994, Schneider et al 2000), possibly secondary to transient venous outflow obstruction (Arnoldi 1991). Osteotomies of the patella provided short-term relief in a number of patients (Arnoldi 1991, Schneider et al 2000). Studies that have investigated the damage to subchondral bone as a source of patellofemoral pain include descriptive human cadaveric studies (Abernathy et al 1978), animal studies that induce mechanical loads (Newberry et al 1997, Radin et al 1973) and in vivo studies using imaging (Dye & Chew 1993, Leppala et al 1998, Lindberg et al 1986, Outerbridge & Dunlop 1975).

Lateral retinaculum

The lateral retinaculum has been implicated as a potent source of patellofemoral pain. A number of quantitative and qualitative histological studies have found evidence of nerve damage in the lateral retinaculum of patients with patellofemoral pain, including nerve fibrosis (Fulkerson & Gosling 1980), neuroma formation (Fulkerson et al 1985, Sanchis-Alfonso et al 1998), increased number of myelinated and unmyelinated nerve fibers with a predominant nociceptive component (Bierdert et al 2000, Sanchis-Alfonso & Rosello-Sastre 2000, Witonski & Wagrowska-Danielewicz 1999) and increased vascularity (Sanchis-Alfonso & Rosello-Sastre 2000, Sanchis-Alfonso et al 1998, Witonski & Wagrowska-Danielewicz 1999). Based on this information, it was hypothesized that division of the lateral retinaculum could improve pain, independent of its effect on patellar tilt, by effectively denervating an area of chronic nerve injury (Fulkerson et al 1985). There were more substance-P positive nerve fibers in the medial and lateral retinacula and in the fat pad of patients with patellofemoral pain syndrome (PFPS), compared with patients undergoing surgery for ACL reconstruction or with knee joint osteoarthritis (OA).

Synovium

Since large amounts of free nerve endings (IVa) were found in the synovia of fresh cadaver knees (Bierdert et al 1992) peripatellar synovitis must be considered as one of the main causes for patellofemoral pain. This was confirmed by Dye et al (1998) who observed that both knees exhibited severe pain in the anterior synovium during arthroscopic palpation. Therefore it is likely that the synovium is a potential cause of patellofemoral pain. Despite the evidence supporting the synovium as a potential pain source, it appears that the histological changes in the synovium of patients with patellofemoral pain are moderate (Arnoldi 1991, Insall et al 1976, Vaatainen et al 1998). The potential for the synovium to be a source of pain appears to increase with progressive joint disease.

Examination

Clinical examination

Subjective examination (history)

In the history, the clinician needs to elicit the area of pain, the type of activity precipitating the pain, the history of pain onset, the behavior of the pain and any associated clicking, giving way or swelling. This gives an indication of the structure involved and the likely diagnosis.

The patient usually complains of a diffuse ache in the anterior knee, which is exacerbated by activities that load the knee (e.g. stair climbing, squats) (Brukner & Khan 2001, Fulkerson & Hungerford 1997, Jacobson & Flandry 1989). The knee may ache during prolonged sitting with the knee flexed (movie sign). Some may have crepitus, which may be present in 62% of the population (Abernathy et al 1978). Some patients experience 'giving way' or 'locking' of their knee, which must be differentiated from similar symptoms associated with an anterior cruciate deficient knee, loose body or meniscal locking (Brukner & Khan 2001). The reader is referred to Chapter 20 for further information on ACL and meniscal injuries.

Objective examination

Observation

Clinical examination establishes the diagnosis and determines the underlying contributing factors so that the appropriate treatment can be implemented. The patient is initially examined in the standing position for assessment of static lower extremity alignment. The patient can be viewed from the front, back and

Table 22.1 Observation of static lower limb alignment

Observation	Implication
Front	
Internal femoral rotation	Femoral anteversion or soft tissue adaptation
– 'Squinting patella'	As above
– No 'squinting patellae'	As above with tight lateral patellar structures
VMO muscle bulk	Size, especially asymmetry may indicate weakness
Q angle	
Enlarged or 'puffy' fat pad	Possible fat pad impingement
Tibia varus/valgus/torsion	Knee alignment
Subtalar joint	Excessive or inadequate foot pronation
Arch height	Excessive or inadequate foot pronation
Side	
Anterior/posterior pelvic tilt/ sway back	Lumbopelvic mechanics
Knee hyperextension	Presence of enlarged fat pad, possible impingement
Back	
PSIS level	Leg length asymmetry
Gluteal bulk	Size, especially asymmetry may indicate weakness
Resting calcaneal posture	Excessive or inadequate foot pronation

side (see Table 22.1). Thus, from the patient's static alignment, the clinician can anticipate how the patient will move. Any deviations from the anticipated movement provide information about the muscle control of the activity.

Dynamic examination

The aim of dynamic examination is to evaluate the effect of muscle action on the static mechanics and to reproduce the patient's symptoms, thus establishing an objective reassessment activity. The least stressful activity of walking is examined first. If the patient's symptoms are not provoked in walking, then evaluation of more stressful activities such as stair climbing, squats and single leg squat may be examined and used as a reassessment activity. The therapist evaluates the muscle control of the lower limb while the patient performs these activities. Ideally when a patient is ascending and descending steps the pelvis should remain level, the hip should be aligned over the knee and the knee should be centered over the second toe of the foot. Any movement of the knee towards the midline involving adduction and internal rotation of the femur indicates poor gluteal control which needs to be addressed in treatment.

Examination in the lying position

With the patient in a lying position, the clinician begins to confirm the diagnosis. A checklist of the examination procedures is outlined in Table 22.2. Careful palpation will enable the clinician to ascertain areas of tenderness and thus structures under

Table 22.2 Assessment of the patellofemoral joint in the lying position

Tests	Purpose
Supine	
Differential diagnostic tests Joint line palpation Tibiofemoral tests Meniscal tests Ligament tests Hip joint tests	To exclude other causes of knee pain
Muscle length tests Thomas test: psoas, rectus femoris, TFL Hamstrings, gastrocnemius	To assess potential contributing factors
Neuromeningeal tests Slump Femoral nerve tension test (modified Thomas test)	To assess potential contributing factors
Patellar orientation tests Glide Mediolateral tilt Anteroposterior tilt Rotation	To assess position of the patella relative to the femur
Sidelying	
Tests for tightness of lateral structures Medial glide Medial tilt	To assess the contribution of the lateral retinaculum
Ober's test	ITB length
Prone	
Lumbar palpation	To confirm lumbar involvement
Foot posture assessment	To assess potential contributing factors
Femoral nerve mobility	To assess potential contributing factors

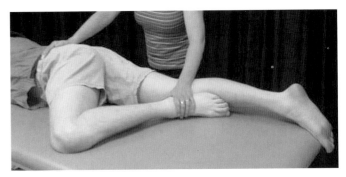

Figure 22.1 • Figure-of-four position used to examine the flexibility of the anterior hip structures.

The retinacular tissue can be specifically tested for compliance and mobility with the patient in a side-lying position and the knee flexed to 20°. Superficial retinacular fiber tightness will prevent a medial patellar glide. An anteroposterior pressure on the medial border of the patella (medial tilt) assesses deep retinacular fiber tightness.

In the prone position, the flexibility of the anterior hip structures is examined using a figure-of-four position, with the underneath foot at the level of the tibial tubercle (Fig. 22.1). The distance of the anterior superior iliac spine from the plinth is measured. Femoral anteversion or internal rotation affects the action of the pelvic musculature and changes the orientation of the femur and the patella (McConnell 2002). A modification of the test position can be used as a treatment technique.

Assessment of patellar position

An integral component of patellofemoral evaluation in the supine position is assessment of the patellar orientation relative to the femur. An optimal patellar position is one where the patella is parallel to the femur in the frontal and the sagittal planes; and the patella is midway between the two condyles when the knee is flexed to 20° (McConnell 1986). The position of the patella is determined in a static and dynamic manner by examining four discrete components: glide, lateral tilt, anteroposterior tilt and rotation. Table 22.3 outlines the optimal alignment and most common abnormalities seen with static and dynamic assessment of patellar position. In addition, during quadriceps contraction, the VMO and the VL should be activated simultaneously, or even slightly earlier for the VMO (Voight & Weider 1991). In patients with patellofemoral pain, the VMO activity may be delayed (Cowan et al 2001a, 2002c, Voight & Weider 1991). Although some investigators have found these tests to be unreliable, recent studies have shown the manual patellar glide test to be both valid and reliable (Herrington 2002, McEwan et al 2006).

Once the PFJ has been thoroughly examined, and the primary problems have been identified the patient is ready for treatment.

Investigations

Different radiological procedures have been recommended to measure patellofemoral alignment. Wide variability in the

stress. In addition, the clinician can get an appreciation of restrictions to optimal movement of the PFJ and surrounding joints by assessing the flexibility of various soft tissues such as hamstrings, gastrocnemius, rectus femoris and iliotibial band.

Pain in the infrapatellar region is difficult to distinguish between infrapatellar fat pad irritation and patellar tendonopathy. If pain is elicited in the infrapatellar region, the clinician should shorten the fat pad by lifting it towards the patella. If on further palpation, the pain is gone, then the clinician may suspect a fat pad irritation. If the pain remains, patellar tendonopathy is the most likely diagnosis. The symptoms of fat pad irritation can often be reproduced with knee extension overpressure.

Table 22.3 Assessment of patellar position

Optimal static alignment	Abnormal static alignment	Abnormal dynamic alignment	Implication
Glide Midpole of the patella is equidistant ($\pm$5 mm) to the medial and lateral femoral epicondyles	Midpole of patella sits closer to the lateral femoral epicondyle (lateral glide)	Patella moves lateral, when the quadriceps contracts	Lateral patellar displacement of the patella decreases VMO tension
Mediolateral tilt Medial and lateral patellar borders equal height and the posterior edge of both borders can be palpated	Medial borders higher than lateral (lateral tilt) Posterior edge of the lateral border will be difficult to palpate	Medial patella displacement results in increased lateral tilt	Tight lateral retinacular structures
Anteroposterior tilt Superior and inferior patellar borders are the same height	Inferior pole is displaced posteriorly Often embedded in the fat pad (posterior tilt)	Quadriceps contraction results in increased posterior tilt, particularly with knee hyperextension	Fat pad irritation, often manifests as inferior patella pain – exacerbated by knee extension
Rotation Long axis of the patella should be parallel to the long axis of the femur	Inferior pole sits lateral to the long axis of the femur (external rotation)		Tightness in retinacular structures

radiographic findings of patients with patellofemoral dysfunction, and the difficulty demonstrating radiographic abnormalities consistent with clinical findings, have contributed to the confusion in the diagnosis and classification of patellofemoral pain disorders. Despite this, numerous authors report that in using certain techniques, the radiological evidence of malposition can be accurately and reliably evaluated.

Studies using computed tomography (CT) or magnetic resonance imaging (MRI) (Powers 2000b, Powers et al 1998, Sheehan & Drace 1999, Witonski & Goraj 1999) noted that in asymptomatic individuals, the patella was laterally tilted at all angles of knee flexion, starting in approximately 5° of lateral tilt, and then gradually increasing the amount of lateral tilt during the first 50° of knee flexion, especially at 35° knee flexion. Also, the sulcus angle demonstrated increasing values as the knee extended from 45° to 0° (Powers 2000b, Powers et al 1998, Schutzer et al 1986, Witonski & Goraj 1999).

Management

Overview of physical therapy management

Most patellofemoral conditions may be successfully managed with physical therapy (i.e. nonsurgical management). Physical therapy interventions aim to reduce the patient's pain, reduce their impairments (e.g. reduced muscle strength or flexibility, poor hip control, altered foot mechanics), and improve their function. For patients with altered patellar tracking, the interventions attempt to restore normal tracking through active (quadriceps or VMO retraining) and/or passive (realignment procedures such as tape, brace, stretching) interventions and/or

improving the pelvic control by muscle training of the gluteals. If necessary, taping the gluteals to facilitate muscle contraction can also decrease the patient's symptoms. The following sections discuss the individual components of generalized strengthening, VMO and gluteal retraining, taping, stretching and orthoses and then discuss the evidence to support or refute the use of physical therapy interventions for PFP.

Generalized strengthening programs

Theory

Reducing the impairments associated with PFP is the common goal of a generalized strengthening program. Mostly, these programs focus on the quadriceps muscle group. The strengthening program is usually a standardized series of exercises, with graduated, progressively increasing resistance. These programs often incorporate some advice and education, generalized conditioning (e.g. exercise bike) and balance training.

Evidence

Controlled clinical trials have evaluated various strengthening programs, including closed kinetic chain, open kinetic chain, proprioceptive neuromuscular facilitation and a progressive resistance brace (McMullen et al 1990, Schneider et al 2001, Stiene et al 1996, Thomee 1997, Timm 1998, Witvrouw et al 2000b, 2004). In these studies, the strengthening programs were mostly conducted in the absence of other physiotherapy interventions (e.g. mobilization, patellar taping, soft tissue techniques). These clinical trials typically compared one type of quadriceps strengthening to another and generally result in significant reductions in pain and disability. Strengthening programs have not been tested, in isolation, against a placebo control. Three systematic reviews (Bizzini et al 2003, Bolga & Malone 2005, Heintjes et al 2003) concluded that there was moderate to strong evidence for strengthening programs for PFP, but that no single approach to strengthening is superior to another and that further research is required to substantiate the efficacy of these programs.

Quadriceps retraining

Theory

Under normal circumstances, the synergistic relationship among the various heads of the quadriceps maintains the alignment of the patella within the femoral trochlea, especially in the first 30° of knee flexion, when stability of the PFJ cannot be provided by its bony configuration.

While it has been proposed that balanced activation of the VMO and VL is disrupted in patients with PFP, the evidence to support imbalance in vasti activation (either decreased activation of VMO or enhanced activation of VL) is contentious (Boucher et al 1992, Coqueiro et al 2005, Mariani & Caruso 1979, Miller et al 1997, Morrish & Woledge 1997, Petschnig et al 1991, Powers 2000a, Powers et al 1996, Sheehy et al 1998, Souza & Gross 1991). Individuals with PFP produce less quadricep torque than those without knee pain (Powers et al 1997, Thomee et al 1995). Differences in methodology (particularly with respect to the use of EMG) and the inherent heterogeneity in the PFP population may account for some of the inconsistencies in study results.

While there is no conclusive evidence to support or refute an imbalance in the magnitude of vasti activation in patients with PFP, disrupted activation of the vasti may take the form of delayed activation of the VMO relative to the VL. It has been hypothesized that the VMO, which has a smaller cross-sectional area than the VL, must receive a feedforward enhancement of its excitation level in order to track the patellar optimally (Grabiner et al 1994, Wickiewicz et al 1983). Many studies that have examined individuals with PFP have supported this hypothesis, by demonstrating that the EMG activity and reflex onset time of the VMO relative to the VL is delayed, when compared with asymptomatic individuals (Cesarelli et al 2000, Cowan et al 2001a, 2001c, 2002c, Mariani & Caruso 1979, Perez et al 1995, Voight & Weider 1991, Witvrouw et al 1997). However, there is some conflict, with a number of authors describing no differences in EMG onsets (Grabiner et al 1992, Karst & Willet 1995, Morrish & Woledge 1997, Powers et al 1996, Sheehy et al 1998). Our research group investigated the onset of EMG activity of the VMO and VL in patients with PFP and asymptomatic controls (Cowan et al 2001a, 2001b, 2002c). We observed that in the PFP population, the EMG onset of VL occurred before that of VMO, while the EMG onsets of VMO and VL occurred simultaneously in the control subjects. More recently, Mellor and Hodges (2005a) have attempted to resolve the debate by investigating the control of the vasti in individuals with PFP at the level of the motor

unit, rather than whole muscle function as has previously been investigated. Their findings support the view that motor control dysfunction is a factor in PFP with their results demonstrating altered motor unit synchronization in the presence of PFP.

Physical therapy interventions for PFP have mostly focused on strengthening the quadriceps without increasing the load on the PFJ. Traditionally, standard quadriceps strengthening consisted of isometric contraction, inner range (non-weightbearing open kinetic chain) contractions and straight leg raises. Often these were progressed through incremental increases in resistance. By exercising the quadriceps in the inner range (30–0°), load on the PFJ is minimized, thus avoiding aggravation of pain. McConnell (1986) proposed that the quadriceps should be retrained using motor learning principles (see Chapter 7). This entails utilizing a weightbearing position (closed kinetic chain), thus enabling motor retraining in activities that are more functional and specific.

There is little evidence to suggest that isolated strengthening of the VMO is possible. The evidence to support or refute the ability to retrain the VMO is presented in the following sections.

Evidence

The effectiveness of VMO retraining may be assessed by studies that investigate whether quadriceps exercises can target VMO activation. It is not possible to measure the strength of the VMO or VL in isolation; therefore EMG has been used to measure the relative activation of these muscles.

There are three main open kinetic chain exercises that are used to strengthen the quadriceps: (1) isometric knee extension, (2) inner range knee extension (terminal or short arc knee extension) and (3) straight leg raises. All three utilize knee flexion less than 30° in order to minimize PFJ contact stress. The available evidence suggests that the VMO is not preferentially activated compared with VL during isometric knee extension (Cerny 1995, Cuddeford et al 1996, Gryzlo et al 1994, Karst & Jewett 1993, Souza & Gross 1991, Zakaria et al 1997), inner range quadriceps (Boucher et al 1992, Cerny 1995, Cuddeford et al 1996, Gryzlo et al 1994, Mirzabeigi et al 1999, Ng & Man 1996) or straight leg raises, regardless of the hip rotation bias (Cuddeford et al 1996, Gryzlo et al 1994, Karst & Jewett 1993, Soderberg & Cook 1983, Wild et al 1982). In fact, all studies evaluating both the straight leg raise and isometric quadriceps setting have shown less EMG activity in the single joint extensors (VL, VML and VMO) during a straight leg raise (even when resistance is applied) than during the isometric quadriceps setting exercise (Wild et al 1982). The addition of hip rotation (internal or external) does not appear to have a beneficial effect on the activation of VMO (Cerny 1995, Mirzabeigi et al 1999, Ng & Man 1996). There are mixed results regarding the addition of hip adduction on the relative activation of VMO and VL, with some authors finding that hip adduction enhances the VMO/VL ratio (Hanten & Schulthies 1990, Hodges & Richardson 1993), while most found no benefits (Cerny 1995, Coqueiro et al 2005, Karst & Jewett 1993, Laprade et al 1998, Zakaria et al 1997).

Closed kinetic chain exercises (step-up, step-down, squats and lunges) may produce a VMO/VL ratio greater than 1.0 (i.e. VMO activity greater than VL). This has been demonstrated for a squat (Cuddeford et al 1996, Gryzlo et al 1994, Hung & Gross 1999, Souza & Gross 1991), for step-up (Cuddeford et al 1996, Miller et al 1997, Sheehy et al 1998, Souza & Gross 1991, Willett et al 1998), step-down (Cerny 1995, Miller et al 1997, Sheehy et al 1998, Souza & Gross 1991) and a lunge (Cerny 1995, Miller et al 1997). Closed kinetic chain exercises have also been found to promote a more balanced initial vasti activation in terms of both onset timing and amplitude of EMG activity (Cowan et al 2002a, 2003, Stensdotter et al 2003), and greater motor unit synchronization of the vasti (Mellor & Hodges 2005b).

Conflicting results from these studies may be partly accounted for by differences in experimental technique (surface electrode vs. fine wire electrodes), methods of quantifying the EMG data (normalized versus non-normalized), specific conditions of the exercises (e.g. hip flexion or extension) and the inherent variability of EMG measurements.

The considerable available evidence does not support the premise that VMO functions independent of the VL, or that the VMO can be selectively recruited relative to the VL. This indicates that isolated recruitment of the VMO does not occur with exercises that are commonly prescribed for the treatment of PFP. Emphasis on selective strengthening of the VMO may result in a balanced activation of the VMO and VL, thus translating into a general quadriceps strengthening effect.

Practice

Weightbearing activities should be commenced early in the retraining program, as long as the therapist can ensure that the activities are pain-free; with or without patellar taping or bracing. Since the patient will be performing weightbearing activities during activities of daily living, it is desirable to do some carefully monitored practice of a functional activity in a pain-free range.

The essential aspect of training in early stages of rehabilitation is that emphasis should be given to the timing and intensity of the contraction. While surface EMG biofeedback devices provide non-normalized data, in clinical practice they appear to be extremely useful (particularly the dual channel device) in facilitating activation because they give patients immediate feedback and reinforcement when the correct pattern is achieved (LeVeau & Rogers 1980, Wild et al 1982).

A useful starting exercise is small range knee flexion and extension movements (the first 30°) in the standing position, with the feet positioned pelvis-width apart, facing forward and with the weight distributed either equally on both feet, or partially through the symptomatic limb. The patient is instructed to maintain the pelvis, hips, knees and feet in a forward-facing alignment while the knees are slowly flexed to 30° and then returned to full extension without locking the knees back. If the patient's pain returns, then patellar tape (see following section) may be applied so the patient can proceed with the training. Muscle stimulation may be used to facilitate a VMO contraction.

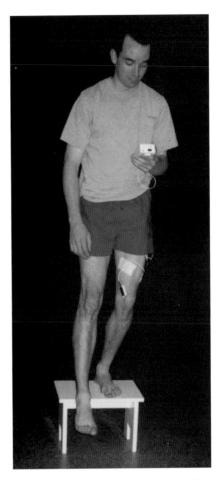

Figure 22.2 • Stepping off a step with adequate pelvic control.

Retraining could progress to small range flexion and extension movements in the walk stance position, with the quadriceps constantly active. This position not only simulates the motion of the knee during the stance phase of walking, but it is also the position where muscle recruitment is poor and the seating of the patella in the trochlea is critical.

Many patients experience pain during stair ascent and descent; therefore one of the aims of treatment is to improve the patient's ability to negotiate stairs without reproducing symptoms. The patients need to practice stepping up and down, initially using a small step. This should be performed slowly, in front of a mirror, so that changes in limb alignment can be observed and deviations can be observed and corrected (Fig. 22.2). Some patients may be able to do only a small number of repetitions with correct lower limb alignment. Since inappropriate practice can be detrimental to learning, using a small number of exercises with correct alignment is sufficient until the patient can perform larger numbers, pain-free and with correct lower limb alignment. Initially, small numbers of exercises should be performed frequently throughout the day and the number of repetitions should be increased as the skill level improves.

For further progression, the patients can move to a larger step, initially decreasing the number of contractions and then slowly increasing them again. As the control improves, patients can alter the speed of their stepping activity and may vary the place on descent where they stop going down. Weights may be introduced in the hands or in a backpack on the back. Initially, the number of repetitions and the speed of the movement should be decreased, then built back up again.

The aim of retraining is to make the transition from functional exercises to functional activities. Training should be applicable to the patient's activities/sport, so that a jumping athlete, for example, should have jumping incorporated in the program. Figure-of-eight running, bounding, jumping off boxes, jumping and turning, and other plyometric routines are particularly appropriate for the high performance athlete.

The quadriceps play an important stabilizing role for the PFJ, therefore endurance training is the ultimate goal. The number of repetitions performed by the patient at a training session will depend upon the onset of muscle fatigue. Initially, it is important to emphasize quality and not quantity, progressing to increase the number of repetitions before the onset of fatigue. Patients should be taught to recognize muscle fatigue or quivering, so that they do not train through the fatigue and risk exacerbating their symptoms.

Improving hip control

A stable pelvis minimizes unnecessary stress on the knee. Recent studies have identified that individuals with PFP have altered hip muscle function (Brindle et al 2003, Ireland et al 2003). Retraining hip external rotation control may reduce the valgus force occurring at the knee. The hip external rotators may be trained in weightbearing with the patient standing side-on to a wall (Fig. 22.3). The leg closest to the wall is flexed at the knee so that the foot is off the ground, and the hip is in a neutral position. All the weight should be on the slightly flexed weightbearing leg. The patient externally rotates the standing leg without moving the foot or the pelvis and at the same time pushes the other leg into the wall. If the patient is doing this exercise correctly, a burning in the posterior hip muscles will be felt, especially if the contraction is sustained for at least 20 s. If the exercise is difficult for a patient to coordinate, then rubber tubing may be used around the ankles as the patient stands on the affected leg, while extending the other leg diagonally at 45°.

Some patients with marked internal femoral rotation will require stretching of anterior hip structures to increase available external rotation range. The patient lies prone with the hip to be stretched in an abducted, externally rotated and extended position, and with the foot of the externally rotated leg underneath the extended leg (Fig. 22.1). The therapist's hands hold the pelvis down. The patient is instructed to flatten the abducted and rotated hip (push the anterior superior iliac spine towards the plinth) and hold the stretch for 5 s. If the patient can achieve this position easily, an instruction is given to lift the knee of the externally rotated leg off the plinth.

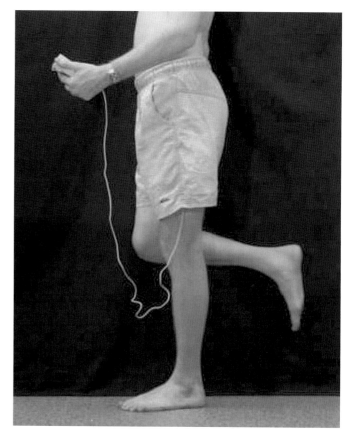

Figure 22.3 • Training of the gluteus medius in weightbearing with the patient standing side-on to a wall. Note the use of EMG biofeedback.

Patellar taping

Theory

Patellar taping aims to change the contact between the patella and the femur (McConnell 1986). Theoretically, using tape to provide a sustained stretch of the tight lateral structures makes use of the creep phenomenon, which occurs in viscoelastic material when a constant low load is applied. Length of soft tissues can be increased with sustained stretching and the magnitude of increased displacement is dependent on the duration of the applied stretch (Mckay-Lyons 1989, Taylor et al 1990).

In addition, it has been proposed that tape may unload painful structures, provide a mechanical advantage to the quadriceps muscle, improve VMO activation and reduce pain (McConnell 1986, 1996). Consequently, taping facilitates recovery, by enabling the patient to participate without pain in activities, while specifically training the VMO. This pain relief is desirable since knee pain and effusion may inhibit the quadriceps (Spencer et al 1984, Stokes & Young 1984).

Patellar taping has four basic components; medial glide, medial tilt, anterior tilt and rotation. Further taping may be required to unload painful structures (e.g. the infrapatellar fat pad) or inhibit the activation of VL. The choice of taping techniques is partly based on assessment of the patellar position and partly on the attainment of pain reduction. Appropriate taping combinations should decrease the patients' pain by at least 50% during provocative activities and may require a number of taping components.

Evidence

The evidence to support or refute the effects of patellar taping has been reviewed by Crossley et al (2001), Bizzini et al (2003) and Aminaka and Gribble (2005). Short-term pain reduction is attained with patellar taping (Aminaka & Gribble 2005, Baker et al 2002, Bockrath et al 1993, Cerny 1995, Christou 2004, Conway et al 1992, Handfield & Kramer 2000, Herrington 2001, Herrington & Payton 1997, Ireland et al 2003, Kenna 1991, Ng & Cheng 2002, Powers et al 1995, Salsich et al 2002, Somes et al 1997, Worrell et al 1994) and research continues to focus on mechanisms to explain this pain relief. A recent randomized clinical trial found a significant benefit on pain relief of using patellar tape in addition to physical therapy intervention (Whittingham et al 2004), which contrasts with the results from earlier trials (Clark et al 2000, Kowall et al 1996). Therefore, while it appears as though taping may play a role in short-term pain reduction, thus promoting effective implementation of quadriceps exercises, this requires further confirmation in controlled trials.

A few studies have evaluated the effects of patellar taping on radiographic patellar alignment in PFP patients with conflicting results. While improvements have been noted in some studies (Pfeiffer et al 2004, Roberts 1989, Somes et al 1997, Worrell et al 1994), other studies failed to find radiological evidence of changed patellar position (Bockrath et al 1993, Gigante et al 2001, Larsen et al 1995, Worrell et al 1998). A number of factors including different measurement procedures (weightbearing versus non-weightbearing), taping techniques and subject attributes may contribute to the disparate results.

Quadriceps function is decreased in subjects with PFP (Bennett & Stauber 1986, Powers et al 1997, Thomee et al 1995), possibly resulting from adaptive mechanisms to decrease quadriceps force and thus reduce PFJ load. Patellar tape significantly increases isokinetic quadriceps torque (Conway et al 1992, Handfield & Kramer 2000, Herrington 2001) and knee extensor moments and power during a vertical jump and lateral step up (Ernst et al 1999).

There is conflicting evidence as to whether patellar tape can change the activation magnitude of the VMO or VL in PFP (Christou 2004, Cowan et al 2006, Herrington et al 2005), but there is evidence to suggest that taping affects EMG onset timing of the VMO and/or VL. VMO EMG activity was found to occur earlier in the movement during stair ambulation when the patella was taped (Gilleard et al 1998). Unfortunately, the authors presented the data on the onset of VMO and VL EMG activity in terms of knee angle at muscle onset rather than as a direct measure of EMG timing. Our research group investigated the effects of patellar tape on the onset timing of VMO and VL during stair ambulation (Cowan et al 2002b). The study used a randomized, crossover design in which participants with PFP

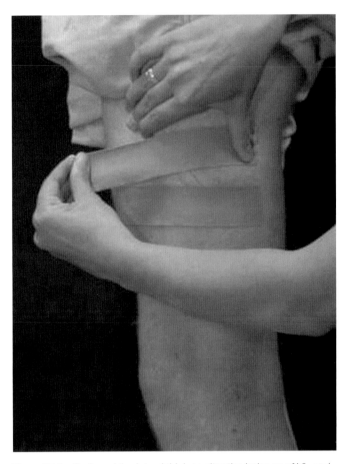

Figure 22.4 • Taping of the lateral thigh to alter the balance of VL and VMO activity. The tape is applied very firmly in a horizontal direction across the VL muscle belly and the mid thigh level to inhibit the activity of VL.

were required to complete their stair-stepping task under three experimental conditions: no tape, therapeutic tape and control tape. During the stair-stepping task, the application of therapeutic tape was found to alter the temporal characteristics of VMO and VL activation, whereas control tape had no effect. These data support the use of patellar taping as an adjunct to treatment in individuals with PFP.

In addition to taping the patella, taping of the lateral thigh has been proposed as a technique that can alter the balance of VL and VMO activity. This tape is applied very firmly in a horizontal direction across the VL muscle belly and the mid thigh level, and is proposed to inhibit the activity of VL (Fig. 22.4). A recent within-subject, placebo-controlled trial found that this inhibitory tape significantly reduced the EMG activity of VL compared with no tape or placebo tape in a stair descent task (Tobin & Robinson 2000). The effects of this inhibitory tape on VMO were inconclusive.

Practice

Patellar taping is unique to each patient. The components corrected, the order of correction, and the tension of the tape is

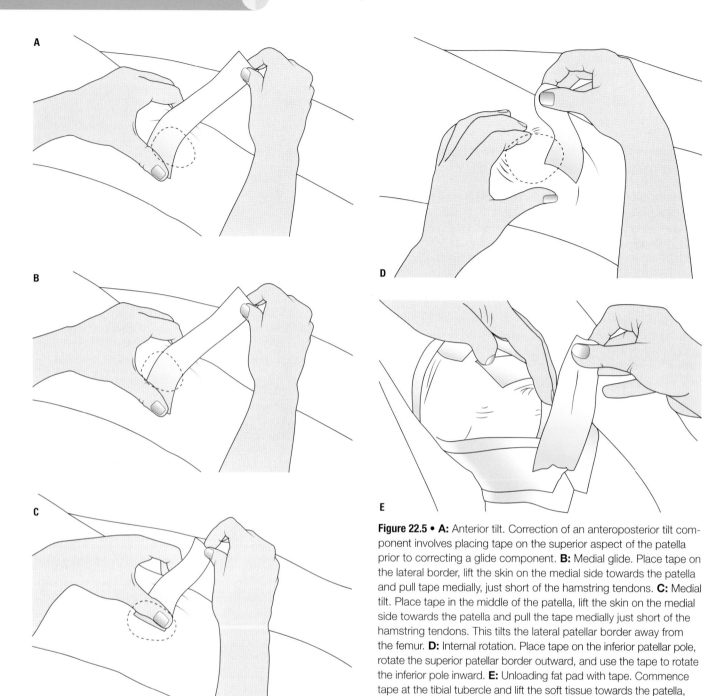

Figure 22.5 • A: Anterior tilt. Correction of an anteroposterior tilt component involves placing tape on the superior aspect of the patella prior to correcting a glide component. **B:** Medial glide. Place tape on the lateral border, lift the skin on the medial side towards the patella and pull tape medially, just short of the hamstring tendons. **C:** Medial tilt. Place tape in the middle of the patella, lift the skin on the medial side towards the patella and pull the tape medially just short of the hamstring tendons. This tilts the lateral patellar border away from the femur. **D:** Internal rotation. Place tape on the inferior patellar pole, rotate the superior patellar border outward, and use the tape to rotate the inferior pole inward. **E:** Unloading fat pad with tape. Commence tape at the tibial tubercle and lift the soft tissue towards the patella, while firmly pulling the tape to the medial and lateral joint lines.

tailored for each individual, based on the assessment of patellar position. The worst component is always corrected first and the effect of each piece of tape on the patient's symptoms should be evaluated by reassessing the painful activity. It may be necessary to correct more than one component. The tape should always improve a patient's symptoms immediately. If not, then the order in which the tape was applied or the components corrected should be re-examined. In most cases, hypoallergenic tape is placed underneath the rigid sports tape to provide a protective layer for the skin. If skin problems persist, a plastic coating (applied as either a spray, roll-on or plastic film) may be applied to the skin prior to the tape. The patient must be taught how to apply the tape with the leg fully extended and the quadriceps relaxed.

If a posterior tilt problem has been ascertained on assessment, it must be corrected first, as taping over the inferior pole of the patella will aggravate the fat pad and exacerbate the patient's pain. The posterior component is corrected together with glide or lateral tilt but the tape is placed on the superior aspect of the patella to lift the inferior pole out of the fat pad (Fig. 22.5A).

If there is no posterior tilt problem, glide may be corrected by placing a piece of nonstretch tape from the lateral patellar border, and firmly pulling it, to just past the medial femoral condyle (Fig. 22.5B). At the same time, the soft tissue on the medial aspect of the knee is lifted towards the patella to create a tuck or fold in the skin superomedially. This provides a more effective correction of the glide component and also minimizes the friction rub (friction between the tape and the skin), which can occur when patients have extremely tight lateral structures.

The mediolateral tilt component is corrected by placing a piece of tape firmly from the middle of the patella to the medial femoral condyle (Fig. 22.5C). The object is to lift the lateral border anteriorly so that the patella becomes parallel with the femur in the frontal plane. Again the soft tissue on the medial aspect of the knee is lifted towards the patella.

External rotation is the most common rotation problem and to correct this, the tape is positioned at the inferior pole and pulled upwards and medially towards the opposite shoulder while the superior pole is rotated laterally. Care must be taken so that the inferior pole is not displaced into the fat pad (Fig. 22.5D). Internal rotation, on the other hand, is corrected by taping from the superior pole downwards and medially.

The principle of unloading is based on the premise that inflamed soft tissue does not respond well to stretch. For example, if a patient presents with a sprained medial collateral ligament, applying a valgus stress to the knee will aggravate the condition, whereas a varus stress will decrease the symptoms. To unload the fat pad, the tape commences at the tibial tubercle and comes out in a wide 'V' to the medial and lateral joint lines. As the tape is being pulled towards the joint line, the skin is lifted towards the patella, thus shortening the fat pad (Fig. 22.5E).

The tape is kept on all day, every day, until patients have learnt how to activate their VMO. The tape is removed with care in the evening, allowing the skin time to recover. The tape can cause a breakdown in the skin either through a friction rub or as a consequence of an allergic reaction. Table 22.4 summarizes the problems related to, and possible solutions for skin irritation due to taping.

If the patient experiences a return of the pain, then the patient should readjust the tape. If the activity is still painful, the patient should cease the activity immediately. The tape will loosen quickly if the lateral structures are extremely tight or the patient's job or sport requires extreme amounts of knee flexion. The patient needs to wear the tape until the muscles have adequate endurance, which may take a considerable time for some. Box 22.1 includes a suggested test sequence that the therapist can give the patient to determine if the patient is ready to be without the tape for daily activities.

In some cases the gluteal muscles are not firing well, so the patient exhibits adduction and internal rotation of the femur during weight bearing activities, so gluteal taping can improve the stability of the pelvis (Fig. 22.6). Kilbreath and co-workers (2006) recently demonstrated improved hip extension in a group of stroke patients following gluteal taping. The subjects who had experienced a stroke between two and eleven

Table 22.4 Skin problems associated with taping, and solutions

Problem	Solution
Friction rub	
On the medial aspect of the knee due to friction between tape and skin	Lift the skin on the medial aspect of the knee during taping
Occurs within 1 week; becomes less of a problem as skin toughens	Remove tape carefully, peel back slowly and use the other hand to decrease the pull on the skin
Common (up to 80% of patients)	Use a tape remover
	Rub hand cream into medial aspect of the knee after tape removal
	Use skin preparation (spray, roll-on or plastic film) to provide a barrier
Allergic reaction	
Raised itchy rash where the tape has been	Leave tape off. Apply ice to relieve the itch
Occurs within 1 day if there is previous exposure; may take 10 days if no previous exposure	If severe, may need to seek medical advice
Rare (5%)	If possible, identify high-risk individuals (previous allergies to tape or adhesive plasters)
	Use hypoallergenic tape only
	Tape for very short periods

Box 22.1 Example of progression of weaning from tape use

The patient should be able to perform the following exercises pain-free to determine if they are ready to discontinue taping for daily activities:

- 5 sets of 10 steps performed slowly and controlled with a 10 s rest between each set
- 1 min quarter squat against the wall
- 1 min half squat against the wall
- A further 5 sets of 10 continuous steps

If the tape is ready to come off, then the patient wears the tape alternate days for 1 week.

If the knee has survived 1 week with no recurrence of symptoms, the patient may take the tape off for daily activities, but keep it on for sport.

If the patient has been pain-free for a month and is not taped for daily activities, the tape may be removed for sport, provided the patient is able to do the test described above, being untaped and pain-free during the test.

years ago, walked at two different speeds (self selected and fast) under three different conditions (control, therapeutic and placebo tape). With the therapeutic tape in situ subjects went from 3° of hip flexion in the control situation to 11° extension

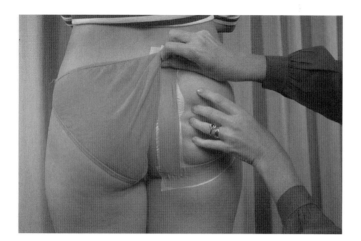

Figure 22.6 • Gluteal taping.

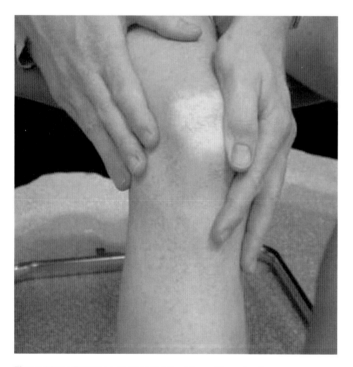

Figure 22.7 • Patient self-stretching of the retinacular tissue.

in self selected walking speed and 8° in fast walking. No difference was found with sham tape.

Other

Stretching

Appropriate flexibility exercises must be included in the treatment regimen. The involved muscles may include the hamstrings, gastrocnemius, rectus femoris and tensor fascia lata/iliotibial band. Stretching tight lateral soft tissue structures may be achieved passively by therapist mobilization of the lateral retinaculum and iliotibial band and by patient self-stretching of the retinacular tissue (Fig. 22.7).

Correcting abnormal foot pronation

Patients exhibiting prolonged pronation during mid-stance in gait may be shown how to train the supinators of their feet. This should improve the stability of the foot for push off and decrease the increased valgus vector force created at the knee by the abnormal foot pronation.

The position of training is mid-stance, the patient is instructed to lift the arch while keeping the great toe on the ground, and then to push the first metatarsal and great toe into the ground. The rationale behind this exercise is that, if the base of the first metatarsal is lifted using the tibialis posterior muscle, the line of action of the peroneus longus is improved. The peroneus longus can then efficiently act on the first metatarsal and improve the stability of the first ray in preparation for push off. If the patient is unable to keep the first metatarsophalangeal joint on the ground when the arch is lifted, then the foot deformity is too large to correct with training alone and orthotics will be necessary to control the excessive pronation.

Efficacy of multimodal physical therapy management

Efficacy of physical therapy management is determined by well-controlled clinical trials. Similar to other musculoskeletal conditions, there are few trials that have evaluated the effectiveness of physical therapy for PFP. Currently, physical therapy in clinical practice generally includes a number of the treatment components described above (e.g. generalized strengthening, specific VMO retraining, stretching, mobilization, hip muscle training, taping/bracing or foot orthoses). Therefore it is appropriate to test a multimodal physical therapy intervention. There are five trials that have examined multimodal physical therapy interventions for PFP and the results of these trials indicate a positive benefit of such an intervention (Clark et al 2000, Crossley et al 2002, Eburne & Bannister 1996, Harrison et al 1999, Whittingham et al 2004). Furthermore, the systematic reviews that have included trials of multimodal physical therapy treatments also support their use to decrease the pain and disability in PFP (Bizzini et al 2003, Bolga & Malone 2005, Crossley et al 2001, Heintjes et al 2003).

We completed a randomized, double-blind, placebo-controlled trial of a McConnell-based physical therapy program in 71 PFP patients (Cowan et al 2001a, 2002a). Standardized treatments consisted of six treatments, once weekly for both the physical therapy and placebo groups. Sixty-seven (33 physical therapy; 34 placebo) subjects completed the trial. The physical therapy group demonstrated significantly better response to treatment and greater improvements in average pain, worst pain and functional activities. Sixty-five subjects were included for EMG testing. At baseline, the EMG onset of VL occurred before that of VMO during a stair-stepping task. Following the 6-week treatment program, the physical therapy group demonstrated greater change in their EMG onset timing of VMO compared to VL. This change resulted in the simultaneous onset of VMO and VL in the concentric phase of the stair-stepping task, and in the eccentric phase the onset of VMO actually preceded VL. However, in the placebo group at the follow-up assessment, the onset of VL still occurred before that of VMO in both phases of the stair-stepping task (Cowan et al 2002a). This study demonstrates that a McConnell-based physical therapy program significantly improves pain and function and can alter EMG onset of VMO relative to VL compared with placebo treatment.

Summary

It is unclear which structure is predominantly implicated as the pathological cause of pain associated with PFP. Despite this, nonsurgical treatment options have evolved, based on decreasing the load on the PFJ through improved patellar tracking and lower limb alignment. A multi-modal approach to the treatment of patellofemoral pain is recommended. This should include an exercise component (including vasti retraining and hip muscle training) and patellar taping or stretching. There appears to be a consistent improvement in short-term pain and function due to such multi-modal treatment. However, studies that have evaluated interventions in isolation are inconclusive.

References

Abernathy P J, Townsend P, Rose R et al 1978 Is chondromalacia patella a separate entity? Journal of Bone and Joint Surgery (Br) 60B:205–210

Ahmed A, Burke D, Yu A 1983 In vitro measurement of static pressure distribution in synovial joints: II. Retropatellar surface. Journal of Biomechanical Engineering 105:226–236

Ahmed A M, Burke D L, Hyder A 1987 Force analysis of the patellar mechanism. Journal of Orthopaedic Research 5:69–85

Almeida S A, Trone D W, Leone D M et al 1998 Gender differences in musculoskeletal injury rates: a function of symptom reporting. Medicine and Science in Sports and Exercise 31:1807–1812

Almeida S, Williams K M, Shaffer R A et al 1999 Epidemiological patterns of musculoskeletal injuries and physical training. Medicine and Science in Sports and Exercise 31:1176–1182

Aminaka N, Gribble P A 2005 A systematic review of the effects of therapeutic taping on patellofemoral pain syndrome. Journal of Athletic Training 40:341–351

Arnoldi C C 1991 Patellar pain. Acta Orthopaedica Scandinavia 62 (suppl 224):1–29

Baecke J A H, Burema J, Frijters J E R 1982 A short questionnaire for the measurement of habitual physical activity in epidemiological studies. American Journal of Clinical Nutrition 36:936–942

Baker V, Bennell K, Stillman B et al 2002 Abnormal knee joint position sense in individuals with patellofemoral pain syndrome. Journal of Orthopaedic Research 20:208–214

Baquie P, Brukner P 1997 Injuries presenting to an Australian sports medicine centre: a 12 month study. Clinical Journal of Sports Medicine 7:28–31

Bennett J G, Stauber W T 1986 Evaluation and treatment of anterior knee pain using eccentric exercise. Medicine and Science in Sports and Exercise 18:526–530

Bennell K, Hodges P, Mellor R et al 2004 The nature of anterior knee pain following injection of hypertonic saline into the infrapatellar fat pad. Journal of Orthopaedic Research 22:116–121

Bierdert R, Stauffer E, Niklaus N F 1992 Occurrence of free nerve endings in the soft tissue of the knee joint. A histologic investigation. American Journal of Sports Medicine 20:430–433

Bierdert R, Lobenhoffer P, Lattermann C et al 2000 Free nerve endings in the medial and posteromedial capsuloligamentous complexes: occurrences and distribution. Knee Surgery, Sports Traumatology and Arthroscopy 8:68–72

Bizzini M, Childs J D, Piva S R et al 2003 Systematic review of the quality of randomized controlled trials for patellofemoral pain. Journal of Orthopaedic and Sports Physical Therapy 33:4–20

Bockrath K, Wooden C, Worrell T et al 1993 Effects of patella taping on patella position and perceived pain. Medicine and Science in Sports and Exercise 25:989–992

Bolga L, Malone T 2005 Exercise prescription and patellofemoral pain: evidence for rehabilitation. Journal of Sports Rehabilitation 14:72–88

Bose K, Kanagasuntheram R, Osman M B H 1980 Vastus medialis obliquus; an anatomic and physiologic study. Orthopedics 3:883–880

Boucher J P, King M A, Lefebvre R et al 1992 Quadriceps femoris muscle activity in patellofemoral pain syndrome. American Journal of Sports Medicine 20:527–532

Brindle T J, Mattacola C, McCrory J 2003 Electromyographic changes in the gluteus medius during stair ascent and descent in subjects with anterior knee pain. Knee Surgery, Sports Traumatology, Arthroscopy 11:244–251

Brownstein B A, Lamb R L, Mangine R E 1985 Quadriceps torque and integrated eletromyography. Journal of Orthopaedic and Sports Physical Therapy 6:309–314

Brukner P, Khan K 2001 Clinical sports medicine, 2nd edn. McGraw-Hill, Sydney

Bull A M J, Senavongse W W, Taylor A R et al 1998 The effect of the oblique portions of the vastus medialis and lateralis on patellar tracking. Proceedings of the 11th Conference of the ESB, Toulouse, France

Cerny K 1995 Vastus medialis oblique/vastus lateralis muscle activity ratios for selected exercises in persons with and without patellofemoral pain syndrome. Physical Therapy 75:672–682

Cesarelli M, Bifulco P, Bracale M 2000 Study of the control strategy of the quadriceps in anterior knee pain. IEEE Transactions on Rehabilitation Engineering 8:330–341

Chew J T, Stewart N J, Hanssen A D et al 1997 Differences in patellar tracking and knee kinematics among three different total knee designs. Clinical Orthopaedics and Related Research 345:87–98

Christou E A 2004 Patellar taping increases vastus medialis oblique activity in the presence of patellofemoral pain. Journal of Electromyography and Kinesiology 14:495–504

Clark D I, Downing N, Mitchell J et al 2000 Physiotherapy for anterior knee pain: a randomised controlled trial. Annals of the Rheumatic Diseases 59:700–704

Clement D B, Taunton J E, Smart G W et al 1981 A survey of overuse injuries. Physician and Sportsmedicine 9:47–58

Conlan T, Garth W P, Lemons J E 1993 Evaluation of the medial soft-tissue restraints of the extensor mechanism of the knee. Journal of Bone and Joint Surgery (Am) 75A:682–693

Conway A, Malone T, Conway P 1992 Patellar alignment/tracking alteration: effect on force output and perceived pain. Isokinetics and Exercise Science 2:9–17

Coqueiro K, Bevilaqua-Grossi D, Berzin F et al 2005 Analysis on the activation of the VMO and VLL muscles during semisquat exercises with and without hip adduction in individuals with patellofemoral pain syndrome. Journal of Electromyography and Kinesiology 15:596–603

Cowan S M 2002 Motor control of the vasti in patellofemoral pain syndrome. PhD thesis, University of Melbourne

Cowan S M, Bennell K L, Hodges P W et al 2001a Delayed onset of electromyographic activity of vastus medialis obliquus relative to vastus lateralis in subjects with patellofemoral pain syndrome. Archives of Physical Medicine and Rehabilitation 82:183–189

Cowan S M, Hodges P W, Bennell K L 2001b Anticipatory activity of vastus lateralis and vastus medialis obliquus occurs simultaneously in voluntary heel and toe raising. Physical Therapy in Sport 2:71–79

Cowan S M, Bennell K L, Crossley K M et al 2002a Physiotherapy treatment alters the recruitment of the vasti in patellofemoral pain syndrome. Medicine and Science in Sports and Exercise 34(12):1879–1885

Cowan S M, Bennell K L, Hodges P W 2002b Therapeutic patellar taping changes the timing of vasti muscle activation in people with patellofemoral pain syndrome. Clinical Journal of Sports Medicine 12(6):339–347

Cowan S M, Hodges P W, Bennell K L et al 2002c Altered vasti recruitment when people with patellofemoral pain syndrome complete a postural task. Archives of Physical Medicine and Rehabilitation 83(7):989–995

Cowan S M, Bennell K L, Hodges, P W 2003 Simultaneous feedforward recruitment of the vasti in untrained postural tasks can be restored by specific training. Journal of Orthopaedic Research 21:553–558

Cowan S M, Hodges P W, Crossley J M et al 2006 Patellar taping does not change the amplitude of electromyographic activity of the vasti in a stair stepping task. British Journal of Sports Medicine 40:30–34

Crossley K, Bennell K, Green S et al 2001 A systematic review of physical interventions for patellofemoral pain syndrome. Clinical Journal of Sports Medicine 11:103–110

Crossley K, Bennell K, Green S et al 2002 Physical therapy for patellofemoral pain: a randomized, double-blinded, placebo-controlled trial. American Journal of Sports Medicine 30:857–865

Cuddeford T, Williams A K, Medeiros J M 1996 Electromyographic activity of the vastus medialis oblique and vastus lateralis muscles during selected exercises. Journal of Manual and Manipulative Therapy 4:10–15

DeHaven K E, Lintner D M 1986 Athletic injuries: comparison by age, sport and gender. American Journal of Sports Medicine 14:218–224

Desio S M, Burks R T, Bachus K N 1998 Soft tissue restraints to lateral patellar translation in the human knee. American Journal of Sports Medicine 26:59–65

Devereaux M, Lachmann S 1984 Patellofemoral arthralgia in athletes attending a sports injury clinic. British Journal of Sports Medicine 18:18–21

Duri Z A, Aichroth P M, Dowd G 1996 The fat pad. Clinical observations. American Journal of Knee Surgery 9:55–66

Dye S F, Chew M H 1993 The use of scintigraphy to detect increased osseous metabolic activity about the knee. Journal of Bone and Joint Surgery (Am) 75A:1388–1406

Dye S F, Vaupel G L 1994 The pathophysiology of patellofemoral pain. Sports Medicine and Arthroscopy Review 2:203–210

Dye S F, Vaupel G L, Dye C C 1998 Conscious neurosensory mapping of the internal structures of the human knee without intraarticular anaesthesia. American Journal of Sports Medicine 26:773–777

Eburne J, Bannister G 1996 The McConnell regimen versus isometric quadriceps exercises in the management of anterior knee pain. A randomised prospective controlled trial. Knee 3:151–153

Ernst G P, Kawaguchi J, Saliba E 1999 Effect of patellar taping on knee kinetics of patients with patellofemoral pain syndrome. Journal of Orthopaedic and Sports Physical Therapy 29:661–667

Farahmand F, Tahmasbi M N, Amis A A 1998 Lateral force-displacement behaviour of the human patella and its variation. Journal of Biomechanics 31:1147–1152

Fulkerson J, Hungerford D 1997 Disorders of the patellofemoral joint. Williams and Wilkins, Baltimore, MD

Fulkerson J P, Shea K P 1990 Current concepts review: disorder of patellofemoral alignment. Journal of Bone and Joint Surgery (Am) 72A:1424–1429

Fulkerson J P, Tennant R, Jaivin J S et al 1985 Histological evidence of retinacular nerve injury associated with patellofemoral malalignment. Clinical Orthopaedics and Related Research 197:196–205

Gigante A, Pasquinellii F M, Palodini P et al 2001 The effects of patellar taping on patellofemoral incongruence: a computerised tomography study. American Journal of Sports Medicine 29:88–92

Gilleard W, McConnell J, Parsons D 1998 The effect of patellar taping on the onset of vastus medialis obliquus and vastus lateralis muscle activity in persons with patellofemoral pain. Physical Therapy 78:25–32

Goh J C H, Lee P Y C, Bose K 1995 A cadaver study of the function of the oblique part of vastus medialis. Journal of Bone and Joint Surgery (Br) 77B:225–231

Goodfellow J, Hungerford D S, Woods C 1976 Patello-femoral joint mechanics and pathology: 2. Chondromalacia patellae. Journal of Bone and Joint Surgery (Br) 58B:291–299

Grabiner M D, Koh T J, Miller G F 1991 Fatigue rates of vastus medialis oblique and vastus lateralis during static and dynamic knee extension. Journal of Orthopaedic Research 9:391–397

Grabiner M D, Koh M A, Andrish J T 1992 Decreased excitation of vastus medialis oblique and vastus lateralis in patellofemoral pain. European Journal of Experimental Musculoskeletal Research 1:33–39

Grabiner M D, Koh T J, Draganich L F 1994 Neuromechanics of the patellofemoral joint. Medicine and Science in Sports and Exercise 26:10–21

Grelsamer R P, Klein J R 1998 The biomechanics of the patellofemoral joint. Journal of Orthopaedic and Sports Physical Therapy 28: 286–297

Gryzlo S M, Patek R M, Pink M et al 1994 Electromyographic analysis of knee rehabilitation exercises. Journal of Orthopaedic and Sports Physical Therapy 20:36–43

Handfield T, Kramer J 2000 Effect of McConnell taping on perceived pain and knee extensor torques during isokinetic exercise performed by patients with patellofemoral pain syndrome. Physiotherapy Canada Winter:39–44

Hanten W P, Schulthies S S 1990 Exercise effect on electromyographic activity of the vastus medialis oblique and the vastus lateralis. Physical Therapy 70:39–43

Harrison E L, Sheppard M S, McQuarrie A M 1999 A randomized controlled trial of physical therapy treatment programs in patellofemoral pain syndrome. Physiotherapy Canada Spring:93–106

Hautamaa P V, Fithian D C, Kaufman K R et al 1998 Medial soft tissue restraints in lateral patellar instability and repair. Clinical Orthopaedics and Related Research 349:174–182

Heegard J, Leyvraz P, van Kampen A et al 1994 Influence of soft structures on patellar three dimensional tracking. Clinical Orthopaedics and Related Research 299:235–243

Heintjes E, Berger M Y, Bierma-Zeinstra S M A et al 2003 Exercise therapy for patellofemoral pain syndrome. Cochrane Database of Systematic Reviews 4:CD003472

Heir T, Glomsaker P 1996 Epidemiology of musculoskeletal injuries among Norwegian conscripts undergoing basic military training. Scandinavian Journal of Medicine and Science in Sports 6:186–191

Herrington L 2001 The effect of patella taping on quadriceps peak torque and perceived pain: a preliminary study. Physical Therapy in Sport 2:23–28

Herrington L C 2002 The inter-tester reliability of a clinical measurement used to determine the medial-lateral orientation of the patella. Manual Therapy 7:163–167

Herrington L, Payton C J 1997 Effects of corrective taping of the patella on patients with patellofemoral pain. Physiotherapy 83:566–572

Herrington L, Malloy S, Richard J 2005 The effect of patella taping on vastus medialis oblique and vastus lateralis EMG activity and knee kinematic variables during stair descent. Journal of Electromyography and Kinesiology 15:604–607

Hodges P, Richardson C A 1993 The influence of isometric hip adduction on quadriceps femoris activity. Scandinavian Journal of Rehabilitation Medicine 25:57–62

Hung Y-J, Gross M T 1999 Effect of foot position on electromyographic activity of the vastus medialis oblique and vastus lateralis during lower-extremity weight-bearing activities. Journal of Orthopaedic and Sports Physical Therapy 29:93–105

Hungerford D S, Barry M 1979 Biomechanics of the patellofemoral joint. Clinical Orthopaedics and Related Research 144:9–15

Insall J, Falvo K A, Wise D W 1976 Chondromalacia patellae: a prospective study. Journal of Bone and Joint Surgery (Am) 58A:1–8

Ireland M L, Wilson J D, Ballantyne B T et al 2003 Hip strength in females with and without patellofemoral pain. Journal of Orthopaedic and Sports Physical Therapy 33:671–676

Isear J A, Erickson J C, Worrell T W 1997 EMG analysis of lower extremity muscle recruitment patterns during an unloaded squat. Medicine and Science in Sports and Exercise 29:532–539

Jacobson K E, Flandry F C 1989 Diagnosis of anterior knee pain. Clinics in Sports Medicine 8:179–195

James S L, Bates B T, Osternig L R 1978 Injuries to runners. American Journal of Sports Medicine 6:40–50

Jones B H, Cowan D N, Tomlinson J R et al 1993 Epidemiology of injuries associated with physical training among young men in the army. Medicine and Science in Sports and Exercise 25:197–203

Kannus P, Aho H, Järvinen M et al 1987 Computerised recording of visits to an outpatient sports clinic. American Journal of Sports Medicine 15:79–85

Karst G M, Jewett P D 1993 Electromyographic analysis of exercises proposed for differential activation of medial and lateral quadriceps femoris muscle components. Physical Therapy 73:286–299

Karst G M, Willet G M 1995 Onset timing of electromyographic activity in the vastus medialis oblique and vastus lateralis muscles in subjects with and without patellofemoral pain syndrome. Physical Therapy 75:813–823

Karst G M, Willett G M 1997 Reflex response times of vastus medialis oblique and vastus lateralis in normal subjects and in subjects with patellofemoral pain. [Letter to editor.] Journal of Orthopaedic and Sports Physical Therapy 26:108–109

Kenna M 1991 The effect of patellofemoral joint taping on pain during activity. Paper presented at the Manipulative Physiotherapists Association of Australia 7th Biennial Conference, Blue Mountains, Australia

Kilbreath S L, Perkins S, Crosbie J et al 2006 Gluteal taping improves hip extension during stance phase of walking following stroke. Australian Journal of Physiotherapy 52:53–56

Kowal D M 1980 Nature and cause of injuries to women resulting from an endurance training program. American Journal of Sports Medicine 8:265–269

Kowall M G, Kolk G, Nuber G W et al 1996 Patellar taping in the treatment of patellofemoral pain. A prospective randomized study. American Journal of Sports Medicine 24:61–66

Lange G W, Hintermeister R A, Schlegel T et al 1996 Electromyographic and kinematic analysis of graded treadmill walking and the implications for knee rehabilitation. Journal of Orthopaedic and Sports Physical Therapy 23:294–301

Laprade J, Culham E, Brouwer B 1998 Comparison of five isometric exercises in the recruitment of the vastus medialis oblique in persons with and without patellofemoral pain syndrome. Journal of Orthopaedic and Sports Physical Therapy 27:197–204

Larsen B, Adreasen E, Urfer A et al 1995 Patellar taping: a radiographic examination of the medial glide technique. American Journal of Sports Medicine 23:465–471

Leppala J, Kannus P, Natri A et al 1998 Bone mineral density in the chronic patellofemoral pain syndrome. Calcified Tissue International 62:548–553

LeVeau B F, Rogers C 1980 Selective training of the vastus medialis muscle using EMG biofeedback. Physical Therapy 60:1410–1415

Lieb F J, Perry J 1968 Quadriceps function. An anatomical and mechanical study. Journal of Bone and Joint Surgery (Am) 50A:1535–1548

Lieb F J, Perry J 1971 Quadriceps function: an electromyographic study under isometric conditions. Journal of Bone and Joint Surgery (Am) 53A:749–758

Lindberg U, Lysholm J, Gillquist J 1986 The correlation between arthroscopic findings and the patellofemoral pain syndrome. Arthroscopy 2:103–107

McConnell J 1986 The management of chondromalacia patellae: a long term solution. Australian Journal of Physiotherapy 32:215–223

McConnell J 1996 Management of patellofemoral problems. Manual Therapy 1:60–66

McConnell J 2002 The physical therapist's approach to patellofemoral disorders. Clinics in Sports Medicine 21:363–387

McEwan I, Herrington L, Thom J 2006 The validity of clinical measures of patella position. Manual Therapy doi:10.1016/j.math.2006.06.013

Macintyre J G, Taunton J E, Clement D B et al 1991 Running injuries: a clinical study of 4173 cases. Clinical Journal of Sports Medicine 1:81–87

Mckay-Lyons M 1989 Low-load, prolonged stretching the treatment of elbow contractures secondary to head trauma. Physical Therapy 69:292

McMullen W, Roncarati A, Koval P 1990 Static and isokinetic treatments of chondromalacia patella: a comparative investigations. Journal of Orthopaedic and Sports Physical Therapy 12:256–266

Mariani P, Caruso I 1979 An electromyographic investigation of subluxation of the patella. Journal of Bone and Joint Surgery (Am) 61A:169–171

Matheson G O, Macintyre J G, Taunton J E et al 1989 Musculoskeletal injuries associated with physical activity in older ages. Medicine and Science in Sports and Exercise 21:370–385

Mellor R, Hodges P W 2005a Motor unit synchronization is reduced in anterior knee pain. Journal of Pain 6:550–558

Mellor R, Hodges P W 2005b Motor unit synchronization of the vasti muscles in closed and open chain tasks. Archives of Physical Medicine and Rehabilitation 86:716–721

Milgrom C, Kerem E, Finestone A et al 1991 Patellofemoral pain caused by overactivity. A prospective study of risk factors in infantry recruits. Journal of Bone and Joint Surgery (Am) 73A:1041–1043

Miller J P, Sedory D, Croce R V 1997 Vastus medialis obliquus and vastus lateralis activity in patients with and without patellofemoral pain syndrome. Journal of Sport Rehabilitation 6:1–10

Mirzabeigi E, Jordan C, Gronley J K et al 1999 Isolation of the vastus medialis oblique muscle during exercise. American Journal of Sports Medicine 27:50–53

Moller B N, Moller-Larsen F, Frich L H 1989 Chondromalacia induced by patellar subluxation in the rabbit. Acta Orthopaedica Scandinavia 60:188–191

Morrish G M, Woledge R C 1997 A comparison of the activation of muscles moving the patella in normal subjects and in patients with chronic patellofemoral problems. Scandinavian Journal of Rehabilitation Medicine 29:43–48

Nagamine R, Otani T, White S E et al 1995 Patellar tracking measurements in the normal knee. Journal of Orthopaedic Research 13:95–96

Newberry W N, Zukosky D K, Haut R C 1997 Subfracture insult to a knee joint causes alterations in the bone and in the functional stiffness of overlying cartilage. Journal of Orthopaedic Research 15:450–455

Ng G Y, Cheng J M 2002 The effects of patellar taping on pain and neuromuscular performance in subjects with patellofemoral pain syndrome. Clinical Rehabilitation 16:821–827

Ng G Y F, Man V Y 1996 EMG analysis of vastus medialis obliquus and vastus lateralis during static knee extension with different hip and ankle positions. New Zealand Journal of Physiotherapy 4:7–10

Ohno O, Naito J, Iguchi T et al 1988 An electron microscopic study of early pathology in chondromalacia of the patella. Journal of Bone and Joint Surgery (Am) 70A:883–899

Outerbridge R E 1961 The etiology of chondromalacia patellae. Journal of Bone and Joint Surgery (Br) 43B:752–757

Outerbridge R, Dunlop J 1975 The problem of chondromalacia. Clinical Orthopaedics and Related Research 110:177–196

Pagliano J W, Jackson D W 1987 A clinical study of 3000 long distance runners. Annals of Sports Medicine 3:88–91

Perez P L, Gossman M R, Lechner D et al 1995 Electromyographic temporal characteristics of the vastus medialis oblique and the vastus lateralis in women with and without patellofemoral pain. Paper presented at the12th International Congress of the World Confederation for Physical Therapy, Washington, DC

Petschnig R, Baron R, Engel A et al 1991 Objectivation of the effects of knee problems on vastus medialis and vastus lateralis with EMG and dynamometry. Physical Medicine and Rehabilitation 2:50–54

Pfeiffer R P, DeBeliso M, Shea K G et al 2004 Kinematic MRI assessment of McConnell taping before and after exercise. American Journal of Sports Medicine 32:621–628

Powers C M 2000a Patellar kinematics, Part I: the influence of vastus muscle activity in subjects with and without patellofemoral pain. Physical Therapy 80:956–964

Powers C M 2000b Patellar kinematics, Part II: the influence of the depth of the trochlear groove in subjects with and without patello-femoral pain. Physical Therapy 80:965–973

Powers C M, Landel R, Carpenter T et al 1995 The effects of patel-lar taping on loading characteristics in subjects with patellofemoral pain. Paper presented at the12th International Congress of the World Confederation for Physical Therapy, Washington, DC

Powers C M, Landel R F, Perry J 1996 Timing and intensity of vastus muscle activity during functional activities in subjects with and with-out patellofemoral pain. Physical Therapy 76:946–955

Powers C M, Perry J, Hsu A et al 1997 Are patellofemoral pain and quadriceps femoris muscle torque associated with locomotor function? Physical Therapy 77:1063–1075

Powers C M, Shellock F G, Pfaff M 1998 Quantification of patellar tracking using kinematic resonance imaging. Journal of Magnetic Resonance Imaging 8:724–732

Radin E L, Parker H G, Pugh J W et al 1973 Response of joints to impact loading: III. Relationship between trabecular microfractures and cartilage degeneration. Journal of Biomechanics 6:51–57

Raimondo R A, Ahmad C S, Blankevoort L et al 1998 Patellar stabiliza-tion: a quantitative evaluation of the vastus medialis obliquus muscle. Orthopaedics 21:791–795

Reider B, Marshall J L, Koslin D et al 1981a The anterior aspect of the knee joint. Journal of Bone and Joint Surgery (Am) 63A:351–356

Reider B, Marshall J L, Ring B 1981b Patellar tracking. Clinical Orthopaedics and Related Research 157:143–148

Reilly D T, Martens M 1972 Experimental analysis of the quadriceps muscle force and patellofemoral joint reaction forces for various activi-ties. Acta Orthopedica Scandinavia 43:126–137

Reynolds L, Levin T, Medeiros J et al 1983 EMG activity of vastus medialis obliquus and vastus lateralis and their role in patella align-ment. American Journal of Physical Medicine 62:61

Roberts J M 1989 The effect of taping on patellofemoral alignment: a radiological pilot study. Paper presented at the Manipulative Therapists Association of Australia Biennial Conference, Adelaide

Salsich G B, Brechter J H, Farwell D et al 2002 The effects of patellar taping on knee kinetics, kinematics and vastus lateralis muscle activity during stair ambulation in individuals with patellofemoral pain. Journal of Orthopaedic and Sports Physical Therapy 32:3–10

Sanchis-Alfonso V, Rosello-Sastre E 2000 Immunohistochemical analy-sis for neural markers of the lateral retinaculum in patients with isolated symptomatic patellofemoral malalignment. American Journal of Sports Medicine 28:725–731

Sanchis-Alfonso V, Rossello-Sastre E, Monteagudo-Castro C et al 1998 Quantitative analysis of nerve changes in the lateral retinaculum in patients with isolated symptomatic patellofemoral malalignment. American Journal of Sports Medicine 26:703–709

Scharf W, Weinstable R, Othrner E 1985 Anatomical separation and clinical importance of two different parts of the vastus medialis muscle. Acta Anatomy 123:108–111

Schneider F, Labs K, Wagner S 2001 Chronic patellofemoral pain syndrome: alternatives for cases of therapy resistance. Knee Surgery Traumatology and Arthroscopy 9:290–295

Schneider U, Wenz W, Breusch S J et al 2000 A new concept in the treatment of anterior knee pain: patellar hypertension syndrome. Orthopedics 23:581–586

Schutzer S F, Ramsby G R, Fulkerson J P 1986 Computed tomographic classification of patellofemoral pain patients. Orthopedic Clinics of North America 17:235–248

Schwellnus M P, Jordaan G, Noakes T D 1990 Prevention of common overuse injuries by the use of shock absorbing insoles. A prospective study. American Journal of Sports Medicine 18:636–641

Sheehan F T, Drace J E 1999 Quantitative MR measures of three-dimensional patellar kinematics as a research and diagnostic tool. Medicine and Science in Sports and Exercise 31:1399–1405

Sheehy P, Burdett R G, Irrgang J J et al 1998 An electromyographic study of vastus medialis oblique and vastus lateralis activity while ascending and descending steps. Journal of Orthopaedic and Sports Physical Therapy 27:423–429

Shwayhat A F, Linenger J M, Hofherr L K et al 1994 Profiles of exer-cise history and overuse injuries among United States Navy sea, air, and land (SEAL) recruits. American Journal of Sports Medicine 22:835–840

Signorile J F, Kacsik D, Perry A et al 1995 The effect of knee and foot position on the electromyographical activity of the superficial quadriceps. Journal of Orthopaedic and Sports Physical Therapy 22:2–9

Smith G P, Howe T E, Oldham J A et al 1995 Assessing quadri-ceps muscles recruitment order using rectified averages. Clinical Rehabilitation 9:40–46

Soderberg G, Cook T 1983 An electromyographic analysis of quadri-ceps femoris muscle setting and straight leg raise. Physical Therapy 63:1434–1438

Somes S, Worrell T W, Corey B et al 1997 Effects of patellar taping on patellar position in the open and closed kinetic chain: a preliminary study. Journal of Sports Rehabilitation 6:299–308

Souza D R, Gross M 1991 Comparison of vastus medialis obliquus: vastus lateralis muscle integrated electromyographic ratios between healthy subjects and patients with patellofemoral pain. Physical Therapy 71:310–320

Spencer J, Hayes K, Alexander I 1984 Knee joint effusion and quadri-ceps inhibition in man. Archives of Physical Medicine 65:171–177

Stensdotter A, Hodges P, Mellor R et al 2003 Quadriceps activation in closed and in open kinetic chain exercise. Medicine and Science in Sports and Exercise 35:2043–2047

Stiene H A, Brosky T, Reinking M F et al 1996 A comparison of closed kinetic chain and isokinetic joint isolation in patients with patellofemoral dysfunction. Journal of Orthopaedic and Sports Physical Therapy 24:136–141

Stokes M, Young A 1984 Investigations of quadriceps inhibition: implica-tions for clinical practice. Physiotherapy 70:425–428

Taylor D, Dalton J, Seaber A 1990 Visco-elastic properties of muscle-tendon units. The biomechanical effect of stretching. American Journal of Sports Medicine 18:300

Terry G C, Hughston J C, Norwood L A 1986 The anatomy of the iliopatellar band and iliotibial tract. American Journal of Sports Medicine 14:39–45

Thiranagama R 1990 Nerve supply of the human vastus medialis muscle. Journal of Anatomy 170:193–198

Thomee R 1997 A comprehensive treatment approach for patellofemoral pain syndrome in young women. Physical Therapy 77:1690–1703

Thomee R, Renstrom P, Karlsson J et al 1995 Patellofemoral pain syn-drome in young women: II. Muscle function in patients and healthy controls. Scandinavian Journal of Medicine and Science in Sports 5:245–251

Timm K E 1998 Randomized controlled trial of protonics on patellar pain, position, and function. Medicine and Science in Sports and Exercise 30:665–670

Tobin S, Robinson G 2000 The effect of McConnell's vastus lateralis inhibition taping technique on vastus lateralis and vastus medialis obliquus activity. Physiotherapy 26:173–183

Vaatainen U, Lohmander L S, Thonar E et al 1998 Markers of carti-lage and synovial metabolism in joint fluid and serum of patients with chondromalacia. Arthritis and Cartilage 6:115–124

van Kampen A, Huiskes R 1990 The three-dimensional tracking pattern of the human patella. Journal of Orthopaedic Research 8:372–382

Voight M, Weider D 1991 Comparitive reflex response times of the vastus medialis and the vastus lateralis in normal subjects with extensor mechanism dysfunction. American Journal of Sports Medicine 19:131–137

Whittingham M, Palmer S, Macmillan F 2004 Effects of taping on pain and function in patellofemoral pain syndrome: a randomized controlled trial. Journal of Orthopaedic and Sports Physical Therapy 34:504–510

Wickiewicz T L, Roy R R, Powell P L et al 1983 Muscle architecture of the human lower limb. Clinical Orthopaedics and Related Research 179:275–283

Wild J J, Franklin T D, Woods G W 1982 Patellar pain and quadriceps rehabilitation: an EMG study. American Journal of Sports Medicine 10:12–15

Willett G M, Karst G M, Canney E M et al 1998 Lower limb EMG activity during selected stepping exercise. Journal of Sport Rehabilitation 7:102–111

Williams P L, Warrick R 1989 Gray's anatomy. Churchill Livingstone, Edinburgh

Witonski D, Goraj B 1999 Patellar motion analyzed by kinematic and dynamic axial magnetic resonance. Archives of Orthopaedic and Trauma Surgery 119:46–49

Witonski D, Wagrowska-Danielewicz M 1999 Distribution of substance-P nerve fibers in the knee joint of patients with anterior knee pain. A preliminary report. Knee Surgery Traumatology and Arthroscopy 7:177–183

Witvrouw E, Delvaux K, Lysens R et al 1997 Reflex response times of vastus medialis oblique and vastus lateralis in normal subjects and in subjects with patellofemoral pain-response. Journal of Orthopaedic and Sports Physical Therapy 26:109–110

Witvrouw E, Lysens R, Bellemans J et al 2000a Intrinsic risk factors for the development of anterior knee pain in an athletic population. A two year prospective study. American Journal of Sports Medicine 28:480–489

Witvrouw E, Lysens R, Bellemans J et al 2000b Open versus closed kinetic chain exercises for patellofemoral pain syndrome. A prospective, randomized study. American Journal of Sports Medicine 28:687–694

Witvrouw E, Danneels L, Van Tiggelen D et al 2004 Open versus closed kinetic chain exercises in patellofemoral pain: a 5-year prospective randomized study. American Journal of Sports Medicine 32:1122–1130

Worrell T W, Ingersoll C D, Farr J 1994 Effect of patellar taping and bracing on patellar position: an MRI case study. Journal of Sport Rehabilitation 3:146–153

Worrell T, Ingersoll C D, Bockrath-Pugliese K et al 1998 Effect of patellar taping and bracing on patellar position as determined by MRI in patients with patellofemoral pain. Journal of Athletic Training 33:16–20

Zakaria D, Harburn K L, Kramer J F 1997 Preferential activation of the vastus medialis oblique, vastus lateralis, and hip adductor muscles during isometric exercises in females. Journal of Orthopaedic and Sports Physical Therapy 26:23–28

Foot, ankle and lower leg

D. S. Blaise Williams III and Jack Taunton

CHAPTER CONTENTS

Introduction 420

Arthrology 420

Examination 423

Common sport-related injuries 426

Less common injuries 433

Summary 437

Introduction

Ankle injuries are the most common acute injury in the athletic population (Adamson & Cymet 1997, Lofvenberg et al 1995, Lynch & Renstom 1999). Lateral ankle injuries account for 15–25% of all sports injuries (Adamson & Cymet 1997). Because the foot is the contact with the ground during sports activities, it is subjected to very high forces. Finally, because the talus is tightly coupled with motion in the tibia, forces are transferred directly to the tibia and muscles of the lower leg. Overuse injuries are common at the foot and ankle complex and even more so in the lower leg as a result of the need to eccentrically control motion during landing activities. This chapter outlines the functional anatomy of the foot and ankle complex and lower leg, gives a complete discussion of functional evaluation and describes current physical therapy approaches to treatment of common pathologies in the athletic population.

Arthrology

Proximal tibiofibular joint

The proximal tibiofibular joint is the articulation between the lateral condyle of the tibia and the head of the fibula. The joint is a plane synovial joint. The flat facet of the fibula faces anterior and medial and articulates closely with the posterior lateral facing surface of the lateral tibial condyle. Slight movement occurs at the joint during dorsiflexion. With full dorsiflexion, the lateral portion of the talus will press the lateral maleolus superior on the tibia. When the talocrural joint returns to neutral, the fibula slides inferiorly. There is less inferior motion of the fibula when moving from neutral to plantarflexion. Controversy exists regarding the medial-lateral and rotational motion of the tibia (Soavi et al 2000). This is likely due to the variability that is present in the articular surfaces of the joint. A fibrous and synovial capsule surround the proximal tibiofibular joint. The fibrous capsule is thickened by the anterior and posterior ligaments of the head of the fibula. Although not often diagnosed, synovitis of the proximal tibiofibular joint may be more common than previously thought (Bozkurt et al 2004).

Distal tibiofibular joint

The distal tibiofibular joint is the articulation between the inferior ends of the tibia and fibula. The joint is a syndesmotic fibrous joint and has little to no movement. The only motion that is available is a slight opening which accommodates the anterior portion of the talus during dorsiflexion. The convex surface of the fibula articulates with the concave surface of the tibia. A portion of the synovial membrane from the talocrural joint covers a small portion of the distal tibiofibular joint but does not encompass it. The primary connection between the distal tibia and fibula is a thickening of the interosseus membrane known as the interosseus ligament. The interosseus ligament is just superior to the anterior and posterior tibiofibular ligaments. These ligaments extend as far laterally as the maleolus on the fibula. The posterior tibiofibular ligament is much stronger than the anterior tibiofibular ligament and can create an avulsion fracture of the posterior tibia in severe ankle injuries. A great deal of the strength of the ankle joint is dependent on the stability provided by the distal tibiofibular joint.

Talocrural joint

The talocrural joint is the articulation between the distal ends of the tibia and fibula (mortise) and the superior surface of the talus (trochlea). The joint is a diarthrodial or synovial joint and is classified as a hinge joint. This joint is typically referred to as the ankle joint. The joint allows for dorsiflexion and plantarflexion, which occurs with slight amounts of secondary plane motion. This is a result of the orientation of the talocrural joint axis, which essentially passes through the maleoli. In a static condition, this corresponds to approximately 20–30° of external rotation and 10° down and lateral in the frontal plane (Barnett & Napier 1952, Hicks 1953, Lundberg et al 1989). It is important to note that, in a dynamic condition, the axis of the joint changes its orientation as individuals move through the dorsiflexion/plantarflexion range of motion (Lundberg et al 1989) (Fig. 23.1). The concave surface of the mortise articulates with the convex surface of the talus when viewed in the sagittal plane. However, there is a slightly concave shape to the talus when viewed anteriorly. The joint is encompassed by a thin synovial membrane.

There are thickenings of the membrane medially and laterally, which provide the primary support at the ankle. Medially, the deltoid ligament is comprised of three separate parts named for their attachments (tibionavicular, posterior tibiotalar and tibiocalcaneal). The deltoid ligament is thicker and stronger than the lateral ligaments. The lateral ligaments are separate from one another and are, again, named for their bony attachments. The anterior talofibular ligament is the weakest and most often injured. The remaining two lateral ligaments, the calcaneofibular ligament and posterior talofibular ligament, are stronger and injured less. The primary motions occurring at this joint are plantarflexion and dorsiflexion. The joint is most stable in dorsiflexion as the talus locks between the tibia and the fibula due to the larger anterior portion of the talus. The

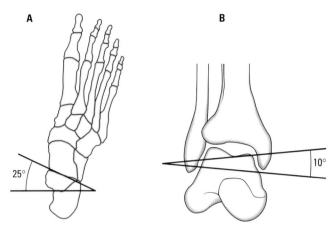

Figure 23.1 • Axis of the talocrural joint in the transverse plane (**A**) and frontal plane (**B**).

joint becomes less stable in the plantarflexed position as the smaller posterior surface of the talus moves forward allowing for more lateral movement of the talus within the mortise.

Subtalar joint

The subtalar joint is the articulation between the inferior surface of the talus and the superior surface of the calcaneus. The joint is a diarthrodial joint and is classified as a plane joint. This joint is often referred to as the 'keystone of the foot' because the subtalar joint transfers motion from the foot to the lower leg in closed kinetic chain situations. The joint allows for triplanar motion dominated by inversion and eversion. The axis for motion at the subtalar joint sits approximately 42° from horizontal in the sagittal plane and 16° laterally in the transverse plane. A significant amount of abduction and adduction is also present as a result of the orientation of the joint axis in the sagittal plane. Finally, a small amount of dorsiflexion and plantarflexion is possible at this joint based on the orientation of the joint axis (Fig. 23.2). There are three articulations between the calcaneus and the talus. The large posterior talar facet on the calcaneus is convex and it articulates with the concave surface of the talus. The middle and anterior facets of the calcaneus have a concave orientation and arthrokinematically function opposite of the posterior facet. The structure of the subtalar joint, therefore, acts to stabilize the joint dynamically (Fig. 23.3). The joint is further encompassed by its own capsule and is supported by the medial, lateral and posterior talocalcaneal ligaments. Additionally, the joint is supported anteriorly by the strong interosseus talocalcaneal ligament.

Midtarsal joint

The midtarsal joint is a complex articulation between four bones: the calcaneus, talus, navicula and cuboid. The joint is a diarthrodial joint and is classified as a plane joint. There are two joint capsules: one surrounding the talus, calcaneus and

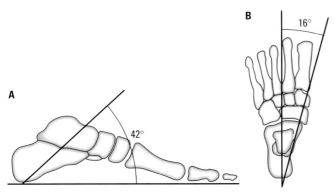

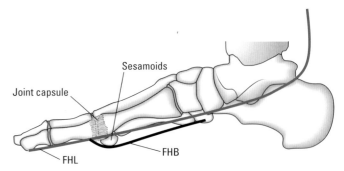

Figure 23.2 • Axis of motion at the subtalar joint. **A**: The lateral view demonstrates how almost equal amounts of frontal plane (inversion/eversion) and transverse plane (adduction/abduction) can occur about this joint. **B**: The superior view shows the axis almost in line with the long axis of the foot, resulting in primarily frontal plane motion.

Figure 23.4 • A synovial capsule encompasses the first metatarsalphalangeal joint while the sesamoid bones are outside the capsule. The sesamoids provide a greater moment arm for the flexor hallucis brevis (FHB) muscle and provide protection for the flexor hallucis longus (FHL) muscle, which passes between the sesamoids and the metatarsal head.

calcaneocuboid articulation. Dorsolaterally, the bifurcate ligament supports the joint.

Tarsometatarsal joints

The tarsometatarsal joints are the articulation between the cuboid, the three cuneiforms and the five metatarsals. The joints are diarthrodial and classified as plane joints. The three joint capsules are named for their positions in the foot: medial, intermediate and lateral tarsometatarsal joints. The medial joint is the articulation between the medial cuneiform and the base of the first metatarsal and is the most mobile of the three tarsometatarsal joints. Motion occurs about a joint axis, which allows primarily for plantarflexion and dorsiflexion at the joint. The joints also abduct and invert with dorsiflexion. The most stable of the three tarsometatarsal joints is the intermediate joint. Due to the bony architecture, the second and third metatarsals create a rigid central pillar in the foot. The second and third metatarsals articulate with the three cuneiforms. The lateral tarsometatarsal joint is the articulation between the fourth and fifth metatarsals and the cuboid. A small amount of motion is available at this joint, primarily consisting of plantarflexion and dorsiflexion. All three joints are supported by the dorsal, plantar and interosseus tarsometatarsal ligaments.

Metatarsalphalangeal joints

The metatarsalphalangeal (MTP) joints are articulations between the heads of the metatarsals and the bases of the proximal phalanges. Discussion will be limited to the first as most information is available. The joint is a diarthrodial joint and is classified as a condyloid joint. The joint capsule surrounds the first metatarsal and the proximal phalanx. The medial and lateral sesamoid bones are extracapsular (Fig. 23.4). The joint allows for dorsiflexion and plantarflexion as well as abduction and adduction. The joint is supported medially and laterally by collateral ligaments and by a strong plantar ligament.

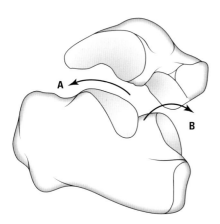

Figure 23.3 • As the subtalar joint everts (in an open kinetic chain), the distal end of the calcaneus moves laterally. At the joint surfaces, the posterior facet glides medially while the anterior and medial facets glide laterally. This provides a screw-like mechanism that effectively locks the joint and provides stability even without the ligaments.

navicular, and one surrounding the lateral portion of the calcaneus and the cuboid. The joint is highly mobile and motion occurs about two primary joint axes: a longitudinal axis and an oblique axis. Inversion and eversion is the primary motion about the longitudinal axis while motion about the oblique axis is truly triplanar. The mobility of the midtarsal joint increases as the subtalar joint pronates and becomes less mobile as it supinates. The medial side of the joint is supported by the dorsal talonavicular ligament and more significantly by the plantar calcaneonavicular or spring ligament. The spring ligament plays an important role in maintaining the medial longitudinal arch of the foot. On the lateral side of the midtarsal joint, the long plantar ligament is the most superficial and helps to support the calcaneocuboid articulation and maintain the arches of the foot. The short plantar ligament is deep and only supports the

Calcaneal fat pad

The plantar aspect of the heel is made up of connective and specialized fat tissue, which is between 10 and 20 mm in thickness (Whittle 1999). The pad is attached to the medial calcaneal tuberosity with the fat being divided into chambers. The heel pad acts to absorb between 47 and 66% of the shock when the plantar surface of the foot is in contact with the ground (Aerts et al 1995). Injuries and pain in the calcaneus are often attributed to decreased ability of the calcaneal fat pad to absorb shock. Injuries to the calcaneal fat pad are often the result of trauma to the area. Fortunately, due to the adequate blood supply, fat pad injuries often heal well with rest and anti-inflammatory intervention. Compressive heel cups may also provide support and increase the resting thickness of the fat pad allowing for compression without further damage to the tissue.

Metatarsal fat pad

A fat pad also protects the plantar aspect of the metatarsal heads. The pad is attached to the plantar fascia and the metatarsal heads themselves. The fat pad acts to absorb shock and provide lubrication when the plantar surface of the metatarsal heads is in contact with the ground. Injuries to the metatarsal are often attributed to atrophy or dislocation of the fat pad. However, recent evidence suggests that metatarsal fat pad atrophy is not associated with metatarsalgia (Waldecker 2001). Metatarsal fat pad injuries respond to similar treatment as calcaneal fat pad injuries. Relieving the pressure on the metatarsal head with a metatarsal pad may also be an effective treatment.

Extrinsic muscles

The primary plantarflexors of the ankle are the gastrocnemius and soleus, both innervated by the tibial nerve S1–S2. Several other muscles cross posterior to the maleoli and act as secondary plantarflexors of the ankle. The tibialis posterior (tibial nerve [L4]–L5), and flexor digitorum longus and flexor hallucis longus (both tibial S2–S3) are found on the medial side while the peroneus longus and brevis (both superficial peroneal L5–S1) pass posterior to the lateral maleolus. Dorsiflexion is mainly provided by the tibialis anterior (deep peroneal [L4]–L5) and supported by the extensor digitorum longus and extensor hallucis longus (both deep peroneal L5–S1). Inversion is provided by the posterior and anterior tibialis muscles. Eversion is accomplished by the peroneus longus and brevis muscles. Additionally, the medial longitudinal arch is supported externally by the anterior tibialis, posterior tibialis and the peroneus longus.

Intrinsic muscles

There is little evidence to support the idea that the intrinsic muscles of the foot act as stabilizers of the arch during ambulation (Fiolkowski et al 2003, Mann & Hagy 1979). Quantitative analyses (Kura et al 1997, Silver et al 1985) have revealed the potential for these muscles to produce force in the toes especially for flexion. These conclusions are based on the structure and orientation of the intrinsic muscles of the foot and not upon electromyographic (EMG) data. Recent EMG data confirms that loss of activity of the abductor hallucis muscle results in a lowering of the height of the navicular and hence the medial longitudinal arch (Fiolkowski et al 2003). However, it is difficult to clinically justify the training of these muscles (i.e. towel crunches) especially when there is no method of quantifying the progression of strength in these muscles and no current data confirms that strengthening of these muscles will help maintain the medial longitudinal arch.

Examination

A thorough history is especially important when evaluating the athlete with an injury of the foot, ankle or lower leg. The therapist should ask the athlete if they have had any previous injuries to the lower extremities. Previous injuries to other lower extremity joints, even on the contralateral side, can provide crucial information for the possibility of the mechanical development of foot, ankle and lower leg pathology. The mechanism of injury as described by the athlete can often provide enough information to determine the structure involved in the pathology. The therapist should ask the athlete to describe the exact location and the nature of the pain. Pain as it relates to time of day or activity level can also help determine the exact course of injury development. Neuropathic pain such as numbness, tingling or burning into the foot may be related to an entrapment such as tarsal tunnel syndrome or posterior compartment syndrome. The level of current and previous function should be determined first through history and then through physical examination.

Observation of the patient in both static and dynamic conditions will give the therapist information about mechanical alignment, ability to move, and willingness to move. It is important to observe the patient from anterior, posterior and side views in order to establish a complete picture of their posture as it relates to their pathology. When viewing the athlete from the anterior and posterior, comparisons should be made between sides for symmetry.

There are several structures that should be evaluated from the anterior view. The angle of gait refers to the amount of external rotation of the feet. This is approximately 5–18° in normal individuals (McGee 1992) (Fig. 23.5). The therapist should also observe symmetry between sides. The base of gait or base of support is how far apart the medial borders of the feet are during stance. A narrow or wide base of support can be predictors of mechanical imbalances leading to pathology. Hallux position whether neutral or valgus can give some indication about dynamic function during gait. Midfoot position can be directly measured, preferably through an arch ratio (Saltzman et al 1995, Williams & McClay 2000) or can be visually assessed as normal high or low (Giladi et al 1985).

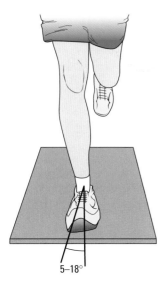

5–18°

Figure 23.5 • The angle of gait can be observed in standing, walking or running. In the athlete, observing the angle of gait during running may give information that is more beneficial to the pathology than the angle during standing or walking. The angle of gait most often decreases as the speed of locomotion is increased.

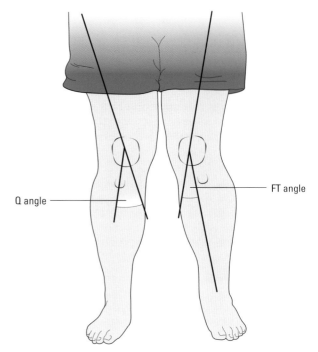

Q angle — — FT angle

Figure 23.6 • The Q-angle measures the alignment of the patella relative to the tibial tuberosity and ASIS but gives no information about frontal plane knee joint alignment. The femoral tibial (FT) angle represents the angle formed between the long axis of the tibia and the long axis of the femur.

Symmetry should be observed in this measurement also. Patellar position (alta, baja, medial, lateral, internal or external rotation) should be assessed in standing as well as supine. Q-angle may also be evaluated in conjunction with patellar position in order to further assess patellar position relative to the entire lower extremity (Fig. 23.6). Q-angle only assesses the relationship of the patella to the entire lower extremity. It does not evaluate knee joint valgus. Directly measuring the angle between the long axes of the femur and tibia will measure frontal plane knee joint orientation (Fig. 23.6). Femoral internal or, less often, external rotation can be evaluated from the anterior. The position of the patella is often a partial indicator of femoral rotation as the patella should be nested between the femoral condyles during stance. Finally, the anterior superior iliac spine (ASIS) symmetry should be evaluated for possible differences in leg length.

Most of the information gained from observation from the side relates to range of motion and alignment issues primarily in the sagittal plane. Resting knee angle should be evaluated for the presence of hyperextension (recurvatum) or slight knee flexion. These could be related to changes in foot, ankle or even hip orientation. In the same way, resting hip angle may be increased or decreased. Pelvic tilt and lumbar position should also be evaluated. Changes in lumbar or pelvic orientation can relate to differences in muscle extensibility and have effects at the knee, tibia and subsequently the foot and ankle complex.

Many of the structures viewed from the posterior can help confirm observations made from the anterior. However, most of the information gathered from the posterior will relate to alignment and motion in the frontal plane. Tibial position, whether varum or valgum, helps give an indication of how much rearfoot (tibia relative to calcaneus) pronation may occur. Resting calcaneal stance position (RCSP) is the relationship of the calcaneus to the floor. Again, this measure alone may be important but becomes more meaningful when compared to the tibial position. For instance, a rearfoot angle of 20° could be the result of 20° of calcaneal eversion and 0° of tibial angle or from 10° of calcaneal and 10° of tibial varum. Neutral calcaneal stance position (NCSP) is the relationship of the calcaneus to the floor with the joint held in a subtalar neutral position. The difference between this position and the RCSP provides a measurement of the motion of the subtalar joint (Fig. 23.7). Lateral toe sign is related to angle of gait and can be compared for symmetry and excessive external rotation of the entire lower extremity. Typically we would like to see only the fourth and fifth toes when viewed from behind. However, individual assessment of femoral rotation, tibial rotation and foot abduction should be completed to determine which contributes to the position of toe-out. The popliteal fossa can also be viewed as a representation of internal or external rotation of the hips. This should be referenced to the patella. If the patella is neutral and the fossa is internally rotated then it is likely the femur is internally rotated. However, if the patella is lateral and the fossa is neutral, the patella is likely laterally tracking. Posterior superior iliac spine and iliac crest symmetry are evaluated for inominate rotations or leg length discrepancies. Scapular asymmetry may indicate spinal curvatures or muscular imbalances.

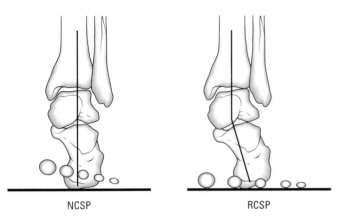

NCSP   RCSP

Figure 23.7 • Subtalar joint motion can be assessed in standing by comparing the difference between the calcaneal position when the subtalar joint is placed in its neutral position (left) and when it is allowed to relax in normal weightbearing (right).

Non-weightbearing assessment

Non-weightbearing evaluation of foot and ankle begins in the prone position. The subtalar neutral position was first introduced by Root et al (1977) as a reference position for measuring motion at the ankle and subtalar joint. In order to accurately attain the neutral position of the subtalar joint, the hip should be held in a neutral (internal/external rotation) position. The calcaneus should then be bisected and marked with pen. The distal third of the tibia is also bisected. The calcaneus is then rocked between full inversion to full eversion until the talar heads are felt to be congruent beneath the thumb and index finger of the evaluating therapist (Fig. 23.8). This is the neutral position of the subtalar joint and it used as a reference point around which other measurements of the rearfoot are taken. Assessment of passive inversion and eversion allow the therapist to evaluate position as well as mobility of the subtalar joint. Forefoot orientation relative to the rearfoot can be measured with a goniometer projected up from the forefoot. Forefoot varus deformity is a medially facing position of the forefoot relative to the rearfoot. A varus position of the forefoot in subtalar neutral will result in compensatory pronation. Forefoot valgus is a lateral forefoot relative to the rearfoot and results in compensatory supination (Fig. 23.9). First ray orientation and mobility will dictate or be the result of pronation or supination. Fifth ray orientation and mobility should be assessed and evaluated for stress reactions. Lack of ankle dorsiflexion may lead to hypermobility in the midfoot and plantar fasciitis. The forefoot may also rest in an abducted or adducted position and lead to compensatory pronation or supination, respectively. Muscle strength should be evaluated, especially of the peroneals and posterior tibialis. Functional strength must be evaluated through single leg standing tests or balance activities. Manual muscle testing may not be enough to determine functional strength.

In supine, leg length should be assessed. If there is an asymmetry, this may result in pronation on the longer side and

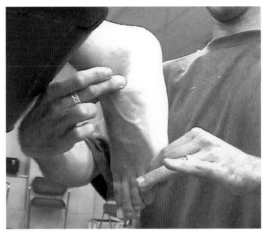

Figure 23.8 • Subtalar neutral is obtained with the patient in the prone position and the foot hanging off the end of the table. The foot is in a relaxed to slightly plantarflexed position and the foot is moved from full inversion to full eversion with the outside hand holding just below the heads of the forth and fifth metatarsals. The inside hand palpates the neck of the talus as it protrudes medially into the thumb and laterally into the index finger. When the pressure on the thumb and index finger are equal, the ankle is pushed toward dorsiflexion until slight resistance is felt. Forcing the ankle into dorsiflexion may change the natural alignment of the forefoot relative to the rearfoot.

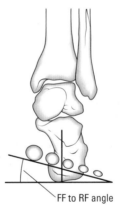

FF to RF angle

Figure 23.9 • The forefoot (FF) to rearfoot (RF) alignment is measured with the athlete in prone and the subtalar joint in neutral. The measurement is the angle formed between the plane of the second through fifth metatarsal heads and the perpendicular to the calcaneal bisection. The axis of the goniometer should be placed laterally for a varus forefoot and medially for a valgus forefoot.

supination on the shorter side during weightbearing. Leg length differences whether functional or structural can result in compensatory pronation or supination. While these changes have not been found to be significant in the past (Bloedel & Hauger 1995), small differences in leg length are likely to cause asymmetrical mechanics. These asymmetries, in conjunction with changes in exposure, shoes or fatigue, may lead to injury. The midtarsal joint axes (longitudinal and oblique) can be evaluated for mobility while holding the talocrural joint in dorsiflexion.

First metatarsalphalangeal joint range of motion should be 70°. Hallux rigidus or hallux limitus can be the cause or the result of pronation during gait. The popliteal angle is the amount of available knee extension with the hip in 90° of flexion and it assesses hamstring length. The Thomas test measures hip flexion range of motion. In sidelying, hip abduction and external rotation strength should be assessed. Ober's test measures iliotibial band extensibility. Again, these are important because changes at the hip will result in possible compensations at the foot and ankle.

Dynamically, the individual segments of the pelvis, thigh, lower leg and foot should be evaluated in the sagittal, frontal and transverse planes. This can be difficult unless the segments are evaluated systematically. Athletes should be asked to walk or run on a treadmill if possible. For more thorough evaluation, a videotape or digital video should be made and viewed frame-by-frame. The motion should be evaluated either from the ground up or from the pelvis down and the segments should be compared for symmetry and normal motion. Evaluate the athlete both during the swing phase and stance phase. Segment and joint motion should be evaluated.

Common sport-related injuries

Lateral ankle sprain

Lateral ankle sprains are one of the most common injuries sustained in sport and exercise activities. Lateral ligament injuries account for 15 to 25% of all sports injuries (Adamson & Cymet 1997). The most common mechanism of injury occurs with the ankle in a plantarflexed and inverted position. The anterior talofibular ligament (ATFL) has been found to be the weakest ligament in tensile strength when compared to other ligaments around the ankle (Pincivero et al 1993). Risk factors have been defined as intrinsic or extrinsic. Extrinsic factors include training errors, sport type, competition level, equipment and environmental conditions. Intrinsic factors refer to structural malalignment, strength deficits, range of motion limitations and ligamentous laxity. After the ATFL, the calcaneofibular ligament is the next most commonly injured and the posterior talofibular ligament is least often injured and the strongest.

The most common way of assessing a lateral ankle injury is by grading the sprain (Nicholas & Hershman 1986). A grade I sprain is microscopic tearing of the ligament with no loss of function. Grade II is partial disruption or stretching of the ligament with some loss of function. Finally, grade III sprains involve a complete tear of the ligament with complete loss of function.

Management of lateral ankle sprains is usually conservative especially when the sprain is grade I or II. Grade III ankle sprains can be treated surgically but research suggests that patients managed conservatively return to function faster than those managed surgically (Kaikkonen et al 1996). A positive anterior drawer or inversion stress test will indicate that the lateral structures are involved. The talar tilt tests inversion with the foot in a dorsiflexed position and is thought to test the calcaneofibular ligament.

The functional approach to ankle rehabilitation has been advocated by a number of researchers (Adamson & Cymet 1997, Clanton & Porter 1997, Lynch & Renstom 1999, Molnar 1988, Seto & Brewster 1994). It is generally agreed that the acute or initial phase of rehabilitation should include management of effusion, pain control and range of motion. The ankle should be placed in as much dorsiflexion as possible to keep the joint initially stable and decrease capsular distention. During the first three weeks the ankle should be protected from inversion to prevent formation of type III collagen, which leads to elongation of the ligament (Lynch & Renstom 1999). Exercises should be focused in the sagittal plane. Regaining range of motion in all planes is important early to stimulate collagen type I formation as it responds best to tension (Buckwalter & Cooper 1987).

Once pain and effusion are managed, rehabilitation should focus on return of full range of motion, weightbearing status and strength as tested with a manual muscle test. Elastic band or tubing exercises and modalities are common during this phase.

Functional strengthening and proprioception should be the focus of rehabilitation once the transition from open to closed kinetic chain exercises has begun. Activities in the weightbearing position have been shown to be of greater benefit to the patient in regaining functional stability of the joint (Stormont et al 1985). Exercises that induce motion in all planes are most likely to be of the highest benefit to the athlete.

Wobble boards and single leg standing tests have been used to increase proprioception and balance (Adamson & Cymet 1997, Clanton & Porter 1997, Lynch & Renstom 1999, Molnar 1988, Seto & Brewster 1994). Balancing on the minitramp while throwing a ball both toward and away from the affected limb is a high-level functional activity (Fig. 23.10). Low load, high repetition tension exercises help most with healing of ligament while figure-of-eight runs, single leg hops, carioca crossovers and shuttle runs train functional stability at the joint. Sport-specific tests should also be performed. Return to function time has been suggested to decrease with a progressive loading approach to rehabilitation (Kern-Steiner et al 1999). Proprioceptive training is also found to be an important factor in ankle rehabilitation. Patients who have trained with wobble boards have shown increased proprioceptive ability and fewer recurrent ankle sprains (Hoffman & Payne 1995, Wester et al 1996). Additionally, balance and coordination training has been shown to decrease perceived ankle instability and increase proprioception (Bernier & Perrin 1998, Rozzi et al 1999).

Shoe wear, bracing and taping may also be important adjuncts to treatment of the lateral ankle sprain. Braces have been shown to reduce inversion velocity, while taping and high-top shoes have been shown to decrease the inversion moment when the ankle is placed in varying degrees of plantarflexion (Ottaviani et al 1995, Shapiro et al 1994a, Vaes et al 1998). Everter strength has been shown to be important in the decrease of

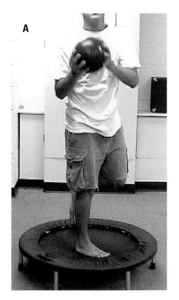
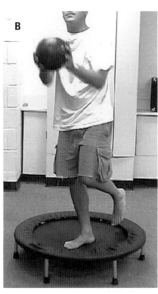

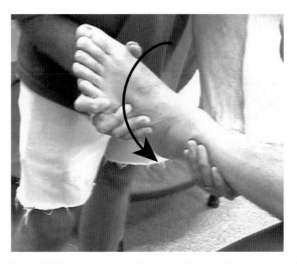

Figure 23.11 • External rotation test will be positive in the individual with a high ankle sprain, as the abduction motion will act to separate the tibia and fibula placing stress on the distal tibiofibular ligaments.

Figure 23.10 • **A:** Catching the ball toward the side of the affected limb requires eccentric activity and control of the inverters and plantarflexors primarily. **B:** Eccentric control of the everters and dorsiflexors is required when the athlete is facing away from the affected side. All activities on the minitrampoline require balance and coactivation of the muscles around the ankle joint.

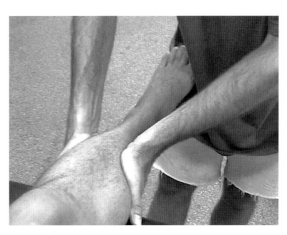

Figure 23.12 • The compression test acts to separate the tibia and fibula and places stress on the injured ligaments at the distal tibiofibular joint.

the inversion moment during weightbearing activities (Ashton-Miller et al 1996).

High ankle sprain

A high ankle sprain is a sprain involving the distal tibiofibular syndesmosis and/or the anterior inferior tibiofibular ligament. This injury is much less common than a lateral ankle sprain and is often seen in conjunction with lateral ankle ligament injuries. The mechanism of injury at this joint is usually one of external rotation of the foot and internal rotation of the tibia. The recovery of the athlete with this type of injury is usually longer than that of an athlete with a lateral ligament injury (Boytim et al 1991).

Management of high ankle sprains is usually conservative as is the case with the lateral ankle sprain. Proper management of this injury begins with proper diagnosis of the sprain. Tenderness to palpation is usually present in the distal tibiofibular joint with associated effusion and ecchymosis. Dorsiflexion in a loaded condition will also be painful. The external rotation stress test (Fig. 23.11) and the tibiofibular compression tests (Fig. 23.12) may also be positive with high ankle sprains.

The acute phase of rehabilitation should include management of effusion, pain control and range of motion. While dorsiflexion is encouraged in the patient with lateral ankle sprain, dorsiflexion, even in an open chain, should be avoided early in order to keep the distal tibiofibular joint from separating. Gait training should progress only up to 50% weightbearing during this stage.

Once the acute phase of rehabilitation is complete, full range of motion in an open chain and progressive resistive exercises should be the focus. Weightbearing should still progress slowly as separation of the tibiofibular joint is still possible with dorsiflexion or foot external rotation in a closed chain. Taping or bracing may help advance weightbearing while limiting distal tibiofibular joint separation. Elastic band or tubing exercises in an open chain will help prepare for functional activities.

Transition to closed kinetic chain activities and return to function are the goals of the final stage of rehabilitation. Single leg standing exercises with a wedge under the heel (plantarflexion = 20°) has been suggested as a method of training proprioception and minimizing dorsiflexion stress (Brosky et al 1995). Wobble boards in a clockwise direction (for the right foot) will aid with normal foot progression during walking. Retrograde walking with slight elevation may help to decrease dorsiflexion stress on the joint. Minitramp, figure-of-eight runs, single leg hopping, carioca cross over and shuttle run can be initiated toward the end of treatment. Proprioceptive training is also important in high ankle sprain rehabilitation. All of the above activities should be performed without pain or 'giving way'. If necessary, shoes, braces and/or taping may be employed to provide stability.

Spring ligament sprain

The spring ligament runs from the sustentaculum tali on the medial side of the calcaneus to the navicular tuberosity. This injury is common in runners and is often seen in conjunction with posterior tibialis tendonitis or dysfunction. The mechanism of injury of this structure is usually traumatic but can also be related to pronation. It is important to differentially diagnose this structure from the posterior tibialis tendon or peroneus longus tendon as they both insert on the navicular.

Management of spring ligament sprains is usually conservative and can be difficult if the true cause of the pathology is not determined. The injury is usually traumatic and the athlete will describe a hard landing on an uneven surface, which forces the forefoot into dorsiflexion or pronation. The patient will be tender directly over the spring ligament with deep palpation. Superficial palpation may not illicit complaints. The patient will likely have no pain with resisted plantarflexion when the rearfoot is neutral, everted or inverted. Direct tension placed on the spring ligament through passive dorsiflexion of the midtarsal joint may also be painful. Finally, patients will usually complain of discomfort during single leg standing. These athletes often present with a pronated midfoot posture.

The acute phase of rehabilitation should include management of any effusion and pain. Any activity that causes pain should be avoided and weightbearing status should be monitored. The patient may benefit from a short period of non-weightbearing if symptoms persist. Lack of motion is not an issue in these patients. In fact, these athletes usually present with an increased amount of midfoot motion and further treatment should focus on stabilization of the midfoot.

Once the acute phase of rehabilitation is complete, progressive resistive exercises should be the focus. Special attention should be paid to the strength of the anterior tibialis, posterior tibialis and peroneus longus. Arch taping or foot orthoses may decrease tension to the structures supporting the medial longitudinal arch. Taping and orthotic management should focus on placing the forefoot in an adducted and plantarflexed position relative to the rearfoot.

Closed kinetic chain activities and return to full function are the goals of the final stage of rehabilitation. Activities that focus on the functional strength of the posterior tibialis and peroneus longus muscles should be included. Single leg standing on uneven surfaces or on the minitramp will aid in training these muscles. Balance beam activities focusing on eccentric control of pronation may also be beneficial (Fig. 23.13).

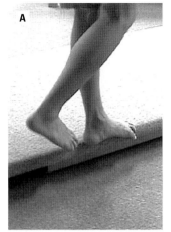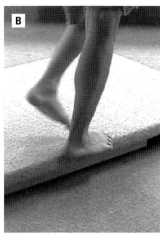

Figure 23.13 • Walking on a balance beam or side of a step requires eccentric control of the inverters **(A)** or everters **(B)**.

Posterior tibialis tendonitis

Posterior tibialis tendonitis is an overuse injury usually related to an inability to adequately control some aspect of pronation. Posterior tibialis tendonitis is the injury typically referred to as 'shin splints'. This injury is seen often in runners or in athletes whose sport requires a great deal of running. This is due to the need of the posterior tibialis to control pronation eccentrically during the loading phase of gait. This becomes especially demanding during running as the joint excursions, velocities and forces are significantly increased (Mann & Hagy 1980). Posterior tibialis tendonitis may also result after the tendon has remained in a shortened position for a period of time such as in an individual with a plantarflexed posture of the rearfoot or in an individual with a cavus medial longitudinal arch.

The patient will usually be tender just posterior to the medial malleolus and often tender on the posterior–medial distal third of the tibia. If the patient is especially painful along the tibia, the pathology should be differentially diagnosed from medial tibial stress syndrome (Mubarak et al 1982). Additionally, the presence of paresthesia or radicular pain in the foot may indicate the presence of tarsal tunnel syndrome. The patient with posterior tibialis tendonitis may also complain of pain with palpation over the navicular, pain with resisted plantarflexion and inversion and pain with passive eversion and dorsiflexion. Passive dorsiflexion and eversion can be accomplished functionally with relaxed single-leg stance. Management of posterior tibialis tendonitis can be challenging. Because the athlete must pronate, even during normal ambulation, decreasing stress on the tendon may be impossible without immobilization or casting. However, this is usually not a necessary measure.

The acute phase of rehabilitation should include management of pain and any swelling. Rest or complete cessation of activity appears to be the best for the athlete in the acute stage. The athlete may still remain active during this stage through cross-training as long as the activity does not increase

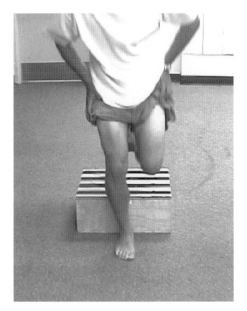

Figure 23.14 • During controlled landing exercises, the athlete should be instructed to maintain their knee over the second toe of the foot. Restrictions on degrees and excursions of knee flexion can also be placed on the exercise.

the symptoms at the posterior tibialis tendon. Nonsteroidal anti-inflammatory drugs, ice and other inflammation reducing modalities are also beneficial during this stage.

Passive range of motion for eversion and dorsiflexion should be the focus of the next stage of treatment. Regaining a normal resting length of the tendon is imperative in restoring the athlete to normal function. Although deterioration of pain and other symptoms should guide treatment, increasing passive range of motion is important, as decreased tendon length will likely be a main limiting factor to progress if not gained early. If increased pronation is a major mechanical problem leading to symptoms, this is a good time in the treatment to introduce some support to the medial longitudinal arch. Heel wedges or over-the-counter orthoses may help temporarily while custom-molded orthoses are being fabricated.

Closed kinetic chain activities and eccentric strengthening are the goals of the final stage of rehabilitation. Single leg standing toe raises with controlled lowering eccentrically loads the posterior tibialis tendon in a functional situation. Wobble boards in both a clockwise and counterclockwise direction provides training of multidirectional control of pronation and supination. Sidestepping and cariocas away from the effected side place increased eccentric demand on the posterior tibialis tendon. Finally, controlled landing activities from progressively increasing step heights train the athlete to control pronation during running, which is a landing activity (Fig. 23.14). Since posterior tibialis pathology is so often associated with pronation, external devices such as shoes or custom-molded orthoses may be necessary to control excess motion in the midfoot and rearfoot.

Peroneal tendonitis

Peroneal tendonitis is a result of overuse of either the peroneus longus or peroneus brevis tendons. This injury is often seen in conjunction with lateral ankle sprains and may be the cause or the result of lateral ankle instability. Peroneal tendonitis differs in its mechanism of injury depending on whether the longus or the brevis is involved. Peroneus brevis involvement is more commonly associated with supinatory overuse as it is stressed in the inverted position of the foot and ankle. A slightly different mechanism is usually attributed to peroneus longus tendonitis. Like the brevis, the longus plantarflexes and everts the foot. However, the longus runs beneath the plantar surface of the foot to attach to the first metatarsal. Hypermobility of the first ray allows for excessive dorsiflexion, which forces the forefoot into pronation during weightbearing activities. Therefore, the inability to control pronation by the peroneus longus often results in tendonitis.

Tenderness to palpation distal and posterior to the lateral maleolus is most common in peroneal tendonitis (Mann & Coughlin 1993). The athlete may also be tender proximal to the maleolus and, depending on the structure involved, at the base of the first or fifth metatarsal. Regardless of the specific structure, the athlete will experience pain with resisted plantarflexion and eversion. Passive eversion and dorsiflexion will be painful for the brevis and likely the longus. Passive first metatarsal dorsiflexion will be painful if the longus is involved.

The acute phase of rehabilitation should include management of any swelling and pain. Taping or bracing may help prevent the tendon from further tension injury especially if any instability or weakness is present. After the acute phase, passive range of motion and concentric resistive exercises should follow. Often, a muscle imbalance has developed so stretching and strengthening antagonists such as the anterior and posterior tibialis muscles may be necessary, especially in the athlete with a cavus foot. Concentric training of first ray plantarflexion may also be beneficial. However, it is likely that the athlete with a hypermobile first ray will not be able to gain enough dynamic strength to control forefoot pronation and orthoses or metatarsal support may be necessary.

Functional activities should complete the rehabilitation of the athlete with peroneal tendonitis. Single leg standing exercises should be the focus in this patient, as they must regain eccentric control of frontal plane activities. This is especially important in the athlete with associated lateral ankle sprains, as they will have decreased proprioceptive ability (Beckman & Buchanan 1995). Wobble boards and minitramp standing with a ball toss will help control eccentric supination or pronation. If instability or decreased proprioception remains toward the end of rehabilitation, taping or orthoses may be necessary in order for the athlete to return to play safely.

Plantar fasciitis

Plantar fasciitis is usually caused by progressive collagen degradation at the medial calcaneal tubercle. This injury is common in athletes in all sports, especially those involving running. However, dancers and gymnasts have some of the highest incidences of plantar fasciitis (Kamenski & Fu 1994, Weiss 1994). The mechanism of injury at this joint is usually one of overuse. The plantar fascia is placed on constant stretch and is often seen in the athlete with a pronated foot type. Athletes with supinated foot types are also prone to the development of plantar fasciitis where a short resting fascia is susceptible to any outside stretch placed on it. A tight gastrocsoleus complex may also be present in individuals with plantar fasciitis (Marshall 1978) and seems to be commonly associated with the cavus foot (Franco 1987).

Tenderness to palpation directly over the medial calcaneal tubercle is most common in these athletes, although some patients complain of pain along the entire plantar surface of the foot and into the fascial insertion at the metatarsal heads. Classic symptoms also include pain with the first few steps in the morning or during the first five to ten minutes of running. The pain usually subsides with activity and increases after periods of rest. Athletes may also have increased symptoms when walking barefoot.

Management of plantar fasciitis can be difficult as the pathology is often described as self-limiting. The acute phase of rehabilitation focuses on pain management. Typical modalities at this point include ice massage, deep friction massage and non-steroidal anti-inflammatory drugs. Stretching and decreasing stress on the fascia should be the focus of the next phase of treatment. Stretching the gastrocnemius and soleus are important as they are proximally attached to the calcaneus and would increase tension on the fascia by means of this attachment. The athlete should be instructed to prevent stretch on the fascia itself especially in the pronated foot. Locking the foot into supination during stretching can be accomplished by placing a wedge or towel under the medial surface of the foot during wall stretches (Fig. 23.15). Stretching of the fascia in the supinated foot can be accomplished by deep friction massage or passive toe extension. Using a low dye taping technique may also relieve tension on the plantar fascia.

As always, functional weightbearing activities should be the focus of the final stage of rehabilitation. Training of extrinsic muscles, which support the medial longitudinal arch, is important to help take passive tension off the fascia. These muscles include the anterior and posterior tibialis muscles, as well as the peroneus longus. Although it is often suggested that the intrinsic muscles of the foot be trained (e.g. with towel crunches), there is little evidence to support that these muscles are even active in controlling foot posture (Mann & Hagy 1979). If increased midfoot mobility is present, a custom-molded orthotic may be necessary. Often a semirigid orthosis with good midfoot support can be helpful in the athlete with plantar fasciitis.

Sesmoiditis

The sesmoid bones are imbedded within the tendon of the flexor hallucis brevis. Sesmoiditis does not refer to the direct inflammation of the bones themselves but rather the soft tissue

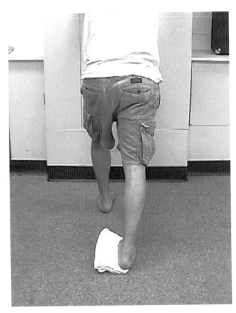

Figure 23.15 • Placing a towel under the medial side of the foot places the subtalar joint in inversion and therefore locks the midtarsal joint, preventing it from pronating. The stretch is then focused on the posterior calf musculature without placing stress on the soft tissues of the arch.

surrounding the bones. Most individuals with sesmoid pain are those with a cavus foot. These individuals usually present with a rigid midfoot and forefoot and a plantarflexed first ray (Axe & Ray 1988). However, individuals who pronate and place excess force on the medial side of the first MTP joint during push off are also susceptible to sesmoiditis. The pathology can result from repetitive trauma as described above or an acute incident of high impact (i.e. landing from a jump).

As the medial sesmoid is most often involved, radiographs may be inconclusive as to whether a fracture is present and contributing to symptoms. Tenderness to palpation over the involved sesmoid is most often present and may also present with a thickening or swelling of the tendinous sheath. The athlete will be painful upon weightbearing especially with the shoes off. Passive or active dorsiflexion of the first MTP joint will be painful. Additionally, rising onto the toes may be painful or difficult for this patient.

The acute phase of rehabilitation should include pain control and decreasing first MTP dorsiflexion range of motion. Taping the joint in neutral or slight plantarflexion decreases stress on the tendons and weightbearing on the sesmoids. Additionally, plantarflexion of the first ray should be minimized as this imparts a relative dorsiflexion at the first MTP joint (Mann & Coughlin 1993). Therefore, a metatarsal pad placed just proximal to the first metatarsal head will limit plantarflexion of the first ray. Decreasing heel height, especially in women's shoes, will also decrease the amount of first MTP dorsiflexion.

Management of sesmoiditis is usually handled with orthoses or shoe inserts. Because the symptoms are often a result of a structural deviation, support of the first ray in either a supinated or pronated foot is important. A metatarsal pad under the first ray may be enough to support the medial column. However, in more severe cases, a full custom-molded orthotic device with significant medial midfoot support may be necessary. Cutouts in the orthosis under the first metatarsal head may also decrease pressure on the sesamoids (White 1996).

Achilles tendonitis

Achilles tendonitis is a common injury among athletes, especially those involved in sports which require constant eccentric loading of the posterior calf muscles (e.g. American football quarterbacks or basketball players). The tendon is especially susceptible to injury based on its reduced blood supply (Smart et al 1980) and the possible wringing effect of this tendon during pronation (Gross 1992). Older athletes may be more predisposed to this injury based on a further decreased blood supply and decreased extensibility of collagen.

Athletes are usually painful with direct palpation over the Achilles tendon but not over the gastrocnemius or soleus muscles. The tendon may also feel fibrous upon palpation. The patient will likely have pain with passive dorsiflexion and resisted plantarflexion of the talocrural joint. Going down steps or walking backwards will also increase symptoms.

The acute phase of rehabilitation should include management of effusion and pain control. Range of motion should be minimized or at least kept within a pain free range of motion. A heel lift in the shoe will decrease passive dorsiflexion and the need for eccentric muscle activity during ambulation. Deep friction massage may also be beneficial, as soft tissue mobilization has been shown to aid in fibroblast formation during healing (Davidson et al 1997). Rest is also recommended to decrease stress on the tissue.

Once the acute phase of rehabilitation is complete, full range of motion in an open chain and progressive resistive exercises should be the focus. Passive dorsiflexion range of motion will increase formation and alignment of collagen. Resistive exercises should begin with isometrics and advance to concentric exercises in an open chain. Eccentrics will be the final stage of strengthening as these exercises place the most tension of the tendon.

Closed kinetic chain activities and functional activities are the goals of the final stage of rehabilitation. Toe walking and single leg standing exercises with toe walking are functional activities with a strong eccentric component. Standing exercises on a wobble board will also help with muscle balance around the joints of the foot and ankle. Retrograde walking focusing on sagittal plane progression is important for specific eccentric training. Minitramp, figure-of-eight runs, single leg hopping and carioca cross-overs on the toes would be exercises utilized toward the end of treatment. Modification of shoewear (i.e. increasing heel height in the shoe) or orthotic management can be beneficial in these patients if intrinsic methods do not return the athlete to full function.

Fractures

Classification of ankle fractures can be difficult based on the large number of mechanisms for injuring the ankle. The most comprehensive system of classifying ankle injuries has been presented by Lauge-Hansen (1950). In general, he categorizes these fractures by the nature of the forces that cause the injury. For instance, a lateral maleolar fracture is most likely the result of a supinatory force.

Because of the large body of literature on ankle fractures, a general outline of postinjury rehabilitation will be discussed here. Fractures of the distal third of the lower leg are considered 'ankle' fractures and can involve the tibia, fibula and talus. The mechanism of injury for the tibia and fibula is usually torsional while it is compressive for the talus.

The severity of the injury will dictate how rehabilitation will progress. Obviously, a simple fibular fracture in a 10-year-old boy will likely be easier to manage than a compound fracture with open reduction/internal fixation in an older person. Even so, the general guidelines for treatment should be the same. Most likely, as physical therapists, we will not see the athlete with the lower leg fracture until after the cast has been removed. However, if we are fortunate enough, early range of motion of adjacent joints should be implemented. Muscle setting and isometrics of muscles surrounding the area should begin as soon as pain allows. Cross-training with an upper body ergometer will help keep the athletes cardiovascular status high while the ankle is immobilized. Weightbearing should be encouraged as soon as possible to stimulate bone healing and regrowth.

Once the cast is removed, range of motion and strengthening should be the primary goals of rehabilitation. Full weightbearing should be achieved very soon after the removal of the cast. Strengthening should progress from concentrics to eccentrics and should not only focus on the previously immobilized muscles but also on the muscles of the adjacent joints. Full range of motion may not be an option after a surgical intervention where surgical hardware remains near the joint. Tendonitis is not an uncommon associated problem in the athlete with a recent fracture. Muscle atrophy and shortening contribute to the development of the pathology, especially once weightbearing activities begin. Passive range of motion and eccentric activities should continue through all stages of physical therapy treatment.

Jones fracture

The Jones fracture is a fracture involving the proximal portion of the fifth metatarsal just distal to the insertion of the peroneus brevis. This fracture is the most common fracture of the fifth metatarsal and should be differentiated from a Dancer's fracture or an avulsion fracture. Jones fractures have a high propensity for nonunion and for this reason are often managed with early surgical insertion of an intermedullary rod (Mindrebo et al 1993). Conservative management is most successful when a non-weightbearing cast is applied for up to six weeks.

Management of the Jones fracture after immobilization should follow a similar course to that of lower leg fractures. Since Jones fractures are often thought to be the result of increased stress to the fifth metatarsal, changing the alignment of the foot and therefore the forces may help decrease the chances of future injury to the lateral side of the foot. Orthoses that redistribute the forces across the entire forefoot and away from the lateral side are an appropriate intervention in the athlete with a biomechanical dysfunction.

Tibial stress fracture

While there is a large range of incidence reported for stress fractures (Milner et al 2006), the incidence in the average adult population is relatively low. Runners, military recruits and women are often reported to have the highest incidence of tibial stress fractures (Pester & Smith 1992). Differential diagnosis is the key element for successful management of the individual with a tibial stress fracture. Obtaining an accurate and complete history in combination with a good physical examination will greatly improve the ability to diagnose and treat the injury early.

Stress fractures are usually diagnosed with imaging techniques. Although a plain film radiograph will show a severe stress fracture, bone scans and recently magnetic resonance imaging (Ruohola et al 2006) have been demonstrated to be more sensitive in the early stages. Patients most often describe their pain as an ache that comes on with increased activity and goes away with rest. However, if gone untreated, the pain begins to occur earlier and will remain even after rest. The pain is usually focal and palpable especially when the fracture is located on the anterior–medial portion of the tibial crest.

A stress fracture is an overuse injury of bone and is likely related to tibial accelerations and therefore some level of loading (Hennig et al 1993). However, there are many other factors thought to be related to stress fractures including muscle fatigue (Mizrahi et al 2000), bone structure (Milgrom et al 1989), joint structure (Krivickas 1997) and joint biomechanics (Milner et al 2006). Finally, there are many pathological factors resulting in osteopenia which may add to the susceptibility to stress fractures.

The physical therapy evaluation will often result in pain upon palpation over anterior medial tibial crest. However, if the fracture is on the posterior medial portion of the tibia, palpation will not be possible. A 'Bump test' or percussion to the plantar surface of the calcaneus may elicit pain if the patient has posterior shin splints. Although rare in the athletic population, pain in the posterior calf may also be related to a deep vein thrombosis.

Although stress fractures may be complex in their etiology, initial treatment is relatively simple. Cessation or modification of the activity will help the healing process to begin. Depending on the severity of the stress fracture, patients may be in an active rest period from 6 to 8 weeks. If the patient is noncompliant or unable to comply completely, a walking boot may be used. It is important during this time that the physical therapist

and the athlete begin to modify other risk factors that may have contributed to the injury. Training techniques, equipment (shoes/cleats, foot orthoses), nutrition and exposure hours are some of the key areas to address.

Because of the modification of activity, muscle strength and range of motion on both lower extremities may be compromised. Strengthening of the proximal muscles of the hip and knee should continue even before full weightbearing is achieved. Non-weightbearing cardiovascular activities should also be included. These activities will help maintain proper mechanics in the lower extremities once the athlete returns to their sport and will help reduce the muscle fatigue which may be related to stress-related injury.

Once healing is confirmed through diagnostic imaging, the athlete may begin to slowly return to loading activities. The intensity and amount of loading should be gradually progressed and monitored. It is also important that the athlete be trained with proper mechanics and equipment. Sport-specific training and evaluation are also important in an attempt to limit future risk factors.

Compartment syndrome

Compartment syndrome is a condition occurring in the lower leg and is characterized by an increased intramuscular pressure that decreases or eliminates arterial blood flow to local tissues, including muscle and nerve. There are four main compartments, with corresponding nerves, in the lower leg where compartment syndromes can occur: anterior compartment (deep peroneal nerve), lateral compartment (superficial peroneal nerve), superficial posterior compartment (saphenous nerve) and deep posterior compartment (tibial nerve) (Fig. 23.16).

Compartment syndrome can present as an acute or traumatic problem with rapid onset or as a chronic exertional problem with the symptoms developing over a longer period.

Acute compartment syndrome

Acute compartment syndrome most frequently occurs with trauma lower leg fractures, crush injuries or occlusion. It has also been reported that burns, drug overdoses and intense exercise may also play a role. With exercise, acute compartment syndrome usually occurs in the unconditioned individual performing strenuous exercise or in athletes with chronic exertional compartment syndrome who are exposed to a higher intensity and/or duration of exercise (Fehlandt & Micheli 1995, Leach et al 1967, Shrier 1991, Stollsteimer & Shelton 1997).

History and physical examination
Severe lower leg pain, swelling over the involved compartment, weakness such as foot drop or foot slapping for the anterior compartment and numbness/tingling are symptoms consistent with acute compartment syndrome.

On examination, there is may be an antalgic gait, severe pain on passive stretch of the involved muscles, poor active contraction, paresthenia/hypesthesia in the distribution of the

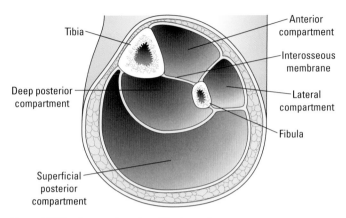

Tibia

Anterior compartment

Interosseous membrane

Deep posterior compartment

Lateral compartment

Fibula

Superficial posterior compartment

Figure 23.16 • Compartments of the lower leg.

involved nerve and a possible impression of the presence of pain that is out of proportion to the physical findings. Pulses are usually diminished, but a normal pulse does not rule out the presence of the syndrome.

Chronic extertional compartment syndrome

Chronic exertional compartment syndrome (CECS) has an uncertain etiology. It is normal for exercise to result in a 20% increase in compartment volume due to myofiber swelling and increased intracompartmental blood volume (Amendola & Rorabeck 1985). It has been suggested that the development of the abnormal increase in compartment pressure that characterizes compartment syndrome is due to: (1) the muscle hypertrophy that occurs with exercise (Amendola & Rorabeck 1985), (2) fascial hypertrophy becoming tight and unyielding from exercise (Amendola & Rorabeck 1985, Detmer 1986, Martens et al 1984), and (3) eccentric muscle contraction causing myofiber damage with release of protein-bound ions and an increase in osmotic pressures in the compartment (Edwards & Myerson 1996). The increase in compartment pressure causes ischemia due to: (1) the increase in osmotic pressure which results in increased capillary relaxation pressure, then decrease in blood flow (Edwards & Myerson 1996); (2) arterial spasm, then decrease in arterial inflow (Matsen 1975); and/or (3) arteriolar or venous collapse due to transmural pressure (Raneman 1975). It is interesting that the best available techniques for detection of ischemia have been unsuccessful, although new infrared spectroscopy may show a decrease in muscle oxygenation (Amendola et al 1990, Blackman 2000, Breit et al 1997, Mohler et al 1997). The use of phosphofructose as a reflection of anaerobic metabolism has demonstrated that phosphofructose within the muscle decreased after fasciotomy (Embrec 1996).

The anterior compartment is involved in 45% of CECS, the deep posterior in 40%, the lateral in 10%, and the superficial posterior in 5% (Edwards & Myerson 1996). Some have suggested that the anterior compartment is involved in 70–80% of CECS (Korkola & Amendola 2001). The posterior tibial compartment (the fifth compartment) involvement in CECS is rare.

History and physical findings

The characteristic symptoms of CECS include an achy, sharp or dull pain or tightness that comes on predictably with exercise and settles within 30 min of rest. The symptoms are bilateral in 50–70% of athletes and tend to occur with running or repetitive stress sports. The athletes are usually young (less than 30 years old) (Edwards & Myerson 1996).

The physical examination is usually unremarkable. There may be the reproduction of characteristic symptoms with repetitive, manually resisted ankle movement, particularly for anterior CECS. Also, examining the athlete after sport participation that caused the symptoms may reveal swelling, tenderness and weakness of the compartment, and hypesthesia to light touch of the involved nerve.

Treatment

The treatment of CECS is seemingly straightforward. Generally there is the impression that the only successful treatment is surgery (Howard et al 2000). There have been few reports of successful non-operative treatment of CECS (Hutchison & Ireland 1994). There may be some athletes with CECS who institute a conservative treatment program early in the disease process, settle their symptoms and successfully return to their activities. They may not have had the condition long enough to prompt the compartment pressure measurements/fasciotomy path. The average duration of symptoms prior to diagnosis and fasciotomy can be 16 months for posterior CECS and 6.8 months for anterior CECS (Schepsis et al 1993).

A conservative treatment program would address extrinsic factors of training, footwear and surface, and intrinsic factors of alignment (from leg length to foot function; pronation/supination), flexibility and strength (core, hip, leg muscles).

The success rate of fasciotomy for anterior CECS is much higher (90% good to excellent) than for posterior CECS (50–65% good to excellent). This may reflect an inadequate release, a persistent soleus bridge, scarring over the fasciotomy defect, entrapment neuropathy in the scar or incorrect diagnosis (Edwards & Myerson 1996, Howard et al 2000, Rorabeck et al 1983, 1988, Schepsis et al 1993, Wiley et al 1987).

The postoperative treatment plan is assisted to full weight-bearing active and passive leg exercise during the first week, cycling in the second week, strengthening through the 3rd and 4th weeks, running in the 5th and 6th weeks, speed/agility drills by the 8th week and back to sport for the 8th to 12th week (Edwards & Myerson 1996). Athletes with fasciotomy for posterior CECS often take longer to progress through the treatment plan.

Less common injuries

Sinus tarsi syndrome

Sinus tarsi syndrome is a complicated problem that falls under the 'less common injuries' portion of this chapter probably because it has been underdiagnosed. This injury is often referred

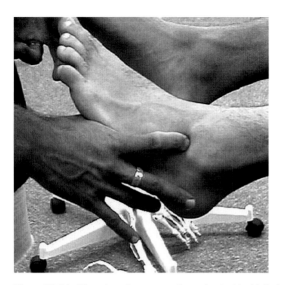

Figure 23.17 • The sinus tarsus can be palpated just inferior and anterior to the lateral maleolus, inferior and slightly posterior to the anterior talofibular ligament, and superior and anterior to the peroneal tubercle on the lateral side of the foot.

to as a chronic ankle sprain or chronic lateral ankle pain (Brown 1960, O'Conner 1958, Taillard et al 1981). These athletes most commonly present with a significant pronated posture of the rearfoot. However, athletes with a supinated foot posture make up 20% of the individuals with sinus tarsi syndrome.

Sinus tarsi syndrome is a result of repetitive trauma to the lateral articulation between the talus and calcaneus. An inflammatory response develops and may exacerbate to the point of compression within the entire sinus tarsus. Pain is most often on the lateral side just posterior to the anterior talofibular ligament. Athletes will complain of pain with forced eversion and palpation over the sinus tarsi laterally (Fig. 23.17). Swelling will likely be present laterally and may progress medially through the sinus tarsus.

The acute phase of rehabilitation should include management of effusion and pain control. Dorsiflexion and eversion should be avoided early in order to keep the subtalar joint separated on the lateral side. This can be accomplished with taping or an over-the-counter orthotic. Once the acute phase of rehabilitation is complete, a thorough biomechanical analysis should be employed to determine the source of the sinus tarsi syndrome. Supinatory patients are more difficult to manage but are also less common. Joint mobilizations to encourage pronation and midfoot mobility with plantarflexion stretching may be enough to decrease the lateral stress in these individuals.

Athletes with sinus tarsi syndrome who pronate should be managed in a way that will decrease the forces on the lateral side of the subtalar joint. Posterior tibialis dysfunction or weak plantarflexors may be contributing to the excessive pronation and can be rehabilitated with strengthening and functional activities. More than likely, these athletes will need to be managed extrinsically by maintaining the subtalar joint away from

full eversion thus decompressing the lateral joint space. This can be achieved with a standard orthotic or may require a more aggressive prescription of an inverted orthotic (Blake 1986).

Lisfranc dislocation

A Lisfranc dislocation is a dislocation of any one or several of the tarsometatarsal joints. Dislocation without fracture at these joints usually occurs as a result of indirect trauma such as pronation of the rearfoot while the forefoot is plantarflexed and fixed to the ground (Shapiro et al 1994b). A dislocation, even if it is severe, will often reduce itself after an injury. This injury is much less common than a lateral ankle sprain and is often seen in conjunction with lateral ankle ligament injuries. The mechanism of injury at this joint is usually one of external rotation of the foot and internal rotation of the tibia. The recovery of the athlete with this type of injury is usually longer than that of an athlete with a lateral ligament injury.

Depending on the severity of the dislocation, the patient may be tender along the dorsal and plantar surface of the joints. Management of the Lisfranc dislocation is not difficult if all pathology has been recognized. There is often an associated fracture with a Lisfranc dislocation, which can significantly slow rehabilitation if gone undiagnosed. Care should be taken to begin physical therapy treatment only after fractures have begun to heal. Even without a fracture, internal fixation of the joint(s) is often necessary for stability after significant dislocation.

If swelling and pain are still present after injury, modalities and NSAIDs will help to reduce symptoms. Weightbearing should be monitored closely as the tarsometarsal joint accepts a great deal of the force during weightbearing activities. Athletes with a Lisfranc injury will likely need good midfoot and forefoot support after physical therapy treatment. Additionally, shoes with firm soles and decreased toe break will help minimize mobility in the joint after injury.

Nerve entrapment

Nerve entrapments commonly occur in the lower leg and diagnosis is often a challenge. Nerve entrapment injuries are often not immediately recognized. Symptoms depend on the function of the injured peripheral nerve. Injured motor nerves present more commonly with pain (even if they lack a sensory component) and weakness, and injured sensory nerves present with pain, numbness and/or tingling. Physical examination should identify any motor or sensory deficits. A lidocaine (lignocaine) injection test into the area of maximal tenderness can often facilitate muscle strength assessment if guarding is present. Abnormal reflexes are usually not found since a reflex is comprised of more than one nerve root. Light tapping over a nerve close to the skin surface that results in radiating tingling, numbness, or an electrical sensation can identify an entrapped nerve (a positive Tinel's sign). Nerve conduction studies conducted by a neurologist or physiatrist localize the nerve injury and provide a prognosis for recovery.

Common peroneal nerve

The common peroneal nerve, a branch of the sciatic nerve, passes through the lateral popliteal fossa, wraps around the head of the fibula and descends 10 cm before passing through the peroneus longus tendon. The nerve then divides into the deep and superficial peroneal nerve. The superficial peroneal nerve innervates the muscles of the lateral compartment (peroneus longus and brevis) as well as the skin of the dorsum of the foot. The deep peroneal nerve innervates the muscles of the anterior compartment (tibialis anterior, peroneus tertius, extensor digitorum longus, extensor hallucis longus and extensor digitorum brevis) and the skin of the first webspace.

The common peroneal nerve is more commonly injured than its superficial and deep branches. Injury can occur by traction, compression, laceration and ischemia. Stretching of the common peroneal nerve occurs following ankle inversion injuries, major knee ligamentous injuries (anterior cruciate ligament, posterior cruciate ligament and lateral collateral ligament injury), fractures or dislocations, and bungee jumping (Feinberg et al 1997).

Direct compression can be caused by isolated traumas to the proximal fibula. This may also cause posterolateral subluxation of the superior tibiofibular joint. This is often seen in contact sports via hockey pucks, soccer kicks, football helmets and falls on a minimally flexed knee. Other more insidious causes are tight ski boots, ice skates, braces and casts. An accessory ossicle in the lateral gastrocnemius muscle (fabella syndrome) and a tight fascial band at the edge of the peroneus longus muscle, which is most often symptomatic in runners, can compress the common peroneal nerve (Feinberg et al 1997).

Compartment syndromes are associated with compression of the superficial (lateral and occasionally anterior compartments) and deep peroneal (anterior compartment) nerve entrapments. Sensory function of the nerve is more commonly affected, though motor manifestations are possible in more extreme cases.

Nerve injury of common peroneal tendon results in:

- pain, numbness and/or tingling over the dorsum of the foot
- weakness in the ankle dorsiflexors and evertors as well as toe extensors
- no change in ankle jerk reflex.

This is distinct from superficial peroneal nerve injury, where there is only weakness of the ankle evertors and no sensory changes in the first webspace.

Tarsal tunnel syndrome

The tibial nerve, a continuation of the sciatic nerve, travels through the popliteal fossa into the posterior compartment of the leg and then resurfaces in the tarsal tunnel. The tarsal tunnel, which lies posterior to the medial malleolus, is formed by bones of the foot and roofed by the flexor retinaculum. Its contents include the posterior tibial nerve, artery and vein as well as the tendon sheaths of tibialis posterior, flexor digitorum longus and flexor hallucis longus. Beyond the tarsal tunnel, the tibial nerve branches further into the lateral plantar, medial plantar and calcaneal nerves, which supply sensation to the sole of the foot and innervate all intrinsic foot muscles.

Tibial nerve injuries are uncommon owing to protection by the calf muscles. Severe trauma, such as tibial fractures and deep lacerations, would be the most common injury scenario.

Reported mechanisms include the following:

- Compression by a synovial cyst, ganglion, or os trigonum (accessory ossicle of the posterior talus present in 10% of the population).
- Repetitive ankle flexion and extension that results in tenosynovitis of the adjacent tunnel occupants.
- Fibrosis following ankle sprains.
- Local trauma or overuse in individuals with excessive pronation (Lau & Daniels 1999).

The diagnosis of tarsal tunnel syndrome is common in runners and mountain climbers. Symptoms of tarsal tunnel nerve entrapment include the following:

- Pain, tingling and numbness over the sole of the foot, which can be worsened with weightbearing.
- Weakness of the intrinsic muscles of the foot, which can result in a weak push-off phase of gait.
- Clawing of the toes in longstanding injury.

Tarsal tunnel nerve entrapment is likely to be overdiagnosed since suspected clinical cases of tarsal tunnel syndrome often yield no abnormalities on nerve conduction studies (NCG) and electromyography (EMG).

Treatment of nerve injuries

The first step is to identify and correct contributing factors to the nerve injury. If inflammation is believed to contribute to the injury, treatment can include the use of oral anti-inflammatories or local corticosteroid injection from the treating physician. Footwear should be modified if it is too constrictive and orthotics may be prescribed if there is excessive pronation.

Decompressive surgery is indicated acutely in peroneal nerve sheath hematoma. It is also useful in cases resistant to conservative treatment, such as compartment syndromes, as well as impingement from osteophytes, accessory ossicles, ganglions, cysts or soft tissue strictures.

If all contributing factors are corrected, time becomes the determining factor in recovery, provided the damage is not too extensive. Nerves regenerate at a rate of 1–7 mm per day.

Deep vein thrombosis

Deep vein thrombosis (DVT) must be considered in individuals with increasing calf pain and swelling. The occurrence rate in healthy active individuals is very rare, but thrombosis may occur with increased activity and has been described by Harvey (1978) as effort thrombosis. The major concern regarding thrombus formation in a vein is that of embolization resulting in pulmonary emboli. The risk of pulmonary emboli is significantly reduced with anticoagulation. Following DVT, venous insufficiency may occur, and the venous stasis itself may be another uncommon cause of exertional leg pain in the older athlete. This can also be seen in incompetent veins with increased varicosities, which are improved with the use of support stockings.

Thromboembolic disorders have been recognized with increasing regularity over the past two decades. More and more vigilence in terms of identification has taken place because of the morbidity and mortality associated with DVT. As mentioned already, the major complication of DVT is that of pulmonary emboli. It is a major concern and complication in the postoperative state, particularly following trauma or surgery to the hip or pelvis or with individuals immobilized in bed for any period of time. In addition, ambulatory patients may also develop DVT. Pulmonary embolism is one of the most common causes of morbidity and mortality among the adult population and it is estimated that some 600,000 cases occur annually with a mortality of 10%. In addition, DVT and pulmonary emboli have been recognized as important complications of pregnancy and oral contraceptive use in individuals who are not ambulatory and in the postsurgical or traumatic state (Speroff 1998). Speroff (1998) states further that the estimated risk of pulmonary emboli among women using oral contraceptives is three to four times greater than in non-users.

DVT occurs in a setting with platelet aggregation and further adhesion to the venous endothelium. Fibrin then forms around the platelets and allows the further entrapment of more platelets as well as red and white blood cells. This process causes the growth of a thrombus, which forms a head that slows the flow of blood in the vessel, and a tail that extends downstream. Venous thrombi form in areas of slower blood flow, particularly at valve pockets and venous sinuses. Virchow first described the triad of factors responsible for facilitating the formation of a blood clot: (1) an abnormal vessel wall, (2) blood stagnation (venous stasis) and (3) increased coagulation. Venous stasis occurs when blood remains confined by or in contact with the venous wall for longer periods of time than normal. In terms of intramuscular veins, the most prevalent area where DVT occurs is in the soleus plexus of veins. These larger valveless veins drain anteriorly and their emptying depends on the rate of arterial flow as well as the pressure gradient between the sinuses in the deeper veins to which they empty. These veins are primarily dependent on the calf muscle pump for emptying. The role of the calf pump here is to increase the pressure and rate of arterial flow. Calf vein thrombosis is seen particularly with prolonged rest due to inactivity of the calf muscle, allowing for an increase in the time that the blood pools in the lower extremity. Abnormalities of the vessel wall occur with changes in the venous intima caused by tissue injury. This results in chemotactic factors being released and diffusing across the venous wall and activating clotting factors. There is a resultant cascade of migration of leukocytes to the venous intima and

adhesion and aggregation of the platelets. A thrombus 3–5 cm in length can be formed, anchored to the vessel wall by fibrin strands. An additional theory describing vessel wall damage focuses on the role of stasis in sites at soleal veins and valve pockets. These areas are believed to be sites for platelet accumulation and activating clotting factors. These two theories can address both the role of stasis and the role of the venous intima in the process of thrombosus. States of increased coaguability have been well known to initiate a clotting sequence. This can occur with so called effort thrombosis and following fever and infection. It is also involved in the role of oral contraceptives in stimulating the coagulation cascade. Reduced levels of antithrombin 3, an anticoagulant found in the blood, were noted in women using oral contraceptives. Lower levels of antithrombin 3 may be necessary to begin the process of thrombosis (Stewart 1975, Strandness et al 1977).

Mackie & Webster (1981) described a marathon runner with gastrocnemius cramping in the final stages of a marathon. In the week after the marathon, this runner developed DVT in the calf. Williams & Williams (1994) described a case of DVT in a 65-year-old individual after a day of telemark skiing. The authors suggested that minor muscle trauma, dehydration and possibly an exercise-induced state might be the factors initiating clot formation in the otherwise healthy active athlete.

Signs and symptoms

Unfortunately, clinical signs are absent or unreliable in DVT, with up to two-thirds of the cases of DVT being missed on examination. However, DVT of the lower leg intramuscular vein often presents with edema, localized warmth over the calf and a tight sensation or pain, particularly with walking or running. There may or may not be local deep tenderness and pain with forced dorsiflexion with positive Homan's sign. Some cases of DVT, uncomplicated by a pulmonary embolism, may be associated with fever or tachycardia. Pulmonary embolism, should it occur, is associated with shortness of breath and chest pain. Other symptoms can include hemoptysis, faintness, anxiety and light-headedness. Calf swelling is often present with DVT.

Differential diagnosis

The differential diagnosis of DVT is extensive and includes strains of the gastrocnemius–soleus complex, hematoma following contusion, a popliteal cyst from an intra-articular knee mechanism, compartment syndromes, popliteal artery entrapment and the post-thrombotic phlebitic syndrome.

Treatment

The treatment of DVT is aimed at the prevention of pulmonary emboli and starts with immediate hospitalization, followed by intravenous heparin administration. Heparin acts immediately to catalyze the cascade of clotting factors and is continued for at least 5–7 days. In addition, within the first 24 h, an oral anticoagulant of warfarin (coumadin) is also initiated to inhibit the synthesis of coagulant proteins. Hirsch et al (1996) emphasized the importance of a period of overlap between heparin and warfarin to ensure that the full effects of warfarin are exhibited. The oral anticoagulants should be continued for 3–6 months for a first-occurrence patient. The reoccurrence rate is 4–7%. For the female, oral contraceptives should be stopped immediately upon diagnosis. When athletes are taking anticoagulants, they can continue non-contact endurance activities, gradually returning at a progressive increase in intensity, and being careful not to suffer any acute gastrocnemius-soleus strains. It should be obvious that individuals who are anticoagulated are not involved in contact sports. The level of anticoagulation with warfarin is monitored by the international normalized ratio (INR) with a level to be achieved between 2.02 and 3.00 for the INR therapeutic range. The INR should be monitored daily initially, then three times per week, and on a weekly basis thereafter. The INR can fluctuate with fever and other forms of stress and travel, so the level of warfarin (coumadin) needs to be adjusted accordingly.

Prevention

In the surgical setting, low dose heparin has been universally used as a means of reducing the likelihood of DVT. In addition, regular calf exercises to improve the calf muscle pump should be utilized in any situation of immobilization. Long car trips and flights are notorious for producing sufficient venous stasis to lead to the formation of a DVT. Regular stops with walking during a car trip, and regular walking and toe raises, either sitting or walking, in the aisles on long flights are strongly recommended. In addition, in the postoperative setting, or in individuals with known varicose veins or previous venous stasis sigvarus, support stockings are recommended. In trauma to the calf with contusion or in the setting of gastrocnemius–soleus strains, early activation, calf support through taping and increased exercise through pool running or cycling are essential to prevent DVT. These situations are enhanced with the older athlete, as age has been identified as a risk factor for both DVT and pulmonary emboli. A family history of DVT should lead to a search for forms of contraception other than oral contraceptives. Suissa et al (1997) reported an increased risk of venous thromboembolism with the use of the newer third generation of oral contraceptives than with the second generation agents. This was contradicted in a subsequent study by Farmer et al (1998), which showed no significant difference in the risk of venous thromboemboli between the users of second and third generation oral contraceptives. Any family history of DVT should stimulate an analysis of the coagulation factors, particularly looking for reduced levels of antithrombin 3 and Factor V Leiden.

Due to the serious consequence of pulmonary embolism associated with DVT in known states of high risk, any athlete presenting with calf pain and swelling must be considered a potential case of DVT with appropriate investigation.

Summary

The ankle is the most commonly injured body part in sport and exercise. Due to the complex makeup of the foot and ankle a thorough anatomical understanding is necessary in order to accurately diagnose and manage injuries in this region. Examination and assessment of foot and ankle injuries should consider all associated joints and soft tissue structures, and should incorporate functional and sport-specific tests. Management of foot and ankle injuries should consider the high-level demands placed on the foot and ankle in many sport and exercise activities.

References

Adamson C, Cymet T 1997 Ankle sprains: evaluation, treatment, rehabilitation. Maryland Medical Journal 46:530–537

Aerts P, Ker R F, deClerq D et al 1995 The mechanical properties of the human heel pad: a paradox resolved. Journal of Biomechanics 28:1299–1308

Amendola A, Rorabeck C H 1985 Chronic exertional compartment syndrome. In: Welsh R P, Shephard R J et al (eds) Current therapy in sports medicine. BC Decker, Toronto

Amendola A, Rorabeck C H, Vellett D et al 1990 The use of magnetic resonance imaging in exertional compartment syndromes. American Journal of Sports Medicine 18:29–34

Ashton-Miller J A, Ottaviani R A, Hutchinson C et al 1996 What best protects the inverted weightbearing ankle against further inversion? Evertor muscle strength compares favorably with shoe height, athletic tape, and three orthoses. American Journal of Sports Medicine 24:800–809

Axe M J, Ray R L 1988 Orthotic treatment of sesamoid pain. American Journal of Sports Medicine 16:411–416

Barnett C H, Napier J R 1952 The axis of rotation at the ankle joint in man: its influence upon the form of the talus and mobility of the fibula. Journal of Anatomy 86:1–9

Beckman S M, Buchanan T S 1995 Ankle inversion injury and hypermobility: effect on hip and ankle muscle electromyography onset latency. Archives of Physical Medicine and Rehabilitation 76:1138–1143

Bernier J N, Perrin D H 1998 Effect of coordination training on proprioception of the functionally unstable ankle. Journal of Orthopedic and Sports Physical Therapy 27:264–275

Blackman P G 2000 A review of chronic exertional compartment syndrome in the lower leg. Medicine and Science in Sports and Exercise 32(3 suppl): S4–S10

Blake R L 1986 Inverted functional orthosis. Journal of the American Pediatric Medical Association 76:275–276

Bloedel P K, Hauger B 1995 The effects of limb length discrepancy on subtalar joint kinematics during running. Journal of Orthopedic and Sports Physical Therapy 22:60–64

Boytim M J, Fischer D A, Neumann L 1991 Syndesmotic ankle sprains. American Journal of Sports Medicine 19:294–298

Bozkurt M, Yilmaz E, Akseki D et al 2004 The evaluation of the proximal tibiofibular joint for patients with lateral knee pain. Knee 11:307–312

Breit G A, Gross J H, Watenpaugh D E et al 1997 Near-infrared spectroscopy for monitoring of tissue oxygenation of exercising skeletal muscle in a chronic compartment syndrome model. Journal of Bone and Joint Surgery (Am) 79A:838–843

Brosky T, Nyland J, Nitz A et al 1995 The ankle ligaments: consideration of syndesmotic injury and implications for rehabilitation. Journal of Orthopedic and Sports Physical Therapy 21:197–205

Brown, J F 1960 The sinus tarsi syndrome. Clinical Orthopedics 18:231–233

Buckwalter J A, Cooper R R 1987 The cells and matrices of skeletal connective tissues. In: Albright J A, Brand R A (eds). The Scientific basis of orthopaedics. Appleton and Lange, Norwalk, CT

Clanton T O, Porter D A 1997 Primary care of foot and ankle injuries in the athlete. Clinics in Sports Medicine 16:435–466

Davidson C J, Ganion L R, Gehlsen G M et al 1997 Rat tendon morphologic and functional changes resulting from soft tissue mobilization. Medicine and Science in Sports and Exercise 29:313–319

Detmer D E 1986 Chronic shin splints. Sports Medicine 3:436–446

Edwards P, Myerson M S 1996 Exertional compartment syndrome of the leg: steps for expedient return to activity. Physician and Sportsmedicine 24(4):31–46

Embrec M J 1996 Chronic compartment syndrome: an analysis at the cellular level. Thesis Faculty of Graduate Studies. The University of Western Ontario, Canada

Farmer R, Todd J, Lewis M et al 1998 The risk of venous thromboembolism among German women using oral contraceptives: a data base study. Contraception 57:67–70

Fehlandt A, Micheli L 1995 Acute exertional anterior compartment syndrome in an adolescent female. Medicine and Science in Sports and Exercise 27:3–7

Feinberg J H, Nadler S F, Krivickas L S 1997 Peripheral nerve injuries in the athlete. Sports Medicine 24(6):385–408

Fiolkowski P, Brunt D, Bishop M et al 2003 Intrinsic pedal musculature support of the medial longitudinal arch: an electromyography study. Journal of Foot and Ankle Surgery 42:327–333

Franco A H 1987 Pes cavus and pes planus, analysis and treatment. Physical Therapy 67:688–694

Giladi M, Milgrom C, Stein M et al 1985 The low arch, a protective factor in stress fractures. Orthopedic Review 14:709–712

Gross M T 1992 Chronic tendonitis: pathomechanics of injury, factors affecting the healing response, and treatment. Journal of Orthopedic and Sports Physical Therapy 16:248–261

Harvey J S 1978 Effort thrombosis in the lower extremity of a runner. American Journal of Sports Medicine 6:400–402

Hennig E, Milani T, Lafortune M 1993 Use of ground reaction force parameters in predicting peak tibial accelerations in runners. Journal of Applied Biomechanics 9:306–314

Hicks J H 1953 Mechanics of the foot: joints. Journal of Anatomy 87:345–357

Hirsh D, Mikkola K, Marks P et al 1996 Pulmonary embolism and DVT during pregnancy and oral contraceptive use. Prevalence of factor V leidin. American Heart Journal 131:1145–1148

Hoffman M, Payne V G 1995 The effects of proprioceptive ankle disk training on healthy subjects. Journal of Orthopedic and Sports Physical Therapy 21:90–93

Howard J L, Mohtadi N G H, Wiley J P 2000 Evaluation of outcomes in patients following surgical treatment of chronic exertional compartment syndrome in the leg. Clinical Journal of Sport Medicine 10:176–184

Hutchison M R, Ireland M L 1994 Common compartment syndrome in athletes: treatment and rehabilitation. Sports Medicine 17:200–208

Kaikkonen A, Kannus P, Jarvinen M 1996 Surgery versus functional treatment in ankle ligament tears. a prospective study. Clinical Orthopedics 326:194–202

Kamenski R, Fu F H 1994 Dance and the arts. In: Fu FH, Stone DA (eds). Sports injuries: mechanisms prevention treatment. Williams and Wilkins, Baltimore, MD

Kern-Steiner R, Washecheck H S, Kelsey D D 1999 Strategy of exercise prescription using an unloading technique for functional rehabilitation of an athlete with an inversion ankle sprain. Journal of Orthopedic and Sports Physical Therapy 29:282–287

Korkola M, Amendola A 2001 Exercise-induced leg pain: shifting through a broad differential. Physician and Sportsmedicine 29(6):35–50

Krivickas L S 1997 Anatomical factors associated with overuse sports injuries. Sports Medicine 24:132–146

Kura H, Luo Z-P, Kitaoka H B et al 1997 Quantitative analysis of the intrinsic muscles of the foot. Anatomical Record 249:143–151

Lau J T C, Daniels T R 1999 Tarsal tunnel syndrome: a review of the literature. Foot and Ankle International 20(3):201–209

Lauge-Hansen N 1950 Fractures of the ankle: II. Combined experimental-surgical and experimental-roentgenological investigation. Archives of Surgery 60:957–972

Leach R E, Hammond G, Stryker W S 1967 Anterior tibial compartment syndrome. Acute and chronic. Journal of Bone and Joint Surgery (Am) 49A:451–462

Lofvenberg R, Karrholm J, Sudelin G et al 1995 Prolonged reaction time in patients with chronic lateral instability of the ankle. American Journal of Sports Medicine 23:414–417

Lundberg A, Svensson OK, Nemeth G et al 1989 The axis of rotation of the ankle joint. Journal of Bone and Joint Surgery (Br) 71B:94–99

Lynch S A, Renstom A F H 1999 Treatment of acute lateral ankle ligament rupture in the athlete. Journal of Sports Medicine 21:61–71

McGee D J 1992 Orthopedic physical assessment, 2nd edn. WB Saunders, Philadelphia, PA

Mackie J A, Webster M A 1981 Deep vein thrombosis in marathon runners. Physician and Sportsmedicine 9(5):91–98

Mann R A, Coughlin, M J 1993 Surgery of the foot and ankle, 6th edn. Mosby, St Louis, MO

Mann R A, Hagy J L 1979 The function of the toes in walking, jogging and running. Clinical Orthopedics 142:24–29

Mann R A, Hagy J 1980 Biomechanics of walking, running, and sprinting. American Journal of Sports Medicine 8:345–350

Marshall R N 1978 Foot mechanics and joggers' injuries. New Zealand Medical Journal 88:288–290

Martens M A, Backaert M, Vermont G et al 1984 Chronic leg pain in athletes due to a recurrent compartment syndrome. American Journal of Sports Medicine 12:148–151

Matsen F A 1975 Compartment syndrome: a unified concept. Clinical Orthopaedics and Related Research 113:8–14

Milgrom C, Giladi M, Simkin A et al 1989 The area moment of inertia of the tibia: a risk factor for stress fractures. Journal of Biomechanics 22:1243–1248

Milner C E, Ferber R, Pollard C D et al 2006 Biomechanical factors associated with tibial stress fracture in female runners. Medicine and Science in Sports and Exercise 38:323–328

Mindrebo N, Shelbourne K D, Van Meter C D et al 1993 Outpatient percutaneous screw fixation of the acute Jones fracture. American Journal of Sports Medicine 21:720–723

Mizrahi J, Verbitsky O, Isakov E 2000 Fatigue-related loading imbalance on the shank in running: a possible factor in stress fractures. Annals of Biomedical Engineering 28:463–469

Mohler L R, Styf J R, Pedowitz R A et al 1997 Intramuscular deoxygenation during exercise in patients who have chronic anterior compartment syndrome of the leg. Journal of Bone and Joint Surgery (Am) 79A:844–849

Molnar M E 1988 Rehabilitation of the injured ankle. Clinics in Sports Medicine 7:193–204

Mubarak S J, Gould R N, Lee Y F et al 1982 The medial tibial stress syndrome. A cause of shin splints. American Journal of Sports Medicine 10:201–205

Nicholas J, Hershman E B 1986 The lower extremity and spine in sports medicine. CV Mosby, St Louis, MO

O'Conner, D 1958 Sinus tarsi syndrome. A clinical entity. Journal of Bone and Joint Surgery (Am) 40A:720–729

Ottaviani R A, Ashton-Miller J A, Kothari S U et al 1995 Basketball shoe height and the maximal muscular resistance to applied ankle inversion and eversion moments. American Journal of Sports Medicine 23:418–423

Pester S, Smith P C 1992 Stress fractures in the lower extremities of soldiers in basic training. Orthopaedic Review 21:297–303

Pincivero D, Gieck J H, Saliba E N 1993 Rehabilitation of a lateral ankle sprain with cryokinetics and functional progressive exercise. Journal of Sport Rehabilitation 2:200–220

Raneman R S 1975 The anterior and the lateral compartmental syndrome of the leg due to intensive use of muscles. Clinical Orthopaedics and Related Research 113:69–80

Root M L, Orien W P, Weed J H 1977 Normal and abnormal function of the foot. Clinical Biomechanics Corporation, Los Angeles, CA

Rorabeck C H, Bourne R B, Fowler P J 1983 The surgical treatment of exertional compartment syndrome in athletes. Journal of Bone and Joint Surgery (Am) 65A:1245–1251

Rorabeck C H, Fowler P J, Nott L 1988 The results of fasciotomy in the management of chronic exertional compartment syndrome. American Journal of Sports Medicine 16:224–227

Rozzi S L, Lephart S M, Sterner R et al 1999 Balance training for persons with functionally unstable ankles. Journal of Orthopedic and Sports Physical Therapy 29:478–486

Ruohola J P, Kiuru M J, Pihlajamaki H K 2006 Fatigue bone injuries causing anterior lower leg pain. Clinical Orthopedics and Related Research 444:216–223

Saltzman C L, Nawoczenski D A, Talbot K D 1995 Measurement of the medial longitudinal arch. Archives of Physical Medicine and Rehabilitation 76:45–49

Schepsis A A, Martini D, Corbett M 1993 Surgical management of exertional compartment syndrome of the lower leg. American Journal of Sports Medicine 21:811–817

Seto J L, Brewster C E 1994 Treatment approaches following foot and ankle injury. Clinics in Sports Medicine 13:695–718

Shapiro M S, Kabo J M, Mitchell P W et al 1994a Ankle sprain prophylaxis: an analysis of the stabilizing effects of braces and tape. American Journal of Sports Medicine 22:78–82

Shapiro M S, Wascher D C, Finerman G A 1994b Rupture of Lisfranc's ligament in athletes. American Journal of Sports Medicine 22:687–691

Shrier 1991 Exercise-induced acute compartment syndrome: a case report. Clinical Journal of Sports Medicine 1:202–204

Silver R L, de la Garza J, Rang M 1985 The myth of muscle balance. A study of relative strengths and excursions of normal muscles about the foot and ankle. Journal of Bone and Joint Surgery (Am) 67A:432–437

Smart G W, Taunton J E, Clement D B 1980 Achilles tendon disorders in runners: a review. Medicine and Science in Sports and Exercise 12:231–243

Soavi R, Girolami M, Loreti I et al 2000 The mobility of the proximal tibio-fibular joint. A roentgen stereophotogrammetric analysis on six cadaver specimens. Foot Ankle International 21:336–342

Speroff L 1998 Oral contraceptives and arterial and venous thromboses: a clinicians formulation. American Journal of Obstetrics and Gynaecology 179:525–536

Stewart G A 1975 The role of the vessel wall in deep vein thrombosis. In: Nicolaides A N (ed) Thromboembolism. University Press, Baltimore, MD

Stollsteimer G T, Shelton W R 1997 Acute atraumatic compartment syndrome in an athlete: a case study. Journal of Athletic Training 32:248–250

Stormont D M, Morrey B F, An K N 1985 Stability of the loaded ankle. Relation between articular restraint and primary and secondary static restraints. American Journal of Sports Medicine 13:295–300

Strandness D E, Ward K, Krugmire R Jr 1977 The present state of acute deep venous thrombosis. Surgical Gynaecology and Obstetrics 145:433–445

Suissa S, Blais L, Spitzer W et al 1997 First time use of new oral contraception. Contraceptives and the risk of venous thromboembolism Contraception 56:141–146

Taillard W, Meyer J M, Garcia J et al 1981 The sinus tarsi syndrome. International Orthopedics 5:117–130

Vaes P H, Duquet W, Casteleyn P P et al 1998 Static and dynamic roentgenographic analysis of ankle stability in braced and nonbraced stable and functionally unstable ankles. American Journal of Sports Medicine 26:692–702

Waldecker U 2001 Plantar fat pad atrophy: a cause of metatarsalgia? Journal of Foot and Ankle Surgery 40:21–27

Weiss, J R 1994 Gymnastics. In: Fu FH, Stone DA (eds) Sports injuries: mechanisms prevention treatment. Williams and Wilkins, Baltimore, MD

Wester J U, Jespersen S M, Nielsen K D et al 1996 Wobble board training after partial sprains of the lateral ligaments of the ankle: a prospective randomized study. Journal of Orthopedic and Sports Physical Therapy 23:332–336

White, S C 1996 Padding and taping techniques. In: Valmassey R L (ed) Clinical biomechanics of the lower extremities. Mosby, St Louis, MO

Whittle M W 1999 Generation and attenuation of transient impulsive forces beneath the foot: a review. Gait and Posture 10:264–275

Wiley J P, Doyle D L, Taunton J E 1987 A primary care perspective of chronic compartment syndrome of the leg. Physician and Sportsmedicine 15:111–120

Williams D S, McClay I S 2000 Measurements used to characterize the foot and the medial longitudinal arch: reliability and validity. Physical Therapy 80:864–871

Williams J S Jr, Williams J S Sr 1994 Deep vein thrombosis in a skier's leg. Did exertion contribute to clotting. Physician and Sportsmedicine 22(1):79–84

Rehabilitation of lower limb muscle and tendon injuries

24

Thomas C. Windley, Suzanne Werner,

Nicola Maffulli and Jack Taunton

CHAPTER CONTENTS

Introduction 440

Sport-specific applied anatomy 440

Musculotendinous injuries 441

General rehabilitation principles for musculotendinous
injuries to the lower extremity 444

Clinical features and rehabilitation of common
sport-related musculotendinous injuries to the
lower extremity 449

Summary 454

Introduction

The musculotendinous unit allows for dynamic power generation during sport activities, and as such, is constantly at an elevated risk for injury caused by the high intrinsic forces created during athletic performance (Brewer 1962). A range of musculotendinous injuries including muscle contusions, strains and tendinopathies can result in functional limitations and time loss from sport. This chapter will discuss the relevant anatomy, types of lower extremity musculotendinous injuries and the examination, investigation and rehabilitation of those injuries. The discussion will focus on injuries to the musculotendinous units of the thigh and lower leg. Specific injuries to the hip, knee, foot and ankle and those involving the bones, ligaments or cartilage of the lower extremity are beyond the scope of this chapter, and are covered in other chapters of this book.

Sport-specific applied anatomy

The sport-specific anatomy relative to this chapter is the musculotendinous units in the thigh and lower leg. The majority of discussion will focus on the clinical significance of the quadriceps, hamstrings and the gastrocnemius/soleus complex. Other smaller muscles will also be discussed as they relate to specific musculotendinous injuries of the lower extremity.

Muscle–tendon complexes of the thigh and lower leg

Quadriceps femoris

Knee extension is performed by the quadriceps femoris on the anterior aspect of the thigh. It is the biggest muscle group of the body, with a weight of approximately 1.5 kg, and consists of four components including the rectus femoris, vastus medialis, vastus lateralis and vastus intermedius (Kendall et al 1993). These four components converge through a conjoined tendon at the superior pole of the patella and insert into the tibial tuberosity via the patellar tendon. The vastus medialis, vastus intermedius and vastus lateralis all originate on the proximal one-third of the femur. The vastus medialis and vastus lateralis are the most prominent of the quadriceps muscles, with the medialis extending slightly more inferiorly, while the intermedius lies between the vastus medialis and vastus lateralis. Vastus medialis can be functionally classified into two distinct portions. These are vastus medialis longus, having more vertically oriented fibers, and vastus medialis obliquus, with an oblique fiber orientation of 40° to 60° medially from the longitudinal femoral axis (Lieb & Perry 1968). The rectus femoris is a bi-articular muscle, originating from the anterior superior iliac spine and inserting at the superior pole of the patella. Since the rectus femoris crosses the hip and knee joints, its function is not only knee extension but also hip flexion. This dual role has been reported to result in an increased risk for injury (Sash 1981, Wilson 1972). The quadriceps muscle group is innervated by the femoral nerve (L2, L3, L4).

Sartorius

Sartorius is the longest muscle in the body, originating from the anterior superior iliac spine (Kendall et al 1993). It crosses the anterior aspect of the thigh medially, in an oblique vertical direction, and continues along the medial side of the thigh and knee joint to insert at the anteromedial, superior portion of the tibia at the pes anserinus. It can be visualized by combined resistance of flexion, abduction and external rotation of the hip with flexion of the knee (Kendall et al 1993). Sartorius is most easy to palpate at the proximal anteromedial aspect of the thigh just distal to its origin. The function of sartorius is to flex, externally rotate and abduct the hip joint and to flex and assist in internal rotation of the knee joint. It is innervated by the femoral nerve (L2, L3).

Hamstrings

The hamstring muscle group, on the posterior aspect of the thigh, consists of the biceps femoris (long and short head) on the lateral side, and semitendinosus and semimembranosus on the medial side (Kendall et al 1993). The long head of biceps femoris, semitendinosus and semimembranosus all originate from the ischial tuberosity while the short head of the biceps femoris originates on the linea aspera and posterior femur. The long and short heads of the biceps femoris insert on the lateral side of the head of fibula, the lateral condyle of tibia and the deep fascia on lateral side of the leg. The short head of biceps femoris is the most frequently strained hamstring muscle. It has two motor points, one innervated by the tibial portion of the sciatic nerve (L5, S1, S2) and the other by the peroneal portion of the same nerve (L5, S1, S2). The dual innervation may cause problems as the short head may contract at the same time as the quadriceps resulting in a hamstring strain (Burkett 1976). Semimembranosus inserts at the posteromedial aspect of medial condyle of tibia. On the anteromedial aspect of the knee, just inferior to the medial tibial plateau, is the pes anserinus. Semitendinosus inserts here along with the gracilis and sartorius. By definition of their origins, with the exception of the short head of the biceps, the hamstrings cross both the hip and knee joints, and are thereby functioning as both hip extensors and knee flexors. This dual function makes them more

prone to injury (Sash 1981, Wilson 1972). With the exception of the dual innervation discussed regarding the short head of the biceps femoris, the rest of the hamstrings are innervated solely by the tibial branch of the sciatic nerve (L5, S1, S2).

Iliotibial band

The iliotibial band is not a muscle, but plays an important role in the mechanics of the lower extremity and does sustain soft tissue injury. It is a thickened band of fascia extending from the iliac crest distally along the lateral side of the thigh to insert at Gerdy's tubercle on the lateral tibial condyle (Moore & Dalley 1999). Proximally, near the greater trochanter, it receives the insertion of the tensor fasciae lata muscle anteriorly, and superficial layer of gluteus maximus posteriorly. It then attaches to the linea aspera of the femur through the lateral intermuscular septum, thus being free in its distal part while it crosses the lateral femoral condyle before attaching to the tibial condyle. It lies anterior to the lateral femoral condyle, with the knee fully extended, and at 30° of knee flexion it lies behind the lateral femoral condyle. Thus it has a dual function in knee extension and flexion depending on the knee angle.

Gastrocnemius–soleus complex

The gastrocnemius–soleus complex, or triceps surae, is in the posterior compartment of the lower leg. Both muscles come together distally to form the conjoined Achilles tendon that inserts into the posterior calcaneous (Moore & Dalley 1999). The gastrocnemius is a two-headed, two-joint muscle that originates on both the lateral and medial femoral condyles, while the deeper soleus is a large flat muscle that originates on the posterior fibula and upper portion of the medial tibia. The two-joint gastrocnemius both flexes the knee and plantarflexes the ankle when the knee is extended. The single-joint soleus plantarflexes the ankle, independent of knee position. They are both innervated by the tibial nerve (S1 and S2).

Musculotendinous injuries

Muscle strain

A muscle strain is a partial or complete tear of the musculotendinous junction (Burkett 1970). Muscle strains are due to dynamic overload causing the strength of the musculotendinous unit to be exceeded, often during an explosive movement in sport when a strong eccentric muscle action is necessary to control joint motion (Glick 1980, Zarins & Ciullo 1983). Typically this is characterized by a violent muscle contraction occurring simultaneously with an excessively forced stretch (Arner & Lindholm 1958, Fuller 1984, Garrett 1983, Garrett et al 1984, Zarins & Ciullo 1983) usually at the musculotendinous junction (Garrett et al 1987, Garrett et al 1988, Norfray et al 1980, Safran et al 1988). The vast majority of muscle strains involve muscles that pass over two joints or more or occur in muscles with complex architecture (Brewer 1962). In the anterior thigh, the rectus femoris is most vulnerable to strains, while in the posterior

Table 24.1 Treatment protocol for mild, moderate and severe muscle strains

	Mild muscle strain	Moderate muscle strain	Severe muscle strain
Days 1–3	Compression Ice Elevation Active range of motion Isometric training Electrical muscle stimulation	Compression Ice Elevation Pain-free active range of motion Electrical muscle stimulation Crutch walking	Compression Ice Elevation Crutch walking
From day 4	Pool training Pain-free stretching Isotonic training (progress from light to heavier weights and from concentric to eccentric actions) Bicycle training Functional exercises	Pain-free isometric training	Electrical muscle stimulation
From day 7	Isokinetic training (progress from fast to slow angular velocities and from concentric to eccentric actions) Plyometric training Sport-specific exercises	Pool training Pain-free stretching Isotonic training (progress from fast to slow angular velocities and from concentric to eccentric actions) Bicycle training Functional exercises	Pain-free active range of motion Pain-free isometric training
From week 2		Isokinetic training (progress from fast to slow angular velocities and from concentric to eccentric actions) Plyometric training Sport-specific exercises	Pool training Pain-free stretching Isotonic training (progress from fast to slow angular velocities and from concentric to eccentric actions) Bicycle training Functional exercises
From week 3			Isokinetic training (progress from fast to slow angular velocities and from concentric to eccentric actions) Plyometric training Sport-specific exercises

thigh the hamstring group, especially the short head of biceps femoris, usually is the one where strains occur.

Muscle strains may range from a small separation of muscle fibers to a complete muscle rupture, and are clinically classified into mild (grade I), moderate (grade II) and/or severe, complete tears (grade III) (Kirkendall et al 2001). A grade I muscle strain is a mild injury that normally results in mild pain and minimal swelling with full joint range of motion. The muscle fibers have been stretched or torn, and there is pain and tenderness during a resisted active contraction and during passive stretching. A localized muscle spasm may also be palpable at the site of pain. The athlete might not be aware of the moment of injury and may not notice symptoms until they have cooled down. Grade II strains are moderate injuries, and are painful with palpation, have a small muscle defect that is usually palpable, moderate swelling, reduced joint range of motion, and cause gait deviations. The muscle fibers have been torn, and

the athlete complains of significant pain on passive stretching and on opposed active contraction. The athlete generally ceases the physical activity at the moment of being injured. Grade III strains are major injuries and are the result of a complete rupture of the muscle belly, muscle tendon junction or tendon insertion. The athlete will have significant pain, a moderate to large defect with palpation, moderate to severe swelling, a 50% or more loss of range of motion, a significant loss of muscle function and significant gait deficits. See Table 24.1 for treatment protocols for mild, moderate and severe muscle strains.

Muscle contusion

The most common muscle contusion is to the quadriceps (Kirkendall et al 2001). A muscle contusion to the quadriceps, or any other muscle, is usually the result of a direct blow to the muscle. At the time of impact, the contracted muscle is compressed against the underlying bone, often causing a deep rupture and bleeding. This direct blow results in formation of an intra- or intermuscular hematoma characterized by hemorrhaging and an inflammatory response, with subsequent formulation of granulation tissue, and, eventually, collagenous scar tissue (Wilson 1972). In the case of intra-muscular hematoma, the first 48 hours is accompanied by tenderness, pain and reduced mobility, with osmosis drawing fluid from the surrounding tissue. If swelling persists, the muscle may become completely impaired (Peterson & Renstrom 2001). Alternatively, intermuscular hematoma results in bruising and swelling distal to the damaged tissue 24–48 hours after the injury, with no increase in pressure. Muscle function is usually restored quickly (Peterson & Renstrom 2001). Muscle contusions mainly occur deep in the muscle, adjacent to the bone (Peterson & Renstrom 2001, Ryan 1969, Walton & Rothwell 1983), but can also be superficial or occur anywhere within the muscle (Peterson & Renstrom 2001).

Like muscle strains, muscle contusions are graded on a scale from grade I to grade III based on severity of the injury and the presenting signs and symptoms (Jackson & Feagin 1973, Kirkendall et al 2001). Grade I muscle contusions rarely result in swelling, loss of motion or strength, or functional deviations, but there may be pain with palpation. Grade II contusions are characterized by voluntary muscle splinting, abnormal gait, a muscle defect causing pain with palpation and a significant loss of motion and muscle strength. In the case of a grade III contusion, there is severe disability, bleeding, and sometimes a herniation of the muscle through the fascia. The associated symptoms include a significant loss of motion and an inability to tolerate resisted muscle strength testing. An objective classification of muscle contusion injuries according to Jackson & Feagin (1973) is given in Table 24.2.

Tendinopathy

Tendon disease, or tendinopathy, covers a wide range of conditions, most of which are chronic in nature. These conditions include tendinitis (an inflammation of the tendon), tenosynovitis or paratendinitis (an inflammation of surrounding tissues), tendinosis (focal degenerative lesions) and partial or complete tendon rupture. However, the majority of tendinopathies are chronic and degenerative rather than inflammatory in nature, with pain being associated with tissue damage in overuse tendinopathy (Leadbetter 1992). Figure 24.1 illustrates the relationship between pain and tissue damage in overuse tendinopathy.

Unfortunately little is known about the etiology and pathogenesis of chronic tendon pain. Recent research, however, has uncovered some of the mystery. A series of studies conducted by a group of investigators in Sweden has evaluated the structure and neurovascular makeup of tendons with clinically diagnosed tendinopathy (Alfredson 2004, Alfredson 2005, Alfredson & Lorentzon 2000, Alfredson & Ohberg 2005, Gisslen & Alfredson 2005, Gisslen et al 2005, Ohberg & Alfredson 2002). Interestingly, there is an absence of inflammatory cell infiltration in and around pathological tendons, thereby rendering anti-inflammatory agents ineffective as a treatment modality (Alfredson 2005). Instead, with the use of ultrasound, color Doppler and biopsy techniques, their work has illustrated that pathological tendons exhibit structural changes in the collagen

Table 24.2 Classification of quadriceps contusions based on the classification suggested by Jackson & Feagin (1973)

Severity	Symptoms	Range of movement	Functional ability
Mild	Local tenderness	>90°	Normal gait Normal knee bend
Moderate	Tender muscle mass Swelling	<90°	Antalgic gait Pain on climbing stairs Pain on rising from chair
Severe	Marked tenderness Marked swelling	<45°	Severe limp (crutches needed) Ispilateral knee pain

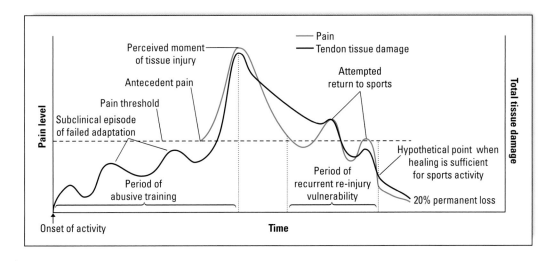

Figure 24.1 • Illustration of pain and tissue damage in overuse tendinopathy. (Reproduced with permission from Leadbetter 1992.)

443

matrix (usually a thickening of the tendon), neovascular changes and a vasculoneural ingrowth pattern in and around the tendon (Alfredson 2004, Alfredson 2005, Alfredson & Lorentzon 2000, Gisslen & Alfredson 2005, Lind et al 2006).

General rehabilitation principles for musculotendinous injuries to the lower extermity

Examination

When examining musculotendinous injuries of the lower extremity it is important to obtain an accurate and thorough subjective history from the patient. Like other examinations, examination of musculotendinous injuries to the lower extremity is based on similar principles as other areas of the body (i.e. inspection, palpation, evaluation of movement). Paying attention to the history combined with the clinical examination, which establishes the diagnosis, will aid the clinician in making an accurate assessment of the athlete's condition. Based on the assessment, the clinician can design an appropriate rehabilitation program.

Clinical examination

The site of pain and the injury mechanism are the most important factors in clinical examination of musculotendinous injuries to the lower extremity. The aim of the clinical examination is to reveal the exact site of pain, and to assess range of motion and muscle strength. Furthermore, sports-related functional tests should be used in order to evaluate the athlete from a sport-specific point of view. It is also important to keep in mind that presentation of pain in the thigh may be indicative of referred or radicular pain. Hence, all examinations of the lower extremity should include ruling out the influence of the lumbar spine, pelvis, sacroiliac joint, hip joint and gluteal muscles. Specific foci of clinical examination of musculotendinous injuries to the lower extremity are listed below:

- *Inspection* should be performed in supine (anterior thigh or lower leg injuries), prone (posterior thigh or lower leg injuries), standing, walking and sport-specific positions or activities.

- *Palpation* of the anterior and posterior muscles of the lower extremity should be performed in supine and prone positions, respectively. Special attention should be paid to possible tenderness and swelling. When dealing with posterior muscle injuries, palpation of the ischial tuberosity and the gluteal muscles, where trigger points may refer pain to the hamstrings, is advisable.

- *Active range of motion* of the ankle, knee and hip joints as well as the mobility of the lumbar spine and the sacroiliac joints should be examined.

- *Muscle flexibility/tightness* of the muscle groups of the thigh and lower leg should be examined.

- *Concentric and eccentric muscle action* should be examined for all muscle groups of the lower extremity.

- *Activities of daily living* can be checked by the single-leg squat test, the single-leg chair test (raise–sit down), the single-leg step test (up–down) and the stair climbing test (up–down) (Magee 1997). Special attention should be paid to reproducing a comparable sign and pain levels, which can be evaluated using Borg's pain scale (Borg et al 1981) or the visual analogue scale (VAS) (Price et al 1983).

- *Sports activities* can be checked by jumping, kicking and different running exercises involving acceleration as well as deceleration movements.

Special tests

Special tests are designed to narrow the scope of focus during the clinical examination. This will allow for an accurate determination of the differential diagnosis, with the result being a focused treatment protocol.

Rectus femoris contracture test

The rectus femoris contracture test assesses rectus femoris inflexibility or restriction (Magee 1997). The athlete is placed supine on a table with the knees bent and hanging off one end of the table. The athlete then pulls one knee to the chest. If the contralateral lower leg extends the test is positive for rectus femoris tightness.

Ely's test

Ely's test is a flexibility test of the rectus femoris (Magee 1997). It is performed with the athlete lying supine with the knee of the symptomatic leg hanging over the edge of the bench. The hip and knee joints of the asymptomatic leg are maximally flexed and the leg is held by the hands toward the chest. Extension of the symptomatic knee joint is a sign of rectus femoris tightness.

Ober's test

Ober's test is specific for iliotibial band inflexibility or restriction (Magee 1997). The athlete is placed on a table in side-lying with the lower leg flexed at the hip and knee. The upper leg is then passively abducted and extended with the knee flexed to 90°. The limb is then lowered. If the limb remains adducted, the test is positive for iliotibial band tightness.

Noble compression test

The noble compression test is specific for iliotibial band friction syndrome (Magee 1997). The athlete is placed supine on a table. The tester then passively flexes the knee to 90° along with hip flexion. The tester then applies pressure to the lateral portion of the patella while the knee is passively extended. Pain at approximately 30° of flexion indicates a positive test for iliotibial band friction syndrome.

Action of the quadriceps muscle group

The action of the quadriceps muscle group is tested by having the patient sitting with the legs hanging over the edge of the bench (Magee 1997). With one hand the examiner stabilizes the thigh by holding it firmly down on the bench. A test of concentric muscle action is performed when the patient is instructed to extend the knee, while the examiner applies a pressure in the direction of flexion with the other hand above the ankle. A test of eccentric muscle action is performed when the patient is instructed to try to maintain the knee in a chosen knee flexion angle, while the examiner applies a pressure and moves the leg in the direction of flexion with the other hand above the ankle.

When comparing the symptomatic leg with the asymptomatic one, this test may give the examiner a rough measure of whether there is a side difference in quadriceps strength. However, it should be pointed out that a more appropriate way of evaluating quadriceps strength is by performing an isokinetic or isometric measurement.

When performing this test of quadriceps strength we must also be aware that painful resisted knee extension, in particular eccentrically, might be due to patellofemoral pain and/or patellar tendinosis, so called jumper's knee. Subsequently, due to pain inhibition these subjects cannot produce a proper test of muscle strength, meaning that this test might give an answer of pain instead of muscle strength. In order to control for pain or inhibition, one can use the isokinetic method with twitch interpolation technique by adding electrical muscle stimulation (McKenzie et al 1992). However, to some extent the Borg's pain scale (Borg et al 1981) or the visual analogue scale (VAS) (Price et al 1983) can also be used.

Wallace test

The Wallace test is an appropriate test for flexibility of the hamstrings muscle group (Wallace 1979). The athlete is lying supine with extended hips and knees. The athlete flexes the hip and knee to be tested to 90°, while stabilizing the thigh in that position with the hands, and from this position tries to fully extend the knee with the hip maintained in 90° of flexion. Decreased hamstrings flexibility is demonstrated by the number of degrees that are lacking from complete knee extension. A tightness of the hamstrings will appear either when there is a restriction of knee extension when the hip is flexed, or when there is a restriction of hip flexion when the knee is extended. This is due to those muscles crossing the knee joint as well as the hip joint.

Straight leg raise test

The straight leg raise test for hamstrings length is a combination of hip flexion and flexion of the lumbar spine (Magee 1997). Having the subject lying supine on the bench, with one hand the examiner passively raises the 'test-leg', with the knee maintained in extension, to an angle of 80–90° of hip flexion. The contralateral leg is held down with the other hand, to stabilize the pelvis and prevent excessive flexion of the lumbar spine. For accurate testing, the low back must be flat on the bench in a posterior pelvic tilt position. To find out whether the athlete's symptom is caused by tight hamstrings, or is of a neurogenic origin, the examiner can raise the leg up to the subject's pain threshold. When slightly lowering the leg, the pain should decrease or disappear. A passive ankle dorsiflexion that causes pain in this slightly lowered leg position reveals a neurogenic pain, while no pain means tight hamstrings muscles.

Slump test

The slump test, which is a neural tension test, can be used to differentiate between hamstring injuries and referred pain to the hamstrings from the lumbar spine (Magee 1997). The athlete is sitting on the edge of the bench, thighs fully supported and the hands behind the back. The athlete slumps forward making a kyphosis of the lumbar and thoracic spine and a maximal flexion of the cervical spine (chin to chest), while maintaining the sacrum vertical. In this position the athlete extends one knee and dorsiflexes the ankle of the same leg, and then slowly releases the flexion of the cervical spine. The test is positive when the athlete's hamstring pain is reproduced and relieved with reduction of the neural tension by releasing the flexion of the cervical spine.

Action of the lateral hamstrings

To test the action of the lateral hamstrings (biceps femoris), the athlete is placed prone on the bench with the 'test-leg' in somewhat less than 90° of knee flexion and the hip externally rotated (Magee 1997). The examiner holds the thigh down firmly on the bench with one hand and pressures with the other hand against the leg proximal to the ankle in the direction of knee extension.

Action of the medial hamstrings

To test the action of the medial hamstrings (semitendinosus and semimembranosus), the athlete is placed prone on the bench with the 'test-leg' in somewhat less than 90° of knee flexion and the hip internally rotated (Magee 1997). The examiner holds the thigh down firmly on the bench with one hand and pressures with the other hand against the leg proximal to the ankle in the direction of knee extension.

Action of gracilis

To test the action of gracilis, the muscle is activated during knee flexion and internal rotation of the knee (Kendall et al 1993). It will be activated by the same test position and pressure as used for the medial hamstrings as explained above. The difference in knee flexion action between the medial hamstrings and the gracilis is due to the fact that the medial hamstrings originate from the ischium, while the gracilis originates from the pubis.

General rehabilitation principles for musculotendinous injuries to the lower extremity

The acute management of musculotendinous injuries is important in order to limit the likelihood of the development of a severe hematoma, and thereby to promote the return to sport. The repair mechanism following a muscle injury is unstable during the first 24–36 hours (Peterson & Renstrom 2001). Hence, further bleeding may occur as a result of another impact, violent muscle contraction or unprotected weightbearing when dealing with moderate or severe injuries. A precise diagnosis can be difficult in the acute phase, and therefore a muscle injury should be considered as potentially serious the first 2 to 3 days.

Acute management should focus on protecting the injured tissues from further damage while controlling the inflammatory response. Treatments may include rest, ice, compression, elevation, immobilization for short periods of time, crutch ambulation and non-steroidal anti-inflammatory agents (Agre 1985).

After the first few days, it may be easier to accurately diagnose a musculotendinous injury and determine the level of its severity. Intramuscular bleeding may still be active if the swelling has not resolved, the bleeding has spread and caused bruising at some distance from the injured area and the muscle contraction capability has not improved. If these signs are present the acute phase is still active, and the muscle–tendon unit should still be protected from loading. In this case it is likely that the injury is severe in nature and may take an extended period of time to be rehabilitated (Peterson & Renstrom 2001).

Once bleeding has stopped, swelling is beginning to resolve and muscle contraction capability is improving, a gradual progressive rehabilitation protocol may be initiated. This progression usually involves a combination of the following activites: electrical stimulation of the muscle belly (Fig. 24.2), most often used for quadriceps strength augmentation (Snyder-Mackler et al 1994); stretching of anterior muscle groups (Fig. 24.3); stretching of the posterior muscle groups (Fig. 24.4); open chain strengthening with no weight applied through a limited range of motion (Fig. 24.5); open chain strengthening with weight applied through a full range of motion (Fig. 24.6); closed chain isotonic resistance strengthening (Fig. 24.7); open chain isotonic resistance strengthening (Fig. 24.8); functional weight-bearing exercises (Fig. 24.9); functional eccentric weightbearing exercises (Fig. 24.10); functional aerobic activities (Fig. 24.11); isokinetic strength training (Fig. 24.12); and functional plyometric exercises (Fig. 24.13).

Return to sport

The goal of rehabilitation is to return the athlete to sport participation in the least amount of time. Sports activity puts

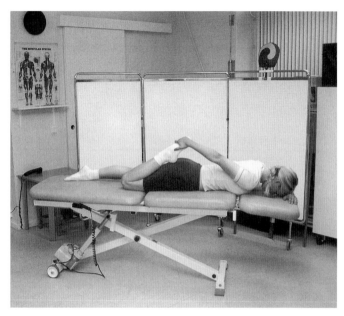

Figure 24.3 • Stretching of anterior muscle groups.

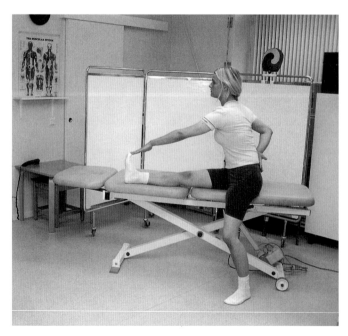

Figure 24.4 • Stretching of the posterior muscle groups.

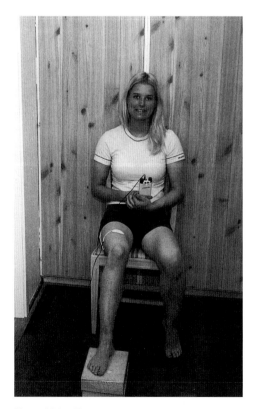

Figure 24.2 • Electrical stimulation of the muscle belly.

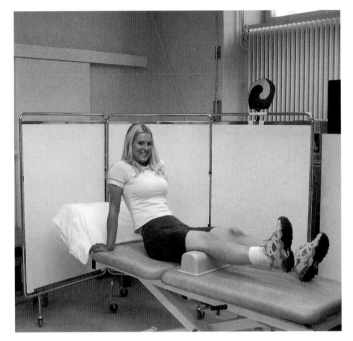

Figure 24.5 • Open chain strengthening with no weight applied through a limited range of motion.

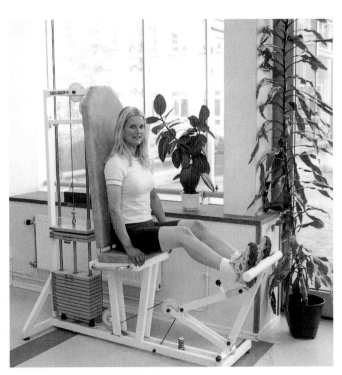

Figure 24.7 • Closed chain isotonic resistance strengthening.

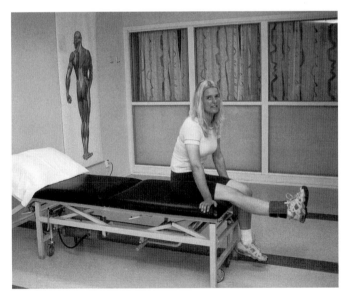

Figure 24.6 • Open chain strengthening with weight applied through a full range of motion.

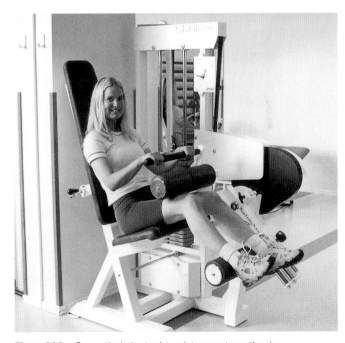

Figure 24.8 • Open chain isotonic resistance strengthening.

heavy demands on physical fitness and conditioning, which is critical when a recently injured athlete is returning to sport. Therefore, the rehabilitation should progress the athlete back to normal function prior to return to sporting activities. The following criteria are suggested to be fulfilled before allowing the athlete with a musculotendinous injury of the lower extremity to return to sport participation:

- Full range of motion throughout the hips, knees, and ankles.

- Appropriate muscle flexibility of the anterior and posterior muscle groups of the thigh and lower leg.

- Appropriate muscle strength of the anterior and posterior muscle groups of the thigh and lower leg ($<$10% side to side differences) (Heiser et al 1984).

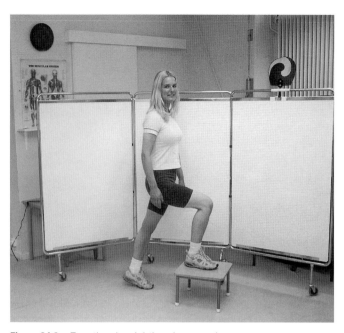

Figure 24.9 • Functional weightbearing exercises.

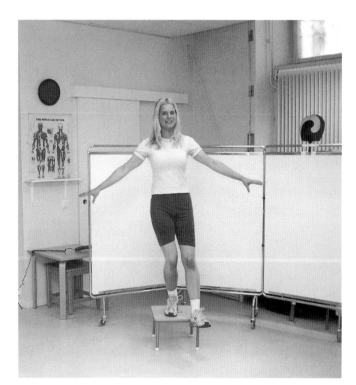

Figure 24.10 • Functional eccentric weightbearing exercises.

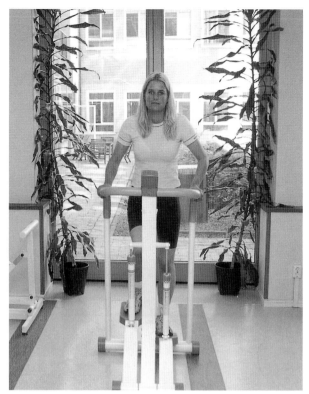

Figure 24.11 • Functional aerobic activities.

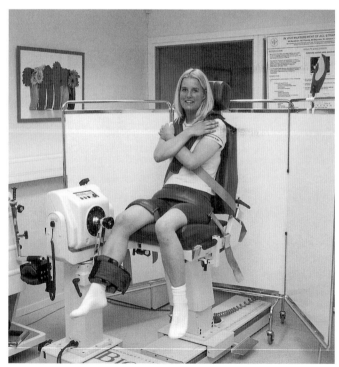

Figure 24.12 • Isokinetic strength training.

- Appropriate muscle strength balance between the anterior and posterior muscle groups (hamstring/quadriceps ratio ≥60%) (Devan et al 2004, Heiser et al 1984).

- Sports-related functional tests, such as running tests with acceleration and deceleration, sprint and hop tests,

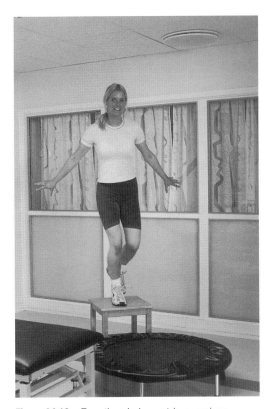

Figure 24.13 • Functional plyometric exercises.

performed at full speed without residual symptoms (Heiser et al 1984).

- The ability to complete a simulated game without functional limitations, soreness or pain during or following (Axe et al 2001, Axe et al 2002).

Prevention of musculotendinous injuries

Different preventive strategies for developing musculotendinous injuries of the lower extremity have been suggested. Authors recommend that athletes routinely practice stretching (Beaulieu 1981, Cross & Worrell 1999, Glick 1980, Hartig & Henderson 1999, Petersen & Holmich 2006). Hamstrings stretches have been shown to, not only increase hamstrings flexibility (Hartig & Henderson 1999), but also to reduce the risk of overuse injuries (Hartig & Henderson 1999) and musculotendinous strains in the lower extremity (Cross & Worrell 1999). A careful warm-up program is also cited as a way of preventing muscle injuries (Wiktorsson-Moller et al 1983), and an appropriate level of muscle strength can protect a musculotendinous unit from injury (Garrett et al 1987, Safran et al 1988). Furthermore, a strength imbalance between the anterior and posterior muscle groups of the lower extremity has been reported to be related to the risk of lower extremity injury (Devan et al 2004). Specifically, hamstrings-to-quadriceps isokinetic strength ratios below 60% are related to iliotibial band friction syndrome, patellar tendonitis

and patellofemoral syndrome. Careful attention to the overall physical conditioning of athletes including the factors listed here will reduce the overall risk of lower extremity injuries.

Clinical features and rehabilitation of common sport-related musculotendinous injuries to the lower extremity

Thigh muscle strains

Clinical features of quadriceps strains

Strains in the quadriceps muscle occur during high-velocity knee extension activities in sport, and the majority of injuries are to the rectus femoris at the musculotendinous junction (Cross et al 2004, Palmer et al 1999). The susceptibility of the rectus femoris to frequent injury is due to its superficial location in the thigh, its high percentage of fast twitch muscle fibers, its often eccentric muscle action and its extension across two joints. At the time of injury, the athlete reports sudden pain in the anterior thigh during an activity that requires a vigorous quadriceps muscle contraction (e.g. during sprinting, jumping or kicking).

Magnetic resonance imaging (MRI) (see Chapter 30) rapidly reveals the anatomical location and size of quadriceps muscle strains, but is not thought to be cost effective, and generally does not influence or change the treatment (Bencardino et al 2000, Brunet & Hontas 1994, Cross et al 2004). An X-ray may only be helpful if treatment is not progressing, and may therefore highlight an avulsion fracture at the proximal attachment. Strain of the rectus femoris can be confirmed by eliciting pain when the hip joint is extended and the knee joint is flexed. Because the muscle is subcutaneous and overlies the remainder of the quadriceps, a localized swelling or a defect is readily apparent. This can be confirmed with the athlete lying supine flexing the hip with the knee held in approximately 45° of flexion. If injury is present, a localized swelling or defect will be apparent in this position.

Clinical features of hamstrings strains

Hamstrings strains and ruptures are the most common muscle injuries in the thigh, and rank second in all injuries in sports (Kuland 1982). The biceps femoris is the most commonly injured muscle of the hamstrings group (DeSmet & Best 2000, Koulouris & Connell 2003, Petersen & Holmich 2006). The etiology of hamstrings strains in athletes is complex, and many factors have been reported as being responsible for this injury. These include inadequate warm-up, low hamstrings-to-quadriceps muscle strength ratio, muscle fatigue, poor hamstrings flexibility, poor technique, poor posture, previous incomplete injury and an abnormal muscle contraction at the time of injury (Agre 1985, Bencardino & Mellado 2005, Burkett 1970, Casperson 1982, Dornan 1971, Garrett 1983, Heiser et al 1984, Kuland 1982, Liemohn 1978, Oakes 1984, O'Neil 1976, Petersen & Holmich 2006, Stafford & Grana 1984).

Hamstrings strains result from overstretching or a rapid contraction causing different degrees of tearing within the musculotendinous unit. The hamstrings muscles have been shown to have a relatively high proportion of 'fast twitch' muscle fibers (Garrett et al 1984). The hamstrings group crosses two joints, leading to greater changes in length when compared to muscles that cross only one joint. Therefore, the high levels of intrinsic tensions produced by the 'fast twitch' fibers, combined with the extrinsic stretch, involved with length changes over two joints, might make the hamstrings prone to injury during high intensity sprinting and jumping activities.

At the time of hamstrings strain injury, the athlete usually experiences a sudden onset of pain in the posterior thigh (Garrett et al 1984). Occasionally, the athlete will report an audible 'pop', identifying a grade II or III strain. As is the case with quadriceps strains, MRI may be an effective tool in determining the extent of damage to the musculotendinous unit (Bencardino & Mellado 2005, Bencardino et al 2000, DeSmet & Best 2000, Koulouris & Connell 2003), and in determining if an avulsion from the ischial tuberosity exists that may necessitate surgery (Koulouris & Connell 2003). Clinically, localized tenderness is identified over the injured area with palpation of the hamstrings, with the athlete lying prone and the knee slightly flexed against resistance.

Treatment of thigh muscle strains

Recent research has indicated that traditional physical therapies may not be as effective as once thought for rehabilitation of acute thigh muscle strains (Sherry & Best 2004). In this study, 11 athletes sustaining acute hamstrings strains participated in a traditional rehabilitation program that included static stretching, isolated progressive hamstrings resistance exercise and cryotherapy. Of those 11 athletes, 6 reinjured their hamstrings within two weeks of returning to their sport, and 7 out of 10 available for a one-year follow-up had sustained reinjury within one year of returning to their sport. Thirteen athletes concurrently participated in a rehabilitation program that consisted of progressive agility and trunk stabilization exercises in addition to cryotherapy. Of those 13 athletes, none had reinjured their hamstrings two weeks after returning to sport and only one had reinjured their hamstrings one year after returning to their sport. Hence, considering the stability of the trunk and a focus on agility training may improve traditional therapies for acute muscle strains.

Regardless of the muscle injured and the therapeutic protocol, return to sport criteria following acute muscle strains of the thigh muscles should focus on simulating the conditions in which the muscle strains occur. Recent evidence shows that mean return to play intervals for rectus femoris strains range from 9.2 days (injury to the muscle belly) to 26.9 days (injury to the central tendon) (Cross et al 2004). Dancers with hamstrings strains, however, have been shown to take approximately 16 weeks to return to their previous level of function, while sprinters may take up to 50 weeks (Askling et al 2006).

Quadriceps contusion and myositis ossificans

Clinical features and rehabilitation of quadriceps contusions

Quadriceps contusions occur as the result of blunt force trauma to the anterior thigh, and tissue damage is proportional to the magnitude of compression, the area over which the compression is applied and the relative tissue resistance in the area (Zarins & Ciullo 1983). Muscle injury is likely to be more extensive if the contusion occurred during a muscle contraction. In most cases the athlete is capable of continuing to participate, at least initially. However, by the next day swelling, pain and stiffness will limit function.

The clinical signs and symptoms of mild, moderate and severe quadriceps contusions are discussed above, and the recommendations for the rehabilitation can be found in Table 24.3.

Clinical features of myositis ossificans of the quadriceps

Occasionally, after a thigh contusion with an intramuscular bleeding, the hematoma calcifies developing myositis ossificans (Zarins & Ciullo 1983). The onset of myositis ossificans has been shown to be related to the severity of the contusion (Jackson & Feagin 1973). Specifically, myositis ossificans has been shown to develop in 72% of athletes with moderate or severe contusions, but not to develop in those with a mild contusion.

Development of myositis ossificans is a possible complication of deep muscle contusions, especially to the anterior thigh and the quadriceps muscle (Walton & Rothwell 1983). The exact mechanism of onset still remains unknown. It may start with a muscle trauma leading to inflammation, cellular proliferation, concentration of growth factors, induction of bone forming cells and ossification.

Several studies have examined the most effective diagnostic techniques for the diagnosis of myositis ossificans. Early after injury, ultrasound (see Chapter 30) may detect myositis ossificans, but it has been reported to be nonspecific, with differential diagnoses including hematoma, abscess and tumor (Fornage & Eftekhori 1989, Kirkpatrick et al 1987). Intramuscular calcification can generally be visualized with an X-ray 10 days to 10 weeks after onset of calcification (Cushner & Morwessel 1992, Estwanik & McAlister 1990).

Clinically, pain, a palpable mass and a flexion contracture following a muscle injury strongly suggest the possibility of myositis ossificans (Cushner & Morwessel 1992). Localized tenderness and warmth may also be present over the injured area. To the athlete, myositis ossificans can be a source of a long-term considerable disability due to inflammatory pain and contracture (Estwanik & McAlister 1990, Garrett 1990). When the diagnosis is still in doubt, a biopsy may be indicated to rule out the presence of an osteosarcoma (Cushner & Morwessel 1992). In patients with myositis ossificans, the pain and size of the mass decrease as the lesion matures, but increase as time progresses in patients with osteosarcoma (Cushner & Morwessel

Table 24.3 Treatment protocol for mild, moderate and severe muscle contusions

	Mild muscle contusion	Moderate muscle contusion	Severe muscle contusion
Day 1	Compression Ice Gentle stretching	Compression Ice Electrical muscle stimulation Crutch walking	
Day 1–3			Compression Ice Rest Electrical muscle stimulation Crutch walking
Days 2 and 3	Strengthening exercises progressing from isometric through to isotonic training (light to heavy weights), and then to isokinetic training (fast to slow angular velocities, concentric to eccentric actions)	Pain-free isometric training Pain-free active range of motion	
Days 5–7		Pool training Isotonic training (progress from light to heavy weights and from concentric to eccentric actions) Bicycle training	Pain-free isometric training Pain-free active range of motion
Days 7–10		Isokinetic training (progress from fast to slow angular velocities and from concentric to eccentric actions)	
Day 10		Stretching exercises	Pool training Isotonic training (progress from light to heavy weights and from concentric to eccentric actions) Bicycle training
Day 14			Isokinetic training (progress from fast to slow angular velocities and from concentric to eccentric actions) Stretching exercises

1992). Young patients engaging in sports can develop malignant tumors (Dudkiewicz et al 2001, Maffulli et al 1990). Hence, osteosarcoma is the most important differential diagnosis, and should be ruled out in every young athlete that presents with a soft tissue mass (Kirkendall et al 2001).

Rehabiliation of myositis ossificans

There is very little that can be done to accelerate the resorptive process of myositis ossificans. Rest and immobilization may prevent further calcification, and most modalities such as heat and ultrasound should be avoided (Zarins & Ciullo 1983). Instead, gentle pain-free range of motion exercises and cryotherapy might help reduce symptoms (Kirkendall et al 2001). Non-steroidal anti-inflammatory drugs are known to decrease calcification, and irradiation has also been suggested for prevention of calcification. Surgery should be delayed until bone formation has reached its maturity, given that surgery may induce greater

ossification (Estwanik & McAlister 1990). If necessary, surgical excision of the calcification one year after injury followed by a slow progressive rehabilitation may restore function to the muscle.

Patellar and Achilles tendinopathy

Clinical features of patellar tendinopathy

Patellar tendinopathy commonly develops in people who, as a part of their sports and/or recreational activity, place excessive strain on the extensor apparatus (Alfredson 2005). The majority of overloading of the extensor mechanism occurs in jumping and landing sports such as long jump, high jump, basketball and volleyball. Lower extremity malalignments, inflexibility, weakness or training on hard surfaces have been postulated to contribute to the development of this condition (Brukner & Khan 2006). Pain and reduced function are the main clinical features. Patients usually complain of pain near the inferior pole of the patella that is aggravated by activities that involve high quadriceps demand, such as squatting. Usually, there is an associated weakness in the quadriceps, with possible poor vastus medialis oblique control, and a possible weakness in the gastrocnemius. In the initial stages of the disease, the pain mainly occurs following activity, but with disease progression pain may become persistent, occurring even at rest. The pain may be elicited on palpation of the abovementioned sites or by extending the knee against resistance. Long periods of sitting with the knee flexed, as while driving or watching a movie, may result in pain. Rarely, continued strain while ignoring the pain may result in rupture of the patellar tendon.

Clinical features of Achilles tendinopathy

Achilles tendinopathy is most common among recreational male runners between the ages of 35 and 45 (Alfredson & Lorentzon 2000). However, it is also commonly associated with basket-ball, cycling, cross-country skiing, dance and figure skating, or other activities in which there is high demand or pressure on the Achilles tendon. Training methods such as repetitive loading of the Achilles tendon, abrupt changes in running mileage and a history of similar injury in the past 12 months may increase the likelihood of Achilles tendon injury. Calf weakness, gastroc-nemius/soleus inflexibility, high arches, improper footwear, age and being of male gender may also contribute to the likelihood of Achilles tendinopathy (Alfredson & Lorentzon 2000).

The classification of Achilles tendinopathy and clinical findings are in Table 24.4. Patients with chronic pathology usually note a long-standing history of heel pain with a progressive magnification of symptoms if untreated. Patients with complete Achilles tendon rupture usually report an audible pop or snap at the time of injury, with a sense of feeling as though they have been kicked. Pain is usually immediate but resolves quickly. Interestingly, asymptomatic rupture has been reported to exist in 30% of patients, leading to a delay in diagnosis (Leppilahti & Orava 1998).

Upon clinical examination, patients with Achilles tendinopathy report pain with palpation of the musculotendinous junction. Often times, a defect can be palpated and a prominence at the posterosuperior aspect of calcaneus may be noted. Tendinosis and partial tendon ruptures are difficult to differentiate, since they usually coexist. When the tendon has ruptured completely, significant swelling and bruising persist. In addition, a palpable gap may be noted in the Achilles tendon. In this case reduced or absent plantar flexion strength and absent plantar flexion following a squeeze of the calf muscle (Thompson's test) are almost universal (Magee 1997). The differential diagnoses of Achilles tendon injuries are listed in Box 24.1.

Rehabilitation of patellar and achilles tendinopathy

Rehabilitation of chronic tendinopathy is traditionally very difficult. However, the findings regarding the structural tendon changes and neovascularization that exist in pathological tendons have spawned an interest in nonsurgical treatments that may be more effective than traditional therapies. Given the noninvasive diagnostic capabilities discovered with ultrasound (determining structural changes) and color Doppler (observing neovascular changes), a Swedish group of researchers has investigated the use of a sclerosing agent, Polidocanol, for treatment of the neovascularization. Studies have shown that in both patellar and Achilles tendinopathy, ultrasound guided injections of Polidocanol is successful in reducing neovascularization (Alfredson 2004, Alfredson 2005, Alfredson & Ohberg 2005, Gisslen et al 2006, Lind et al 2006, Ohberg & Alfredson 2002). A double-blind randomized controlled trial was designed to evaluate the effectiveness of Polidocanol injections for the treatment of chronic Achilles tendinosis in patients with structural collagen changes and neovascularization (Alfredson & Ohberg 2005). Twenty patients received two ultrasound-guided Polidocanol injections, 3–6 weeks apart, and 20 patients received two injections of lidocaine and adrenaline, 3–6 weeks apart. At a 3-month follow-up, 5 of 10 patients in the Polidocanol group reported decreased pain levels with patellar tendon loading, while no patient in the Lidocaine group reported decreased pain levels. Furthermore, the painful tendons still had structural changes and neovascularization, but the nonpainful tendons did not. After conclusion of the study, the patients who still had pain in both groups were treated with Polidocanol, and 19/20 reported complete satisfaction with the treatments and decreased pain levels. To build on those results, in a study without a control group, it has been shown that three injections of Polidocanol, 6–8 weeks apart, has resulted in return to full activity and treatment satisfaction in 37 of 42 patients at a 2-year follow-up (Lind et al 2006). While these results need to be demonstrated in a study with a control group, this line of research indicates that Polidocanol may be an effective treatment for chronic tendinopathy.

Recent research has also illustrated that painful eccentric training of the calf muscles and quadriceps may be beneficial in restoring function and reducing pain in patients with tendinopathy (Alfredson et al 1998, Jonsson & Alfredson 2005, Jonsson et al 2006, Ohberg et al 2004, Young 2005). In patients with chronic patellar tendinopathy, eccentric quadriceps training while standing on a 25° decline board was shown to be effective in treating patellar tendinopathy (Jonsson & Alfredson 2005, Jonsson et al 2006, Young 2005). Specifically, painful eccentric strengthening of the quadriceps was more effective in restoring knee function in those with patellar tendinopathy if conducted on a 25° decline board rather than on a flat step, and that eccentric training was more effective than concentric training. Furthermore, athletes with chronic Achilles tendinopathy who participated in a 12-week eccentric calf strengthening program demonstrated reduced tendon thickness and normalized tendon structure as well as the ability to return to preinjury athletic levels with an increase in calf strength and a decrease in pain (Alfredson et al 1998, Ohberg et al 2004).

In conjunction with these treatments, a conservative approach to rehabilitation should be followed. Conservative treatment typically consists of symptomatic relief and correction of etiologic

Table 24.4 Classification of Achilles tendinopathy and clinical findings (reproduced from Brukner & Khan 1993 with the permission of McGraw Hill)

Classification	Pathology	History	Examination findings
Tendinitis	Local tissue edema Disruption of ground substance rather than damage to tendon fibers Focal degeneration of tendon fibers may develop	Gradual onset of symptoms Pain worse in morning Pain worse on commencing activity and some time after ceasing activity	Marked swelling Extending over several centimeters Thickening of site of pain extending a variable number of centimeters along tendon Decreased extensibility of tendon
Paratendinitis, acute	Acute inflammatory swelling within paratendon	Sudden onset (e.g. pressure from shoes)	Swelling edema and crepitus in paratendon
Paratendinitis, chronic	Chronic inflammation with fibrosis and scarring	Repeated trauma	Firm scarred bands within paratendon
Focal degeneration	Granulomatous changes Loss of normal wavy alignment of collagen	Gradual onset of symptoms Significant pain	Local tenderness May have good function, little swelling
Partial tear	Variable size and site of tear Longitudinal or traverse tear Deep or superficial	Sudden onset of symptoms Pain often increases with activity	Local tenderness and swelling Palpable defect in tendon Pain on resisted plantarflexion (associated with paratendinitis)
Complete rupture	Complete rupture of tendon complex ?Related to degeneration ?Related to corticosteroid injection	Single incident Feel (hear) snap in tendon Immediate weakness and disability	Palpable (visible) defect in tendon when acute Thomson's test positive Some active plantarflexion may be possible
Mixed lesions	Combinations (e.g. paratendinitis and tendonitis or partial tear)	Combination of symptoms	Combination of signs makes diagnosis difficult

Box 24.1 Differential diagnoses of Achilles tendon injuries (reproduced from Kvist 1994 with the permission of Adis Press International)

- Calcaneal apophysitis (Sever's disease)
- Posterior tibial stress syndrome, soleus syndrome (shin splints)
- Tenosynovitis or dislocation of the peroneal tendons
- Tenosynovitis of the plantar flexors of the foot (tibialis posterior, flexor hallucis longus, flexor digiti)
- Plantar fasciitis
- Stress fractures at the ankle region
- Tarsal tunnel syndrome (entrapment of medial calcaneal branch of posterior tibial nerve)
- Neuroma/neuritis of the sural nerve near the Achilles tendon
- Calcaneal periostitis (often post-traumatic bone bruise)
- Spontaneous rupture of the posterior tibial tendon muscle
- Tennis leg (medial gastrocnemius tear)
- Inflammation of ankle ligaments in the calcaneal insertion
- Bone anomalies (painful large os trigonum)
- Calf muscle and Achilles tendon anomalies: anomalous soleus muscle
- Post-traumatic pain syndromes in the ankle and leg (direct and indirect)
- Arthritic conditions (rheumatic arthritis, Rieter syndrome, gout, ankylosing spondylitis, 'fibrositis')
- Tumors of the Achilles tendon (e.g. ossification, xanthomas)
- Systemic or local alterations in the tendon tissue (e.g. infections, vascular diseases, calcifying tendonitis)
- Diseases of the calcaneal bone (e.g. osteomyelitis, osteoid osteoma)

factors. Interventions include activity modifications designed to minimize stress on the patellar or Achilles tendons, local modalities, orthotic or proper footwear prescription, stretching and strengthening throughout the lower extremity and a progressive return to sport.

Surgery is only recommended for individuals who have not improved with conservative treatment. This happens in approximately 20–25% of patients initially diagnosed with Achilles tendinopathy (Ohberg et al 2001). In prospective studies with follow-up over several years, good to excellent results have been seen in approximately 80% of patients (Maffulli et al 1997, Rolf & Movin 1997); however, while function seems to be restored, asymmetrical calf strength differences still seem to persist (Ohberg et al 2001).

Iliotibial band friction syndrome

Clinical features of iliotibial-band friction syndrome

Iliotibial band friction syndrome (ITBFS) is the second most common injury in runners, with the incidence being higher in females than in males, and higher in marathon runners compared to recreational runners (Taunton et al 2002). It is an overuse inflammatory condition associated with overuse and theorized to be elicited by excessive friction between the iliotibial band and the lateral femoral epicondyle (Fairclough et al 2006). ITBFS occurs during repetitive flexion and extension movements of the knee, when the band experiences repeated friction, thus causing inflammation of the band or of the underlying tissues. The etiology is multifactorial, with lower extremity anatomical malalignment, thigh muscle strength imbalances, hip muscle weakness, training changes or errors and changes in activity and/or exercise considered to be significant (Devan et al 2004, Fairclough et al 2006, Fredericson & Weir 2006, Fredericson & Wolf 2005, Krivickas 1997).

Pain at the lateral aspect of the knee and the lateral femoral condyle is the main presenting feature (Brukner & Khan 2006). The pain is often described as stinging in nature, and is usually located 2 cm proximal to the lateral knee joint line, at the lateral femoral condyle. However, it may be present along the whole length of the band. The disease process is graded according to the severity of the pain and its relation to activity.

Treatment of iliotibial band friction syndrome

The mainstay of management of ITBFS is conservative treatment. Initial treatment has been recommended to include cessation and/or modification of offending activities, therapeutic modalities such as cryotherapy to reduce inflammation, non-steroidal anti-inflammatory medications and corticosteroid injections (Fredericson & Weir 2006, Fredericson & Wolf 2005). Recent research has illustrated that local corticosteroid injections, where the iliotibial band crosses the lateral femoral epicondyle, effectively reduce pain during running (Gunter & Schwellnus 2004). As treatment progresses, and inflammation is under control, stretching exercises (especially of the iliotibial band) and myofascial treatments may begin (Fredericson & Weir 2006, Fredericson & Wolf 2005, Gunter & Schwellnus 2004). As flexibility is being restored, strengthening of the lower extremities with a focus on hip musculature may be initiated, and it is appropriate to integrate strengthening during various movement patterns and integrated sport movements. Given the overuse nature of the injury, the final progression back to sport should be slow and progressive in nature. In rare resistant cases, partial surgical release of the band at the level of the femoral condyle, with or without excision of the underlying bursa may provide symptom relief.

Summary

This chapter provides an outline of a range of musculotendinous injuries to the lower extremity. Muscle strains, contusions, hematomas and tendinopathies are the common injuries that cause time loss from sport activity. The rehabilitation of these injuries includes a broad spectrum of mostly conservative treatments that range from exercise and modalities to functional sport training. In all cases, the final goal is a progressive return to sport with an ultimate focus on preventing a recurring injury.

References

Agre J C 1985 Hamstring injuries. Proposed aetiological factors, prevention, and treatment. Sports Medicine 2:21–33

Alfredson H 2004 Chronic tendon pain: implications for treatment. Current Drug Targets 5:407–410

Alfredson H 2005 The chronic painful Achilles and patellar tendon: research on basic biology and treatment. Scandinavian Journal of Medicine and Science in Sports 15:252–259

Alfredson H, Lorentzon R 2000 Chronic Achilles tendinosis: recommendations for treatment and prevention. Sports Medicine 29:135–146

Alfredson H, Ohberg L 2005 Sclerosing injections to areas of neovascularisation reduce pain in chronic Achilles tendinopathy: a double-blind randomised controlled trial. Knee Surgery, Sports Traumatology, and Arthroscopy 13:338–344

Alfredson H, Pietila T, Jonsson P et al 1998 Heavy-load eccentric calf muscle training for the treatment of chronic Achilles tendinosis. American Journal of Sports Medicine 26:360–366

Arner O, Lindholm A 1958 What is tennis leg? Acta chirurgica Scandinavica 116:73–75

Askling C, Saartok T, Thorstensson A 2006 Type of acute hamstring strain affects flexibility, strength, and time to return to pre-injury level. British Journal of Sports Medicine 40:40–44

Axe M J, Windley T C, Snyder-Mackler L 2001 Data-based interval throwing programs for baseball position players from age 13 to college level. Journal of Sport Rehabilitation 10:267–286

Axe M J, Windley T C, Snyder-Mackler L 2002 Data-based interval throwing programs for collegiate softball players. Journal of Athletic Training 37:194–203

Beaulieu M A 1981 Developing a stretching program. Physician and Sportsmedicine 9:59–69

Bencardino J T, Mellado J M 2005 Hamstring injuries of the hip. Magnetic Resonance Imaging Clinics of North America 13:677–690

Bencardino J T, Rosenberg Z S, Brown R R et al 2000 Traumatic musculotendinous injuries of the knee: diagnosis with MR imaging. Radiographics 20:S103–S120

Blatz D J 1981 Bilateral femoral and tibial shaft stress fractures in a runner. American Journal of Sports Medicine 9:322–325

Borg G, Holmgren A, Lindblad I 1981 Quantitative evaluation of chest pain. Acta Medica Scandinavica 644:43–45

Brewer B J 1962 Athletic injuries: musculotendious unit. Clinical Orthopaedics 23:30–38

Brukner P, Khan K 2006 Clinical sports medicine. McGraw-Hill, Sydney

Brunet M E, Hontas R B 1994 The thigh. In: DeLee J C, Drez D (eds) Orthopaedic sports medicine. WB Saunders, Philadelphia, PA, p 1086–1112

Burkett L N 1970 Causative factors in hamstrings strains. Medicine and Science in Sports and Exercise 2:39–42

Burkett L N 1976 Investigation into hamstring strains: the case of the hybrid muscle. Journal of Sports Medicine 3:228–231

Casperson P C 1982 Groin and hamstrings injuries. Athletic Training 17:43–45

Cross K M, Worrell T W 1999 Effects of a static stretching program on the incidence of lower extremity musculotendinous strains. Journal of Athletic Training 34:11–14

Cross T M, Gibbs N, Houang M T et al 2004 Acute quadriceps muscle strains: magnetic resonance imaging features and prognosis. American Journal of Sports Medicine 32:710–719

Cushner F D, Morwessel R M 1992 Myositis ossificans traumatica. Orthopaedic Review 21:1319–1326

DeSmet A A, Best T M 2000 MR imaging of the distribution and location of acute hamstring injuries in athletes. American Journal of Roentgenology 174:393–399

Devan M R, Pescatello L S, Faghri P et al 2004 A prospective study of overuse knee injuries among female athletes with muscle imbalances and structural abnormalities. Journal of Athletic Training 39:263–267

Dornan P 1971 A report on 140 hamstring injuries. Australian Journal of Sports Medicine 4:30–36

Dudkiewicz I, Salai M, Chechik A 2001 A young athlete with myositis ossificans of the neck presenting as a soft-tissue tumour. Archives of Orthopaedic Trauma and Surgery 121:234–237

Estwanik J J, McAlister J A 1990 Contusions and the formation of myositis ossificans. Physician and Sportsmedicine 18:53–64

Fairclough J, Hayashi K, Toumi H et al 2006 Is iliotibial band syndrome really a friction syndrome? Journal of Science and Medicine in Sport doi:10.1016/j.jsams.2006.05.017

Fornage B D, Eftekhori G 1989 Sonographic diagnosis of myositis ossificans. Journal of Ultrasound and Medicine 8:463–466

Fredericson M, Weir A 2006 Practical management of iliotibial band friction syndrome in runners. Clinical Journal of Sports Medicine 16:261–268

Fredericson M, Wolf C 2005 Iliotibial band syndrome in runners: innovations in treatment. Sports Medicine 35:451–459

Fuller P J 1984 Musculotendinous leg injuries. Australian Family Physician 13:495–498

Garrett W E J 1983 Strains and sprains in athletes. Postgraduate Medicine 73:200–209

Garrett W E J 1990 Muscle strain injuries: clinical and basic aspects. Medicine and Science in Sports and Exercise 22:436–443

Garrett W E J, Califf J C, Bassett F H I 1984 Histochemical correlates of hamstring injuries. American Journal of Sports Medicine 12:98–103

Garrett W E, Safran M R, Seaber A V et al 1987 Biomechanical comparison of stimulated and nonstimulated skeletal muscle pulled to failure. American Journal of Sports Medicine 15:448–454

Garrett W E J, Nikolaou P K, Ribbeck B M et al 1988 The effect of muscle architecture on the biomechanical failure properties of skeletal muscle under passive extension. American Journal of Sports Medicine 16:7–12

Gisslen K, Alfredson H 2005 Neovascularization and pain in jumper's knee: a prospective clinical and sonographic study in elite junior volleyball players. British Journal of Sports Medicine 39:423–428

Gisslen K, Gyulai C, Soderman K et al 2005 High prevalence of jumper's knee and sonographic changes in Swedish elite junior volleyball players compared to matched controls. British Journal of Sports Medicine 39:298–301

Gisslen K, Ohberg L, Alfredson H 2006 Is the chronic painful tendinosis tendon a strong tendon? A case study involving an Olympic weightlifter with chronic painful jumper's knee. Knee Surgery, Sports Traumatology, and Arthroscopy 14:897–902

Glick J M 1980 Muscle strains. Prevention and treatment. Physician and Sportsmedicine 8:72–77

Gunter P, Schwellnus M P 2004 Local corticosteroid injection in iliotibial band friction syndrome in runners: a randomised controlled trial. British Journal of Sports Medicine 38:269–272

Hartig D E, Henderson J M 1999 Increasing hamstrings flexibility decreases lower extremity overuse injuries in military basic trainees. American Journal of Sports Medicine 27:173–176

Heiser T M, Weber J, Sullivan G et al 1984 Prophylaxis and management of hamstring muscle injuries in intercollegiate football players. American Journal of Sports Medicine 12:368–370

Jackson D W, Feagin J A 1973 Quadriceps contusions in young athletes. Journal of Bone and Joint Surgery (Am) 55(A):95–105

Jonsson P, Alfredson H 2005 Superior results with eccentric compared to concentric quadriceps training in patients with jumper's knee: a prospective randomised study. British Journal of Sports Medicine 39:847–850

Jonsson P, Wahlstrom P, Ohberg L et al 2006 Eccentric training in chronic painful impingement syndrome of the shoulder: results of a pilot study. Knee Surgery, Sports Traumatology, and Arthroscopy 14:76–81

Kendall F P, McCreary E K, Provance P G 1993 Muscles: testing and function. Williams and Wilkins, Baltimore, MD

Kirkendall D T, Prentice W E, Garrett W E 2001 Rehabilitation of muscle injuries. In: Puddu G, Giombini A, Selvanetti A (eds) Rehabilitation of sports injuries. Springer-Verlag, Berlin, p 185–193

Kirkpatrick J S, Koman L A, Revere G P 1987 The role of ultrasound in the early diagnosis of myositis ossificans. American Journal of Sports Medicine 15:179–180

Koulouris G, Connell D 2003 Evaluation of the hamstring muscle complex following acute injury. Skeletal Radiology 32:582–589

Krivickas L S 1997 Anatomical factors associated with overuse sports injuries. Sports Medicine 24:132–146

Kuland D N 1982 The injured athlete. Lippincott, Philadelphia, PA

Leadbetter W B 1992 Cell matrix response in tendon injury. Clinics in sports medicine 11:533–578

Leppilahti J, Orava S 1998 Total achilles tendon rupture: a review. Sports Medicine 25:79–100

Lieb F J, Perry J 1968 Quadriceps function. An anatomical and mechanical study using amputated limbs. Journal of Bone and Joint Surgery (Am) 50:1535–1548

Liemohn W 1978 Factors related to hamstring strains. Journal of Sports Medicine and Physical Fitness 18:71–76

Lind B, Ohberg L, Alfredson H 2006 Sclerosing polidocanol injections in mid-portion Achilles tendinosis: remaining good clinical results and decreased tendon thickness at 2-year follow up. Knee Surgery, Sports Traumatology, and Arthroscopy 14(2):1327–1332

Maffulli N, Pintore E, Petricciuolo F 1990 Tumours mimicking sports injury in two young athletes. British Journal of Sports Medicine 24:207–208

Maffulli N, Testa V, Capasso G et al 1997 Results of percutaneous longitudinal tenotomy for Achilles tendinopathy in middle- and long-distance runners. American Journal of Sports Medicine 25:835–840

McKenzie D K, Bigeland-Ritchie B, Gorman R B et al 1992 Central and peripheral fatigue of human diaphragm and limb muscles assessed by twitch interpolation. Journal of Physiology 454:643–656

Magee D J 1997 Orthopedic physical assessment. WB Saunders, Philadelphia, PA

Moore K L, Dalley A F 1999 Clinically oriented anatomy. Lippincott Williams and Wilkins, Philadelphia, PA

Norfray J F, Schlachter L, Kernahan W T J et al 1980 Early confirmation of stress fractures in joggers. Journal of the American Medical Association 243:1647–1649

Oakes B W 1984 Hamstring muscle injuries. Australian Family Physician 13:587–591

Ohberg L, Alfredson H 2002 Ultrasound guided sclerosis of neovessels in painful chronic Achilles tendinosis: pilot study of a new treatment. British Journal of Sports Medicine 36:173–177

Ohberg L, Lorentzon R, Alfredson H 2001 Good clinical results but persisting side-to-side differences in calf muscle strength after surgical treatment of chronic achilles tendinosis: a 5 year follow up. Scandinavian Journal of Medicine and Science in Sports 11:207–212

Ohberg L, Lorentzon R, Alfredson H 2004 Eccentric training in patients with chronic Achilles tendinosis: normalised tendon structure and decreased thickness at follow up. British Journal of Sports Medicine 38:8–11

O'Neil R 1976 Prevention of hamstring and groin strain. Athletic Training 11:27–31

Palmer W E, Kuong S J, Elmadbouh H M 1999 MR imaging of myotendinous strain. American Journal of Roentgenology 173:703–709

Petersen J, Holmich P 2006 Evidence based prevention of hamstring injuries in sport. British Journal of Sports Medicine 39:319–323

Peterson L, Renstrom P 2001 Sports injuries: their prevention and treatment. Human Kinetics, Champaign, IL

Price D D, McGrath P A, Rafii A et al 1983 The validation of visual analogue scales as ratio scale measures for chronic and experimental pain. Pain 17:46–56

Rolf C, Movin T 1997 Etiology, histology, and outcome of surgery in achillodynia. Foot and Ankle International 18:565–569

Ryan A J 1969 Quadriceps strain, rupture, and charlie horse. Medicine and Science in Sports and Exercise 1:106–111

Safran M R, Garrett W E J, Seaber A V et al 1988 The role of warmup in muscular injury prevention. American Journal of Sports Medicine 16:123–129

Sash L 1981 Medical problems in association football. Practitioner 225:1047–1050

Sherry M A, Best T M 2004 A comparison of 2 rehabilitation programs in the treatment of acute hamstring strains. Journal of Orthopaedic and Sports Physical Therapy 34:116–125

Snyder-Mackler L, Delitto A, Stralka S W et al 1994 Use of electrical stimulation to enhance recovery of quadriceps femoris muscle force production in patients following anterior cruciate ligament reconstruction. Physical Therapy 74:9–15

Stafford M G, Grana W A 1984 Hamstring/quadriceps ratios in college football players: a high velocity evaluation. American Journal of Sports Medicine 12:209–211

Taunton J E, Ryan A J, Clement D B et al 2002 A retrospective case-control analysis of 2002 running injuries. British Journal of Sports Medicine 36:95–101

Wallace L 1979 Flexibility measurement. In: Blackburn T A, Milne M, DoHollow J (eds) Guidelines for pre-season athletic participation evaluation. Diversified Printing Services, Columbus, GA

Walton M, Rothwell A G 1983 Reactions of thigh tissues of sheep to blunt trauma. Clinical Orthopaedics and Related Research 176:273–281

Wiktorsson-Moller M, Oberg B, Ekstrand J et al 1983 Effects of warming up, massage, and stretching on range of motion and muscle strength in the lower extremity. American Journal of Sports Medicine 11:249–252

Wilson J N 1972 Specific injuries of sport. Physiotherapy 58:194–199

Young M A 2005 Eccentric decline squat protocol offers superior results at 12 months compared with traditional eccentric protocol for patellar tendinopathy in volleyball players. British Journal of Sports Medicine 39:102–105

Zarins B, Ciullo J V 1983 Acute muscle and tendon injuries in athletes. Clinics in Sports Medicine 2:167–182

Section Four

The role of sport and exercise physical therapies in active groups

25   Children and adolescents 459
26   Older exercise participants 484
27   The active female 499
28   Athletes with disability 525

Children and adolescents

25

Heather Southwick, Christine Ploski, Lyle J. Micheli,

Elly Trepman and Lizanne Backe Barone

CHAPTER CONTENTS

Introduction 459

Risk factors 460

Growth and maturation 461

Principles of rehabilitation 462

Spine 462

Hip and pelvis 465

Knee 467

Foot and ankle 470

Shoulder and shoulder girdle 472

Elbow 475

Forearm, hand and wrist 476

Summary 477

Introduction

The popularity of organized sports activities for children and adolescents in recent years has been associated with an increased risk of musculoskeletal injury. Estimates are that 25 million children regularly engage in organized sports in the USA (Micheli et al 2000). The most rapid rise in participation is currently seen among high school girls and children younger than 10 years of age (Metzl 2000). Young athletes often begin their competitive careers as early as age 7 and organized sports participation as early as age 4 (Micheli et al 2000). Athletics is currently considered the number one cause of injuries in children aged 5 to 17 years (Damore et al 2003).

Traditionally, males are more commonly injured than females (Backx et al 1991, Kvist et al 1989, Zaricznyj et al 1980). However, with the recent rise in female sports participation (Warren & Shantha 2000), the discrepancy is lessening. The National Athletic Trainers' Association (NATA) high school injury data show that girls in soccer and softball have statistically significantly higher injury rates than boys in soccer and baseball, while rates in basketball are equal (Rice 2000).

One cause of sports injuries in the young is single impact macrotrauma, in which a single force exceeds the failure threshold of a tissue or bone. Injuries such as fractures, dislocations, ligament sprains and musculotendinous strains occur in children and adolescents, but the nature of these injuries differs significantly from adults as a result of differences in musculoskeletal physiology. The majority of single impact injuries occur in organized sports activity (Backx et al 1989).

Athletic participation can also result in overuse injuries, which presently seem to be the most prevalent sports-related injury mechanisms (Micheli et al 2000). The stresses and strains on the musculoskeletal system resulting from sustained exercise, such as running or swimming, are usually below the threshold of macroscopic tissue failure, but may result in microscopic injury. The body may heal this microscopic injury, and also adapt by strengthening the musculoskeletal components in response to the applied stresses. For example, cortical thickening of the metatarsals, tibia and femur in ballet dancers (Pelipenko 1973, Schneider et al 1974) is a result of many years of repetitive activity during childhood and adolescence. This 'musculoskeletal adaptation' may be analogous to the cardiopulmonary adaptation which occurs in response to aerobic exercise, but occurs more slowly and is more difficult to quantify. If the rate of repetitive microtrauma resulting from intensive training and competition in a single sport exceeds the rate of tissue healing or musculoskeletal adaptation, then clinical overuse injury occurs (Herring & Nilson 1987).

While this chapter cannot provide a comprehensive coverage of pediatric sports injuries across all sports, it will highlight the common injuries in the child and adolescent age group across the major regions of the body. The reader is referred to Caine & Maffulli (2005) and Maffulli & Caine (2005) for details of sport-specific pediatric injury.

Risk factors

Etiological risk factors for sports injury in children have been identified and are helpful in diagnosis and treatment (Micheli et al 2000) (Box 25.1). Many youth sports coaches are well-meaning parents with little knowledge of youth sports, health and injury. There is a growing national and international awareness of the need for youth sports education and credentialing. While some sports have instituted some type of formal training for coaches, it is generally voluntary.

An abrupt increase in training intensity, frequency or duration may cause a greater rate of repetitive microtrauma, exceeding that of either musculoskeletal adaptation or tissue healing (van Mechelen 1992). Therefore, overuse injuries are commonly seen during or after an intensive summer camp or off-season program in which the young athlete abruptly increases activity level in a single sport. Other training errors, such as inadequate warm-up, may result in injuries such as muscle strains (Rodenburg 1994).

Previous injury and inadequate rehabilitation may result in altered mechanics of extremity use, placing greater demand on other, uninjured structures. For example, the pitcher who has

---

Box 25.1 Risk factors for sports injury in children and adolescents

Lack of certified coach

Inadequate or no preparticipation physical examination

Training error
• abrupt increase in training
  – intensity
  – duration
  – frequency
• inadequate warm-up
• improper technique
• tired, injured, or inadequately rehabilitated

Musculotendinous imbalance
• strength
• flexibility

Anatomical malalignment/intrinsic structure
• lumbar hyperlordosis
• lower limb length discrepancy
• abnormal hip rotation
• patellar malalignment
• genu varum
• genu valgum
• pronated pes planus
• cavus foot

Footwear
• poor fit
• inadequate impact absorption
• excessive sole stiffness
• insufficient hindfoot support/heel counter
• arch support
• excessive wear

Playing surface characteristics
• poor shock absorption (e.g. concrete)
• poor resiliency

Genetics
• sex – cercival instability (e.g. Down syndrome)

Hormonal status
• delayed menarche
• amenorrhea

Growth
• prepubescent porous bone
• vulnerable growth cartilage
  – physis
  – articular cartilage
  – traction apophysis
• relative weakness of prepubescent growth plates
• decrease in flexibility during growth spurt
• abnormal development (e.g. diskoid lateral meniscus)

General
• poor nutrition/hydration
• psychological stress
• poor fitness (overall/sport-specific)
• size/weight differences among same age
• inclement weather

Activity-specific factors
• hyperextension of lumbar spine (gymnastics, dance)
• shoulder overuse (swimming, pitching)
• Little league elbow (pitching)
• wrist/distal radius overuse (gymnastics)
• lower extremity (running)
• 'spearing' (football)
• body checking (ice hockey)

shoulder pain with overhead delivery may compensate with a more horizontal ('sidearm') pitch, which may result in injury to the elbow (Albright et al 1978).

Musculotendinous imbalances and anatomical malalignment may accentuate the stresses on specific structures (Micheli & Fehlandt 1994). For example, young runners with genu valgum and tibia vara may develop patellofemoral stress syndrome, and dancers with excessive femoral anteversion may force the turn-out at the knee or foot, resulting in strains of the medial knee and foot structures. Poor shoe or playing surface characteristics may aggravate repetitive stresses on the lower extremities, resulting in overuse injury. Softer running surfaces such as grass or dirt are more forgiving than concrete.

Underlying disease states or certain genetic compositions can increase the risk of both overuse and single impact injury. For example, limited hip motion secondary to previous Legg–Calvé–Perthes disease may result in increased stresses on other lower extremity structures during sports activity. Hormonal imbalances, such as those seen with amenorrhea, increase a woman's risk for stress fracture (Warren & Shantha 2000). The female athlete triad can be a more serious issue for the adolescent age female (Tanner 1998). Delayed menarche, defined as no menses by age 16, has been associated with prepubertal exercise. Delayed menarche results in prolongation of hypoestrogenism and may lead to osteoporosis at an age when bone density should be increasing.

General risk factors for sports injury include poor nutrition and hydration, psychological stress, poor overall or sport-specific fitness and size and weight differences among same age athletes (Micheli & Jenkins 2001).

Injury patterns in different sports are directly related to sport-specific biomechanics. For example, acromioclavicular sprains and separations are common in contact sports such as gridiron football, rugby and hockey, as a result of lateral stresses on the upper torso. Gymnasts, figure skaters and dancers frequently hyperextend the lumbar spine, and can develop symptomatic spondylolysis, which is a stress fracture of the pars interarticularis (Constantini & Warren 1994).

The key to management of sport injuries in children and adolescents is prevention. The preparticipation physical examination is an important precursor to sports participation (see Chapter 12). A standard examination and form has been created through the joint efforts of five medical academies/societies (Smith et al 1997). Primary care practitioners should include preparticipation physical examinations in the patient's regular check-up approximately 6 weeks prior to the sport season. The purpose of this preseason assessment is to determine the general health of the athlete, identify medical contraindications to participation, assess overall fitness and to educate the athlete. A complete preparticipation examination can help provide a clear definition of any limitations. An individualized exercise program should be implemented by a physical therapist to address the particular problems of the athlete as they relate to the requirements of the sport. This allows for potential adequate rehabilitation of identified problems. Emphasis is on safe sports participation and not elimination.

Growth and maturation

Injury patterns in the young athlete vary significantly from those in the adult because of several important differences in musculoskeletal structure and physiology (Fig. 25.1). Changes in bone and soft tissue structure during growth and maturation may result in age-dependent patterns of injury.

Bone tissue undergoes changes in mechanical properties during growth and maturation. The bones of the young child are more porous than those of adults, and may fail in compression. The buckle or torus metaphyseal compression fracture which commonly occurs in children is not seen in adults (Rang 1983). An angulating force may cause a greenstick fracture, which consists of failure of the tension side and bending (plastic deformation) of the compression side. In adolescents, the hormonal responsiveness of bone is particularly important; female athletes with hypoestrogenism resulting from delayed menarche or amenorrhea have a greater incidence of stress fractures and scoliosis (Warren et al 1986).

The growth cartilage of the young athlete is another structure that can be injured, as in fractures of the growth plate (Larson & McMahan 1966, Salter & Harris 1963, Wascher & Finerman 1994) (Fig. 25.2). The fracture pattern of the growth plate changes with age. For example, the Salter–Harris III fracture of the lateral part of the distal tibia physis of the ankle ('juvenile Tillaux') occurs in a narrow age range (12–14 years), after closure of the middle and medial portion of the physis (Dias 1984, Kleiger & Mankin 1964). The evaluation of growth arrest after physeal injury may be facilitated with magnetic resonance imaging (MRI) (Havranek & Lizler 1991).

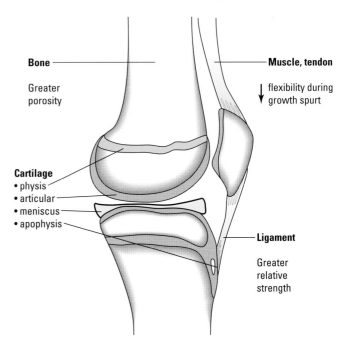

Bone
Greater porosity

Cartilage
• physis
• articular
• meniscus
• apophysis

Muscle, tendon
↓ flexibility during growth spurt

Ligament
Greater relative strength

Figure 25.1 • Factors related to musculoskeletal growth and development modulate sports injury patterns in children and adolescents.

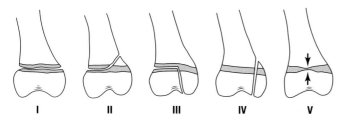

Figure 25.2 • Salter–Harris classification of growth plate fractures.

Joint problems specific to the young athlete include osteochondritis dissecans (OCD) (Stanitski 1994a) and diskoid lateral meniscus (Stanitski 1994b). The ligaments of children can be stronger than the growth plate at certain phases of growth, and excessive forces applied to joints may result in growth plate fracture (Rang 1983, Sanders et al 1980, Wascher & Finerman 1994). However, ligament sprains and tears may be more common in children than previously believed. The growth plate is stronger before the onset of puberty (Bright et al 1974), and ligament tears have been documented in prepubescent children without injury to the growth plate (Bradley et al 1979, Clanton et al 1979, DeLee & Curtis 1983). Ligament tears have also been documented in adolescents (Lipscomb & Anderson 1986).

Joint laxity has been shown to decrease with increasing age during childhood (Cheng et al 1991). Furthermore, the adolescent growth spurt is associated with a loss of flexibility (Gurewitsch & O'Neill 1944). Some pediatric athletic injuries can result from increased tightness of the soft tissues, or muscle imbalances during and after the pubescent growth period. Sport-specific adaptation in flexibility occurs in adolescents because of different biomechanical demands, such as shoulder flexibility changes observed in tennis players (Kibler & Safran 2000).

The traction apophyses, which consist of columns of growth cartilage that unite tendon to bone, can be subject to macroscopic avulsion or repetitive microscopic avulsions with secondary inflammation. These injuries, referred to as traction apophysitises, commonly occur at the tibial tubercle (Osgood–Schlatter disease), inferior patella (Sinding–Larsen–Johansson syndrome), calcaneus (Sever's disease) and iliac crest (Peck 1995). Musculotendinous tightness and associated loss of flexibility, during a growth spurt, can cause or aggravate these conditions, and a directed flexibility program may alleviate the symptoms until growth is completed (Micheli 1987).

Principles of rehabilitation

The focus on sports in the life of today's child seems to be constantly increasing with specialization in specific sports occurring at earlier ages. Increased training hours have led to repetition that can cause overuse injuries. The younger athlete often receives appropriate initial treatment, but inadequate rehabilitation. Most adolescents will return to their sport or competition too quickly following an injury which can cause a recurrence of the injury and can place the athlete at increased risk to develop a new injury. A comprehensive rehabilitation program that is sport specific, includes the young athlete's goals, and emphasizes education and communication with the athlete, parents and coaches is essential to ensure a safe and effective return to the sport.

The focus of a comprehensive rehabilitation program should be to safely maximize the athlete's abilities while protecting the existing injury. The rehabilitation program needs to incorporate ways to maintain the athlete's level of physical fitness during healing. The goals of the program need to include reduction of inflammation and pain, promotion of healing, restoration of function, safe return to sports training and/or competition and prevention of future injury. When reducing inflammation the principles of RICE (rest, ice, compression, elevation) are always effective. Ultrasound is rarely used on the child over a growth plate due to concerns for physeal injury. High intensities of ultrasound to epiphyseal areas can result in demineralization of bone, damage to epiphyseal plates and retardation of long bone growth (Irrgang & Sawhney 1994).

Physical therapy should be focused on attaining full range of motion and strength within 10% of the opposite extremity. Stretching may need to be discontinued while an athlete is recovering from a specific injury. Teaching the young athlete how and when to stretch is critical to improve flexibility and prevent injury. Current evidence indicates that both children and adolescents can increase muscular strength as a consequence of strength training. This increase in strength is largely related to the intensity and volume of loading and appears to be the result of increased neuromuscular activation and coordination, rather than muscle hypertrophy (Guy & Micheli 2001).

Having a strategy to return the athlete to play that is well communicated, accepted and realistic is imperative for full recovery from an injury. Sport-specific activities can be inserted into the rehabilitation program when the athlete demonstrates adequate healing, range of motion, flexibility and strength, and may improve motivation. Functional testing can help determine the athlete's readiness to return to a specific sport. Evaluating sport-specific skills and assessing agility, balance, coordination, reaction time, speed and power can be helpful in demonstrating readiness. Medical clearance needs to be obtained before a young athlete returns to his or her sport.

Spine

Acute spinal injuries can be among the most serious of sports injuries since they can cause long-term disability or even death. Fortunately, these instances are rare. More common is the chronic back injury related to overuse, muscle weakness and tightness, as well as spinal misalignments. Examination of the back in the young athlete should include an assessment for scoliosis or other spinal deformity. Preparticipation physical examination provides a screening opportunity for spinal conditions (Smith et al 1997). Persistent back pain in the child or adolescent may be a result of infection or tumor, and should never be attributed to a sports injury without thorough investigation (Fig. 25.3).

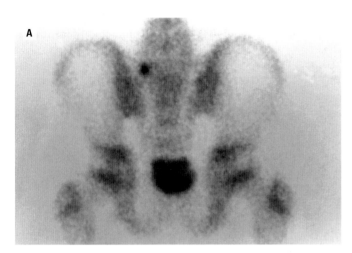 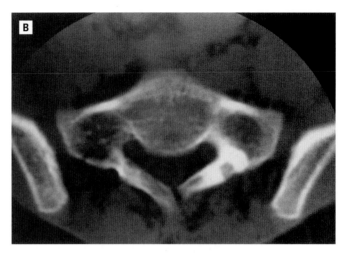

Figure 25.3 • Persistent low back pain may be a result of a pathological process independent of injury or mechanical factors. This 13-year-old boy complained of left low lumbar back pain and stiffness of several years duration, which became progressively worse during the previous year. Examination revealed an antalgic gait and dramatic tightness of the low back on forward bending. Although plain radiographs were normal, **(A)** technetium-99 bone scan and **(B)** computed tomography revealed an osteoid osteoma in the left arch of the S1 vertebra. After resection, the symptoms resolved completely.

Cervical spine

Acute neck injury in the young athlete must be treated with caution (Cantu 2000). A 5-year study utilizing the National Pediatric Trauma Registry revealed that 16% of pediatric cervical spine injuries were sports-related (Kokoska et al 2001). The four youth sports with the highest risk for head and spine injury are football, gymnastics, ice hockey and wrestling (Proctor & Cantu 2000). However, rule changes, such as the prohibition of spearing in football, ball heading in young soccer players and recreational usage of high school trampolines have been effective in reducing the rate of catastrophic neck injury (Proctor & Cantu 2000).

When an acute neck injury occurs, the athlete should be removed from the event on a back board with the neck immobilized in the neutral position, utilizing a collar, sandbags or rolled-up towel. Physical examination should include a detailed neurological examination. Evidence of head injury or facial trauma should raise the suspicion of an occult neck injury, particularly in the unconscious athlete. Radiographic evaluation should consist of plain anteroposterior, lateral and oblique views of all seven cervical vertebrae, including an odontoid view. If pain is elicited with cervical flexion or extension, then lateral radiographs in flexion and extension may be obtained to assess ligamentous stability. MRI, computed tomography (CT) and bone scans may also be useful (Connolly 2001). Although ligament instability may occur, a physiological pseudosubluxation of C2 on C3 may be encountered in the young, and may be incorrectly identified as a sequela of trauma (Jackson et al 1995, Micheli & d'Hemecourt 1998).

If the cervical spine is stable, without evidence of fracture, ligament disruption or neurological abnormalities, then initial treatment should consist of rest, a soft cervical collar, local ice and heat and mild analgesics. As the pain and muscle spasm subside, progressive rehabilitation is started with gentle isometric exercises in the six directions of motion, followed by dynamic range of motion and strengthening exercises through the painless arc of motion in all directions (Micheli & Jenkins 1995).

Thoracic spine

Injury to the upper back and thoracic spine is relatively uncommon because the rib cage partially stabilizes and splints the thoracic spine from the sudden stresses of most sports (Schnebel 2000). Strains of the upper back and periscapular muscles may occur in lifting activities (d'Hemecourt et al 2000), and diagnosis is made by careful physical examination and radiographs to exclude the possibility of fracture. Vertebral body compression fracture can result from sudden flexion of the spine, as in a fall during an equestrian event, and may be demonstrated on radiographs with loss of vertebral body height. Treatment of a compression fracture is usually non-operative and includes initial rest, bracing and subsequent rehabilitation to restore strength and range of motion, once stable bony union has been attained (d'Hemecourt et al 2000).

A common adolescent condition is Scheuermann's disease, which consists of painful dorsal kyphosis, loss of anterior vertebral body height and 'wedging' of the body as seen on the lateral radiograph. This condition may be an overuse syndrome, resulting from repetitive microfracture of the vertebral body end plates, and is often associated with tight pectoral and hamstring muscles (d'Hemecourt et al 2000). Postural issues include increased thoracic kyphosis with a compensatory increased lumbar lordosis and forward head. Associated scoliosis is present in 30–40% of children with Scheuermann's disease (Patrick 1995).

Treatment of Scheuermann's disease includes exercise, orthotic management and, occasionally, surgical management. If significant kyphosis is present (with a Cobb angle greater than 50°), extension bracing for 9–12 months has been shown to result in improvement of both pain and deformity (Ali et al 1999) and should include a comprehensive physical therapy program. Exercises emphasize strengthening and stretching of the trunk extensors and general postural re-education. Abdominal strengthening for pelvic control is important to help maintain improved posture and decrease lumbar lordosis.

Lumbar spine

The lumbar spine in the young athlete is susceptible to either single impact or overuse injury (d'Hemecourt et al 2000). Pain in the lumbar area can be associated with periods of rapid growth. The increase in tightness of the lumbodorsal fascia and quadriceps during the adolescent growth spurt (d'Hemecourt et al 2000) can cause a tight lumbar lordosis or swayback. Tight hamstrings may be associated with a relatively flat back. Tightness in these areas may increase susceptibility to injury (d'Hemecourt et al 2000). Therapy should focus on flexibility of the iliopsoas, rectus femoris, iliotibial band, quadriceps and back extensors and strengthening of abdominal and perispinal muscles (d'Hemecourt et al 2000).

Mechanical low back pain in children and adolescents is associated with increased lumbar lordosis, tight lumbodorsal fascia and hamstrings and a lack of an anatomical lesion suggesting fracture, herniation or narrowing of the spinal canal (Zetaruk 2000). This diagnosis should be made with caution in the young athlete, and only after other causes of low back pain, including infection or malignancy, have been excluded with appropriate radiographic and radioisotopic imaging studies.

Historically, children with mechanical low back pain report pain with extension. The specific finding on examination is pain on provocative extension, similar to spondylolysis (Zetaruk

2000). However, no lesion of the posterior elements is identified with advanced imaging. It has been hypothesized that facet derangement is the origin of mechanical low back pain.

Injury to the posterior spinal elements may occur in activities which involve repetitive lumbar hyperextension such as gymnastics, figure skating or dance (d'Hemecourt et al 2000, Zetaruk 2000). Symptomatic spondylolysis is a stress fracture of the pars interarticularis, which is often demonstrated on oblique radiographs of the lumbar spine. Stress reaction of the pars interarticularis can occur without changes being evident on plain radiography, and a single photon emission computer tomographic (SPECT) bone scan is usually necessary to confirm the diagnosis (d'Hemecourt et al 2000) (see Chapter 30). The pain associated with this condition is reproduced with lumbar hyperextension (d'Hemecourt et al 2000).

Spondylolisthesis is the forward displacement of one vertebra over another, and is associated with bilateral pars defects (Fig. 25.4). This condition, which usually occurs at L5–S1 or L4–L5, is often asymptomatic, but severe displacement or progression may be indications for spinal fusion (d'Hemecourt et al 2000).

Treatment for mechanical low back pain and posterior element problems is similar and includes a lumbar antilordotic strengthening and flexibility exercise program. This should consist of pelvic stabilization and abdominal strengthening as well as postural alignment. Antilordotic bracing may result in resolution of symptoms and may also be used during early return to sports activity (Micheli et al 1980). Bracing should be done in conjunction with a comprehensive physical therapy program. For spondylolysis in younger athletes, radiographic evidence of healing of the pars defect (as seen on CT scan) can be seen after 6 months (d'Hemecourt et al 2000). The athlete may be permitted to return to sports in the brace after 4–6

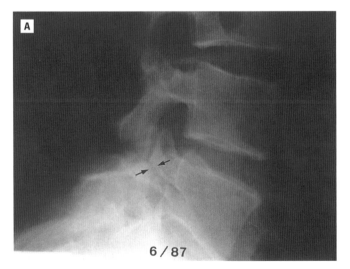
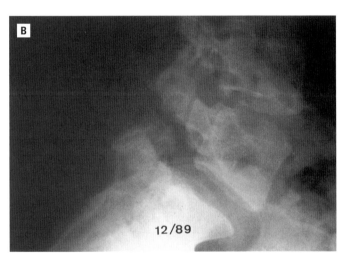

Figure 25.4 • Spondylolysis and spondylolisthesis in an adolescent female athlete. **A:** At the age of 14 years, this athlete developed low back pain with basketball activity. Spondylolysis at L5, without spondylolisthesis, was visible on the lateral radiograph. She was treated with a Boston brace, with resolution of her pain over several months. She subsequently had intermittent episodes of low back pain and occasionally used her brace during these periods. **B:** Two and a half years later, at the age of 16 years, she reinjured her back in a basketball incident. She complained of localized low back pain without radicular symptoms. Radiographs revealed bilateral L5 spondylolysis with grade I spondylolisthesis. She resumed use of the brace, with improvement of her pain.

weeks of bracing if there is no pain on examination. The athlete with persistent symptoms and non-union at 4–6 months can be offered external electrical stimulation, or ultimately, spinal fusion (d'Hemecourt et al 2000).

Flexion injuries to the lumbar spine have been associated with gymnastics, running, football, weightlifting, basketball, soccer and tennis and are usually caused by repetitive flexion with axial loading to the lumbar area (Yancey & Micheli 1994). Flexion injuries can result in vertebral body or end-plate fracture, or intervertebral disk herniation (Yancey & Micheli 1994). Localized neurological symptoms and signs can be present with lateral disk herniation as a result of specific nerve root impingement. However, a central disk bulge or herniation without nerve root impingement can occur in the young athlete, resulting in localized low back pain and hamstring tightness (Zetaruk 2000). Diagnosis can be confirmed with MRI.

The differential diagnosis of sciatica in children and adolescents is broad, and includes spinal problems such as disk herniation or tumor. Furthermore, sciatica can result from extraspinal causes such as piriformis syndrome, in which the sciatic nerve is compressed by a tight piriformis muscle (Roos & Renstrom 1998). Proximal hamstring syndrome is another cause of sciatic nerve compression (Roos & Renstrom 1998). Scarring of an injured hamstring may cause the muscle and nerve to become adhered and, therefore, cause compression symptoms. Occasionally, long-standing spondylolysis may present with low back pain and L5 radiculopathy due to tethering of this nerve root by the hypertrophic pseudoarthosis tissue (Micheli & d'Hemecourt 1998).

Treatment for flexion injuries consists of an exercise program for abdominal and lumbar extension strengthening and posterior flexibility, being cautious not to increase radiculopathy (Zetaruk 2000). Occasionally, a low back brace may improve symptoms by immobilizing the lumbar spine, and may allow early return-to-sports activity (Micheli et al 1980). For more recalcitrant cases, a series of epidural corticosteroid injections to selective nerve roots may be helpful (d'Hemecourt et al 2000). Diskectomy is rarely required in the young athlete, but has been used when symptoms include progressive neurological involvement, bowel or bladder involvement, or pain unresponsive to nonoperative treatment (Yancey & Micheli 1994).

Hip and pelvis

Risk of injury in the hip and pelvis is high, as there are complex ossification patterns and fusion late in childhood. The circular vascularity of the femoral head and neck also creates risk for injury in the growing child (Waters & Millis 1988). A good differential diagnosis is imperative in the growing athlete, as not all complaints of pain are due to trauma or overuse in sports.

Slipped capital femoral epiphysis

Hip pain or limp in the young athlete may be the first symptom or sign of Legg–Calvé–Perthes disease, slipped capital femoral epiphysis, infection or a tumor such as osteosarcoma (Waters & Millis 1994). A coincident history of sports injury may delay the diagnosis of these conditions if thorough evaluation, including radiography, is not performed.

A high clinical index of suspicion of slipped capital femoral epiphysis (SCFE) should be maintained in the young adolescent who presents with complaints of hip or knee pain (Fig. 25.5). This problem can be an acute slip or may occur without any

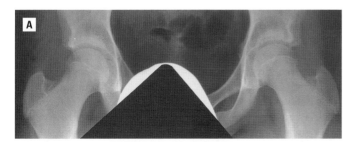

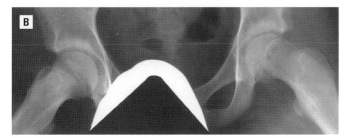

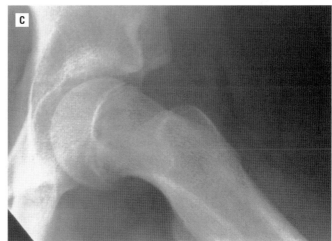

Figure 25.5 • Slipped capital femoral epiphysis. This 11-year-old female complained of diffuse left hip pain of three months duration, without any history of injury. Menarche was 2 months after onset of hip pain. Physical examination revealed a short, moderately overweight black female who walked with a left Trendelenburg limp, with the left lower extremity externally rotated at the hip. She had only 5° of left hip internal rotation in flexion, in contrast with 20° on the other side; external rotation in flexion was 80° on the left and 45° on the right. The anteroposterior radiograph (A) appeared normal; however, frog-lateral radiographs (B, C) revealed slipped capital femoral epiphysis. She underwent epiphysiodesis. A high clinical index of suspicion of this problem is important to avoid delay in diagnosis.

history of trauma. SCFE may be more common in physically active adolescents, and may contribute to the premature onset of osteoarthritis of the hip in later life (Carney et al 1991, Murray & Duncan 1971).

Risk factors for SCFE include obesity, puberty, hypothyroidism and tall, thin individuals (Karlin 1995). Physical examination reveals limitation of internal rotation in flexion, and the diagnosis is confirmed by radiography. Treatment is operative and consists of pinning the slipped femoral neck to the femoral head. Initially weight bearing is limited. Approximately 50% of cases of SCFE are seen bilaterally (Waters & Millis 1994) so contralateral hip pain should be evaluated urgently.

Overuse injuries

Snapping hip

Gymnasts, dancers and sprinters often complain of anterior or lateral snapping and/or popping at the hip, which may be painful. Lateral snapping is usually a result of a tight iliotibial band moving over the greater trochanter and can cause bursitis. Anterior snapping is thought to be related to the iliopsoas tendon snapping over a bony prominence near its insertion on the femur. Tendonitis of the rectus femoris or iliopsoas may also occur. Treatment is similar to that of snapping hip syndromes.

Physical therapy consists of evaluation of the alignment of the pelvis and hip, muscle flexibility and strength. Treatment often includes relative rest and stretching of the tight iliotibial band, iliopsoas, rectus femoris and hamstrings. Muscle strengthening of the abdominal and other core muscles should be addressed to provide a stable base for hip joint mechanics (Micheli 1983, Waters & Millis 1988). Improper athletic technique may also be a causative factor and should be assessed and corrected.

Acute injuries

Muscle strains

Muscle strains around the hip and thigh generally involve multi-joint muscles, such as the hamstrings or rectus femoris, but can occur in any muscle that undergoes a forceful contraction or stretch which is beyond its physiological limits.

Treatment for acute strains should include education in order to decrease the risk of further injury and prevent chronic strains. Some activities such as gymnastics, dance and skating require maximum muscle length for performance. Participants often try to stretch the area in an effort to relieve the perceived tightness and maintain their flexibility after a strain. However, stretching in the acute phase should be avoided. Modification of activities may be necessary for at least 4–6 weeks depending on the severity of the injury.

Contusions

Thigh contusions occur from direct impact in such sports as ice hockey and soccer. Occasionally, they are severe and cause significant thigh pain, swelling, and limitation of knee motion. The most commonly contused thigh sites are the anterior and

antereolateral thigh (Javin & Fox 1995). Treatment normally consists of initial rest, ice and gentle compression. Heat modalities and massage are avoided in the early rehabilitation of this injury to minimize muscular hemorrhage and swelling (Javin & Fox 1995). Gentle progressive knee flexion is commenced early to disperse the hematoma. A strengthening and flexibility program may begin when the athlete is comfortable. A severe thigh contusion may cause disability for over 1 year, particularly if it is complicated by the development of myositis ossificans or abscess (Gross 1994b). Myositis ossificans is a lesion of hypertrophic bone localized in soft tissue. Return to sports may be facilitated by the use of neoprene shorts which provide support and warmth to the injured tissues.

Acetabular labral tear

Intra-articular causes of anterior hip pain can include acetabular labral tears, a condition that has been recorded in children as young as 6 years old (Lage et al 1996). With the advent of magnetic resonance arthrograms and hip arthroscopy, diagnosis and management of acetabular labral tears has been facilitated (Fitzgerald 1995, Keeney et al 2004).

The mechanism of injury is repetitive flexion, flexion/abduction or extension/external rotation and is frequently seen in dancers, gymnasts and skaters (Kocher et al 2005). The most frequent location of the injury is in the anterior superior portion of the labrum. The injury can either be traumatic or have an insidious onset (Lage et al 1996). Risk factors for labral tears can include femoral anterversion and acetabular retroversion. Femoral acetabular impingment (FAI) is a condition of abnormal contact between the proximal femur and acetabulum as a result of bony deformity or excessive motion (Ganz et al 2003). Labral tears are associated with FAI as well as developmental dysplasia of the hip and osteoarthritis (Peele et al 2005, Tanzer & Noiseux 2004, Wenger et al 2004).

Symptoms can include hip pain with activity, painful anterior hip snapping and pain with provocative maneuvers such as flexion, internal rotation and adduction. Often the diagnosis is delayed, but should be considered whenever anterior hip pain is prolonged in spite of appropriate conservative treatment such as rest, or activity restrictions and physical therapy (McCarthy & Lee 2004).

Surgical treatment consists of arthroscopic debridement (Kocher et al 2005). Early postoperative rehabilitation involves limited weight bearing and avoidance of activities which cause pain. External rotation and exercises with long lever arms, such as straight leg raising is generally avoided in the early postoperative period. Physical therapy should focus on decreasing anterior joint forces, improving alignment and re-educating muscles (Lewis & Sahrmann 2005). Long-term outcomes have yet to be reported, but outcome appears positive in the short term (Kocher et al 2005).

Avulsion fractures

The hip and pelvis is a common site of avulsion fracture secondary to sudden muscle contraction, with seven different sites at risk (Waters & Millis 1988) (Table 25.1). Apophysitis may cause pain and limitation of activity, particularly during the adolescent growth spurt (Clancy & Foltz 1976, Pueschel & Scola 1987). The muscle groups involved are commonly treated with rest and ice to decrease inflammation. Physical therapy includes a progressive stretching program of the iliopsoas, rectus femoris and iliotibial band. Strengthening is initiated once acute inflammation is resolved (Metzmaker & Pappas 1985). Neoprene shorts may be helpful during rehabilitation and in the early return-to-sports phase. While most of these avulsions are treated by first stage healing in situ, some do require operative fixation.

Fractures and dislocations

Fractures and dislocations of the hip are associated with high-energy trauma, and can occur in sports activities such as football, motocross and skiing (Fig. 25.6). Stress fractures of the

Table 25.1 Apophyseal avulsion fracture sites about the hip/pelvis

Apophyseal avulsion fracture	Muscle involved
Anterior superior iliac spine	Sartorius
Ichial tuberosity	Hamstring
Lesser trochanter	Iliopsoas
Anterior inferior iliac spine	Rectus femoris
Iliac crest	External oblique abdominus Transverse abdominus Gluteus medius Tensor fascia lata Latissimus dorsi Gluteus maximus
Acetabular rim	
Symphysis pubis	Adductor insertion

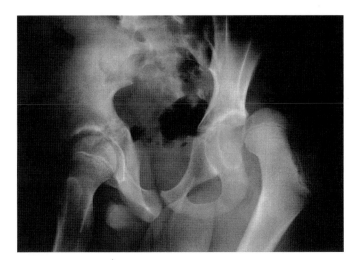

Figure 25.6 • This posterior hip dislocation on an 11-year-old male occurred during vigorous football activity.

femoral neck can be the result of repetitive microtrauma in runners or dancers, but are rare before the growth plate is closed (Karlin 1995, Puddu et al 1998). A SPECT bone scan or MRI may be necessary to make the diagnosis if plain radiographs are normal yet other symptoms indicate a stress reaction or stress fracture (Pirnay & Crielaard 2001).

Knee

The knee is a common site of single-impact and overuse injuries in the young athlete (Steiner & Grana 1988). The types of knee injuries that occur in the child and adolescent differ from those in the adult as a result of the different tissue characteristics associated with age and growth (Iobst & Stanitski 2000).

Overuse injuries

Patellofemoral pain

Patellofemoral pain is a frequent problem in the young athlete (Outerbridge & Micheli 1995). The symptoms are similar to that of chondromalacia patellae in adults. However, the pathophysiology of patellofemoral pain in the young athlete differs from that in the adult because the articular surface is often normal on arthroscopic examination (Griffiths & Pinder 1981, Steiner & Grana 1988). Macrotrauma, repetitive microtrauma and growth can all contribute to patellofemoral complaints. The pain is believed to result from an increase in patellofemoral joint pressure associated with lateral malalignment (Outerbridge & Micheli 1995). Weakness of the vastus medialis in conjunction with tightness of the iliotibial band, rectus femoris and lateral retinaculum are contributing issues that can be addressed with physical therapy (Outerbridge & Micheli 1995).

More than 80% of young athletes with patellofemoral pain improve with physical therapy (see Chapter 22). Therapy includes a static progressive resistance strengthening exercise program focused on strengthening the vastus medialis. Flexibility exercises for the quadriceps, hamstrings and iliotibial band are also incorporated. Activities which increase patellofemoral pressure should be minimized (Micheli & Jenkins 2001). McConnell taping or use of a tracking brace may be beneficial for the short term (Crossley et al 2001). Patellar taping improves proprioception and the sense of mechanical stability, and allows for more effective pain-free strengthening of the vastus medialis (Aminaka & Gribble 2005).

If pain persists despite this program, lateral retinacular release with a medial thermal plication has been shown to be successful in relieving symptoms (Micheli 1999, Micheli & Stanitski 1981). Occasionally, medial realignment of the infrapatellar tendon insertion, with medial retinaculum plication and vastus medialis advancement, is indicated for refractory patellofemoral pain associated with malalignment or recurrent lateral patellar dislocation (Fondren et al 1985, Insall et al 1983). Custom orthotics should be considered for the athlete with malalignment or foot formation issues.

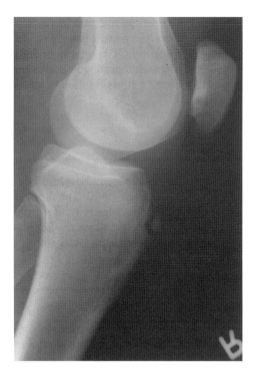

Figure 25.7 • Osgood–Schlatter disease. This male developed persistent pain at the right tibial tubercle at the age of 10 years. This radiograph at 21 years of age revealed a non-union of the tibial tubercle apophysis. Fourteen years later, at the age of 35 years, the discomfort and radiographic appearance were unchanged.

On occasion, anterior knee pain may progress to lateral subluxation of the patella. Anterior knee pain with the onset of subluxation symptoms, usually associated with radiographic criteria, suggests that therapy alone will be unsuccessful in relieving symptoms (Outerbridge & Micheli 1995). Surgical realignment of the extensor mechanism is usually necessary in such cases.

Traction apophysitis

The extensor mechanism of the knee in adolescents can be the site of traction apophysitis, such as Osgood–Schlatter disease (tibial tubercle) (Ogden & Southwick 1976) (Fig. 25.7) or Sinding–Larsen–Johansson syndrome (inferior pole of patella) (Fig. 25.8). These problems are associated with tightness of the extensor mechanism, demonstrated clinically with a positive Ely test, and may be exacerbated by repetitive jumping activities. Treatment consists of a program of pain-free quadriceps strengthening and stretching exercises to the quadriceps and iliotibial band (Micheli 1987). The cornerstone of rehabilitation remains static progressive resistance exercises (PRE), including straight leg raises.

Osteochondritis dissecans

Osteochondritis dissecans (OCD) is another condition that may affect the knee of younger athletes (Fig. 25.9). It can affect either the distal femur or the patella, and it is associated

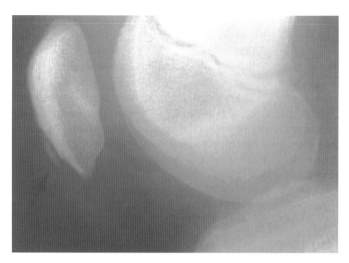

Figure 25.8 • Sinding–Larsen–Johansson syndrome. This 9-year-old gymnast developed bilateral infrapatellar knee pain during a period of intensive springboard activity. Physical examination was remarkable for localized tenderness at the inferior pole of the patella, and radiography revealed evidence of Sinding–Larsen–Johansson traction apophysitis at the right knee. The symptoms resolved several weeks after starting a quadriceps flexibility program.

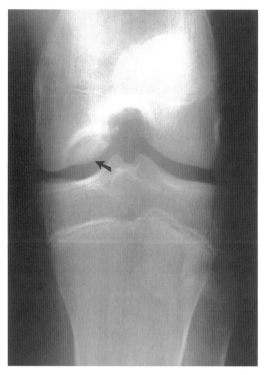

Figure 25.9 • Osteochondritis dissecans of the medial femoral condyle in an adolescent. This lesion may be missed if a tunnel view is not obtained.

with intense physical training in young athletes. However, some studies debate this relationship, finding no association between high level sports and trauma in affected patients (Wong & Mafulli 2006).

The child or adolescent with OCD of the knee may be asymptomatic or may complain of low-grade aching pain and intermittent swelling. Locking may occur if the lesion is displaced. Radiographs are usually diagnostic and a tunnel view should be obtained (Fig. 25.9). Treatment is controversial and may vary depending on the presence of symptoms, age and skeletal maturity of the patient, and status of the lesion (loose or intact articular cartilage) (Kocher et al 2001). Relative rest alone may be the only treatment needed to attain healing. With advanced maturity, large lesion size or partial detachment, drilling of the lesion, with or without pinning in an attempt to revascularize the bony fragment and promote union to the underlying bony bed, may be indicated (Kocher et al 2001). In larger lesions, where the detached fragment has not been reimplanted and healed, cartilage transplant can be used (Kocher et al 2001).

If the lesion is loose and does not involve a major part of the weight bearing surface, it is occasionally excised. If OCD is diagnosed before skeletal maturity, and is left untreated, it is associated with a high incidence of subsequent osteoarthritis, especially if the defect is large or involves the lateral femoral condyle (Twyman et al 1991).

Acute injuries

Ligament injuries

The knee ligaments of the young athlete are relatively stronger than in adults, and the anterior cruciate ligament (ACL) in children is usually avulsed at the tibial spine rather than torn (Rang 1983). Nevertheless, ligament tears have been observed in prepubescent children (Bradley et al 1979, Clanton et al 1979, DeLee & Curtis 1983, Micheli et al 1999b), and surgical reconstruction may be indicated (Lipscomb & Anderson 1986, Micheli et al 1999b). The medial collateral ligament (MCL) may also be torn in children, as on occasion, stress radiographs can reveal MCL avulsion with physeal fracture of the distal femur or proximal tibia (Steiner & Grana 1988). Posterior cruciate ligament (PCL) injury is relatively rare in the young athlete (DeLee 1994, Mayer & Micheli 1979, Sanders et al 1980).

Physical therapy for knee ligament injuries consists of closed chain strengthening with progressive range of motion and weight bearing as indicated by tissue healing (Cassella et al 2006). Water therapy or use of a Pilates reformer can allow for closed chain activities with reduced impact and stress to the joint.

Young female athletes have a 2–8 times greater chance of tearing their ACL compared to young males (Micheli et al 1999b). ACL injuries are more prevalent in running sports that involve quick changes in direction, such as basketball or soccer, but are also common with skiing. ACL sprains do not present at significantly different rates in boys and girls before puberty (Andrish 2001, Buehler-Yund 1999). After the onset of puberty, female athletes may not have a neuromuscular spurt to match their rapid increase in growth and development. The neuromuscular spurt is defined as increased power, strength and coordination that occur with increasing chronologic age and maturation stage in adolescent boys (Myer et al

2004). The lack of neuromuscular adaptation in females during puberty seems to facilitate the development of neuromuscular imbalances, increasing the risk for ACL injury. Neuromuscular imbalances that have been identified in young females include relying on ligaments rather than knee musculature for shock absorption, imbalance between the quadriceps and hamstring recruitment patterns, and differences in muscular strength, flexibility and coordination between the dominant and non-dominant leg (Myer et al 2004).

Much of the current research in this field has been focused on proper jumping and landing techniques for protection of injury (Hewett et al 2000, Micheli et al 1999a). Specifically addressing neuromuscular imbalances is essential for prevention of ACL injuries in females. Progressing from proper mechanics and technique with two-foot landings before single-leg landings are introduced is imperative as most non-contact ACL injuries occur when landing or decelerating on a single limb (Boden et al 2000). In addition, balance and proprioceptive training have been shown to be important elements in the reduction of ACL injuries, especially for female athletes (Hewett et al 2005). A neuromuscular training program that consisted of basic 'warm-up' activities, stretching for the trunk and lower extremity, quadriceps strengthening, plyometric activities and specific agility drills demonstrated 88% less ACL injuries in the first year and 74% in the second year of a study on female soccer players age 14 to 18 years (Mandelbaum et al 2005).

Meniscal injuries

Tears of the meniscus may occur in the young athlete in association with twisting injuries or ACL tears. MRI is valuable for diagnosis of such conditions and arthroscopy is useful in both diagnosis and treatment (Iobst & Stanitski 2000). Repair of meniscal tears is preferable to preserve the protective articular cartilage in an effort to reduce the risk of future osteoarthritis. Postoperatively, these patients are partial weight bearing with a brace that limits their range of motion for 4 weeks. Isometric quadriceps setting and hamstring and quadriceps strengthening within the limits of the brace can begin immediately after surgery. Athletes with simple partial meniscectomies may progress more rapidly.

Another meniscal problem of the young athlete is the diskoid lateral meniscus. These large, redundant lateral menisci may or may not have an intact posterior peripheral attachment. They tend to cause a prominent snapping sensation in the lateral compartment as the flexed knee is extended (Dickhaut & DeLee 1982) (Fig. 25.10). Treatment is operative and a more extensive meniscectomy may be required if the posterior horn is detached or additional tears are present (Aichroth et al 1991, Dickhaut & DeLee 1982, Steiner & Grana 1988).

Fractures

Fractures about the knee in the young athlete have a high complication rate (Johnson 1998). The Salter–Harris II fracture of the distal femur is frequently followed by growth disturbance, particularly if displacement is present (Jiffin & Briard

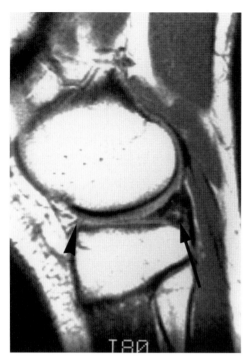

Figure 25.10 • Diskoid lateral meniscus. This 15-year-old female had a 'clunking' sensation in the right knee from the age of 2 years, associated with pain. Physical examination revealed a loud, painful 'snap' during extension of the knee with valgus stress applied. MRI revealed a complex tear of the posterior horn of the lateral meniscus (large arrow), with absence of the anterior horn (arrowhead). Arthroscopic findings consisted of a large, complex tear of a diskoid lateral meniscus. The pain and snapping resolved after arthroscopic partial lateral meniscectomy.

1998). Open reduction and internal fixation may be necessary to achieve an anatomical position, and the patient should be followed with radiographs, even after the fracture is healed, in order to detect growth disturbance early.

In the proximal tibia, collateral ligament insertion sites are distal to the physis. Therefore, varus and valgus stresses are usually transmitted to the metaphysis, and physeal fractures of the proximal tibia are rare (Burkhart & Peterson 1979). Nevertheless, proximal tibia growth plate fractures can occur from higher velocity trauma, or in association with avulsion of the tibial tubercle physis (Chow et al 1990). These fractures may be complicated by popliteal artery injury or compartment syndrome (Jiffin & Briard 1998) (Fig. 25.11). Early treatment should include careful observation, and circumferential plaster should be avoided during the first few days following injury (Steiner & Grana 1988).

Foot and ankle

The foot and ankle are susceptible to injury in almost every sport. Foot and ankle problems are the second most common

musculoskeletal problem facing primary care physicians in children under 10 years of age next to acute injury (Omey & Micheli 1999). Due to the influences of growth, children are susceptible to injuries in the foot and ankle that are not present in the adult.

Overuse injuries

Tendinitis and apophysitis

Achilles tendonitis is a common complaint among young athletes in almost any sport. It is generally associated with tight heel cords and pronation. Complaints of Achilles tendon pain often occur during a preadolescent growth spurt. Heel pain in younger athletes can be a result of calcaneal apophysitis (Sever's disease) (Micheli & Ireland 1987). This condition is a traction apophysitis of the calcaneal insertion of the tendo-Achilles. Physical examination reveals tenderness at this site. Radiographs should be obtained because acute fracture or stress fracture may also be a cause of heel pain in the child (Dowdy et al 1998). Treatment for both Achilles tendonitis and calcaneal apophysitis is directed at stretching of the gastrocnemius, soleus and hamstring along with dorsiflexion strengthening exercises (Sullivan 1994). When pronation is also present, strengthening of foot extrinsic and intrinsic muscles can be helpful along with orthotics when indicated. Early symptomatic relief may be provided with improved shoe wear, heel cups, a temporary heel lift, intermittent ice and anti-inflammatory medication (Sullivan 1994). Traction apophysitis can also occur at the base of the fifth metatarsal (Fig. 25.12).

Stress fractures

Stress fractures that occur in the tibia, lateral and medial malleolus, and metatarsal bones are often due to repetitive stress from sudden increased training, poor biomechanics of the foot or change in foot wear (Brukner et al 1999). Occasionally, a bone scan may be necessary to confirm the diagnosis of a stress fracture in the young athlete (Rosen et al 1982). Chapters 5 and 23 contain further details of such injuries. Activity restriction and immobilization are often required to allow for proper healing.

Physical therapy can be beneficial to address biomechanical issues. For example, stretching of the gastrocnemius/soleus and plantar fascia can be beneficial to an athlete who has been running or jumping on his or her toes without proper heel strike. Tightness in these areas predisposes an athlete to increased stress and shock to the anterior tibial bone with impact. Stress fractures of the navicular bone or the sesamoid bones are of particular concern in the school age athlete. Both of these sites benefit from early diagnosis with bone scan and non-weightbearing immobilization initially to allow for healing (Micheli & d'Hemecourt, 1998).

Acute injuries

Ligaments and associated injuries

Single impact injuries of the ankle in the young athlete are determined by the greater strength of ligaments relative to

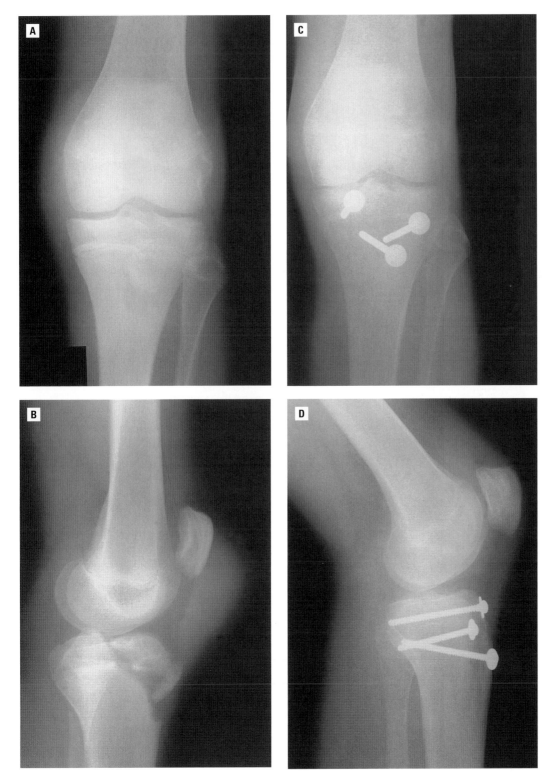

Figure 25.11 • Avulsion of the tibial tubercle, with Salter IV fracture of the proximal tibia, in a 16-year-old male (**A**, **B**). An acute compartment syndrome developed several hours after injury, as a result of extensive bleeding into the compartments of the leg. Emergency fasciotomy, with open reduction and internal fixation, was performed. The fracture healed without sequelae (**C**, **D**).

growth cartilage. In contrast to the adult, lateral ankle ligament sprains are unusual in the young athlete. Inversion injuries more commonly cause a minimally displaced avulsion fracture or fracture of the distal fibular growth plate. Careful physical

examination may localize the structure injured, with maximal point of tenderness at the ligaments, ligament origin or growth plate. If a Salter–Harris I fracture of the distal fibula is present, radiographs may be normal except for some soft tissue

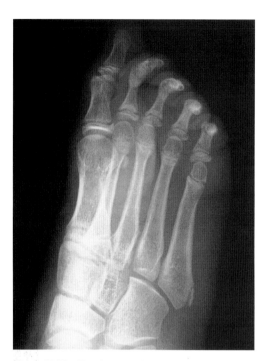

Figure 25.12 • Traction apophysitis of the base of the fifth metatarsal. This 10-year-old female had gradually progressive pain at the base of the fifth metatarsal without any history of injury. Physical examination revealed hindfoot pronation, flexible flatfoot and localized tenderness at the base of the fifth metatarsal. Treatment included peroneal stretching and metatarsal pads, and the pain resolved within 2 months.

swelling. Treatment of this kind of fracture consists of a short leg cast for 3–4 weeks, or longer if tenderness persists. The distal tibia may also sustain growth plate fractures, and these may be complicated by subsequent growth disturbances (Fig. 25.13) or degenerative changes (Spiegel et al 1978, Taunton et al 1998).

Lateral ankle sprains are treated with initial rest, ice, compression and elevation. Painless active range of motion with avoidance of inversion should begin as early as possible. Progressive peroneal strengthening exercises should be introduced when pain and swelling have been reduced. More severe ankle sprains may require short-term immobilization such as a walking boot or stirrup until the athlete is comfortable. Early rehabilitation, including tendoachilles stretching, dorsiflexion and eversion strengthening, and modalities to control inflammation are essential for prompt return to safe activity.

Return to sports may be facilitated with braces or taping to protect the lateral ligaments by preventing inversion, but allowing dorsiflexion and plantarflexion (Stover 1980, Taunton et al 1998). Additionally, exercises to restore proprioception and balance are essential for all sports (Taunton et al 1998). Use of a wobble board as part of a home program, can improve static and dynamic balance (Emery et al 2005).

Other foot and ankle injuries

Tarsal coalitions can occur in young athletes. A tarsal coalition is a bony or fibrocartilaginous connection of two or more tarsal bones of unknown etiology. A calcaneonavicular bar may be seen on the oblique radiograph of the foot (O'Neill & Micheli 1989) (Fig. 25.14). Talonavicular bars are also seen in this younger population. In the young athlete, excision of the bar may alleviate symptoms and improve function (O'Neill & Micheli 1989). The postoperative regimen usually includes a period of 2–4 weeks of immobilization to decrease inflammation and the chance of bone reformation.

The child or adolescent can develop foot or ankle pain from accessory ossicles (Sullivan 1994). The painful accessory navicular, associated with the insertion of the tibialis posterior tendon, can be aggravated by pronation and repetitive activity (Fig. 25.15). If pain relief is not achieved with orthotics, tibialis posterior stretching and foot instrinsic and extrinsic strengthening exercises, then short-term immobilization or, ultimately, excision of the accessory navicular may be indicated (Sella et al 1986).

Another common accessory ossicle is the os trigonum at the posterior aspect of the talus (Kadel et al 2000). This ossicle may cause posterior ankle pain as a result of impingement of the ossicle between the posterior tibia and calcaneus in activities such as dance and gymnastics, which involve repetitive pointing of the ankle and foot (Hamilton 1982, Kadel et al 2000). Excision is occasionally required.

Shoulder and shoulder girdle

Sports activities which involve repetitive overhead use of the shoulder are common causes of problems of the shoulder region in the young athlete. These problems include subacromial impingement, instability and fracture. The accuracy of diagnosis of glenohumeral and subacromial derangements has been improved with MRI and MRI arthrograms, as well as with shoulder arthroscopy (Gross 1994a).

Overuse injuries

Impingement

Subacromial impingement problems are common in throwing athletes and swimmers, and include subacromial bursitis, rotator cuff tendinitis and partial or full-thickness rotator cuff tears (Berkowitz et al 1998). Arthroscopy can sometimes show associated glenohumeral derangements (Andrews & Gidumal 1987, Ireland & Andrews 1988).

Shoulder dislocation and subluxation

Glenohumeral dislocation is uncommon in the prepubescent, but may occur in the adolescent. Anterior dislocation is the most common type of instability, but posterior subluxation and dislocation can also occur (Kocher et al 2000, Norwood & Terry 1984,

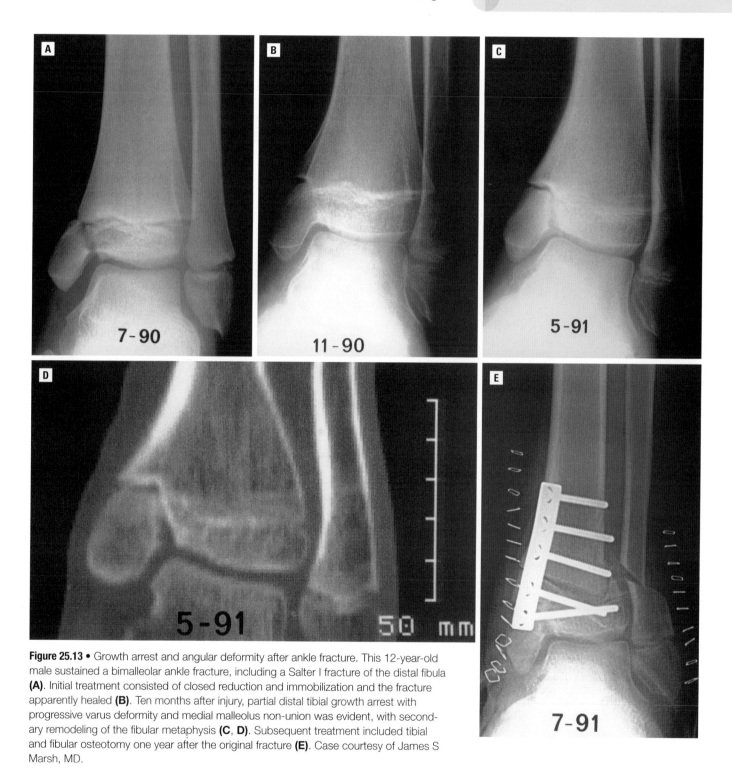

Figure 25.13 • Growth arrest and angular deformity after ankle fracture. This 12-year-old male sustained a bimalleolar ankle fracture, including a Salter I fracture of the distal fibula **(A)**. Initial treatment consisted of closed reduction and immobilization and the fracture apparently healed **(B)**. Ten months after injury, partial distal tibial growth arrest with progressive varus deformity and medial malleolus non-union was evident, with secondary remodeling of the fibular metaphysis **(C, D)**. Subsequent treatment included tibial and fibular osteotomy one year after the original fracture **(E)**. Case courtesy of James S Marsh, MD.

Samilson & Prieto 1983). In individuals with anterior shoulder instability requiring surgery, contralateral shoulder instability is more common if the initial dislocation occurred before the age of 15 years (O'Driscoll & Evans 1991). Therefore, bilateral shoulder complex conditioning programs are important.

Shoulder pain in the young swimmer or thrower can be a sign of anterior glenohumeral subluxation. These athletes may develop progressive anterior capsular laxity, reflected on examination by an increase in external rotation. Multidirectional glenohumeral instability in the growing athlete is relatively rare,

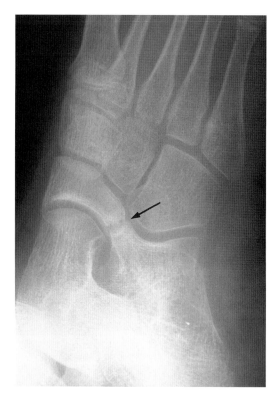

Figure 25.14 • A calcaneonavicular coalition is often most clearly revealed in the oblique radiograph of the foot. This 14-year-old male had midfoot pain associated with this bar. Excision resulted in resolution of symptoms.

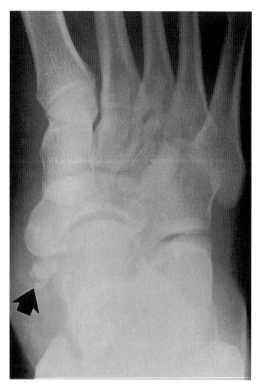

Figure 25.15 • Painful accessory navicular in a skeletally mature aerobics dancer.

but may occur (Kocher et al 2000, Neer & Foster 1980). In contrast, physical signs of instability may be common in normal, asymptomatic adolescents, even in the absence of generalized joint laxity (Emery & Mullaji 1991). In contrast to the adult, early detection of subluxation or multidirectional instability in the adolescent can often be successfully treated by physical therapy (Kocher et al 2000).

General principles of physical therapy treatment for shoulder complex problems include restoration of normal biomechanics (Pappas et al 1995). Scapular position and mechanics are usually altered and must be addressed in order to have optimal function of the glenohumeral joint (Borsa et al 2003, Borstad 2006).

Assessment should include postural assessment, as well as range of movement, manual muscle tests and observation of mechanics and scapulohumeral rhythm. Soft tissue imbalances, such as posterior capsule tightness, occur as a result of the repetitive motions incurred during training and playing. Stretching of tight structures to facilitate improved scapular position should occur before strengthening (Voight & Thomson 2000). Strengthening of the rotator cuff muscles should also include eccentric training in throwing athletes (Pappas et al 1995).

Acute injuries

Fractures

Proximal humerus stress fractures are common in throwing sports (Kocher et al 2000). 'Little League shoulder' is a stress fracture of the proximal humeral physis resulting from the cumulative effects of repetitive microtrauma secondary to vigorous pitching activity (Cahill et al 1974, Kocher et al 2000). Treatment consists of the suspension of throwing activities for 6–8 weeks (Cahill et al 1974, Kocher et al 2000). Prevention of subsequent injury includes a vigorous preseason conditioning program, limits on the frequency of pitching during the subsequent year and proper throwing mechanics. Ball control should be emphasized over velocity (Kocher et al 2000).

Single-impact fracture of the proximal humerus physis in adolescents is usually a Salter–Harris II fracture, and remodeling may occur despite displacement. Treatment can include closed reduction and sling or spica cast. Operative treatment is rarely required (Rang 1983). Fracture of the base of the coracoid process is less common, and is also usually treated non-operatively (Fig. 25.16).

Other joints of the shoulder girdle

Acromioclavicular sprains and separations are less common in the prepubescent, but may occur in the adolescent in contact sports such as gridiron football, rugby, lacrosse, Australian football and hockey. Treatment is usually symptomatic, and open reduction is rarely required.

Sternoclavicular separation can also occur in contact sports as a result of lateral stress on the upper torso. In the young athlete, this injury is usually an epiphyseal separation of the medial

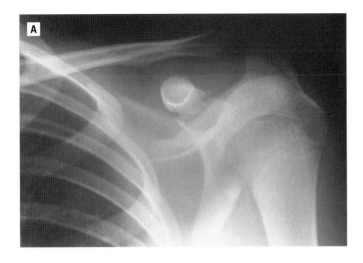

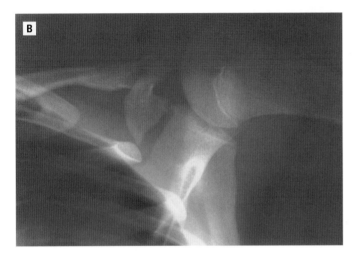

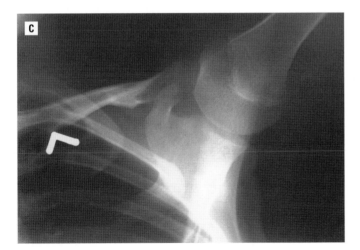

Figure 25.16 • Fracture of the base of the coracoid. This 15-year-old male fell off a bicycle, landing on the posterior aspect of his shoulder. Maximal tenderness was at the coracoid process, and radiography (**A**, **B**) revealed a fracture of the base of the coracoid. Treatment included a sling and early motion, and the fracture healed without sequelae (**C**).

clavicle (Curtis 1994), because the physis does not fuse until the age of 23–25 years. With anterior displacement, the medial clavicle is prominent; posterior displacement of the medial clavicle may result in tracheal compression and dyspnea requiring emergency intervention. Treatment may be non-operative, but internal fixation is required in some cases (Curtis 1994).

Clavicle shaft fracture is common in the child, either from direct trauma (blow or fall) or indirect forces (fall on outstretched hand) (Curtis 1994). Treatment consists of a sling or figure-of-eight brace for comfort, and open reduction is rarely required. Parents should be instructed that the fracture callus may cause a prominent 'bump' because of the subcutaneous location of the bone.

Elbow

Pediatric elbow injuries are common and patterns are related to age-related stage of elbow development and the sport-specific mechanism of injury (Kocher et al 2000).

Overuse injuries

Little League elbow is a group of overuse injuries of the elbow joint resulting from repetitive lateral compression and medial traction secondary to valgus and sheering stresses on the elbow from pitching (Kocher et al 2000). The young pitcher complains of progressive medial or lateral elbow pain and tenderness over the medial epicondyle; pain increases with pitching and is relieved with rest. Little League elbow can be categorized into three disorders: medial epicondylitis, capitellar OCD and premature arrest of the proximal radial physis. Young pitchers are subject to these injuries due to the presence of physeal tissue at the joint surface and medial epicondyle (Kocher et al 2000). As overtraining seems to be the common denominator for most of these injuries, young baseball players should limit their skilled throws (Kocher et al 2000) to 300 per week (Micheli & Jenkins 2001).

Lateral elbow pain, catching or locking may be signs of OCD of the capitellum, which may be associated with loose bodies in the joint (Fig. 25.17). If detected early, this condition can improve with rest and strengthening exercises, and recurrence can be prevented by proper throwing mechanics (Albright et al 1978, Kocher et al 2000). However, occasionally this condition may require elbow arthroscopy or arthrotomy, with excision of loose bodies and curettage of the base of the lesion (McManama et al 1985). Premature arrest of the proximal radial physis can be seen in conjunction with the two other conditions of 'Little League elbow' (Bradley 1994).

Traction apophysitis of the triceps insertion to the olecranon can be caused by rapid growth (Ireland & Andrews 1988, Micheli 1987). Also, medial and lateral epicondylitis can occur in the young athlete (Leach & Miller 1987, Renstrom 1998). Lateral epicondylitis is rare in young throwers and occurs more in tennis players (Gerbino 2003).

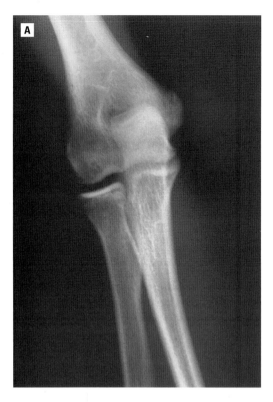

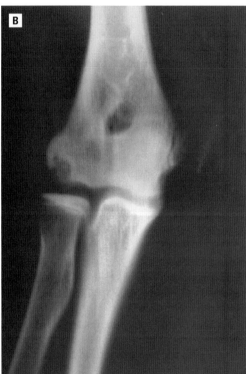

Figure 25.17 • Osteochondritis dissecans of the capitellum, as demonstrated by **(A)** plain radiography and **(B)** tomography.

Medial epicondylitis can progress to a significant widening of the growth plate followed by fracture and displacement of the epicondyle (Kocher et al 2000). Treatment for the overuse injury to the medial epicondylar apophysis includes relative rest, followed by progressive strengthening exercises, as well as education regarding throwing mechanics (Kocher et al 2000). There is often an associated flexion contracture of the elbow with this overuse injury and therapy must be directed to address this abnormality. Medial collateral ligament (MCL) tears at the elbow may occur in adolescents, and may be difficult to diagnose (Ireland & Andrews 1988, Norwood et al 1981). Radiographs with valgus stress may reveal widening of the medial compartment, and arthrography can be helpful (Ireland & Andrews 1988). Primary surgical repair has been recommended in these high-demand athletes (Ireland & Andrews 1988).

Acute injuries

Fractures

In children and adolescents, the elbow can also be injured in sports involving upper extremity weightbearing. Gymnastic activity can result in fractures about the elbow, dislocations and capitellar OCD (Bradley 1994, Priest & Weise 1981). An acutely injured and swollen elbow in a child is an emergency. Some single-impact injuries, such as a displaced supracondylar fracture, may result in permanent disability or loss of the extremity because of neurovascular compromise.

Other fractures of the elbow in the young athlete may be less likely to cause vascular compromise than a displaced supracondylar fracture. Nevertheless, circumferential bandages or casts should be avoided in any acute elbow injury associated with swelling. Early range of motion is an essential component of elbow injury rehabilitation.

Throwing athletes, most commonly baseball pitchers, sustain single-impact and overuse injuries of the elbow as a result of valgus stresses (Kocher et al 2000). Avulsion of the medial collateral ligament from the medial epicondyle may occur secondary to throwing alone (Fig. 25.18), or may be associated with elbow dislocation sustained in contact sports (Ireland & Andrews 1988). Internal fixation of the medial epicondyle may be required to ensure anatomical reduction, in order to minimize subsequent laxity or instability, and may allow early protected motion to minimize stiffness (Ireland & Andrews 1988).

Forearm, hand and wrist

Hand and wrist injuries are common during athletic competition, accounting for up to 14% of all athletic injuries (McCue et al 1998). Typically, the hand is in front of the athlete and often absorbs the initial contact or repetitive stress. Injuries range from dislocations and fractures to overuse syndromes. Most injuries are treated in a nonoperative fashion. Proper protection and appropriate rehabilitation are key to optimal healing (McCue et al 1998).

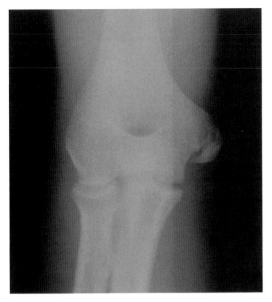

Figure 25.18 • Medial epicondyle avulsion fracture in a 15-year-old Little league pitcher. The fracture was treated with open reduction and screw fixation because of the high demand on this elbow.

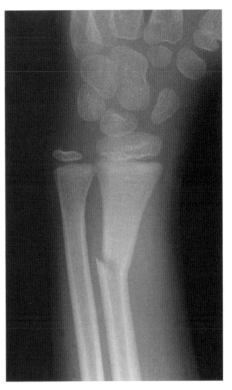

Figure 25.19 • Greenstick fracture of the distal radius in a 6-year-old female who fell on her outstretched hand. The dorsal apex of the deformity resulted from pronation at the time of injury, and closed reduction required a supination maneuver.

Acute injuries

Fractures

Evaluation of a forearm injury should include an examination of the entire extremity, and radiographs should include both the elbow and wrist. Pain with forearm rotation can be a sign of injury. A Monteggia fracture is a fracture of the ulna shaft associated with a radial head dislocation, and the latter may be overlooked if the elbow is not included in the examination or radiographic studies. Neurovascular assessment is important as displaced fractures about the wrist can lead to median nerve injury.

Fractures of the distal radius vary in an age-related pattern which is determined by the changing mechanical properties of bone with age (Rang 1983). The younger child can sustain a minimally displaced metaphyseal buckle or torus fracture. Treatment consists of a short arm cast for 4 weeks. A greenstick forearm fracture may be associated with significant malrotation, and reduction is usually necessary, occasionally under anesthesia (Fig. 25.19). Adolescents can sustain Salter–Harris II fractures through the distal radius growth plate with significant displacement (Fig. 25.20).

Many gymnastic maneuvers require weightbearing on the upper extremities. Ground reaction forces put stresses on the wrist up to 2.37 times the gymnast's body weight in movements such as the back handspring (Zetaruk 2000). As a result of weight bearing on hyperdorsiflexed wrists, often with rotational forces, wrist injuries are common among young gymnasts (d'Hemecourt et al 2000). Salter–Harris type I microfractures of the growth plate are commonly incurred (Zetaruk 2000). Pain is usually localized to the dorsum of the radial aspect

of the wrist. Treatment includes rest for 2–4 weeks, ice and anti-inflammatory medication. Severe cases require splinting. Flexibility and strength should be maintained during the rehabilitation phase while avoiding axial loading and torsion of the physis. Early recognition of pain and reduction of training may reduce the incidence of these types of fractures.

Fractures and other problems of the carpal bones are less common in the young athlete than in the adult (Kocher et al 2000, Simmons & Lovallo 1988). However, fractures of the digits are common in children and adolescents (Kocher et al 2000). An apparent dislocation or sprain of the finger in the child may actually be a fracture through the growth plate, and reduction must be performed with care to minimize further injury to the physis (Simmons & Lovallo 1988) (Figs 25.21 and 25.22).

Summary

With the rise in youth participation in organized sports, there has been a subsequent increase in sport-related injury patterns in young athletes. Many youth injuries differ from adult injuries because of differing stages of physical development. Children have different structural and physiologic components

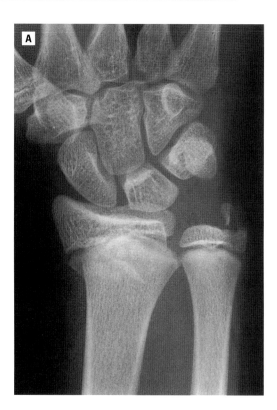

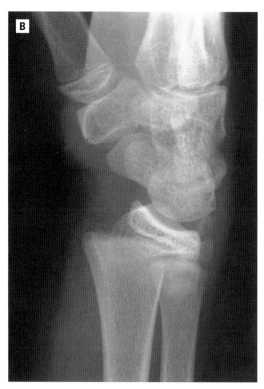

Figure 25.20 • Anterior–posterior **(A)** and lateral **(B)** views of a Salter–Harris II fracture of the distal radius. This 13-year-old male fell on ice during a football activity, and landed on his outstretched hand. Closed reduction was performed after hematoma block, and the fracture healed without sequelae.

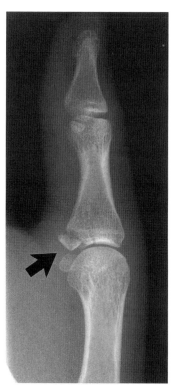

Figure 25.21 • Avulsion fracture of the ulnar collateral ligament of the thumb metacarpophalangeal joint. This 15-year-old cheerleader fell on her thumb, with forceful thumb abduction. The Salter–Harris III ulnar collateral ligament avulsion fracture was treated with a thumb spica cast. Thumb stability was normal after the fracture had healed.

that must be specifically addressed. A knowledge of risk factors which predispose or contribute to musculoskeletal injury facilitates the clinical evaluation of the injured child and adolescent athlete (Box 25.1) (Micheli & Jenkins 1995).

Information based on risk factors can also be used in developing an approach to injury prevention (Faigenbaum 2000). Preparticipation clinical assessment of the young athlete can identify areas at risk for injury in an individual (Micheli 1984, Rooks & Micheli 1988). Specific recommendations can be made for the improvement of physical characteristics such as strength and flexibility, which may increase safety and improve performance (Rooks & Micheli 1988). Preseason conditioning, as well as the amount and content of practice sessions during the season, appears to correlate with a lower incidence of injury (Cahill & Griffith 1978, Ekstrand et al 1983, Smith et al 1997). Attention to sport-specific technique may also prevent injury in the young.

While prevention of injuries is paramount for young athletes, a comprehensive and effective rehabilitation program following an injury is also imperative. Incorporating sport specific activities is not only essential in assisting the young athlete's ability to safely return to sports, but also helps to motivate the athlete while building confidence.

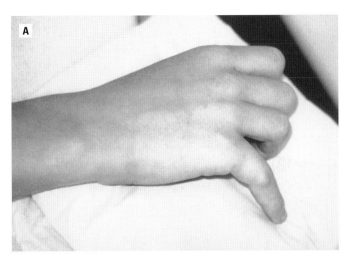

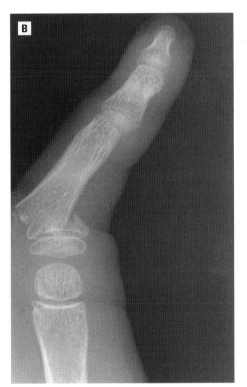

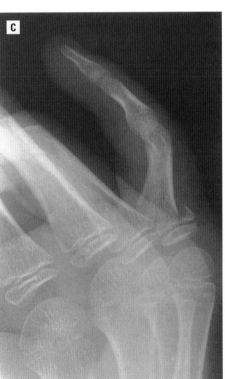

Figure 25.22 • Salter–Harris II fracture of the base of the proximal phalanx. This 11-year-old male jammed his little finger against a baseball, with hyperextension of the digit. The abduction and supination deformity **(A)** was a result of a Salter–Harris II fracture of the base of the fifth proximal phalanx **(B, C)**. Closed reduction was performed after hematoma block, and the fracture healed after 8 weeks of immobilization. It is important to correct the rotational deformity during the reduction, in order to prevent crossover with the ring finger during grasping activities.

The most successful rehabilitation program includes a team approach. Communication between the physician, physical therapist or athletic trainer, coach, athlete and parents is essential for a safe and successful return to play. Approaching the injury as an opportunity to assist the athlete in returning to his or her sport better than before the injury occurred can maximize motivation, compliance and performance. Clinical research is essential in order to identify the specific risks and benefits of organized sports for children and adolescents. There is a growing interest in the research of young athletes, and with this focus, further gains in injury prevention and rehabilitation are anticipated.

References

Aichroth P M, Patel D V, Marx C L 1991 Congenital discoid lateral meniscus in children. A follow-up study and evolution of management. Journal of Bone and Joint Surgery (Br) 73B:932–936

Albright J A, Jokl P, Shaw R et al 1978 Clinical study of baseball pitchers: correlation of injury to the throwing arm with method of delivery. American Journal of Sports Medicine 6:15–21

Ali R M, Green D M, Patel T C 1999 Scheuermann's kyphosis. Current Opinion in Pediatrics 11:65–66

Aminaka N, Gribble P A 2005 A systematic review of the effects of therapeutic taping on patellofemoral pain syndrome. Journal of Athletic Training 40:341–351

Andrish J T 2001 Anterior cruciate ligament injuries in the skeletally immature patient. American Journal of Orthopedics 30:103–110

Andrews J R, Gidumal R H 1987 Shoulder arthroscopy in the throwing athlete: perspectives and prognosis. Clinics in Sports Medicine 6:565–571

Backx F J G, Erich W B M, Kemper A B A et al 1989 Sports injuries in school-aged children. An epidemiologic study. American Journal of Sports Medicine 17:234–240

Backx F J G, Beijer H J M, Bol E et al 1991 Injuries in high risk persons and high-risk sports. American Journal of Sports Medicine 19:124–130

Berkowitz M M, Bowen M K, Warren R F 1998 Injuries of the rotator cuff. In: Harries M, Williams C, Stanish W D et al (eds) Oxford textbook of sports medicine. Oxford University Press, Oxford, p 517–533

Boden B P, Dean G S, Feagin J A Jr et al 2000 Mechanisms of anterior cruciate ligament injury. Orthopedics 23:573–578.

Borsa P A, Timmons M K, Sauers E L 2003 Scapular-positioning during humeral elevation in unimpaired shoulders. Journal of Athletic Training 38:12–17

Borstad J D 2006 Resting position variables at the shoulder: evidence to support a posture-impairment association. Physical Therapy 86:549–557

Bradley G W, Shives T C, Samuelson K M 1979 Ligament injuries in the knees of children. Journal of Bone and Joint Surgery (Am) 61A:588–591

Bradley J P 1994 Upper extremity: elbow injuries in children and adolescents. In: Stanitski C L, DeLee J C, Drez D (eds) Pediatric and adolescent sports medicine. WB Saunders, Philadelphia, PA, p 254–261

Bright R W, Burstein A H, Elmore S M 1974 Epiphyseal-plate cartilage: a biomechanical and histological analysis of failure modes. Journal of Bone and Joint Surgery (Am) 56A:688–703

Bruckner P, Bennell K, Matheson G 1999 Stress fractures. Blackwell Science Asia, Melbourne, p 41–82

Buehler-Yund C 1999 A longitudinal study of injury rates and risk factors in 5 to 12 year old soccer players. Environmental Health. University of Cincinnati, OH, p 161

Burkhart S S, Peterson H A 1979 Fractures of the proximal tibial epiphysis. Journal of Bone and Joint Surgery (Am) 61A:996–1002

Cahill B R, Griffith E H 1978 Effect of preseason conditioning on the incidence and severity of high school football knee injuries. American Journal of Sports Medicine 6:180–184

Cahill B R, Tullos H S, Fain R H 1974 Little league shoulder. Journal of Sports Medicine 2:150–153

Caine D J, Maffulli N 2005 Epidemiology of children's individual sports injuries. An important area of medicine and sport science research. Medicine and Science in Sports and Exercise 48:1–7

Cantu R C 2000 Cervical spine injuries in the athlete. Seminars in Neurology 20:173–178

Carney B T, Weinstein S L, Noble J 1991 Long-term follow-up of slipped capital femoral epiphysis. Journal of Bone and Joint Surgery (Am) 73A:667–674

Cassella M, Richards K, Gustafson C 2006 Physical therapy/rehabilitation. In: Micheli L J, Kocher, M The pediatric and adolescent knee. Saunders & Elsevier, Philadelphia, PA, p 131–145

Cheng J C Y, Chan P S, Hui P W 1991 Joint laxity in children. Journal of Pediatric Orthopedics 11:752–756

Chow S P, Lam J J, Leong J C Y 1990 Fracture of the tibial tubercle in the adolescent. Journal of Bone and Joint Surgery (Br) 72B:231–234

Clancy W G, Foltz A S 1976 Iliac apophysitis and stress fractures in adolescent runners. American Journal of Sports Medicine 4:214–218

Clanton T O, DeLee J C, Sanders B et al 1979 Knee ligament injuries in children. Journal of Bone and Joint Surgery (Am) 61A:1195–1201

Connolly P J 2001 Physician decision making in return to play following cervical spine injury. Paper presented at the 68th Annual Meeting of the American Academy of Orthopedic Surgeons

Constantini N W, Warren M P 1994 Special problems of the female athlete. Baillière's best practice and research. Clinical Rheumatology 8:199–219

Crossley K, Bennell K, Green S et al 2001 A systematic review of physical interventions for patellofemoral pain syndrome. Clinical Journal of Sports Medicine 11:103–110

Curtis R J 1994 Skeletal injuries. In: Harries M, Williams C, Stanish WD et al (eds) Oxford textbook of sports medicine. Oxford University Press, Oxford, p 68–85

Damore D T, Metzl J D, Ramundo M et al 2003 Patterns in childhood sports injury. Pediatric Emergency Care 19:65–67

DeLee J C 1994 Ligamentous injuries of the knee. In: Harries M, Williams C, Stanish W D et al (eds) Oxford textbook of sports medicine. Oxford University Press, Oxford, p 129–131

DeLee J C, Curtis R 1983 Anterior cruciate ligament insufficiency in children. Clinical Orthopaedics and Related Research 172:112–118

d'Hemecourt P A, Gerbino P G, Micheli L J 2000 Back injuries in the young athlete. Clinics in Sports Medicine 19:663–679

Dias L S 1984 Fractures of the tibia and fibula. In: Rockwood C A, Wilkins K E, King R E (eds) Fractures in children. JB Lippincott, Philadelphia, PA, p 647–657

Dickhaut S C, DeLee J C 1982 The discoid lateral-meniscus syndrome. Journal of Bone and Joint Surgery (Am) 64A:1068–1073

Dowdy P A, Miller M D, Fu F H 1998 Ankle and foot. In: Johnson R J, Lombardo J (eds) Current review of sports medicine, 2nd edn. Butterworth Heinemann, Philadelphia, PA, p 103–120

Ekstrand J, Gillquist J, Moller M et al 1983 Incidence of soccer injuries and their relation to training and team success. American Journal of Sports Medicine 11:63–67

Emery C A, Cassidy J D, Klassen T P et al 2005 Effectiveness of a home-based balance-training program in reducing sports-related injuries among healthy adolescents: a cluster randomized controlled trial. Canadian Medical Association Journal 172:749–754

Emery R J, Mullaji A B 1991 Glenohumeral joint instability in normal adolescents. Journal of Bone and Joint Surgery (Br) 73B:406–408

Faigenbaum A D 2000 Strength training for children and adolescents. Clinics in Sports Medicine 19:593–619

Fitzgerald R H 1995 Acetabular labral tears. Clinical Orthopedics and Related Research 311:60–68

Fondren F B, Goldner J L, Bassett F H 1985 Recurrent dislocation of the patella treated by the modified Roux–Goldthwait procedure. Journal of Bone and Joint Surgery (Am) 67A:993–1005

Ganz R, Parvizi J, Beck M et al 2003 Femoraoacetabular impingement: a cause for osteoarthritis of the hip. Clinical Orthopedics and Related Research 417:112–120

Gerbino P 2003 Elbow disorders in throwing athletes. Orthopedic Clinics of North America 34:417–426

Griffiths I D, Pinder I M 1981 Chondromalacia patellae: a clinical and arthroscopic study. Annals of the Rheumatic Diseases 40:617

Gross G W 1994a Imaging. In: Stanitski C L, DeLee J C, Drez D (eds) Pediatric and adolescent sports medicine. WB Saunders, Philadelphia, PA, p 456–497

Gross R H 1994b Acute musculotendinous injuries. In: Stanitski C L, DeLee J C, Drez D (eds) Pediatric and adolescent sports medicine. WB Saunders, Philadelphia, PA, p 131–143

Gurewitsch A D, O'Neill M A 1944 Flexibility of healthy children. Archives of Physical Therapy 25:216–221

Guy J A, Micheli L J 2001 Strength training for children and adolescents. Journal of the American Academy of Orthopaedic Surgeons 9:29–36

Hamilton W G 1982 Stenosing tenosynovitis of the flexor hallucis longus tendon and posterior impingement upon the os trigonum in ballet dancers. Foot and Ankle International 3:74–80

Havranek P, Lizler J 1991 Magnetic resonance imaging in the evaluation of partial growth arrest after physeal injuries in children. Journal of Bone and Joint Surgery (Am) 73A:1234–1241

Herring S A, Nilson K L 1987 Introduction to overuse injuries. Clinics in Sports Medicine 6:225–239

Hewett T E, Lindenfeld T N, Riccobene J V et al 2000 The effects of neuromuscular training on the incidence of knee injury in female athletes. A prospective study. American Journal of Sports Medicine 28:615–616

Hewett T E, Myer G D, Ford K R 2005 Biomechanical measures of neuromuscular control and valgus loading of the knee predict anterior cruciate ligament injury risk in female athletes: a prospective study. American Journal of Sports Medicine 33:492–501

Insall J N, Aglietti P, Traino A J 1983 Patellar pain and incongruence: II. Clinical application. Clinical Orthopaedics and Related Research 176:225–232

Iobst C A, Stanitski C L 2000 Acute knee injuries. Clinics in Sports Medicine 19:621–635

Ireland M L, Andrews J R 1988 Shoulder and elbow injuries in the young athlete. Clinics in Sports Medicine 7:473–494

Irrgang J J, Sawhney R 1994 Rehabilitation for childhood and adolescent orthopaedic sports related injuries. In: Stanitski C L, DeLee J C, Drez D (eds) Pediatric and adolescent sports medicine. WB Saunders, Philadelphia, PA, p 498–519

Jackson D W, Lowery W D, Ciullo J V 1995 Injuries of the spine. In: Nicholas J A, Hershman E B (eds) The lower extremity and spine in sports. Mosby, St Louis, MO, p 1307–1344

Javin J S, Fox J M 1995 Thigh injuries. In: Nicholas J A, Hershman E B (eds) The lower extremity and spine in sports medicine. Mosby, St Louis, MO, p 999–1024

Jiffin J R, Briard J L 1998 Fractures and dislocations. In: Harries M, Williams C, Stanish W D et al (eds) Oxford textbook of sports medicine. Oxford University Press, Oxford, p 477–472

Johnson R J 1998 Acute knee injuries: an overview. In: Harries M, Williams C, Stanish W D et al (eds) Oxford textbook of sports medicine. Oxford University Press, Oxford, p 411–419.

Kadel N, Micheli L J, Solomon R 2000 Os trigonum impingement syndrome in dancers. Journal of Dance Medicine and Science 4:1–4

Karlin L I 1995 Injuries to the hip and pelvis. In: Nicholas J A, Hershman E B (eds) The lower extremity and spine in sports medicine. Mosby, St Louis, MO, p 1277–1306

Keeney J A, Peelle M W, Jackson J et al 2004 Magnetic resonance arthrography versus arthroscopy in the evaluation of articular hip pathology. Clinical Othopedics and Related Research 429:163–169

Kibler W B, Safran M R 2000 Musculoskeletal injuries in the young tennis player. Clinics in Sports Medicine 19:781–792

Kleiger B, Mankin H J 1964 Fracture of the lateral portion of the distal tibial epiphysis. Journal of Bone and Joint Surgery (Am) 46A:25–32

Kocher M S, Waters P M, Micheli L J 2000 Upper extremity injuries in the paediatric athlete. Sports Medicine 30:117–135

Kocher M S, Yaniv M, Adrignolo A A et al 2001 Functional and radiographic outcome of juvenile osteochondritis dissecans of the knee treated with antegrade arthroscopic drilling. American Journal of Sports Medicine 29:562–566

Kocher M S, Kim Y, Millis M et al 2005 Hip arthroscopy in children and adolescents. Journal of Pediatric Orthopedics 25:680–686

Kokoska E R, Keller M S, Rallo M C et al 2001 Characteristics of pediatric cervical spine injuries. Journal of Pediatric Surgery 36:100–105

Kvist M, Kujala U M, Heinonen O J et al 1989 Sports-related injuries in children. International Journal of Sports Medicine 10:81–86

Lage L A, Patel J G, Villar R N 1996 The acetabular labral tear: An arthroscopic classification. Arthroscopy 12:269–272

Larson R L, McMahan R O 1966 The epiphyses and the childhood athlete. Journal of the American Medical Association 196:607–612

Leach R E, Miller J K 1987 Lateral and medial epicondylitis of the elbow. Clinics in Sports Medicine 6:259–272

Lewis C L, Sahrmann S A 2005 Acetabular labral tears. Physical Therapy 86:110–121

Lipscomb A B, Anderson A F 1986 Tears of the anterior cruciate ligament in adolescents. Journal of Bone and Joint Surgery (Am) 68A:19–28

McCarthy J C, Lee J 2004 Arthroscopic intervention in early hip disease. Clinical Orthopedics and Related Research 429:157–162

McCue F C, Dinsmore H H, Kowalk D L 1998 Athletic injuries to the hand and wrist. In: Johnson R J, Lombardo J (eds) Current review of sports medicine, 2nd edn. Butterworth Heinemann, Philadelphia, PA, p 43–54.

McManama G B, Micheli L J, Berry M V et al 1985 The surgical treatment of osteochondritis of the capitellum. American Journal of Sports Medicine 13:11–21

Maffulli N, Caine D 2005 The epidemiology of children's team sports injuries. Medicine and Science in Sports and Exercise 49:1–8

Mandelbaum B R, Silvers H J, Watanabe D S et al 2005 Effectiveness of neuromuscular training and proprioceptive training in preventing anterior cruciate ligament injuries in female athletes: two year follow-up. American Journal of Sports Medicine 33:1003–1011

Mayer P J, Micheli L 1979 Avulsion of the femoral attachment of the posterior cruciate ligament in an eleven-year-old boy. Journal of Bone and Joint Surgery (Am) 61A:431–432

Metzl J D 2000 Sports medicine in pediatric practice: keeping pace with the changing times. Pediatric Annals 29:146–148

Metzmaker J N, Pappas A M 1985 Avulsion fractures of the pelvis. American Journal of Sports Medicine 13:349–358

Micheli L J 1983 Overuse syndromes in children in sport: the growth factor. Orthopedic Clinics of North America 14:337–360

Micheli L J 1984 Preparticipation evaluation for sports competition: musculoskeletal assessment of the young athlete. In: Kelley V C (ed) Practice of pediatrics. Harper and Row, Philadelphia, PA, p 1–9

Micheli L J 1987 The traction apophysitises. Clinics in Sports Medicine 6:389–404

Micheli L J 1999 Pediatric lateral retinacular release with medial plication under arthroscopic control. Oratec Interventions Case Report K3

Micheli L J, d'Hemecourt P A 1998 Spine and chest wall. In: Johnson RJ, Lombardo J (eds) Current review of sports medicine, 2nd edn. Butterworth Heinemann, Philadelphia, PA, p 2–18

Micheli L J, Fehlandt A F 1994 Stress fractures. In: Letts R M (ed) Management of pediatric fractures. Churchill Livingstone, Edinburgh, p 973–987

Micheli L J, Ireland M L 1987 Prevention and management of calcaneal apophysitis in children: an overuse syndrome. Journal of Pediatric Orthopedics 7:34–38

Micheli L J, Jenkins M 1995 The sports medicine bible. Harper Perennial, New York

Micheli L J, Jenkins M 2001 The sports medicine bible for young athletes. Sourcebooks, Naperville, IL

Micheli L J, Stanitski C L 1981 Lateral patellar retinacular release. American Journal of Sports Medicine 9:330–336

Micheli L J, Hall J E, Miller M E 1980 Use of modified Boston brace for back injuries in athletes. American Journal of Sports Medicine 8:351–356

Micheli L J, Metzl J D, DiCanzio J et al 1999a Anterior cruciate ligament reconstructive surgery in adolescent soccer and basketball players. Clinical Journal of Sports Medicine 9:138–141

Micheli L J, Rask B, Gerberg L 1999b Anterior cruciate ligament reconstruction in patients who are prepubescent. Clinical Orthopaedics and Related Research 364:40–47

Micheli L J, Glassman R, Klein M 2000 The prevention of sports injuries in children. Clinics in Sports Medicine 19:821–834

Murray R O, Duncan C 1971 Athletic activity in adolescence as an etiological factor in degenerative hip disease. Journal of Bone and Joint Surgery (Br) 53B:406–419

481

Myer G D, Ford K R, Hewett T E 2004 Rationale and clinical techniques for anterior cruciate ligament injury prevention among female athletes. Journal of Athletic Training 39:352–364

Neer C S, Foster C R 1980 Inferior capsular shift for involuntary inferior and multidirectional instability of the shoulder. Journal of Bone and Joint Surgery (Am) 62A:897–908

Norwood L A, Terry G C 1984 Shoulder posterior subluxation. American Journal of Sports Medicine 12:25–30

Norwood L A, Shook J A, Andrews J R 1981 Acute medial elbow ruptures. American Journal of Sports Medicine 9:16–19

O'Driscoll S W, Evans D C 1991 Contralateral shoulder instability following anterior repair. Journal of Bone and Joint Surgery (Br) 73B:941–946

Ogden J A, Southwick W O 1976 Osgood-Schlatter's disease and tibial tuberosity development. Clinical Orthopaedics and Related Research 116:180–189

Omey M L, Micheli L J 1999 Foot and ankle problems in the young athlete. Medicine and Science in Sports and Exercise 3l (7 suppl): S470–476

O'Neill D B, Micheli L J 1989 Tarsal coalition: a followup of adolescent athletes. American Journal of Sports Medicine 17:544–549

Outerbridge A R, Micheli L J 1995 Overuse injuries in the young athlete. Clinics in Sports Medicine 14:503–516

Pappas A M, McCarthy C F, Zawacki R M 1995 Care and rehabilitation of the throwing shoulder. In: Pappas A M (ed) Upper extremity injuries in the athlete. Churchill Livingstone, New York, p 277–301

Patrick C 1995 Spinal conditions. In: Campbell S K (ed) Physical therapy for children. WB Saunders, Philadelphia, PA, p 239–259

Peck D M 1995 Apophyseal injuries in the young athlete. American Family Physician 51:1897–1898, 1981–1985

Peele M W, Della Rocca G J, Maloney W J et al 2005 Acetabular and femoral radiographic abnormalities associated with labral tears. Clinical Orthopedics and Related Research 441:327–333

Pelipenko V I 1973 On peculiarities of the development of the foot skeleton in the pupils of a choreographic school. Archives of Anatomy Gistol Embryology 64:46–50

Pirnay L, Crielaard J M 2001 Stress fractures and sports. Review Medicale de Liege 56:369–374

Priest J D, Weise D J 1981 Elbow injury in women's gymnastics. American Journal of Sports Medicine 9:288–295

Proctor M R, Cantu R C 2000 Head and neck injuries in young athletes. Clinics in Sports Medicine 19:693–715

Puddu G C, Cerullo G, Selvanetti A et al 1998 Stress fractures. In: Harries M, Williams C, Stanish W D et al (eds) Oxford textbook of sports medicine. Oxford University Press, Oxford, p 649–668

Pueschel S M, Scola F H 1987 Atlantoaxial instability in individuals with Down syndrome: epidemiologic, radiographic, and clinical studies. Pediatrics 80:555–560

Rang M 1983 Children's fractures, 2nd edn. JB Lippincott, Philadelphia, PA

Renstrom P A 1998 An introduction to chronic overuse injuries. In: Harries M, Williams C, Stanish W D et al (eds) Oxford textbook of sports medicine. Oxford University Press, Oxford, p 633–648

Rice S G 2000 Risks of injury during sports participation. In: Sullivan J A, Anderson S J (eds) Care of the young athlete. American Academy of Orthopaedics, Oklahoma City, OK, p 9–18

Rodenburg J B 1994 Warm-up, stretching and massage diminish harmful effects of eccentric exercise. International Journal of Sports Medicine 15:414–419

Rooks D S, Micheli L J 1988 Musculoskeletal assessment and training: the young athlete. Clinics in Sports Medicine 7:641–677

Roos H P, Renstrom P A 1998 Pain about the groin, hip and pelvis. In: Harries M, Williams C, Stanish W D et al (eds) Oxford textbook of sports medicine. Oxford University Press, Oxford, p 911–924

Rosen P R, Micheli L J, Treves S 1982 Early scintigraphic diagnosis of bone stress and fractures in athletic adolescents. Pediatrics 70:11–15

Salter R B, Harris W R 1963 Injuries involving the epiphyseal plate. Journal of Bone and Joint Surgery (Am) 45A:587–622

Samilson R L, Prieto V 1983 Posterior dislocation of the shoulder in athletes. Clinics in Sports Medicine 2:369–378

Sanders W E, Wilkins K E, Neidre A 1980 Acute insufficiency of the posterior cruciate ligament in children. Journal of Bone and Joint Surgery (Am) 62A:129–131

Schnebel B E 2000 Spine. In: Sullivan J A, Anderson S J (eds) Care of the young athlete. American Academy of Orthopaedics, Oklahoma City, OK, p 129–131

Schneider H J, King A Y, Bronson J L et al 1974 Stress injuries and developmental change of lower extremities in ballet dancers. Radiology 113:627–632

Sella E J, Lawson J P, Ogden J A 1986 The accessory navicular synchondrosis. Clinical Orthopaedics and Related Research 209:280–285

Simmons B P, Lovallo J L 1988 Hand and wrist injuries in children. Clinics in Sports Medicine 7:495–512

Smith D S, Kovan J R, Rich B S et al 1997 In: Preparticipation Physical Evaluation Task Force (eds) Preparticipation physical evaluation, 2nd edn. Monograph published by the Physician and Sportsmedicine, McGraw Hill, New York

Spiegel P G, Cooperman D R, Laros G S 1978 Epiphyseal fractures of the distal ends of the tibia and fibula. Journal of Bone and Joint Surgery (Am) 60A:1046–1050

Stanitski CL 1994a Osteochondritis dissecans of the knee. In: Stanitski C L, DeLee J C, Drez D (eds) Pediatric and adolescent sports medicine. WB Saunders, Philadelphia, PA, p 387–405

Stanitski C L 1994b Meniscal lesions. In: Stanitski C L, DeLee J C, Drez D (eds) Pediatric and adolescent sports medicine. WB Saunders, Philadelphia, PA, p 371–386

Steiner M E, Grana W A 1988 The young athlete's knee: recent advances. Clinics in Sports Medicine 7:527–546

Stover C N 1980 Air stirrup management of ankle injuries in the athlete. American Journal of Sports Medicine 8:360–365

Sullivan J A 1994 Ankle and foot injuries in the pediatric athlete. In: Stanitski C L, DeLee J C, Drez D (eds) Pediatric and adolescent sports medicine. WB Saunders, Philadelphia, PA, p 441–455

Tanner S M 1998 The young female athlete In: Chan K M, Micheli L J (eds) Sports and children. Human Kinetics, Champaign, IL, p 249–257

Tanzer M, Noiseux N 2004 Osseous abnormalities and early arthritis: The role of hip impingement. Clinical Orthopedics and Related Research 429:170–177

Taunton J E, Robertson L S, Fricker P A 1998 Acute and overuse ankle injuries. In: Harries M, Williams C, Stanish W D et al (eds) Oxford textbook of sports medicine. Oxford University Press, Oxford, p 555–570

Twyman R S, Desai K, Aichroth P M 1991 Osteochondritis dissecans of the knee. Journal of Bone and Joint Surgery (Br) 73B:461–464

Voight M L, Thomson B C 2000 The role of the scapula in the rehabilitation of shoulder injuries. Journal of Athletic Training 35:329–337

Van Mechelen W 1992 Running injuries: a review of the epidemiologic literature. Sports Medicine 14:320–335

Warren M P, Shantha S 2000 The female athlete. Baillière's best practice and research. Clinical Endocrinology and Metabolism 14:37–53

Warren M P, Brooks-Gunn J, Hamilton L H et al 1986 Scoliosis and fractures in young ballet dancers: relation to delayed menarche and secondary amenorrhea. New England Journal of Medicine 314:1348–1353

Wascher D C, Finerman G A 1994 Physeal injuries in young athletes. In: Stanitski C L, DeLee J C, Drez D (eds) Pediatric and adolescent sports medicine. WB Saunders, Philadelphia, PA, p 144–161

Waters P M, Millis M B 1988 Hip and pelvic injuries in the young athlete. Clinics in Sports Medicine 7:513–526

Waters P M, Millis M B 1994 Hip and pelvic injuries in the young athlete. In: Stanitski C L, DeLee J C, Drez D (eds) Pediatric and adolescent sports medicine. WB Saunders, Philadelphia, PA, p 279–293

Wenger D E, Kendell K R, Miner M R et al 2004 Acetabular labral tears rarely occur in the absence of bony abnormalities. Clinical Orthopedics and Related Research 426:145–150

Wong J, Maffulli N 2006 Epidemiology of pediatric knee injuries. In: Micheli L, Kocher M (eds) The pediatric and adolescent knee. Saunders, Philadelphia, PA, p 10–11

Yancey R A, Micheli L J 1994 Thoracolumbar spine injuries in pediatric sports. In: Stanitski C L, DeLee J C, Drez D (eds) Pediatric and adolescent sports medicine. WB Saunders, Philadelphia, PA, p 592–591

Zaricznyj B, Shattuck L J M, Mast T A et al 1980 Sports-related injuries in school-aged children. American Journal of Sports Medicine 8:318–324

Zetaruk M 2000 The young gymnast. Clinics in Sports Medicine 19:757–780

Older exercise participants

26

Jennifer E. Stevens

CHAPTER CONTENTS

Introduction 484

Physiological effects of aging 484

Aging and body function 486

Benefits of exercise throughout the aging process. . . 488

Guidelines for exercise 489

Exercise and chronic illness 493

Summary 495

Introduction

Aging is accompanied by inevitable deterioration of many physiological parameters. Research has sought to prevent the effects of aging and the decline that comes with increasing age. Joint crepitus, muscle atrophy, slowing down, failing eyesight, loss of hearing and thinning hair and skin are a few examples of changes with aging.

From a physiological prime in the third decade of life, changes occur in almost every cell in the body including bones, muscle and soft tissue. These cellular changes affect almost every function. We do not, of course, notice this gradual physiological decline unless we measure it. Athletes know when their performances slip: training becomes more difficult and they have to work harder to maintain their fitness. But most people are unaware of their declining fitness until it begins to affect their everyday life. We can track the decline over years by measuring various physiological parameters, monitoring gross changes using X-ray and magnetic resonance imaging (MRI), and examining the changes at tissue level using microscopy and electron microscopy.

Although there is no single intervention able to prevent age-related deterioration in function, exercise, especially strength training, can help slow some of the inevitable decline (Mazzeo et al 1998). This chapter will outline the effect of age on tissue and function, its influence on physical fitness and wellbeing and how physical activity may help delay some of the effects of aging.

Physiological effects of aging

Understanding the source of age-related declines in the neuromuscular system provides a basis for the goals of rehabilitation aimed at countering these changes. Many impairments in mobility stem from the cumulative effect of physiological changes in bone, muscle, articular cartilage, ligaments and tendons, as well as alterations in the central and peripheral nervous system. By examining the physiological basis for age-related impairments, the mechanisms for successful interventions that slow the progression of age-related changes in the neuromuscular system can be better understood.

Bone and articular cartilage

Bone is an active tissue with constant turnover that relies on a balance between bone resorption and bone formation (see Chapter 5). With increasing age, the balance between these two processes can shift, resulting in greater bone loss than formation. This progressive loss of bone mineral density, which occurs to a greater extent in women, leads to a disruption in the micro-architecture of the bone that makes bone more susceptible to fracture (Kohrt et al 2004). On average, as people get older, they lose almost 1% of bone per year after the age of 35 years (World Health Organization 1994). This is especially difficult for women where there is an increase in bone loss after the menopause of 2–3% per year that may lead to osteoporosis (World Health Organization 1994). Osteoporosis is defined as bone mass density that is ≥2.5 standard deviations below the mean bone density for young adults. Osteoporosis is a silent disease: bone loss often goes unnoticed until an individual experiences a compression fracture, most commonly in the vertebrae or the hips.

Prevention is essential to minimize the amount of bone loss that can occur in older adults, especially since bone loss is not often diagnosed until a fracture occurs (Siris et al 2001). Weightbearing exercise can help prevent or slow the age-related loss of bone mineral density, but exercise must be of sufficient intensity to load the musculoskeletal system adequately to promote an increase in bone mineral density (Kohrt et al 2004).

Articular cartilage also changes with increasing age, and erosion and deformation of articular cartilage can result in osteoarthritis (Felson et al 2000). The primary role of articular cartilage is to protect the ends of bone from forces transmitted at the joints and to provide friction-free surfaces for joints to articulate. With increasing age, degenerative changes affect the ability of articular cartilage to perform this role. Changes in the chondrocytes, collagen fibers and proteoglycans that comprise articular cartilage account for much of the deformation of articular cartilage. Progressive articular cartilage degeneration can eventually cause joint pain, swelling and stiffness, and often profoundly impacts on function.

Ligament and tendon

The majority of research examining age-related changes in connective tissue, such as ligaments and tendons, relies on animal models (Buckwalter 1997). The advantage of using animal models is that more precise measurements of connective tissue can be made, but the disadvantage is that assumptions are made that age-related changes in connective tissue are similar between animals and humans.

The compliance and flexibility of ligaments and tendons decreases with increasing age, such that connective tissue is less able to stretch with large loads. Collagen plays a large role in connective tissue changes because it provides much of the structure and tensile strength to connective tissue (Kjaer 2004). With increasing age, collagen becomes more cross-linked, which results in greater stiffness of ligaments and tendons. Another major component of connective tissue is elastin, which allows tissue to stretch and react to loads (Uitto 1986). Structural and compositional changes in elastin also contribute to an increased stiffness in connective tissue. Decreased water content, secondary to a decrease in the proteoglycan content, adds to the loss of flexibility in the connective tissue of older adults (Buckwalter 1997). The overall result is that injuries of ligaments, tendons and other soft tissues occur more easily because they lose the dynamic ability to respond to loads (Buckwalter 1997, Kjaer 2004) when proper warm-up and stretching routines are not integrated with exercise programs. Regular exercise can mitigate the risk for injury by keeping soft tissue more supple and less susceptible to damage (Menard 1996).

Muscle

Aging is associated with a loss of muscle mass and muscle strength. Cross-sectional and longitudinal studies have documented the loss of muscle mass as a part of the normal aging process (Frontera et al 2000, Metter et al 1999). Muscle mass decreases at a rate of 1% per year in both men and women after the age of 60 years (Evans 1995, Lexell 1995). The changes in muscle mass are the result of a reduction in the total number of muscle fibers and a preferential atrophy of fast, type II muscle fibers, which results in slower muscle contractile properties.

Other age-related morphological changes in muscle include a decreased total number of motor units and a concurrent increased size of the remaining motor units (Vandervoort 2002). Fewer motor units, now larger in size, compromise the precision of force control in older adults. Less precision may affect fine motor skills and may alter an older adult's response to unexpected perturbations.

Nervous system

Changes in the peripheral and central nervous system affect nerve conduction velocity, sensory discrimination, muscle strength and autonomic responses.

Peripheral nervous system

With aging, nerves undergo structural, functional and biochemical changes (Verdu et al 2000). There is a loss of myelinated nerve fibers and a decrease in the size and myelin of the remaining myelinated fibers, both of which contribute to decreased nerve conduction velocities. Increasing age also decreases the ability of nerves to regenerate and reinnervate muscle after injury.

Central nervous system

Deficits in the ability of older adults to activate muscles fully (central activation) may contribute to age-related losses in strength. Some research has found that central activation deficits exist in healthy, older adults (Stevens et al 2001), while other studies have not found deficits (Connelly et al 1999). The discrepancy in findings may be a result of the sensitivity of the techniques used to assess muscle activation deficits.

Aging and body function

Strength

Muscle strength declines with age, although the decline in strength can be delayed by maintaining a physically active lifestyle or accelerated by illness or medication (Hurley & Roth 2000). In general, strength is maintained until the age of 45–50 years, after which, there is a subsequent pronounced decline. After the age of 50 years, muscular strength decreases at a rate of about 1.5–3.0% per year (Porter et al 1995, Vandervoort & McComas 1986). The loss of muscle strength with aging, however, is even greater than the loss of muscle mass. Muscle mass only decreases at the rate of 1% per year in both men and women after the age of 60 years (Evans 1995, Lexell 1995). The greater loss of strength than of muscle mass suggests that factors other than muscle mass (e.g. decreased central activation of muscle) must also account for some age-related muscle weakness (Stackhouse et al 2001, Stevens et al 2001).

Loss of strength may reach a critical level, below which there is a decline in function during tasks of daily living. If the physiological load remains the same but the amount of muscle mass is reduced, a larger percentage of the muscle will need to be recruited to perform a particular task (Chandler et al 1998). For example, an older adult might perceive that climbing a set of stairs is a harder task than it was 10 years ago. Even though individuals report being out of breath at the top of the stairs, their cardiovascular system may be taxed because of diminished lower extremity strength rather than a lack of endurance. Ascending a 6-inch step might require a greater percentage demand of each muscle group than would be required of a younger adult. As a result, it seems reasonable that older adults may report increasing difficulty with performing certain tasks.

Older muscle can be trained with high-intensity strength training programs, and although the inevitable decline in strength cannot be stopped, it is possible to slow the speed of progression and help maintain sufficient strength for daily living (Nadel & DiPietro 1995, Symons et al 2005). Older adults have less muscle tissue, but the remaining muscle tissue responds well to training. Even adults aged 86–96 years had an average increase in quadriceps strength of 174% after 8 weeks of high-intensity strength training (Fiatarone et al 1990). The intensity of strength training was measured as a percentage of an individual's one Repetition Maximum (1 RM). A 1 RM is the maximum amount of weight an individual can lift once, while maintaining proper technique (Evans 1999). In Fiatarone et al's study, subjects performed 3 sets of 8 repetitions at 50% of their 1 RM for the first week of exercise. By the end of the second week, the intensity was increased to 80% of the 1 RM. The 1 RM was remeasured every 2 weeks and weights for strength training were adjusted accordingly.

A similar study in adults, aged 72–98 years, found that strength training of the hip and knee extensors resulted in an average strength gain of 113% (Fiatarone et al 1994). Strength training was performed at 80% of the 1 RM, 3 times a week for 10 weeks. Lower extremity strength gains translated to improved gait velocities and stair-climbing power.

Endurance

There are inevitable changes in endurance capacity with increasing age. Changes in endurance capacity can be attributed to changes in both the cardiovascular system and in muscle energetics.

Cardiovascular system

Cardiovascular fitness, as measured by maximal oxygen consumption (VO_2max), declines with age. Even in elite athletes, an individual decline in cardiovascular fitness with age is evident (Ashworth et al 1994, Brooks et al 1994). On average, VO_2max decreases 4–5.5 ml/min/kg/decade in older men and 2–3.5 ml/min/kg/decade in older women, which translates to around a 12–13% decrease per decade (Holloszy & Kohrt 1995). Even active, lean older adults have a 9% decrease in VO_2max/decade and master athletes (who maintain a very vigorous activity level) have a 5% decrease in VO_2max/decade (Holloszy & Kohrt 1995).

The age-related declines in cardiovascular function occur largely because of a decrease in maximal heart rate (HR), although other changes in the cardiovascular system contribute as well (Bouvier et al 2001, Whaley 2006). Maximal HR can be calculated using the following formula: HR max = 220 − age. This formula only provides a crude calculation of maximal HR because it may underestimate maximal HR by ~10 bpm (Guccione 2000). Regardless of the exact decrement in HR, if HR decreases and the size of the chambers of the heart remain the same, there has to be a reduction in the maximum flow (cardiac output). In fact, cardiac output has been shown to decrease by 2–30% (Menard 1996). Reduced cardiac output limits endurance capacity because the older heart has to work harder in response to a given workload (Astrand & Rodahl 1977).

Other age-related changes in the cardiovascular system include an increase in the total peripheral vascular resistance (Hankey et al 2006, Nichols 2005). This occurs largely because of a decrease in arterial wall elasticity and an increase in the accumulation of fatty deposits on the vessel walls. The result is higher blood pressure with increasing age.

Age-related changes in hormone regulation may also affect cardiovascular performance, in particular, the HR (Guccione 2000). The release of adrenaline (epinephrine) and noradrenaline (norepinephrine) is less during exercise in older adults compared to younger adults. Changes in the release of these catecholamines may, in part, explain the decreases in HR with increasing age. Additional age-related changes to the cardiovascular system may affect endurance, but the majority of evidence indicates that the reduction in pump efficiency (i.e. HR) is arguably the most important (McArdle et al 2006).

Although regular exercise cannot completely counter all the changes in the cardiovascular system with increasing age, there is ample evidence to suggest that exercise attenuates the progression of some of the age-related changes. In particular, older adults still retain the ability to increase VO$_2$max with prolonged endurance exercise to the same extent as younger adults (Kohrt et al 1991, Mazzeo et al 1998).

Muscle endurance

There is less consensus regarding changes in muscle energetic pathways, but it appears that muscle endurance in older, healthy muscle is comparable to that of younger muscle (Guccione 2000, Stevens et al 2001). When healthy, older adults participate in voluntary and electrically elicited isokinetic or isometric fatigue protocols, there are no differences in the rate of fatigue compared to younger adults (Stevens et al 2001). Although the absolute strength of older adults is less, the rate of fatigue is comparable to that of younger adults. Most of these studies have been performed in healthy adults, so it is possible that the findings may not be generalized to all older adult populations.

Flexibility

Soft tissues require greater effort with increasing age to maintain the same degree of mobility and flexibility that is present in younger adults (Buckwalter 1997, Chen et al 2005), yet there are few studies that have explored interventions to improve flexibility in older adults (Mazzeo et al 1998). The small number of studies that have focused on improving flexibility with exercise are somewhat inconclusive because they have not systematically determined a dose–response relationship for flexibility training (Mazzeo et al 1998). Yet there is no question that older adults would benefit from increased flexibility; the question is how to effectively increase flexibility. Most studies have indirectly focused on flexibility by enrolling older adults in regular exercise programs and monitoring changes in range of motion (Mazzeo et al 1998). At least from these studies, we can conclude that exercise offers one possibility for increasing flexibility in older adults, but more research is necessary to design interventions specifically intended to improve flexibility.

Mobility and balance

Balance is impaired with increasing age secondary to a variety of changes in strength and postural control. Increasing age is accompanied by changes in the vestibular ocular reflex, increased joint stiffness, decreased tissue flexibility, increased static sway, a greater number of steps necessary to respond to a perturbation and an increased cocontraction of antagonist muscle groups (Guccione 2000). In addition, older adults have slower postural responses (20–30 ms delay), which may be caused by a slower processing of sensory information, combined with a decrease in nerve conduction velocity (Studenski et al 1991).

The combination of these sensorimotor changes and decreased muscle strength predisposes older adults to an increased risk of falling. In fact, falls are a major cause of morbidity and mortality in adults over the age of 65 years and often result in hospitalization (Rose & Maffulli 1999). Even falls that do not lead to injury have profound consequences because as little as one fall may encourage an older adult to avoid situations that may increase the risk of falling (Sattin et al 2005). Yet, decreasing the exposure to falls does not necessarily result in fewer falls (Gregg et al 2000). The tendency for older adults to avoid activities that put them at risk perpetuates the inability to respond appropriately to an impending fall. Consequently, a fear of falling may promote social isolation and greater dependence.

One of the most devastating consequences of falling is a hip fracture, which almost always necessitates hospitalization. Research indicates that a 50-year-old Caucasian female has a 17% risk of sustaining a hip fracture during her remaining lifetime (Rose & Maffulli 1999). After the age of 50 years, the risk of sustaining a hip fracture has been estimated to double every 5 years. By the age of 90, 1 in 4 women and 1 in 8 men will have had a hip fracture (Rose & Maffulli 1999). A third of patients who sustain a hip fracture die within a year of the fracture. Of patients who live past the first year, only 66% return home after a hip fracture (Rose & Maffulli 1999). Unfortunately, the total number of hip fractures in older adults is increasing each year because of a growing proportion of older adults in the population (Rose & Maffulli 1999, Wehren & Magaziner 2003).

In addition to the sensorimotor changes that impair balance in older adults, other factors also partially account for the incidence of falls each year. Muscle weakness, especially of the knee and ankle, is significantly related to recurrent falls in older adults (Whipple et al 1987). In addition, medications that cause sedation or affect vestibular function can result in dizziness and potentially a fall. Environmental factors can also contribute to an increased risk of falling because environmental hazards, like carpets, increase this risk (Campbell et al 2005).

Prevention has been shown to be the most important factor in reducing the incidence of falls. In addition to carefully monitoring medication use, physical activity plays a very important role in decreasing fall risk (Campbell et al 2005, Gregg et al 2000). O'Loughlin et al (1993) suggested that those who remain active can maintain balance, flexibility, reflexes, muscle strength, coordination and appropriate reaction times required to avoid imbalance. Paradoxically, physical activity increases exposure to falls, and yet physical activity is related to a decreased risk of falls.

Exercise interventions for older adults often involve a multifaceted approach that makes it difficult to identify the specific components of each program that contribute to a decreased fall risk. Nevertheless, there is evidence that exercise interventions that incorporate balance and lower extremity strength training appear to be most effective in decreasing the risk of falls (Campbell et al 2005, Gregg et al 2000). In a major US study (Province et al 1995), older people who took part in an exercise intervention were 10% less likely to fall. People who followed an individualized exercise program that included resistance, flexibility, and balance training, reduced their risk of falling. The greatest benefit was found with exercise programs that had a balance retraining component and, in particular, those that included Tai Chi (discussed later in this chapter) (Sattin et al 2005, Wolfson et al 1996).

Other studies have also shown positive results for reducing fall risk with exercise programs. Tinetti et al (1994) demonstrated that patients who participated in an intervention with medication monitoring, patient education, and exercise prescription had 31% fewer falls than with those who did not receive the intervention. Similarly, a randomized controlled trial of home safety modifications compared to an exercise program for strength and balance retraining in participants over 75 years old showed that both programs were effective in reducing the rate of falls (Campbell et al 2005).

Epidemiological studies of physical activity in older adults

Epidemiological studies around the world give us some indication of the levels of physical fitness of the general population. It is difficult to make direct comparisons because studies use different instruments and criteria, but some general observations can be made. The American College of Sports Medicine (ACSM), in their Position Stand on exercise and physical activity for older adults (Mazzeo et al 1998), emphasized how participation in a regular exercise program is an effective means of reducing some of the functional decline associated with aging.

Recently, it was reported that the prevalence of leisure-time physical inactivity declined in older adults in 2004 compared to 1994 (Trends in Leisure-Time Physical Inactivity by Age, Sex, and Race/Ethnicity: CDC 2004). Still, only 10% of those over the age of 65 years engage in vigorous activity in the USA (Elward & Larson 1992) and only 36% engage in moderate intensity activities, such as walking 30 minutes per day for 5 days of the week (Centers for Disease Control and Prevention 2003). Studies from the UK also showed that a large proportion of older adults are relatively inactive, and more importantly, have poor physical fitness (Allied Dunbar National Fitness Survey 1992, MacAuley et al 1994). Comparative data from Australia show a similar pattern to that of the UK and US studies; a national cardiovascular risk factor study in 1991 classified 32% of respondents as inactive, 54% as moderately active and 15% as aerobic (Bauman & Owen 1991). A further study by the same group showed that those who were inactive were more likely to be older, less well educated, and to have lower incomes (Owen & Bauman 1992). In a more recent study, Booth et al (2000) found that more males than females in Australia were physically active and that physical activity participation was related to age. Specifically, a greater proportion of those aged 65–69 were active than those aged 60–64 or 70 years or older. The factors most associated with being active were high self-efficacy, regular participation in exercise with friends and family, finding footpaths safe for walking, and access to local facilities (Booth et al 2000). A Canadian study also found that the proportion of people who exercise decreases with increasing age, such that 20% of adults ages 65–74 exercise and only 6% of adults older than 84 years of age exercised (Rockwood et al 2004).

Benefits of exercise throughout the aging process

In light of the plethora of changes in physical functioning associated with aging, exercise becomes increasingly important with advancing age. The effects of exercise on strength, balance and endurance are key factors in reducing falls, minimizing ill health and maintaining independence (Gill et al 1995). When physical activity is promoted to those in their older years, it is often done so as to improve physical fitness in order to maintain functional independence (Wagner 1997) or to enhance already existing levels of athletic performance. The main objectives of exercise for older adults are to improve strength, agility and cardiovascular fitness by promoting physiological adaptations to exercise (Guccione 2000, Mazzeo et al 1998, Tipton 2006).

If physical fitness can be maintained, even if we do not prolong life, we may theoretically delay 'dependency'. Delaying and shortening the time period of illness and dependency is an interesting concept that has been called the 'compression of morbidity' (Fries 1998, Vita et al 1998). Similarly, the Medical Research Council Topic Review on the elderly uses the term 'Healthy Active Life Expectancy' (HALE) with the emphasis on extending the active period within one's life rather than the actual duration of life (Medical Research Council 1994).

Strength training in older adults has a myriad of benefits, aside from the most obvious one: increasing muscle strength. Strength training improves insulin action, increases bone density, helps maintain metabolically active tissue mass, decreases blood pressure, reduces body fat, decreases pain from arthritis, increases levels of physical activity, improves the quality of sleep, enhances functional performance and decreases the risk of falls (Borst 2004, Brill et al 1995, Mazzeo et al 1998, Taylor et al 2004). Being older, inactive or unfit is not a contraindication to strength training and age is no barrier (Fiatarone et al 1990).

Endurance training enhances cardiovascular function. In particular, aerobic exercise promotes an increase in VO_2max and cardiac output (Coudert & Van Praagh 2000, McArdle et al 2006). The degree of increase depends on the baseline level of fitness and the intensity of training. Endurance exercise is also associated with lower blood pressure, improved plasma lipoprotein profiles, and decreased overall percentage of body fat. Endurance training especially benefits individuals with poor glucose tolerance or insulin sensitivity, as aerobic exercise improves both (Borghouts & Keizer 2000, Ryan 2000).

Balance training improves postural stability and decreases the risk of falls (Maffulli et al 2001, Province et al 1995, Sherrington et al 2004). Balance training also reduces the fear of falling, which encourages older adults to increase their physical activity levels (Sattin et al 2005, Wolf et al 1996). Tai Chi has recently become one of the most popular and effective means of enhancing balance.

Physical activity also has a positive effect on psychological wellbeing in older adults. Physical activity improves depression in older adults, although the mechanism for the improvement is not yet understood (Barbour & Blumenthal 2005, Butler et al 1998, Tsutsumi et al 1997). In a randomized clinical trial involving progressive resistance strength training, 14 of 16 initially depressed individuals were no longer clinically depressed at the end of a 10-week strength training program. Interestingly, the intensity of strength training was related to the degree of improvement in depression scores. Tsutsumi et al (1997) also found strength training programs improved psychological status. Training was performed three times a week for 12 weeks and included either high (75–85% 1 RM) or low intensity (55–65% 1 RM) strength training. For both training intensities, there were improvements in mood, anxiety and perceived confidence for physical capability, compared to controls. In addition, exercise appears to have a positive impact on the cognitive status of older adults (Heyn et al 2004).

Guidelines for exercise

Assessing risks of exercise participation in older adults

As people get older, they are more likely to experience chronic medical conditions where vigorous exercise requires more supervision (Guccione 2000, Mazzeo et al 1998). Although the contraindications for exercise and the warning signs to cease exercising are the same for younger and older adults (Boxes 26.1 and 26.2), the likelihood of experiencing health-related problems during exercise increases with advancing age. All older adults should seek medical advice before commencing an exercise program, but whether they need to undergo extensive pre-exercise testing is more controversial. The American College of Sports Medicine (Evans 1999, Whaley 2006) recommends an exercise stress test for anyone over the age of 50 years who wants to initiate a vigorous exercise program, and anyone who has a history of ischemic heart disease, angina, diabetes or hypertension. Others contend that adults over the age of 50 years who do not have significant cardiovascular disease risk factors may not necessitate a stress test. In fact, among 14 studies that used high-intensity strength training programs for older adults, only three included exercise stress tests in the prescreening (American Geriatrics Society Panel on Exercise and Osteoarthritis 2001). Alternatives to physician-supervised stress tests may be appropriate for many relatively healthy older adults who wish to initiate an exercise program (Evans 1999). Evans (1999) proposed a weightlifting stress test where patients perform 3 sets of 8 repetitions at around 80% 1 RM. Meanwhile, electrocardiographic (ECG) and blood pressure measurements are used to gauge responses to exercise.

There are aspects of a medical history that may indicate risks of falling and particular care needed for physical activity participation. For example, if a patient lost consciousness on a previous fall, they may have an underlying medical condition (Puisieux et al 2000). Prescribed drugs should be reviewed, and lying and standing blood pressure measured. Simple tests of balance and muscle strength can be important but a history

of previous falls is consistently the strongest risk factor for further falls (Bloem et al 2001).

Increased risks with exercise and medications

Older adults have a two- to threefold greater risk of experiencing an adverse drug reaction than younger adults (Nolan & O'Malley 1988). Older adults not only ingest a larger number of drugs, but they also have an altered response to drugs (Naranjo et al 1995, Tsujimoto et al 1989) and this can therefore affect exercise tolerance. Medications can affect older adults differently than younger adults because of changes in drug distribution to tissues, drug metabolism and drug excretion (Guccione 2000, Naranjo et al 1995). Those taking medication should consult their physician, particularly those taking medication for hypertension, diabetes or any heart condition.

Some medications used for blood pressure regulation and cardiac disease management can adversely affect activity tolerance (Brukner & Khan 2001, Guccione 2000) (Table 26.1). With congestive heart failure, medications are frequently used to increase the strength of myocardial contraction and also affect heart rate (HR) (e.g. digitalis and beta blockers). With

---

Box 26.1 Contraindications to exercise in older adults

Absolute contraindications
- Acute myocardial infarction
- Unstable angina
- Uncontrolled arrhythmias
- Third degree heart block
- Acute congestive heart failure

Relative contraindications
- Uncontrolled blood pressure
- Cardiomyopathy
- Valvular heart disease
- Uncontrolled metabolic disease

Box 26.2 Warning signs to stop exercise in older adults

- Chest pain – always stop exercise with chest pain. Heart-related chest pain is usually described as a tightness or weight in the central chest, often radiating to the neck or left arm. If in doubt, stop exercising and seek help
- Palpitations – if the heart rate is excessive or irregular
- Feeling of weakness, pale, clammy, fainting
- Dizziness or light-headedness – this may simply be due to exercise intensity, but if there is an associated risk of falling, cease exercise
- Other reasons to stop exercising include sickness, nausea, vomiting, becoming short of breath or wheezy

Table 26.1 Possible drug side effects with exercise

Drug	Primary intended use	Possible side effects with exercise
Cardiovascular drugs		
Beta blockers	↓ HR	Hypotension Greater fatigue HR is not a good indicator of exercise intensity
Digitalis	↑ contraction force of heart ↓ HR	Cardiac arrhythmias, gastrointestinal symptoms, confusion, sedation and blurred vision with digitalis toxicity
ACE inhibitors	↓ BP	Hypotension
Diuretics	↓ fluid volume ↓ HR	Hypotension Confusion, mood changes, weakness and fatigue with extreme fluid and electrolyte imbalance
Psychotropic drugs		
Sedative-hypnotic	Improve sleep	Drowsiness, sluggishness
Anti-anxiety	↓ anxiety	Sedation
Antidepressants	Treat depression	Sedation and confusion
Antipsychotics	Normalize behavior and treat mental illness	Sedation Extrapyramidal symptoms
Drugs for pain and inflammation		
Glucocorticoids	Reduce inflammation	With prolonged use: Ligament or tendon rupture Muscle strain Osteoporotic bone fracture
Non-opiate analgesics (NSAIDs and acetominophen)	Reduce pain and inflammation	Minimal side effects with exercise
Opiate analgesics	Reduce severe pain	Sedation Mood changes Gastrointestinal problems Confusion
Drugs for diabetes		
Insulin or hypoglycemic drugs	Control blood sugar levels	Headaches, dizziness, confusion, sweating, fatigue or nausea from hypoglycemia

both hypertension and congestive heart failure, medications are used to decrease fluid volume and vascular resistance (e.g. angiotensin converting enzyme (ACE) inhibitors and diuretics). Each of these medications can alter responses to exercise (Guccione 2000). For example, one effect of beta blockers is to reduce resting HR and stabilize the HR, which interferes with the normal HR response to exercise. This means that patients taking beta blockers may have more difficulty with exercise and may fatigue easily. Those taking beta blockers should be aware that HR will no longer be an adequate guide to exercise intensity, and that perceived exertion is a more relevant indication of intensity than HR (Table 26.1). Patients with cardiac conditions may also be taking diuretics to reduce fluid volume in order to decrease cardiac workload. Usually, diuretics do not affect exercise tolerance unless there is significantly altered fluid and electrolyte balance. Warning signs include confusion, mood changes, weakness and fatigue. In these situations, electrolyte balance should be carefully monitored. Additionally, ACE inhibitors can also affect electrolyte levels and they decrease cardiac workload because they decrease peripheral vascular resistance by decreasing the formation of angiotensin II, a potent vasoconstrictor. One of the most important side effects of many drugs used to improve cardiovascular per-for-mance is postural hypotension, especially when standing suddenly or initiating exercise.

Psychotropic drugs have been associated with a greater risk of falling in a growing number of studies (Campbell et al 1999, Leipzig et al 1999, Salgado et al 2004, Schwab et al 2000). These medications include agents that affect mood, behavior or cognition and can be described as sedative-hypnotic agents, antianxiety agents, antidepressants, antipsychotics and anti-convulsants (Guccione 2000, Leipzig et al 1999, Naranjo et al 1995) (Table 26.1). All of these drugs can alter alertness and perceptions and contribute to an increased risk of falls. In particular, the sedative-hypnotic agents that are often used to treat sleep disorders can be the most dangerous for falling (Guccione 2000). They produce drowsiness and sluggishness in the morning, which can predispose an individual to a greater risk of falling, especially with exercise. For this reason, individuals taking sedative-hypnotic agents should exercise in the afternoon when they are alert, or use shorter acting alternatives. Antidepressants can also be associated with sedation and even confusion, as can antianxiety and antipsychotic drugs, although not as often (Guccione 2000, Leipzig et al 1999).

Medication for pain and inflammation remains a focal point of research because of the growing number of older adults who are afflicted with arthritis. There are three main classes of drugs used to treat pain and inflammation: opioid analgesics, non-opioid analgesics and glucocorticoids (Fine 2001, Guccione 2000) (Table 26.1). Opioid analgesics are narcotics that are used to treat severe pain (Fine 2001). Side effects that can affect exercise include sedation, mood changes and gastrointestinal problems. Non-opioid analgesics include non-steroidal anti-inflammatory drugs (NSAIDs) and acetaminophen and do not typically interfere with exercise, but, rather, may enhance the ability of individuals to carry out an exercise program. Finally, glucocorticoids are steroids that effectively reduce inflammation, but they do so at the expense of catabolic effects on the body. Prolonged use of glucocorticoids may contribute to gradual breakdown of bones, ligaments, tendons, skin and muscle. This is especially important during exercise because an individual may have a greater risk of rupturing a tendon or ligament, developing a muscle strain, or suffering from an osteoporotic fracture.

Older adults with diabetes may take hypoglycemic drugs or insulin to control blood sugar levels (Rosenstock 2001) (Table 26.1). These drugs may cause blood glucose levels to drop too much, resulting in hypoglycemia. Warning signs may include headaches, dizziness, confusion, fatigue, nausea and sweating. Hypoglycemia is most likely to manifest itself when older adults increase their activity level or initiate exercise programs without monitoring their blood sugars appropriately.

General exercise guidance for the older person

In general, exercise-training principles are the same in older and younger athletes (Evans 1999, Mazzeo et al 1998, Whaley 2006). The most effective training involves structured, goal-directed exercise regimens. It is important to establish why an older person wishes to exercise and what level of exercise they seek to advance towards, in order to design an exercise program to meet their needs. Some older adults may have decided to become active and attend a specific exercise class and others may already be active, but seek to improve their peak physical performance. Other older adults may have participated in athletic activities throughout their lives, but now find it increasingly difficult to maintain their previous level of physical performance. With all older adults, it is important to discuss the importance of strength, balance, and cardiovascular fitness, with evidence for why each is essential for minimizing long-term health problems. Although information should be presented in a way that will not intimidate older adults who may have just begun to think about exercise, follow-up discussions should soon be aimed at increasing the intensity of exercise.

Routinely, older adults underestimate their exercise capacity for fear of injury from excessively increasing the intensity of exercise. Patient education regarding the proven safety of higher intensity levels of physical activity, after proper warm-up and stretching, is imperative (Fig. 26.1). Warm-up should include a low-intensity activity that slowly increases the HR (Guccione 2000). For example, activities such as walking and swimming should begin with a slower-paced warm-up, with a gradual increase in the intensity of activity during the first 5–10 min of exercise. Once the tissues and joints have been warmed-up, stretching should be initiated. Stretching should avoid ballistic or jerky movements that can cause injury. Instead, each stretch should be performed to the point of mild discomfort, but not pain, and held for 10–30 s (Pollock et al 1998). Each stretch should be performed at least twice. Older adult athletes may have been able to skip warm-ups and stretching when they were younger, but tissue changes with advancing age necessitate the inclusion of proper warm-up and stretching in order to minimize injury. A cool-down phase at the end of an exercise session is equally important because if one stops exercising suddenly, there may be a sudden drop in blood pressure, or arrhythmia, with dizziness, fainting and a fall (Mazzeo et al 1998).

Many older adults are able to successfully engage in higher level athletic activities, such as running, tennis or skiing without significant limitations (Maffulli et al 2001). Many of these individuals have been active all their lives, but now require modification of existing exercise programs to continue to engage in high-level athletic activities. Cross-training is one such modification that offers advantages because it reduces the risk of overuse injury, prevents boredom and conditions a greater variety of muscles (Guccione 2000). Individuals who have pain with high-level activities, such as running or tennis, may find that swimming offers some relief by minimizing joint impact. A program that alternates between swimming and walking or tennis offers

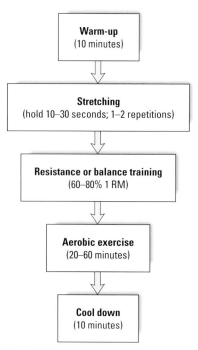

Figure 26.1 • Recommended exercise progression.

an ideal combination because of the preservation of bone density with weightbearing exercise, while minimizing repeated stress to lower extremity joints (O'Grady et al 2000).

Adherence to exercise programs can be increased by encouraging older adults to join a local fitness center where they can interact with other adults who are engaged in comparable activities. By making exercise a social activity, older adults are much more likely to continue to exercise (Kirkby et al 1999). Alternatively, a spouse or 'exercise buddy' can be equally effective in encouraging compliance with a regular exercise program.

Strength training principles

A common misconception regarding the intensity of strength training with older adults is that the training intensity should be less than that used for younger adults, especially for frail older adults. In fact, a growing body of literature advocates the use of high-intensity strength training (above 60% of 1 RM), 3 times a week, for active older adults, as well as frail older adults (Brill et al 1995, Evans 1999, Fiatarone et al 1990, Whaley 2006) (Box 26.3). Injury with high-intensity strength training is not common, and several studies have demonstrated that high-intensity strength training can be performed safely when adequate warm-up and stretching are incorporated into an exercise program (Brill et al 1995, Evans 1999, Fiatarone et al 1990, Whaley 2006). Exercise with elastic bands or tubing, light weights, light manual resistance or against body weight is not likely to result in strength gains for the majority of older adults. For example, asking a healthy older adult to perform a sitting knee extension exercise with a 5 lb cuff weight is not likely to overload the quadriceps muscle sufficiently to promote hypertrophy of the muscle.

Box 26.3 Resistance training exercise guidelines for older adults

Goal:	Increase muscle strength
Frequency:	3 days per week
Intensity:	60–80% of 1 RM[a]
Sets/repetitions:	3 sets of 8 to 12 repetitions[b]
Rest between sets:	60 s

[a] Weight should produce fatigue by the last repetition in each set. 1 RM is the greatest amount of weight that can be lifted one time with proper form. If an individual's 1 RM was 10 lb with biceps curls, then exercise should be initiated with 6 lb (60% of 1 RM) and progressed to 8 lb within the first week of strength training.
[b] More than 12 repetitions will not increase strength, but rather endurance. If an individual can perform more than 12 repetitions, the weight should be increased if increasing muscle strength is the goal.

With any high-intensity strength training program, some muscle soreness is inevitable (McArdle et al 2006). Patients must be informed that they should expect muscle soreness 24–48 h after exercise, especially when initiating new exercises. Adherence to any exercise program is related to an understanding of what to expect, and unexplained muscle soreness may discourage older adults from complying with their prescribed exercise regimen.

If time does not permit measurement of an individual's 1 RM, a general rule of thumb can be substituted to facilitate adequate overload of muscle: at the end of each set of 8–12 repetitions of an exercise (maintaining proper form), an individual should feel fatigued to the point they cannot perform another repetition (Mazzeo et al 1998). At least 1 min of rest should separate each set of 8–10 repetitions. Ideally, 2 to 3 sets of each exercise should be performed (Fig. 26.2).

Endurance training principles

Aerobic exercise should follow strength and balance training (Mazzeo et al 1998) and can include activities such as walking, bicycling, swimming, dancing, rowing and playing tennis. Aerobic exercise should be performed 3–5 days per week for 20–60 min each day, at an intensity of 55–65% of the estimated maximum HR (Mazzeo et al 1998) (Box 26.4). This is a level of exercise that should leave an individual slightly out of breath, but still able to carry on a conversation. Another means of quantifying exercise intensity is with a rating of perceived exertion (RPE), which correlates well with exercise HRs and work rates (Guccione 2000, Whaley 2006) (Table 26.2). The RPE is also known as the Borg scale and it allows individuals to subjectively rate their level of exertion with exercise. It is especially useful for individuals who cannot depend on HR monitoring, secondary to a heart transplant or medications that artificially control HR (Guccione 2000).

Balance training – Tai Chi

In recent years, Tai Chi has been shown to be an effective, low-cost means of improving balance and functional status in older adults (Province et al 1995, Sattin et al 2005, Wolf et al 1996).

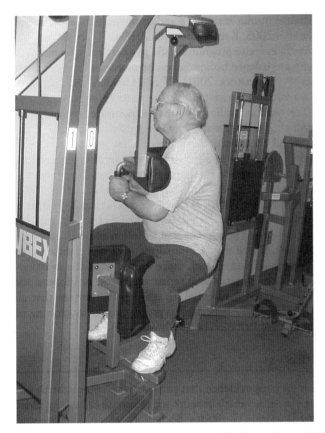

Figure 26.2 • High-intensity strength training has been shown to be safe and effective for older adults.

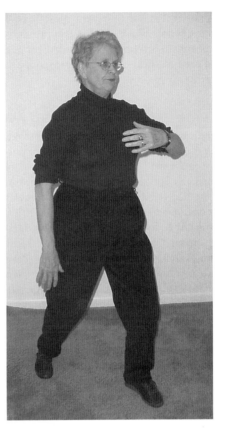

Figure 26.3 • Tai Chi has become an increasingly popular form of balance training for older adults.

Box 26.4 Aerobic exercise guidelines for older adults

Goal:	Increase cardiovascular fitness
Frequency:	3–5 days per week
Mode:	Walking, cycling, swimming, rowing, dancing
Duration:	20–60 min
Intensity:	55–65% of HR max

Table 26.2 Relationships among methods of quantifying exercise intensity during endurance exercise

Relative intensity		Rating of perceived exertion	Classification of intensity
HR max (%)	VO$_2$max (%)		
<3.5	<30	<10	Very light
35–59	30–49	10–11	Light
60–79	50–74	12–13	Somewhat hard
80–89	75–84	14–16	Hard
>89	>84	>16	Very hard

When combined with a strength training program, it offers tremendous benefits for older adults of various levels of physical health (Wolfson et al 1996). Tai Chi is a martial art that developed in China and it combines a series of postures and slow movements with deep breathing and meditation. It has been shown to improve balance, to lower blood pressure and to give older adults an overall sense of wellbeing (Mazzeo et al 1998). A study conducted by Wolf et al (1996) found that older people taking part in a 15-week Tai Chi program reduced their risk of multiple falls by 47.5%. Subjects also demonstrated a reduction in their fear of falling with Tai Chi (Sattin et al 2005).

Tai Chi conditions individuals to move more slowly through an enhanced body awareness, which is one of the biggest reasons why it may successfully reduce fall risk in older adults (Fig. 26.3). The movements of Tai Chi are less jarring than those of a low-impact exercise class, so patients with arthritis may benefit tremendously from Tai Chi. Tai Chi classes can be found at health clubs, martial arts schools, hospitals and community centers. Video instruction is also available, but hands-on instruction is invaluable for maximizing the potential of Tai Chi.

Exercise and chronic illness

Patients with chronic illness often avoid exercise for fear of making their condition worse or overexerting themselves, yet these patients are the ones that stand to benefit most from a regular exercise program. Chronic illness is not a contraindication to exercise when adequate attention is provided for the medical management of each medical condition in response to exercise (Mazzeo et al 1998).

Cardiac disease

Exercise is not contraindicated in cardiac disease, but rather, exercise is an integral part of both primary and secondary prevention of future cardiac problems (Ades 1999, Lavie & Milani 1996, Volaklis & Tokamakidis 2005). Patients with a previous myocardial infarction, cardiac failure, valve disease, irregular heart rhythm or angina can benefit from exercise (Ades 1999, Lavie & Milani 1996, Volaklis & Tokamakidis 2005). The decision to exercise is often precipitated by a cardiac event. Most patients now undergo an exercise stress test before they leave the hospital, following a myocardial infarction, and are given guidance on the appropriate level of exercise. The main principle of exercise programs in such patients is to train the peripheral muscles effectively without producing great cardiovascular stress (Bjarnason-Wehrens et al 2004, Volaklis & Tokamakidis 2005). To accomplish this goal, new modes of training use dynamic resistance training, based on the principles of interval training. Patients perform dynamic strength exercises slowly, at an intensity usually in the range of 50–60% of one repetition maximum.

Exercise intensity may be restricted by angina, but those with angina may exercise within the limits of their symptoms (Bjarnason-Wehrens et al 2004, DeGroot et al 1998). For some, this may mean walking only short distances on level ground, but most individuals should be able to engage in regular exercise. Anti-angina medication, usually in the form of a spray or sublingual medication, should be used in advance of exercise and patients should carry their medication with them while exercising.

Hypertension

Aerobic and resistance training are not only safe for individuals with high blood pressure, they also help reduce resting systolic and diastolic blood pressure (Dickey & Janick 2001, Ehsani 2001, Hurley & Roth 2000). Although some health professionals are reluctant to prescribe resistance training for individuals with elevated blood pressure, when a proper technique is used, strength training does not result in substantial increases in systolic blood pressure (Evans 1999). In particular, patients should be cautioned not to hold their breath during any phase of weight training. Patients should be instructed to inhale before lifting a weight, exhale when lifting the weight, and inhale as they lower the weight (Evans 1999, Whaley 2006). Even moderate aerobic activity that helps to control blood pressure can be an important part of medical management of hypertension (Ehsani 2001, Hurley & Roth 2000).

Diabetes mellitus

Exercise is particularly indicated for the medical management of non-insulin-dependent diabetes mellitus because exercise can increase insulin sensitivity and improve glucose tolerance (Ibanez et al 2005, Katz & Lowenthal 1994). Diabetic patients initiating an exercise program should pay particular attention to their glucose balance because exercise increases the utilization of glucose (Rosenstock 2001). If an individual with diabetes exercises without understanding the need to increase glucose intake, or reduce insulin, they may experience hypoglycemia (Rosenstock 2001). Patients who inject insulin should be especially careful about injection sites. If they inject insulin into a muscle, blood flow will increase with exercise, giving more rapid insulin absorption and hypoglycemia.

Foot care is also very important in diabetic patients who exercise (Springett 2000). If there is neurological impairment, there may be some loss of sensation in the feet so that patients may be unaware of blisters, or skin irritation and cause damage to their feet. There may be impairment of the circulation to both large blood vessels and, more importantly, the microcirculation which inhibits tissue repair and recovery (Rosenstock 2001). Prevention is essential, so it is very important that all diabetic patients are educated regarding proper monitoring of feet for signs of irritation or skin breakdown.

Arthritis

There is growing evidence that patients with osteoarthritis can achieve the same health benefits with exercise as healthy, older adults (American Geriatrics Society Panel on Exercise and Osteoarthritis 2001, Mazzeo et al 1998, O'Grady et al 2000), yet patients with advanced osteoarthritis should seek medical advice before initiating an unsupervised exercise program. Many older adults with osteoarthritis are afraid to exercise for fear of exacerbating their arthritis, yet randomized clinical trials have found that exercise training does not exacerbate pain or accelerate disease progression (American Geriatrics Society Panel on Exercise and Osteoarthritis 2001). In fact, exercise improves mobility, reduces pain and improves function in patients with arthritis (Fisher et al 1991). Although exercise may not actually slow the pathological disease process of osteoarthritis, many benefits are still conferred with exercise in arthritic patients (O'Grady et al 2000). Exercise may increase muscle strength and decrease the stress at arthritic joints, which may explain the decreased arthritic pain and improved function in arthritic patients who initiate an exercise program. In addition, weight loss from regular exercise also decreases the stress at lower extremity joints afflicted with arthritis. Of course, the same general health benefits of exercise seen in healthy, older adults are also conferred to patients with arthritis.

An exercise program for patients with osteoarthritis should emphasize options that minimize excessive compression of arthritic joints, while promoting strength gains and endurance (O'Grady et al 2000). Such activities include, but are not limited to, bicycling, swimming, dance, water aerobics, walking, Tai Chi and rowing. Cross-training is advocated in any older adult population, but in particular, patients with arthritis benefit the most from alternating different forms of exercise in order to vary the compressive forces across their joints.

The intensity and mode of exercise should be determined by how much pain they feel with the activity.

Exercise prescription for resistance training requires creativity for patients with arthritis. Patients with arthritis may not be able to perform resistance training at the same intensities as non-arthritic patients, if severe joint pain limits them, but every attempt should be made to experiment with various resistance exercises to find those that allow patients to maximize their strength gains (O'Grady et al 2000). For example, patients may have knee pain with a closed chain, leg press activity performed at 60% of their 1 RM, but when they perform an open chain sitting knee extension exercise, they may be able to surpass 60% of their 1 RM and achieve higher training intensities. Alternatively, patients may be able to perform exercises pain-free throughout their entire range of motion, but strength gains can still be achieved with exercise through partial ranges of motion (Evans 1999).

Patient education is essential for adherence to any long-term exercise program (O'Grady et al 2000). Patients with arthritis should be aware that physical performance and arthritic symptoms may vary from day to day. They should also understand that the warning signs for excessive exercise include joint pain for more than 1–2 h after exercise, swelling and excessive fatigue. Patients should limit their exercise if their joints become acutely inflamed, until the inflammation returns to baseline. Exercise may be most comfortable in the afternoon, as morning stiffness and pain are common features of osteoarthritis.

In addition to resistance and aerobic exercise, patients with arthritis should understand the importance of stretching and joint mobilization to maintain their range of motion, since the persistent joint swelling and stiffness that accompany arthritis can lead to a progressive loss of joint range of motion (O'Grady et al 2000). Treatment aimed at restoring joint range of motion should begin in conjunction with resistance and aerobic exercise programs.

Peripheral vascular disease

Exercise has been shown to be of value in people with peripheral vascular disease (Ciaccia 1993, Hankey et al 2006, Tan et al 2000). Long-standing atherosclerosis may result in narrowing of the main arteries, and in particular those providing blood supply to the lower limbs. When exercise raises the oxygen needs of the muscle, but the arteries are unable to supply sufficient oxygen-rich blood, muscles become painful. With rest, the muscles recover. This occurs most often in the calf muscles and can cause problems when someone undertakes an exercise program (Creager 2001). Evidence exists that exercise itself can help in this condition (Tan et al 2000). With exercise there may be minor changes in the blood vessels, but more importantly, the muscles become more efficient and patients can tolerate a greater level of exercise (Tan et al 2000). Those with peripheral vascular disease are encouraged to exercise but within the level of comfort. For example, it is better to walk slowly for a longer distance than to set off too fast and have to stop because of muscle pain.

Osteoporosis

Older women should be especially aware of the risks associated with osteoporosis (see Chapters 5 and 27). Depending on the severity of the osteoporosis, many individuals with osteoporosis can still engage in high-intensity strength training. Extreme care must be taken to perform all exercises with proper postural alignment to minimize the risk of fractures. In particular, individuals should avoid exercises that put excess pressure on the spine (Hertel & Trahiotis 2001). Some individuals may have such severe osteoporosis that even daily activities put them at risk for fracture, which makes strength training contraindicated with severe osteoporosis.

Weightbearing exercise plays an important role in increasing bone mass. Even brisk walking for 30 min a day, 3 times a week, has been found to increase bone density in older women (Hatori et al 1993). Other studies have shown that exercise training (endurance and strength) combined with ongoing hormone replacement therapy increases bone mineral density in physically frail elderly women (Villareal et al 2003).

Summary

Exercise mitigates the physical deterioration that occurs with increasing age, yet many older adults engage in little to no physical activity. As our population ages worldwide, more attention must be directed towards encouraging older adults to exercise regularly to prevent many health-related problems.

Exercise programs must combine strength, endurance and balance training to optimally protect older adults from developing functional deficits. A common misconception is that exercise interventions for older adults should be performed at lower intensities. Until recently, high-intensity strength training was often avoided for fear of injury. Now, research indicates it is one of the most important parts of an exercise program. Numerous studies have safely carried out high-intensity strength training programs with even the oldest of adults, and have produced substantial strength gains. Not only does strength training improve muscle strength, it also decreases risk of falling and improves functional performance.

Exercise is one of the most effective ways to reduce the chances of falling, which is a major cause of morbidity in older adults. Exercise that improves balance and coordination (e.g. Tai Chi) has received increasing popularity, as increasing evidence indicates that the health benefits from Tai Chi are numerous. Although more recent attention has been focused on strength and balance training, the cardiovascular benefits of regular aerobic exercise cannot be overlooked.

Older adults with chronic medical conditions often avoid exercise, yet these adults are the most likely to benefit from a regular exercise program. Health professionals must educate all older adults regarding the importance of exercise and physical activity and attempt to counter the perception that certain patient populations should avoid exercise.

References

Ades P A 1999 Introduction: the elderly in cardiac rehabilitation. American Journal of Geriatric Cardiology 8:61–62

Allied Dunbar National Fitness Survey 1992 Activity and health research. Health Education Authority and Sports Council, London

American Geriatrics Society Panel on Exercise and Osteoarthritis 2001 Exercise prescription for older adults with osteoarthritis pain: consensus practice recommendations. A supplement to the AGS Clinical Practice Guidelines on the management of chronic pain in older adults. Journal of the American Geriatric Society 49:808–823

Ashworth J B, Reuben D V, Benton L A 1994 Functional profiles of healthy elder persons. Age and Ageing 23:34

Astrand P-O, Rodahl K 1977 Textbook of work physiology. McGraw Hill, New York

Barbour K A, Blumenthal J A 2005 Exercise training and depression in older adults. Neurobiology of Aging 26 (suppl 1):119–1123

Bauman A, Owen N 1991 Habitual physical activity and cardiovascular risk factors. Medical Journal of Australia 154:22–28

Bjarnason-Wehrens B, Mayer-Berger W, Meister E R et al 2004 Recommendations for resistance exercise in cardiac rehabilitation. Recommendations of the German Federation for Cardiovascular Prevention and Rehabilitation. European Journal of Cardiovascular Prevention and Rehabilitation 11:352–361

Bloem B R, Boers I, Cramer M et al 2001 Falls in the elderly. I. Identification of risk factors. Wiener Klinische Wochenschrift 113(10):352–362

Booth M L, Owen N, Bauman A et al 2000 Social-cognitive and perceived environment influences associated with physical activity in older Australians. Preventive Medicine 31:15–22

Borghouts L B, Keizer H A 2000 Exercise and insulin sensitivity: a review. International Journal of Sports Medicine 21:1–12.

Borst S E 2004 Interventions for sarcopenia and muscle weakness in older people. Age and Ageing 33:548–555

Bouvier F, Saltin B, Nejat M et al 2001 Left ventricular function and perfusion in elderly endurance athletes. Medicine and Science in Sports and Exercise 33:735–740

Brill P A, Drimmer A M, Morgan L A et al 1995 The feasibility of conducting strength and flexibility programs for elderly nursing home residents with dementia. Gerontologist 35:263–266

Brooks S V, Larsson L, Woledge R et al 1994 Impairments in the structure and function of skeletal muscle with aging. Medicine and Science in Sports and Exercise 26:S27

Brukner P, Khan K 2001 Clinical sports medicine, 2nd edn. McGraw Hill, Sydney, p 702–703

Buckwalter J A 1997 Maintaining and restoring mobility in middle and old age: the importance of the soft tissues. Instructional Course Lectures 46:459–469

Butler R N, Davis R, Lewis C B et al 1998 Physical fitness: benefits of exercise for the older patient: 2. Geriatrics 53:46, 49–52, 61–62

Campbell A J, Robertson M C, Gardner M M et al 1999 Psychotropic medication withdrawal and a home-based exercise program to prevent falls: a randomised controlled trial. Journal of the American Geriatric Society 47:850–853

Campbell A J, Robertson M C, La Grow S J et al 2005 Randomised controlled trial of prevention of falls in people aged > or =75 with severe visual impairment: the VIP trial. British Medical Journal 331:817

Centers for Disease Control and Prevention: US Physical Activity Statistics, 2001–2003 State physical activity comparisons by demographic group. Retrieved from http://www.cdc.gov/nccdphp/dnpa/physical/stats/index.htm

Chandler J M, Duncan P W, Kochersberger G et al 1998 Is lower extremity strength gain associated with improvement in physical performance and disability in frail, community-dwelling elders? Archives of Physical Medicine and Rehabilitation 79:24–30

Chen A L, Mears S C, Hawkins R J 2005 Orthopaedic care of the aging athlete. Journal of the American Academy of Orthopaedic Surgeons 13:407–416

Ciaccia J M 1993 Benefits of a structured peripheral arterial vascular rehabilitation program. Journal of Vascular Nursing 11:1–4

Connelly D M, Rice C L, Roos M R et al 1999 Motor unit firing rates and contractile properties in tibialis anterior of young and old men. Journal of Applied Physiology 87:843–852

Coudert J, Van Praagh E 2000 Endurance exercise training in the elderly: effects on cardiovascular function. Current Opinion in Clinical Nutrition and Metabolic Care 3:479–483

Creager M A 2001 Medical management of peripheral arterial disease. Cardiology in Review 9:238–245

DeGroot D W, Quinn T J, Kertzer R et al 1998 Circuit weight training in cardiac patients: determining optimal workloads for safety and energy expenditure. Journal of Cardiopulmonary Rehabilitation 18:145–152

Dickey R A, Janick J J 2001 Lifestyle modifications in the prevention and treatment of hypertension. Endocrine Practice 7:392–399

Ehsani A A 2001 Exercise in patients with hypertension. American Journal of Geriatric Cardiology 10:253–259, 273

Elward K, Larson E B 1992 Benefits of exercise for older adults: a review of existing evidence and current recommendations for the general population. Clinics in Geriatric Medicine 8:35–50

Evans W J 1995 What is sarcopenia? Journal of Gerontology SOA (special issue):S8

Evans W J 1999 Exercise training guidelines for the elderly. Medicine and Science in Sports and Exercise 31:12–17

Felson D T, Lawrence R C, Dieppe P A et al 2000 Osteoarthritis – new insights: 1: The disease and its risk factors. Annals of Internal Medicine 133:635–646

Fiatarone M A, Marks E C, Ryan N D et al 1990 High intensity strength training in nonagenarians: effects on skeletal muscle. Journal of the American Medical Association 263:3029–3034

Fiatarone M A, O'Neill E F, Ryan N D et al 1994 Exercise training and nutritional supplementation for physical frailty in very elderly people. New England Journal of Medicine 330:1769–1775

Fine P G 2001 Opioid analgesic drugs in older people. Clinics in Geriatric Medicine 7:479–487

Fisher N M, Pendergast D R, Gresham G E et al 1991 Muscle rehabilitation: its effect of muscular and functional performance of patients with knee osteoarthritis. Archives of Physical Medicine and Rehabilitation 72:367–374

Fries J P 1998 Reducing cumulative lifetime disability: the compression of morbidity. British Journal of Sports Medicine 32:193

Frontera W R, Hughes V A, Fielding R A et al 2000 Aging of skeletal muscle: a 12-yr longitudinal study. Journal of Applied Physiology 88:1321–1326

Gill T M, Williams C S, Tinetti M E 1995 Assessing risk for the onset of functional dependence among older adults: the role of physical performance. Journal of the American Geriatric Society 43:603–609

Gregg E W, Pereira M A, Caspersen C J 2000 Physical activity, falls, and fractures among older adults: a review of the epidemiologic evidence. Journal of the American Geriatric Society 48:883–893

Guccione A A 2000 Geriatric physical therapy, 2nd edn. Mosby, St Louis, MO

Hankey G J, Norman P E, Eikelboom J W 2006 Medical treatment of peripheral arterial disease. Journal of the American Medical Association 295:547–553

Hatori M, Hasegawa A, Adachi H et al 1993 The effects of walking at the anaerobic threshold level on vertebral bone loss in postmenopausal women. Calcified Tissue International 52:411–414

Hertel K L, Trahiotis M G 2001 Exercise in the prevention and treatment of osteoporosis. Nursing Clinics of North America 36:441–453

Heyn P, Abreu B C, Ottenbacher K J 2004 The effects of exercise training on elderly persons with cognitive impairment and dementia: a meta-analysis. Archives of Physical Medicine and Rehabilitation 85:1694–1704

Holloszy J O, Kohrt W M 1995 Exercise. In: Masoro E J (ed) Handbook of physiology: aging. University Press, Oxford, p 633–658

Hurley B F, Roth S 2000 Strength training in the elderly: effects of risk factors for age-related diseases. Sports Medicine 30:249–268

Ibanez J, Izquierdo M, Arguelles I et al 2005 Twice-weekly progressive resistance training decreases abdominal fat and improves insulin sensitivity in older men with type 2 diabetes. Diabetes Care 28:662–667

Katz M S, Lowenthal D T 1994 Influences of age and exercise on glucose metabolism: implications for management of older diabetics. Southern Medical Journal 87:S70–73

Kirkby R J, Kolt G S, Habel K et al 1999 Exercise in older women: motives for participation. Australian Psychologist 34:122–127

Kjaer M 2004 Role of extracellular matrix in adaptation of tendon and skeletal muscle to mechanical loading. Physiological Review 84:649–698

Kohrt W M, Malley M T, Coggan A R et al 1991 Effects of gender, age, and fitness level on response of VO_2max to training in 60–71 year olds. Journal of Applied Physiology 71:2004–2011

Kohrt W M, Bloomfield S A, Little K D et al 2004 American College of Sports Medicine Position Stand: physical activity and bone health. Medicine and Science in Sports and Exercise 36:1985–1996

Lavie C J, Milani R V 1996 Effects of nonpharmacologic therapy with cardiac rehabilitation and exercise training in patients with low levels of high-density lipoprotein cholesterol. American Journal of Cardiology 78:1286–1289

Leipzig R M, Cumming R G, Tinetti M E 1999 Drugs and falls in older people – a systematic review and meta-analysis: I. Psychotropic drugs. Journal of the American Geriatric Society 47:30–39

Lexell J 1995 Human aging, muscle mass, and fiber type composition. Journal of Gerontology Series A 50A:11–16

McArdle W D, Katch F I, Katch V L 2006 Essentials of exercise physiology. 3rd edn. Lippincott Williams & Wilkins, Baltimore, MD

MacAuley D, McCrum E E, Stott G et al 1994 The Northern Ireland health and activity survey. Her Majesty's Stationery Office, London

Maffulli N, Chan K M, Macdonald R et al 2001 Sports medicine for specific ages and abilities. Churchill Livingstone, Edinburgh

Mazzeo R S, Cavanagh P, Evans W J et al 1998 American College of Sports Medicine Position Stand: exercise and physical activity for older adults. Medicine and Science in Sports and Exercise 30:992–1008

Medical Research Council 1994 The health of the UK's elderly people. Medical Research Council, London

Menard D 1996 The aging athlete. In: Harries M, Williams C, Stanish W D et al (eds) Oxford textbook of sports medicine. Oxford University Press, Oxford, p 596–620

Metter E J, Lynch N, Conwit R et al 1999 Muscle quality and age: cross-sectional and longitudinal comparisons. Journals of Gerontology. Series A, Biological Sciences and Medical Sciences 54:B207–218

Nadel E R, DiPietro L 1995 Effects of physical activity on functional ability in older people: translating basic science findings into practical knowledge. Medicine and Science in Sports and Exercise 25:S36

Naranjo C A, Herrmann N, Mittmann N et al 1995 Recent advances in geriatric psychopharmacology. Drugs and Aging 7:184–202

Nichols W W 2005 Clinical measurement of arterial stiffness obtained from noninvasive pressure waveforms. American Journal of Hypertension 18(1 Pt 2):3S–10S

Nolan L, O'Malley K 1988 Prescribing for the elderly: I. Sensitivity of the elderly to adverse drug reactions. Journal of the American Geriatric Society 36:142–149

O'Grady M, Fletcher J, Ortiz S 2000 Therapeutic and physical fitness exercise prescription for older adults with joint disease. Rheumatic Disease Clinics of North America 26:617–646

O'Loughlin J L, Robitaille Y, Boivin J F et al 1993 Incidence and risk factors for falls and injurious falls among the community dwelling elderly. American Journal of Epidemiology 137:342–354

Owen N, Bauman A 1992 The descriptive epidemiology of a sedentary lifestyle in adult Australians. International Journal of Epidemiology 21:305–310

Pollock M L, Gaesser G A, Butcher J D et al 1998 The recommended quantity and quality of exercise for developing and maintaining cardiorespiratory and muscular fitness, and flexibility in healthy adults. Medicine and Science in Sports and Exercise 30:975–991

Porter M M, Vandervoort A A, Lexell J 1995 Aging of human muscle: structure, function and adaptability. Scandinavian Journal of Medicine and Science in Sports 5:129–142

Province M A, Hadley E C, Hornbrook M C et al 1995 The effects of exercise on falls in elderly patients. A pre planned meta-analysis of the FICSIT trials. Journal of the American Medical Association 273:1341–1347

Puisieux F, Bulckaen H, Fauchais A L et al 2000 Ambulatory blood pressure monitoring and postprandial hypotension in elderly persons with falls or syncopes. Journals of Gerontology. Series A, Biological Sciences and Medical Sciences 55:M535–540

Rockwood K, Howlett S E, MacKnight C et al 2004 Prevalence, attributes, and outcomes of fitness and frailty in community-dwelling older adults: report from the Canadian study of health and aging. Journals of Gerontology. Series A, Biological Sciences and Medical Sciences 59:1310–1317

Rose S, Maffulli N 1999 Hip fractures. An epidemiological review. Bulletin (Hospital for Joint Diseases) 58:197–201

Rosenstock J 2001 Management of type 2 diabetes mellitus in the elderly: special considerations. Drugs and Aging 18:31–44

Ryan A S 2000 Insulin resistance with aging: effects of diet and exercise. Sports Medicine 30:327–346

Salgado R I, Lord S R, Ehrlich F et al 2004 Predictors of falling in elderly hospital patients. Archives of Gerontology and Geriatrics 38:213–219

Sattin R W, Easley K A, Wolf S L et al 2005 Reduction in fear of falling through intense tai chi exercise training in older, transitionally frail adults. Journal of the American Geriatric Society 53:1168–1178

Schwab M, Roder F, Aleker T et al 2000 Psychotropic drug use, falls and hip fracture in the elderly. Aging (Milan) 12:234–239

Sherrington C, Lord S R, Finch C F 2004 Physical activity interventions to prevent falls among older people: update of the evidence. Journal of Science and Medicine in Sport 7 (1 suppl):43–51

Siris E S, Miller P D, Barrett-Connor E et al 2001 Identification and fracture outcomes of undiagnosed low bone mineral density in post-menopausal women: results from the national osteoporosis risk assessment. Journal of the American Medical Association 286:2815–2822

Springett K 2000 Foot ulceration in diabetic patients. Nursing Standard 14:65–68, 70–71

Stackhouse S K, Stevens J E, Pearce K M et al 2001 Maximum voluntary activation in fresh and fatigued muscle of young and elder individuals. Physical Therapy 81:1102–1109

Stevens J E, Binder-Macleod S, Snyder-Mackler L 2001 Characterization of the human quadriceps muscle in active elders. Archives of Physical Medicine and Rehabilitation 82:973–978

Studenski S A, Duncan P W, Chandler J M 1991 Postural responses and effector factors in persons with unexplained falls: results and methodologic issues. Journal of the American Geriatric Society 39:229–234

Symons T B, Vandervoort A A, Rice C L et al 2005 Effects of maximal isometric and isokinetic resistance training on strength and functional mobility in older adults. Journals of Gerontology. Series A, Biological Sciences and Medical Sciences 60:777–781

Tan K H, De Cossart L, Edwards P R 2000 Exercise training and peripheral vascular disease. British Journal of Surgery 87:553–562

Taylor A H, Cable N T, Faulkner G et al 2004 Physical activity and older adults: a review of health benefits and the effectiveness of interventions. Journal of Sport Sciences 22:703–725

Tinetti M E, Baker D I, McAvay G et al 1994 A multifactorial intervention to reduce the risk of falling among elderly people living in the community. New England Journal of Medicine 331:821–827

Tipton C M 2006 ACSM's advanced exercise physiology. Lippincott Williams and Wilkins, Philadelphia, PA

Tsujimoto G, Hashimoto K, Hoffman B B 1989 Pharmacokinetic and pharmacodynamic principles of drug therapy in old age. International Journal of Clinical Pharmacology, Therapy, and Toxicology 27:13–26

Tsutsumi T, Don B M, Zaichkowsky L D et al 1997 Physical fitness and psychological benefits of strength training in community dwelling older adults. Applied Human Science 16:257–266

Uitto J 1986 Connective tissue biochemistry of the aging dermis. Age-related alterations in collagen and elastin. Dermatologic Clinics 4:433–446

Vandervoort A A 2002 Aging of the human neuromuscular system. Muscle and Nerve 25:17–25

Vandervoort M, McComas A J 1986 Contractile changes in opposing muscles of the human ankle joint with aging. Journal of Applied Physiology 61:361–367

Verdu E, Ceballos D, Vilches J J et al 2000 Influence of aging on peripheral nerve function and regeneration. Journal of the Peripheral Nervous System 5:191–208

Villareal D T, Binder E F, Yarasheski K E et al 2003 Effects of exercise training added to ongoing hormone replacement therapy on bone mineral density in frail elderly women. Journal of the American Geriatric Society 51:985–990

Vita A J, Terry R B, Hubert H B et al 1998 Aging, health risks and cumulative disability. New England Journal of Medicine 338:1035–1041

Volaklis K A, Tokmakidis S P 2005 Resistance exercise training in patients with heart failure. Sports Medicine 35:1085–1103

Wagner E H 1997 The effect of strength and endurance training on gait, balance, fall risk and health services use in community living adults. Journal of Gerontology 52:M218–224

Wehren L E, Magaziner J 2003 Hip fracture: risk factors and outcomes. Current Osteoporosis Reports 1:78–85

Whaley M H 2006 ACSM's Guidelines for exercise testing and prescription. 7th edn. Lippincott Williams & Wilkins, Philadelphia, PA

Whipple R, Wolfson L, Amerman P 1987 The relationship of knee and ankle weakness to falls in nursing home residents. An isokinetic study. Journal of the American Geriatric Society 35:13–20

Wolf S L, Barnhart H X, Kutner N G et al 1996 Reducing frailty and falls in older persons: an investigation of Tai Chi and computerized balance training. Atlanta FICSIT Group. Frailty and injuries: cooperative studies of intervention techniques. Journal of the American Geriatric Society 44:489–497

Wolfson L, Whipple R, Derby C 1996 Balance and strength training in older adults: intervention gains and Tai Chi maintenance. Journal of the American Geriatric Society 44:498–506

World Health Organization 1994 Assessment of fracture risk and its application to screening for osteoporosis. Technical services report 843. World Health Organization, Geneva

The active female

Amanda Weiss-Kelly and Martin Kilbane

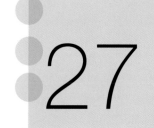

CHAPTER CONTENTS

Introduction 499

Anatomical and physiological considerations
for athletic women. 499

Oral contraceptive use and performance 503

Menstrual cycle phase and performance 503

The female athlete triad 503

Pregnancy and exercise. 512

Summary 516

Introduction

The role of women in sport has changed dramatically over the last century. Forbidden from participation in the first modern Olympic Games in 1896, over 4000 women participated in the 2004 Olympic Games in Athens and women made up 41% of the competitors at these games.

Historically, women were discouraged from participation in physical activity for fear that exertion would harm the reproductive system and because it was not felt to be feminine (Lutter 1994). More recently, the growing realization of the significant health and social benefits that sport and exercise has for girls and women has led physicians, physical therapists and parents to encourage girls to participate in sports. Girls who play sport are less likely to become pregnant during their adolescent years, smoke or experience depression than their non-athletic counterparts (Aaron et al 1996, Colton & Gore 1991, Women's Sports Foundation Report 1998). Furthermore, females involved in sports participation are more likely to graduate from high school and college (National Collegiate Athletic Association 1997, Wilson Report 1989).

As the number of girls and women participating in sport rises, it becomes increasingly important to understand the health effects and benefits that exercise has for women (Fig. 27.1).

Anatomical and physiological considerations for athletic women

Height and weight

Females are, in general, both shorter and lighter than males. For example, mature women are 13 cm shorter and 18–22 kg lighter than men (Ebben & Jensen 1998). Women also have a larger surface area to mass ratio than men (Wells 1985). When exercising in a warm dry environment, this may offer an advantage for women; however, it may also allow for increased heat loss during exercise in a cold environment (Sanborn & Jankowski 1994).

Body composition

On average, women have 8–10% more body fat than men (Chardoukian & Joyner 2004, Sanborn & Jankowski 1994). This higher proportion of body fat could adversely affect

With resistance training, women experience similar relative gains in strength as men (Cureton et al 1988, Lemmer et al 2000). In addition, during periods of detraining, women maintain strength gains as well as men do (Lemmer et al 2000). Strength training can offer significant health and performance benefits for women. For example, when added to aerobic training activities, resistance training has been shown to improve aerobic capacity beyond that found with aerobic training alone (Kraemer et al 2001). This combination of activities can also decrease the percentage of body fat and improve work economy, both of which may enhance performance (Ebben & Jensen 1998, Hoff et al 1999, Stone et al 2001, Wilmore 1983). Since connective tissue strength is enhanced with resistance training, such exercise could help prevent injury during other activities (Ebben & Jensen 1998, Fleck & Falkel 1986, Lehnhard et al 1996, Stone et al 2001). Resistance training can also lead to increased bone density at the sites of mechanical loading, improving overall bone health (Ayalon et al 1987, Ebben & Jensen 1998, Marcus et al 1992, Snow-Harter et al 1992). Improvements in strength have been shown to reduce the physiological stresses encountered during daily activities that require strength, allowing trained women to perform such activities more easily (Ebben & Jensen 1998, Stone et al 2001). In aging women, this is especially important since strength gains made from training may improve functional mobility and allow for longer independent living (Ramsbottom 2004). Finally, aside from physiological changes, women who participate in strength training have also reported an improvement in self-esteem and confidence (Ebben & Jensen 1998).

Investigators have also demonstrated that women tend to demonstrate less muscle tightness than men. There is significant disagreement in the literature, however, about whether or not this increased flexibility can help prevent injury. Two recent reviews of both the clinical and basic science literature concluded that there was not sufficient evidence to state that stretching or flexibility significantly influenced risk for injury (Thacker 2004, Shrier 1999).

Aerobic performance

Maximal aerobic power is measured as VO_2max. VO_2max is considered to be the best measure of an athlete's cardiovascular fitness (Wells 1985). Before puberty, boys and girls have similar VO_2max. After puberty, however, women have 40–60% lower VO_2max than men (Eisenmann et al 2001). When VO_2max is expressed relative to body mass, the difference is decreased to 20–30% (Charkoudian 2004, Eisenmann et al 2001). Furthermore, when VO_2max is expressed relative to fat free mass, the difference is reduced to only 8–10% (Sady & Freedson 1984). Thus, body composition (specifically the amount of fat-free mass) is important in explaining much of the difference in VO_2max between genders. This means that the higher fat content of females will place them at a disadvantage in weightbearing aerobic activities where VO_2max plays an important role in performance (Berg 1984). In an early study, Cureton & Sparling (1980) simulated the effect of the

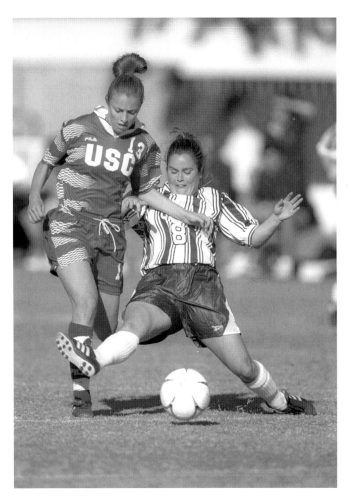

Figure 27.1 • Female soccer players. (Reproduced with the permission of UCLA Athletic Department.)

the performance of women during weightbearing activities (O'Toole & Douglas 1994). Excess fat increases the energy cost of activities like running, cycling and cross-country skiing (Fahey 1994). Contrary to this, however, increased body fat can enhance swimming performance since it adds buoyancy that raises female swimmers out of the water and decreases drag (Mirkin 1994, Sanborn & Jankowski 1994).

Muscle tissue

Until the onset of puberty, girls exhibit about 90% of the muscular strength of boys. By the age of 15–16 years, girls have 75% of the strength of boys and mature women have about 67% of the strength of men (Beim & Stone 1995, Komi 1992, Sanborn & Jankowski 1994). These strength differences are more pronounced for upper body strength than lower body strength (Stone et al 2001, Wells 1985). Despite these strength differences, the muscle composition of men and women is similar, with each having the same relative proportion of fast and slow twitch fibers (Cureton et al 1988).

increased body fat load with which women exercise by having a group of men exercise with external weights. This decreased the men's VO_2max and the differences in VO_2max between men and women were reduced to insignificant levels. This further illustrates the importance that the increased body fat found in women plays in the maximal aerobic power attainable by female athletes.

Differences in oxygen transport and oxygen carrying capacity also help to explain the gender difference in VO_2max. Cardiac output, stroke volume, blood volume, hemoglobin and hematocrit all contribute to an individual's ability to transport oxygen to the body. Women have both smaller heart and stroke volumes than men, resulting in lower maximal cardiac outputs (Sanborn & Jankowski 1994). Women also have lower blood volumes and concentrations of hemoglobin and hematocrit than men, which limits their oxygen carrying capacity (Charkoudian 2004, Green et al 1999, Sanborn & Jankowski 1994, Wiebe et al 1998). With training, women of all ages experience increases in VO_2max which are comparable to men undergoing similar training regimens (Charkoudian 2004).

Anaerobic power

Anaerobic activities are those performed at a high intensity for a short duration. Lactic acid is produced during the anaerobic breakdown of glucose and glycogen (Wells 1985). Lactic acid concentrations reflect the degree of anaerobic metabolism occurring (Nattiv et al 2001). The concentrations of lactic acid found in the blood during anaerobic activities are determined by lactic acid production from anaerobic breakdown of glucose and glycogen, and lactic acid removal from oxidation (Wells 1985). The lactate threshold is defined as the level of exercise needed to produce blood lactate levels above 4 mM (Wells 1985). Exercise beyond the lactate threshold is difficult, secondary to fatigue (Wells 1985).

In females, the lactate threshold is reached at a lower absolute workload than in males (Helgerud 1994, Wells 1985). These differences in lactate threshold between men and women, however, are insignificant when expressed as a percentage of VO_2max (Helgerud 1994, Wells 1985). Also, when comparing well-trained athletes, there is less absolute difference in anaerobic threshold between men and women. Scaling anaerobic power for body mass also reduces the differences in anaerobic power between men and women (Weber et al 2006). Thus, the difference in anaerobic threshold between men and women is less than initially believed (Serresse et al 1989).

Heat tolerance

The findings of several investigations suggested that women were less tolerant of heat stress than men (Shephard 2000, Wells 1985). However, in these studies, the female subjects were not as physically fit as the males (Griffin 1994, Wells 1985). When men and women exercise at the same relative intensity, it has been shown that they tolerate heat equally well (Stephenson & Kolka 1993, Wells 1985). In temperatures

higher than body temperature, women may be at a small disadvantage compared to men, since their higher surface to mass ratio will allow women to gain heat by convection faster than men (Shephard 2000, Wells 1985). The more current literature indicates that level of fitness and acclimatization are more important than gender in terms of heat tolerance (Shephard 2000, Wells 1985). Women acclimatize to exercise in warm environments as well as men (Nunneley 1979, Shapiro 1980, Frye 1983, Keatisuwan 1996).

Skeletal considerations

Women have a different lower extremity alignment to men. For example, their wider pelvis and increased femoral anteversion result in higher Q angles in women. Although increased Q angles have been implicated as a predisposing factor for patellofemoral pain, a clear consensus on the importance of the Q angle in patellofemoral pain has not been established (Baker & Juhn 2000). The role of the Q angle has been questioned because Q angle values have not been found to vary significantly between symptomatic and asymptomatic subjects. Also, there are wide variations in Q angles with significant overlap between values found in men and women (Baker & Juhn 2000). See Chapter 22 for a complete discussion of patellofemoral pain.

Women have also been found to have a narrower femoral notch, increased genu valgum and external tibial torsion compared to men (Ireland 1994) (Fig. 27.2). The importance of these factors in terms of predisposition to injury, however, has not been established.

Injury rates

Many military studies have indicated that female recruits suffer injuries 2–4 times more often than male recruits (Bensel & Kish 1983, Jones et al 1996, Knapik et al 2001, Neely 1998, Ross & Woodward 1994, Yates & White 2004). However, a recent study indicated that when aerobic fitness is controlled for, the difference in injury rate between men and women is not significant (Canada et al 2003). In another study, female recruits were found to be more likely to voluntarily report injuries and when unreported injuries from male recruits were accounted for, injury rates were not significantly different (Almeida et al 1999). The civilian literature is less clear, with some studies indicating that women are more likely to incur musculoskeletal injuries than men (Gilchrist et al 2000, Powell & Barber-Foss 2000, Roberts 2000), while others reported no difference (McHugh et al 2006, Sallis et al 2001) or fewer injuries in female athletes (Knowles et al 2004, Stevenson et al 2000).

Despite the fact that overall injury risk is probably not much greater in women than men, it has become clear that the risk for anterior cruciate ligament (ACL) injury is much greater in female athletes (Arendt & Dick 1995, Malone et al 1993, Zelisko et al 1982). Several theories have been posed to explain the increased incidence of ACL injury in female athletes. Some have suggested that increased levels of estrogen may reduce the strength of the ACL. Some studies have evaluated timing of ACL injuries in

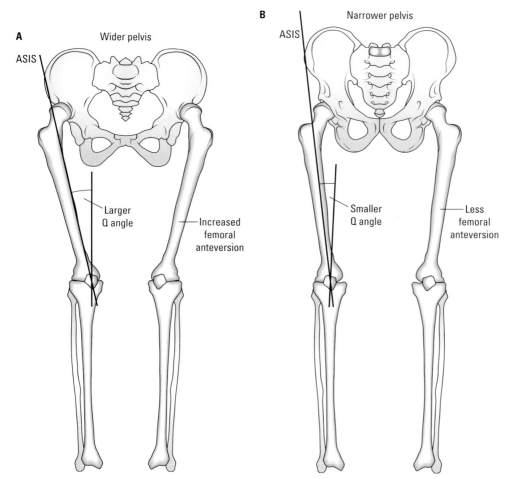

A Wider pelvis

ASIS

Larger
Q angle

Increased
femoral
anteversion

B Narrower pelvis

ASIS

Smaller
Q angle

Less
femoral
anteversion

Figure 27.2 • Women (**A**) have a different lower extremity alignment from men (**B**). A wider pelvis and increased femoral anteversion result in increased Q angles in women compared with men.

relationship to menstrual phase, and no clear relationship has been established; however, the follicular, ovulatory and luteal phases have all been implicated in different studies (Moller-Nielsen & Hammer 1989, Myklebust et al 1998, Slauterbeck et al 2002, Wojtys et al 1998). Other investigators have evaluated the effect of estrogen on ACL laxity and some have found significantly increased laxity at the time of peak estrogen and progesterone concentrations while others have not found significant differences in ACL laxity based on menstrual phase (Belanger et al 2004, Deie et al 2002, Heitz et al 1999). At this point, there is no convincing evidence that any one portion of the menstrual cycle predisposes female athletes to ACL injury, although further studies with improved, more accurate, documentation of menstrual cycle phase may help elucidate the issue.

Another theory is that anatomic factors such as the smaller intercondylar notch found in women may increase the risk for ACL injury. The ACL may become impinged on the medial border of the lateral femoral condyle with valgus stress (Harner et al 1994). The increased Q-angle in women has also been implicated as a predisposing factor for ACL injury in women, with Nisell (1985) noting that quadriceps contractions at knee flexion angles less than 60° place a greater strain on the ACL in women than men.

Finally, a growing body of recent research has focused on neuromuscular elements that may increase ACL injuries in female athletes. Women have been found to land from jumps and pivot with knees in a slightly flexed, valgus position, an unstable position that places the ACL at risk (Hewett et al 1999, Noyes et al 1992). In addition, female athletes tend to rely more on the quadriceps muscle during landing, have weaker hamstrings and take longer to generate peak hamstring muscle torque on landing (Ahmad et al 2006, Hewett et al 1996, Huston & Wojtys 1996). Since the hamstrings are important in stabilizing the knee joint, weaker hamstrings and slow hamstring activation may increase ACL injury risk (Baratta et al 1988, More et al 1993, Tibone et al 1986). Several groups have undertaken plyometric training programs to teach proper landing technique and maximize hamstring strength and function. These programs have successfully decreased ACL injuries by up to 74% in the trained group compared to the untrained athletes (Hewett et al 1999, Mandelbaum et al 2005). In addition, significant improvements in speed and vertical jump height have been documented with plyometric training programs, making these programs beneficial from an injury prevention and performance enhancement perspective (Hewett et al 1996).

Oral contraceptive use and performance

Athletes often choose to use oral contraceptive pills (OCP) to prevent pregnancy, regulate menstrual cycles or decrease premenstrual symptoms. Since use by athletes is rising, interest in the potential effect of OCP on performance has increased (Bennell et al 1999).

Some beneficial effects have been noted. Since OCP use can decrease menstrual blood loss significantly, the risk of iron deficiency anemia is decreased for women using OCP (Bennell et al 1999). As iron deficiency anemia and possibly even decreased iron stores have been shown to adversely affect performance, this is an important benefit (Friedmann et al 2001, Hinton et al 2000, Nattiv et al 2001). Also, the OCP allows athletes to manipulate their menstrual cycle around competition.

Some investigators have found that OCP use has negative effects on VO_2max. In an early study Daggett et al (1983) found an 11% decrease in VO_2max with OCP use. After discontinuation of OCP, VO_2max returned to previous levels. In a prospective study of trained women, Notelovitz et al (1987) found a 7% decrease in VO_2max in the group using OCP, while controls demonstrated a slight increase in VO_2max over the study period. Again, VO_2max returned to normal with discontinuation of the OCP. More recently, Lebrun et al (2003) performed a double blind placebo controlled trial evaluating the effects of a tri-phasic OCP on aerobic capacity and found that women taking the OCP had small decreases in aerobic capacity while women in the placebo group actually had a small improvement in VO_2max (Lebrun et al 2003). Cassaza et al (2002) also found that OCP use increased body weight and fat mass and decreased VO_2max. Other investigators have failed to demonstrate any change in VO_2max with OCP use (Bryner et al 1996, Frankovich & Lebrun 2000, Lynch & Nimmo 1998). Thus, the effects of OCP use on VO_2max and aerobic performance are not clear.

Menstrual cycle phase and performance

The potential effects that the cyclical endogenous hormonal variations associated with the menstrual cycle may have on performance have been a topic of great interest for female athletes. The increased level of progesterone during the luteal phase of the menstrual cycle has been associated with increased minute ventilation at rest and with increased hypoxic and hypercapnic respiratory drives (Brutsaert et al 2002, Dombovy et al 1987). This has led to speculation that performance may be decreased during the luteal phase (Dombovy et al 1987).

Some investigators have found changes in athletic performance with different menstrual phases. Nicklas et al (1989) and Jurkowski et al (1978) studied trained women and found small but significant improvements in endurance during the luteal phase. Contrary to this, Williams & Krahenbuhl (1997) found that running economy during the luteal phase was decreased at 85% VO_2max, but not at 55% VO_2max. Lebrun et al (1995) found a small, statistically insignificant, decrease in VO_2max during the luteal phase. No significant differences in aerobic endurance or maximum minute ventilation were noted, despite the change in VO_2max. Furthermore, Schoene et al (1981) found that untrained women had significant decreases in maximal exercise performance during the luteal phase.

Many other investigators have failed to demonstrate any difference in performance during the phases of the menstrual cycle. In a study of eight untrained women, Dombovy et al (1987) failed to find any difference in VO_2max, perceived exertion or maximal workload during the luteal or follicular phase. De Souza et al (1990) included amenorrheic and eumenorrheic athletes in their investigation of the effects of menstrual phase and amenorrhea on exercise performance. No differences were found between early follicular and midluteal phases, or among amenorrheic and eumenorrheic athletes for VO_2max, maximum minute ventilation, maximum heart rate or perceived exertion (De Souza et al 1990). More recently, Beidleman et al (1999) investigated the effects of menstrual cycle phase on minute ventilation and physical performance at altitude and at sea level. Neither of these factors was affected by menstrual cycle phase at sea level or high altitude (Beidleman et al 1999). A more recent study evaluated exercise performance in women during hormonally confirmed cycle phases and found no difference in VO_2max or lactate threshold during the early follicular, mid follicular or midluteal portions of the menstrual cycle (Dean et al 2003). Finally, during exercise in a hot environment, Sunderland & Nevill (2003) did not find any difference in performance when comparing mid-follicular and mid-luteal phases.

Giacomoni et al (2000) and Lebrun et al (1995) both investigated the influence of menstrual cycle phase on anaerobic performance and found that no significant changes in anaerobic performance occurred during different menstrual cycle phases, while Masterson (1999) and Redman and Weatherby (2004) both found that anaerobic performance was enhanced during the luteal phase in moderately active women. Most investigators have not noted changes in muscular strength in relationship to menstrual cycle phase (Birc 2002, Birch & Reilly 1999, Constantini et al 2005, Friden et al 2003, Janse de Jonge et al 2001); however in a study by Birc (2002), an increase in heart rate in response to a lifting task was noted during the luteal phase even though task performance was no different than during the follicular phase. Thus, some variation exists in the literature concerning the effects of menstrual cycle phase on performance. It does not seem that menstrual cycle phase can be consistently related to alterations in aerobic or anaerobic exercise performance or muscle strength in athletic women.

The female athlete triad

The female athlete triad consists of three interrelated components: disordered eating, amenorrhea and osteoporosis (Nattiv et al 1994). These components are intimately associated in etiology, pathogenesis and health consequences (American College

Box 27.1 Diagnostic criteria for anorexia nervosa (data from American Psychiatric Association 1994, p 544–545)

1. Refusal to maintain body weight at or above a minimally normal weight for age and height (e.g. weight loss leading to maintenance of body weight less than 85% of that expected; or failure to make expected weight gain during period of growth, leading to body weight less than 85% of that expected).
2. Intense fear of gaining weight or becoming fat, even though underweight.
3. Disturbance in the way in which one's body weight or shape is experienced; undue influence of body weight or shape on self-evaluation, or denial of the seriousness of the current low body weight.
4. In postmenarcheal females, amenorrhea (i.e. the absence of at least three consecutive menstrual cycles). A woman is considered to have amenorrhea if her periods occur only following hormone (e.g. estrogen) administration.

Specify type:

Restriction type: the person has not regularly engaged in binge eating or purging behavior (self-induced vomiting or the misuse of laxatives, diuretics or enemas) during the current episode of anorexia nervosa.

Binge eating/purging type: the person has regularly engaged in binge eating or purging behavior during the current episode of anorexia nervosa.

Box 27.2 Diagnostic criteria for bulimia nervosa (data from American Psychiatric Association 1994, p 549–550)

1. Recurrent episodes of binge eating. An episode of binge eating is characterized by both of the following:
   - eating in a discrete period of time (e.g. within any 2-hour period) an amount of food that is definitely larger than most people would eat during a similar period of time and under similar circumstances.
   - sense of lack of control over eating during the episode (e.g. a feeling that one cannot stop eating or control what or how much one is eating).
2. Recurrent, inappropriate compensatory behavior in order to prevent weight gain, such as self-induced vomiting; misuse of laxatives, diuretics, enemas or other medications; fasting; or excessive exercise.
3. The binge eating and inappropriate compensatory behaviors both occur, on average, at least twice a week for 3 months.
4. Self-evaluation is unduly influenced by body shape and weight.
5. The disturbance does not occur exclusively during episodes of anorexia nervosa.

Specify type:

Purging type: during the current episode of bulimia nervosa, the person has regularly engaged in self-induced vomiting or the misuse of laxatives, diuretics or enemas.

Non-purging type: during the current episode of bulimia nervosa, the person has used other inappropriate compensatory behaviors, such as fasting or excessive exercise, but has not regularly engaged in self-induced vomiting or the misuse of laxatives, diuretics or enemas.

of Sports Medicine 1997). While early studies established these links by demonstrating associations between two of the three components at a time, a recent study by Cobb et al (2003) more firmly established the link between disordered eating, menstrual dysfunction, and decreased bone mineral density by evaluating all three components simultaneously in one study population. Another recent study evaluating all three components concurrently found a prevalence of 4.3% of the triad in female athletes (Torstveit & Sundgot-Borgen 2005b). The female athlete may adopt disordered eating patterns as she strives to lose weight in order to achieve the thin appearance or low body weight deemed necessary for excellence in her sport. These disordered eating patterns can then lead to menstrual dysfunction and osteoporosis (Nattiv et al 1994). Athletes involved in sports that emphasize leanness for the purposes of appearance (e.g. ballet), performance (e.g. rhythmic gymnastics) or inclusion in a specific weight class (e.g. rowing) are at increased risk for development of the triad (Sundgot-Borgen 1993a). However, it is important to remember that the triad can affect athletes involved in any sport, and can also affect recreational athletes (Torstveit & Sundgot-Borgen 2005b).

Disordered eating

Most athletes with disordered eating do not meet the criteria for anorexia nervosa or bulimia nervosa. Severe restriction of food intake and an intense fear of gaining weight are characteristics of anorexia nervosa (Box 27.1). Bulimia nervosa is characterized by binge eating followed by purging to prevent weight gain (Box 27.2).

The fact that many athletes do not meet the strict criteria for anorexia or bulimia nervosa, but still have significant problems associated with disordered eating, has led some authors to propose a classification of disordered eating called anorexia athletica. Criteria for this disorder were originally set by Pugliese et al (1983) and were modified by Sundgot-Borgen (1993a) (Box 27.3).

The Diagnostic and Statistical Manual of Mental Disorders-IV (DSM-IV) (American Psychiatric Association 1994) also acknowledges that this issue exists and has a category of eating disorders not otherwise specified (EDNOS), which includes disorders that do not meet the criteria for anorexia or bulimia nervosa. Some athletes with anorexia athletica meet the criteria for EDNOS (Box 27.4).

The reported prevalence of disordered eating among athletes varies among studies from 10 to 62% (Cobb et al 2003, Marshall & Harber 1996, O'Connor et al 1995, Sundgot-Borgen 1993a, Taub & Blinde 1992, Torstveit & Sundgot-Borgen 2005a). An explanation for the large variance in reported prevalence lies in the different methods used to collect data, definitions used to define disordered eating, and athletic populations included in each of the studies. While athletes competing in sports that emphasize leanness are believed to be at increased risk for

Box 27.3 Criteria for anorexia athletica (data from Sundgot-Borgen 1993a, p 29–40)

Absolute criteria (all must be present)
1. Weight loss: >5% of expected body weight
2. Gastrointestinal complaints
3. Absence of medical illness or affective disorder explaining the weight reduction
4. Excessive fear of becoming obese
5. Restriction of food (<1200 kcal/day)

Relative criteria (one or more must be met)
1. Delayed puberty: lack of menstruation at age 16 (primary amenorrhea)
2. Menstrual dysfunction: primary amenorrhea, secondary amenorrhea or oligomenorrhea
3. Distorted body image
4. Use of purging methods: self-induced vomiting, laxatives and diuretics
5. Bingeing
6. Compulsive exercise

Box 27.4 Criteria for eating disorders not otherwise specified (EDNOS) (data from American Psychiatric Association 1994, p 550)

1. For females, all of the criteria for anorexia nervosa are met except that the individual has regular menses.
2. All of the criteria for anorexia nervosa are met except that, despite significant weight loss, the individual's current weight is in the normal range.
3. All of the criteria for bulimia nervosa are met except that the binge eating and inappropriate compensatory mechanisms occur at a frequency of less than twice a week or for a duration of less than 3 months.
4. The regular use of inappropriate compensatory behavior by an individual of normal body weight after eating small amounts of food (e.g. self-induced vomiting after the consumption of two cookies).
5. Repeatedly chewing and spitting out, but not swallowing, large amounts of food.
6. Binge eating disorder: recurrent episodes of binge eating in the absence of the regular use of inappropriate compensatory behaviors characteristic of bulimia nervosa.

disordered eating and the female athlete triad, athletes involved in any sport can be affected (Fig. 27.3).

Most investigators used surveys, including the Eating Disorders Inventory (EDI) and Eating Attitudes Test (EAT), to assess an athlete's risk for disordered eating behaviors. The EDI (Garner et al 1983, 1984), EDI-2, an updated version of the EDI (Garner 1991), and EAT (Garner & Garfinkel 1979) are standardized measures that have been tested for reliability and validity in the general population, but not in athletes. They are intended for use as screening, not diagnostic, tools (Garner et al 1998). Scores on these tests have been correlated with disordered eating in athletes (O'Connor et al 1995, Sundgot-Borgen 1993a).

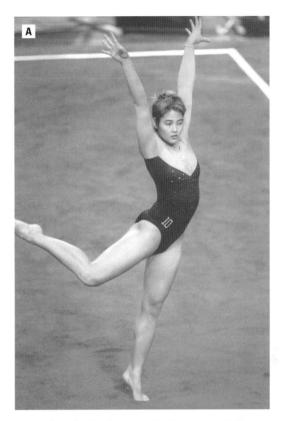

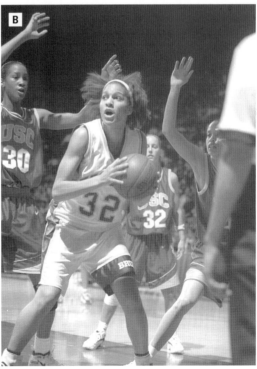

Figure 27.3 • While athletes competing in sports that emphasize leanness (e.g. gymnastics) **(A)** are believed to be at increased risk for disordered eating and the female athlete triad, athletes involved in any sport (e.g. basketball) **(B)** can be affected. (Reproduced with the permission of UCLA Athletic Department.)

The use of surveys alone to assess risk for disordered eating is problematic. Sundgot-Borgen (1993a) demonstrated that significant under-reporting of disordered eating symptoms occurred when only screening questionnaires were used, compared to when surveys were combined with clinical interviews and physical examinations as assessment tools. Also, O'Connor et al (1995) showed that athletes can fake the EDI-2.

Some studies have found that elite athletes and athletes involved in sports that emphasize leanness are at increased risk for disordered eating. For example, Sundgot-Borgen (1993) and Sundgot-Borgen and Torstveit (2004) found that elite athletes in all sport groups were at increased risk for disordered eating compared to controls. Also, the prevalence of disordered eating was significantly higher in sports that emphasized leanness (esthetic, weight dependent, and endurance sports) in comparison to other sports (technical and ball game sports) and controls. More recently, Torstveit and Sundgot-Borgen (2005a) demonstrated that elite athletes competing in non-leanness sports may actually be less at risk for disordered eating and the female athlete triad than athletes competing in leanness sports and active controls.

Prevalence estimates for the use of pathogenic weight control techniques or preoccupation with weight in the college athlete range from 0 to 62% (Dummer et al 1987, Johnson et al 1999, O'Connor et al 1995, Rosen & Hough 1986, Warren et al 1990). As in elite athletes, college women participating in sports that emphasize leanness are at increased risk for preoccupation with weight and use of pathogenic weight control techniques (Warren et al 1990). Some investigators have, however, found that some groups of college athletes are not at increased risk for disordered eating compared to controls (Ashley et al 1996, O'Connor et al 1995, Torstveit & Sundgot-Borgen 2005a, Warren et al 1990).

Studies of eating disorders in high school athletes are limited. The prevalence of the use of pathogenic weight control techniques by high school female athletes is estimated to be between 15 and 25% (Dummer et al 1987, Rhea 1999). However, in studies that included a control group, an increased risk for disordered eating among female athletes was not found (Fulkerson et al 1999, Rhea 1999, Taub & Blinde 1992). In fact, female athletes have been found to have higher self-efficacy and self-esteem compared to controls, which might actually provide a protective effect against the development of disordered eating behaviors (Fulkerson et al 1999, Rhea 1999).

Many triggers for the onset of disordered eating in athletes have been identified (Rosen & Hough 1986, Sundgot-Borgen 1994). Rosen & Hough (1986) found that 75% of gymnasts who were told by coaches that they were overweight resorted to pathogenic weight control techniques to lose weight. Sundgot-Borgen (1994) found that prolonged periods of dieting, weight fluctuations, coaching changes, injury and casual comments made about weight by coaches, parents and friends were the most common reasons given by athletes for the development of disordered eating. Personal stressors including leaving home, problems in a relationship, family trouble, death of a significant other and sexual abuse were also identified as triggers.

Beginning sport-specific training at a younger age was identified as another risk factor (Sundot-Borgon 1994).

Disordered eating and pathogenic weight loss can lead to serious medical complications for athletes. The changes in fluids and electrolytes that accompany purging and starvation behaviors can lead to dehydration, electrolyte abnormalities, hypotension and cardiac dysrrythmias (Becker et al 1999, Palla & Litt 1988, Pomeroy & Mitchell 1992). Clearly, these sequelae pose a particular risk to the competitive athlete. Boxes 27.5 and 27.6 provide a more complete list of medical complications associated with disordered eating.

Disordered eating may also have detrimental effects on athletic performance such as decreased endurance, strength and coordination (Fogelholm 1994, Webster et al 1990). Webster et al (1990) demonstrated decreased VO_2max, upper body strength and coordination in athletes who had rapid weight loss due to the accompanying dehydration. Gradual weight loss has also been associated with decreased VO_2max in some studies (Fogelholm et al 1993).

Box 27.5 Symptoms and physical examination findings in disordered eating

Head and neck
  Face edema
  Enlargement of parotid glands
  Erosion of dental enamel

Heart
  Bradycardia
  Hypotension
  Arrhythmia

Gastrointestinal
  Constipation
  Esophagitis
  Rectal prolapse

Skin
  Dry skin
  Lanugo
  Carotenemia
  Russel's sign: callused knuckles from scraping teeth with induced vomiting

Thermoregulation
  Hypothermia
  Cold intolerance

Box 27.6 Laboratory findings in disordered eating

EKG abnormalities
  Prolonged QTc

Electrolyte abnormalities
  Hypokalemia
  Hypoglycemia

Hematological abnormalities
  Anemia
  Leukopenia
  Thrombocytopenia

Evaluation of the athlete with disordered eating includes measurement of serum electrolytes and glucose, and a complete blood investigation. Also, since arrhythmias and prolonged Q–T intervals can be found in athletes with disordered eating, an electrocardiogram should be obtained.

Usually, athletes with disordered eating can be effectively treated as outpatients. Inpatient management should, however, be considered in patients who have cardiac arrhythmias, electrolyte disturbances, weight loss to 75% expected body weight, suicidal ideation or a history of rapid weight loss (Becker et al 1999).

Proper treatment of disordered eating requires recognition of the problem, identification and resolution of psychosocial precipitants and establishment of healthy eating patterns (Becker et al 1999). When caring for athletes with disordered eating, physicians usually act as part of a multidisciplinary team (Nattiv et al 1994). The role of the team physician is to ensure that the athlete's medical condition is stable and to coordinate care. A nutritionist provides nutritional guidance and a psychologist or psychiatrist should address the psychosocial issues using individual, group and family therapy as needed (Becker et al 1999, Currie & Morse 2005). Sundgot-Borgen & Sundgot-Schnieder (2001) highlighted the importance of the psychiatric component of treatment in a recent study. They found that cognitive behavioral therapy was more effective than nutrition counseling or no counseling in reducing the pursuit of thinness and use of pathogenic weight control techniques. Nutritional counseling was more helpful than no treatment. Coaches, physical therapists and athletic trainers can often help identify athletes with signs of disordered eating and facilitate treatment, since they have the most contact with the athletes.

Pharmacotherapy is not usually indicated in the initial stages of treatment for anorexia nervosa, but fluoxetine may stabilize the patient during the recovery period once 85% of expected weight has been reached (Becker et al 1999). Fluoxetine, desipramine and imipramine have all been used in the treatment of bulimia (Becker et al 1999).

Amenorrhea

The prevalence of amenorrhea in the athletic woman has been reported to range up to 66% (Johnson et al 1999, Loucks & Horvath 1985, Otis 1992, Sundgot-Borgen & Larsen 1993, Torstveit & Sundgot-Borgen 2005c). The prevalence in the general population is estimated to be 2–5% (Bachmann & Kemmann 1982, Loucks & Horvath 1985).

Secondary amenorrhea is defined as the cessation of menstrual periods for three or more consecutive menstrual cycles in a woman who has achieved menarche (Shangold et al 1990). A spectrum of menstrual disorders occurs in the female athlete. Hypoestrogenic amenorrhea is at one end of the spectrum and periods of oligomenorrhea are at an intermediate point (Nattiv 2001). Oligomenorrhea is defined as infrequent menstrual cycles that are greater than 35 days in length (Loucks & Horvath 1985, Nattiv 2001). Ovulatory and luteal dysfunction also occurs in athletes. Athletes with these disorders may remain unrecognized

since they can continue to have cycles at normal intervals, making it difficult to estimate the prevalence of these conditions (Bullen et al 1985, Loucks et al 1989). Luteal phase dysfunction is manifested by a shortened luteal phase with inadequate progesterone production (Shangold et al 1990).

Primary amenorrhea or delayed menarche is defined as the absence of menses by the age of 16 years (Loucks & Horvath 1985). While sports participation has been associated with delayed menarche in girls, a causal relationship has not been established (Loucks 1990, Malina et al 1994, Torstveit & Sundgot-Borgen 2005c).

Investigators have shown that menstrual history and dysfunction are significant predictors for decreased bone mineral density (BMD) (Cann et al 1988, Cobb et al 2003, Drinkwater et al 1990, Grimston et al 1990, Myburgh et al 1993, Wolman et al 1990). Amenorrheic and oligomenorrheic athletes have decreased BMD compared to their eumenorrheic peers (Cann et al 1984, Drinkwater et al 1984, Marcus et al 1985). Also, some evidence suggests that athletes with luteal phase dysfunction may also be at increased risk for low bone density (Drinkwater et al 1990).

Loss of bone mineral density can have serious health consequences for the female athlete. Lower peak BMD in the athlete with menstrual dysfunction can predispose her to osteoporosis and fractures later in life (Drinkwater et al 1990, Snow-Harter 1994) (Figs 27.4 and 27.5). Also, amenorrhea and low bone density have been identified as risk factors for stress fractures in young athletes, which are not only a serious medical issue, but can have consequences for the athlete's performance (Bennell et al 1995, 1996, Lloyd et al 1986, Myburgh et al 1990). Drinkwater et al (1990) demonstrated a linear relationship between degree of menstrual dysfunction and degree of bone loss.

The normal menstrual cycle is characterized by pulsatile secretion of gonadotrophin releasing hormone (GnRH) from the hypothalamus. GnRH stimulates the pulsatile release of luteinizing hormone (LH) and follicle stimulating hormone (FSH) from the pituitary gland. FSH stimulates the granulosa cell to produce estrogen, which promotes proliferation of the

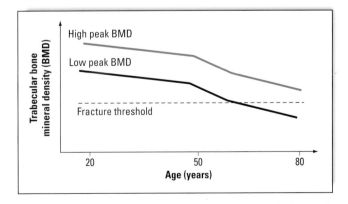

Figure 27.4 • The individual who enters adulthood with a higher peak bone mass may lose similar amounts of bone to an individual with lower peak bone mass, but may still remain above a critical fracture threshold. (Reproduced with permission from Snow-Harter 1994.)

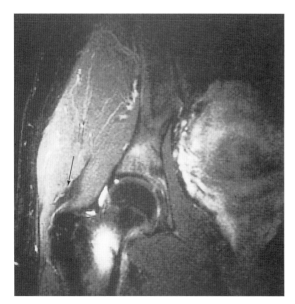

Figure 27.5 • MRI demonstrating a stress fracture of the femoral neck in an amenorrheic athlete.

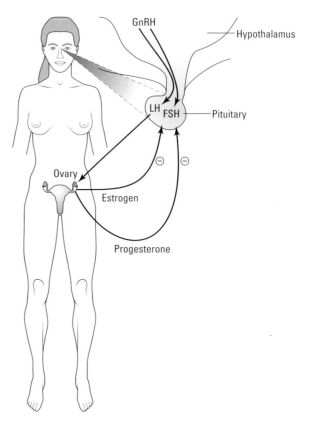

Figure 27.6 • Basic physiology of the menstrual cycle. Pulsatile release of GnRH from the hypothalamus stimulates the release of FSH and LH from the pituitary. LH and FSH stimulate the release of estrogen and progesterone in the ovaries.

endometrium during the follicular phase. LH stimulates the corpus luteum to produce progesterone, which stimulates the endometrium to mature into a secretory lining suitable for implantation of the fertilized egg (Fig. 27.6).

The pulse pattern of LH secretion varies with the phases of the menstrual cycle (Harber 2000). During the follicular phase, LH is secreted in a low-amplitude, high-frequency fashion (Harber 2000). At ovulation, a surge of LH occurs. Finally, during the luteal phase, LH is released in a high-amplitude, low-frequency pattern (Harber 2000) (Fig. 27.7).

In athletes with menstrual dysfunction, the normal monthly phasic changes in LH do not occur (Loucks et al 1989, 1994, Williams et al 1995). LH patterns in amenorrheic athletes demonstrate a decreased frequency of pulses and variable interpulse intervals (Loucks et al 1989). Athletes with luteal phase dysfunction have LH patterns characterized by reduced frequency of pulses and increased pulse amplitude (Loucks et al 1989). These changes in LH pattern are due to alterations in the hypothalamic pituitary ovarian axis, with reduced GnRH release (Loucks et al 1989). Thus, exercise-associated amenorrhea is hypothalamic in origin (Fig. 27.8).

While many mechanisms for the disruption of normal menstrual function have been proposed, the energy availability hypothesis is the most widely accepted (Loucks 2003, Zanker & Cooke 2004). This hypothesis states that insufficient energy availability, defined as the difference between dietary caloric intake and energy expenditure from exercise, is responsible for alterations in menstrual function. The observation that athletes, both amenorrheic and cyclic, take in fewer calories than expected for their level of activity without a resultant decrease

in body weight provided the initial evidence for this hypothesis (Drinkwater et al 1984, Loucks et al 1989, Marcus et al 1985, Myerson et al 1991).

Bullen et al (1985) demonstrated that increasing energy expenditure in untrained eumenorrheic women by the introduction of a strenuous exercise routine could lead to a reversible disruption in normal menstrual cycle. Further investigations have revealed that exercise alone will not disrupt LH pulsatility; a failure to replace the increased energy expenditure with increased dietary intake and a resultant energy imbalance must also occur (Loucks et al 1998, Williams et al 1995).

Amenorrheic athletes have endocrine signs of energy deficiency, which support the energy drain hypothesis (Loucks et al 1989, 1998). Low levels of serum tri-iodothyronine (T_3) are found in amenorrheic athletes but not in athletes with regular menses (Loucks & Heath 1994, Loucks et al 1992b).

Zanker & Swaine (1998b) attempted to demonstrate the relationship between estradiol concentration and multiple indices of energy balance in young female distance runners. They found that estradiol concentrations were more strongly related to calculated energy imbalance, T_3 and insulin-like growth factor (IGF) than to body mass index or body fat (Zanker & Swaine 1998c). As expected, T_3 and IGF were closely related to energy balance. Specifically, T_3 and IGF were more highly correlated

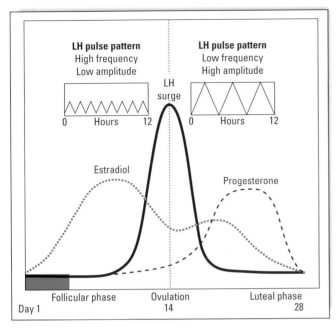

Figure 27.7 • Patterns of hormone secretion across the normal menstrual cycle. An LH surge occurs at the time of ovulation and marks the division between the follicular phase (days 1–14) and the luteal phase (days 15–28). LH pulse pattern also changes across the menstrual cycle; pulse frequency decreases from the follicular phase (~65- to 80-min intervals) to the luteal phase (~185- to 200-min intervals), whereas pulse amplitude increases from the follicular phase (~5 mIU/mL) to the luteal phase (~12 mIU/mL).

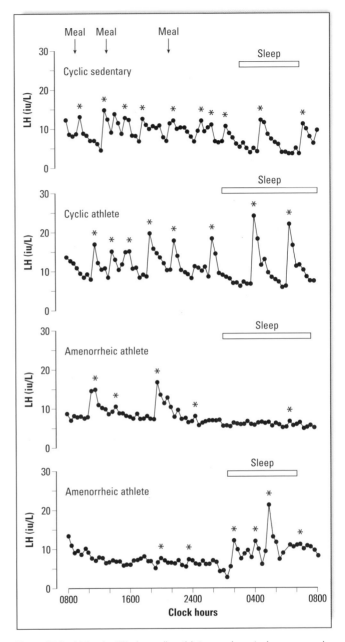

Figure 27.8 • LH pulsatility in cyclic athletes and controls compared to amenorrheic athletes. In amenorrheic athletes, a range of pulse patterns with decreased frequency and variable interpulse intervals are found. (Reproduced with permission from Loucks A B, Mortola J F, Girton L, Yen S S 1989 Alterations in the hypothalamic–pituitary–ovarian and the hypothalamic–pituitary–adrenal axes in athletic women. Journal of Clinical Endocrinology and Metabolism 68:402–411, © The Endocrine Society.)

with energy intake than energy expenditure. These relationships between estradiol and energy imbalance further support the idea that reproductive dysfunction in female athletes is associated with an energy deficit (Zanker & Swaine 1998c).

Research on IGF-1 indicates that it may play an important role in the disturbance of bone turnover in the setting of energy deficiency (Heer et al 2002, Hotta et al 2000, Zanker & Cooke 2004). IGF-1 promotes bone formation by acting on osteoblasts and preosteoblasts to stimulate the synthesis of osteocalcin and Type 1 collagen (Chevalley et al 1998, Zanker & Cooke 2004). Reduced serum concentrations of IGF-1 have been associated with decreased bone formation (Chevalley et al 1998, Grinspoon et al 1996, Hotta et al 2000), and refeeding of anorexic patients is accompanied by increased serum levels of IGF-1 and markers of bone formation (Hotta et al 2000, Zanker & Cooke 2004). The reduced serum IGF-1 concentrations associated with conditions of energy deficit may be due to related decreased serum insulin levels which are associated with resistance of the tissue to growth hormone (GH), thus slowing IGF-1 synthesis (Counts et al 1992, Zanker & Cooke 2004). This, in turn, leads to an impairment of IGF-1 production (Counts et al 1992, Zanker & Cooke 2004).

Leptin, a protein product of the obesity gene, may also be important in regulating bone loss in situations of energy deficiency. Investigators have attempted to identify the specific metabolic signal that leads to the disruption of normal hypothalamic GnRH release in response to decreased energy availability. Evidence suggests that leptin may be an important metabolic signal that integrates nutritional status and reproductive function (Laughlin & Yen 1997). Also, receptors for leptin are found in both the hypothalamus and ovary (Laughlin & Yen 1997). Leptin levels are correlated with the percentage of body fat and they decrease with weight loss. In amenorrheic athletes, the normal diurnal variation of leptin is absent (Considine et al 1996, Laughlin & Yen 1997). In the study by Laughlin & Yen (1997), compared to controls, both amenorrheic and athletes within a normal cycle had lower 24 h leptin levels. Hilton & Loucks (2000) demonstrated that exercise must be associated with low energy availability in order for changes in diurnal pattern of leptin to occur. Further, in vitro investigations have demonstrated that leptin can enhance osteoblast differentiation and inhibit osteoclast generation (Holloway et al 2002, Thomas & Gurguera 2002). Finally, like IGF-1, leptin concentrations increase during refeeding of anorexic patients (Heer et al 2002). These findings highlight the connection between leptin and energy availability, diet and reproductive function in the athlete.

Prevention plays an important role in the management of the female athlete triad. It has been found that providing education about the female athlete triad to coaches and athletes leads to decreases in the prevalence of eating disorders.

Initial evaluation of the amenorrheic athlete usually includes a pregnancy test, thyroid studies and FSH and prolactin level tests. If polycystic ovarian syndrome is suspected or features of androgen excess are noted on examination, laboratory studies for LH, free testosterone and dihydroepiandosterone sulfate levels should be obtained.

The main goal in the treatment of exercise-associated amenorrhea is to restore normal menstrual patterns and to prevent associated osteoporosis. Successful return of menses in the amenorrheic athlete should occur if the existing energy imbalance is treated. Hilton & Loucks (2000) demonstrated that an improvement in nutritional status will lead to return of normal LH patterns, even with continued exercise.

Treatment of the decreased BMD found in amenorrheic athletes is a challenging issue. As these athletes are often found to have inadequate calcium and vitamin D intake (Kirchner et al 1995, Sundgot-Borgen 1993b), appropriate supplementation should be provided. Also, athletes with stress fractures have been found to have lower calcium intakes than athletes without stress fractures (Myburgh et al 1990). Drinkwater et al (1993) observed an increase in tibial BMD in amenorrheic athletes taking supplemental calcium compared to those not taking supplemental calcium. Another study demonstrated a positive linear correlation between dietary calcium and spinal trabecular bone density (Wolman et al 1990). The recommended calcium intake for athletes with menstrual dysfunction is 1200–1500 mg/day and the recommended intake for vitamin D is 400–800 IU/day. Improved caloric intake and weight gain have been found to improve BMD in athletes (Drinkwater et al 1986). In a recent case study, a young amenorrheic runner with osteoporosis showed an improvement in BMD up to the normal range when she improved caloric intake and body weight, suggesting that a potential for 'catch-up' in BMD in athletes with osteoporosis may exist (Fredericson & Kent 2005).

The usefulness of estrogen replacement, whether in the form of the OCP or as estrogen replacement therapy (ERT), in the treatment of menstrual dysfunction and decreased BMD in young amenorrheic athletes is a controversial issue. Prospective data involving the effects of estrogen on bone density in young athletes with menstrual disturbances is quite limited. Several cross-section investigations have demonstrated an association between estrogen use and increased bone density. Lloyd et al (1986) and Myburgh et al (1990) found that athletes without stress fractures were more likely to have used the OCP. In another retrospective study, Cumming (1996) found that amenorrheic athletes using estrogen replacement had significantly higher BMD at the lumbar spine and femoral neck compared to amenorrheic controls who received no therapy.

In a randomized controlled trial study of amenorrheic women, Hergenroeder et al (1997) found significant increases in BMD at the lumbar spine and in the total body in amenorrheic subjects taking the OCP in comparison to controls using medroxyprogesterone or placebo. Athletes with amenorrhea were included in this study, but the study group was not composed entirely of athletes. In another study following 52 women with amenorrhea of various etiologies, Gulekli et al (1994) found a significant increase in bone mass with the use of various types of estrogen therapy. Of note was that the authors found that weight gain was more effective than any type of estrogen therapy in increasing BMD. Haenggi et al (1994) also found a small positive effect on BMD with OCP treatment.

Some prospective studies have found that estrogen replacement had either no effect or a negative effect on BMD. In a study of 40 women with hypothalamic amenorrhea, Warren et al (1994) found no difference in BMD in the spine, wrist or foot in women treated with estrogen compared to nontreated controls. However, in three subjects who gained weight during the study period, a significant increase in BMD was noted. Polatti et al (1995) followed 200 healthy women who were either receiving the OCP or no estrogen therapy and found that the group of women who were not taking the OCP had a significant increase in BMD over the study period, while those taking the OCP did not. This led them to suggest that OCP use may prevent peak bone mass in healthy young women (Polatti et al 1995). In another prospective study, Klibanski et al (1995) evaluated the effects of estrogen therapy on anorexic women with amenorrhea. The group treated with estrogen did not show significant improvement in BMD compared to controls. However, women in the control group who had weight gain and spontaneous resumption of menses did have a significant increase in BMD compared to other subjects.

The mixed findings in these studies suggest that estrogen deficiency may not be the only, or even the most important, etiology for the loss of BMD in amenorrheic athletes. The energy deficit associated with amenorrhea in athletes might play a role in decreased BMD (Zanker & Swaine 1998b).

More recently, Grinspoon et al (2002) demonstrated that subcutaneous recombinant IGF-1 administered with an oral contraceptive can lead to significant improvements in spinal BMD. However, research on the therapeutic use of IGF-1 in osteoporotic anorexics and athletes is limited and it is not currently a regularly used therapy (Zanker & Cooke 2004).

Cyclic medroxyprogesterone has also been studied as a treatment for decreased BMD in active women with menstrual dysfunction. Prior et al (1994) found that treatment with cyclic medroxyprogesterone led to significant increases in bone density in active women with menstrual disturbances. Hergenroeder et al (1997), however, did not demonstrate an improvement in BMD with medroxyprogesterone therapy.

Osteoporosis

Osteoporosis has been defined as a disease characterized by low bone mass, microarchitectural deterioration of bone tissue leading to enhanced skeletal fragility and an increased risk for fracture (Consensus Development Conference 1991) (also see Chapter 5). The World Health Organization (WHO) developed diagnostic criteria for osteoporosis in postmenopausal women, based on bone density measurements; however, criteria using bone density have not been established for young women (Box 27.7).

The osteoporosis found in female athletes with menstrual dysfunction has been attributed to the hypoestrogenic state that accompanies hypothalamic amenorrhea (Drinkwater et al 1984, Loucks et al 1992a, Marcus et al 1985). Support for this conclusion comes from the documentation of the causal relationship between hypoestrogenemia and osteoporosis in postmenopausal women. In postmenopausal women, loss of BMD is associated with increased bone turnover and exaggerated bone resorption, demonstrated by evidence from measurement of serum markers of bone turnover (Delmas 1992).

In amenorrheic runners Zanker & Swaine (1998a) demonstrated that bone turnover is actually decreased. They measured serum markers of bone formation in amenorrheic athletes and found evidence of decreased bone formation. The different patterns of bone turnover between amenorrheic runners and postmenopausal women led Zanker & Swaine (1998a) to propose that hypoestrogenemia is not the sole factor responsible for the decreased BMD found in amenorrheic athletes. They suggested that the negative energy balance found in amenorrheic athletes plays a significant role in decreased BMD (Loucks 1990, Loucks & Callister 1993, Zanker & Swaine 1998b). The fact that estrogen replacement did not lead to improvement in BMD in some studies supports the idea that hypoestrogenemia

may not be the only factor responsible for loss of bone density in these athletes.

The prognosis for the young amenorrheic athlete with osteoporosis is guarded. With weight gain and the return of normal menses, these athletes do have a significant increase in BMD. However, several investigators have demonstrated that, in comparison to cyclic controls, previously amenorrheic athletes continue to have significantly lower BMD even after weight gain (Drinkwater et al 1986, Herzog et al 1993, Iketani et al 1995, Jonnavithula et al 1993, Keen & Drinkwater 1997, Rigotti et al 1991). Thus, the loss of bone density in amenorrheic athletes may be partially irreversible. Nevertheless, a recent case study of a 22-year-old amenorrheic, osteoporotic runner demonstrated that, with improved nutrition and weight gain, some athletes may be capable of attaining normal BMD for age (Fredericson & Kent 2005).

If osteoporosis is suspected in an athlete, dual energy X-ray absorptiometric scan (DXA) is useful for evaluating BMD. If the athlete is found to be osteopenic or osteoporotic, bone markers can be measured. Urine N-telopeptide is used to assess bone resorption and serum osteocalcin to assess bone formation (Nattiv 2001).

The treatment of decreased BMD with the OCP in amenorrheic athletes is discussed above. A more in-depth discussion of osteoporosis can be found in Chapter 5.

Bone health

The factors that determine bone mass in postmenopausal women are peak bone mass and age-related bone loss (Nichols et al 2000). Maximizing peak bone mass and minimizing age-related bone loss will decrease the risk for osteoporosis and fragility fractures.

Bone mass gains during childhood are important for the attainment of an optimal peak bone mass. The maximum rate of bone formation occurs between the ages of 10–14 years and peak bone mass is attained between the ages of 20 and 30 years (Bonjour et al 1991, Sabatier et al 1996). By the end of adolescence, almost 90% of adult bone mass has been obtained (Sabatier et al 1996). Genetics, participation in weightbearing activities and diet all influence bone mass in children (Pollitzer & Anderson 1989, Ruiz et al 1995, Slemenda et al 1991).

Bone loss in adult women is most rapid in the 3–4 years following menopause. The marked hypoestrogenemia associated with this time period is felt to be the cause of this bone loss, and it can be prevented with estrogen replacement (Ettinger et al 1985, Prestwood et al 1994). Evidence indicates that increased bone turnover and resorption is occurring during this phase of rapid bone loss (Delmas 1992). After this period of rapid bone loss, a phase of gradual bone loss takes over.

Strategies to minimize adult bone loss include optimizing nutrition, pharmacotherapy and exercise programs. Calcium supplementation may slow bone loss in women after the first 5 years of menopause (Dawson-Hughes et al 1990); and, in combination with estrogen replacement or vitamin D, calcium supplementation may help increase BMD in postmenopausal

---

Box 27.7 WHO guidelines for osteoporosis

Normal: BMD ≤ 1 SD[a] below mean peak bone mass[b]

Osteopenia: BMD > 1 and ≤ 2.5 SD below the mean peak bone mass

Osteoporosis: BMD > 2.5 SD below the mean peak bone mass

Severe osteoporosis: osteoporosis criteria plus one or more fragility fractures

[a] SD=standard deviation
[b] These measurements are compared with the mean value of peak bone mass in normal young women

women (Nichols et al 2000). Estrogen replacement therapy has been proven to increase BMD and to decrease risk for fracture in postmenopausal women (Ettinger et al 1985, Nichols et al 2000). However, all women may not experience improvement in BMD with estrogen replacement (Nichols et al 2000, Stevenson et al 1993).

Calcitonin is another medication that has been shown to increase BMD and to decrease fracture risk. Other, newer classes of drugs for the treatment of osteoporosis include bisphosphonates and selective estrogen receptor modulators.

While the results of exercise intervention are variable, resistance exercise and high impact training do seem to lead to site-specific increases in bone mass at the areas of greatest stress (Bassey et al 1998, Dook et al 1997, Drinkwater 1996, Friedlander 1995, Pruitt et al 1992, Simikin et al 1987, Taaffe et al 1995). Mature women with a history of participation in high impact sports (e.g. basketball) and medium impact sports (e.g. running) exhibit greater bone density than those who had a history of participation in low impact sports (e.g. swimming) or who were non-athletic (Dook et al 1997). Children and adolescents participating in significant impact loading activities have been found to have higher levels of bone density than children in non-impact activities (Grimston et al 1993, Taaffe et al 1995). In a randomized controlled trial, Snow-Harter et al (1992) found that young women who did weight training or jogging had significantly greater gains in lumbar BMD than controls over an 8-month study period. Creighton et al (2001) used markers of bone formation to demonstrate that athletes participating in high impact sports had more bone formation than those in non-impact sports. The high impact sports athletes also had increased BMD. Premenopausal women may have larger BMD responses to impact activities than postmenopausal women, although postmenopausal women have been shown to have some increases in BMD with impact and resistance exercise (Bassey et al 1998, Maddalozzo & Snow 2000).

Secondary prevention of osteoporotic fractures is another important issue. One in five women with a vertebral fracture will experience another vertebral fracture within one year (Lindsay et al 2001). Vertebral compression fractures are often recognized as the hallmark of osteoporosis (Nevitt et al 1998) and affect approximately 25% of all postmenopausal women in the USA (Melton 1997). Many osteoporotic fractures, particularly those of the long bones, result from falls, which typically occur during activities of daily living (Campbell 2002). Many agree that the best way to prevent osteoporotic fractures is to prevent falls (Arnold et al 2005, Bennell et al 2000, Campbell 2002, Koike 2005, Lange et al 2005, Old & Calvert 2004, Swanenburg et al 2003, Tinetti 2003, Werle & Zimber 1999, Wilkins & Birge 2005).Women aged 65–75 with osteoporosis who participated in a community-based exercise program experienced improvements in dynamic balance and strength, both of which are important determinants in decreasing risk for falls (Carter et al 2002). Aquatic therapy has also been shown to be successful at improving balance in women 65 years and older with osteoporosis (Devereux et al 2005). Other studies have explored the effect of excessive kyphosis and its

negative effect on balance in women with osteoporosis and the improvement of balance with dynamic postural exercises and strengthening of spinal extensors (Sinaki & Lynn 2002, Sinaki et al 2005a, 2005b). Physical therapists can play a key role in treating women with osteoporosis by proper evaluation and treatment of both active and sedentary females at high risk for fractures. Treatment programs consisting of strengthening, balance and gait training should be designed to improve posture and reduce the risk of falls.

Pregnancy and exercise

Exercise and other forms of physical activity have become an essential part of life for many women. That a large proportion of women wish to continue a regular exercise routine during pregnancy raises questions about the safety of exercise during pregnancy (Fig. 27.9).

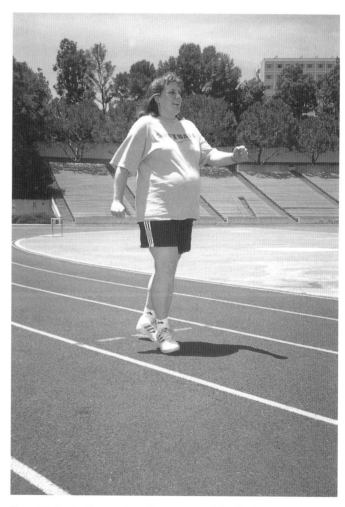

Figure 27.9 • As the number of women participating in regular exercise rises, more women are continuing to exercise during pregnancy. (Reproduced with permission of Suzanne Hecht.)

Physiological considerations and theoretical concerns

It has been suggested that physiological responses to exercise in pregnant women could lead to poor pregnancy outcomes including abortion, fetal malformations, poor fetal growth, fetal injury and premature labor. There are concerns that exercise and pregnancy-induced changes in hemodynamics, body temperature, circulating stress hormones, caloric expenditure and the musculoskeletal system could lead to poor maternal or fetal outcomes (Clapp 2000, Clapp & Rizik 1992). Fortunately, most of these concerns have not been validated in the literature. In the following sections, each of these areas of theoretical concern will be addressed.

Hemodynamics

The hemodynamic responses to exercise, especially alterations in splanchnic blood flow, have raised concern that adequate uterine blood flow may not be maintained during exercise. Decreased uterine blood flow could decrease oxygen and nutrient availability to the fetus, inhibiting growth and development (Clapp 1994). Also, there is a concern that decreased myometrial oxygen delivery to the uterus could stimulate uterine contractions, leading to premature labor and delivery (Clapp 2000). In non-pregnant women, weightbearing exercise causes splanchnic flow to decrease to 40–50% of normal resting levels (Clapp 1994). Fortunately, the cardiovascular changes associated with both pregnancy and regular exercise offer protection against large decreases in splanchnic flow during exercise. A 40–50% increase in blood volume typically occurs during pregnancy (Capeless & Clapp 1989, Clapp 2000, Pivarnik et al 1992). In exercising pregnant women, this increase may be as much as 35% more than in sedentary controls (Hale & Milne 1996, Pivarnik et al 1993, 1994). In addition, trained pregnant women have significantly higher cardiac outputs than their sedentary counterparts (Clapp 2000, Pivarnik et al 1993). These changes in the cardiovascular system result in decreases in splanchnic flow with exercise that are 20–30% less in trained pregnant women than in sedentary controls (Clapp 2000). Ultrasound studies have been performed to assess uteroplacental blood flow before and after exercise in pregnant women. These studies have yielded mixed results, some showing no difference in uteroplacental blood flow with exercise, and others showing decreased uterine circulation with exercise (Baumann et al 1989, Rauramo & Forss 1988). Definitive evidence of decreased uteroplacental flow during exercise in pregnant women is not available. Results similar to splanchnic flow have been obtained with assessment of umbilical artery flow during exercise (Baumann et al 1989, Veille 1996, Veille et al 1989).

In order to assess fetal distress with maternal exercise, some studies have monitored fetal heart rate before and immediately after exercise. The results are mixed, but even in studies where changes in fetal heart rate are documented, the changes are transient and no prolonged adverse fetal effects have been documented as a result, indicating that adequate blood flow to the fetus is maintained (Carpenter et al 1988, Clapp 1985, Clapp et al 1992, Collings et al 1983, O'Neill 1996, Veille 1996).

Body temperature

The increased body temperatures associated with exercise have led to concerns about the potential for fetal malformations. In women who are not pregnant, body temperature can be elevated above 39.2°C with exercise, a level felt to have teratogenic potential (American College of Obstetrics and Gynecology 1994). Studies indicating an increase in neural tube defects or miscarriage due to hot tub use by pregnant women added to these concerns (Li 2003, Milunsky et al 1992). Both pregnancy and regular exercise improve heat dissipation, which helps prevent increased body temperatures during exercise (Clapp et al 1987). Clapp (1991) demonstrated that, during pregnancy, maternal body temperature decreased by 0.3°C in the first trimester, and continued to decrease 0.1°C each month until the 37th week. Also, trained pregnant woman demonstrate an even better ability to dissipate heat than untrained pregnant women (Clapp 1990, 1994, Clapp et al 1987). Several investigators have measured the rectal temperatures of trained pregnant women during exercise and found that the body temperatures of these women do not reach levels felt to have teratogenic potential (Clapp et al 1987, Lindqvist et al 2003, O'Neill 1996). Finally, prospective studies involving women who exercise during pregnancy have failed to demonstrate an increased risk for congenital anomalies or early pregnancy loss, compared to controls (Clapp 1989, Clapp & Dickstein 1984).

Caloric expenditure

As glucose is the main fetal substrate, there is concern that glucose use by exercising muscles might limit fetal substrate availability. It has been shown that maternal blood glucose levels do fall during exercise (Clapp 1991, Clapp et al 1987, Soultanakis et al 1996). In spite of this, investigations of fetal growth have provided mixed results, most showing no difference in the growth of fetuses of exercising women compared to sedentary women (Bell et al 1995, Clapp 1990, 2000, Clapp & Dickstein 1984, Clapp & Little 1995, Clapp et al 1992, Collings et al 1983, Hatch et al 1993, Jackson et al 1995, Klebanoff et al 1990, Lokey et al 1991, Sternfeld et al 1995). Compensatory mechanisms to improve substrate delivery to the fetus may develop in the exercising pregnant woman, including increased placental size and increased glucose delivery after bouts of exercise (Clapp 2000, Clapp et al 1992, Jackson et al 1995). Also, since exercise performance tends to decrease late in pregnancy, the amount of glucose used by working muscles is limited during this time (Clapp et al 1987).

While women who continue to exercise during pregnancy do tend to gain less weight than sedentary women, their level of weight gain does fall within acceptable ranges (Clapp & Little 1995). Women who continue to exercise during pregnancy may require increased energy intake in order to achieve appropriate weight gains during pregnancy.

Stress hormones

Exercise leads to a stress response with increased levels of cate-cholamines (Artal et al 1981, Bonds & Delivoria-Papadopoulos 1985). Noradrenaline (norepinephrine) has been shown to increase strength and frequency of contractions, leading to concerns that exercise might lead to uterine contractions (Artal et al 1981). Subjectively, some women note contractions during exercise. However, assessment with tocodynamometry immediately after exercise has not demonstrated that increased uterine activity occurs with exercise (Veille et al 1985).

Musculoskeletal

There is concern that the increases in maternal weight, changes in center of gravity and increased ligamentous laxity associated with pregnancy may cause maternal injury with exercise during pregnancy (Clapp et al 1992, Clapp 1994). Despite these changes, very few maternal injuries have been associated with exercise during pregnancy (Clapp 2000). This may be due to the decrease in performance that occurs late in pregnancy when weight is highest and ligamentous laxity is most profound (Clapp 1990, 2000, Clapp et al 1987).

Maternal effects

The effects of exercise during pregnancy on pregnancy length, course of labor and symptoms of pregnancy have all been investigated (Clapp & Dickstein 1984, Clapp 1990, Hatch et al 1993). Exercise during pregnancy has been associated with many beneficial effects for the mother.

Exercise has been related to a decrease in some of the symptoms associated with pregnancy. Women who exercise during pregnancy may have fewer complaints of low back pain and other musculoskeletal complaints than sedentary women (Kihlstrand et al 1999, Sternfeld et al 1995). Back pain is very common during pregnancy, with up to 72% of pregnant women complaining of back pain, and one-third of these women finding that back pain is a severe problem (MacEvilly 1996, Mogren & Pohjanen 2005, Wang et al 2004). In addition, back pain accounts for the majority of sick leave among pregnant women (Ostgaard et al 1994). History of back pain prior to pregnancy has been found to be an important predictive factor for back pain during pregnancy (Mogren & Pohjanen 2005, Padua et al 2002, Wang et al 2004). Several investigators have documented reduced complaints of low back pain in women who exercise during pregnancy (Garshasbi & Zedeh 2005, Kihlstrand et al 1999, Sternfeld et al 1995). The results of physical therapy for treatment of back pain during pregnancy are inconsistent. A recent review of nine studies did not find strong evidence that physical therapy interventions can prevent and treat low back and pelvic pain in pregnancy (Stuge et al 2003). However, other groups have demonstrated that personalized physical therapy programs may help treat low back pain during pregnancy (Ostgaard et al 1994, Suputtitada et al 2002). Despite this lack of consensus in the literature, many pregnant women may seek physical therapy intervention to alleviate low back pain, and it is important to thoroughly evaluate each patient in order to determine possible biomechanical causes of pain that may have been present prior to pregnancy and those that are a result of pregnancy to help develop a personalized treatment plan for each woman (Ostgaard et al 1994). It is also important to note that women may continue to have pelvic girdle and back pain after pregnancy. Physical therapy utilizing specific stabilizing exercises was found to be more effective in reducing pain in women with pelvic girdle pain after pregnancy than physical therapy without specific stabilizing exercises (Stuge et al 2004).

Pregnant women who exercise also report improved self-image and fewer depressive symptoms, both during pregnancy and the postpartum period, compared to those who do not (Hall & Kaufmann 1987, Sternfeld et al 1995).

Exercise has not been associated with increased risk of premature delivery (Clapp 1990, Clapp & Dickstein 1984, Hatch et al 1993, Kulpa et al 1986, Lokey et al 1991, Sternfeld et al 1995). However, Clapp (1990) found that exercising women tend to deliver about 1 week earlier than women who do not exercise, an effect that the women in the study found to be beneficial.

Investigations examining the effects of maternal exercise on the course of labor have produced inconsistent results (Clapp 1990, Collings et al 1983, Kardel & Kase 1998, Kulpa et al 1986, Lokey et al 1991). While most studies suggest that maternal exercise has no effect on the course of labor, some have demonstrated a shorter active phase and second stage of labor in exercising women (Clapp 1990, Kulpa et al 1986). In contrast, an observational study of exercising military women noted a longer first stage of labor in exercising women (Magann et al 2002). Finally, some investigators have found that women who exercise during pregnancy have a lower incidence of operative deliveries and episiotomies (Clapp 1990, Hall & Kaufmann 1987, Sternfeld et al 1995).

It has been suggested that the increased blood volume gained by women who exercise during pregnancy may offer some protection in the event of a hemorrhage during delivery (Clapp 2000). Also, exercise during pregnancy may protect against problems with loss of bladder control, both in the immediate postpartum period and 1 year after delivery (Clapp 2000).

Women who continue to exercise during and after pregnancy may return to their prepregnancy weight faster than sedentary women, since they have lower overall weight gain and subcutaneous fat deposition (Clapp 2000). During lactation, however, exercise does not increase the rate of weight loss without concomitant caloric restriction (Clapp 2000, 2001, Clapp & Little 1995, Dewey 1998). Despite concerns to the contrary, exercise, dieting, and gradual weight loss in the postpartum period do not seem to adversely affect lactation or infant growth (Dewey 1998, Lovelady et al 2000, McCrory et al 1999).

Exercise during pregnancy may have additional benefits for prevention and treatment of gestational diabetes. The American Diabetes Association has endorsed exercise 'as a helpful adjunctive therapy' for treatment of gestational diabetes mellitus (American College of Obstetrics and Gynecology 2002). A moderate exercise program may improve postprandial blood glucose levels and insulin sensitivity (American Diabetes Association 2004, Artal 2003, Langer 2006).

Fetal effects

Studies investigating the effects of maternal exercise on birth weight are numerous and have provided mixed results. Most investigators have found no difference in birth weight of offspring born to exercising mothers compared to sedentary controls, but some have found either increased or decreased weight in the offspring of exercising mothers (Bell et al 1995, Clapp 1990, 1996, 2000, Clapp & Dickstein 1984, Clapp & Little 1995, Clapp et al 1992, 1998, Collings et al 1983, Hall & Kaufmann 1987, Hatch et al 1993, Jackson et al 1995, Klebanoff et al 1990, Kulpa et al 1986, Lokey et al 1991, Sternfeld et al 1995). The level of exercise performance may influence birth weight. Studies involving women who participated in low intensity, non-weightbearing exercise routines tend to show either no change or a slight increase in birth weight (Bell et al 1995, Clapp 2000, Clapp et al 1992, Collings et al 1983, Hall & Kaufmann 1987, Hatch et al 1993, Jackson et al 1995, Klebanoff et al 1990, Kulpa et al 1986, Lokey et al 1991, Sternfeld et al 1995). It has been hypothesized that the increased birth weight observed in these infants may be due to alterations in placental growth and blood flow induced by exercise (Clapp 1990, 2000, Clapp et al 1992, Hatch et al 1993, Jackson et al 1995). High intensity exercise may be associated with a decrease in birth weight, especially if maternal weight gain is limited (Bell et al 1995, Clapp 1990, 1996, Clapp & Dickstein 1984, Clapp & Little 1995, Clapp et al 1998). Clapp (1990) found that the decreased birth weight in these infants could be attributed to lower fat mass and slightly decreased gestational age. Little or no change has been demonstrated in head circumference, length or lean body mass in infants born to exercising versus sedentary mothers (Clapp 1990). A recent review concluded that the available data are reassuring that exercise during pregnancy does not lead to a clinically important reduction in length of gestation (Kramer 2005).

During labor, infants of mothers who exercised during pregnancy show fewer signs of distress (Clapp 1990). They have a decreased incidence of meconium stained amniotic fluid and abnormal fetal heart rate patterns (Clapp 1990). APGAR scores of infants born to exercising mothers are similar to or higher than those of infants born to sedentary mothers (Clapp 1990, Kardel & Kase 1998, Lokey et al 1991, Sternfeld et al 1995).

Finally, maternal exercise during pregnancy may have an effect on newborn activity level and later development. During the early postnatal period, Clapp et al (1999) found that infants born to exercising mothers are more alert and more able to quieten themselves after exposure to stimuli than infants born to sedentary mothers. This may be the result of learned fetal responses to intermittent arousal stimulus produced by maternal exercise during gestation (Clapp et al 1999). Later in development, Clapp et al (1998) demonstrated that children of mothers who exercised during pregnancy had slightly better motor skills at 1 year of age. Further, at 5 years of age,

they were leaner and performed better on standardized tests of intelligence than controls (Clapp 1996).

Placental effects

Maternal exercise has been shown to have effects on placental growth and composition (Clapp 2000, Clapp et al 1992, Jackson et al 1995). Ultrasound studies indicate that women who exercise during pregnancy have larger placentas (Clapp 2000, Clapp et al 1992). Jackson et al (1995) found that sustained exercise during pregnancy led to changes in placental composition and enhanced villous growth. These changes may increase placental perfusion and improve transport of nutrients and oxygen in the placentas of exercising women, enhancing fetal substrate availability during the periods of decreased uterine blood flow associated with exercise.

Guidelines for exercise during pregnancy

Current data suggest that healthy women with an uncomplicated pregnancy may safely continue or begin a regular exercise program during pregnancy (American College of Obstetrics and Gynecology 2002, Clapp 2000). Maternal symptoms should dictate the intensity of exercise (American College of Obstetrics and Gynecology 1994, 2002, Hartmann & Bung 1999). Sedentary women who wish to begin a regular exercise program during pregnancy may be encouraged to do so as long as they do so in a gradual fashion (American College of Obstetrics and Gynecology 2002, Kelly 2005). Typically, starting with about 15 minutes of light aerobic exercise three days each week and gradually increasing to 30 minutes of continuous exercise 4 days each week is a reasonable goal (Kelly 2005). Women should be encouraged to participate in a variety of activities at a moderate intensity to decrease risk for overuse injury; walking, dancing, stationary cycling and water aerobics are usually well tolerated (Artal & O'Toole 2003). Women who are already active can often continue current exercise regimens, using comfort levels to alter level of activity (Kelly 2005). It is important for elite and highly competitive athletes to recognize that it may be difficult to maintain current training volumes during pregnancy and to set reasonable expectations for training during pregnancy, such as maintenance of fitness levels rather than attainment of peak fitness (Artal & O'Toole 2003, Kelly 2005). Certain positions and types of sports should be avoided. For example, the supine position should be avoided as it may lead to decreased cardiac output (American College of Obstetrics and Gynecology 1994, 2002). Also, activities which may cause abdominal trauma, like the martial arts, gymnastics, horseback riding and some ball sports, should be avoided (American College of Obstetrics and Gynecology 2002, Hartmann & Bung 1999). During the postpartum period, resumption of prepregnancy levels of exercise should be done gradually. Some women may be physically and medically able to begin safely exercising within days of delivery, while others may not be ready for several weeks (American College of Obstetrics and Gynecology 2002). There are no identified maternal complications associated with resumption

Box 27.8 Contraindications to exercise during pregnancy (adapted from American College of Obstetricians and Gynecologists 1994, Davies et al 2003, Kelly 2005)

Absolute	Relative
Incompetent cervix	Extremely underweight
Intrauterine growth restriction	Maternal eating disorder
Multiple gestation (≥triplets) Persistent bleeding	Maternal arrhythmia or cardio vascular disorder
Placenta previa after 25–28 weeks gestation	Mild to moderate respiratory disorder
Preeclamsia	Previous spontaneous abortion
Pregnancy-induced hypertension	Severe anemia
History of premature labor	Twin pregnancy after 28th week of gestation
Premature labor in current pregnancy	
Risk for premature labor	
Premature rupture of membranes	

of training in the postpartum period (American College of Obstetrics and Gynecology 2002).

Since pregnancy itself is associated with increased energy requirements, pregnant women who choose to exercise must be very conscious about replacing calories expended with exercise with appropriate dietary intake (American College of Obstetrics and Gynecology 1994, Kelly 2005).

Contraindications to exercise during pregnancy include premature rupture of membranes, uterine bleeding, preterm labor and incompetent cervix (American College of Obstetrics and Gynaecology 1994, Hartmann & Bung 1999). See Box 27.8 for a complete list of absolute and relative contraindications to aerobic exercise during pregnancy.

Stress urinary incontinence (SUI), the loss of urine following a sudden increase in intra-abdominal pressure, is a common problem for female athletes, especially after giving birth. It is important to remember that SUI is quite common in nulliparous athletes as well, with as many as 28% of nulliparous athletes experiencing SUI (Bo & Sundgot-Borgen 2001, Nygaard et al 1994). It does not seem that athletes are at increased risk for SUI in comparison to controls; Bo and Sundgot-Borgen (2001) found that 41% of elite athletes and 39% of controls reported SUI. Active females suffering from stress incontinence may be susceptible to involuntary loss of urine during exercise that limits the ability to run, jump, participate in aerobics, lift weights and perform abdominal exercises.

Fortunately for women experiencing SUI there has been increased interest and specialization by physical therapists in the area of urinary incontinence and pelvic floor dysfunction. Physical therapy intervention may consist of but is not limited to Kegel exercises, manual tactile cues, biofeedback and electrical stimulation. Pelvic floor exercises performed twice a week under the supervision of a therapist for a period of 12 weeks was considered to be an effective and low cost treatment for urinary stress incontinence (Moreno et al 2004). Research studies have demonstrated that physical therapy programs focusing on pelvic floor exercises in conjunction with other modalities have been successful in the short term (Bo 2003, Turkan et al 2005), at 5-year follow-up (Parkkinen et al 2004) and at 10-year follow-up when initial therapy is successful (Cammu et al 2000). In addition, therapy intervention was found to be successful at decreasing postpartum stress incontinence (Harvey 2003). Pelvic floor exercises done antenatally may even prevent postpartum SUI; women performing pelvic floor exercises under the supervision of a physical therapist at monthly intervals from 20 weeks until delivery reported less postpartum stress incontinence compared to control groups (Reilly et al 2003).

Summary

As more women become active participants in sports and exercise, it becomes increasingly important to understand the health effects of such involvement. There are many health benefits associated with regular exercise in women. Sports participation can lead to improvements in strength, heat tolerance and aerobic and anaerobic performance in women. Regular exercise can also improve the physical and psychological symptoms associated with pregnancy. Also, regular weightbearing exercise may improve bone density and overall bone health.

Despite these many benefits, female athletes participating at the elite level or in sports that emphasize leanness are at particular risk for disordered eating and the female athlete triad. Since this can have important consequences for the female athlete's overall health, and bone health in particular, medical professionals and coaches should be aware of these issues. Athletes with signs of disordered eating or amenorrhea should be referred to a physician for a complete evaluation.

Finally, available evidence suggests that regular exercise is not only safe during pregnancy, but can offer important benefits for both mother and child. Exercise during pregnancy has not been associated with premature delivery, retardation of fetal growth or problems with lactation. Women who exercise during pregnancy have fewer musculoskeletal complaints and depressive symptoms associated with pregnancy. Children born to exercising mothers demonstrate fewer signs of distress during labor and are more alert in the early postnatal period.

References

Aaron D J, Dearwater S R, Anderson R et al 1996 Physical activity and the initiation of high risk activities in adolescents. Medicine and Science in Sports and Exercise 27:1639–1645

Ahmad C S, Clark A M, Heilmann N et al 2006 Effect of gender and maturity on quadriceps-to-hamstring strength ration and anterior cruciate ligament laxity. American Journal of Sports Medicine 34:370–374

Almeida S A, Trone D W, Leone D M et al 1999 Gender differences in musculoskeletal injury rates: a function of symptom reporting? Medicine and Science in Sports and Exercise 31:1807–1812

American College of Obstetrics and Gynecology (ACOG) 1994 Technical bulletin number 189. ACOG Press, Washington, DC

American College of Obstetrics and Gynecology (ACOG) 2002 Exercise during the pregnancy and the postpartum period. ACOG Committee opinion no. 267. Obstetrics and Gynecology 99:171–173

American College of Sports Medicine 1997 The female athlete triad. Medicine and Science in Sports and Exercise 26:i–ix

American Diabetes Association 2004 Position statement on gestational diabetes mellitus. Diabetes Care 27 (suppl 1):S88–S90

American Psychiatric Association 1994 Diagnostic and statistical manual of mental disorders, 4th edn (DSM-IV). American Psychiatric Association, Washington, DC

Arendt E, Dick R 1995 Knee injury patterns among men and women in collegiate basketball and soccer. NCAA data and review of literature. American Journal of Sports Medicine 223:694–701

Arnold C M, Busch A J, Schachter C L et al 2005 The relationship of intrinsic fall risk factors to a recent history of falling in older women with osteoporosis. Journal of Orthopedic and Sports Physical Therapy 35:452–460

Artal R 2003 Exercise: the alternative therapeutic intervention for gestational diabetes. Clinics in Obstetrics and Gynecology 46:479–487

Artal R, O'Toole M 2003 Guidelines of the American College of Obstetricians and Gynecologists for exercise during pregnancy and the postpartum period. British Journal of Sports Medicine 37:6–12

Artal R, Platt L D, Sperling M et al 1981 Maternal cardiovascular and metabolic responses in normal pregnancy. American Journal of Obstetrics and Gynecology 140:123–127

Ashley C D, Smith J F, Robinson J B et al 1996 Disordered eating in female collegiate athletes and collegiate females in an advanced program of study: a preliminary investigation. International Journal of Sports Nutrition 6:391–401

Ayalon J, Simkin A, Leichter I et al 1987 Dynamic bone loading exercises for post menopausal women: effect on the density of the distal radius. Archives of Physical Medicine and Rehabilitation 68:280–283

Bachmann G A, Kemmann E 1982 Prevalence of oligomenorrhea and amenorrhea in a college population. American Journal of Obstetrics and Gynecology 144:98–102

Baker M M, Juhn M S 2000 Patellofemoral pain syndrome in the female athlete. Clinics in Sports Medicine 19:315–329

Baratta R, Solomonow M, Zhou B H et al 1988 Muscular coactivation. The role of the antaonist musculature in maintaining knee stability. American Journal of Sports Medicine 16:113–122

Bassey E J, Rothwell M C, Littlewood J J et al 1998 Pre- and postmenopausal women have different bone mineral density responses to the same high-impact exercise. Journal of Bone and Mineral Research 13:1805–1813

Baumann H, Hutch A, Huch R 1989 Doppler sonographic evaluation exercise-induced blood flow velocity and changes in fetal, uteroplacental and large maternal vessels in pregnant women. Journal of Perinatal Medicine 17:279–287

Becker A E, Grinspoon S K, Klibanski A et al 1999 Eating disorders. New England Journal of Medicine 340:1092–1098

Beidleman B A, Rock P B, Muza S R et al 1999 Exercise V_E and physical performance at altitude are not affected by menstrual cycle phase. Journal of Applied Physiology 86:1519–1526

Beim G, Stone D A 1995 Issues in the female athlete. Sports Medicine 26:443–451

Bell R J, Palma S M, Lumley J M 1995 The effect of vigorous exercise during pregnancy on birth-weight. Australia and New Zealand Journal of Obstetrics and Gynecology 35:46–51

Belanger M J, Moore D C, Crisco J J 3rd et al 2004 Knee laxity does not vary with the menstrual cycle, before or after exercise. American Journal of Sports Medicine 32:1150–1157

Bennell K L, Malcolm S A, Thomas S A et al 1995 Risk factors for stress fractures in female track-and-field athletes: a retrospective analysis. Clinical Journal of Sports Medicine 5:229–235

Bennell K L, Malcolm S A, Thomas S A 1996 Risk factors for stress fractures in track and field athletes: a twelve-month prospective study. American Journal of Sports Medicine 24:810–818

Bennell K, White S, Crossley K 1999 The oral contraceptive pill: a revolution for sportswomen? British Journal of Sports Medicine 33:231–238

Bennell K, Khan K, McKay H 2000 The role of physiotherapy in the prevention and treatment of osteoporosis. Manual Therapy 5:198–213

Bensel C K, Kish R N 1983 Lower extremity disorders among men and women in army basic training and effects of two types of boots. Unites States Army Natick Research and Development Laboratories Report TR83/026, Massachusetts

Berg K 1984 Aerobic function in female athletes. Clinics in Sports Medicine 3:779–789

Birc K 2002 The diurnal rhythm in isometric muscular performance differs with eumenorrheic menstrual cycle phase. Chronobiology International 19:731–742

Birch K M, Reillly T 1999 Manual handling performance: the effects of menstrual cycle phase. Ergonomics 42:1317–1332

Bo K 2003 Pelvic floor muscle strength and response to pelvic floor muscle training for stress urinary incontinence. Neurourology and Urodynamics 22:654–658

Bo K, Sundgot-Borgen J 2001 Prevalence of stress and urge urinary incontinence in elite athletes and controls. Medicine and Science in Sports and Exercise 33:1797–1802

Bonds D R, Delivoria-Papadopoulos M 1985 Exercise during pregnancy: potential fetal and placental metabolic effects. Annals in Clinical and Laboratory Science 15:91–99

Bonjour J P, Theintz G, Buchs B et al 1991 Critical years and stages of puberty for spinal and femoral bone mass accumulation during adolescence. Journal of Clinical Endocrinology and Metabolism 73:555–563

Brutsaert T D, Spielvogel H, Caceres E et al 2002 Effect of menstrual cycle phase on exercise performance of high-altitude native women at 3600m. Journal of Experimental Biology 205:233–239

Bryner R W, Toffle R C, Ullrich I H et al 1996 Effect of low dose oral contraceptives on exercise performance. British Journal of Sports Medicine 30:30–36

Bullen B A, Skrinar G S, Beitins I Z et al 1985 Induction of menstrual disorders by strenuous exercise in untrained women. New England Journal of Medicine 312:1349–1353

Canada S, Knapik J, Toney E et al 2003 Injury risks in relation to gender and aerobic endurance in US Army ordnance school students. Medicine and Science in Sports and Exercise 35:S28

Campbell J A 2002 Preventing fractures by preventing falls in older women. Canadian Medical Association Journal 167:1005–1006

Cammu H, Van Nylen M, Amy J J 2000 A 10 year follow-up after Kegel pelvic floor muscle exercises for genuine stress incontinence. BJU International 85:655–658

Cann C E, Martin M C, Genant H K et al 1984 Decreased spinal mineral content in amenorrheic women. Journal of the American Medical Association 251:626–629

Cann C E, Cavanaugh D J, Schnurpfiel K et al 1988 Menstrual history is the primary determinant of the trabecular bone density in women. Medicine and Science in Sports and Exercise 20:S59

Capeless E L, Clapp J F 1989 Cardiovascular changes in early phase of pregnancy. American Journal of Obstetrics and Gynecology 161:1449–1453

Carpenter M W, Saddy S P, Hoegsberg B 1988 Fetal heart rate response to maternal exertion. Journal of the American Medical Association 259:3006–3009

Carter C D, Khan K M, McKay H A et al 2002 Community-based exercise program reduces risk factors for falls in 65 to 75 year-old women with osteoporosis: randomized controlled trial. Canadian Medical Association Journal 167:997–1004

Cassaza G A, Suh S, Miller B F et al 2002 Effects of oral contraceptives on peak exercise capacity. Journal of Applied Physiology 93:1698–1702

Chardoukian N, Joyner M J 2004 Physiologic considerations for exercise performance in women. Clinics in Chest Medicine 25:247–255

Chevalley T R, Rizzoli D, Manen J et al 1998 Arginine increases insulin-like growth factor 1 production and collagen synthesis in osteoblast-like cells. Bone 23:103–109

Clapp J F 1985 Fetal heart rate response to running in midpregnancy and late pregnancy. American Journal of Obstetrics and Gynecology 153:251–252

Clapp J F 1989 The effects of maternal exercise on early pregnancy outcome. American Journal of Obstetrics and Gynecology 161:1453–1457

Clapp J F 1990 The course of labor after endurance exercise during pregnancy. American Journal of Obstetrics and Gynecology 163:1799–1805

Clapp J F 1991 The changing thermal response to endurance exercise during pregnancy. American Journal of Obstetrics and Gynecology 165:1684–1689

Clapp J F 1994 A clinical approach to exercise during pregnancy. Clinics in Sports Medicine 13:443–458

Clapp J F 1996 Morphometric and neurodevelopmental outcome at age five years of the offspring of women who continued to exercise regularly throughout pregnancy. Journal of Pediatrics 129:856–863

Clapp J F 2000 Exercise during pregnancy: a clinical update. Clinics in Sports Medicine 19:273–286

Clapp J F 2001 Exercise during pregnancy and lactation. In: Garret W E, Lester G E, McGowan J et al (eds) Women's health in sports and exercise. American Academy of Orthopaedic Surgeons, Maryland, p 357–368

Clapp J F, Dickstein S 1984 Endurance exercise and pregnancy outcome. Medicine and Science in Sports and Exercise 16:556–562

Clapp J F, Little K D 1995 Effect of recreational exercise on pregnancy weight gain and subcutaneous fat deposition. Medicine and Science in Sports and Exercise 27:170–177

Clapp J F, Rizk K H 1992 Effect of recreational exercise on midtrimester placental growth. American Journal of Obstetrics and Gynecology 167:1518–1521

Clapp J F, Wesley M, Sleamaker R H 1987 Thermoregulatory and metabolic responses to jogging prior to and during pregnancy. Medicine and Science in Sports and Exercise 19:124–130

Clapp J F, Rokey R, Treadway J L et al 1992 Exercise in pregnancy. Medicine and Science in Sports and Exercise 24:S294–S300

Clapp J F, Simonian S, Lopez B et al 1998 The one-year morphometric and neurodevelopmental outcome of the offspring of women who continued to exercise regularly throughout pregnancy. American Journal of Obstetrics and Gynecology 178:594–599

Clapp J F, Lopez B, Harcar-Sevcik R 1999 Neonatal behavioral profile of the offspring of women who continued to exercise regularly throughout pregnancy. American Journal of Obstetrics and Gynecology 180:91–94

Cobb D L, Bachrach L K, Greensdale G et al 2003 Disordered eating, menstrual irregularity, and bone mineral density in female runners. Medicine and Science in Sports and Exercise 35:711–719

Collings C A, Curet L B, Mullin J P 1983 Maternal and fetal responses to a maternal aerobic exercise program. American Journal of Obstetrics and Gynecology 145:702–707

Consensus Development Conference 1991 Prophylaxis and treatment of osteoporosis. American Journal of Medicine 90:107–110

Considine R V, Sinha M K, Heiman M L 1996 Serum immunoreactive-leptin concentrations in normal-weight and obese humans. New England Journal of Medicine 334:292–295

Constantini N W, Dubnov G, Lebrun C M 2005 The menstrual cycle and sport performance. Clinics in Sports Medicine 24:e51–e82

Counts D R, Gwirtsman H, Carlsson L M et al 1992 The effects of anorexia nervosa and re-feeding on growth hormone-binding protein, the insulin-like growth factors and the IGF-binding proteins. Journal of Clinical Endocrinology and Metabolism 75:762–766

Creighton D L, Morgan A L, Boardley D et al 2001 Weight-bearing exercise and markers of bone turnover in female athletes. Journal of Applied Physiology 90:565–570

Cumming D C 1996 Exercise-associated amenorrhea, low bone density and estrogen replacement therapy. Archives of Internal Medicine 156:2193–2195

Cureton K J, Sparling P B 1980 Distance running performance and metabolic responses to running in men and women with excess weight experimentally equated. Medicine and Science in Sports and Exercise 12:288–294

Cureton K J, Collins M A, Hill D W et al 1988 Muscle hypertrophy in men and women. Medicine and Science in Sports and Exercise 20:338–344

Currie A, Morse E 2005 Eating disorders in athletes: managing the risks. Clinics in Sports Medicine 24:871–883

Daggett A, Davis B, Boobis L 1983 Physiological and biochemical responses to exercise following oral contraceptive use [abstract]. Medicine and Science in Sports and Exercise 15:174

Davies G A, Wolfe L A, Mottola M F et al 2003 Exercise in pregnancy and the postpartum period. Journal of Obstetrics and Gynaecology Canada 25:516–529

Dawson-Hughes B, Harris S S, Krall E A et al 1990 A controlled trial of the effect of calcium supplementation on bone density in postmenopausal women. New England Journal of Medicine 323: 878–883

Dean T M, Perreault L, Mazzeo R S et al 2003 No effect of menstrual cycle phase on lactate threshold. Journal of Applied Physiology 95:2537–2543

Deie M, Sakamaki Y, Sumen Y et al 2002 Anterior knee laxity in young women varies with their menstrual cycle. International Orthopedics 26:154–156

Delmas P D 1992 Clinical use of biochemical markers of bone remodeling in osteoporosis. Bone 13:S17–S21

De Souza M J, Maguire M S, Rubin K R et al 1990 Effects of menstrual phase and amenorrhea on exercise performance in runners. Medicine and Science in Sports and Exercise 22:575–580

Dewey K G 1998 Effects of maternal caloric restriction and exercise during lactation. Journal of Nutrition 128:S386–S389

Devereux K, Robertson D, Briffa N K 2005 Effects of water-based program on women 65 years and over: a randomized controlled trial. Australian Journal of Physiotherapy 51:102–108

Dombovy M L, Bonekat H W, Williams T J et al 1987 Exercise performance and ventilatory response in the menstrual cycle. Medicine and Science in Sports and Exercise 19:111–117

Dook J E, Henderson N K, Price R I 1997 Exercise and bone mineral density in mature female athletes. Medicine and Science in Sports and Exercise 29:291–296

Drinkwater B L 1996 Exercise and bones lessons learned from female athletes. American Journal of Sports Medicine 24:S33–S35

Drinkwater B L, Nilson D, Chesnut C H et al 1984 Bone mineral content of amenorrheic and eumenorrheic athletes. New England Journal of Medicine 311:277–281

Drinkwater B L, Nilson K, Ott S et al 1986 Bone mineral density after resumption of menses in amenorrheic athletes. Journal of the American Medical Association 256:380–382

Drinkwater B L, Bruemner B, Chesnut C H 1990 Menstrual history as a determinant of current bone density in young athletes. Journal of the American Medical Association 263:545–548

Drinkwater B L, Healy N L, Rencken M L et al 1993 Effectiveness of nasal calcitonin in preventing bone loss in young amenorrheic women [abstract]. Journal of Bone and Mineral Research 8:S264

Dummer G M, Rosen L W, Heusner W W et al 1987 Pathogenic weight-control behaviors of young competitive swimmers. Physician and Sportsmedicine 15:75–78

Ebben W P, Jensen R L 1998 Strength training for women debunking myths that block opportunity. Physician and Sportsmedicine 26:86–97

Eisenmann J C, Pivarnik J M, Malina R M 2001 Scaling peak VO$_2$ to body mass in young male and female distance runners. Journal of Applied Physiology 90:2172–2180

Ettinger B F, Genant H K, Cann C E 1985 Long term estrogen replacement therapy prevents bone loss and fractures. Annals of Internal Medicine 102:319–324

Fahey T D 1994 Endurance training. In: Shangold M M, Mirkin G (eds) Women and exercise: physiology and sports medicine, 2nd edn. FA Davis, Philadelphia, PA, p 73–88

Fleck S J, Falkel J E 1986 Value of resistance training for the reduction of sports injuries. Sports Medicine 3:61–68

Fogelholm G M, Koskinen R, Laakso J et al 1993 Gradual and rapid weight loss: effects on nutrition and performance in male athletes. Medicine and Science in Sports and Exercise 25:371–377

Fogelholm M 1994 Effects of bodyweight reduction on sports performance. Sports Medicine 18:249–267

Frankovich R J, Lebrun C M 2000 Menstrual cycle, contraception and performance. Clinics in Sports Medicine 19:251–271

Fredericson M, Kent K 2005 Normalization of bone density in a previously amenorrheic runner with osteoporosis. Medicine and Science in Sports and Exercise 37:1481–1486

Friden C, Saartok T, Backstrom et al 2003 The influence of premenstrual symptoms on postural balance and kinesthesia during the menstrual cycle. Gynecological Endrocrinology 17:433–440

Friedlander A L 1995 Two-year program of aerobics and weight training increases bone mineral density in young women. Journal of Bone and Mineral Research 10:574–585

Friedmann B, Weller E, Mairbaurl H et al 2001 Effects of iron repletion on blood volume and performance capacity in young athletes. Medicine and Science in Sports and Exercise 33:741–746

Frye A, Kamon E 1983 Sweating efficiency in acclimated men and women exercising in humid and dry heat. Journal of Applied Physiology: Respiratory Environmental Exercise Physiology 54:972–977

Fulkerson J A, Keel P K, Leon G R et al 1999 Eating-disordered behaviors and personality characteristics of high school athletes and nonathletes. International Journal of Eating Disorders 26:73–79

Garner D M 1991 The Eating Disorders Inventory-2. Psychological Assessment Resources, Odessa, FL

Garner D M, Garfinkel P E 1979 An index of symptoms of anorexia nervosa. Psychological Medicine 2:273–279

Garner D M, Olmstead M P, Polivy J 1983 Development and validation of a multidimensional eating disorder inventory for anorexia and bulimia. International Journal of Eating Disorders 2:15–34

Garner D M, Olmstead M P, Polivy J 1984 Manual of eating disorder inventory EDI. Psychological Assessment Resources, Odessa, FL

Garner D M, Rosen L W, Barry D 1998 Eating disorders among athletes: research and recommendations. Sport Psychiatry 7:839–857

Garshasbi A, Zedeh S F 2005 The effect of exercise on the intensity of low back pain in pregnant women. Gynecology and Obstetrics 88:271–275

Giacomoni M, Bernard T, Gavarry O et al 2000 Influence of the menstrual cycle phase and menstrual symptoms on maximal anaerobic performance. Medicine and Science in Sports and Exercise 32:486–492

Gilchrist J, Jones B H, Sleet D A et al 2000 Exercise-related injuries among women: strategies for prevention from civilian and military studies. Morbidity and Mortality Weekly Report 49(RR02):13–33

Green H J, Carter S, Grant S et al 1999 Vascular volumes and hematology in male and female runners and cyclists. European Journal of Applied Physiology and Occupational Physiology 79:244–250

Griffin L Y 1994 The female athlete In: DeLee J C, Drez D Jr (eds) Orthopedic sports medicine principles and practices. WB Saunders, Philadelphia, PA, p 356–373

Grimston S K, Sanborn C F, Miller P D et al 1990 The application of historical data for evaluation of osteopenia in female runners: the menstrual index. Clinical Sports Medicine 2:108–118

Grimston S K, Willows N D, Hanley D A 1993 Mechanical loading regime and its relationship to bone mineral density in children. Medicine and Science in Sports and Exercise 25:1203–1210

Grinspoon S, Baum H, Lee K et al 1996 Effects of short-term recombinant human insulin-like growth factor 1 administration on bone turnover in osteopenic women with anorexia nervosa. Journal of Clinical Endocrinology and Metabolism 81:3864–3870

Gulekli B, Davies M C, Jacobs H S 1994 Effect of treatment on established osteoporosis in young women with amenorrhea. Clinical Endocrinology 41:275–281

Haenggi W, Casez J P, Birkhaeuser M H et al 1994 Bone mineral density in young women with long-standing amenorrhea: limited effect of hormone replacement therapy ethinylestradiol and desogestrel. Osteoporosis International 4:99–103

Hale R W, Milne L 1996 The elite athlete and exercise in pregnancy. Seminars in Perinatology 20:277–284

Hall D C, Kaufmann D A 1987 Effects of aerobic and strength conditioning on pregnancy outcomes. American Journal of Obstetrics and Gynecology 157:1199–1203

Harber V J 2000 Menstrual dysfunction in athletes: an energetic challenge. Exercise and Sport Sciences Reviews 28:19–22

Harner C D, Paulos L E, Greenwald A E et al 1994 Detailed analysis of patients with bilateral anterior cruciate ligament injuries. American Journal of Sports Medicine 22:37–43

Hartmann S, Bung P 1999 Physical exercise during pregnancy: physiological considerations and recommendations. Journal of Perinatal Medicine 27:204–215

Harvey M A 2003 Pelvic floor exercises during and after pregnancy: a systematic review of their role in preventing pelvic floor dysfunction. Journal of Obstetrics and Gynaecology Canada 25:451–453

Hatch M, Shu X O, McLean D E et al 1993 Maternal exercise during pregnancy, physical fitness and fetal growth. American Journal of Epidemiology 137:1105–1114

Heer M, Mika C, Grzella I et al 2002 Changes in bone turnover in patients with anorexia nervosa during eleven weeks of inpatient dietary treatment. Clinical Chemistry 48:754–760

Heitz N A, Eisenman P A, Beck C L et al 1999 Hormonal changes throughout the menstrual cycle and increased anterior cruciate ligament laxity in females. Journal of Athletic Training 34:144–149

Helgerud J 1994 Maximal oxygen uptake, anaerobic threshold and running economy in women and men with similar performances level in marathons. European Journal of Applied Physiology and Occupational Physiology 68:155–161

Hergenroeder A C, Smith E O, Shyailo R et al 1997 Bone mineral changes in young women with hypothalamic amenorrhea treated with oral contraceptives, medroxyprogesterone, or placebo over 12 months. American Journal of Obstetrics and Gynecology 176:1017–1025

Herzog W, Minne H, Deter C et al 1993 Outcome of bone mineral density in anorexia nervosa patients 11.7 years after first admission. Journal of Bone and Mineral Research 8:597–605

Hewett T E, Stroupe A L, Nance T A et al 1996 Plyometric training in female athletes. Decreased impact forces and increased hamstring torques. American Journal of Sports Medicine 24:765–773

Hewett T E, Lindenfeld T N, Riccoben J V et al 1999 The effect of neuromuscular training on the incidence of knee injury in female athletes. American Journal of Sports Medicine 27:699–706

Hilton L K, Loucks A B 2000 Low energy availability, not exercise stress, suppresses the diurnal rhythm of leptin healthy young women. Endocrinology and Metabolism 278:E43–E49

Hinton P S, Giordano C, Brownlie T et al 2000 Iron supplementation improves endurance after training in iron-depleted, nonanemic women. Journal of Applied Physiology 88:1103–1111

Hoff J, Helegerud J, Wisloff U 1999 Maximal strength training improves work economy in trained female cross-country skiers. Medicine and Science in Sports and Exercise 31:807–877

Holloway W R, Collier F M, Aitkin C J et al 2002 Leptin inhibits osteoclast generation. Journal of Bone and Mineral Research 17:200–209

Hotta M, Fukuda I, Sato K et al 2000 The relationship between bone turnover and body weight, serum insulin-like growth factor, and serum IGF-binding protein levels in patients with anorexia nervosa. Journal of Clinical Endocrinology and Metabolism 85:200–206

Huston L J, Wojtys E M 1996 Neuromuscular performance characteristics in elite female athletes. American Journal of Sports Medicine 24:427–436

Iketani T, Kiriike N, Nakanishi S et al 1995 Effects of weight gain and resumption of menses on reduced bone density in patients with anorexia nervosa. Biological Psychiatry 37:521–527

Ireland M L 1994 Special concerns of the female athlete. In: Fu F H, Stone D A (eds) Sports injuries: mechanism, prevention, and treatment, 2nd edn. Williams and Wilkins, Baltimore, MD

Jackson M R, Gott P, Lye S J et al 1995 The effects of maternal aerobic exercise on human placental development: placental volumetric composition and surface areas. Placenta 16:179–191

Janse de Jonge XA, Boot C R L, Thom J M et al 2001 The influence of menstrual cycle phase on skeletal muscle contractile characteristics in humans. Journal of Physiology 530:161–166

Johnson C, Powers P S, Dick R 1999 Athletes and eating disorders: the national collegiate athletic association study. International Journal of Eating Disorders 26:179–188

Jones B H, Knapik J J, Pollard J A 1996 Frequency of training and past injuries as risk factors for injuries in infantry soldiers. Medicine and Science in Sports and Exercise 235:S40

Jonnavithula S, Warren M P, Fox R P et al 1993 Bone density is compromised in amenorrheic women despite return of menses: a 2-year study. Obstetrics and Gynecology 81:669–674

Jurkowski J E, Jones N I, Walker C et al 1978 Ovarian hormonal responses to exercise. Journal of Applied Physiology 44:109–114

Keatisuwan W, Ohnaka T, Tochihara Y 1996 Physiological responses of men and women during exercise in hot environments with equivalent WBGT. Applied Human Science Journal of Physiological Anthropology 15:249–258

Kardel K R, Kase T 1998 Training in pregnant women: effects on fetal development and birth. American Journal of Obstetrics and Gynecology 178:280–286

Keen A D, Drinkwater B L 1997 Irreversible bone loss in former amenorrheic athletes. Osteoporosis International 4:311–315

Kelly A W K 2005 Practical exercise advice during pregnancy: guidelines for active and inactive women. Physician and Sports Medicine 33(6):24–30

Kihlstrand M, Steman B, Nilsson S et al 1999 Water-gymnastics reduced the intensity of back/low back pain in pregnant women. Acta Obstetricia et Gynecologica Scandinavia 78:180–185

Kirchner E M, Lewis R D, O'Connor P J 1995 Bone mineral density and dietary intake of female college gymnasts. Medicine and Science in Sports and Exercise 27:543–549

Klebanoff M A, Shiono P H, Carey J C 1990 The effect of physical activity during pregnancy on preterm delivery and birth weight. American Journal of Obstetrics and Gynecology 163:1450–1456

Klibanski A, Biller B M, Schoenfeld D A et al 1995 The effects of estrogen administration on trabecular bone loss in young women with anorexia nervosa. Journal of Clinical Endocrinology and Metabolism 80:898–904

Knapik J J, Sharp M A, Canham-Chervak M et al 2001 Risk factors for training-related injuries among men and women in basic combat training. Medicine and Science in Sports and Exercise 33:946–954

Koike T 2005 Evaluation of exercise as a preventive therapy for osteoporosis. Clinical Calcium 15:673–677

Komi P V (ed) 1992 Strength and power in sport. Blackwell Scientific, Oxford

Knowles S B, Marshall S W, Yang J et al 2004 A gender comparison of injuries in North Carolina varsity high school athletes. Medicine and Science in Sports and Exercise 36:S275

Kraemer W J, Keuning M, Ratamess N A et al 2001 Resistance training combined with bench-step aerobics enhances women's health profile. Medicine and Science in Sports and Exercise 33:259–269

Kulpa P J, White B M, Visscher R 1986 Aerobic exercise in pregnancy. American Journal of Obstetrics and Gynecology 156:1395–1403

Lange U, Teichmann J, Uhlemann C 2005 Current knowledge about physiotherapeutic strategies in osteoporosis prevention and treatment. Rheumatology International 26:99–106

Langer O 2006 Management of gestational diabetes: pharmacologic treatment options and glycemic control. Endocrinology and Metabolism Clinics of North America 35:53–78

Laughlin G A, Yen S S 1997 Hypoleptinemia in women athletes: absence of a diurnal rhythm with amenorrhea. Journal of Clinical Endocrinology and Metabolism 82:318–321

Lebrun C M, McKenzie D C, Prior J C et al 1995 Effects of menstrual cycle phase on athletic performance. Medicine and Science in Sports and Exercise 27:437–444

Lebrun C M, Petit M A, McKenzie D C et al 2003 Decreased maximal aerobic capacity with use of a triphasic oral contraceptive in highly active women: a randomised controlled trial. British Journal of Sports Medicine 37:315–320

Lehnhard R A, Lehnard H R, Young R et al 1996 Monitoring injuries on a college soccer team: the effect of strength training. Journal of Strength and Conditioning Research 10:115–119

Lemmer J T, Hurlbut D E, Martel G F et al 2000 Age and gender responses to strength training and detraining. Medicine and Science in Sports and Exercise 32:1505–1512

Li D K, Janevic T, Odouli R et al 2003 Hot tub use during pregnancy and the risk of miscarriage. American Journal of Epidemiology 158:931–937

Lindqvist P G, Marsal K, Merlo J et al 2003 Thermal response to submaximal exercise before, during and after pregnancy: a longitudinal study. Journal of Maternal-Fetal and Neonatal Medicine 13:152–156

Lindsay R, Silverman S L, Cooper C et al 2001 Risk of new vertebral fracture in the year following a fracture. Journal of the American Medical Association 285:320–323

Lloyd T, Triantafyllou S J, Baker E R et al 1986 Women athletes with menstrual irregularity have increased musculoskeletal injuries. Medicine and Science in Sports and Exercise 18:374–379

Lokey E A, Tran Z V, Wells C L et al 1991 Effects of physical exercise on pregnancy outcomes: a meta-analytic review. Medicine and Science in Sports and Exercise 23:1234–1239

Loucks A B 1990 Effects of exercise training on the menstrual cycle: existence and mechanisms. Medicine and Science in Sports and Exercise 22:275–280

Loucks A B 2003 Energy availability not body fatness, regulates reproductive function in women. Exercise and Sports Science Reviews 31:144–148

Loucks A B, Callister R 1993 Induction and prevention of low-T_3 syndrome in exercising women. American Journal of Physiology 264:R924–R930

Loucks A B, Heath E M 1994 Induction of low-T_3 syndrome in exercising women occurs at a threshold of energy availability. American Journal of Physiology 35:R817–R823

Loucks A B, Horvath S M 1985 Athletic amenorrhea: a review. Medicine and Science in Sports and Exercise 17:56–72

Loucks A B, Mortola J F, Girton L et al 1989 Alterations in the hypothalamic–pituitary–ovarian and the hypothalamic–pituitary–adrenal axes in athletic women. Journal of Clinical Endocrinology and Metabolism 68:402–411

Loucks A B, Vaitukaitis J, Cameron J L et al 1992a The reproductive system and exercise in women. Medicine and Science in Sports and Exercise 24:S288–S292

Loucks A B, Laughlin G A, Mortola J F et al 1992b Hypothalamic–pituitary–thyroidal function in eumenorrheic and amenorrheic athletes. Journal of Clinical Endocrinology and Metabolism 75:514–518

Loucks A B, Heath E M, Law T et al 1994 Dietary restriction reduces luteinizing hormone pulse frequency during waking hours and increases LH pulse amplitude during sleep in young menstruating women. Journal of Clinical Endocrinology and Metabolism 78:910–915

Loucks A B, Verdun M, Heath E M 1998 Low energy availability, not stress of exercise, alters LH pulsatility in exercising women. Journal of Applied Physiology 84:37–46

Lovelady C A, Garner K E, Moreno K L et al 2000 The effect of weight loss in overweight, lactating women on the growth of their infants. New England Journal of Medicine 17:449–453

Lutter J M 1994 History of women in sports: societal issues. Clinics in Sports Medicine 13:263–279

Lynch N J, Nimmo M A 1998 Effects of menstrual cycle phase and oral contraceptive use on intermittent exercise. European Journal of Applied Physiology and Occupational Physiology 78:565–572

McCrory M A, Nommsen-Rivers L A, Mole P A et al 1999 Randomized trial of the short-term effects of dieting compared with dieting plus aerobic exercise on lactation performance. American Journal of Clinical Nutrition 69:959–967

MacEvilly 1996 Back pain and pregnancy: a review. Pain 64:405–414

McHugh M P, Tyler T, Tetro D T et al 2006 Risk factors for noncontact ankle sprains in high school athletes. The role of hip strength and balance ability. American Journal of Sports Medicine 34:464–467

Maddalozzo G F, Snow C M 2000 High intensity resistance training: effects on bone in older men and women. Calcified Tissue International 66:399–404

Magann E F, Evans S F, Weitz B et al 2002 Antepartum, intrapartum and neonatal significance of exercise on healthy low-risk pregnant working women. Obstetrics and Gynaecology 99:466–472

Malina R M, Ryan R C, Bonci C M 1994 Age at menarche in athletes and their mothers and sisters. Annals of Human Biology 21:417–422

Malone T R, Hardaker W T, Barrett W E 1993 Relationship of gender to anterior cruciate ligament injuries in intercollegiate basketball players. Journal of the Southern Orthopedic Association 2(1):36–39

Mandelbaum B R, Silvers H J, Watanabe D S et al 2005 Effectiveness of a neuromuscular and proprioceptive training program in preventing anterior cruciate ligament injuries in female athletes. 2-year follow-up. American Journal of Sports Medicine 33:1003–1010

Marcus R, Cann C, Madvig P et al 1985 Menstrual function and bone mass in elite women distance runners. Annals of Internal Medicine 102:158–163

Marcus R T, Drinkwater B, Dalsky G et al 1992 Osteoporosis and exercise in women. Medicine and Science in Sports and Exercise 24: S301–S307

Marshall J D, Harber V J 1996 Body dissatisfaction and drive for thinness in high performance: field hockey athletes. International Journal of Sports Medicine 17:541–544

Masterson G 1999 The impact of menstrual phases on anaerobic power performance in collegiate women. Journal of Strength and Conditioning Research 13:325–329

Melton L J 1997 Epidemiology of spinal osteoporosis. Spine 22(24 Suppl):2S–11S

Milunsky A, Ulcickas M, Rothman K J et al 1992 Maternal heat exposure and neural tube defects. Journal of the American Medical Society 268:882–885

Mirkin G 1994 Nutrition for Sports. In: Shangold M, Mirkin G (eds) Women and exercise physiology and sports medicine, 2nd edn. FA Davis, Philadelphia, PA

Mogren I, Pohjanen A I 2005 Low back pain and pelvic pain during pregnancy: prevalence and risk factors. Spine 30:983–991

Moller-Nielsen J, Hammer M 1989 Women's soccer injuries in relation to the menstrual cycle and oral contraceptive use. Medicine and Science in Sports and Exercise 21:126–129

More R C, Karras B T, Neiman R et al 1993 Hamstrings: an anterior cruciate ligament protagonist. An in vitro study. American Journal of Sports Medicine 21:231–237

Moreno A L, Benitez C M, Castro R A et al 2004 Urodynamic alterations after pelvic floor exercises for treatment of stress urinary incontinence in women. Clinical and Experimental Obstetrics and Gynecology 31:194–196

Myburgh K H, Hutchins J, Gataar A B et al 1990 Low bone density is an etiologic factor for stress fractures in athletes. Annals of Internal Medicine 113:754–759

Myburgh K H, Bachrach L K, Lewis B et al 1993 Low bone mineral density at axial and appendicular sites in amenorrheic athletes. Medicine and Science in Sports and Exercise 25:1197–1202

Myerson M, Gutin B, Warren M P 1991 Resting metabolic rate and energy balance in amenorrheic and eumenorrheic runners. Medicine and Science in Sports and Exercise 23:15–22

Myklebust G, Maehlum S, Holm I et al 1998 A prospective cohort study of anterior cruciate ligament injuries in elite Norwegian team handball. Scandinavian Journal of Medicine, Science and Sports 8:149–153

National Collegiate Athletic Association 1997 NCAA Division I Graduation Rates Report 1997. National Collegiate Athletic Association, Indianapolis, IN

Nattiv A 2001 The female athlete triad. In: Garrett W E, Lester G E, McGowan J et al (eds) Women's health in sports and exercise. American Academy of Orthopaedic Surgeons, Laurel, MD

Nattiv A, Agostini R, Drinkwater B et al 1994 The female athlete triad. The inter-relatedness of disordered eating, amenorrhea and osteoporosis. Clinics in Sports Medicine 13:405–418

Nattiv A, Arendt E A, Hecht S S 2001 The female athlete. In: Garrett W E, Kirkendall D T, Squire D L (eds) Principles and practice of primary care sports medicine. Lippincott Williams and Wilkins, Philadelphia, PA

Neely F G 1998 Intrinsic risk factors for exercise-related lower limb injuries. Sports Medicine 28:253–263

Nevitt M C, Ettinger B, Black D M et al 1998 The association of radiographically detected vertebral fractures with back pain and function: a prospective study. Annals of Internal Medicine 128:793–800

Nichols D L, Bonnick S L, Sandborn C F 2000 Bone health and osteoporosis. Clinics in Sports Medicine 19:233–249

Nicklas B J, Hackney A C, Sharp R L 1989 The menstrual cycle and exercise: performance, muscle glycogen, and substrate responses. International Journal of Sports Medicine 10:264–269

Nisell R 1985 Mechanics of the knee. A study of joint and muscle load with clinical applications. Acta Orthopaedica Scandinavica 21 (suppl):1–42

Noyes F R, Schipplein O D, Andriacchi T P et al 1992 The anterior cruciate ligament-deficient knee with varus alignment. An analysis of gait adaptations and dynamic joint loadings. American Journal of Sports Medicine 20:707–716

Notelovitz M, Zauner C, McKenzie L et al 1987 The effect of low-dose oral contraceptives on cardiorespiratory function, coagulation, and lipids in exercising young women: a preliminary report. American Journal of Obstetrics and Gynecology 156:591–598

Nunneley S A 1979 Physiological responses of women to thermal stress: a review. Medicine and Science in Sports and Exercise 10:250–255

Nygaard I E, Thompson F L, Svengalis S L et al 1994 Urinary incontinence in elite nulliparous athletes. Obstetrics and Gynecology 84:183–187

O'Connor P J, Lewis R D, Kirchner E M 1995 Eating disorder symptoms in female college gymnasts. Medicine and Science in Sports and Exercise 27:550–555

Old J L, Calvert M 2004 Vertebral compression fractures in the elderly. American Family Physician 69:111–116

O'Neill M E 1996 Maternal rectal temperature and fetal heart rate responses to upright cycling in late pregnancy. British Journal of Sports Medicine 30:32–35

Ostgaard H C, Zetherstrom G, Roos-Hansson E et al 1994 Reduction of back and posterior pelvic pain in pregnancy. Spine 19:894–900

O'Toole M L, Douglas P S 1994 Fitness: definition and development. In: Shangold M, Mirkin G (eds) Women and exercise. Physiology and sports medicine, 2nd edn. FA Davis, Philadelphia, PA

Otis C L 1992 Exercise-associated amenorrhea. Clinics in Sports Medicine 11:351–362

Palla B, Litt I F 1988 Medical complications of eating disorders in adolescents. Pediatrics 81:631–623

Parkkinen A, Karjalainen E, Penttinen J 2004 Physiotherapy for female stress urinary incontinence: individual therapy at the outpatient clinic versus home-based pelvic floor training. A 5-year follow-up study. Neurology and Urodynamics 23:643–648

Pivarnik J M, Marichal C J, Spillman T et al 1992 Menstrual cycle phase affects temperature regulation during endurance exercise. Journal of Applied Physiology 72:543–548

Pivarnik J M, Ayres N A, Mauer M B et al 1993 Effects of maternal aerobic fitness on cardiorespiratory responses to exercise. Medicine and Science in Sports and Exercise 25:993–998

Pivarnik J M, Mauer M B, Ayres N A et al 1994 Effects of chronic exercise on blood volume expansion and hematologic indices during pregnancy. Obstetrics and Gynecology 83:265–269

Polatti F, Perotti F, Filippa N et al 1995 Bone mass and long-term monophasic oral contraceptive treatment in young women. Contraception 51:221–224

Pollitzer W S, Anderson J B 1989 Ethnic and genetic differences in bone mass: a review with a hereditary versus environmental perspective. American Journal of Clinical Nutrition 50:1244–1259

Pomeroy C, Mitchell J E 1992 Medical issues in the eating disorders. In: Brownell K D, Rodin J, Wilmor J H (eds) Eating, body weight and performance in athletes. Disorders in modern society. Lea and Febiger, Philadelphia, PA, p 202–221

Powell J W, Barber-Foss 2000 Sex-related injury patterns among selected high school sports. American Journal of Sports Medicine 28:385–391

Prestwood K M, Pilbeam C C, Burleson J A et al 1994 The short term effects of conjugated estrogen on bone turnover in older women. Journal of Clinical Endocrinology and Metabolism 79:366–371

Prior J C, Vigna Y M, Barr S I et al 1994 Cyclic medroxyprogesterone treatment increases bone density: a controlled trial in active women with menstrual cycle disturbances. American Journal of Medicine 96:521–530

Pruitt L A, Jackson R D, Bartels R L 1992 Weight training effects on bone mineral density in early postmenopausal women. Journal of Bone and Mineral Research 7:179–185

Pugliese M T, Lipshitz F, Grad G et al 1983 Fear of obesity: a cause of short stature and delayed puberty. New England Journal of Medicine 309:513–518

Ramsbottom R, Ambler A, Potter J et al 2004 The effect of 6 months of training on leg power, balance, and functional mobility of independently living adults over 70 years old. Journal of Aging and Physical Activity 12:497–510

Rauramo J, Forss M 1988 Effect of exercise on maternal hemodynamics and placental blood flow in healthy women. Acta Obstetricia et Gynecologica Scandinavia 67:21–25

Redman L M, Weatherby R P 2004 Measuring performance during the menstrual cycle: a model using oral contraceptives. Medicine and Science in Sports and Exercise 36:130–136

Reilly E T, Freeman R M, Waterfield M R et al 2003 Prevention of postpartum stress incontinence in primigravidae with increased bladder neck mobility: a randomized controlled trial of antenatal pelvic floor exercises. British Journal of Obstetrics and Gynaecology 109:68–76

Rhea D J 1999 Eating disorder behavior of ethnically diverse urban female adolescent athletes and non-athletes. Journal of Adolescence 22:379–388

Rigotti N A, Neer R M, Skates S J et al 1991 The clinical course of osteoporosis in anorexia nervosa: a longitudinal study of cortical bone mass. Journal of the American Medical Association 265:1133–1138

Roberts W O 2000 A 12-year profile of medical injury and illness for the Twin Cities marathon. Medicine and Science in Sports and Exercise 32:1549–1555

Rosen L W, Hough D O 1986 Pathogenic weight-control behavior of female college gymnasts. Physician and Sportsmedicine 16:141–144

Ross J, Woodward A 1994 Risk factors for injury during basic military training: is there a social element to injury pathogenesis? Journal of Occupational Medicine 36:120–126

Ruiz J C, Mandel C, Garabedian M 1995 Influence of spontaneous calcium intake and physical exercise on the vertebral and femoral bone mineral density of children and adolescents. Journal of Bone and Mineral Research 10:675–682

Sabatier J P, Guaydier-Souquieres G, Laroche D et al 1996 Bone mineral acquisition during adolescence and early adulthood: a study in 574 healthy females 10–24 years of age. Osteoporosis International 6:141–148

Sady S P, Freedson P S 1984 Body composition and structural comparisons of female and male athletes. Clinics in Sports Medicine 3:755–777

Sallis R E, Jones K, Sunshine S et al 2001 Comparing sports injuries in men and women. International Journal of Sports Medicine 22:420–423

Sanborn C F, Jankowski C M 1994 Physiologic considerations for women in sport. Clinics in Sports Medicine 13:315–327

Schoene R B, Robertson H T, Pierson D J et al 1981 Respiratory drives and exercise in menstrual cycles of athletic and nonathletic women. Journal of Applied Physiology 50:1300–1305

Schultz D 1991 Risk, resiliency, and resistance: current research on adolescent girls. Ms Foundation for Women and the National Council for Research on Women, New York

Serresse O, Ama P F, Simoneau J A et al 1989 Anaerobic performances of sedentary and trained subjects. Canadian Journal of Sport Science 14:46–52

Shangold M, Rebar R, Wetz A C et al 1990 Evaluation and management of menstrual dysfunction in athletes. Journal of the American Medical Association 263:1665–1669

Shapiro Y, Pandolf K, Avellini B, Pimental N, Goldman R 1980 Physiological responses of men and women to humid and dry heat. Journal of Applied Physiology: Respiratory Environmental Exercise Physiology 49:1–8

Shephard R J 2000 Exercise and training in women: I. Influence of gender on exercise and training responses. Canadian Journal of Applied Physiology 25:19–34

Shrier I 1999 Stretching before exercise does not reduce the risk of local muscle injury: a critical review of the clinical and basic science literature. Clinical Journal of Sports Medicine 9:221–227

Simikin A, Ayalon J, Leichter I 1987 Increased trabecular bone density due to bone loading exercises in postmenopausal osteoporotic women. Calcified Tissue International 40:59–63

Sinaki M, Lynn S G 2002 Reducing the risk of falls through proprioceptive dynamic posture training in osteoporotic women with kyphotic posturing: a randomized pilot study. American Journal of Physical Medicine and Rehabilitation 81:241–246

Sinaki M, Brey R, Hughes C A et al 2005a Significant reduction in risk of falls and back pain in osteoporotic-kyphotic women through a Spinal Proprioceptive Extension Exercise Dynamic (SPEED) program. Mayo Clinic Proceedings 80:847–848

Sinaki M, Brey R, Hughes C A et al 2005b Balance disorder and increased risk of falls in osteoporosis and kyphosis: significance of kyphotic posture and muscle strength. Osteoporosis International 16:1004–1010

Slauterbeck J R, Fuzie S F, Smith M P et al 2002 The menstrual cycle, sex hormones, and anterior cruciate ligament injury. Journal of Athletic Training 37:275–278

Slemenda C, Christian J, Williams C 1991 Genetic determinants of bone mass in adult women: a reevaluation of the twin model and the potential importance of gene interaction on heritability estimates. Journal of Bone and Mineral Research 6:561–567

Snow-Harter C M 1994 Bone health and prevention of osteoporosis in active and athletic women. Clinics in Sports Medicine 13:389–404

Snow-Harter C, Bouxsein ML, Lewis BT et al 1992 Effects of resistance and endurance exercise on bone mineral status of young women: a randomized exercise intervention trial. Journal of Bone and Mineral Research 7:761–769

Soultanakis H N, Artal R, Wiswell R A 1996 Prolonged exercise in pregnancy: glucose homeostasis, ventilatory and cardiovascular responses. Seminars in Perinatology 20:315–327

Stephenson L A, Kolka M A 1993 Hemoregulation in women. Exercise and Sport Science Review 21:231–262

Sternfeld B, Quesenberry C P, Eskenazi B et al 1995 Exercise during pregnancy and pregnancy outcome. Medicine and Science in Sports and Exercise 27:634–640

Stevenson J C, Hillard T C, Lees B et al 1993 Postmenopausal bone loss: does HRT always work? International Journal of Infertility and Menopausal Study 28 (suppl):88–91

Stevenson M R, Hamer P, Finch C F et al 2000 Sport, age, and sex specific incidence of sports injuries in Western Australia. British Journal of Sports Medicine 34:188–194

Stone M H, Triplett-McBride T, Stone M E 2001 Strength training for women: intensity, volume and exercise selection factors. In: Garrett W E, Lester G E, McGowan J et al (eds) Women's health in sports and exercise. American Academy of Orthopaedic Surgeons, Laurel, MD

Stuge B, Hilde G, Vollestad N 2003 Physical therapy for pregnancy-related low back and pelvic pain: a systematic review. Acta Obstetricia et Gynecologica Scandinavica 82:983–890

Stuge B, Laerum E, Kirkesola G et al 2004 The efficacy of a treatment program focusing on specific stabilizing exercises for pelvic girdle pain after pregnancy: a randomized controlled trial. Spine 29:351–359

Sunderland C, Nevill M 2003 Effect of the menstrual cycle on performance of intermittent, high-intensity shuttle running in a hot environment. European Journal of Applied Physiology 88:345–352

Sundgot-Borgen J 1993a Prevalence of eating disorders in elite female athletes. International Journal of Sport Nutrition 3:29–40

Sundgot-Borgen J 1993b Nutrient intake of female elite athletes suffering from eating disorder. International Journal of Sport Nutrition 3:431–442

Sundgot-Borgen J 1994 Risk and trigger factors for the development of eating disorders in female elite athletes. Medicine and Science in Sports and Exercise 26:414–419

Sundgot-Borgen J, Larsen S 1993 Preoccupation with weight and menstrual function in female elite athletes. Scandinavian Journal of Medicine and Science in Sports and Exercise 3:156–163

Sundgot-Borgen J, Sundgot-Schneider L 2001 The long term effect of CBT and nutritional counseling in treating bulimic elite athletes: a randomized controlled study. Medicine and Science in Sports and Exercise 33:S97

Sundgot-Borgen J, Torstveit M K 2004 Prevalence of eating disorders in elite athletes is higher than in the general population. Clinical Journal of Sports Medicine 14:25–32

Suputtitada A, Wacharapreechanont T, Chaisayan P 2002 Effect of the 'sitting pelvic tilt exercise' during the third trimester in primigravidas on back pain. Journal of the Medical Association of Thailand 85 (suppl 1):S170–S179

Swanenburg J, Mulder T, De Bruin E D et al 2003 Physiotherapy interventions in osteoporosis. Zeitschrift für Rheumatologie 62:522–526

Taaffe D R, Snow-Harter C, Connolly D A et al 1995 Differential effects of swimming versus weight-bearing activity on bone mineral status of eumenorrheic athletes. Journal of Bone and Mineral Research 10:586–593

Taub D E, Blinde E M 1992 Eating disorders among adolescent female athletes: influence of athletic participation and sport team membership. Adolescence 27:832–848

Thacker S, Gilchrist, Stroup D, Kimsey C 2004 The impact of stretching on sports injury risk: a systematic review of the literature. Medicine and Science in Sports and Exercise 36:371–378

Thomas T, Gurguera G 2002 Is leptin the link between fat and bone mass? Journal of Bone and Mineral Research 17:1563–1569

Tibone J E, Antich T J, Fanton G S et al 1986 Functional analysis of anterior cruciate ligament instability. American Journal of Sports Medicine 14:276–284

Tinetti M E 2003 Preventing falls in elderly persons. New England Journal of Medicine 348:40–49

Torstveit M K, Sundgot-Borgen J 2005a The female athlete triad: are elite athletes at increased risk? Medicine and Science in Sports and Exercise 37:184–193

Torstveit M K, Sundgot-Borgen J 2005b The female athlete triad exists in both elite athletes and controls. Medicine and Science in Sports and Exercise 37:1449–1459

Torstveit M K, Sundgot-Borgen 2005c Participation in leanness sports but not training volume is associated with menstrual dysfunction: a national survey of 1276 elite athletes and controls. British Journal of Sports Medicine 39:141–147

Turkan A, Yuksel I, Fazli D 2005 The short term effects of physical therapy in different intensities of urodynamic stress incontinence. Gynecologic and Obstetric Investigation 59:43–48

Veille J C 1996 Maternal and fetal cardiovascular response to exercise during pregnancy. Seminars in Perinatology 20:250–262

Veille J C, Hohimer A R, Burry K et al 1985 The effect of exercise on uterine activity in the last eight weeks of pregnancy. American Journal of Obstetrics and Gynecology 151:727–730

Veille J C, Bacevice A E, Wilson B et al 1989 Umbilical artery waveform during bicycle exercise in normal pregnancy. Obstetrics and Gynecology 73:957–960

Wang S M, Dezinno P, Maranets I et al 2004 Low back pain during pregnancy. Obstetrics and Gynecology 104:65–75

Warren B J, Stanton A L, Blessing D L 1990 Disordered eating patterns in competitive female athletes. International Journal of Eating Disorders 9:565–569

Warren M P, Fox R P, DeRogatis A J et al 1994 Osteopenia in hypothalamic amenorrhea: a 3 year longitudinal study [abstract]. Program of the Endocrine Society Annual Meeting, Anaheim, CA

Weber C L, Chia M, Inbar O 2006 Gender difference in anaerobic power of the arms and legs: a scaling issue. Medicine and Science in Sports and Exercise 38:128–137

Webster S, Rutt R, Weltman A 1990 Physiological effects of a weight loss regimen practiced by college wrestlers. Medicine and Science in Sports and Exercise 22:229–234

Werle J, Zimber A 1999 Prevention of falls in elderly osteoporotic women: conception and effects of an intervention program. Zeitschrift fur Gerontologie Geriatrie 32:348–357

Wells C 1985 Physiologic differences and similarities. In: Wells C (ed) Women, sports and performance: a physiological perspective. Human Kinetics, Champaign, IL, p 19–34

Wiebe C G, Gledhill N, Warburton D E et al 1998 Exercise cardiac function in endurance-trained males versus females. Clinical Journal of Sports Medicine 8:272–279

Wilkins C H, Birge S J 2005 Prevention of osteoporotic fractures in the elderly. American Journal of Medicine 118:1190–1195

Williams N I, Young J C, McArthur J W et al 1995 Strenuous exercise with caloric restriction: effect on luteinizing hormone secretion. Medicine and Science in Sports and Exercise 27:1390–1398

Williams T J, Krahenbuhl G S 1997 Menstrual cycle phase and running economy. Medicine and Science in Sports and Exercise 29:1609–1618

Wilmore J H 1983 Body composition in sport and exercise: directions for future research. Medicine and Science in Sports and Exercise 15:21–31

Wilson Report 1989 Moms, dads, daughters and sports. Women's Sports Foundation, East Meadow, NY

Wolman R L, Clark P, NcNally E et al 1990 Menstrual state and exercise as determinants of spinal trabecular bone density in female athletes. British Journal of Sports Medicine 301:516–518

Women's Sports Foundation Report 1998 Sport and teen pregnancy. Women's Sport Foundation, East Meadow, NY

Wojtys E M, Huston L J, Lindenfeld T N et al 1998 Association between the menstrual cycle and anterior cruciate ligament injuries in female athletes. American Journal of Sports Medicine 26:614–619

Yates B, White S 2004 The incidence and risk factors in the development of medial tibial stress syndrome among naval recruits. American Journal of Sports Medicine 32:772–780

Zanker C L, Cooke C B 2004 Energy balance, bone turnover, and skeletal health in physically active individuals. Medicine and Science in Sports and Exercise 36:1372–1381

Zanker C L, Swaine I L 1998a Bone turnover in amenorrhoeic and eumenorrhoeic women distance runners. Scandinavian Journal of Medicine Science and Sports 8:20–26

Zanker C L, Swaine I L 1998b Relation between bone turnover, oestradiol, and energy balance in women distance runners. British Journal of Sports Medicine 32:167–171

Zanker C L, Swaine I L 1998c The relationship between serum oestradiol concentration and energy balance in young women distance runners. International Journal of Sports Medicine 19:104–108

Zelisko J A, Noble H B, Porter M 1982 A comparison of men's and women's professional basketball injuries. American Journal of Sports Medicine 10:297–299

Athletes with disability

Zoë Hudson and Amy Brown

28

CHAPTER CONTENTS

Introduction 525
Benefits of exercise for people with disability 526
Sports. 526
Classification for competition 527
Athletes with cerebral palsy 529
Athletes with learning disabilities. 529
Athletes with visual impairment 530
Amputee athletes 531
Wheelchair athletes 532
Other general issues. 534
Summary 535

Introduction

The history of sport and disability lies in the field of medical rehabilitation. Dr Ludwig Guttmann is generally recognized as one of the main pioneers and is known as 'the father of disabled sport'. As a neurosurgeon at Stoke Mandeville hospital in the UK towards the end of the Second World War, he saw that sport had a valuable role to play in the rehabilitation of physically disabled servicemen, and specifically those with spinal cord-related injuries who were confined to wheelchairs. In 1948, the first 'games' took place at Stoke Mandeville and by 1960 the first Paralympic Games were held in Rome following the Olympic Games. Since Seoul in 1988, the Paralympics have always been held in the same place as the Olympic Games, with the athletes using the same venues and competition sites. Since 1960 there has been an exponential rise in both the number of countries and the number of athletes competing. At the Athens 2004 Paralympic Games there were 3806 competitors representing 136 countries (www.paralympic.org). This increase reflects the growing interest and participation of people with a disability in sport. This growth has developed, in part, through an increased public awareness and participation in physical activity and recreational sports. Indeed, events for elite athletes with a disability have begun to be incorporated into able-bodied games. The Commonwealth Games in Manchester in 2002 was the first mainstream multi-sport event to do this, and subsequently this incorporated approach has been used in world championships in individual sports such as athletics in Helsinki in 2005. Whilst these events are restricted to a limited program, integration into able-bodied sport has helped to maintain and raise the profile gained during the high media coverage of the Paralympics. At the same time, a myriad of sports organizations now exist that provide information, coordination and support for people with all levels of physical and mental impairment who wish to participate in sporting activity.

The International Paralympic Committee (IPC) reported that over 500 million people worldwide are affected by disabilities (Sydney Paralympic Organizing Committee 2000). The Paralympic Games are a good reflection of the progression and development of sport and disability. The significance of the Paralympic Games, so-called because they are parallel to the Olympic Games, for disabled-bodied athletes is similar to that of the Olympic Games to the able-bodied. Competition at the 2004 Games involved 19 events, 15 of which were conducted under the same rules as their Olympic counterparts.

The majority of these contests were seen in the same stadiums and venues. The Paralympic athletes shared parallel stories of dedication, sacrifice, past failure or injury and, at times, controversy in arriving at the elite level of their sport. For this reason, this chapter will describe sport and disability in the context of elite athletes at the Paralympic Games. This is not intended to diminish other events such as the Special Olympics, which is a large international sporting organization for people with learning disabilities. There are many thousands of disabled-bodied athletes competing at the non-elite level and it is due to the lack of available literature that they are not covered in this chapter.

Benefits of exercise for people with disability

The physiological and psychological benefits of exercise for those with and without disability have been well documented (Durstine et al 2000). Physical benefits of exercise include improved cardiopulmonary function, strength, muscle coordination and balance. In some cases, functional ability of the disabled may improve through physical training; for example, gait quality and speed improved with strength training in a study of those with spastic cerebral palsy (Damiano & Abel 1998). Preliminary findings of the effect of an aerobic training program on lower extremity amputee subjects suggested a decrease in the metabolic cost of ambulation (Ward & Meyers 1995). A strength and flexibility training program has been shown to decrease the prevalence of shoulder pain in long-time wheelchair users (Curtis et al 1999b). The physically active disabled population may also enjoy decreased comorbidities such as diabetes, heart disease and obesity (Rimmer 1999). Psychologically, too, exercise can enhance mood, self-confidence and self-esteem (Shephard 1991). Labronici et al (2000) studied the effects of sport participation over a 2-year period and found that those involved in sport showed higher levels of vigor, lower levels of depression and improved social integration. Improved community integration that included satisfaction with leisure activities, social contacts and relationships with partners was reported in wheelchair athletes, in comparison to predisability levels of function (Pluym et al 1997). Along with the benefits of exercise, however, there is also an inherent risk of injury. Injury patterns in athletes with disability have been shown to be similar to their able-bodied counterparts, but the location of injuries appears to be disability and sport dependent (Ferrara & Peterson 2000). Much of the data collected to date have been facilitated by increasing numbers of participants at competition and records kept of those seeking medical attention. Some predictable patterns of injury related to sport, disability, or adaptive equipment were identified in the 1996 Summer Paralympic Games (Nyland et al 2000). The injury experience for the disabled ski athlete was also found to be similar to the able-bodied athlete in terms of extremity involvement and total injury history (Ferrara et al 1992). A further study by Laskowski & Murtaugh (1992) found that disabled skiers incur less severe injuries than the able-bodied.

Table 28.1 Disability associations in the USA and internationally

Disability	National organization	International organization
Amputee	Disability Sports USA	International Sport Organization for the Disabled
Cerebral palsy	US Cerebral Palsy Athletic Association	Cerebral Palsy Sport and Recreation Association
Intellectual disability	Special Olympics[a]	International Sports Federation for People with Intellectual Disability
Visual impairment	US Association of Blind Athletes	International Blind Sport Association
Wheelchair sport	Wheelchair Sports USA	International Stoke Mandeville Wheelchair Sport Federation

[a] Not under the auspices of the International Paralympic Committee

Much information has also been gained by self-report of injury and retrospective study. One such valuable source was the Athletes with Disabilities Injury Registry that detailed risk and severity of injury to disabled athletes from 1990 to 1992 (Ferrara & Buckley 1996). Formation by the IPC of the biennial VISTA Conferences provides an international forum for discussion and sharing of information and research between sports scientists and experts in the field of sport for athletes with disability. The management of medical problems specific to the physically challenged athlete is an important consideration for all those working in this field (Dec et al 2000). This chapter will describe the different sports and disabilities and how different impairments are classified.

Sports

There are five main categories of disability with respect to sport: visual impairment, cerebral palsy, intellectual disability, amputees and wheelchair athletes. Each disability or impairment has its own organization for registration, governing rules and regulation of sporting events at local, regional and national levels of competition (Table 28.1). The United States Olympic Committee (USOC) and the IPC oversee sanctioned events for Paralympic qualification. The International Olympic Committee (IOC) is the top of this organizational structure presiding over both the USOC and the IPC at all Olympic sanctioned international sporting events.

Disabled athletes participate in a variety of sports that can either be described as the same as or a modified version of the able-bodied counterpart, or as a disability-specific sport. Boccia, for example, is a disability-specific sport. It has been adapted from boules or petanques, and is played by people

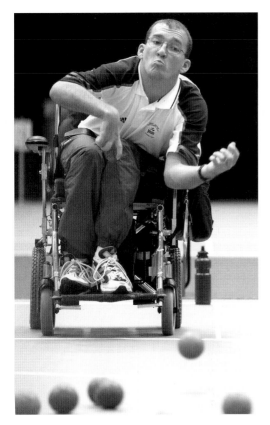

Figure 28.1 • Boccia player. (Reproduced with permission of ©Allsport, UK Ltd.)

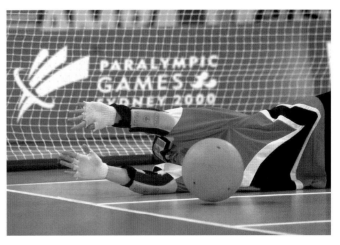

Figure 28.2 • Goalball player attempting to block the ball. (Reproduced with permission of © Allsport, UK Ltd.)

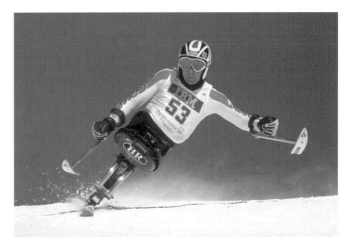

Figure 28.3 • Alpine skiing at the Winter Paralympic Games. (Reproduced with permission of © Allsport, UK Ltd.)

with cerebral palsy using a wheelchair during competition. It is a game of precision whereby the athlete attempts to throw leather balls as close to the jack as possible, down a long, narrow playing field (Fig. 28.1). Boccia can be played in an individual or team format.

Goalball is a sport designed to be played by athletes with a visual impairment. Two teams of six players compete, with only three from each team allowed on the court at any one time. The aim is to score by getting the ball over the opponent's goal line; the athletes defend their goal line by trying to block the ball using their body (Fig. 28.2). The ball has a bell inside and can only be thrown underarm. The players need to concentrate on the sound from the ball, therefore requiring all spectators to be silent.

While these are two examples of disability-specific sports, most sports are the same as, or adapted from, able-bodied sport (Fig. 28.3). Box 28.1 shows the sports that are currently sanctioned at Paralympic competition. This list has continued to evolve and does not reflect the numerous other sporting events or recreational activities that are available to the disabled athlete at the local and regional level. Although no exhibition sports were included at the Sydney 2000 Paralympic Games, increasing participation in yachting and wheelchair rugby was the force behind the move to include these competitions in Sydney after they were non-medal events in Atlanta 1996. Basketball was added as an exhibition sport to the 2004 Games in Athens. The

Winter Paralympic Games in 2006 saw the addition of wheelchair curling. With this trend, the addition of more sports may be anticipated in future Paralympic Games.

Classification for competition

It is often hard for a layperson to comprehend the complex classification system within the various disabled-bodied competitions. The purpose of any classification system is an attempt to create parity in competition, and to this effect, it is no different to classification systems that exist in able-bodied sport, such as different weight categories in boxing. Classification in disability sport has traditionally been structured by the disability. However, in several sports, a change of emphasis is developing away from the medical disability towards the athlete's level of function. Each sport has a different classification structure. Sports that utilize a functional classification system commonly have a classification team that conducts examinations

Box 28.1 Medal sports at the most recent Summer and Winter Paralympic Games

Summer Olympic sports	Winter Olympic sports
Archery	Alpine ski racing
Athletics	Biathlon
Basketball (exhibition 2004)	Cross country skiing
Boccia[a]	Ice sledge race
Cycling	Ice sledge hockey
Equestrian	Wheelchair curling
Fencing	
Football, 5-a-side	
Football, 7-a-side	
Goalball[a]	
Judo	
Powerlifting	
Sailing	
Shooting	
Swimming	
Table tennis	
Tennis	
Volleyball	
Wheelchair basketball[a]	
Wheelchair rugby[a]	
Wheelchair fencing[a]	
Wheelchair tennis[a]	

[a] Unique to Paralympic Games

Table 28.2 Classification for athletes competing in track and field events

Class	Description
Class 11–13	Different levels of visual impairment
Class 20	Learning disability
Class 32–38	Athletes with cerebral palsy (with and without wheelchairs)
Class 40–46	Ambulant athletes with different levels of amputation and other disabilities
Class 51–58	Wheelchair athletes with different levels of spinal cord injury and amputations

Table 28.3 Classification for athletes competing in swimming events

Class	Description
1–10	Wheelchair athletes, amputees and those with cerebral palsy
11–13	Different levels of visual impairment
14	Learning disability

on the athletes. A classification team may typically include a physician, physical therapist or athletic trainer and a sports technician. Range of motion, strength, balance and motor coordination are evaluated and assigned a point value in phase one of the evaluation. The second phase is actual assessment of sport performance with point values assigned for biomechanics and sport-specific abilities. The sum of these points is used to determine classification. Most athletes with cerebral palsy are typically classified by this manner, although again, it is sport dependent. The medical model is typically utilized for classification of amputee athletes, the visually impaired and those with spinal lesions. Readers are referred to www.paralympic. org for a complete account of classification systems for disabled-bodied sports. Tables 28.2 and 28.3 illustrate the differences between the classification structures in track and field, and swimming, respectively.

For track and field classification, the letters 'T', 'F' or 'P' indicate whether the event is on the track, field or pentathlon. These letters will precede class numbers in the classification system. In swimming, the prefix 'S' is used for backstroke, butterfly and freestyle, 'SB' for breaststroke and 'SM' for the individual medley. Therefore, a swimmer with no light perception at all in either eye, and who is competing in the 200 m individual medley, will race in class 200 m SM11. Swimmers within the same class and event may dive or start from the water. In classes 1 to 10, the higher the number, the greater the degree of functional ability.

Team sports such as wheelchair basketball and wheelchair rugby operate on a points system, whereby each player is given a points rating according to their level of physical function. For example, an athlete with a lower spinal lesion who has better trunk control and upper limb function would have a higher rating than someone with a higher lesion and less function. In wheelchair basketball, the points range from 1 (the lowest) to 4.5, and a team is not allowed more than 14 points between the five players on court at any one time.

The classification process has often come under criticism, partly due to the subjectivity in the functional classification process. While the functional process seeks to create an equal ground for competition, there has been concern that training effects may be confused with functional ability. In this system, those athletes who may have improved through training alone may be penalized if they 'over-perform' during testing and be reclassified to compete against athletes with lesser disability. Athletes can be classified many times during their sporting career, and it is not unusual to move up or down a class. It has been suggested that classification could be exploited by athletes wishing to gain an unfair advantage, and that this is the disability sports' equivalent of doping (Firth 1999). The lengths that some athletes go to achieve success has been illustrated by the Spanish team who won the gold medal in the intellectual disability basketball game at the Sydney 2000 Paralympic Games. It was subsequently discovered that there were members in the team who were not at all intellectually disabled. As a consequence of this, all competition for athletes in this group has been banned at the Paralympic Games and there were no competitors at Athens 2004.

Athletes with cerebral palsy

Cerebral palsy (CP) is the term used to refer to a non-progressive group of brain disorders resulting from a lesion or developmental abnormality in fetal life or early infancy. CP is characterized by altered muscle tone, adaptive length changes in muscles, poor coordination and control of movement and, in some cases, skeletal deformity (Shepherd 1995). Disorders of movement are typically differentiated and classified clinically in terms of tone and involuntary movement. There are five main descriptors:

- Spastic: involving tight muscles and limited range of motion
- Athetoid: involving slow writhing and purposeless movement
- Hypotonic: having low tone of extremities and/or poor trunk control
- Ataxic: involving balance and gait deficits
- Mixed lesions: involving multiple factors as above.

CP can be further classified depending on the part of the body involved, using terms such as monoplegia, diplegia, triplegia, hemiplegia, paraplegia or quadriplegia. CP can also be associated with cognitive deficits, deafness, visual impairment, dysphagia, seizures and speech and communication disorders. According to the degree of impairment, athletes may be ambulant or wheelchair dependent.

The physiological benefits of exercise and CP have been well documented. Hutzler et al (1998) showed a 65% increase in the baseline vital capacity of children with CP who embarked on a 6-month exercise program that included swimming, in comparison to an increase of 23% in the control group. Energy consumption is higher in CP athletes and is dependent on the extent of impairment. Duffy et al (1996) examined the energy expenditure in ambulant children with and without CP. The rate of oxygen consumption was significantly higher in those with CP, and higher in those with diplegia as opposed to hemiplegia. Duffy and colleagues attributed abnormal equilibrium reactions to the increased expenditure in those with diplegia. Barfield et al (2005) compared disability type and exercise response during power wheelchair soccer and found that those with CP had significantly greater heart rate (12 beats per minute more) compared to athletes with spinal cord injury. Furthermore, 71% of the athletes with CP exceeded 55% of the estimated heart rate max for at least 30 minutes during the competition (Barfield et al 2005). Use of orthoses or appropriate bracing for those with spastic CP may help to lower ambulatory energy expense (Maltais et al 2001). Cocontraction of lower extremity muscle groups has also been implicated as a significant factor in increased energy cost in gait of those with spastic CP (Unnithan et al 1996). Due consideration, therefore, must be made to the intensity of training programs and recovery times needed for an athlete with CP. As the motor impairment is the result of an alteration of the descending pathways, the concept of trying to alter movement patterns in terms of training and technique is contentious. It was previously believed that strengthening programs may create increased negative tone in those with spasticity. Recent research, however, has demonstrated that strength programs improve both motor function and gait quality in children (Blundell et al 2003, Damiano & Abel 1998, Morton et al 2005). In adults with cerebral palsy a 10 week progressive strength program resulted in improved walking velocity and Gross Motor Function Measure (GMFM) with no increase in spasticity (Andersson et al 2003). Use of hippotherapy, or equine riding programs, has been documented as beneficial for improving symmetry of muscle activity in children with spastic CP (Benda et al 2003). Use of botulinum toxin A has played a significant role in antispasticity management. Other advances in medical management continue.

Massage is commonly used in practice both before and after sporting activity for able-bodied athletes. Theoretically, massage can have either an excitatory or an inhibitory effect on muscle tone. Therefore athletes with CP must be cautious with the utilization of massage in the training program, especially if the athlete is reliant on tone for sport performance. Massage has been advocated in those with hypotonic muscles, but contraindicated in spastics and athetoids (Levitt 1982). There have been some anecdotal reports of the benefits of massage for athletes with CP (Clews 1995, Stewart 2000), but otherwise there is a paucity of research in the available literature. As with able-bodied athletes, it is important that the inclusion of massage in an athlete's schedule has been explored in training and not just introduced at a competition when it may be more readily available.

Maintaining flexibility is important for those with spasticity, and proprioceptive neuromuscular facilitation techniques can be employed by the therapist to address the muscle groups affected. As with massage, this may also affect the tone that the athlete relies on for stability and function, and thus the effect of stretching techniques must be assessed on an individual basis. The physical therapist also needs to consider the positioning of these athletes during assessment and treatment, from both a safety and tone aspect. Narrow portable treatment couches may be unsafe, and lying in the prone position may increase tone and therefore be inappropriate.

In competition, CP athletes are susceptible to a wide variety of injury. At the 1996 Summer Paralympic Games, CP athletes were treated most frequently for soft tissue injuries or muscle strains of the low back, lower extremities, foot and ankle (Nyland et al 2000). Those who compete in wheelchairs sustain injuries common to all wheelchair athletes, largely to the upper extremities. Standing athletes are harder to pattern, largely because CP athletes are the least homogeneous group. For those athletes who use ankle–foot orthoses or other orthoses, special attention should be paid to skin for signs of redness or breakdown. Some athletes who compete in standing events utilize crutches; these should be appropriately padded to avoid friction and pressure injury.

Athletes with learning disabilities

Athletes with learning disabilities may or may not present the physical therapist with any different physical problems from those of able-bodied athletes. For many individuals, the physiological potential is independent of the mental deficit. However, in some conditions such as Down syndrome and other forms of mental disability, the maximal heart rate is lower and may impact on training programs (Fernhall et al 2001). Target heart rate during intense training should be adjusted appropriately. Exercise has been shown to have some positive effects on both gait and bone metabolism in people with profound mental disability (Lancioni et al 2000). Athletes with intellectual disability have also been found to have a high prevalence of uncorrected visual or ocular deficits (Woodhouse et al 2003). Therapists should be cognizant of visual needs of the athlete and encourage eye exams if not previously screened in this group of athletes. The physical therapist must understand the limitations of cognitive impairment and have realistic expectations both of physical and mental ability. Management must be tailored to account for the cognitive impairments that may exist. If dysarthria or expressive deficits exist, the therapist should allow appropriate time for the athlete to communicate. Signboards, gesture or written communication may be utilized. Second party communication by the athlete's family or assistant should be utilized only as necessary to avoid miscommunications with the athlete. Athletes with learning disabilities may have difficulties understanding injury processes and explanations for the rationale behind therapeutic interventions. Problems with retention and recollection are often exhibited. The physical therapist on subsequent treatments should repeat an explanation for an intervention that was given at the initial instigation. Reiteration is very important with this group of athletes to facilitate comprehension and understanding. For example, in order to ensure adequate hydration during training and competition, checks may need to be made that all athletes have their own water bottles. The athletes may also need to be reminded to consume fluid at regular intervals. Prophylactic exercise-based programs, such as core stability work or rehabilitation programs postinjury, may need to be formally supervised to ensure compliance and correct technique.

An athlete with learning disabilities has to meet minimum disability criteria, which in accordance with the World Health Organization (WHO) definition is determined by:

- An IQ score below 75

- Limitations in regular skills areas (e.g. communication, self care, social skills, etc.)

- Onset of learning disability before the age of 18 years.

Athletes with visual impairment

Athletes with visual impairment are normally classified under one of three categories from B1 to B3 according to the International Blind Sports Association (IBSA) (Table 28.4).

The effect of visual impairment and musculoskeletal dysfunction is an area that to date has been poorly researched. In competition, visually impaired athletes have been found to

Table 28.4 Classification of visually impaired athletes (International Blind Sport Association)

Class	Description
B1	No light perception at all in either eye, or may have some light perception but an inability to recognize the shape of a hand at any distance or in any direction
B2	Can recognize the shape of a hand, and has the ability to perceive clearly up to 2/60. The visual field is less than 5°
B3	Can recognize the shape of a hand, and has the ability to perceive clearly from 2/60 to 6/60. The visual field is more than 5° and less than 20°

have higher numbers of lower extremity injuries (Ferrara & Peterson 2000) which are often attributed to an increased risk of accidents and inadvertent collisions. Further investigation may also implicate gait mechanics as a possible factor for increased incidence of lower extremity injury. Compared to those with sighted gait, the visually impaired demonstrate shorter stride length, slower walking speed and longer stance phase (Nakamura 1997). When attention is diverted to another task, gait quality may be significantly and potentially negatively altered (Ramsey et al 1999). These factors have the potential to create a higher incidence in overuse type injuries in the lower extremities.

Cervicothoracic complaints were also commonly reported by visually impaired athletes during the 1996 Summer Paralympic Games (Nyland et al 2000). This was suggested to be related to higher velocity injuries such as falls or rapid direction changes. However, the nature of visually impaired gait adaptation may also predispose this population to increased cervicothoracic stresses. Many visually impaired people find the use of a long cane helpful in daily mobility and obstacle avoidance. Long cane users were found to lack normal intersegmental movement of the neck, trunk and shoulder during gait (Mount et al 2001). This could lead to an increase in posture-related spinal problems, especially at the cervical and lumbar levels. Morioka & Maeda (1998) studied the effect of cane-transmitted vibration to the hand and upper extremity and determined that potentially detrimental effects may exist. Athletes with visual impairment who use the assistance of a cane or guide dog have the inherent potential to become overdeveloped on the side that the cane or dog is used. This could be problematic in a sport that relies on limb symmetry. For example, if a freestyle swimmer has muscle imbalance in the upper limb, this could manifest itself in an unequal arm pull, resulting in a less efficient stroke. Conversely, those who do not use a cane or the assistance of a guide dog, may adopt a kyphotic or poorer posture, and flex much more at the neck in order to judge the ground for distance.

A common strategy for those with tunnel vision or significant loss of peripheral vision is a 'scanning' approach that utilizes the central visual field for obstacle detection. The adaptation is typically seen as a persistent movement of the cervical spine, which consists of rotation usually, and some degree of side-bending. This constant, repeated movement has the potential to lead to cervical dysfunction. Those who rely on vision from one eye only may develop abnormal cervical alignment. The resultant effects on the rest of their postural alignment could potentially lead to upper limb overload and neuromusculo-skeletal dysfunction.

The protocol for the use of guides during competition is sport and Games specific. In some sports, such as tandem cycling and alpine skiing, a guide is necessary. Track and field events also utilize sighted pilots. In these events, every effort should be made to appropriately match the athlete gait and pace with that of the pilot to maximize potential and prevent injury.

Amputee athletes

Limb deficiency in the amputee athlete category may be of a congenital or traumatic origin. It occurs more commonly in the lower than upper limb, and the athlete may need to compete with a prosthesis in certain sports such as athletics (sprinting), standing volleyball and cycling. In other sports such as swimming, a prosthesis is not necessary. Classification of the athlete is dependent on the use of prostheses, wheelchair or other adaptive equipment during competition, as well as the location and extent of the amputation(s) (Webster et al 2001). For those athletes who compete with a prosthesis, the development of strong, lightweight materials (carbon fiber, titanium and Kevlar), using advanced technology and design, have all contributed to the potential for increased levels of performance. For example, the current 100 m world record (Class T43) is 11.16 seconds held by bilateral amputee Oscar Pistorius from South Africa.

There are many considerations for the type and design of a prosthesis for athletic use. For example, the socket design, fit and interface are of paramount importance for the amputee runner. The use of interface materials such as silicone liners, gel liners or hypobaric socks provides added padding and helps to absorb and disperse potentially damaging pressure and shear forces (Webster et al 2001). For transfemoral amputees, a flexible inner liner may be used to decrease the weight of the prosthesis and to accommodate the changing shape of the thigh during muscular contraction. For an above knee amputee, an ultra-lightweight pylon is usually used to connect the knee unit to the foot. Several options may enhance function, but at the same time, add expense and weight to the prosthesis. Torque absorbers, placed between the knee and the pylon, can absorb rotational forces and thus reduce shear at the socket/residual limb interface. This allows a certain amount of twisting between the foot and the knee (Huang et al 2001). The advent of high-profile elastic-response-type feet are now the choice of those athletes involved in sprinting sports (Fig. 28.4).

Cycling is a very popular sport for amputee athletes, and the prosthetic design considerations differ greatly from the running athlete. Athletes with a limb deficiency above the

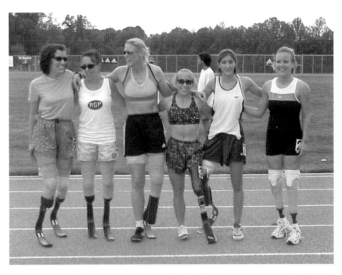

Figure 28.4 • Examples of high-profile elastic-response type feet (athletes on the left). (Reproduced with permission of Ossur/Flex-Foot, Aliso Viejo, CA.)

midtransfemoral level will not usually use a prosthesis as they cannot gain sufficient power to drive the pedal. Those who do use a prosthesis can have a problem keeping the foot component on the pedal. To counteract this, the component can be locked onto the pedal, although this raises injury potential in the event of falls or collisions.

Upper limb prostheses are also highly specialized and can be designed for those involved in throwing, swinging or catching sports. There are many devices available for holding hockey sticks, rackets, golf clubs, bowling balls, fishing rods, baseball bats and ski poles (Webster et al 2001).

With such a vast array of different components and materials, other considerations such as the location of the limb deficiency, the demand of the sport and the expectation of the athlete, mean that the prosthetist must work closely with the athlete, physical therapist and coach through all phases of the assessment, design, fitting and follow-up to ensure the optimal outcome.

The main problems encountered by amputee athletes are:

- Skin breakdown
- The consequence of limb asymmetry
- Component failure.

Skin breakdown at the socket/residual limb interface is common (Levy 1995). Shear forces and abnormal pressures on the residual limb within the prosthesis can contribute to skin breakdown. Silicon liners and total contact sockets have been found to considerably decrease pressure related pain; however, they have also been associated with increased problems with dermatitis secondary to increased perspiration, residual moisture and folliculitis (Hachisuka et al 2001). Skin irritation and pain can result in decreased tolerance to prosthesis use and subsequent loss of training days for the amputee athlete. Some considerations in the design of the prosthesis, to reduce the forces at this interface, and therefore decrease the risk of skin breakdown, have already been discussed. Athletes may encounter problems with adapting to a new prosthesis and training may have to be modified or reduced in order to overcome this. A tight socket will impede vascular performance. Problems may also develop as a prosthesis or socket wears out and a loose-fitting socket will cause areas of friction. The stump is very sensitive to overload, which can cause stump soreness. Sweating during activity can lead to pressure sores and stump breakdown. The therapist must be aware of the causes and implications, and regular inspection of the stump is recommended. This is particularly important when the athlete is more vulnerable, such as after training and during competition.

Limb asymmetry can cause a unique set of problems. For example, in order for an athlete with an above-knee amputation to swim in a straight line, there may be a need to pull more with the contralateral upper limb, thereby creating muscle imbalance and musculoskeletal problems as a consequence. This could cause a dilemma for the physical therapist who may not want to address the imbalance, but concentrate on injury prevention strategies on the side that is prone to overload.

Energy expenditure during gait is increased in lower limb amputees, dependent on the level of amputation (Waters et al 1976), and therefore they are likely to fatigue more quickly compared to an able-bodied athlete on a comparable training program. The sound limb on a unilateral below-knee amputee or above-knee amputee may also experience increased workload and moments of force resulting in potential for overuse type injuries (Czerniecki & Gitter 1992, Czerniecki et al 1996, Seroussi et al 1996). Data from a recent Paralympic Games indicated that sound side lower extremity injuries were common in the running athlete. Measured moments of the amputated side hip and reattached musculature were also significantly increased in ambulation and running gait of both transtibial and transfemoral subjects with possible implications for overuse injury (Buckley 1999, Jaegers et al 1996). Different weights of the prosthesis do impact on the work capacity and kinematics of both the sound and amputated sides. Attempts to match limb weight of the sound side with the weight of the prosthesis actually worsened the energy expense of gait and created a larger differential in limb loads (Mattes et al 2000). The lighter prosthesis (50% of the sound side) decreased energy expenditure and limb load suggesting that anatomical recreation is not the biomechanical advantage. Rehabilitation of a prosthetic-sided injury using the rest, ice, compression, elevation (RICE) principles are difficult to apply for the amputee athlete, for whom the loss of use of the prosthesis means the loss of functional mobility. Alerting the prosthetist to any area of concern may not only prevent days lost from training but also avoid the frustration of altered mobility and ability to carry out normal daily activities.

Wheelchair athletes

Athletes competing in the wheelchair category are most often associated with those who have a spinal cord injury (SCI), but

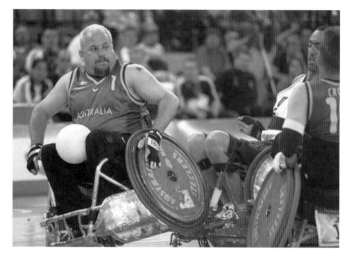

Figure 28.5 • Quad rugby in action, illustrating upper extremity weight-bearing demands. (Reproduced with permission of www.quadrugby.com and photographer Dariyoosh Hariri.)

they also include those with spina bifida, postpoliomyelitis and limb deficiency. Wheelchair athletes compete in a wide variety of sports, the most popular being track and field, basketball and swimming. However, there is a vast array of other sports, such as archery, table tennis, tennis, rugby, sailing and winter sports, to name but a few. Whilst the relationship between aerobic and anaerobic training and speed/sprint racing and endurance performance in able-bodied athletes is well established, the correlation is yet to be proven in this group of athletes. Anecdotal evidence would indicate that training and performance profiles match those of the demands of the sport; however, further research is warranted in this area (Bhambhani 2002).

Wheelchair designs have changed dramatically over the last 20 years, and just as prostheses have become sport-specific for athletes with limb deficiency, so too have wheelchairs. For example, the design of a chair used in basketball or quad rugby (Fig. 28.5) has demands for high maneuverability, and rapid acceleration and deceleration that differ greatly from the design of a chair used in track racing (Fig. 28.6).

Most chairs will be further adapted in accordance with the athlete's degree of trunk control. The biomechanical efficiency of wheelchair propulsion has been studied in order to maximize performance and reduce the risk of injury (Vanlandewijck et al 2001). It is not surprising that upper limb injuries predominate in this group of athletes (Ferrara & Peterson 2000). Common injuries include soft tissue injuries (33%), blisters (18%) and skin lacerations and abrasions (17%), and 5% reported symptoms of hand weakness or numbness (Curtis & Dillon 1985). Repetitive and forceful hand movements and pressure of the heel of the hand on the push rim of the chair may contribute to peripheral nerve entrapments. Burnham & Steadward (1994) reported a 23% incidence of peripheral nerve entrapment in wheelchair athletes. The median nerve at the carpal tunnel was most frequently affected, followed by the ulnar nerve at the wrist and forearm. Gloves and tape are often used to try and prevent the onset of symptoms (Fig. 28.6).

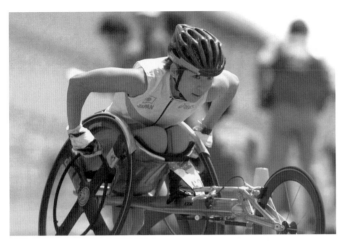

Figure 28.6 • A track-racing wheelchair. The athlete is wearing extensive hand protection. (Reproduced with permission of © Allsport, UK Ltd.)

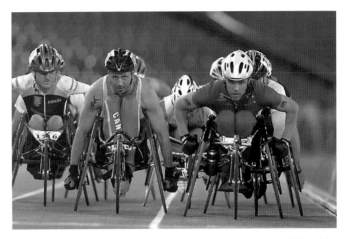

Figure 28.7 • Wheelchair track racers showing the amount of shoulder abduction required during different phases of the propulsion technique. (Reproduced with permission of © Allsport, UK Ltd.)

A high incidence of shoulder pain has also been reported in wheelchair athletes. In a study of 46 female wheelchair basketball players, only 14% reported shoulder pain prior to using a wheelchair (Curtis & Black 1999). This incidence rose to 72% since using a chair, with 52% reporting current symptoms. Furthermore, in another study, the prevalence and intensity of shoulder pain was reported as significantly higher in subjects with tetraplegia than in subjects with paraplegia (Curtis et al 1999a). However, these findings must be considered in light of the fact that they are based on self-reporting and/or retrospective questionnaires. Webborn & Turner (2000) also found that shoulder symptoms were the most common presentation in the British squad before and during the Atlanta Paralympic Games in 1996. On clinical assessment, however, cervicothoracic dysfunction was by far the most common source, and accounted for 59% of those reporting shoulder symptoms. Wheelchair athletes who are involved with overhead activities such as tennis, basketball and field throwing sports are more likely to incur shoulder pathology than those who are not. Wheelchair propulsion alone does not necessitate sufficient levels of abduction to give rise to symptoms such as impingement (Fig. 28.7). The additive stressors of the sport are compounded by the use of the upper extremities for activities of daily living, weightbearing in transfers and daily mobility.

Despite careful consideration of seating needs, poor flexed sitting posture is common in wheelchair users. In addition, during sports such as track racing, athletes adopt a flexed posture in order to achieve greater speed and to improve aerodynamics (Fig. 28.7). This position will force the cervical spine into protraction and stress the cervicothoracic junction. If wheelchair athletes present with pain in the shoulder area (C5 dermatome), it is important to determine the origin of the symptoms. Preventative measures may be identified in screening programs, and postural re-education implemented. Due to the repetitive nature and overload of wheelchair propulsion and transfers, these athletes are prone to muscle imbalance with a tendency to develop overactive latissimus dorsi, trapezius and pectoralis major muscles. Any imbalance/flexibility issues should also be incorporated into the athlete's training program. Testament to such an approach was seen in a 6-month exercise protocol, which was effective in decreasing the intensity of shoulder pain in wheelchair users during functional activities in a randomized controlled study (Curtis et al 1999b). The protocol involved five shoulder exercises that were performed daily over the 6-month period. Two exercises involved stretching the anterior structures, whilst the other three addressed muscle strengthening of the posterior structures.

While upper extremity complaints are the most commonly reported in the wheelchair athlete, the potential for lower extremity injury is especially high in contact or collision sports such as rugby and basketball. Athletes with sensory deficits may not be aware of the injury. Additionally, drag injuries to the lower extremity may occur if the leg is displaced off a footrest after contact or collision. A sensory areas should be appropriately protected and checked for signs of abrasions or contusions after training or competition. Lack of protective sensation also puts the wheelchair user at risk of developing abnormal pressures over weightbearing surfaces, which if left untreated, could lead to ulceration and potential infection. Pressure injuries should be avoided with appropriate seating systems, cushioning and frequent weight shifting (Minkel 2000).

Wheelchair athletes are also more prone to other medical conditions. Autonomic dysreflexia (ADR) is a potentially dangerous condition that can affect anyone with a SCI at the T6 level or above (Ericksson 1980). It can result from a variety of noxious stimuli, which in turn trigger sympathetic hyperactivity. Patients usually present with elevated blood pressure and bradycardia due to stimulation of the cranial nerve X (vagus) below the level of the injury. The body's attempt to reduce blood pressure causes vasodilation above the level of the injury. The common signs and symptoms of autonomic dysreflexia are shown in Box 28.2. This condition must be properly assessed and treated quickly and efficiently at the earliest signs or symptoms to prevent a potentially life-threatening crisis (Ericksson

Box 28.2 Common signs and symptoms of autonomic dysreflexia

- A sudden and significant increase in both systolic and diastolic blood pressure
- Pounding headache
- Profuse sweating above the level of the lesion
- Goose bumps above the level of the lesion
- Blurred vision
- Nasal congestion

1980). The elevated blood pressure is of most concern, and the blood pressure will drop with the removal of the stimulus. If the stimulus is not removed immediately, seizures, stroke and death can occur (Ericksson 1980). ADR is commonly triggered by an obstructed bowel or bladder (Ericksson 1980).

There have been reports of athletes self-inflicting ADR in order to elevate the blood pressure and enhance performance. This is a doping method unique to disability sport and is known as 'boosting' (Webborn 1999). Boosting may be achieved by using cutaneous, visceral or proprioceptive stimuli below the level of the cord lesion or by consuming large quantities of fluids with a clamped catheter drain. Boosting is considered a widespread and effective practice by wheelchair athletes, with improvements in mean race time reported to be as much as 9.7% (Burnham et al 1994). It is a dangerous practice that has been banned by the IPC. No athlete exhibiting signs of ADR is allowed to participate in competition. A systolic blood pressure of 180 mmHg or above over two examinations will result in the withdrawal of the athlete from the competition (www.paralympic.org).

Other general issues

Several general issues that relate to athletes with disability are important for physical therapists to be aware of. These include environmental considerations, drugs and doping and travel issues.

Environmental issues

A change of climate, whether related to temperature, humidity, or altitude will pose problems for any athlete. For example, the selection of Atlanta for the Olympic and Paralympic Games in 1996, where the average temperature in August was 85°F and with 60% humidity (Webborn 1996), posed problems for able- and disabled-bodied athletes alike. However, athletes with SCI are particularly vulnerable because their normal thermoregulation is affected. SCI above the level of T1 will compromise the parasympathetic nervous system, affecting the circulating blood volume and sweat production. As a result, quadriplegics do not perspire below the site of the lesion and therefore cannot effectively cool the body. In effect, such athletes have a decreased functional surface area by which to control thermoregulation. These athletes are equally at risk from heat and cold-related

conditions. Progressively higher levels of paraplegics were also found to have higher body core temperatures during comparable exercise in a hot environment due to lack of perspiration below the level of the lesion (Yamasaki et al 2001). Thermoregulation in temperatures below 50°F is also compromised in those with SCI lesions above T1 who lack circulatory shunting, reflexive shivering or goosebump production. Winter sport participants should have adequate clothing and access to indoor shelter in these conditions.

The same principles regarding fluids and rehydration apply for disabled-bodied athletes as for able-bodied athletes in both hot and cold weather environments. All athletes should be encouraged to maintain fluid intake. Intellectually impaired athletes may need particular attention in this area. Monitoring of athlete weight during intense training may be an effective way to track fluid replacement. In hot conditions, additional water should be sprayed frequently on the skin for the cooling effect of evaporation. The Atlanta Games found the utilization of misting booths for athletes particularly helpful. Water bottles are typically mounted onto wheelchairs. Athletes who are catheterized typically utilize a collection bag strapped to the leg. Because of the added weight of the filling bag, some athletes may defer taking on water to prevent competing with the filling bag or the interruption of draining the bag close to start of competition. This practice may predispose them to dehydration and the subsequent effects this has on performance. Athletes with SCI are also particularly vulnerable to the harmful effects of sun exposure. Circulatory changes and decreased sensory input put this population at greater risk, and therefore, the appropriate preventative precautions of adequate sun block and shaded shelters are recommended. Certain medications have the potential to affect thermoregulatory ability and some magnify the effect of sun exposure. Athletes should be advised when the medications may alter typical body response and take appropriate precautions with their training program.

Change of setting can have a great impact on both visually impaired athletes and those dependent on wheelchairs. For those dependent on wheelchairs, there are issues of access to accommodation, such as width of doors, and space in the bedroom to maneuver the wheelchair. Sport chairs, particularly, can have cambered wheels that exceed normal doorway frames or entries. The terrain to be covered, access to the training and competition venues, transport, etc., all need to be considered; for example, the Paralympic Village in the Sydney 2000 Paralympic Games was built on a fairly steep bank that was quite difficult for wheelchair athletes to negotiate. A regular bus service ensured that the athletes could avoid this difficulty.

A change of setting for athletes with visual impairment can also be very disorienting. For those with low vision, different lighting at the competition venue may impact on their visual acuity (Kuyk et al 1996) and subsequently their performance. The use of a guide may help the athlete make the transition into the new setting, both in the competition arena and in residents' accommodation. As discussed above, these athletes are more vulnerable to inadvertent collisions and avoidance of injury is a priority.

Drugs and doping

As the level of competition rises, so does the potential for an athlete to attempt to utilize means to gain the competitive edge that is not provided by training alone. Use of ergogenic aids and doping are not exclusive to able-bodied sports. At the 2004 Athens Paralympics there were ten positive drug tests during the games indicating a rise in prevalence nearing that of the able-bodied counterparts.

The list of prohibited classes of substances and prohibited methods of doping for disabled-bodied athletes are the same as for their able-bodied counterparts. In testing for drugs and doping, the primary difference between able- and disabled-bodied athletes is the fact that more disabled-bodied athletes may be on medication for underlying medical conditions. For example, 10% of the British swimming team at the European Championships in 1995 had some form of epilepsy (Webborn 1996). Exemptions allowing the use of drugs on the list for medical purposes can be sought by medical certification. The World Anti-Doping Agency (WADA) was enlisted in 2004 to initiate an out-of-competition testing program for athletes. 'Therapeutic use exemption' for medically necessary substances is approved by the Medications Advisory Panel reviewing by case and sport.

An official attending with any athlete who is to be drug tested must be familiar with the procedures and regulations (see Chapter 29). The main difference in procedures for the disabled, rather than able-bodied, sport is for athletes who are catheterized. Their leg bags must be emptied prior to testing and a fresh specimen obtained.

In terms of cheating for advantage, trying to deceive the classification procedure may be perceived, at present, as an easier route than taking performance-enhancing drugs. As classification systems develop further, this may change.

Travel issues

Since the advent of the Americans with Disabilities Act, and similar legislation in other countries, accessibility for the disabled has been the buzzword for all businesses, including the travel and tourism industry. Transportation difficulties have previously deterred the disabled from enjoying recreational travel. Today, there exist no less than 50 organizations that facilitate disabled travel worldwide (see www.routesinternational. com). The Air Carrier Access Act, implemented in 1986, stipulates that no airline may discriminate against persons with disabilities. The airline must supply an appropriate van or shuttle ground service, aircraft stowing procedures for power or specialized wheelchairs, collapsible boarding chairs and an appropriate environment to allow for safe boarding. Advance notice to the airline is necessary to detail all specific needs. Arrangements may need to be made in advance to accommodate some assistive devices, special seating or boarding assistance. However, even the most careful of planning can succumb to unexpected airline schedule changes or delays. This may present itself as the accessible aircraft being unavailable at the scheduled time. While able-bodied travelers are not inconvenienced by traveling on another aircraft, the disabled traveler may be in for significant delays. The disabled traveler may not be able to be rerouted onto non-jet planes or those that need to be boarded by stairwell rather than jetwalks. For travel delay reasons, the disabled flyer may be wise to carry on all medications as well as all pertinent emergency contact information, physicians' names, and numbers.

Hotel accommodation also needs to be carefully researched in advance of booking. The advent of the Americans with Disabilities Act has prompted numerous changes in building codes to accommodate the needs of the disabled; however, compliance is still an issue even in healthcare facilities (Sanchez et al 2000). 'Handicapped accessible' can encompass a very broad range of descriptors, or include only the minimum to meet legal requirements. Other countries may have different regulations regarding building codes for accessibility. Obtaining a complete description of shower facilities, grab bars, lowered sink measurements, raised toilet seats, doorway widths, closet facilities and other facility accommodations may avoid potential pitfalls. The facility may need to know some information regarding wheelchair dimensions, and weight or type of tires to further determine barriers to accessibility. Cambered chairs, as frequently used in wheelchair sports, add width and may be a consideration in planning for both hotel accommodation and ground transport. Hotel facilities may also need advance notice to accommodate guide dogs or assistive pets.

Another consideration during travel is special dietary needs. When planning the trip, the disabled athlete will want to ensure that at all stages during the travel process, appropriate nutrition is available, making advance plans as necessary. Delays in travel should also be anticipated and supplies planned ahead for this. Water consumption in some countries is not advised and careful planning is needed to avoid inadvertent ingestion during bathing, tooth brushing or use of water for cooling in hot weather competition. Medications, as discussed above, should be carried on the person or assistant at all times. A physician-issued card may be necessary to allow travel with syringes, and also in the case of metal implants that may set off airport and other security metal detectors; carrying of these documents can prevent untimely delays in travel.

Travel for the able-bodied can be wrought with frustration, but even more consideration and planning are required for the disabled traveler to minimize travel difficulties. Careful planning can eliminate unnecessary inconveniences and lessen the effects of problems from typical travel woes.

Summary

This chapter illustrates many of the considerations of therapy in disabled sport, and provides a description of the scope of the needs of athletes with disability. From the social and psychological benefits to the health-enhancing aspects of exercise, the physical therapist can have an important role in helping the athlete minimize days lost from training or activity. With the steady rise of participants in disabled sports, physical therapists will need increased awareness of rehabilitation considerations and will need to be able to identify potential risks inherent in this population. Few therapists or facilities work regularly with the disabled athlete, making expertise in the field a rarity. However, with knowledge of disability-specific issues, the therapist can provide the highest standard of care to the athlete. In addition, the therapist has a role of promoting sport and exercise to all disabled patients who may not be aware of the opportunities that exist. Referring patients to the appropriate sport association or club may be paramount to any therapy otherwise provided. Further research is needed in all aspects of disabled sport to advance the role of therapy, injury prevention and rehabilitation. Some topics, such as athlete classification, are expected to continue to evolve. Ever advancing biotechnology, as seen in prosthetics and wheelchair design, may also influence therapy consideration. Increasing visibility of disabled competition, local through international, will result in a rise of disabled sport participants. Physical therapists will have an ever-increasing role in education, health promotion and rehabilitation of this population.

Acknowledgments

Thanks go to Chris Holmes MBE, nine times Paralympic gold medallist, for his help in the preparation of this chapter for the first edition.

References

Andersson C, Grooten W, Hellsten M et al 2003 Adults with cerebral palsy: walking ability after progressive strength training. Developmental Medicine and Child Neurology 45:220–228

Barfield J P, Malone L A, Collins J M et al 2005 Disability type influences heart rate response during power wheelchair sport. Medicine and Science in Sports and Exercise 37:718–723

Benda W, McGibbon N H, Grant K L 2003 Improvements in muscle symmetry in children with cerebral palsy after equine-assisted therapy (hippotherapy). Journal of Alternative and Complementary Medicine 9:817–825

Bhambhani Y 2002 The physiology of wheelchair racing in athletes with spinal cord injury. Sports Medicine 32:23–51

Blundell S W, Shepherd R B, Dean C M et al 2003 Functional strength training in cerebral palsy: a pilot study of a group circuit training class for children aged 4–8 years. Clinical Rehabilitation 17:48–57

Buckley J G 1999 Sprint kinematics of athletes with lower limb amputations. Archives of Physical Medicine and Rehabilitation 80:501–508

Burnham R S, Steadward R D 1994 Upper extremity peripheral nerve entrapments among wheelchair athletes: prevalence, location, and risk factors. Archives of Physical Medicine and Rehabilitation 75:519–524

Burnham R, Wheeler G, Bhambhani Y et al 1994 Intentional induction of autonomic dysreflexia among quadriplegic athletes for performance enhancement: efficacy, safety and mechanism of action. Clinical Journal of Sports Medicine 4:1–10

Clews W 1995 Cerebral palsied athletes: massage benefits. Sport Health 13(4):22–23

Curtis K A, Black K 1999 Shoulder pain in female wheelchair basketball players. Journal of Orthopaedic and Sports Physical Therapy 29:225–231

Curtis K A, Dillon D A 1985 Survey of wheelchair athletic injuries: common patterns and prevention. Paraplegia 23:170–175

Curtis K A, Drysdale G A, Lanza R D et al 1999a Shoulder pain in wheelchair users with tetraplegia and paraplegia. Archives of Physical Medicine and Rehabilitation 80:453–457

Curtis K A, Tyner T M, Zachary L et al 1999b Effect of a standard exercise protocol on shoulder pain in long-term wheelchair users. Spinal Cord 37:421–429

Czerniecki J M, Gitter A 1992 Insights into amputee running. A muscle work analysis. American Journal of Physical Medicine and Rehabilitation 71:209–218

Czerniecki J M, Gitter A J, Beck J C 1996 Energy transfer mechanisms as a compensatory strategy in below knee amputee runners. Journal of Biomechanics 29:717–722

Damiano D L, Abel M F 1998 Functional outcomes of strength training in spastic cerebral palsy. Archives of Physical Medicine and Rehabilitation 79:119–125

Dec K L, Sparrow K J, McKeag D B 2000 The physically challenged athlete: medical issues and assessment. Sports Medicine 29:245–258

Duffy C M, Hill A E, Cosgrove A P et al 1996 Energy consumption in children with spina bifida and cerebral palsy: a comparative study. Developmental Medicine and Child Neurology 38:238–243

Durstine J L, Painter P, Franklin B A et al 2000 Physical activity for the chronically ill and disabled. Sports Medicine 30:207–219

Eriksson R P 1980 Autonomic hyperreflexia: pathophysiology and medical management. Archives of Physical Medicine and Rehabilitation 61:431–440

Fernhall B, McCubbin J A, Pitetti K H et al 2001 Prediction of maximal heart rate in individuals with mental retardation. Medicine and Science in Sports and Exercise 33:1655–1660

Ferrara M S, Buckley W E 1996 Athletes with Disabilities Injury Registry. Adapted Physical Activity Quarterly 13:50–60

Ferrara M S, Peterson C L 2000 Injuries to athletes with disabilities: identifying injury patterns. Sports Medicine 30:137–143

Ferrara M S, Buckley W E, Messner D G et al 1992 The injury experience and training history of the competitive skier with a disability. American Journal of Sports Medicine 20:55–60

Ferrara M S, Palutsis G R, Snouse S et al 2000 A longitudinal study of injuries to athletes with disabilities. International Journal of Sports Medicine 21:221–224

Firth F Y 1999 Seeking misclassification: 'doping' in disability sport. British Journal of Sports Medicine 33:152

Hachisuka K, Nakamura T, Ohmine S et al 2001 Hygiene problems of residual limb and silicone liners in transtibial amputees wearing the total surface bearing socket. Archives of Physical Medicine and Rehabilitation 82:1286–1290

Huang M E, Levy C E, Webster J B 2001 Acquired limb deficiencies: 3. Prosthetic components, prescriptions, and indications. Archives of Physical Medicine and Rehabilitation 82 (3 suppl 1):S17–S24

Hutzler Y, Chacham A, Bergman U et al 1998 Effects of a movement and swimming program on vital capacity and water orientation skills of children with cerebral palsy. Developmental Medicine and Child Neurology 40:176–181

Jaegers S M, Arendzen J H, de Jongh H J 1996 An electromyographic study of the hip muscles of transfemoral amputees in walking. Clinical Orthopedics 328:119–128

Kuyk T, Elliott J L, Biehl J et al 1996 Environmental variables and mobility performance in adults with low vision. Journal of the American Optometric Association 67:403–409

Labronici R H, Cunha M C, Oliveira A D et al 2000 [Sport as integration factor of the physically handicapped in our society.] Arquivos de Neuro-psiquiatria 58:1092–1099

Lancioni G E, Gigante A, O'Reilly M F et al 2000 Indoor travel and simple tasks as physical exercise for people with profound multiple disabilities. Perceptual and Motor Skills 91:211–216

Laskowski E R, Murtaugh P A 1992 Snow skiing injuries in physically disabled skiers. American Journal of Sports Medicine 20:553–557

Levitt S 1982 Outline of treatment approaches. In: Levitt S (ed) Treatment of cerebral palsy and motor delay. Blackwell Scientific, Oxford

Levy S W 1995 Amputees: skin problems and prostheses. Cutis 55:297–301

Maltais D, Bar-Or O, Galea V et al 2001 Use of orthoses lowers the O_2 cost of walking in children with spastic cerebral palsy. Medicine and Science in Sports and Exercise 33:320–325

Mattes S J, Martin P E, Royer T D 2000 Walking symmetry and energy cost in persons with unilateral transtibial amputations: matching prosthetic and intact limb inertial properties. Archives of Physical Medicine and Rehabilitation 81:561–568

Minkel J L 2000 Seating and mobility considerations for people with spinal cord injury. Physical Therapy 80:701–709

Morioka M, Maeda S 1998 Measurement of hand-transmitted vibration of tapping the long cane for visually handicapped people in Japan. Industrial Health 36:179–190

Morton J F, Brownlee M, McFayden A K 2005 The effects of progressive resistance training for children with cerebral palsy. Clinical Rehabilitation 19:283–289

Mount J, Howard P D, Dalla Palu A L et al 2001 Postures and repetitive movements during use of a long cane by individuals with visual impairment. Journal of Orthopaedic and Sports Physical Therapy 31:375–383

Nakamura T 1997 Quantitative analysis of gait in the visually impaired. Disability and Rehabilitation 19:194–197

Nyland J, Snouse S L, Anderson M et al 2000 Soft tissue injuries to USA paralympians at the 1996 summer games. Archives of Physical Medicine and Rehabilitation 81:368–373

Pluym S M, Keur T J, Gerritsen J et al 1997 Community integration of wheelchair-bound athletes: a comparison before and after onset of disability. Clinical Rehabilitation 11:227–235

Ramsey V K, Blasch B B, Kita A et al 1999 A biomechanical evaluation of visually impaired persons' gait a long-cane mechanics. Journal of Rehabilitation Research and Development 36:323–332

Rimmer J H 1999 Health promotion for persons with disabilities: the emerging shift from disability prevention of secondary conditions. Physical Therapy 79:495–502

Sanchez J, Byfield G, Brown T T et al 2000 Perceived accessibility versus actual physical accessibility of healthcare facilities. Rehabilitation Nursing 25:6–9

Seroussi R E, Gitter A, Czerniecki J M et al 1996 Mechanical work adaptations of above knee amputee ambulation. Archives of Physical Medicine and Rehabilitation 77:1209–1214

Shephard R J 1991 Benefits of sport and physical activity for the disabled: implications for the individual and for society. Scandinavian Journal of Rehabilitation Medicine 23:51–59

Shepherd R B 1995 Cerebral palsy. In: Shepherd R B (ed) Physiotherapy in paediatrics. Butterworth Heineman, Oxford

Stewart K 2000 Massage for children with cerebral palsy. Nursing Times 96:50–51

Sydney Paralympic Organizing Committee 2000 Sydney 2000 Paralympic Games official programme. News Custom Publishing, Southbank, Victoria

Unnithan V B, Dowling J J, Frost G et al 1996 Role of cocontraction in the O_2 cost of walking in children with cerebral palsy. Medicine and Science in Sports and Exercise 28:1498–1504

Vanlandewijck Y, Theisen D, Daly D 2001 Wheelchair propulsion biomechanics: implications for wheelchair sports. Sports Medicine 31:339–367

Ward K H, Meyers M C 1995 Exercise performance of lower-extremity amputees. Sports Medicine 20:207–214

Waters R L, Perry J, Antomelli D et al 1976 Energy cost of walking of amputees: influence of level of amputation. Journal of Bone and Joint Surgery (Am) 58A:42–46

Webborn A D 1996 Heat-related problems for the Paralympic Games, Atlanta 1996. British Journal of Therapy and Rehabilitation 3:429–434

Webborn A D 1999 'Boosting' performance in disability sport. British Journal of Sports Medicine 33:74–75

Webborn A D J, Turner H M 2000 The aetiology of shoulder pain in elite Paralympic wheelchair athletes: the shoulder or cervical spine. Proceedings from the 5th International Paralympic Committee Scientific Congress, Sydney, Australia

Webster J B, Levy C E, Bryant P R et al 2001 Sports and recreation for persons with limb deficiency. Archives of Physical Medicine and Rehabilitation 82 (3 suppl 1):S38–S44

Woodhouse J M, Adler P M, Duigan A 2003 Ocular and visual defects amongst people with intellectual disabilities participating in Special Olympics. Ophthalmic Physiology 23:231–232

Yamasaki M, Kim K T, Choi S W et al 2001 Characteristics of body heat balance of paraplegics during exercise in a hot environment. Journal of Physiological Anthropology and Applied Human Science 20:227–232

Section Five

Medical considerations for rehabilitation practitioners in sport and exercise

29 Pharmacological agents in sport and exercise 541
30 Medical imaging of injury 558
31 Medical issues in sport and exercise 578

Pharmacological agents in sport and exercise

29

Andrew Garnham

CHAPTER CONTENTS

Introduction 541
Therapeutic agents 541
Legal considerations 550
Performance-enhancing drugs 550
Summary 555

Introduction

Modern medicine to a large degree is dependent on a wide armamentarium of drugs for a great diversity of conditions. Medicine in relation to sport is no exception, with the misuse of drugs, in particular, having assumed a very prominent role. Clinical treatment of sport and exercise injury and sport-associated illness has relied upon a much narrower range of agents, but is not without controversy.

This chapter explores both the drugs commonly used in the treatment of sport and exercise injury and drugs that are used to achieve unfair advantage. The rationale for use, benefits and side effects of each of these two distinct, but not entirely separate, classes of drugs are detailed. While the use of the great majority of these agents is restricted to physicians, it is important for all working in the field of sport and exercise injury to have an understanding of them. Legal considerations regarding drug prescription, regulation of drug use in sport and drug testing are essential knowledge for any practitioner working with athletes.

While reading this chapter, it should be acknowledged that the laws and regulations regarding the prescription and use of pharmacological agents differ between countries.

Therapeutic agents

A range of pharmacological agents have been used in the treatment of sport and exercise injuries. Some of the better known include non-steroidal anti-inflammatory drugs (NSAIDs), corticosteroids, analgesics, rubefacients and thrombolytic agents. While there is a great deal of information on NSAIDs and corticosteroids in the rheumatology literature, in particular, there is a relative paucity of sound evidence-based material on the benefits or otherwise of these agents in the treatment of sports injury (Almekinders 1999, Gotzsche 2005, Leadbetter 1995, Paoloni & Orchard 2005, Stanley & Weaver 1998, Weiler 1992). The majority of studies have focused on the anti-inflammatory effects of these medications in acute injuries. Particularly conspicuous is a lack of evidence of both an inflammatory process and a therapeutic response to anti-inflammatory agents in chronic and overuse sports injuries. Analgesia probably plays a larger part in favorable outcomes than has been generally recognized.

Recently, hyperbaric oxygen therapy and novel antiarthritic drugs have also been used for the management of sports injuries, but are yet to find an established place in mainstream injury management. In the future, agents such as bone and tendon growth factors and their analogs will become more readily available, and may take on an increasingly important role in the management of chronic and overuse injuries in particular.

The inflammatory process

The cardinal features of tissue inflammation are pain (dolor), heat (calor), redness (rubor), swelling (tumor) and inevitable loss of function (functio laesa). These features are particularly evident in rheumatological conditions, such as inflammatory arthritis, with gout being the classical example of acute inflammatory effects. The patient with gouty arthritis is grateful for the swift and often complete relief that anti-inflammatory medications bring. In chronic inflammatory diseases, such as rheumatoid arthritis, the valuable role of anti-inflammatory medications is well established. However, when an athlete sustains an injury, loss of function, pain and, to a lesser extent, swelling are generally the symptoms most important to them, rather than heat or redness. It has been assumed that these changes are the deleterious effects of the inflammatory process, and therefore, reversal of inflammation should expedite recovery. This assumption is founded on very limited and largely anecdotal evidence (Dahners & Mullis 2004, Magra & Maffulli 2006). Whenever anti-inflammatory medication is proposed for treatment of an injury, consideration must be given to both the potential benefits and deleterious effects of the drug.

When tissue is injured, a well-ordered sequence of events follow, extending over 48–72 h in the acute phase, but spanning weeks to months before healing is complete. The three components of the inflammatory process are: first, the acute vascular inflammatory phase; second, the repair and regeneration phase; and third, the maturation phase. Features of the initial vascular inflammatory phase are dilatation of blood vessels (with an increase in blood flow and vascular permeability), exudation of fluids (including plasma proteins), activation and release of immunologically active mediators, activation of humoral response mechanisms and leukocyte migration to the inflammatory focus (Leadbetter 1995).

As part of these processes, a range of chemicals is produced at the site of injury. At the outset, vascular injury results in the liberation of vasoactive amines, anaphylatoxins and kinins. Neutrophil activation results in the production of oxygen-free radicals that attack the phospholipases of cell membranes, leading to breakdown of the cell wall and the generation of arachidonic acid metabolites, including various prostaglandins (Leadbetter 1995). This process is shown in Fig. 29.1, along with the sites at which anti-inflammatory medications inhibit the process.

During repair and regeneration, which is the second phase of the inflammatory process, cellular debris is removed by macrophages, vessels regenerate, and collagen synthesis begins. Fibroblasts and macrophages are the dominant infiltrating cells at this stage.

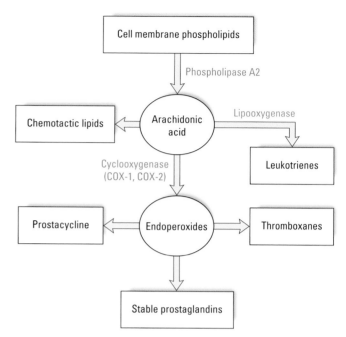

Figure 29.1 • Arachidonic acid metabolism and the influences of corticosteroids and NSAIDs. Corticosteroids inhibit phospholipase A2. NSAIDs inhibit cyclooxygenase. Some NSAIDs also inhibit lipooxygenase.

The third phase of the inflammatory process involves the maturation of collagen. Forces applied to the tissue influence cross-linkages and orientation of collagen fibers, affecting the ultimate tensile strength of the healed tissue (Best & Garrett 1994).

Medications can have an influence at any of the three phases of inflammation. Pain and swelling in the first phase, mediated in part by prostaglandins, is inhibited by the use of anti-inflammatory medications (Almekinders et al 1995, Stanley & Weaver 1998). These medications may then interfere with the repair process of the second phase by impairing DNA synthesis (Almekinders 1993, Almekinders et al 1995). Finally, relief of muscle pain and spasm, mediated by analgesic medication, can facilitate the rehabilitation process as tissue remodeling and maturation proceeds, as well as enhancing protein synthesis (Almekinders et al 1995, Mazanec 1998). Most research attention has been centered on the influence of NSAIDs and corticosteroids on these processes. There is clear evidence that part of the process is impaired, while other parts are enhanced by these drugs, with no major change in tissue healing overall. Whether the ultimate outcome is influenced positively or negatively remains uncertain, and is the subject of continuing investigation. Results vary between studies looking at the healing influences on muscle, tendon, articular cartilage and ligament. Also, much of this information has been based on animal research models which may not be directly applicable to human sporting injuries (Almekinders et al 1995, Best & Garrett 1994, Hanson et al 2005, Leadbetter 1995).

Non-steroidal anti-inflammatory drugs (NSAIDs)

NSAIDs have been widely used, both in prescription and over-the-counter forms, for virtually all types of musculoskeletal injury. They are widely promoted for the relief of spinal and joint pain. It is, however, only relatively recently that their place in sports injury treatment has been scrutinized. There remains much to be learned in this respect, and these drugs should certainly not be regarded as an injury panacea.

Clinical effects of NSAIDs in sports injury

Many recent studies have investigated the benefits of NSAIDs in the treatment of sports injury. From critical reviews of such investigations (Gotzsche 2005, Ogilvie-Harris & Gilbart 1995, Paoloni & Orchard 2005, Weiler 1992) it has been shown that athletes with acute injuries (typically ankle sprains) who are treated with NSAIDs return to sport slightly more quickly, and with lower levels of pain, than control groups. These studies, however, show little difference in terms of overall outcome where swelling and functional capacity are concerned. It has not been possible to determine whether the tissue healing process has been enhanced or impaired through the use of NSAIDs (Dahners & Mullis 2004, Magra & Maffulli 2006, Ogilvie-Harris & Gilbart 1995, Slatyer et al 1997, Stanley & Weaver 1998, Weiler 1992). NSAIDs, when used prophylactically, have been shown to be effective in reducing parameters associated with delayed onset muscle soreness, such as pain, power, swelling and creatine kinase levels (Dudley et al 1997, Hasson et al 1993, O'Grady et al 2000, Sayers et al 2001). However, these findings cannot be translated to most clinical situations, as the experimental model is not typical of sporting injuries for which NSAIDs are commonly used. Most studies involving the use of NSAIDs on ligamentous injury have been methodologically flawed by limitations in injury classification, use of other concurrent therapy modalities, poor randomization and lack of true control groups (Weiler 1992). It can be concluded that individual athlete circumstances are the major determining factor in choosing to employ NSAIDs following injury; for example, a desire to return to sport quickly would encourage their use. Pain, leading to impaired rehabilitative capability is also an indication, although other analgesics may be just as effective (Woo et al 2005). In light of these theoretical concerns regarding whether NSAIDs impair the repair, regeneration and remodeling processes, they should probably only be used for short periods.

Choice of NSAID

There is no evidence to suggest that any one NSAID is more effective in the treatment of sports injury than another (Gotzsche 2005, Ogilvie-Harris & Gilbart 1995, Weiler 1992). As seen in Table 29.1, NSAIDs belong to a range of quite different chemical classes, but this has little effect on their clinical usefulness. NSAIDs that inhibit lipooxygenase in addition to cyclooxygenase (diclofenac, indomethacin and ketoprofen) are arguably more potent, but this contention is not well supported by clinical evidence (Sayers et al 2001). The relative degree

Table 29.1 Commonly used NSAIDs in the management of sport and exercise injuries

Class	Sub class	Generic drug name
Carboxylic acids	Acetic acids	Diclofenac Etodolac Indomethacin Sulindac Tolmetin
	Fenamates	Meclofenamic acid Mefanamic acid
	Propionic acids	Fenoprofen Flurbiprofen Ibuprofen Ketoprofen Naproxen Oxaprozin Tiaprofenic acid
	Salicylates	Aspirin Diflunisal Salsalate Sulfasalazine
Enolic acids	Oxicams	Piroxicam Tenoxicam
	Pyrazoles	Celecoxib Ketorolac Phenylbutazone

of inhibition of cyclooxygenase-1 and cyclooxygenase-2 by different agents may affect the extent of central and peripheral action, and therefore potency. However, clinical evidence for this proposed effect is again lacking in the literature.

Factors determining the choice of an NSAID include side-effect profile, relative cost, onset of action and duration of action. The dosage form (i.e. tablet, capsule, suspension, suppository) may be important to some patients. Dosage frequency, which can vary between 1 and 4 times daily, should be considered. In the treatment of acute injury, an NSAID with a rapid onset of action is probably most suitable. For patients less likely to remember their medication, a longer acting, once daily form may be better suited. Patients should always be reminded to take NSAIDs immediately after meals, and never on an empty stomach, to minimize direct gastric irritation. It should be borne in mind, however, that many gastric side effects are systemic in nature, and are not prevented by taking the medication with food. Ketorolac, an injectable NSAID, while particularly potent, is only indicated for postoperative pain relief, and not for the treatment of sports injury.

In general, a practitioner will become familiar with several different NSAIDs, and prescribe on the basis of their personal experience. Although many NSAIDs are packaged to allow about

4 weeks' supply at normal dosages, it should be explained to patients that this is not a defined course of treatment, and that if no benefit is apparent after 1 week, there is probably no reason to continue the medication. If one NSAID is not having the desired benefit, there is no evidence to suggest that changing to another agent is worthwhile, assuming the initial dosage was adequate. In acute sprains of mild to moderate severity, 3–7 days of use is probably optimal to facilitate recovery (Mazanec 1998, Weiler 1992). In chronic conditions, such as degenerative joint disease in active patients, NSAIDs can be used as required to control symptoms, where the condition itself is unlikely to be modified. For example, NSAIDs may be used for a day or so before and after a weekly sporting activity to minimize pain and potential drug side effects, and to optimize function and enjoyment.

Selective cyclooxygenase-2 (COX-2) inhibitors (e.g. celecoxib, rofecoxib) have been promoted as major advances in NSAID technology. Cyclooxygenase-1 (COX-1) is the constitutional isoenzyme primarily responsible for the production of prostaglandins that regulate normal physiological functions, such as gastric cytoprotection, renal parenchymal function, and platelet activity. COX-2 is an inducible isoenzyme primarily responsible for the production of prostaglandins that regulate pain, inflammation, and fever. Most of the anti-inflammatory benefits of NSAIDs appear to be the result of COX-2 inhibition (Stanley & Weaver 1998). As many of the side effects of NSAIDs are associated with COX-1 inhibition, selective COX-2 inhibitors should have a more favorable side-effect profile, while still maintaining efficacy. This benefit is borne out in a significant reduction in peptic ulceration. However, gastrointestinal side effects do still occur with the selective COX-2 inhibitors, and they may also have prothrombotic effects (Brunton et al 2006). Rofecoxib has been withdrawn from sale because of its strong association with adverse cardiovascular events. Efficacy appears to be similar to established NSAIDs. Overall, COX-2 inhibitors are more expensive and appear to offer no advantage other than a reduction in peptic ulceration in long term users (Paoloni & Orchard 2005, Warden 2005).

Side effects of NSAIDs

A large number of side effects of NSAIDs have been recorded. Although gastrointestinal side effects are common, the great majority of side effects are infrequent, and details are readily available in pharmacology texts (e.g. Brunton et al 2006, Goldman & Ausiello 2003). The use of NSAIDs in pregnancy and lactation is relatively contraindicated. All NSAIDs have been shown to produce a low incidence of teratogenic effects in animal studies, and all are excreted in breast milk. A history of previous side effects with use, or allergy to NSAIDs, including aspirin, should always be sought before prescription. Substitution of a different NSAID may prove satisfactory, but should only be undertaken with great caution.

Major side effects of NSAIDs include the following (Brunton et al 2006):

- Gastrointestinal disturbance, including indigestion, epigastric pain, gastroesophageal reflux, nausea, diarrhea and constipation

- Peptic ulceration, with a risk of bleeding, which may be occult in nature and lead to anemia

- Renal dysfunction, including sodium retention with consequent fluid retention and renal failure

- Impaired platelet aggregation, leading to prolongation of bleeding time. This effect may persist for days, or even weeks after cessation of the medication

- Possible increased risk of cardiovascular events, particularly myocardial infarction

- Precipitation of asthma

- Rash

- Headache

- Tiredness

- Interaction with other drugs, particularly anticoagulants and antihypertensives.

Gastrointestinal symptoms may occur in as many as 25% of patients treated with NSAIDs (Brunton et al 2006, Leadbetter 1995). Serious complications such as peptic ulceration are most likely to occur with long-term use, and in the elderly (Brunton et al 2006). However, peptic ulcer should be considered in any patient using NSAIDs who has persistent or severe gastrointestinal symptoms. Generally, patients who experience symptoms should be advised to cease the medication, as long-term use is most often not required in the treatment of sports injury. If necessary, a different NSAID may not cause symptoms. Various anti-ulcer drugs can be used in combination with NSAIDs to minimize symptoms, but this approach should only be necessary in the presence of chronic disease that is unresponsive to other therapy. Interaction with alcohol is a side-effect concern often raised by athletes who are prescribed NSAIDs. No significant interaction occurs, but athletes should be reminded that both agents can cause gastrointestinal disturbance, and are best not combined. Alcohol consumption soon after injury should be avoided in any case, due to its vasodilatory effects.

The risk of bleeding at the injury site following administration of NSAIDs is a concern often raised in relation to the timing of commencement of dosage. NSAIDs should not precipitate bleeding once clotting has occurred. The standard measures of rest, ice, compression and elevation (RICE) should be commenced as soon as possible following any traumatic injury, and bleeding at the site should then cease within minutes. Therefore, it should be reasonable to commence NSAIDs as soon as 1 hour after initial treatment. However, there is no evidence to suggest when the most suitable time is, and questions remain in relation to beneficial or deleterious effects of NSAIDs in the inflammatory process (Dahners & Mullis 2004, Magra & Maffulli 2006). It should be remembered that many athletes might already be taking NSAIDs at the time of injury, or in the days beforehand. In this situation, extra effort should be made to minimize bleeding.

Topical NSAIDs

A number of well-known NSAIDs are available in topical forms such as creams, gels, slow-release patches and sprays. Their use as topical agents has two major potential advantages over systemic forms. Firstly, side effects, especially gastrointestinal, should be reduced. Secondly, the patient may gain additional therapeutic benefit by the method of administration, such as massage or phonophoresis. Topical NSAIDs are probably most useful for conditions affecting relatively superficial structures, as their depth of penetration is limited at normal dosage levels, and probably extends to 3–4 mm (Burnham et al 1998, Singh & Roberts 1994). Blood concentrations of less than 10% of those achieved with oral medications have been demonstrated with topical agents (Stanley & Weaver 1998). Topical agents have been shown to be effective in reducing pain in acute and chronic sporting injuries (Burnham et al 1998, Mason et al 2004b, 2004c, Stanley & Weaver 1998). Large doses applied over extensive areas of skin can lead to significant systemic absorption, and consequently to the potential side effects associated with oral NSAIDs. Prolonged use of topical NSAIDs is associated with a significant incidence of skin irritation, and some patients develop rashes early in the use of the products (Burnham et al 1998, Mason et al 2004a, 2004b). Use beyond 10–14 days should be avoided, as should application to broken skin.

Corticosteroids

Corticosteroids (referred to as glucocorticosteroids in doping literature), especially in injected forms, are the most notorious drugs commonly used in the treatment of sports injury. Reports of almost immediate and complete relief of pain lead to exaggerated expectations of benefit in some athletes. Other athletes avoid corticosteroids at all costs, fearing permanent tissue damage, long-term systemic illness and severe pain with injection. The truth lies between these two extremes, with corticosteroids certainly having an important and useful place in clinical sports medicine. The potent anti-inflammatory action of corticosteroids is a result of their inhibition of the chemical chain of inflammation almost at its beginning (Fig. 29.1). The inhibition of leukocyte migration to the site of injury is an important distinction between effects of corticosteroids and NSAIDs. This effect is the main reason for the immunosuppression associated with corticosteroid use. Corticosteroids are also important membrane stabilizers, reducing enzyme release from cells (Leadbetter 1995, Stanley & Weaver 1998). By their action, corticosteroids must have some analgesic properties, but the extent of this is uncertain. Athletes often regard corticosteroid injections as painkillers, but this is primarily the effect of the accompanying local anesthetic. The effects of corticosteroids extend well beyond controlling inflammation, and facets of their action remain to be elucidated.

A major concern with the use of corticosteroids is their known inhibition of collagen synthesis and fibroblast proliferation in healing tissue (Best & Garrett 1994, Leadbetter 1995, Stanley & Weaver 1998). These factors lead to concerns about impaired healing and possibly an increased predisposition to new or further injury. The majority of evidence leading to concern is derived from animal models, often in isolated cell cultures, and extrapolation of findings to human sporting injuries must be undertaken with caution (Leadbetter 1995, Stanley & Weaver 1998). Clinical studies of the benefits and hazards of corticosteroid injections are often poorly controlled and rely on subjective and anecdotal evidence (Leadbetter 1995, Nichols 2005, Read 1999, Shrier et al 1996). Well-controlled clinical studies are hampered by the difficulty in recruiting sufficient numbers of patients with similar conditions where corticosteroid injection is appropriate. However, some conclusions can be drawn. Corticosteroids are most effective early in the course of inflammatory conditions such as bursitis, tenosynovitis, paratenonitis and joint synovitis, where they can achieve excellent results. While they are used in conditions such as epicondylitis, tendinopathies, osteoarthritis, spinal facet joint pain and active trigger points, there is no sound evidence that the benefit is more than temporary symptom relief (Alvarez et al 2005, Arroll & Goodyear-Smith 2005, Crawford 2005, Shrier et al 1996, Smidt et al 2002, Snibbe & Gambardella 2005). Nevertheless, anecdotally, reports have indicated that excellent responses are sometimes achieved in these conditions, while other patients with seemingly similar pathology gain no benefit from corticosteroid injection.

The most important determinant in electing to use a corticosteroid injection is a thorough and accurate anatomical and pathological diagnosis. A considered decision can then be made in regard to risks and benefits. As level of knowledge and personal experience of the physician tend to strongly influence decision making, the incidence of corticosteroid use in practice varies greatly. The physician must be confident that the affected structure can be well localized and injected without risk to neurovascular structures and other sensitive tissues. Also, there must be no signs of local infection. Following injection, the area must be rested, or at least excessive load avoided, for a suitable period of time, usually between 2–14 days. The athlete must understand that even if there is very good initial symptom relief following injection, all aspects of rehabilitation such as stretching, strengthening, and technique modification must still be carried out diligently. Too often, injection is seen as a quick fix or short-cut to return to sport, only to fail when the condition recurs and rehabilitation has been neglected. It is accepted practice to avoid injecting the same site of injury more than three times (Stanley & Weaver 1998). Likewise, repeated injections at intervals of less than several weeks are discouraged (Stanley & Weaver 1998). These practices are based on extrapolations of evidence from animal tissue studies, with minimal human clinical basis. Nevertheless, these are sound practices in that the need for repeated injection may imply an inaccurate diagnosis, inadequate treatment in other respects or simply an attempt to ignore a very strong message to reduce activity. Of important consideration is that corticosteroid injections must be notified in competition, and prior permission obtained from the sporting organization if any doubt exists about regulations.

Side effects and complications of corticosteroid injections are relatively uncommon (Nichols 2005). Infection of the injection site must be avoided by good sterile technique. Local subcutaneous atrophy and skin pigmentation or depigmentation can be avoided by ensuring that the injection is more deeply placed. However, in superficial conditions the patient must be warned of this risk. Pain associated with injection can be minimized by the accompanying use of local anesthetic, a narrow-gauge needle and good injection technique (Leadbetter 1995). Postinjection flare of symptoms sometimes occurs, but usually settles within a day or so, and patients should be advised of this risk, and analgesics recommended where necessary. Postinjection flare is said to have been more common in the past when less soluble corticosteroids were used (Leadbetter 1995). In diabetic patients, a short-term rise in blood glucose is likely, but systemic effects are otherwise rare (Leadbetter 1995).

Tendon rupture is the most widely known side effect of corticosteroid injection, but it is in fact rare. Reviews of reported postinjection ruptures confirm that the association of injection with rupture is anecdotal, and no direct relationship is usually present (Leadbetter 1995, Nichols 2005, Shrier et al 1996). It is well accepted that intratendinous injection should be avoided (Leadbetter 1995, Shrier et al 1996). Even if the corticosteroid does not affect tendon structure, the needle tip may lacerate the tendon. If there is any risk of complete or partial tendon rupture being present, this should be established by imaging studies (see Chapter 30), and injection avoided. The only common exception to this rule is pre-existing rotator cuff tear, where symptoms may be largely the result of coexisting bursitis and impingement. It is likely that tendon rupture is the natural outcome of some conditions, and injection is an incidental and unsuccessful attempt to relieve the symptoms of an inevitable tendon failure. Injection around intact tendons appears to be accompanied by minimal risk of tendon rupture (Leadbetter 1995, Read 1999, Tallon et al 2001). Spontaneous rupture of the Achilles tendon, which is sometimes bilateral, is a well-recognized result of the use of oral corticosteroids (Shrier et al 1996). This again, however, may often be an expression of the attrition of diseased tendon, as severe inflammatory disorders are usually the indication for this therapy. Nevertheless, all patients should be warned that a small risk of tendon rupture exists, and a suitable period of reduced activity should be advised.

Long-term articular cartilage damage is a further important concern with respect to the use of corticosteroids. Again, most studies are based on animal models, and clinical evidence is limited (Leadbetter 1995). The use of intra-articular injections should be restricted along the same lines as soft tissue injections, with injections into weightbearing joints, and areas of known articular cartilage injury, being treated with particular caution.

Oral corticosteroids are occasionally used in the management of recalcitrant inflammatory conditions, or in situations where injection may not be physically feasible such as around the pelvis, and in areas close to nerves and arteries. This therapy, however, is not used widely enough in the treatment of sports injury to evaluate its efficacy. Courses of oral corticosteroids should last no longer than 10 days, and should preferably use a tapering dosage regimen to minimize side effects. Potent oral agents such as dexamethasone should be avoided, as high doses have led to avascular necrosis of the hip (Brunton et al 2006). Common side effects include gastrointestinal disturbance, altered fluid balance and insomnia (Brunton et al 2006). Oral corticosteroids are prohibited in competition in sport.

Iontophoresis has been used as an alternative to injection to administer corticosteroids. While possibly useful in those afraid of needles, advantages of this technique are otherwise unclear. Penetration of the agent to the site of injury must be reduced, and systemic absorption increased relative to injection. Short-term pain relief has been demonstrated, but convincing benefits are otherwise lacking (Gudeman et al 1997).

Rubifacients and other topical agents

Heat rubs and liniments, collectively referred to as rubifacients, are one of the oldest forms of sports injury treatment. Their ingredients usually include methyl salicylate and a variety of plant derived essential oils, such as menthol, thymol, camphor, capsaicin and eucalyptus oil, and often a 'secret or unidentified unique' ingredient. They act by encouraging blood flow to the area, and may have a topical analgesic effect. They have been widely used to warm up tight and sore muscles. As a result of their direct warming effect on the skin, and their often pungent aroma, these agents are popular with some athletes. As their depth of penetration is limited, they do not take the place of the normal warming up processes of activity and stretching, but may be a useful adjunct. Evidence of therapeutic benefits in sporting injuries is limited, but a low to moderate level of pain relief has been demonstrated (Mason et al 2004a, 2004d). Allergic reactions can occur, but the most common side effect is the severe burning that can be experienced if applied to broken skin or sensitive areas such as mucous membranes and the eyes. The hands should always be washed thoroughly after applying rubifacients. Olive oil is helpful in displacing these agents from sensitive skin. Experience indicates that rubifacients should never be used simultaneously with heat packs, as subcutaneous necrosis has been reported from excessive tissue heating.

Various anticoagulant and hemolytic topical agents have been employed for the treatment of contusions and muscle strains. In theory, assistance with the removal of blood from tissues is probably beneficial, however, convincing evidence of this benefit is not available, and it is often suggested that the massage used for application of these agents is possibly their greatest virtue.

Analgesics

Pain is a prominent feature of many sporting injuries and its relief is essential to recovery and return to function. The role of NSAIDs in this process has been discussed above, and it may well be that analgesia is the major clinical benefit of these drugs. There is no questioning the benefit of relief of pain following traumatic injury, in assisting early mobilization and progression to rehabilitation. In severe injury such as fracture, where further competition is impossible, injected analgesics such as pethidine and morphine should not be withheld for fear of drug testing or addiction. In less severe injury, where analgesia is used to permit continuing participation, serious consideration must be given to the possibility of the athlete sustaining further harm.

Widely used analgesics such as aspirin, paracetamol (acetaminophen) and codeine are used in standard dosage regimens to relieve the pain of sports injury. These drugs are permitted for use both in and out of competition. Patients should understand that it is good practice to make use of a regular dosage of a relatively mild but safe analgesic such as paracetamol, in order to control pain levels. Practices such as withholding pain relief, or trying to demonstrate a high pain tolerance, are counterproductive, and lead to a greater risk of side effects when more potent agents become necessary.

In chronic pain, agents such as tricyclic antidepressants have a beneficial pain modifying effect (Mazanec 1998). However, these circumstances require the involvement of a physician experienced in pain management, and fall beyond the normal scope of sports injury therapy.

Hyperbaric oxygen

Hyperbaric oxygen therapy is well established as a treatment for a range of medical conditions including various soft tissue injuries. Consequently, it has been assumed that it may be beneficial for the treatment of sports injuries, in particular traumatic soft tissue and joint injuries. This possibility has been embraced by the manufacturers of hyperbaric oxygen equipment, and enthusiastically supported by some athletes in anecdotal reports. These circumstances have resulted in a widespread perception that hyperbaric oxygen therapy is a well-established and effective treatment for sports injury. However, this perception is not supported by sound evidence (see Chapter 14) (Bennett et al 2005).

Hyperbaric oxygen therapy involves the inspiration of 100% oxygen at pressures greater than the ambient barometric pressure at sea level (1 atmosphere). Pressures of between 2 and 3 atmospheres are commonly used. Hyperbaric oxygen can offset local hypoxia by increasing the partial pressure of oxygen in the tissues, which in turn promotes healing and helps to prevent infection. Vasoconstriction results in the reduction of edema, and blood flow is also reduced by the direct compression of increased atmospheric pressure (Babul & Rhodes 2000, Ishii et al 2005). Hyperbaric oxygen is the primary treatment modality for decompression sickness and air embolism associated with underwater diving, and carbon monoxide poisoning. It has also been shown to accelerate the healing process in burns, crush injuries, acute compartment syndromes and osteomyelitis (Babul & Rhodes 2000). These benefits are thought to derive from both the direct pressure effect and the physiological benefit of increased oxygen availability, resulting in both improved wound healing and enhanced tissue survival (Babul & Rhodes 2000, Ishii et al 2005). Consequently, logic suggests that many traumatic sports injuries such as muscle tears should benefit. However, the known benefits occur in situations of severe soft tissue damage and hypoxia, and measurable improvements may not occur in lesser degrees of damage. Experimental human models of delayed onset muscle soreness, induced by eccentric exercise, have failed to show improvement on parameters of soft tissue swelling, isometric strength and creatine kinase levels when treated with hyperbaric oxygen, and participants have experienced increased levels of pain (Bennett et al 2005). Also, no beneficial effect was seen in studies of traumatic ankle and knee sprains (Bennett et al 2005).

Anecdotally, hyperbaric oxygen therapy does have a pronounced, but possibly temporary effect in reducing joint effusions. This is probably a direct compression benefit, and is not related to any improvement in the underlying pathology. Further studies are being carried out, particularly using animal models for bone cartilage and tendon healing, and it may be possible to demonstrate benefits in the future. Hyperbaric oxygen therapy requires expensive equipment and close supervision by a physician. It is a very expensive and time intensive form of treatment. It cannot be widely recommended for use in managing sport and exercise injuries at present.

Other antiarthritic agents

Glucosamine and chondroitin sulfate have become popular as treatments for chronic joint conditions, in particular arthritis. Both agents have been promoted as natural treatments for arthritis, initially being derived from shellfish and sharks respectively. Increasing evidence suggests that they are useful in the treatment of mild to moderate arthritis (McAlindon & Biggee 2005, Richy et al 2003, Towheed et al 2005). It is proposed that both glucosamine and chondroitin sulfate assist the regeneration of articular cartilage, as well as having analgesic benefits. Both products are readily available without prescription, and appear to be relatively free of side effects, but with the proviso that patients allergic to seafood should avoid them. Anecdotally, their use has been proposed for the treatment of intervertebral disc injuries and other soft tissue injury but convincing evidence of any benefits is not yet available.

Hyaluronic acid is a natural constituent of several human tissues, including synovial fluid, the skin and joint cartilage. Osteoarthritis is associated with the breakdown of hyaluronic acid, resulting in increased susceptibility of the articular cartilage to injury. Hyaluronic acid in injectable form is available as a palliative treatment for osteoarthritis, particularly of major joints, such as the knee. It is effective in producing symptom relief, with results similar to corticosteroid injection, but of longer duration (Bellamy et al 2006). Side effects, such as subsequent joint effusion, are not uncommon. It is a relatively expensive form of treatment.

Muscle relaxants

Muscle relaxant agents are sometimes used in addition to NSAIDs and analgesics for acute musculoskeletal injuries such as muscle strains, particularly when the paraspinal muscles are affected. All muscle relaxant agents rely on a central neurological mechanism to modulate stretch reflexes (Mazanec 1998). All muscle relaxants also have a sedative effect, which may account in part for their efficacy (Mazanec 1998). It has not been demonstrated that they are any more effective than analgesics in relieving muscle spasm (Mazanec 1998). Also, it is doubtful that muscle relaxant medications are any more effective than various physical methods such as stretching, heat packs and massage. They may have a short-term role following acute injury.

The use of muscle relaxants should be avoided in sports that require high levels of skill and balance, such as gymnastics, archery and equestrian events. Their effects in terms of prolonged reaction time, reduced balance and sedation make them potentially dangerous (Henderson 1998).

Antibiotics and antiviral agents

Although antibiotics are widely used in the community for the treatment of bacterial infections, there are many concerns about their inappropriate use for non-bacterial or minor infections. Concerns center on the increased risk of bacterial resistance, and the side effects suffered by many patients. Nevertheless, in active bacterial infection, antibiotics remain extremely valuable. In their need for treatment of infection, athletes are no different to other members of the community. However, athletes often blame subsequent poor performances on the fact that they are taking antibiotics. Consequently, many athletes are reluctant to make use of antibiotics when they are indicated, because they believe that they may produce fatigue, or other symptoms of impaired performance. There is no evidence to support this contention and the athlete should always be reminded that it is the illness that is causing the impaired performance, rather than the medication. Notwithstanding, side effects such as gastrointestinal upset and skin reaction are quite common with antibiotic use and would certainly have a negative effect on performance. Whenever antibiotics are required, isolation of the athlete from other team members should always be considered. Prior to prescription of antibiotics, athletes should always be closely questioned about the possibility of allergic reaction. The type of infection, cost, availability and dosage regimen of the drug concerned dictates choice of antibiotic. In athletes, compliance issues are of particular importance, especially with regard to training and travel requirements.

Antibiotics are sometimes used prophylactically for the prevention of traveler's diarrhea (Brukner & Khan 2002, Goldman & Ausiello 2003). Local conditions and safe sources of food and water should always be ascertained prior to travel. The choice to use antibiotics for prevention of traveler's diarrhea will be determined by previous experience, knowledge of the local conditions, and a consideration of the potential benefits in regards to competition versus the possibility of athletes experiencing side effects.

Some antibiotics such as ciprofloxacin and related quinolones have been associated with impaired fibroblast metabolism and consequent tendon rupture (Khaliq & Zhanel 2005). It has been proposed that these antibiotics effectively produce a toxic tendinopathy. This effect may persist for several weeks after cessation of the drug.

Antiviral agents are becoming increasingly available for a variety of infections. Specific antivirals are useful for the treatment of common skin conditions such as herpes simplex and herpes zoster infections. These infections are particularly relevant in sports that require close skin contact, such as wrestling. It is advisable that, along with specific treatment, athletes with active infections be isolated from competition. Antiviral agents have been proposed as prophylaxis for common upper respiratory viral infections in athletes subject to major physical stress, such as severe training and overseas travel for major competition. This therapy is expensive, and demonstrated efficacy and acceptance have not yet been achieved.

Oral contraceptives

Oral contraceptives are widely used by females for contraception, but also for regulation of the menstrual cycle, and relief of premenstrual and menstrual symptoms. In amenorrheic and oligoamenorrheic athletes, oral contraceptives may also provide benefit in improving bone density when this is reduced (Bennell et al 1999, Liu & Lebrun 2006, Rickenlund et al 2004). Oral contraceptives are permitted in all forms of competition. They are effective in regulating the menstrual cycle, which is of particular benefit to female athletes who find that premenstrual or menstrual symptoms impair their training and competition (Constantini et al 2005). It is possible by manipulation of dosage to delay or miss a period altogether without deleterious effects. This is often of particular importance in traveling to major events. Oral contraceptives generally reduce the amount of menstrual blood loss (Bennell et al 1999), which is of benefit in those who tend to suffer from iron depletion.

The effects of the oral contraceptive on performance have been studied quite extensively, but no firm conclusions have been drawn. Various studies (e.g. Bennell et al 1999, Lebrun et al 2003, Quadagno 2000, Rickenlund et al 2004) have suggested that oral contraceptives may result in small reductions, no change, or small gains in laboratory performance measures. No significant pattern of change has been observed in competitive performance. Weight gain is popularly attributed to the oral contraceptive but this is not supported by a number of studies. Any weight gain that occurs when a female athlete commences the oral contraceptive is more likely to be the result of lifestyle and dietary modifications, rather than any true physiological effect of the medication. This is particularly the case with low dose formulations that are now available (Bennell et al 1999, Rickenlund et al 2004).

The menstrual cycle has been associated with increased risk of soft tissue injury, such as ligamentous tears (Bennell et al 1999, Martineau et al 2004). Concerns have also been raised about the potentially increased risk of stress fracture in amenorrheic and oligoamenorrheic athletes, where estrogen levels are low (Bennell et al 1999). In both soft tissue injury and stress fracture, the possibility that the oral contraceptive may offer a protective effect is appealing. However, convincing evidence of this is not available (Bennell et al 1999, Martineau et al 2004).

From a practical point of view, the oral contraceptive certainly offers benefits for many female athletes. Many different preparations are available, allowing choices that optimize convenience of dosage and that minimize side effects. A practitioner experienced in the needs of female athletes should be able to offer an oral contraceptive most suited to the individual's needs.

Asthma medications

Asthma is a common condition in the community, and is similarly common in athletes. Exercise-induced asthma is especially prevalent in the athletic population (Helenius et al 2005, Langdeau & Boulet 2003, Miller et al 2005). Several reasons have been put forward for this. Firstly, many asthmatic children are encouraged to take up sport, especially swimming, in order to help control their respiratory symptoms. Swimming, however, may cause problems because of exposure to high chlorine levels in poorly ventilated pools (Helenius et al 2005, Miller et al 2005). Secondly, intensive exercise, particularly in endurance sports, may expose symptoms that would otherwise go unnoticed in less active people. Thirdly, there are some concerns that exercise-induced asthma is over-diagnosed in athletes, when other conditions may be the cause of their respiratory symptoms. Finally, it has been suggested and observed clinically that some athletes make use of asthma medications, even though they do not suffer asthma, in the hope that they will provide some ergogenic benefit.

Bacterial and viral illnesses, allergens, pollutants, smoking and exercise may provoke asthmatic symptoms. There is evidence that concentrations of these provocative agents may be increased in indoor sporting arenas (Helenius et al 2005, Miller et al 2005). Asthma is also intrinsic in some people with no specific provocative stimuli. In the case of exercise-induced asthma, the relative hyperventilation of exercise prevents the upper airways from adequately warming and humidifying the inhaled air. This results in an influx of cool dry air, which then results in a cascade of events, leading to airways inflammation and bronchoconstriction (Helenius et al 2005, Miller et al 2005). This is particularly relevant when the ambient conditions are cold and dry, and especially so in alpine sports. Training and competition in a polluted environment may also contribute to symptoms. Successful asthma therapy is reliant upon the control of the longer-term inflammation of airways and reversal of the short-term bronchoconstriction that results in the well-recognized symptoms of breathlessness often associated with wheezing and coughing.

Asthma medications fall into two major categories: preventer and reliever medications. Fundamental to successful asthma treatment is the prevention of symptoms. Many athletes tend to rely on reliever medications only, which is likely to result in suboptimal respiratory function. Any athlete who frequently requires use of reliever medication during training or competition should have their asthma management plan reviewed by a physician. Preventer medications commonly used as inhaled agents in athletes include sodium cromoglycate, nedocromil sodium and corticosteroids. Common reliever medications are beta-2 agonists, which in longer acting forms can also be used as preventive medications. Other agents include leukotriene antagonists, oral corticosteroids and theophylline.

Sodium cromoglycate and nedocromil sodium both act by stabilization of the cell membranes of mast cells, which release a number of the mediators causing asthma (Holzer et al 2002, Miller et al 2005). They appear to be particularly beneficial in exercise-induced asthma, and are administered on a regular daily basis. They should be used shortly before exercise, and they act for several hours afterwards. Such agents are of no benefit in relieving acute symptoms. Both drugs are relatively free of side effects and are permitted for use in competition without restriction.

Inhaled corticosteroids are the mainstay of preventive treatment in moderate to severe asthma, whether exercise-induced or not. They are effective in reducing both the inflammation of airways and bronchial hyper-reactivity (Holzer et al 2002, Miller et al 2005). They are only effective on a preventive basis, and are generally not useful in an acute episode. Inhaled corticosteroids are administered on a regular daily basis, and can be taken without regard to the timing of exercise. Side effects are minimal. At the dosages normally used by athletes, systemic corticosteroid side effects are most unlikely to occur. Other preventer and reliever medications can be used in combination with inhaled corticosteroids. They are permitted for use in competition, but some sporting federations may require notification of their use.

Beta-2 agonists, such as salbutamol, have been widely used for the relief of asthma symptoms. Short-acting inhaled beta-2 agonists induce bronchodilation within minutes, and also have some impact on the mediators released by mast cells (Holzer et al 2002, Miller et al 2005). A positive response to beta-2 agonists is a simple tool for the diagnosis of exercise-induced asthma, and can be used for ongoing treatment in milder cases. However, any symptoms not readily controlled by pre-exercise use of an inhaled beta-2 agonist demand review by a physician, and the likely institution of effective preventer medications. Long-term use of beta-2 agonists, both in short- and long-acting forms, leads to a level of tolerance to these medications, and may ultimately reduce respiratory performance, as well as the possibility of increased risk of cardiac events and sudden death (Salpeter et al 2004). Common side effects of short-acting beta-2 agonists are tachycardia and skeletal muscle tremor (Brunton et al 2006). Tolerance to these side effects usually develops in regular users. Longer acting beta-2 agonists such as salmeterol have become increasingly widely used, but similar concerns about their long-term effect on respiratory performance remain.

Beta-2 agonists in both short- and long-acting form are classified as both stimulants and anabolic agents. However, the use of some beta-2 agonists is permitted with specific notification (see later in this chapter). Since 2001, permission to use inhaled beta-2 agonists requires the submission of clinical and laboratory findings confirming the diagnosis of asthma. A range of appropriate tests is available (Holzer et al 2002, Miller et al 2005). Inhaled beta-2 agonists have been shown to have an ergogenic effect in non-asthmatic athletes if taken in large doses (van Baak et al 2004). However, inhaled and injectable forms of beta-2 agonists, which are not widely available, have been shown to have an anabolic effect, and are hence banned (van Baak et al 2000).

Leukotrienes are potent agents given in oral form for asthma management. They are generally reserved for use by severe asthmatics, but have been shown to be beneficial in the management of exercise-induced asthma (Miller et al 2005). Theophylline was once a frequent preventive asthma medication taken in oral form. Its use has declined, but it maintains a place in the management of severe asthma, in combination with other drugs. It has no specific role in the management of exercise-induced asthma.

Oral and intravenous corticosteroids are very effective at relieving severe episodes of asthma (Brunton et al 2006); however, these medications are banned in sport competition. They may, however, occasionally be essential to the management of severely asthmatic athletes. In these circumstances, the relevant national sporting federation should be contacted, as special provision for treatment may be possible, under the supervision of an independent respiratory specialist.

Legal considerations

Many drugs are restricted by law, and can only be prescribed by physicians, and dispensed by physicians and pharmacists. A few minor exceptions exist in relation to specific medications used in dentistry, podiatry and other areas. The prescription or dispensing of restricted medications by other practitioners is specifically prohibited, to avoid dangers to the patient. Physicians and pharmacists receive extensive training in pharmacology, and have a good understanding of the effects, side effects, contraindications and interactions of a wide range of drugs. Other practitioners, in general, do not have this level of training.

Many medications, such as simple analgesics and some NSAIDs are available for over-the-counter purchase in pharmacies, supermarkets and convenience stores. The recommendation and dispensing of these medications by practitioners other than physicians and pharmacists is often not clearly spelled out by the law. Whilst these drugs are generally safer than prescription-only medication, risks of side effects, interaction and allergy remain, and it is good practice to avoid recommendation of any form of medication without the specific advice of a trained practitioner.

Performance-enhancing drugs

Historical perspective of performance-enhancing drugs in sport

Drugs have been used in the hope of enhancing performance ever since the recording of organized sporting competitions began (Verroken 2005). One of the better known classes of performance-enhancing drugs, anabolic steroids, was first developed in 1927 and is first known to have been used at the Olympic Games by Russian weightlifters in 1952. There is, however, some suggestion that they may have been used as early as 1936. At that time, no regulations controlling use, and no effective detection measures were in place. In 1960, the death of a Danish cyclist in the team time trial event at the Rome Olympics was associated with the use of amphetamines. In 1967, champion British cyclist Tom Simpson died during the Tour de France whilst the event was being covered on television. His death was attributed to heat exhaustion and amphetamines, traces of which were found in his jersey pockets. An increasing tide of public concern resulted in the formation of the International Olympic Committee Medical Commission in 1967, and performance-enhancing drugs were banned in Olympic competition. Soon after, a drug-testing program was introduced, initially testing only for stimulants and narcotics. Controls were introduced at the 1968 Olympics, and at that event and every subsequent Olympic Games a number of athletes have tested positive for various drugs and suffered the consequences. With each Olympic Games since 1968 there have been revelations of new drugs being used, and allegations made that many more athletes are using drugs than the number detected. Testing procedures have been continually refined. Out of competition testing was first introduced in 1987. The issue of drugs in sport was brought into sharp international focus in 1988 after Ben Johnson was stripped of his gold medal in the 100 m sprint following a positive test for anabolic steroids. Several countries undertook inquiries into the issue of drugs in sport, and more stringent testing and regulations were introduced. Increasingly stringent controls have been put in place subsequently.

The year 2001 saw the advent of a universal regulation and testing program under the auspices of the International Olympic Committee (IOC) and the World Anti-Doping Agency (WADA). This process culminated in the establishment of the World Anti-Doping Code in 2003, coming into force in 2004. WADA, working in conjunction with the IOC Medical Commission, international sporting federations and national governments, is the peak body in establishing anti-doping regulations. The objective of WADA is to adopt and administer the World Anti-Doping Code uniformly across all sports and countries.

New challenges continue to arise in the battle against drug use in sport. The use of synthetic forms of various hormones, which are almost indistinguishable from the natural products, has presented a major challenge in both drug detection and regulation. New technology will continue to produce new drugs and the requirement for ever more sophisticated testing technology. There is some hope that there will be fewer and fewer avenues by which performance may be enhanced with drugs, and that the battle may then be won. However, gene therapy may generate a whole new range of testing and legislative challenges.

The World Anti-Doping Code

Prohibited classes of substances and prohibited methods are published under the auspices of the World Anti-Doping Code.

Box 29.1 World Anti-Doping Code prohibited classes of substances and prohibited methods

Substances and methods prohibited at all times (in- and out-of-competition)

Prohibited substances
S1. Anabolic agents
S2. Hormones and related substances
S3. Beta-2 agonists
S4. Agents with anti-estrogenic activity
S5. Diuretics and other masking agents

Prohibited methods
M1. Enhancement of oxygen transfer
M2. Chemical and physical manipulation
M3. Gene doping

Substances and methods prohibited in-competition
S6. Stimulants
S7. Narcotics
S8. Cannabinoids
S9. Glucocorticosteroids

Substances prohibited in particular sports
P1. Alcohol
P2. Beta-blockers

Specified substances

Table 29.2 Major side effects of anabolic androgenic steroids

System	Effects
Musculoskeletal	Tendon rupture Premature closure of epiphyses
Endocrine – males	Testicular atrophy Decreased or nil sperm production Prostatic hypertrophy Prostatic carcinoma Reduced hormone production Gynecomastia
Endocrine – females	Masculinization – male pattern hair growth and baldness Breast tissue reduction Voice changes Clitoral hypertrophy Menstrual irregularity
Hepatic	Abnormal liver enzyme function Hepatic carcinoma Jaundice
Cardiovascular	Coronary artery disease Altered lipid profile Hypertension Clotting problems
Renal	Renal tumors Impaired renal function
Central nervous system	Psychosis Aggression Altered libido
Skin	Acne Striae

This code is subject to annual review and update and is published on the WADA website (www.wada-ama.org). Its current details (World Anti-Doping Agency 2005) are included in Box 29.1.

Within the code, examples of prohibited substances are given in each class but it is made clear that no list is exhaustive, and any drug that is deemed to fall within a specific class may be considered banned. Each of these major categories will be considered in turn.

Substances and methods prohibited at all times

S1. Anabolic agents

1. Anabolic androgenic steroids:
   a. Exogenous anabolic androgenic steroids
   b. Endogenous anabolic androgenic steroids
2. Other anabolic agents

Anabolic androgenic steroids (AAS) are all close chemical relations of testosterone, the principal anabolic and androgenic hormone in males, which is also found in lesser concentrations in females. The testes, adrenal glands and ovaries normally produce testosterone. All of these drugs, whether synthetic or natural, have a combination of both anabolic (bodybuilding) and androgenic (masculinizing) effects. The relative proportion and potency of the anabolic and androgenic effect tends to determine the side-effect profile of each drug, and also their usefulness for abusers. Major side effects of AAS are listed in Table 29.2.

Technology to detect the use of AAS has become increasingly sophisticated, and the recent use of all synthetic forms in competition should be readily detected. Evidence of use months before competition can also be obtained from metabolic profiles (Bowers 1998). These techniques rely on the detection of metabolic breakdown products of the synthetic hormones being present in the urine. The proportions of these products can then determine that AAS have been used, even though the specific drug may not be detected.

The major challenge in the fight against the use of AAS is the use of testosterone and related naturally occurring steroids, such as androstenediol, androstenedione, norandrostenedione and dehydroepiandrosterone (DHEA), all of which are naturally occurring in varying levels. All of these AAS, except testosterone, have a very weak anabolic effect, and have doubtful (if any) direct benefit in enhancing performance. However, norandrostenedione, which is naturally occurring and also contained in some food supplements, is metabolized to nandrolone, which in high doses, is well known as a potent synthetic AAS (Baume et al 2005, Bowers 1998). Detection of these drugs currently relies upon variations in the testosterone: epitestosterone ratio, epitestosterone being an inactive isomer of testosterone produced naturally. The normal ratio is subject to variation in some circumstances, and so confirmation of positive test results can be difficult. Athletes have exploited uncertainties relating to testosterone:epitestosterone ratios to avoid suspension following positive tests (Baume et al 2005).

AAS such as norandrostenedione and DHEA may be contained in readily available food supplements, and even in trace amounts, can result in positive tests. Extreme caution in the use of supplements must be taken (Maughan 2005). The potential for contamination of food supplements has been used as a means to avoid suspension following positive tests for these drugs.

The performance-enhancing benefits of AAS were debated for many years. Many clinical trials (George 2005b, Sturmi & Diorio 1998) failed to show the expected performance benefits in terms of strength gains, with or without the presence of changes in muscle bulk. However, it is well recognized that the doses used by athletes have been many times greater than the recommended doses for various medical conditions. Consequently, ethical constraints have prevented the depth of study necessary to fully delineate the performance benefits of AAS. Anecdotally, there is abundant evidence that great improvements in strength and muscle bulk can be achieved. It is now generally accepted that AAS can increase muscle protein synthesis and block the catabolic effects of glucocorticosteroids (George 2005b, Sturmi & Diorio 1998). In order to be effective, the drugs must be used in collaboration with an intensive training program and a high quality diet (George 2005b, Sturmi & Diorio 1998).

AAS abuse has been most closely linked with power sports such as throwing events, weightlifting, power lifting, wrestling and sprinting. However, their benefits can be translated to a wide variety of sports, as many athletes will benefit from measurable gains in strength and speed. AAS are also reputed to enhance recovery and improve endurance (George 2005b, Sturmi & Diorio 1998). There is little evidence to support this, but on a theoretical basis it is plausible. While the common perception of an AAS abuser is of an extremely powerfully built athlete, dosage regimen can be tailored to suit even lightly built athletes in endurance sports, in the hope that specific strength and recovery can be enhanced, without the penalty of weight gain. In prolonged events, AAS could help counter both the catabolic effects of sustained exercise and the lack of appetite for the large amounts of food required (Sturmi & Diorio 1998).

The abuse of AAS has been associated with a wide variety of well-recognized side effects. Many of the well-known side effects are reversible on cessation of the drugs, but there is significant concern about a number of long-term, potentially fatal, side effects. Some of the major side effects are detailed in Table 29.2.

Trade in AAS is either severely restricted or prohibited in most countries. Consequently, the majority of these drugs are obtained illegally and their exact identity and purity must be questioned. Abuse of AAS in activities outside organized competitive sport is widespread, for potential improvement in strength and appearance. The use of injectable forms of AAS raises additional concerns with regard to the potential for infectious disease transmission via the sharing of needles.

Other prohibited anabolic agents include Clenbuterol, Zeranol and Zilpaterol, beta agonists used as growth-promoting agents in animals, and Tibolone, which has mild androgenic properties, normally used for treating menopausal symptoms.

S2. Hormones and related substances

Prohibited substances include the following examples and their analogs and agents with similar effects:

1. Erythropoietin (EPO)
2. Growth hormone (hGH), insulin-like growth factors (e.g. IGF-1), mechano growth factors (MGFs)
3. Gonadotrophin (LH, hCG) prohibited in males only
4. Insulin
5. Corticotrophins

The presence of an abnormal concentration of an endogenous hormone in section S2 or its diagnostic marker(s) in the urine of a competitor constitutes an offence, unless it has been proven to be due to a physiological or pathological condition. In these cases a Therapeutic Use Exemption must be obtained.

Each of the above substances is a naturally occurring human hormone which has a wide variety of metabolic influences. All of these hormones can now be synthesized, and have specific uses in medical practice for a variety of disease conditions; the best known in this respect being insulin for diabetes. Once peptide hormones have been synthesized, active components of the molecules can then be identified, and synthesized as mimetic drugs. Analogs are close chemical relations of the naturally occurring hormones, which have undergone minor chemical modification, resulting in similar effects, increased potency, or a longer or shorter duration of action. This potential to continue producing a wide range of drugs with actions similar to the naturally occurring hormones is the reason for the broad definition of drugs within this class (George 2005c).

These drugs have presented a major challenge to drug testing authorities. It can be very difficult, if not impossible, to distinguish the natural hormone level from doping. In some cases breakthroughs have been made because of minor chemical differences between the natural hormone and synthetic drug. Concurrent blood and urine testing expedites detection of abuse, but further research is necessary before testing can be widely applied and results upheld.

S3. Beta-2 agonists

Beta-2 agonists have been used for many years for the treatment of asthma, but their potential anabolic effect has only been recognized relatively recently (van Baak et al 2000). They have been widely used in animal production to produce rapid gains in muscle bulk. They also have stimulant and other ergogenic effects (van Baak et al 2004). All beta-2 agonists in oral and injectable form are prohibited in competitive sport.

Beta-2 agonist drugs used for the prevention and treatment of asthma and exercise-induced asthma (salbutamol, salmeterol, terbutaline and formoterol) may only be used in inhaled form with lodgment of an abbreviated Therapeutic Use Exemption with the relevant sporting federation. This must be provided by a respiratory physician or team physician confirming that the athlete suffers asthma and/or exercise-induced asthma. At the Olympic Games, an independent medical panel will assess athletes who request permission to use inhaled beta-2 agonists. Regardless of any form of Therapeutic Use Exemption a salbutamol concentration in urine greater than 1000 ng/mL is not permitted unless it can be proved that this was the consequence of therapeutic use of the inhaled drug.

S4. Agents with anti-estrogenic activity

These agents include aromatase inhibitors, selective estrogen receptor modulators and other anti-estrogenic substances. They may be used to disguise side effects of anabolic agents such as gynecomastia. They may also be used to mask abnormal hormonal levels, and may have a direct anabolic or precursory effect.

S5. Diuretics

A wide range of diuretic drugs has been used to increase urinary output. This has two potential benefits to the athlete. Firstly, body weight can be suddenly reduced in order to make weight for sports where specific categories are applied (e.g. weight-lifting, lightweight rowing, fighting sports). Secondly, a large output of very dilute urine makes the presence of other drugs difficult to detect. In this context, diuretics are often used as a masking agent. For making weight, diuretics are often combined with other potentially dangerous practices such as the use of saunas and severe restriction of food and fluids.

Abuse of diuretics can lead to severe dehydration, cramps, fall in blood pressure and electrolyte and metabolic disturbances (Verroken 2005). Fatal events are possible. To extend the dangers, the technique of rapidly infusing large volumes of intravenous fluids to regain weight rapidly following diuresis has been an accepted practice in some sports.

Prohibited methods

The following procedures are prohibited in- and out-of-competition:

M1. Enhancement of oxygen transfer – This includes blood doping, where the blood may be from any source, and products designed to artificially enhance the uptake, transport and delivery of oxygen.

M2. Chemical and physical manipulation – Chemical, and physical manipulation relate to the practices of diluting, adulterating, and substituting urine when a sample is presented for testing. Intravenous infusions are prohibited, except as a legitimate acute medical treatment.

M3. Gene doping – The non-therapeutic use of cells, genes, genetic elements or of the modulation of gene expression, having the capacity to enhance athletic performance, is prohibited (Trent & Alexander 2006).

Substances prohibited in-competition only

S6. Stimulants

Historically, stimulants have been the most widely abused drugs. Well-established detection methods are in place, but athletes continue to test positive for stimulants at each Olympic Games. Various stimulants are widely used in society, both for their stimulant effect (e.g. caffeine) and for other benefits (e.g. the bronchodilating effect of beta-2 agonists and decongestant effects of sympathomimetics such as pseudoephedrine). More potent stimulants such as strychnine and cocaine have been used for many years, and continue to be abused. All stimulants act on the central nervous system and, in so doing, increase alertness and reduce tiredness (George 2005a). They also improve concentration, which is beneficial in many precision events (George 2005a). In theory at least, they may help athletes achieve maximal explosive power, and may also help endurance athletes avoid the normal sensation of fatigue. In everyday life, there is abundant empirical evidence that commonly used stimulants (e.g. caffeine) help overcome tiredness and may improve concentration. However, there is limited experimental evidence to show that improvements can be achieved in the concentration, power generation or endurance of a well-prepared athlete attempting optimal performance (George 2005a). They may be of benefit in prolonged events, but evidence for this is lacking. Whether small improvements achieved in laboratory testing translate to improvements in competition is unknown. Caffeine, which is permitted in competition, has been shown to have some ergogenic benefit, but probably for reasons other than its stimulant effect.

As a result of the widespread use of stimulant drugs in society, outside of sporting competition, a number of specific provisions in regard to their use in sport have been made. Caffeine, its more potent precursor guarana, and common decongestant medications such as pseudoephedrine and phenylpropanolamine, which were formerly banned, are now permitted. However their use is monitored.

Sympathomimetic drugs such as pseudoephedrine and phenylpropanolamine are frequently used to counteract the symptoms of upper respiratory infections. They are most often taken as oral tablets and capsules, but also can be used as nasal drops and inhalers. The trade names for these medications vary greatly from country to country, and a brand that is permissible for sport in one country may not be in another. Also, under the one well-known trade name, a number of different formulations may be marketed. Some related stimulants are banned, but are considered separately as specified substances, and violations may result in reduced sanctions. Ephedrine is banned at a urinary concentration above 10 μg/ml, and Cathine above 5 μg/ml. To avoid inadvertent doping, packaging must be examined with great care, and if any doubt remains, expert advice should be sought, or the medication avoided altogether. Adrenaline when contained in local anesthetic agents, or for use in the eye or nose, is not prohibited. Many so-called social and recreational drugs such as amphetamines, cocaine and ecstasy are potent stimulants, and will result in positive drug tests, even though there may have been no intention to gain a performance enhancing benefit. No reduction in sanction applies to the use of these drugs.

S7. Narcotics

Narcotics are well known and widely used in medicine as potent analgesic agents. There is no evidence that they produce performance-enhancing effects as such, but there are concerns that pre-existing injury and illness may be exacerbated by the use of painkillers during continued participation. Common side effects of the use of narcotics are drowsiness, constipation, nausea and vomiting. Allergic reactions to these drugs are also quite common (Verroken 2005).

Narcotics including morphine, methadone, oxycodone, pethidine and diamorphine (heroin) are not permitted in-competition. However, as very effective analgesics, their use should not be withheld in situations of severe traumatic injury, where continued participation is clearly impossible.

Widely used narcotic analgesics of mild to moderate potency are permitted for use in training and competition. These permitted drugs include codeine, dextromethorphan, dextropropoxyphene, dihydrocodeine, diphenoxylate, ethylmorphine, pholcodine, propoxyphene and tramadol. NSAIDs are not subject to any restriction.

S8. Cannabinoids (marijuana, hashish)

Judgment and motor control may be impaired with the use of cannabinoids and their use may result in a reduced sanction if it can be demonstrated that there was no intention to enhance sporting performance.

S9. Glucocorticosteroids (clinically referred to as corticosteroids)

Systemic use of glucocorticosteroids, whether by oral, rectal, intramuscular or intravenous administration, is prohibited. When medically necessary, local and intra-articular injections of glucocorticosteroids are permitted with the completion of an abbreviated Therapeutic Use Exemption. Inhaled corticosteroids for asthma also require an abbreviated Therapeutic Use Exemption. Preparations for use on the skin, and in the eye, ear, nose and mouth are permitted.

Substances prohibited in particular sports

P1. Alcohol

The dangerous effects of alcohol on judgment and motor control are well recognized in the operation of machinery, especially motor vehicles. Similar risks apply in many sports, particularly those involving high speed. Alcohol is banned in competition for the safety of all participants in aeronautics, archery, automobile sports, billiards, boules, karate, modern pentathlon (shooting), motorcycling and powerboating.

P2. Beta-blockers

These drugs act as membrane stabilizers, slowing the heart rate and reducing muscle tremor (Henderson 1998, Reilly 1996). They may enhance performance in precision sports including aeronautics, archery, automobile, billiards, bobsleigh, boules, bridge, chess, curling, gymnastics, modern pentathlon (shooting), motorcycling, nine-pin bowling, sailing (match race helms), shooting, skiing/snowboarding (ski jumping, freestyle aerials/halfpipe, snowboard halfpipe/big air) and wrestling, and are prohibited in-competition only. They are also prohibited out-of-competition in archery and shooting.

Specified substances

Specified substances include inhaled beta-2 agonists, some stimulants, cannabinoids, glucocorticosteroids, alcohol, and beta-blockers. It is recognized that these substances are generally available in medicinal products, and anti-doping rule violations may be the result of inadvertent use. A reduced sanction may apply if the use of the substance was not intended to enhance sporting performance.

Out-of-competition testing

Unless specifically requested by the responsible authority, out-of-competition testing is directed solely at prohibited substances in classes S1–S5 and prohibited methods M1–M3. There are circumstances where a prohibited substance may be therapeutically necessary for the treatment of uncommon conditions. In this situation, most countries have established a specialist panel to review such circumstances. If a prohibited substance is to be permitted, it must be demonstrated that health would be impaired if the substance was not available, and that there is no therapeutic alternative. The condition and dosage must be monitored by an independent specialist physician. In these circumstances a Therapeutic Use Exemption may be granted.

Drug testing

In the past, there has been a wide range of drug testing procedures utilized by different countries and sporting organizations. This has often led to allegations of inadequate or unfair testing protocols. With the advent of the World Anti-Doping Code, a major goal has been a commitment to universal testing practices, although this has not yet been fully implemented.

An athlete may be selected for testing at any time outside competition, at the conclusion of an event, or during the course of a multiple day event. Athletes may be selected in competition on the basis of their finishing place or randomly. Where an athlete or event is the subject of rumor, selection may be specifically targeted.

It is advisable for team medical staff to be familiar with drug testing protocols, by personally observing the testing process. Staff can then attend with team members who may be chosen for testing, to ensure that all processes are carried out correctly, and that the athlete fully understands all aspects of testing. There is usually provision for the accompanying person to countersign all paperwork as the athlete's representative. As testing protocols can vary between different sports and countries, it is important to ensure that all steps are clearly understood, and that language interpretation is available when necessary. Samples of either or both urine and blood may be required. Normally the representative will be permitted to observe all aspects of the testing process, except the actual passing of urine. When athletes are selected for testing, they are permitted to first complete all necessary victory ceremonies and media commitments. They may also complete a warm-down, change their clothing, and undertake any necessary medical care, prior to presenting at the drug testing facility; however, all of these activities should take place under the direct observation of the chaperone acting for the drug testing authority. Competition testing must always involve the first urine passed after completion of the event.

Essential components of any testing process are the following:

- The athlete must be formally notified in writing of selection for testing.
- The drug testing room must be clearly identified, private and secure.
- All personnel must be clearly identified.
- A choice of sealed drinks must be offered to help with rehydration.
- A choice of clean containers for urine must be provided.
- The chaperone (of the same sex as the athlete) must observe the passage of urine, ensuring that the athlete is naked between chest and knee so that no manipulation of the sample can occur.
- Only the athlete should handle the sample until it has been sealed in the official containers.
- A choice of clean sample containers for both the A and B samples, each individually numbered and recorded, must be provided.
- The athlete must ensure that the container is sealed and tamper proof, and all numbering correctly recorded.
- The urine should be tested for pH and concentration to ensure it is suitable for analysis. If it is not, additional urine will be required, until a suitable sample is obtained.
- All paperwork should be fully completed, and countersigned by the officials of the drug testing authority, and the athlete's representative.
- Paperwork accompanying the sample itself should not identify the athlete by name. Identification should be by code, with details held by the testing authority.
- The athlete should be given a copy of all the paperwork.
- Secure passage of the samples to the laboratory must be ensured.

In the case of a positive test, the athlete is notified and is given the opportunity to attend the opening and testing of the B sample to confirm the result. The athlete may also invite a representative to attend. If the result is confirmed, it is then the responsibility of the relevant sporting federation to hear the case, and impose an appropriate sanction. Results are most often protested on the basis of legal loopholes, and possible breaches of testing protocols, rather than the actual laboratory finding. Protracted and expensive legal proceedings are a further major impediment to the elimination of doping.

Physical therapists and other health-care practitioners involved in sport and exercise injury management should ensure that they maintain current knowledge of drug testing procedures. Individual authorities in each country should be contacted for these details.

Summary

A sound understanding of the inflammatory process should underpin our rationale for many treatment modalities in sport and exercise injuries, particularly the use of pharmacological agents. While this process can be inhibited, the best interest of the patient should be considered. Prior to using anti-inflammatory and analgesic drugs, the anticipated benefits and side effects must be weighed up.

Corticosteroids, especially in injectable form, have long been controversial in sports injury management. Ongoing research is likely to settle some concerns, but again, benefits and risks must be duly considered. A number of newer treatment agents are becoming more widely used. Newness does not necessarily imply efficacy and safety, a fact that athletes often overlook in striving for rapid recovery.

The treatment of illness in athletes is as important as injury management, and regulations affecting drug use in sport must always be considered. Drug abuse to aid sporting performance has become entrenched, but every effort to eliminate it must be made. There is no doubt about the harmful effects of many of the abused drugs. All practitioners should have a sound knowledge of drug side effects, regulations, and testing if drug abuse in sport is to be overcome, and the wellbeing of athletes maintained.

References

Almekinders L C 1993 Anti-inflammatory treatment of muscular injuries in sports. Sports Medicine 15:139–145

Almekinders L C 1999 Anti-inflammatory treatment of muscular injuries in sport. An update of recent studies. Sports Medicine 28:383–388

Almekinders L C, Baynes A J, Bracey L W 1995 An in vitro investigation into the effects of repetitive motion and nonsteroidal anti-inflammatory medication on human tendon fibroblasts. American Journal of Sports Medicine 23:119–123

Alvarez C M, Litchfield R, Jackowski D 2005 A prospective, double-blind, randomized clinical trial comparing subacromial injection of betamethasone and xylocaine to xylocaine alone in chronic rotator cuff tendinosis. American Journal of Sports Medicine 33:255–262

Arroll B, Goodyear-Smith F 2005 Corticosteroid injections for painful shoulder: a meta-analysis. British Journal of General Practice 55:224–228

Babul S, Rhodes E C 2000 The role of hyperbaric oxygen therapy in sports medicine. Sports Medicine 30:395–405

Baume N, Avois L, Sottas P E et al 2005 Effects of high-intensity exercises on 13C-nandrolone excretion in trained athletes. Clinical Journal of Sport Medicine 15:158–166

Bellamy N, Campbell J, Robinson V et al 2006 Viscosupplementation for the treatment of osteoarthritis of the knee. Cochrane Database of Systematic Reviews 2:CD005321

Bennell K, White S, Crossley K 1999 The oral contraceptive pill: a revolution for sportswomen? British Journal of Sports Medicine 33:231–238

Bennett M, Best T M, Babul S et al 2005 Hyperbaric oxygen therapy for delayed onset muscle soreness and closed soft tissue injury. Cochrane Database of Systematic Reviews 4:CD004713.pub2

Best T M, Garrett W E 1994 Basic science of soft tissue. In: DeLee J C, Drez D (eds) Orthopedic sports medicine principles and practice. WB Saunders, Philadelphia, PA, p 1–45

Bowers L D 1998 Athletic drug testing. Clinics in Sports Medicine 17:299–318

Brukner P, Khan K 2002 Clinical sports medicine, 2nd revised edn. McGraw-Hill, Sydney

Brunton L, Lazo J, Parker, K 2006 Goodman and Gilman's: the pharmacological basis of therapeutics, 11th edn. McGraw-Hill, New York

Burnham R, Gregg R, Healy P et al 1998 The effectiveness of topical diclofenac for chronic lateral epicondylitis. Clinical Journal of Sport Medicine 8:78–81

Constantini N W, Dubnov G, Lebrun C M 2005 The menstrual cycle and sport performance. Clinics in Sports Medicine 24:51–82

Crawford F 2005 Plantar heel pain and fasciitis. Clinical Evidence 13:1533–1545

Dahners L E, Mullis B H 2004 Effects of nonsteroidal anti-inflammatory drugs on bone formation and soft-tissue healing. Journal of the American Academy of Orthopedic Surgeons 12:139–13

Dudley G A, Czerkawski J, Meinrod A et al 1997 Efficacy of naproxen sodium for exercise-induced dysfunction muscle injury and soreness. Clinical Journal of Sport Medicine 7:3–10

George A 2005a Central nervous system stimulants. In: Mottram D R (ed) Drugs in sport, 4th edn. Routledge, London, p 64–102

George A 2005b The anabolic steroids and peptide hormones. In: Mottram D R (ed) Drugs in sport, 4th edn. Routledge, London, p 140–190

George A 2005c Peptide and glycoprotein hormones and sport. In: Mottram D R (ed) Drugs in sport, 4th edn. Routledge, London, p 191–206

Goldman L, Ausiello D 2003 Cecil textbook of medicine, 22nd edn. WB Saunders, Philadelphia, PA

Gotzsche P C 2005 Musculoskeletal disorders. Non-steroidal anti-inflammatory drugs. Clinical Evidence 14:1498–1505

Gudeman S D, Eisele S A, Heidt Jr R S et al 1997 Treatment of plantar fasciitis by iontophoresis of 0.4% dexamathasone. American Journal of Sports Medicine 25:312–316

Hanson C A, Weinhold P S, Afshari H M et al 2005 The effect of analgesic agents on the healing rat medial collateral ligament. American Journal of Sports Medicine 33:674–679

Hasson S M, Daniels J C, Divine J G et al 1993 Effect of ibuprofen use on muscle soreness, damage, and performance: a preliminary investigation. Medicine and Science in Sports and Exercise 25:9–17

Helenius I, Lumme A, Haahtela T 2005 Asthma, airway inflammation and treatment in elite athletes. Sports Medicine 35:565–574

Henderson J M 1998 Therapeutic drugs: what to avoid with athletes. Clinics in Sports Medicine 17:229–244

Holzer K, Brukner P, Douglass J 2002 Evidence-based management of exercise-induced asthma. Current Sports Medicine Reports 1:86–92

Ishii Y, Deie M, Adachi N et al 2005 Hyperbaric oxygen as an adjuvant for athletes. Sports Medicine 35:739–746

Khaliq Y, Zhanel G G 2005 Musculoskeletal injury associated with fluoroquinolone antibiotics. Clinics in Plastic Surgery 32:495–502

Langdeau J B, Boulet L P 2003 Is asthma over- or under-diagnosed in athletes? Respiratory Medicine 97:109–114

Leadbetter W B 1995 Anti-inflammatory therapy in sports injury: the role of nonsteroidal drugs and corticosteroid injection. Clinics in Sports Medicine 14:353–410

Lebrun C M, Petit M A, McKenzie D C et al 2003 Decreased maximal aerobic capacity with use of a triphasic oral contraceptive in highly active women: a randomised controlled trial. British Journal of Sports Medicine 37:315–320

Liu S L, Lebrun C M 2006 Effect of oral contraceptives and hormone replacement therapy on bone mineral density in premenopausal and perimenopausal women: a systematic review. British Journal of Sports Medicine 40:11–24

McAlindon T E, Biggee B A 2005 Nutritional factors and osteoarthritis: recent developments. Current Opinion in Rheumatology 17:647–652

Magra M, Maffulli N 2006 Nonsteroidal antiinflammatory drugs in tendinopathy: friend or foe. Clinical Journal of Sport Medicine 16:1–3

Martineau P A, Al-Jassir F, Lenczner E et al 2004 Effect of the oral contraceptive pill on ligamentous laxity. Clinical Journal of Sport Medicine 14:281–286

Mason L, Moore R A, Derry S et al 2004a Systematic review of topical capsaicin for the treatment of chronic pain. British Medical Journal 328:991

Mason L, Moore RA, Edwards JE et al 2004b Topical NSAIDs for chronic musculoskeletal pain: systematic review and meta-analysis. BioMed Central Musculoskeletal Disorders 19:28.

Mason L, Moore RA, Edwards JE et al 2004c Topical NSAIDs for acute pain: a meta-analysis. BioMed Central Family Practice 17:10

Mason L, Moore RA, Edwards JE et al 2004d Systematic review of efficacy of topical rubefacients containing salicylates for the treatment of acute and chronic pain. British Medical Journal 328:995

Maughan R J 2005 Contamination of dietary supplements and positive drug tests in sport. Journal of Sports Science 23:883–889

Mazanec D J 1998 Medication use in sports rehabilitation. In: Kibler B W, Herring S A, Press J M et al (eds) Functional rehabilitation of sports and musculoskeletal injuries. Aspen Publishers, Gaithersburg, MD, p 71–78

Miller M G, Weiler J M, Baker R et al 2005 National athletic trainers' association position statement: management of asthma in athletes. Journal of Athletic Training 40:224–245

Nichols AW 2005 Complications associated with the use of corticosteroids in the treatment of athletic injuries. Clinical Journal of Sport Medicine 15:370–375

Ogilvie-Harris D J, Gilbart M 1995 Treatment modalities for soft tissue injuries of the ankle: a critical review. Clinical Journal of Sport Medicine 5:175–186

O'Grady M, Hackney A C, Schneider K et al 2000 Diclofenac sodium (voltaren) reduced exercise-induced injury in human skeletal muscle. Medicine and Science in Sports and Exercise 32:1191–1196

Paoloni J A, Orchard J W 2005 The use of therapeutic medications for soft-tissue injuries in sports medicine. Medical Journal of Australia 183:384–388

Quadagno D M 2000 Exercise and the female reproductive system: the effect of hormonal status on performance. In: Warren M P, Constantini N W (eds) Sports endocrinology. Humana, Totawa, p 321–334

Read M T F 1999 Safe relief of rest pain that eases with activity in achillodynia by intrabursal or peritendinous steroid injection; the rupture rate was not increased by these steroid injections. British Journal of Sports Medicine 33:134–135

Reilly T 1996 Alcohol, anti-anxiety drugs and sport. In: Mottram D R (ed) Drugs in sport, 2nd edn. E and FN Spon, London, p 144–172

Richy F, Bruyere O, Ethgen O et al 2003 Structural and symptomatic efficacy of glucosamine and chondroitin in knee osteoarthritis: a comprehensive meta-analysis. Archives of Internal Medicine 163:1514–1522

Rickenlund A, Carlstrom K, Ekblom B et al 2004 Effects of oral contraceptives on body composition and physical performance in female athletes. Journal of Clinical Endocrinology and Metabolism 89:4364–4370

Salpeter S R, Ormiston T M, Salpeter E E 2004 Cardiovascular effects of beta-agonists in patients with asthma and COPD: a meta-analysis. Chest 125:2309–2321

Sayers S P, Knight C A, Clarkson P M et al 2001 Effect of ketoprofen on muscle function and sEMG activity after eccentric exercise. Medicine and Science in Sports and Exercise 33:702–710

Shrier I, Matheson G O, Kohl H W 1996 Achilles tendonitis: are corticosteroid injections useful or harmful? Clinical Journal of Sport Medicine 6:245–250

Singh P, Roberts MS 1994 Skin permeability and local tissue concentrations of nonsteroidal anti-inflammatory drugs after topical application. Journal of Pharmacology and Experimental Therapeutics 268:144–151

Slatyer M A, Hensley M J, Lopert R 1997 A randomized controlled trial of piroxicam in the management of acute ankle sprain in Australian regular army recruits. American Journal of Sports Medicine 25:544–553

Smidt N, van der Windt DA, Assendelft WJ et al 2002 Corticosteroid injections, physiotherapy, or a wait-and-see policy for lateral epicondylitis: a randomised controlled trial. Lancet. 2002 359:657–662

Snibbe J C, Gambardella R A 2005 Use of injections for osteoarthritis in joints and sports activity. Clinics in Sports Medicine 24:83–89

Stanley K L, Weaver J E 1998 Pharmacologic management of pain and inflammation in athletes. Clinics in Sports Medicine 17:375–392

Sturmi J E, Diorio D J 1998 Anabolic agents. Clinics in Sports Medicine 17:261–282

Tallon C, Maffulli N, Ewen SW 2001 Ruptured Achilles tendons are significantly more degenerated than tendinopathic tendons. Medicine and Science in Sports and Exercise 33:1983–1990

Towheed T E, Maxwell L, Anastassiades T P et al 2005 Glucosamine therapy for treating osteoarthritis. Cochrane Database of Systematic Reviews 2:CD002946

Trent R J, Alexander I E 2006 Gene therapy in sport. British Journal of Sports Medicine 40:4–5

van Baak M A, Mayer L H J, Kempinski R E S et al 2000 Effect of salbutamol on muscle strength and endurance performance in nonasthmatic men. Medicine and Science in Sports and Exercise 32:1300–1306

van Baak M A, de Hon O M, Hartgens F et al 2004 Inhaled salbutamol and endurance cycling performance in non-asthmatic athletes. International Journal of Sports Medicine 25:533–538

Verroken M 2005 Drug use and abuse in sport. In: Mottram D R (ed) Drugs in sport, 4th edn. Routledge, London, p 29–63

Warden S J 2005 Cyclo-oxygenase-2 inhibitors: beneficial or detrimental for athletes with acute musculoskeletal injuries? Sports Medicine 35:271–283

Weiler J M 1992 Medical modifiers of sports injury: the use of nonsteroidal anti-inflammatory drugs in sports soft-tissue injury. Clinics in Sports Medicine 11:623–644

Woo W W, Man S Y, Lam P K et al 2005 Randomized double-blind trial comparing oral paracetamol and oral nonsteroidal antiinflammatory drugs for treating pain after musculoskeletal injury. Annals of Emergency Medicine 46:352–361

World Anti-Doping Agency 2005 The 2006 Prohibited List International Standard. Online. Available: http://www.wada-ama.org/rtecontent/document/code_v3.pdf (15 June 2006)

Medical imaging of injury

30

Douglas N. Mintz

CHAPTER CONTENTS

Introduction 558

Imaging modalities and techniques 558

Types of injuries 566

Specific disease entities and injuries 570

Complications 573

Therapeutics 574

Future developments 575

Summary 575

Introduction

Imaging of musculoskeletal injury requires a detailed knowledge of normal anatomy and the changes that reflect the pathophysiology of injury. There are many ways to image an injury, and the method chosen depends on the information required. Types of imaging vary in cost, availability, use of radiation, comfort for the patient, expertise required of the performer of the examination and expertise required of the interpreter of the examination. If clinicians understand both the disease processes and the imaging options, they will be able to use the least expensive and least invasive test that will answer the appropriate clinical question.

Imaging modalities and techniques

Plain film

Conventional radiographs are relatively inexpensive, widely available and provide a good starting point for imaging evaluation. Radiographs provide excellent bony, but not very good soft tissue, detail. The usual procedure involves obtaining at least two views of a body part (preferably orthogonal), with additional views, such as oblique views, stress views or special views, added as necessary (Harris & Harris 2000). Specific X-ray positions have been developed to better assess the ankle mortise, the carpal tunnel, the calcaneus, the subtalar joints and even the sesamoid bones at the base of the first metatarsal (Pavlov et al 1999). For example, the Harris heel view is used to evaluate the calcaneus. A carpal tunnel view may be used to look for bony spurs that may contribute to carpal tunnel syndrome and to look for fractures of the hamate or pisiform bone. Using the principle that to evaluate a structure radiographically it should be visible, unencumbered by overlapping structures, and in two orthogonal views, radiologists and clinicians have developed appropriate projections over time. Some bear the name of the inventor (e.g. Broden's view of the subtalar joint, Grashey's view of the glenohumeral joint, Judet's views of the acetabulum), while others are descriptive (e.g. the inlet and outlet views of the pelvis, and the sesamoid view of the great toe).

X-rays are created by passing an electrical current through an X-ray tube, which can be aimed so that the X-rays go into the body (Curry et al 1990). Some of the X-rays are absorbed and those that pass through the body expose a film or detector on the other side of the patient from the tube. More modern techniques produce a digital image rather than an image on film.

Several methods of adding information to the routine radiograph using X-rays include fluoroscopy, tomography, arthrography and myelography.

Fluoroscopy

In fluoroscopy, continuous radiographic images are obtained and viewed on a monitor, enabling a clinician or radiologist to see what is happening while it occurs. Fluoroscopy (as an alternative to ultrasound) is often used to guide joint or bursal injectious or aspirations for therapeutic and diagnostic purposes. The technique is useful to guide procedures such as facet and nerve root injections where real-time examination of contrast injections is useful.

Information can also be recorded, either digitally or with video, to show controlled motion as a cine loop. Whereas this technique is commonly used for other reasons, such as to evaluate patients' swallowing mechanisms, it can be useful in the evaluation of carpal bones for suspected midcarpal instability (Mathoulin et al 1990, Werber et al 1990). It can also be useful when performing an arthrogram, to facilitate the tracking of contrast. For example, if a radiocarpal joint injection is performed, and contrast extends into the midcarpal compartment, there is a tear of either the scapholunate or lunotriquetral ligament. If a video was taken at the time of the injection, it might be possible to better follow the course of the contrast and identify the exact location of the tear.

Tomography

Although rarely used in modern imaging, tomography is a technique that puts one level plane or depth in focus. By moving that plane up or down, one can see one level of a structure, bone or soft tissue, in focus, and the rest out of focus (Fig. 30.1). The level in focus is moved up or down systematically to evaluate the structure in question. This is achieved by moving the X-ray tube and the plate simultaneously so that only one area remains in focus. The patterns of motion can be simple (linear tomography) or complex (e.g. hypocycloidal) depending on the details required. Tomography is useful in assessing for articular step-off in intra-articular fractures and also in looking for fractures that might otherwise be obscured by adjacent bone (e.g. odontoid fractures or pars interarticularis fractures). Plain tomography has, for the most part, been replaced by computed tomography (CT), and so much so that there are few, if any, complex tomography machines that remain in use.

Myelography/arthrography

Myelography is a procedure in which contrast is injected into the subarachnoid space and then examined with radiographs

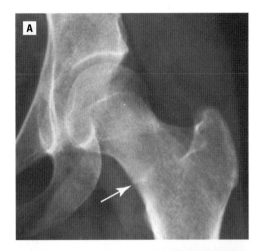

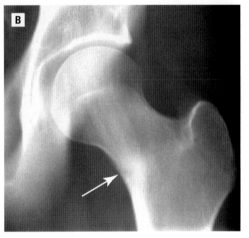

Figure 30.1 • A: Frontal view of the left hip demonstrating stress fracture of the medial femoral neck (arrow). **B:** Tomogram of the same fracture (arrow). Note that the fracture is better seen on the tomogram.

and with CT scans (Fig. 30.2). This can be achieved in the cervical, thoracic or lumbar spine. The injection is performed with a thin needle in the lower lumbar or upper cervical spine in such a way as to limit the risk of contacting the spinal cord. Myelography was formerly the mainstay of imaging of the spine for soft tissue abnormalities such as disk herniations. The technique has been largely replaced, however, by magnetic resonance imaging (MRI), although myelograms are still used as a preoperative tool or in patients who are unable to have MRI examinations.

When performing a myelogram, as much information as possible should be obtained from the examination. For example, when assessing the lumbar spine, images of the patient's spine in flexion and extension should be obtained. These images can be used both to evaluate stability and to look at the effect of the motion on the degree of any stenosis or impingement that is present.

Arthrograms, in which contrast is injected into a joint, were once the most common approach to imaging the shoulder for

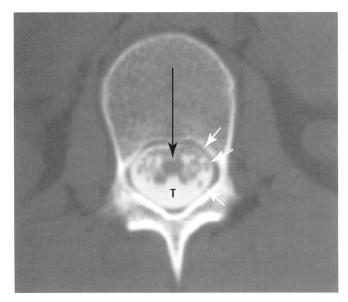

Figure 30.2 • Axial CT image at the L1 level after the subarachnoid administration of iodinated contrast for a myelogram. Note the CSF in the thecal sac (T) is dense from the contrast. The large arrow is on the conus medullaris. The short arrows point to the individual nerve roots of the cauda equina, outlined by contrast.

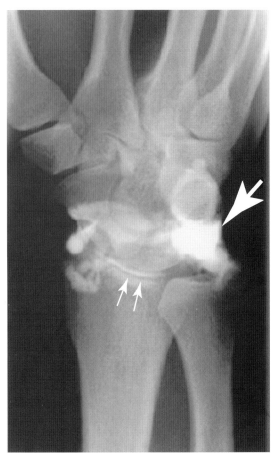

Figure 30.3 • Arthrogram of the wrist. The contrast is white and outlines the radiocarpal joint (small arrows) and collects in the pisiform bursa (large arrow).

rotator cuff tear, the knee for meniscal tear, and the wrist for evaluation of the triangular fibrocartilage (Fig. 30.3). These techniques have been largely replaced by MRI and ultrasound. Many centers perform arthrography in conjunction with MRI (MR arthrography) to help evaluate the glenoid and acetabular labra. Arthrography is still used for patients who are unable to undergo MRI in evaluation of the knee meniscus.

Nuclear medicine

Nuclear medicine is the field of radiology in which radioactive agents, called radionuclides or radiopharmaceuticals, are injected into the body and subsequently imaged using radiation detectors placed over the body. Radionuclides are bioactive substrates so nuclear medicine studies can evaluate physiological properties. This is the only imaging test that evaluates a process or function rather than giving only an anatomic representation.

Bone scan

In nuclear medicine, there are many procedures used to image the body. The procedure that is most common in evaluating injuries is the bone scan, whereby the patient is injected with radioactive technetium-labeled diphosphonate which distributes itself to metabolically active bone. There are three potential phases to imaging. Phase 1 (the vascular phase) involves imaging the patient immediately, while the substance is in the artery. Phase 2 (the blood pool phase) involves imaging when the radionuclide is starting to perfuse the soft tissues.

Phase 3 is the imaging of the bone after the radionuclide has left the soft tissues and been concentrated into the bone. This occurs about 2 hours after injection at which time the patient is imaged under a radiation counter to produce an image (Fig. 30.4). This should be done with the detector close to the body and after the radionuclide has left the soft tissue and become more conspicuous in the bone. Since the bone scanning agent is excreted in the urine, it gets concentrated in the bladder, so that the bladder becomes black on the images (Fig. 30.4). A full bladder can obscure the sacrum thereby requiring patients to empty their bladders before being scanned, especially if the study is done to identify pelvic or sacral fractures.

Bone scans are very sensitive, but not very specific. The lack of specificity means that the clinical setting is very important. In a runner, a stress fracture can be seen on bone scan before it is demonstrated on X-ray. The same appearance in a different location or clinical setting, however, may represent an infection, arthritis or a bone tumor (Levin et al 1967). Another use of bone scan is to identify fractures of the pars interarticularis and to evaluate healing as a function of radionuclide uptake (Anderson et al 2000). Cross-sectional images can be obtained using single photon emission computed tomography (SPECT)

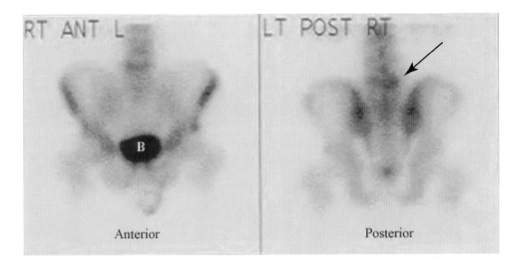

Anterior

Posterior

Figure 30.4 • Bone scan with anterior and posterior views with faint increased uptake in the right lower lumbar region (arrow). The bladder (B) contains concentrated radionuclide.

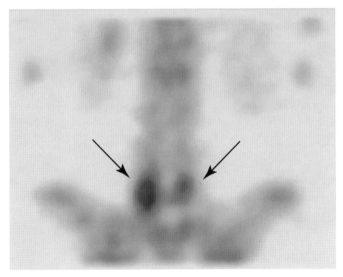

Figure 30.5 • Coronal slice from SPECT of the bone scan in Fig. 30.4, with more conspicuous uptake, seen on the right more than left (arrow). The finding indicates pars fractures, more active on the right. These are seen in the CT scan of Fig. 30.10.

(Fig. 30.5), where the detector passes around the body, as in regular CT, but much more slowly. MRI has also been used for this purpose (Resnick & Kransdorf 2004, Standaert et al 2000).

Bone densitometry

Several methods are available to measure the density of bone. Bone density is correlated to bone mineral content to evaluate for osteopenia/osteoporosis. Statistical comparisons are made to the young healthy general population (T-values) and age-matched controls (Z-values). Osteopenia is defined as having a bone density of 1 standard deviation below the mean and osteoporosis is defined as 2.5 standard deviations below the mean (see Chapters 5 and 27).

Bone density can be determined using many imaging modalities, including X-ray, MRI, CT and ultrasound. In general, radiographs are not sensitive enough to bone loss to be useful for evaluating bone density (Edelstyn et al 1967). The most commonly used method (which is inexpensive, convenient, has a low radiation dose and is reproducible) of measuring bone densitometry is dual emission X-ray absorptometry (DEXA). DEXA quantitatively compares absorption of X-ray beams of two different energies. This test is performed on different parts of the body, including the spine, hip, and wrist. It is useful in identifying and following osteopenia or osteoporosis (Faulkner 2001). In the young injured population, DEXA is used in the presence of stress fractures to identify a more important underlying problem such as osteoporosis and malnutrition (see Chapter 5 for a further account of the use of DEXA).

Ultrasound

Ultrasound is an excellent tool to image musculoskeletal injury. Diagnostic ultrasound uses lower energy than the therapeutic ultrasound (discussed in Chapter 14). Ultrasound scans invoke principles of transmission and reflection of sound waves, as in sonar, to obtain a cross-sectional image of an area. Modern ultrasound uses high frequency transducers to get high-level detail in evaluation of the soft tissues, particularly superficially (Fig. 30.6). Ultrasound technology is available in small machines and can be portable and used to evaluate sports injuries acutely, but since it is somewhat difficult to learn the technique of interpretation of ultrasound, this is not readily done by physical therapists or athletic trainers.

In order to create an ultrasound image, there must be an 'acoustic window', which is an area that does not reflect sound waves and allows them to be transmitted. The internal structures of the knee, such as the cruciate ligaments, are therefore not amenable to ultrasound, nor are the deep structures of the other joints. Imaging of the shoulder and acetabular labra is possible, but limited in its extent, as is the evaluation of the menisci of the knee.

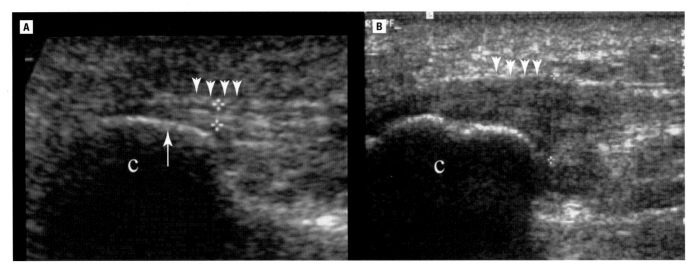

Figure 30.6 • Ultrasound images comparing normal plantar fascia **(A)** with plantar fasciitis **(B)**. The plantar fascia (small arrowheads) is normally a thin echogenic structure arising from the calcaneus **(C)**. Note the white line (large arrow) indicating the reflective cortical surface of the calcaneus. In **B**, the plantar fascia is markedly thickened (calipers) and has decreased echogenicity.

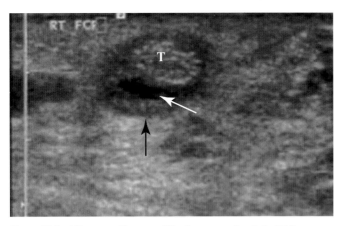

Figure 30.7 • Ultrasound image of the flexor carpi radialis (T) in cross-section. There is tenosynovitis with fluid in the tendon sheath (white arrow) and thickening of the tendon sheath itself (black arrow).

Ultrasound is of great benefit for evaluation of superficial tendons such as in the foot, ankle and wrist (Fig. 30.7), as well as the tendons and ligaments around the shoulder, elbow and knee. Ultrasound has the advantage of being a real-time modality so that an ultrasonographer can manipulate patients and discuss their symptoms with them while the study is being performed and apply force and pressure to further elicit patient symptoms or see if structures are compressible. For example, one can compress vessels. One can also compress the fluid that might fill a tendon tear and confirm that it is indeed a tear. Since it can be used dynamically, ultrasound can also directly diagnose impingement in the shoulder, observing the supraspinatus tendon bunching up at the coracoacromial arch with abduction of the humerus (Read & Perko 1998).

As with every imaging modality, learning to interpret the images is dependent upon knowing normal anatomy and getting used to the way it looks on imaging. In ultrasound, experience is gathered by performing the test. Most imaging is performed by a technologist and interpreted thereafter. In ultrasound, the person performing the test acquires snapshots of what they are looking at to review later. If the performer of the study does not see the pathology, they do not take an image of it. Therefore the person performing the study must be highly experienced, making ultrasound very much a user-dependent test.

As with radiographs (and MRI) the structures are imaged in at least two planes. On ultrasound these are the long and short axes of the anatomy or the longitudal and transverse planes. For the patellar tendon, for example, the cranial–caudal plane would be long axis or longitudinal, and medial–lateral plane would be the short axis or transverse plane. The images must be appropriated labeled.

Because ultrasound uses sound to evaluate structures, structures are called echogenic when they bounce sound back, or echolucent when they allow sound to pass through. Fluid for example is echolucent (dark on usual unconventional ultrasound) and allows sound to easily pass through making structures beyond more echogenic (a property called through-transmission). Structures that reflect sound more strongly (e.g. muscle) are more echogenic. Some substances such as bone completely reflect sound and do not allow sound to continue to go through them. They appear as a bright line with black below them (shadowing). Foreign bodies and calcification have this appearance (Figs 30.6 and 30.8). Cortical disruption, such as in fractures, can be seen, as can spikes of bone (osteophytes) arising from normally smooth surfaces (Hubner et al 2000, Patten et al 1992).

Another valuable tool that ultrasound provides is the ability to look at blood flow. This relates to the way sound reflects off

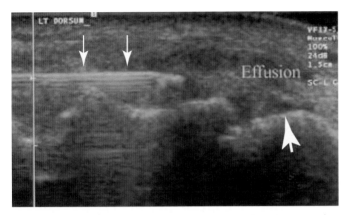

Figure 30.8 • Ultrasound image of a metatarsalphalangeal joint injection. Note the needle (thin arrows) within the joint effusion. The cortex of bone is a white line because it reflects the sound waves (fat arrow).

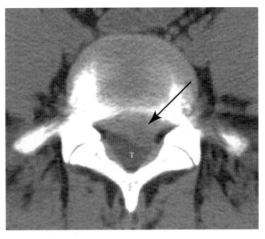

Figure 30.9 • Axial CT image demonstrating moderately large left-sided disk herniation at L5–S1 (arrow), pressing on the thecal sac (T).

moving targets (Doppler effect), and this allows one to look at vessels and blood flow within the structure to gauge the degree of inflammation, and examine arterial and venous structures. On the images one can assign color to blood flowing through a vessel, making it easier to see on the screen. It is by using this technique, in part, that one can identify a deep vein thrombosis: there will be vein, but no flow through it.

Computed tomography

Computed tomography (CT) is an X-ray technique that uses ionizing radiation. Higher doses than with conventional radiography are absorbed (in the order of 1–2 rads in modern imaging) by the body part being imaged. CT shows very clear bony detail but not as good soft tissue contrast. The images are obtained by a rotating X-ray tube contained in a loop (torus) circling a patient who is lying on a radiolucent table. As the patient goes through the middle of the torus, images of cross-sections of the body part in the transverse plane are obtained. These sections can be reformatted so that they can be viewed in any plane. Newer generations of CT scanners exist which comprise multiple detectors, allowing larger areas to be scanned at the same time making scans quite fast, so that scans can now take a matter of seconds, rather than minutes. CT is more available than MRI in most clinical settings (many emergency departments have CT scanners), is less expensive and there are no contraindications to the study.

In trauma, CT is a good screening test for internal organ injury (Harris & Harris 2000). For the musculoskeletal system, fractures can usually be screened for, and evaluated by, radiograph. CT is used for further evaluation such as for inadequate or suspicious radiographs of the cervical spine. Due to the excellent bony detail afforded by CT, it is used for evaluating complex intra-articular fractures, such as those of the tibial plateau, wrist and acetabulum. Another structure amenable to CT examination is the spine, where myelographic and non-myelographic CT is excellent for evaluating disk disease,

particularly in the lumbar spine (Fig. 30.9). Some advocate using CT for evaluating the pars interarticularis for potential lysis (Congeni et al 1997) (Fig. 30.10).

The speed of acquiring images in CT continues to increase and the ability of the information processing has also improved. At the time of this publication scanners with up to 128 slices are available. This allows remarkably fast imaging, not as important in the musculoskeletal system, as for example in cardiac angiography, which can now be done with CT. Newer scanners have allowed for reducing artifact created from orthopedic hardware. Better and faster image processing has allowed quick three-dimensional rendering of body parts complete with different colors for bone, muscles and vessels. Techniques allow virtual navigation of the body, including for example, virtual angiography, bronchoscopy and colonoscopy.

Magnetic resonance imaging

Magnetic resonance imaging (MRI) is the best overall test for imaging sport-related injury. Its excellent soft tissue contrast and multiplanar capabilities make it useful for evaluation of all of the anatomical structures, including articular cartilage (Fig. 30.11), bone, the myotendinous unit (Fig. 30.12) and ligamentous structures (Fig. 30.13). MRI has sensitivity to fracture and bone contusion, that have a typical appearance.

MRI uses a strong magnet and radiofrequency pulses to obtain its image: patients go into a magnetic field (about 25 000 times stronger than the earth's). This magnetic field is created in a tube or long tunnel into which patients are placed. Their bodies' hydrogen ions are aligned in the magnetic field. The hydrogen ions are then deflected by radiofrequency waves. The behavior of the ions in this field is dependent on their local environment and can be exploited by different ways of imparting the radiofrequency waves. Complex mathematical manipulation of the waves that come back from the body allow the creation of an image. Ions other than hydrogen can be used

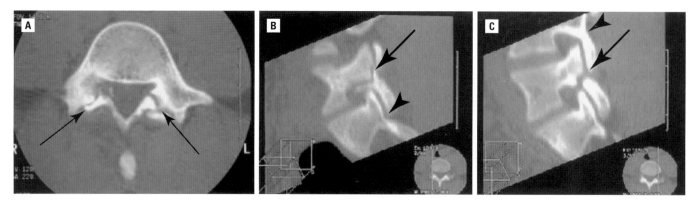

Figure 30.10 • Axial (**A**) and sagitally reformatted (**B** = left, **C** = right) CT scans demonstrating bilateral pars fractures at L5 (arrows). The pars interarticularis of L4 (right) and S1 (left) are intact (arrowheads).

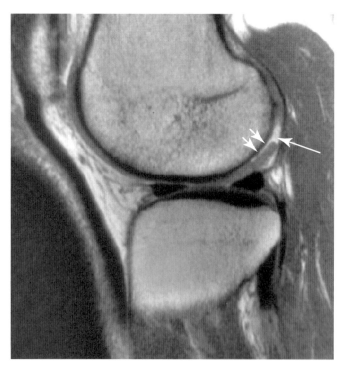

Figure 30.11 • Sagittal MR image demonstrating a focal full-thickness defect in the articular cartilage of the lateral femoral condyle (long arrow), creating a flap (short arrows).

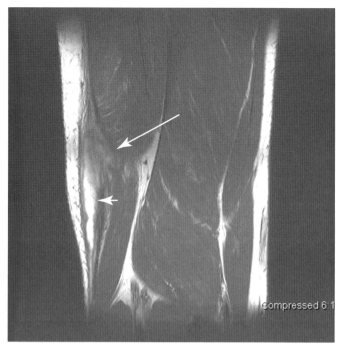

Figure 30.12 • Coronal MR image of the lower thigh indicating tear of the long head of the biceps femoris (long arrow) with adjacent hematoma (short arrow), which was drained under ultrasound guidance.

for imaging (most often sodium); however, since there is such a high concentration of hydrogen in the body, it is easier to use. MRI is dependent on a strong and homogeneous magnetic field. It is dangerous to bring loose ferromagnetic substances (e.g. wheelchairs, oxygen canisters, tools) near the magnetic field because they can be pulled into the magnet; however, immobile metal objects, such as orthopedic instrumentation are safe. Imaging ferromagnetic substances is challenging since they distort the field and thus the image. To some extent, the radiologist can compensate for instrumentation (White et al 2000).

There are contraindications to the use of MRI (Table 30.1). Patients with pacemakers are not allowed near the magnet due to possible inactivation of the pacemaker. Patients with cerebral aneurysm clips, due to the risk of the clip moving, are imaged only if a non-ferromagnetic clip is used, and then only at the discretion of the radiologist. Likewise, patients with intravascular stents should not be put in the MRI magnet for at least 6 weeks after placement of such devices, which gives a chance for the device to be secured by the body's fibrous tissue. Spinal cord and nerve stimulators are not permitted in the magnet due to the risk of causing stimulation/damage to

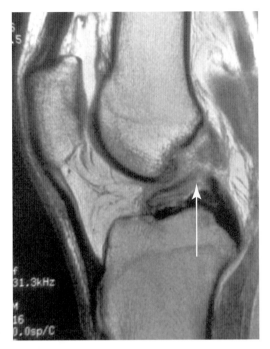

Figure 30.13 • Sagittal MR image demonstrating acute proximal anterior cruciate ligament tear (arrow).

Table 30.1 Some contraindications to magnetic resonance imaging (MRI)

Absolute	Relative
Pacemaker	Claustrophobia
Cerebral aneurysm clip	Aneurysm clip
Implanted nerve stimulator	Pregnancy
Implanted tissue expander	Tremor (inability to remain still)
	Metal worker (ocular foreign body)

the nerves (Shellock 2005). MRI safety is an important issue. Patients should be screened and, if questions arise, they should be answered before a patient gets close to the magnet (Sawyer-Glover & Shellock 2000).

During each MRI examination, a technologist acquires images in sets of data or pulse sequences. Much research had and is being done on designing the best pulse sequences to image that take into account speed, accuracy and clinical importance. Some give anatomic information and are most often used, others give ultrastructural information, while others quantify tissue components. Most of the time, we look at anatomic images, performed in different planes, although one is able now to obtain all planes of information at once as a volume and display in whatever planes are best for interpretation.

Knowledge of some of the terms used in MRI is important. These include spin echo, fast (turbo) spin echo, gradient echo and STIR (short tau inversion recovery). These are all types of pulse sequences used in obtaining images. In a magnetic field, hydrogen ions have their own magnetic dipole and line up facing either toward or away from the direction of the field, which is along the z-axis using Cartesian coordinates. A greater number of hydrogen ions line up toward the field and these are the ions used in MRI. Using radiofrequency pulses, the ions that are lined up are perturbed into the x–y plane. This puts them into higher energy states, so that they want to go back to the z-axis. When they realign, they release energy in the form of radiofrequency waves. A receiver listens for these waves, which are then used to create the MRI image. While the ions are going back to line up along the z-axis, they disperse in the x–y plane. This dispersion reduces the strength of signal so, before listening, another radiofrequency pulse refocuses or realigns the ions in the x–y plane. This sequence of events is called spin echo imaging. If multiple refocusing pulses are used for each perturbing pulse, it is called fast (turbo) spin echo imaging. Gradient echo imaging does not use a refocusing pulse. A STIR sequence is different in that it uses different sequences of perturbing pulses that are timed to be able to take advantage of the protons' characteristic behaviors and remove the signal from the protons in molecules of fat.

T1 and T2 are terms that describe characteristics of a tissue. T1 (presented as a number) is defined as 63% of the length of the time it takes for a proton that is perturbed into the x–y plane to line up with the magnet. T2 (also presented as a number) is defined as the length of time it takes for a proton in the x–y plane to disperse in that plane. Although they do not have to, MRI pulse sequences can accentuate T1 characteristics of a tissue or T2 characteristics of a tissue. These are called T1- and T2-weighted sequences, respectively. Fat has a lot of signal on T1-weighted sequences and is, therefore, 'bright' or white on T1-weighted images. Fluid has high signal on T2-weighted images and is, therefore, 'bright' on T2-weighted images. Musculoskeletal imaging is often performed somewhere between T1 and T2 weighted imaging.

Images can be manipulated to exclude signal from fat. Fat suppression techniques include STIR and frequency-selective fat suppression. Every study should include at least one plane which has fat suppression (Fig. 30.14). Suppressing the fat on an image, or making it dark, makes pathology more conspicuous and allows detection of minor injuries such as bone contusions, which would otherwise be difficult to recognize (Mirowitz et al 1994). On any given system, there are many variables that can be manipulated to obtain an image. The degrees to which imaging centers, hospitals or radiologists optimize these variables for particular studies are considerably different, based on individual preference, bias and expertise.

Not only are there variations in pulse sequence determination by software, there are differences in hardware, such as coil design and magnet strength. The coil can be thought of as the radiofrequency receiver (although some also impart waves). To get the best reception of the information coming back from the tissues, coils can be placed on the patient (surface coils), allowing better signal reception that can translate into high definition images. Different magnets are now available. The traditional long closed tube designs are being replaced by shorter tubes and newer open designs, accommodating claustrophobic

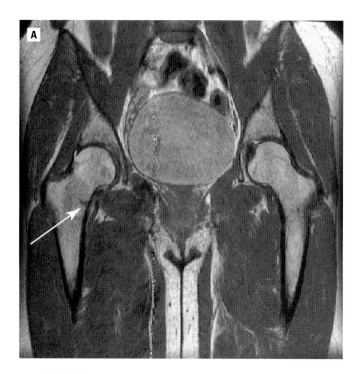

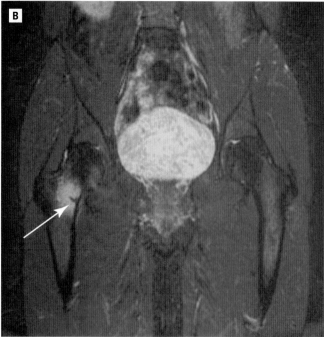

Figure 30.14 • Coronal MRI of the hip in a woman runner demonstrating right medial femoral neck fracture (arrow) as indicated by the low-signal line extending part of the way through the bone (**A** and **B**). Note the surrounding reactive signal on the fat-suppressed image (**B**).

patients. There is also an MRI unit that can perform studies while patients are standing, sitting or bending, allowing one to determine if a disc protrusion is changing with different positions. Also newly available are dedicated extremity magnets which have a small hole where patients can put a foot, ankle, knee, wrist or elbow and be imaged in a much more comfortable position with only that body part being in the magnet.

Types of injuries

Due to the many imaging modalities available and the redundancy of the information that can be obtained through these methods, deciding on the appropriate imaging study for a particular injury can be confusing. There are criteria for imaging developed by the American College of Radiology (2005), but the best way to determine the appropriate test is to discuss the clinical situation with an experienced radiologist. Some guidelines for specific injuries are included in Table 30.2. There is not so much a correct or incorrect way to use imaging to assist diagnosis, as methods that people are more or less comfortable and experienced with. Open communication between the practitioner and radiologist is important to obtain appropriate studies and helps the radiologist to specifically address the clinical problem and target the examination.

The different types of tissues that make up the neuromusculoskeletal system are discussed in Chapters 2–7. The differences of tissue character mean that each tissue type cannot be imaged in the same way, and the challenges created by having to image different types of tissue create one of the more interesting aspects of musculoskeletal radiology. Much of learning how to interpret imaging studies is learning what to expect, that is, the normal anatomy and seeing the differences between what we know as normal from what we see for a given patient. For example, bones should have well-defined cortical lines. When we see a break in this line (e.g. as in a fracture), we identify the pattern as being abnormal anatomy. The recognition of abnormality comes only with an appreciation of normal anatomy. Radiologists learn what is normal through repetition. Non-radiologists are encouraged to do the same by examining all imaging studies that deal with their patients.

Bone

A bone can be evaluated in all imaging modalities, from the fracture seen on radiographs to the contusional pattern seen on MRI. Even ultrasound, which does not penetrate bone, is able to image the cortex and to detect occult greater tuberosity fractures when looking at the rotator cuff (Patten et al 1992). The primary modality for the imaging of bone injury is the conventional radiograph. As mentioned earlier in this chapter, radiographs are very specific, but not as sensitive as other modalities. They are, however, the primary method for diagnosing and following fractures. Radiographs also continue to be the best test to evaluate most bone tumors (Greenspan 2004).

The clearest images of bone are obtained by CT scan, where the windows can be created to accentuate the differences in density between bone and the surrounding soft tissues. Tomographic capabilities allow sections thinner than 1 mm and can define some ultrastructural bone characteristics (Buchman et al 1998).

Table 30.2 Choice of imaging modality

Body part	Suspected problem	First examination	Second examination	Comments
Any	Stress fracture	X-ray	MRI or bone scan	Stress fractures can be readily identified on both MRI and bone scan. MRI has the advantage of better defining the extent of the fracture. If X-ray is positive, further imaging is usually not required
Back pain	Pars fracture, pedicle stress fracture, disk herniation, facet arthrosis or synovitis, sacroiliitis	X-ray	MRI	X-ray can identify some pathologies, obviating the need for further testing. Whereas CT scan is good for pars defects and disk herniations, MRI gives more information without ionizing radiation. Bone scan can be useful for active pars defects but does not look for other etiologies of pain
Shoulder pain (older patient)	Rotator cuff tear, bursitis, arthrosis, fracture	X-ray	MRI or ultrasound	To evaluate the tendons of the rotator cuff and biceps, MRI and ultrasound are both useful and accurate
Shoulder pain (young patient)	Rotator cuff tear, labral or capsular pathology, cartilage abnormality, fracture	X-ray	MRI	In younger patients, MRI can evaluate pathologies such as the labral capsular complex and articular cartilage, as well as the bone marrow, that cannot be seen on ultrasound
Elbow pain	Fracture, tendon/ligament injury, osteochondritis dissecans, overuse syndromes	X-ray	MRI or ultrasound	Medial and lateral epicondylitis can be evaluated with both ultrasound and MRI
Wrist/finger	Ligament tears, ganglion, fracture, tendon pathologies	X-ray	MRI or ultrasound	In trauma, avulsion fractures can define tendon or ligament pain pathology on plain X-ray. Further evaluation of the superficial structures can be done with ultrasound. The deeper structures require MRI for evaluation. Deeper structures include the bony abnormalities. Bone scan and CT can be used to identify occult fractures but provide less information than MRI
Knee pain	Meniscal tear, ligament tear, cartilage injury, tendon abnormality, synovitis, fracture	X-ray	MRI	Ultrasound can be useful for looking at superficial structures around the knee such as the patellar tendon or collateral ligaments. To look at the deeper structures, including the menisci, articular cartilage and cruciate ligaments, MRI is necessary
Ankle pain	Fracture, ligament tears, tendon pathologies, impingement syndromes, nerve pathologies, Achilles tendon and plantar fascia problems	X-ray	MRI or ultrasound	For superficial pathologies such as tenosynovitis or tendon degeneration or tear, ultrasound is a good test. For a global picture including cartilage, ligament, tendons and bone, MRI is a better test. Plantar fascia and Achilles tendon pathologies are excellently seen on ultrasound, which can also guide injections

(Continued)

Table 30.2 (Continued)

Body part	Suspected problem	First examination	Second examination	Comments
Compartment syndrome		Compartment pressures		Exertional compartment syndrome is still evaluated using compartment pressures before and after exercise. Whereas there is a role for other modalities, these are best used in centers experienced with them
Focal pain	Muscle injury, tendon injury, fascial injury, mass, stress fracture, ganglion cyst	MRI or ultrasound		For a general evaluation, MRI is easier to evaluate many structures in a region; however, ultrasound has the advantage of direct interaction with the patient and real time scanning. The choice relies upon clinicians' judgment and radiologists' experience

On MRI, bone gives a similar signal intensity to fat, because of the fat in bone marrow. Abnormalities become low signal on T1-weighted images, making them stand out. Fat suppression techniques make MRI an ideal modality for identifying stress fractures or stress injuries by making them more conspicuous (high signal) than the adjacent bone. The resolution of MRI is similar to that of CT, although thinner images can be obtained routinely in CT. Bone scans provide a sensitive method for looking for global bone injury or tumor, since the whole body can be imaged at the same sitting without additional radiation. Bone scans, however, are dependent on bone being metabolically active and pathology being more active than normal bone. Since they are less expensive than MRI, and almost as sensitive, bone scans can be used to confirm a diagnosis, such as stress fracture (Fig. 30.15), for which there is a high clinical suspicion – a situation where a positive result (increased uptake of radionuclide) will not yield ambiguous interpretation.

Myotendinous unit

The myotendinous unit comprises the muscle, myotendinous junction and the tendon itself, and is best imaged with MRI and ultrasound. When imaging muscle, ideally one looks at three things: muscle size and composition, to look for atrophy and fatty infiltration from disuse or chronic injury; structure, where damage to the structure is the result of direct or indirect injury; and indirect signs of ultrastructural abnormalities, such as denervation or inflammation (myositis). MRI and ultrasound prove better tools than CT (Berquist 1992). Nuclear medicine does not have a strong role in imaging of myotendinous injuries. Contrast tenography, where contrast is injected into the tendon sheath and radiographs are obtained, is rarely used.

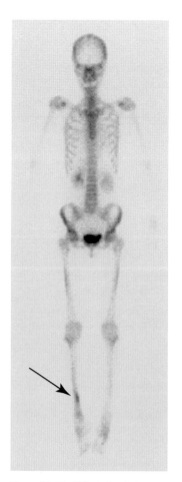

Figure 30.15 • Whole body bone scan, frontal view, demonstrating increased uptake in the medial aspect of the right distal tibia (arrow).

Both ultrasound and MRI are able to evaluate muscle–tendon junction, tendon and insertion of tendon onto bone (van Holsbeeck & Introcaso 2001). On ultrasound, muscle abnormality is evidenced by loss of the normal architecture of the muscle and loss of the normal echo texture. Inflammation can often be seen using Doppler techniques to identify increased blood flow (van Holsbeeck & Introcaso 2001). The anatomical structure can be examined for size, and the presence of fatty infiltration can be determined by increased echogenicity. The structure can be examined along its course in a dynamic setting, and the muscle tendon junction can be carefully examined for tear. In tendons surrounded by a sheath, the first sign of pathology is fluid in the sheath (tenosynovitis). Tendinopathy is evidenced by thickening of a tendon, a loss in the normal increased echogenicity as well as loss of the normal fibrillar architecture (van Holsbeeck & Introcaso 2001). Chronic tendinopathy can lead to calcifications within the tendon (Fornage 1995). Tendon tear is seen as discontinuity of the tendon. Common areas imaged with ultrasound include the tendons of the shoulder (rotator cuff and biceps), wrist and elbow. In the lower extremity, the hamstring origin and the foot and ankle tendons are easy to demonstrate using ultrasound imagery.

It is possible to define muscle size and intrinsic abnormal signal, from denervation, injury or myositis. Injuries to the muscle, tendon or muscle–tendon junction are directly visualized, as are potential secondary hematomas (Fig. 30.12). Only relatively few injuries to the myotendinous unit require imaging. In the case of tear, if surgical repair is considered, imaging is useful to delineate the anatomy. Tears of the tendinous insertions onto bone are more amenable to surgical repair than are the more common muscle–tendon junction injuries (Connell et al 1999). Identification, in acute injuries, of muscle hematomas is also useful, as these can be drained, both to reduce pain and to decrease the chance of developing myositis ossificans (Arrington & Miller 1995). Injuries that are refractory to nonoperative management may be imaged to exclude partial tendon tears that might be more amenable to operative treatment.

For MRI, tendinosis is evidenced by loss of the normal homogenous low signal of the tendon. Normally, a tendon on MRI is a homogeneously low signal structure because of the immobility of the protons in a tendon's regular structure. When a tendon degenerates (tendinosis), it becomes thicker and higher in signal. Tears and partial tears are defined by partial or complete discontinuity of the tendon. Tenosynovitis is evidenced by fluid in the tendon sheath in both MRI and ultrasound. There can be thickening of tendon sheaths. The entity of the calcific tendonitis can be identified on radiographs where a small focus of calcification is seen in the tendinous insertion (Fig. 30.16). This calcification is less conspicuous on MRI but visible and evident on ultrasound by the reflective interface of the calcification.

On ultrasound, tendons are relatively echogenic (white). Degeneration of the tendon results in a decrease in echogenicity with the structure becoming darker. It is important to have the ultrasound positioned appropriately since off-angle positioning can cause artificial echolucency, making the tendon look

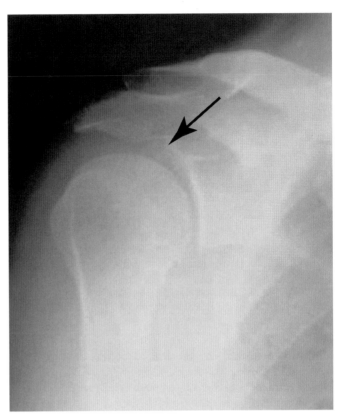

Figure 30.16 • Frontal radiograph of the right shoulder demonstrating calcification at the origin of the long head of the biceps off the glenoid indicating calcific tendinitis (arrow).

artificially dark. This is related to a characteristic of tendon tissue known as anisotropy. When a tendon is torn, such as in the rotator cuff, applied pressure will make the echolucent fluid filling the gap completely disappear.

An entity that involves the muscles but is not an injury per se is exertional compartment syndrome. Various methods have been used to document the entity, most reliably, compartment pressure measurements before and after exercise. Imaging methods have looked at two aspects of such diagnosis: blood flow, done with nuclear medicine studies and ultrasound (Edwards et al 1999); and morphological changes using MRI immediately after exercise (Yao et al 1994).

Ligaments

Ligaments have the same imaging characteristics as tendons, and where an acoustic window is available, ultrasound can be used to evaluate them. MRI is the mainstay of evaluation of ligaments, although ultrasound can be used for the collateral ligaments in the knee and for the talofibular and tibiofibular ligaments of the ankle. In the imaging of ligaments on MRI, frank discontinuity is not always evident. Thus, tears of ligaments (e.g. anterior talofibular ligament) are evidenced as thickening and diffuse high signal, rather than discontinuity. These 'tears' correspond to what may clinically be called a sprain. MRI is accurate in evaluating the integrity of ligaments such as the anterior cruciate ligament (Cotten et al 2000, Ha et al 1998).

Cartilage

The imaging of articular cartilage is an area of great interest. Articular cartilage injury can be difficult to diagnose by physical examination and is important to the outcome of a joint injury. Formerly, arthrography was used to image articular cartilage. Irregularity of the surface or lack of space between cartilage and bone indicated abnormality. More recently, CT arthrography has been used. Currently, however, MRI is the study of choice for evaluating articular cartilage (Fig. 30.11). Ultrasound can evaluate cartilage, but is limited in its ability to visualize both joint services of a given joint. The techniques used in MRI for evaluating cartilage differ. Some radiologists use gradient echo techniques, others use fast spin echo imaging (Disler 1997, Disler et al 2000, McCauley & Disler 2001, Potter et al 1998) and some radiologists make no effort to evaluate articular cartilage. Cartilage is graded by a modified Outerbridge grading scale for articular cartilage, with I indicating softening, II being fibrillation less than 50% of the cartilage thickness, III being fibrillation or fissuring greater than 50% of the cartilage thickness and IV being a full-thickness defect (Outerbridge 1961). Newer techniques of MR imaging such as T2-mapping, T1-rho, sodium imaging and degemric (delayed gadolinium enhanced imaging) can be used for evaluation of ultrastructural abnormalities of articular cartilage. At present, these are done predominately for research but may have clinical applications in the future (as treatments for chondral injuries improve).

Fibrocartilage, such as the menisci of the knee and the labrum of the hip, can best be seen with MRI (Resnick et al 2006), with CT arthrography as the second choice. Patterns and location of meniscal injury can be defined on MRI and can explain symptoms of pain or locking (Green 2001, Resnick et al 2006).

Nerve

Clinicians can augment information gained by electrophysiological tests on peripheral nerves, with images from cross-sectional imaging modalities. Nerve injuries include avulsion of a root from the spinal cord, traumatic laceration, traction injuries and secondary inflammation from an adjacent mass or adjacent inflamed soft tissue (e.g. hamstring tendinosis causing radicular symptoms). An example of this is an osteochondroma causing a mass effect or lesions in closed spaces like soft tissue ganglia in the carpal or tarsal tunnel. High-resolution imaging can define the nerve fascicles and the nerve can be traced on MRI and ultrasound. The named nerves of the extremities can be seen with high-quality cross-sectional MR and ultrasound imaging, extending to the peripheral and even to the digital nerves of the hands and feet (van Holsbeeck & Introcaso 2001). Secondary findings of nerve abnormality (e.g. denervation of muscle) can be apparent as high T2 signal on MRI. Often the goal of imaging peripheral nerves is to exclude treatable pathologies, such as intrinsic nerve problems (schwannomas and neurofibromas)

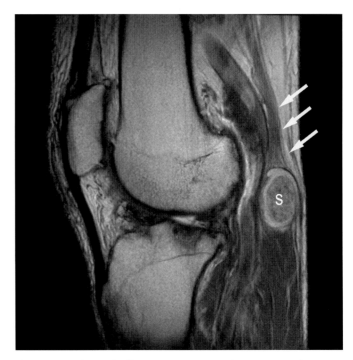

Figure 30.17 • Sagittal MR image of the knee shows a posterior mass (S) in line with the tibial nerve (arrows). This is characteristic of a benign nerve sheath tumor (Schwannoma).

(Fig. 30.17). Some of the masses cause nerve entrapment syndromes, such as paralabral cysts of the shoulder and accessory muscles can be surgically treated (Resnick et al 2006).

Specific disease entities and injuries

There are certain specific injuries or entities that warrant further discussion in a chapter of this nature. In the clinical setting, certain injuries are suspected and imaging is used to confirm those suspicions and to exclude a more sinister cause of patients' symptoms. For example, in a runner with posteromedial tibial pain, the diagnosis of a stress fracture may be clinically apparent. It may still be prudent, however, to obtain a radiograph to exclude the presence of neoplasm in this region with pathological fracture.

Stress fractures

The imaging of stress fractures should begin with a radiograph (Fig. 30.18). If this is normal, a repeated radiograph after 1 week may start to show periosteal reaction, associated with fracture (Berquist 1992). An earlier diagnosis may be sought with the more sensitive nuclear medicine bone scan (Fig. 30.15) or MRI. Radiographs can also miss stress fractures, especially those involving primarily trabecular bone (Berquist 1992). MRI is particularly useful in the hip to guide the need for operative intervention. If a compression-side (medial) stress fracture is present and partial, the decision may be made to treat the

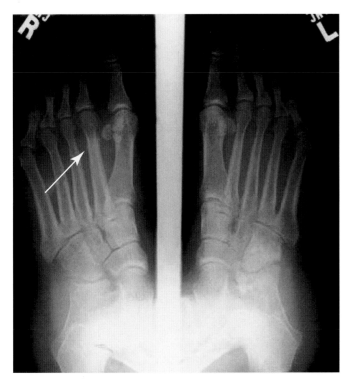

Figure 30.18 • Oblique radiograph of both feet demonstrating a stress fracture of the right second metatarsal (arrow). There is callus forming. Incidental note is made of a bipartite medial sesamoid on the right.

patient non-operatively, with close clinical follow-up (Fig. 30.14). The major concern for stress fractures is that they not go on to become complete fractures that might require more aggressive treatment.

Patellofemoral disease

As discussed in Chapter 22, anterior knee pain is a common complaint. Whereas there can be many causes of anterior knee pain in an athlete (e.g. patellar tendinosis, Osgood–Schlatter disease, prepatellar bursitis) patellofemoral disease is one of the more complex. Sometimes associated with mild knee dysplasia, patellofemoral tracking disorders and chondromalacia patellae (loss or structural abnormality of patellar cartilage) can be evaluated using imaging. The shape of the patella, relative length of the patellar tendon and shape and congruency of the patellofemoral joint can be evaluated on X-ray, CT and MRI. CT can also be used to evaluate the way the patella tracks in the trochlear groove by obtaining images in different degrees of flexion. MRI and, to a lesser extent, ultrasound, can look at the cartilage over the patellofemoral joint to help guide the type of surgical intervention.

Femoroacetabular impingement

Femoroacetabular impingement has become a recent field of interest to ascribe an etiology for hip pain (and potentially of

hip arthrosis) in a subset of patients (Beall et al 2005). The entity suggests that from whatever cause (e.g. undiagnosed prior physeal injury or developmental abnormality) one of two types of motion abnormality can arise. These two types, cam type and pincer type, often coexist and have typical imaging characteristics. The cam type involves an osseous bump at the anterior femoral neck that bumps against the acetabulum and injures articular cartilage and the anterior labrum. The pincer type, associated with acetabular retroversion, impinges the femoral neck against the anterior acetabular lip. Not yet fully understood, both of these can be addressed surgically. Femoroacetabular impingement is a clinical diagnosis that imaging supports. The bony bump can be demonstrated on radiograph (especially using an elongated femoral neck lateral view). It can also be demonstrated on axial CT or MR images.

Internal impingement

Whereas subacromial impingement is often acknowledged as a cause of shoulder pain, and is often ascribed to acromial shape (Berquist 1992), internal impingement is a problem in the throwing athlete. In the late cocking phase, abutment of the humeral head with the posterior superior glenoid (or more correctly the soft tissue structures covering these structures – the infraspinatus tendon with the posterior superior labrum) cause degeneration and pain. The findings are typical on MRI.

Groin pain

Imaging can help to determine the cause of groin pain, a common complaint among athletes (especially soccer players). Unfortunately, there are many causes of groin pain, including adductor muscle strain, rectus abdominus muscle strain, osteitis pubis, hernias and various hip pathologies, making the imaging choice difficult. Some pathologies can be seen with radiograph (e.g. osteitis pubis, adductor avulsion if it includes bone). CT, as well as being sensitive to these pathologies, can also be used to diagnose hernias. The soft tissue abnormalities require MR or ultrasound imaging. Since the treatments of some of these conditions are different, determining the cause of groin pain can be useful, especially in recalcitrant cases. Unfortunately, even with imaging, the cause in not always clear.

Head and neck injuries

Head and neck injuries are of major clinical concern, especially when there is loss of consciousness or neurological symptoms (Feinberg 2000, Proctor & Cantu 2000). Imaging is usually not required for these injuries, but if a reparable nerve avulsion is a clinical consideration, MRI or CT myelogram can confirm or refute this diagnosis (Carvalho et al 1997). In contact sports, concussions are common, and even after brief loss of consciousness, imaging of the head is usually not required (Sturmi et al 1998) (see Chapter 31 for an account of such injuries). If the clinical suspicion of a subdural or epidural hematoma is

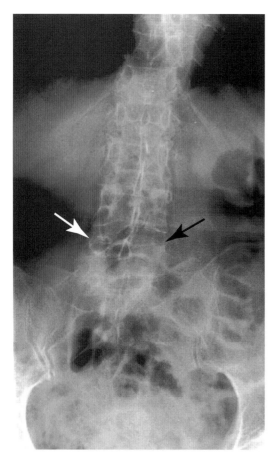

Figure 30.19 • Frontal view of the spine in a patient with congenital absence of the left L5 pedicle (black arrow). There is a normal pedicle on the right, seen with its normal circular appearance (white arrow).

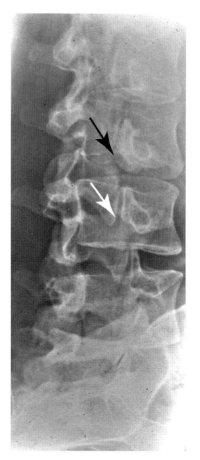

Figure 30.20 • Oblique view of the lumbar spine demonstrating a defect in the pars interarticularis of L3 (black arrow). The pars interarticularis at L4 is intact (white arrow).

present, a CT scan of the brain is a useful method of excluding this diagnosis. MRI of the brain can also be performed but close monitoring of patients in MRI is more difficult.

For severe cervical spine injuries where instability or fracture is suspected, radiographs should be obtained, including the C7–T1 junction on the lateral view. Flexion and extension views can be obtained to look for ligamentous stability (Graber & Kathol 1999). In contact sports, fractures of the posterior spinous process of the lower cervical/upper thoracic spine (clay shoveler's fracture) are not uncommon.

Lumbar spine

Pars defects

The technique used for imaging the lumbar spine is dependent upon the suspected pathology. Congenital anomalies can be excluded with frontal and lateral radiographs (Fig. 30.19) and often defects in pars interarticularis can be excluded by examining the neck of the 'Scottie dog' on oblique views (Fig. 30.20). The activity of the pars defect can be evaluated with

a bone scan (Fig. 30.5) or MRI. CT evaluation can also define the fractures (Fig. 30.10). The presence of a stress injury to the pars or stress fracture of the pedicle can mimic a pars fracture and can be identified on cross-sectional imaging techniques (MRI and CT scan) (Standaert & Herring 2000).

Diskogenic disease

The imaging of suspected diskogenic disease should not be undertaken until symptoms have persisted for 6 weeks or longer, with the patient having failed nonoperative treatments (Deyo et al 1990). Additional indications for the imaging of suspected diskogenic disease are provided in Box 30.1. If imaging is required, unless there is a contraindication, MRI is the study of choice. The second choice would be a CT scan. CT myelography makes the noninvasive CT scan more invasive by requiring subarachnoid contrast injection. The studies are evaluated for acute and chronic abnormalities. In addition to looking for disk herniations, the study is evaluated for degenerative disk disease, facet arthrosis, fractures, masses and paraspinal disease that may mimic disk disease (Cacayorin & Kieffer 1991).

Pediatric injuries

Pediatric injuries merit separate discussion. The injuries that children and younger adolescents incur are slightly different from those of adults and may be missed without special attention to them. In the developing body, tendons and ligaments are sometimes stronger than the bone at their insertion sites (Green 2001). Therefore, bony avulsions are more common (Green 2001). Examples of this phenomenon include the extensor tendon of a mallet finger or an avulsion of the tibial spine at the footprint of the anterior cruciate ligament.

In children, the physes are open; indeed, some physes do not fuse until the late teens or early twenties (e.g. iliac apophysis, medial clavicle). Physeal injuries should be identified and treated to prevent early fusion and subsequent growth disturbance (Fig. 30.21). For example, a slipped capital femoral epiphysis is usually pinned to prevent further deformity and subsequent arthrosis (see Chapter 25). Long bone fractures in children can be very subtle (torus fractures). Indeed, children's bones can 'bend' rather than break (plastic deformity). It is important to maintain a high index of suspicion for pediatric injuries and to look for secondary signs of injury on radiographs, such as joint effusion and soft tissue swelling. Obtaining additional views, obtaining additional tests, or repeating radiographs for persistent symptoms may bring to light a fracture that was previously overlooked (Harris & Harris 2000).

Congenital/developmental mimics of injuries

There are several clinical mimics of injury (entities that can lead to pain or discomfort). These include congenital anomalies such as tarsal coalition (Greenspan 2004), which causes ankle pain while walking on uneven surfaces, and transitional lumbosacral junctions which have been thought to be a cause of pain themselves and that are associated with disk herniations. (Castellvi et al 1984). These entities can be identified radiographically and are among the reasons for obtaining radiographs in patients with persistent symptoms.

Other entities are radiographic mimics of disease. These tend to be developmental, are present in the pediatric population, and can be symptomatic. It is important to be able to identify these entities so as not to be inappropriately aggressive in treatment. Therefore, if a radiographic appearance does not fit the clinical situation, treat the patient, not the radiograph. Keats et al (2001) provides an excellent coverage of these mimics. They include the normal appearance of an epiphysis mimicking fracture,

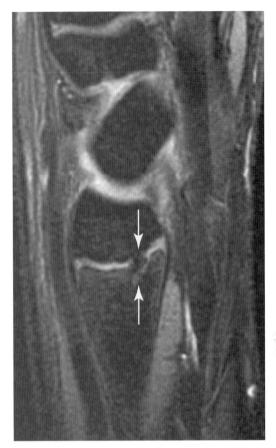

Figure 30.21 • Sagittal MR image in a 15-year-old soccer goalkeeper showing a bony bar (arrows) crossing the normal physis.

and a category of diseases (the osteochondroses), all of which have eponyms. Köhler's disease (tarsal navicular), Legg–Calvé–Perthes disease (proximal femoral apophysis), Blount's disease (medial proximal tibial apophysis), Osgood–Schlatter's disease (tibial tubercle) and Freiberg's infraction (2nd or 3rd metatarsal head) (Fig. 30.22) all have characteristic appearances. These lesions may be symptomatic and resolve (as with Köhler's) or go on to cause deformity that requires treatment (e.g. valgus osteotomy for Blount's). Breck (1971), in his atlas of osteochondrosis, describes 41 named osteochondroses.

Other developmental conditions, such as unfused apophyses or accessory ossicles, can also cause symptoms. These include os acromiale (Ryu et al 1999, Salamon 1999), accessory navicular (Resnick et al 2006) and os trigonum (Jones et al 1999). Although these are not examples of injuries themselves, they do appear during the radiological work-up of injury. It is important to be aware of these entities and the potential for symptoms.

Complications

It is important to be aware of the complications of injuries. For bone, the many complications include non-union of a fracture,

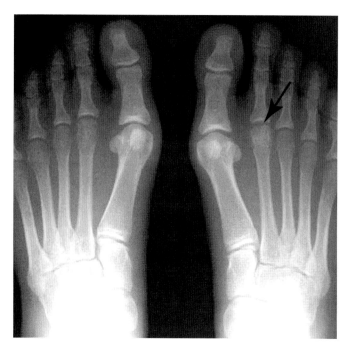

Figure 30.22 • Frontal radiograph of the feet in a teenager demonstrating Freiberg's infraction, or osteonecrosis of the second metatarsal head (black arrow). Note the flattening and sclerosis.

osteonecrosis, early arthrosis and, in the case of ostechondral impaction, osteochondritis dissecans (Rogers 2001).

Osteochondritis dissecans is an osteochondral fracture that occurs in typical locations (Resnick et al 2006). It is most frequently seen in the ankle on the medial talar dome and in the knee at the lateral aspect of the medial femoral condyle (Fig. 30.23) (Cassidy & Petty 2001). It is less often seen on the capitellum and the medial patellar facet. The disorder is believed to be post-traumatic, occurring after one or more traumatic events (Cassidy & Petty 2001). The importance of recognizing osteochondritis dissecans is to explain a patient's symptoms, and because the lesion can become dislodged and present as a foreign body. The role of imaging of this condition is to identify the lesion (commonly done with X-ray) and to evaluate the overlying articular surface, with the goal of surgically intervening if the articular surface is damaged or if the lesion appears loose (De Smet et al 1990a, 1990b). If the lesion is not displaced, loosening is evidenced by fluid extending into the interface between the fragment and native bone (as seen by imaging with MRI or athrographic techniques).

Another complication of injury is osteonecrosis, a condition that can affect fractures, especially in the talus, scaphoid and the humeral and femoral heads (Rogers 2001). The blood supply for these bones is tenuous (Greenspan 2004). Osteonecrosis is suspected when pain persists, and can be a cause for non-union of a fracture (Rogers 2001). The early radiographic sign for this condition is an area of sclerosis or lucency. The necrotic area can progress to the point of collapse and eventual arthrosis (Mazières 2003). Bone scan and MRI can detect osteonecrosis before it is visible on radiograph (Resnick et al 2006). The

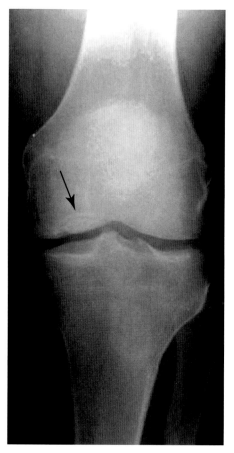

Figure 30.23 • Frontal radiograph of the left knee demonstrating osteochondritis dissecans in the typical location (arrow).

finding on radiograph, termed Hawkins sign in the talus, is the presence of relative osteoporosis. The osteoporosis indicates that the vasculature is intact and normal healing is occurring (Hawkins 1970). If the blood supply was cut off, the bone would remain dense since normal remodeling could not occur.

Therapeutics

In addition to its role in diagnosis, imaging also plays an important and increasing role in guiding therapeutics.

Needle guidance

Image-guided injections can be performed using CT, fluoroscopy and ultrasound. The advantage of using image guidance is that one knows exactly where the injected material is going (e.g. into a joint, tendon sheath, bursa, cyst, neuroma or nerve root sleeve). Despite clinicians' comfort with performing injections without image guidance, the injections are not as accurate in position as one would hope (Partington & Broome 1998). Joint injections can be diagnostic or therapeutic. A joint can be injected with anesthesia and steroid (Fig. 30.8). The anesthesia can determine if a known pathology (such as labral tear of the hip, or subtalar arthrosis) is the cause of a patient's symptoms. If the injection relieves symptoms, the pathology is likely to be intra-articular. The steroid may relieve symptoms for a longer time. Tenosynovitis can be treated in a similar way. The injection of saline can be used to distend the shoulder capsule as a treatment for adhesive capsulitis (Rizk et al 1994). Morton's neuromas can be injected under ultrasound (Sofka et al 2001). The advantage of ultrasound is that the operator can directly see the needle and what is being injected as it is injected. Unlike fluoroscopically guided injections, there is no ionizing radiation involved. Additional ultrasound-guided procedures have proved useful in the treatment of rotator cuff, elbow and ankle tendons (especially the Achilles). These include dry needling to stimulate blood flow and healing (Connell et al 2006). Some clinicians have had moderate success injecting autologous blood into tendons to try to induce and stimulate healing. Pain from Achilles tendinosis has been shown to be associated with blood flow. Sclerosis of the neovessels can reduce pain (although it does not promote healing) (Alfredson & Hohberg 2005).

In using fluoroscopy, one injects contrast and watches its distribution, while injecting. Thereafter, if the distribution is appropriate, the anesthesia/steroid is injected, being careful not to move the needle. Radiofrequency ablations of osteoid osteomas can also be performed percutaneously using image guidance (Rosenthal 1997), as can bone and soft tissue biopsies (Ghelman 1998, van Holsbeeck & Introcaso 2001).

A myriad of spine procedures are done with image guidance. In addition to nerve root, facet and sacroiliac joint injections, medial branch blocks can be performed to confirm the etiology of pain before rhizotomy is performed percutaneously (Dussault et al 2000, Murtagh 1988). Intradiscal electrothermoenucleation (IDET) is a procedure performed percutaneously to seal tears of the annulus fibrosis of a disc. More complex percutaneous spine procedures such as disc fusions also require image guidance (Singh et al 2005).

As the population ages, but remains active, osteoporotic compression fractures have become more common. Vertebral body compression fractures (whether traumatic or not) have started, in some cases, to be treated percutaneously. This is done primarily to alleviate pain but sometimes to reduce the fracture to try to prevent further or adjacent collapse. Two procedures called verebroplasty and kyphoplasty are used for these purposes. They involve injection of cement into the fractured vertebral body, using image guidance. It is performed by physicians in various specialties and is remarkably effective at reducing pain. There is controversy, however, as to whether the technique causes additional adjacent fractures. Sacral fractures can be treated similarly (sacroplasty) (Mathis et al 2002).

Ultrasound therapy

Ultrasound, in the guise of extracorporeal shock wave therapy (see Chapter 14), is available for treating plantar fasciitis (Maier et al 2000, Ogden et al 2001) and calcific tendonitis (Chaudhry 1999, Ebenbichler et al 1999). This, however, does not involve imaging.

Future developments

This short section aims to outline the many potential developments and applications of imaging. Radiology is driven by the need to answer clinical questions and is supported by new technology. Technology will continue to advance and as this happens, two things will be likely to occur: the imaging tools that we have now will improve, and new imaging tools will be developed.

The increase in computer speed and memory capacity has boosted the speed of all cross-sectional imaging modalities and will continue to allow higher resolution imaging. Tube and detector designs in CT, probe designs in ultrasound and coil and magnet designs in MRI are constantly improving.

Magnet improvements have enhanced the comfort and strength of MR machines, allowing only the body part being imaged to be enclosed. New pulse sequences in MRI allow better tissue characterization and can be used to evaluate new treatments such as cartilage and meniscal scaffolds as they become available.

In ultrasound, three-dimensional representation and extended field-of-view imaging allow better representation of the images for easier understanding. Techniques for evaluating the presence and degree of blood flow have become quite sensitive and quantification of blood flow is on the horizon as are additional uses for new intravenous contrast agents.

In nuclear medicine, new radionuclides have recently allowed more accurate evaluation of intravascular thrombi. Antibody tagged agents may foster new agents for nuclear medicine. Combinations of nuclear medicine with CT allow us to combine the physiologic advantages of nuclear medicine with the anatomic detail of CT.

Radiographic manipulation has improved with digital imaging techniques, and it is possible with new film screen combinations to obtain increasingly better images. Computer screens are replacing X-ray film. In some fields, such as mammography and chest radiography, computers can assist in the evaluation of the images, in order to limit human error. Lastly, the burgeoning field of computer-assisted surgery has image-driven aspects.

It is hard to predict new imaging tools. Infrared imaging has been used in vivo for skin and muscle and in vitro for bone and articular cartilage (Kuboki et al 2001, Ou-Yang et al 2001). This general field is called solid-state spectroscopy.

Summary

When imaging is required for a musculoskeletal injury, there are many relevant options available. One must remember the importance of an appropriate history and dedicated physical examination. Imaging should be used only when appropriate and when it will affect patient care. When imaging is deemed necessary, the images should be interpreted in concert with the patient's presentation to guide appropriate therapy. Attention to detail is required in performing and interpreting the studies, with an understanding of the patterns of disease and the musculoskeletal disease processes.

References

Alfredson H, Ohberg L 2005 Sclerosing injections to areas of neo-vascularisation reduce pain in chronic Achilles tendinopathy: a double-blind randomised controlled trial. Knee Surgery, Sports Traumatology, Arthroscopy 13:338–344

American College of Radiology 2005 Appropriateness Criteria, ACR web site edition American College of Radiology. Online. Available: http://www.acr.org/s_acr/sec.asp?CID=1845&DID=16050 (15 June 2006)

Anderson K, Sarwark J F, Conway J J et al 2000 Quantitative assessment with SPECT imaging of stress injuries of the pars interarticularis and response to bracing. Journal of Pediatric Orthopedics 20:28–33

Arrington E D, Miller M D 1995 Skeletal muscle injuries. Orthopaedic Clinics of North America 26:411–422

Beall D P, Sweet C F, Martin H D et al 2005 Imaging findings of femoroacetabular impingement syndrome. Skeletal Radiology 34:691–701

Berquist T H 1992 Imaging of sports injuries. Aspen Publishers, Gaithersburg, MD

Breck L W 1971 An atlas of the osteochondroses. Charles C Thomas, Springfield

Buchman S R, Sherick D G, Goulet R W et al 1998 Use of microcomputed tomography scanning as a new technique for the evaluation of membranous bone. Journal of Craniofacial Surgery 9:48–54

Cacayorin E D, Kieffer S A 1991 The herniated intervertebral disc. In: Taveras J M, Ferrucci J T (eds) Radiology: diagnosis – imaging – intervention, vol 3:105. Lippinncott-Raven, Philadelphia, PA

Carvalho G A, Nikkhah G, Matthies C et al 1997 Diagnosis of root avulsions in traumatic brachial plexus injuries: value of computerized tomography myelography and magnetic resonance imaging. Journal of Neurosurgery 86:69–76

Cassidy J T, Petty R E 2001 Pediatric rheumatology, 4th edn. WB Saunders, Philadelphia, PA

Castellvi A E, Goldstein L A, Chan D P 1984 Lumbosacral transitional vertebrae and their relationship with lumbar extradural defects. Spine 9:493–495

Chaudhry H J 1999 Ultrasound therapy for calcific tendinitis of the shoulder. New England Journal of Medicine 341:1237

Congeni J, McCulloch J, Swanson K 1997 Lumbar spondylolysis. A study of natural progression in athletes. American Journal of Sports Medicine 25:248–253

Connell D A, Potter H G, Sherman M F et al 1999 Injuries of the pectoralis major muscle: evaluation with MRI imaging. Radiology 210:785–791

Connell D A, Ali K E, Ahmad M et al 2006 Ultrasound-guided autologous blood injection for tennis elbow. Skeletal Radiology 35:371–377

Cotten A, Delfaut E, Demondion X et al 2000 MR imaging of the knee at 0.2 and 1.5 T: correlation with surgery. American Journal of Roentgenology 174:1093–1097

Curry T, Dowdey J, Murry R 1990 Christensen's physics of diagnostic radiology, 4th edn. Lea and Febiger, Philadelphia, PA

De Smet A A, Fisher D R, Burnstein M I et al 1990a Value of MR imaging in staging osteochondral lesions of the talus (osteochondritis dissecans): results in 14 patients. American Journal of Roentgenology 154:555–558

De Smet A A, Fisher D R, Graf B K et al 1990b Osteochondritis dissecans of the knee: value of MR imaging in determining lesion stability and the presence of articular cartilage defects. American Journal of Roentgenology 155:549–553

Deyo R A, Loeser J D, Bigos S J 1990 Herniated lumbar intervertebral disk. Annals of Internal Medicine 112:598–603

Disler D G 1997 Fat-suppressed three-dimensional spoiled gradient-recalled MR imaging: assessment of articular and physeal hyaline cartilage. American Journal of Roentgenology 169:1117–1123

Disler D G, Recht M P, McCauley T R 2000 MR imaging of articular cartilage. Skeletal Radiology 29:367–377

Dussault R G, Kaplan P A, Anderson M W 2000 Fluoroscopy-guided sacroiliac joint injections. Radiology 214:273–277

Ebenbichler G R, Erdogmus C B, Resch K L et al 1999 Ultrasound therapy for calcific tendonitis of the shoulder. New England Journal of Medicine 340:1533–1538

Edelstyn G A, Gillespie P J, Grebbell F S 1967 The radiological demonstration of osseous metastases. Experimental observations. Clinical Radiology 18:158–162

Edwards P D, Miles K A, Owens S J et al 1999 A new non-invasive test for the detection of compartment syndromes. Nuclear Medicine Communications 20:215–218

Faulkner K G 2001 Update on bone density measurement. Rheumatic Diseases Clinics of North America 27:81–99

Feinberg J H 2000 Burners and stingers. Physical Medicine and Rehabilitation Clinics of North America 11:771–784

Fornage B D 1995 Musculoskeletal ultrasound. Churchill Livingstone, New York

Ghelman B 1998 Biopsies of the musculoskeletal system. Radiologic Clinics of North America 36:567–580

Graber M A, Kathol M 1999 Cervical spine radiographs in the trauma patient. American Family Physician 59:331–342

Green W B 2001 Essentials of musculoskeletal care, 2nd edn. American Academy of Orthopaedic Surgeons, Rosemont, IL

Greenspan A 2004 Orthopedic radiology: a practical approach, 4th edn. Lippincott Williams and Wilkins, Philadelphia, PA

Ha T P, Li K C, Beaulieu C F et al 1998 Anterior cruciate ligament injury: fast spin-echo MR imaging with arthroscopic correlation in 217 examinations. American Journal of Roentgenology 170:1215–1219

Harris J H, Harris W H 2000 The radiology of emergency medicine, 4th edn. Williams and Wilkins, Philadelphia, PA

Hawkins L G 1970 Fractures of the neck of the talus. Journal of Bone and Joint Surgery (Am) 52A:991–1002

Hubner U, Schlicht W, Outzen S et al 2000 Ultrasound in the diagnosis of fractures in children. Journal of Bone and Joint Surgery (Br) 82B:1170–1173

Jones D M, Saltzman C L, El-Khoury G 1999 The diagnosis of the os trigonum syndrome with a fluoroscopically controlled injection of local anesthetic. Iowa Orthopaedic Journal 19:122–126

Keats T E, Anderson M W, Anderson M 2001 Atlas of normal roentgen variants that may simulate disease, 7th edn. Elsevier Health Sciences, Philadelphia, PA

Kuboki T, Suzuki K, Maekawa K et al 2001 Correlation of the near-infrared spectroscopy signals with signal intensity in T(2)-weighted magnetic resonance imaging of the human masseter muscle. Archives of Oral Biology 46:721–727

Levin D C, Blazena M E, Levina E 1967 Fatigue fractures of the shaft of the femur: simulation of a malignant tumor. Radiology 89:883–885

McCauley T R, Disler D G 2001 Magnetic resonance imaging of articular cartilage of the knee. Journal of the American Academy of Orthopaedic Surgeons 9:2–8

Maier M, Steinborn M, Schmitz C et al 2000 Extracorporeal shock wave application for chronic plantar fasciitis associated with heel spurs: prediction of outcome by magnetic resonance imaging. Journal of Rheumatology 27:2455–2462

Mathis J M, Deramond H, Belkoff S M 2002 Percutaneous vertebroplasty. Springer-Verlag, New York

Mathoulin C, Saffar P, Roukoz S 1990 [Lunar-triquetral instability]. Annales de Chirurgie de la Main et du Membre Superieur 9:22–28

Mazières B 2003 Osteonecrosis. In: Hochberg MC, Silman AJ (eds) Rheumatology. 3rd edn. Mosby, Edinburgh, p 1877–1890

Mirowitz S A, Apicella P, Reinus W R et al 1994 MR imaging of bone marrow lesions: relative conspicuousness on T1-weighted, fat-suppressed T2-weighted, and STIR images. American Journal of Roentgenology 162:215–221

Murtagh F R 1988 Computed tomography and fluoroscopy guided anesthesia and steroid injection in facet syndrome. Spine 13:686–689

Nash C L Jr, Gregg E C, Brown R H et al 1979 Risks of exposure to X-rays in patients undergoing long-term treatment for scoliosis. Journal of Bone and Joint Surgery (Am) 61A:371–374

Ogden J A, Alvarez R, Levitt R et al 2001 Shock wave therapy for chronic proximal plantar fasciitis. Clinical Orthopaedics and Related Research 387:47–59

Outerbridge R 1961 The etiology of chondromalacia patellae. Journal of Bone and Joint Surgery (Br) 43B:752–757

Ou-Yang H, Paschalis E P, Mayo W E et al 2001 Infrared microscopic imaging of bone: spatial distribution of $CO_3(^{2-})$. Journal of Bone and Mineral Research 16:893–900

Partington P F, Broome G H 1998 Diagnostic injection around the shoulder: hit and miss? A cadaveric study of injection accuracy. Journal of Shoulder and Elbow Surgery 7:147–150

Patten R M, Mack L A, Wang K Y et al 1992 Nondisplaced fractures of the greater tuberosity of the humerus: sonographic detection. Radiology 182:201–204

Pavlov H, Burke M, Giesa M et al 1999 Orthopaedist's guide to plain film imaging. Thieme, New York

Potter H G, Linklater J M, Allen A A et al 1998 Magnetic resonance imaging of articular cartilage in the knee. An evaluation with use of fast-spin-echo imaging. Journal of Bone and Joint Surgery (Am) 80A:1276–1284

Proctor M R, Cantu R C 2000 Head and neck injuries in young athletes. Clinics in Sports Medicine 19:693–715

Read J W, Perko M 1998 Shoulder ultrasound: diagnostic accuracy for impingement syndrome, rotator cuff tear, and biceps tendon pathology. Journal of Shoulder and Elbow Surgery 7:264–271

Resnick D, Kransdorf M J 2004 Bone and joint imaging, 3rd edn. WB Saunders, Philadelphia, PA

Resnick D, Kang H S, Pretterklieber M L 2006 Internal derangements of joints: emphasis on MR imaging, 2nd edn. WB Saunders, Philadelphia, PA

Rizk T E, Gavant M L, Pinals R S 1994 Treatment of adhesive capsulitis (frozen shoulder) with arthrographic capsular distension and rupture. Archives of Physical Medicine and Rehabilitation 75:803–807

Rogers L F 2001 Radiology of skeletal trauma, 3rd edn. Churchill Livingstone, New York

Rosenthal D I 1997 Percutaneous radiofrequency treatment of osteoid osteomas. Seminars in Musculoskeletal Radiology 1:265–272

Ryu R K, Fan R S, Dunbar W H 1999 The treatment of symptomatic os acromiale. Orthopedics 22:325–328

Salamon P B 1999 The treatment of symptomatic os acromiale. Journal of Bone and Joint Surgery (Am) 81A:1198

Sawyer-Glover A M, Shellock F G 2000 Pre-MRI procedure screening: recommendations and safety considerations for biomedical implants and devices. Journal of Magnetic Resonance Imaging 12:92–106

Shellock F G 2005 Reference manual for magnetic resonance safety, implants, and devices. Biomedical Research Publishing, CA

Singh K, Ledet E, Carl A 2005 Intradiscal therapy: a review of current treatment modalities. Spine 30(17 suppl):S20–26

Sofka C M, Collins A J, Adler R S 2001 Use of ultrasonographic guidance in interventional musculoskeletal procedures: a review from a single institution. Journal of Ultrasound in Medicine 20:21–26

Standaert C J, Herring S A 2000 Spondylolysis: a critical review. British Journal of Sports Medicine 34:415–422

Standaert C J, Herring S A, Halpern B et al 2000 Spondylolysis. Physical Medicine and Rehabilitation Clinics of North America 11:785–803

Sturmi J E, Smith C, Lombardo J A 1998 Mild brain trauma in sports. Diagnosis and treatment guidelines. Sports Medicine 25:351–358

van Holsbeeck M T, Introcaso J H 2001 Musculoskeletal ultrasound, 2nd edn. Mosby, St Louis, MO

Werber K D, Wuttge-Hannig A, Hannig C 1990 [Cinematography, a new diagnostic procedure in evaluation of the injured painful wrist joint]. Langenbecks Archiv fur Chirurgie. Supplement II. Verhandlungen der Deutschen Gesellschaft fur Chirurgie 727–729

White L M, Kim J K, Mehta M et al 2000 Complications of total hip arthroplasty: MR imaging – initial experience. Radiology 215:254–262

Yao L, Dungan D, Seeger L L 1994 MR imaging of tibial collateral ligament injury: comparison with clinical examination. Skeletal Radiology 23:521–524

Medical issues in sport and exercise

31

Bruce Hamilton and Mark Gillett

CHAPTER CONTENTS

Introduction 578

Asthma 578

Epilepsy 580

Head and neck injuries in sport 582

Cardiac conditions in sport and exercise 585

Diabetes mellitus 587

The tired athlete 590

Travel medicine for the international athlete 592

Infections in athletes 593

Summary 595

Introduction

With the increasing number of individuals involved in both competitive and recreational sport and exercise activities, it is imperative that medical and health care personnel involved in sports medicine have an understanding of the impact that common medical conditions have on such participation, and the impact of exercise on common medical conditions. While professional sports codes may have a physician at their disposal, at most sporting events the most medically qualified person is the physical therapist or athletic trainer. While well prepared to manage musculoskeletal injuries, those involved in the physical therapies often lack the understanding and preparation for the management of common medical problems. This has become of increasing importance now that physical therapists are often the primary contact practitioners in many countries.

In recent years, authors have concentrated entire volumes on medical subspecialties within sports medicine, and it is beyond the scope of this chapter to comprehensively cover all topics in this area. The following chapter aims to provide an up-to-date outline of the presentation and management of common medical conditions, which a medical practitioner, physical therapist or athletic trainer involved in sports medicine may encounter.

Asthma

Asthma is a common condition affecting up to 10% of the population and is associated with a high morbidity (McFadden 1991). It is characterized by intermittent wheeze, shortness of breath, chest tightness and persistent cough. Pathophysiologically, asthma is considered a chronic inflammatory condition resulting in a reversible airways obstruction (Hancock 2001). People with asthma fall into one of three categories: atopic, classical and exercise-induced asthma. Atopic asthma is characterized by seasonal variations in symptom severity. It is associated with both the presence of antigens in the environment, and a history of atopy (Tang et al 1996). By contrast, classical asthma involves perennial symptoms. For example, the airways in classical asthma display persistent low grade inflammation, with intermittent, severe exacerbations (Crimi et al 2001). Exercise-induced asthma (EIA), however, is characterized by symptoms during or after exercise, and while up to 90% of chronic asthmatics will suffer symptoms of EIA (Lacroix 1999), it may also occur in otherwise healthy individuals (Storms 1999). This review will focus on EIA.

EIA is the term used to describe the transient narrowing of the airways that follows vigorous exercise of 6–8 minutes duration (Anderson & Holzer 2000, Spooner et al 2000). EIA may result in symptoms such as stomach pains and nausea, in addition to the classic asthma symptoms of shortness of breath, wheeze, cough and chest tightness. EIA has been shown to limit endurance and prolong recovery from exercise (Spooner et al 2000). EIA is now recognized as being very common, occurring in up to 21% of Olympic athletes (Dickinson et al 2005a, Wilber et al 2000). Exercising in cold, dry air, with a high minute ventilation is considered to be most provocative, and subsequently participants in winter sports have a higher incidence than their summer counterparts (Rundell et al 2000, Zeitoun et al 2004). EIA is provoked more by continuous exercise than intermittent, and exercising in polluted or allergen filled air will also increase its incidence (Beck 1999, Gavett & Koren 2001). As a result, EIA is most common in sports such as running, cross country skiing and ice skating (Provost-Craig et al 1996, Weiler & Ryan 2000, Wilber et al 2000). In the general population, EIA is often unrecognized, untreated and may significantly impair performance (Spooner et al 2000, Storms 1999).

Airway function in mild to moderate asthmatics varies depending on the nature of the exercise. With constant load exercise, there is an initial period of mild bronchodilation, followed by bronchoconstriction after 15–20 minutes of exercise, lasting for the duration of the exercise. By contrast, incremental exercise results in progressive bronchoconstriction, while variable intensity exercise results in relative bronchodilation during higher exercise intensity, and bronchoconstriction at lower intensities (Beck 1999). In non-asthmatic individuals, the airways bronchodilate during exercise or undergo a mild bronchoconstriction. Following the induction of bronchoconstriction secondary to exercise and subsequent recovery, there is a variable period of reduced airway responsiveness, known as a 'refractory period'. This has been found to last up to 2 hours (Anderson & Holzer 2000, Beck 1999). In addition, a second drop in airway function may occur 6–8 hours following exercise and this is thought to be secondary to an increase in inflammatory cell activity following the initial antigenic (exercise) challenge (Beck 1999).

Two classic hypotheses attempt to explain the transient bronchospasm associated with exercise. The thermal hypothesis, first proposed in 1979 (Anderson & Daviskas 2000, Deal et al 1979), suggests that it is the airway cooling and rapid rewarming following exercise that is responsible for the bronchoconstriction. This theory, however, has largely been discredited (Anderson & Daviskas 2000). By contrast, evidence supporting the osmotic hypothesis (Fig. 31.1), which suggests that dehydration and subsequent increases in osmolarity may precipitate EIA, is mounting (Anderson & Daviskas 2000, Anderson & Holzer 2000).

Diagnosis of EIA

There are several ways in which a diagnosis of EIA may be made, depending on the resources one has at their disposal. The simplest means is a clinical trial with an inhaled bronchodilator.

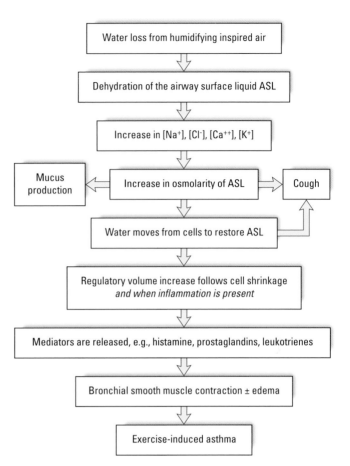

Figure 31.1 • Flow chart describing the events leading to cough, mucus production and exercise induced asthma. (Reproduced from Anderson & Holzer 2000 with the permission of Mosby, Inc.)

With a history consistent with asthma, an improvement in both symptoms and peak expiratory flow rate (PEFR) of approximately 15% following the inhalation of bronchodilator therapy provides a presumptive diagnosis (Fields & Reimer 1997). The use of an exercise challenge is similarly practical. Classically, this involves exercising at an intensity just below anaerobic threshold for 10–12 minutes, with PEFR measurements being taken pre-exercise and 1, 3, 6, 10 and 15 minutes following exercise. A positive test for EIA is most frequently defined as a >10% fall in forced expiratory volume in one second (FEV1) or PEFR (Anderson & Holzer 2000). However, it has been suggested that the lower limit for the fall in FEV1 and PEFR for normal, elite, cold weather athletes may be 6.4 and 12%, respectively (Rundell et al 2000). The benefits of PEFR and field-testing are the relatively inexpensive cost, ease of administration (Tancredi et al 2004), and in addition, it has been found that laboratory testing may underestimate EIA in cold weather athletes (Rundell et al 2000). Typical flow-volume curves for asthmatic and non-asthmatic subjects are shown in Fig. 31.2.

Testing for EIA using either the hyperventilation of dry air containing 4.9% carbon dioxide, or hyperosmolar saline aerosols, has a very high sensitivity for EIA, but requires more

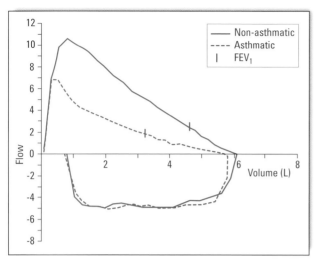

Figure 31.2 • Flow–volume curves for asthmatic and non-asthmatic subject. (Provided by Mr John Dickinson.)

specialized and expensive equipment (Dickinson et al 2006). The use of pharmacological agents for EIA testing, such as methacholine and histamine, has recently been questioned, as elite athletes have been found to show increased bronchial reactivity to such agents (Anderson & Holzer 2000, Helenius et al 1998). Changes in FEV1 as a result of provocation is recognized as the most sensitive method for diagnosis of EIA (Dickinson et al 2005b).

Management of EIA

The management of EIA is multifaceted. All people with EIA should be provided with an asthma action plan, outlining the steps to be taken should their breathing deteriorate (Miller et al 2005). Education of the athlete is mandatory and should be ongoing (Fields & Reimer 1997, Storms 1999). Regular assessment of pulmonary function will allow an athlete and coach to objectively assess the relationship of lung function to performance. Environmental manipulation, such as dietary changes (Mickleborough et al 2005), running with a mask in cool air, using a humidifier when training indoors, nose breathing, maintaining hydration and avoiding exercising in polluted air may assist in minimizing the extent of EIA (Fields & Reimer 1997, Storms 1999). Similarly, the induction of a refractory phase, by using a slower, longer warm-up is proposed to reduce the impact of EIA (Storms 1999). The ability of athletes to utilize this refractory period effectively, however, has been questioned (Rundell et al 2000).

Pharmaceutically, EIA has traditionally been managed with beta 2-agonists, taken either once or twice, 15–30 minutes prior to exercise (Storms 1999). Long acting beta 2-agonists have also been found to be beneficial, should a prolonged duration of coverage be required (Kemp 2000, Storms 1999). The International Olympic Committee (IOC) has restrictions on the use of some beta 2-agonists, requiring formal notification of dose and indications, and has banned several beta 2-agonists as

a result of reported ergogenic effects (see Chapter 29). Hence, care needs to be taken when prescribing for athletes with EIA.

Both mast cell stabilizing agents and leukotriene receptor antagonists have a role in reducing both the duration and severity of EIA (Edelman et al 2000, Knopfli et al 2005, Spooner et al 2000). Inhaled corticosteroids should continue to be used to minimize airway inflammation in the management of classical asthma and refractory EIA (Edelman et al 2000, Thien 1999).

A preferred approach to pharmacological management of uncomplicated EIA is the use of a beta 2-agonist inhaler 30 minutes prior to exercise, followed by a mast cell stabilizer 15 minutes later. Treatment failure with this method may be the result of a number of factors including drug dosage, empty canisters and drug inhalation technique. With continued failure to respond to treatment, misdiagnosis and possible secondary gain should be considered.

Treatment of the acute, severe asthma attack 'on the field', where an individual is clearly in distress, involves the early administration of bronchodilator therapy (e.g. salbutamol) and the immediate transportation to a medical facility. If a nebulizer or oxygen is available then they should be utilized. Similarly, spacer devices can assist in the delivery of inhaled medications. The preferred method of transportation is in an ambulance (Thomas 2001).

Epilepsy

Epilepsy is a neurological disorder characterized by recurrent seizure activity (Sirven & Varrato 1999). A seizure is an abnormal electrical discharge within the cortical and subcortical neurons of the brain, which may or may not result in convulsive activity (Spiegal & Gates 1997). While true epilepsy may affect up to 3% of the population, up to 10% of the population will experience a single seizure in their lifetime (Spiegel & Gates 1997). Of all people who experience epilepsy, most are diagnosed before the age of 30 years (Cantu 1998a). Most cases of epilepsy are idiopathic, but it can also result from cerebrovascular accidents, central nervous system infections, neoplasms, metabolic derangements, birth trauma or anatomical abnormalities such as in Sturge–Weber syndrome (Gates & Spiegel 1993, Sirven & Varrato 1999).

Diagnosis of epilepsy

Up to 25% of patients referred to neurologists with a tentative diagnosis of epilepsy have other causes for their brief, sudden loss of consciousness and muscle tone (syncope) (Williams & Bernhardt 1995), and the most useful diagnostic tool to avoid misdiagnosis is an accurate history (McLaughlin 1999). Seizures that occur only while sitting or standing are more likely to be syncopal in origin (McLaughlin 1999). Brief stiffening of the body may occur in syncope, but can usually be differentiated from epilepsy by its brief duration (usually only a few seconds). Prior to a syncopal episode, a patient may have faintness or dizziness, while in epilepsy the first symptom may be an aura,

Table 31.1 Classification of seizure type (data from McLaughlin 1999 and van Linschoten et al 1990)

Type of seizure	Category	Sub-category
1. Partial (focal, localized seizure)	Simple partial (no altered level of consciousness)	With motor signs (e.g. limb twitching) With somatosensory hallucinations (e.g. taste or smell sensations) With autonomic signs and symptoms With psychic symptoms
	Complex partial (altered level of consciousness)	Simple followed by impairment of consciousness With impaired consciousness from the onset
	Partial evolving to generalized	
2. Generalized (convulsive or non-convulsive seizure)	Absence Atypical absence Myoclonic Clonic Tonic Tonic clonic Atonic	
3. Unclassified seizure		

which is actually the commencement of the seizure. While an aura is often difficult to describe, it will usually be similar on each occasion (McLaughlin 1999). The presence of drowsiness, headache and fatigue following an epileptic seizure are common. Other than in the immediate postictal phase, examination of a patient with epilepsy is usually normal (McLaughlin 1999). However, as the differential diagnosis for seizures includes cardiogenic and vasovagal syncope, transient ischemic attacks, metabolic disturbances and psychological causes, a full physical examination is required (Trost et al 2005).

If epilepsy is suspected, then an electroencephalogram (EEG) should be performed. Ideally, this should be performed as close to the seizure as possible, but despite this, the EEG may still be normal in up to 50% of subsequently diagnosed sufferers. In addition, up to 15% of sufferers may always have a normal EEG. Magnetic resonance imaging (MRI), single photon emission computerized tomography (SPECT) and positron emission tomography (PET) scans are all used to localize the focus of epileptic seizures (McLaughlin 1999, Trost et al 2005).

Seizures are classified on the basis of their external manifestations and EEG findings, and it is important to appropriately classify the seizure in order to ensure optimal management (Trost et al 2005). Table 31.1 illustrates a current classification system for epilepsy.

General management of epilepsy

Management of epilepsy is predominantly pharmacological, with up to 80% of individuals able to be controlled on a single drug. A number of drug classes are used to control epilepsy and the pharmacological options are rapidly evolving (Trost et al 2005). The most common include sodium channel blockers (e.g. phenytoin, carbemazepine), gamma-aminobutyric acid (GABA) release stimulators (e.g. valproic acid) and, more recently, the GABA analogs (vigabatrin, gabapentin) (Quinn et al 2001). Many of the drugs, however, have drowsiness and visual disturbances as potential side effects and these must be considered prior to making exercise recommendations. Exercise has not been found to influence the efficacy of antiepileptic medication (Cantu 1998a)

Exercise and epilepsy

In considering the relationship between exercise and epilepsy, it is important to consider both the effect of epilepsy on exercise and the effect of exercise on epilepsy. It has been found that during exercise there is a reduction in seizure frequency (Nakken 1999) but that immediately following exercise cessation, an increased risk of seizure activity is present (Nakken 1999, van Linschoten et al 1990). It has been postulated that this is a result of the increased concentration of GABA during exercise, which may suppress electrical activity in the brain (Cantu 1998a). Also, a reduction in blood pH levels following exercise could account for an increased risk of seizure immediately following activity (Sirven & Varrato 1999).

If epilepsy is well controlled with medication, it should have no effect on an athlete's performance (van Linschoten et al 1990). However, during the postictal phase (which may last up to a few days) performance may be affected by fatigue, and impaired alertness, balance and coordination (Spiegel & Gates 1997). Similarly, anticonvulsant medication may impair cognition, vision, concentration and coordination, all of which are important in exercise and sport performance. While exercise has not been found to significantly affect serum levels of antiepileptic medications, any abrupt change in body weight or composition as a result of training may alter the distribution of medications. Subsequently, serum levels of medications should be monitored carefully (Nakken 1999).

It is clear that the cardiovascular and psychosocial benefits of exercise outweigh its risks in people experiencing epilepsy. Athletes who are seizure-free and who are well controlled on medication have few contraindications to sport (Sirven & Varrato 1999). Similarly, there is little evidence that repeated minor head trauma will induce seizure activity (Sirven & Varrato 1999, van Linschoten et al 1990). However, some activities are associated with unacceptable risk to both the individual and other participants should a seizure occur, and as a result, are contraindicated for people with epilepsy. Sports that are absolutely contraindicated with epilepsy include rock climbing, scuba diving, flying, hang gliding, parachuting, shooting, archery and boxing. Sports that are relatively contraindicated include swimming and water sports, cross-country skiing, back packing, cycling, skating, horse riding, gymnastics, motor sports and many contact sports (Cantu 1998a, Fallon 1997, Sirven & Varrato 1999, van Linschoten et al 1990). In addition, there are a number of physiological states, commonly encountered in competitive sport, which may precipitate seizure activity (e.g. fatigue, sleep deprivation, hypoxia, hyponatremia, hyperthermia, hypoglycemia) (Sirven & Varrato 1999, Spiegel & Gates 1997, Trost et al 2005, van Linschoten et al 1990). For example, participation in high altitude activities could result in hypoxia and subsequently increase the risk of seizures (Sirven & Varrato 1999). While there is little evidence that exercise-induced physiological changes will necessarily precipitate seizures (Spiegel & Gates 1997), caution is recommended when advising athletes with epilepsy regarding their participation in sports which induce extreme physiological states (van Linschoten et al 1990). Common sense should always prevail and the potential risk to the both the individual and others should a seizure occur, should be carefully assessed (Cantu 1998a).

Management of epileptic seizures

Management of a seizure should follow basic first-aid guidelines. An area should be cleared so the patient does not harm themselves, but do not move the patient unless they are at risk of harming themselves. Do not place objects in the patient's mouth, or try to restrain a convulsing individual (Sirven & Varrato 1999). Attempts should be made to protect the airway, while being careful to avoid damaging the cervical spine. Any medical bracelets should be looked for, and professional assistance be sought should the convulsion not resolve rapidly. Following seizure cessation, ensure pulse and breathing are present. If absent, immediately begin cardiopulmonary resuscitation and enlist medical assistance (Sirven & Varrato 1999). All seizures require medical review, and first time convulsions require assessment by a neurologist. The decision to return to activity following a seizure requires individualized assessment (Spiegel & Gates 1997).

Head and neck injuries in sport

One of the most anxious situations for the physician, physical therapist or athletic trainer to be faced with is the athlete with a head or neck injury. Assessment is often difficult, time is pressured and the consequences of inappropriate initial management of even a minor injury can be devastating (Newcombe et al 1995, Warren & Bailes 1998a). While catastrophic head and neck injuries are rare, mild head and neck injuries are common, accounting, for example, for between 14 and 37% of injuries in elite level football in Australia (Seward et al 1993). It is important that physicians, physical therapists, and athletic trainers have a clear understanding of their role in the management of both severe and mild head and neck injury.

Box 31.1 Definition and features of concussion according to the International Conference on Concussion in Sport 2004

Sports concussion is defined as a complex pathophysiological process affecting the brain, induced by traumatic biomechanical forces. Several common features that incorporate clinical, pathological and biomechanical injury constructs that may be utilized in defining the nature of a concussive head injury include:

1. Concussion may be caused either by a direct blow to the head, face, neck, or elsewhere on the body with an 'impulsive' force transmitted to the head.
2. Concussion typically results in the rapid onset of short-lived impairment of neurological function that resolves spontaneously.
3. Concussion may result in neuropathological changes, but the acute clinical symptoms largely reflect a functional disturbance rather than structural injury.
4. Concussion results in a graded set of clinical syndromes that may or may not involve loss of consciousness (LOC). Resolution of the clinical and cognitive symptoms typically follows a sequential course.
5. Concussion is typically associated with grossly normal structural neuroimaging studies.

Concussion

The definition and management of concussion in sport has been redefined in the last few years by the First International Conference on Concussion in Sport in 2001 (Aubry et al 2002) and a second conference in 2004 (McCrory et al 2005). Defining features of concussion are outlined in Box 31.1.

Concussion is a significant problem with up to 300 000 episodes per year in contact sport in the USA (Johnston et al 2000) and up to 3.9 per 1000 player hours in Australian football (McIntosh et al 2000, Newcombe et al 1995, Seward et al 1993). In a study of rugby union and rugby league players, McIntosh et al (2000) found that 97% of cases of concussion were the result of direct contact. Most head impacts were caused in a tackle situation and involved collision with the upper body or upper limb of an opponent.

Diagnosis and assessment of concussion

Concussion may cause a variety of symptoms, but one must be aware that loss of consciousness (LOC) is not a prerequisite for diagnosis or severity. Other symptoms associated with concussion are memory disorders (both anterograde and retrograde), headache, nausea, poor coordination, dizziness, double/blurred vision and confusion. There are several approaches that have been taken to assess and diagnose concussion. Unfortunately the standard orientation questions regarding time, place and person are unreliable when compared to brief neuropsychological memory batteries assessing memory and attention function (McCrea et al 1997, Maddocks et al 1995). Both the Maddocks' questions (Box 31.2) and the Standardized Assessment of Concussion (SAC) (McCrea et al 1998) are widely used in the assessment of concussion. Both of these batteries have been incorporated into the Sports Concussion Assessment Tool (SCAT) developed

Box 31.2 Maddocks' questions for the assessment of concussion

Maddocks Protocol. The following questions are asked either within 10 minutes of the injury or when the patient becomes conscious. One point for each correct answer.
Items for assessing orientation:

(1) What is your name?
(2) What is your date of birth?
(3) How old are you?
(4) What year is it?
(5) What month is it?
(6) What day of the week is it?
(7) What is the date?
(8) What time of day (morning, afternoon, night) is it?

Items for assessing recent memory:

(1) Where are we playing? (At which ground are we?)
(2) Which period is it? (Which quarter is it?)
(3) How far into the period is it? (How far into the quarter is it, the first, middle, or last 10 minutes?)
(4) Which side scored last? (Which side scored the last goal?)
(5) Which team did we play last week?
(6) Did we win last week?

Response	Points
correct	1
uncertain	0
incorrect	0

Interpretation: minimum scores: 0, maximum total score: 14. The higher the score the better.

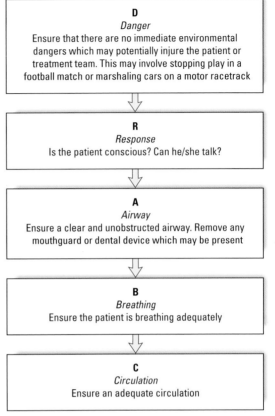

Figure 31.3 • Guide to the initial management of concussion. (Reproduced from McCrory P R 1997 Were you knocked out? A team physician's approach to initial concussion management. Medicine and Science in Sports and Exercise 29:S207–212 with the permission of Lippincott Williams & Wilkins.)

as part of the agreement statement for the Second International Conference on Concussion in Sport in 2004. This document adds to previously validated neuropsychological batteries with a dual role of patient education and clinical assessment.

Previously the assessment of the severity of a concussive episode has involved measurement of the duration of posttraumatic amnesia and loss of consciousness (Cantu 1998c, Moeller 1996). The validity of this approach has been questioned in the past, as these systems are not based on any scientific evidence (McCrory 1999, Johnston et al 2000). The Second International Conference on Concussion in Sport classifies the condition into two groups:

● *Simple concussion:* where the injury resolves progressively over 7–10 days

● *Complex concussion:* where the athlete suffers persistent symptoms, specific sequelae or prolonged cognitive impairment after the injury.

On-field assessment of concussion should involve a primary survey with appropriate interventions (Fig. 31.3). Should cervical spine injuries be suspected, neck immobilization and transport on a long spinal board should be expedited (Warren & Bailes 1998a). In an unconscious patient a spinal injury should be assumed to be present until proven otherwise (Newcombe

et al 1995). Once a patient has been stabilized and removed from the field of play, assessment should continue in the quiet of the dressing room. This is the appropriate time to take a full history, perform a full neurological examination and document the player's response to the cognitive questions and tests favored by the treating physician. If a player has any symptoms or signs of concussion, then that player should not be allowed to return to play, should not be left alone and should be reviewed serially by medical personnel (Johnston et al 2000). The rationale for not allowing an immediate return to play is based on an observed reduction in information processing and reaction times following head injury, which can predispose an individual to further injury.

In children and adolescents, there may also be an increased risk of diffuse brain swelling, known as second impact syndrome (SIS) (Cantu 1998b). More recent literature, however, has suggested that in the past, the risk of SIS following concussion has been over-emphasized (McCrory 1999, 2001b, McCrory & Berkovic 1998a). Indications for urgent referral following concussive incidents include signs of a cervical spine fracture, focal neurology, prolonged LOC or confusion, convulsive movements or a significant medical history (e.g. hemophilia) (McCrory 1997). Discharge home should only be allowed in the supervision of a mature adult, with instructions on how to manage any deterioration in symptoms.

Returning to play after concussion

Return to play guidelines following concussion is an area shrouded in controversy. The most recognized return to play guidelines are based on injury severity grading systems (Cantu 1998c, Johnston et al 2000, McCrory 1999, Moeller 1996). However, many of these systems are not based on sound scientific research (McCrory 1997). Mandatory exclusion criteria, based on a particular grade of injury, are inherently dangerous in that they may lead to under-reporting of concussive events. Further, such criteria could allow a premature return to play. The approach of choice is that based upon neuropsychological testing in conjunction with symptom assessment (McCrory 1997). In the days following a concussive incident regular symptom assessment and examination should be performed. Examination should include a digit symbol substitution test (DSST), which should be compared with a pre-season baseline assessment. The DSST is a simple neuropsychological test which is thought to reflect information processing and psychomotor speed, as well as visual short-term memory. It involves the copying of symbols and matching them with numbers over a 90 s period (Grindel et al 2001). On return of the DSST to baseline levels and with no symptoms at rest, the athlete is allowed to perform light aerobic exercise as part of a stepwise return to play strategy. If this is managed without any symptoms, the following day the athlete should perform non-contact drills, finally returning to contact training, prior to being allowed to return to play (Johnston et al 2000, McCrory 1997, McCrory et al 2005). More recently, computerized assessment techniques have become popular. If symptoms occur at any level of the program, the player should return to the previous asymptomatic level and reattempt progression after another 24 h. Persistence or deterioration of symptoms warrants further investigation by a neurologist or sports physician.

Prevention of concussion

In recent years there has been an increase in the use of headgear and mouthguards with a view to preventing concussive head injury. McIntosh et al (2000) found that the average head impact energy causing concussion in 97 subjects was 56 joules, and that the impact attenuation ability of foam headgear was lost above an impact energy of 20 joules (McIntosh & McCrory 2000). This suggests that the commercially available headgear was unlikely to reduce the risk of concussion. Interestingly, it has been shown that players wearing headgear perceived increased levels of safety and hence an ability to tackle harder (Finch et al 2001). It could be that headgear alters on-field behavior, and subsequently increases the risk of injury.

A further device historically thought to decrease the risk of concussion is mouthguards (Hickey et al 1967, Kerr 1986). However, while mouthguards do offer protection against dental injury, there is only limited evidence that they offer any

protective effect against concussion (McCrory 2001a). Prevention of concussion and other head injury is best achieved by education and enforcement of appropriate rules preventing dangerous play, with severe penalties for breach of these rules (Johnston et al 2000, 2001, McCrory & Berkovic 1998b, Newcombe et al 1995).

Cervical spine injury in sport

Serious spinal cord injuries continue to occur in contact sport despite progressive law and attitude changes (Rotem et al 1998). According to National Sports Injury Center data, sporting events account for approximately 7.5% of all spinal cord injuries in the USA. Such injuries have a significant impact on both individuals' lives and community resources. While conditions such as spinal canal stenosis may predispose to cervical spine injury, the role of screening for such conditions, and their relative risk for spinal cord injury continue to be debated (Cantu 1997, Torg & Glasgow 1991, Torg & Ramsey-Emrhein 1997).

Assessment of cervical spine injuries

Making a safe clinical judgment on an athlete with a suspected cervical spine injury is difficult. There are often confounding pressures from coaches and managers that make the operation of simple 'in-hospital' cervical clearance protocols very difficult on the field of play. The initial care of the patient focuses on preventing any further neurological insult (Warren & Bailes 1998b), and in order to achieve this aim, it is recommended that physical therapists, athletic trainers and medical personnel are competent with the use of cervical collars, long spinal boards and scoop stretchers. These skills need to practiced and recertified regularly.

Often the symptoms and signs of cervical injury are subtle and a high index of clinical suspicion is required. Observation of the mechanism of injury is critical, as this can stratify the index of suspicion appropriately (Newcombe et al 1995). This is particularly evident if the incident involves either hyperflexion or hyperextension of the cervical spine, especially in association with axial loading or rotation (McLatchie & Lloyd-Parry 1997). An unconscious patient must be assumed to have sustained a cervical spine injury (Newcombe et al 1995), until either the player regains consciousness and can be examined appropriately, or definitive imaging has been performed (Marion et al 2000). If breathing is absent, log roll the patient into a supine position, remove the mouthpiece or facemask, and commence cardiopulmonary resuscitation immediately (Warren & Bailes 1998b). Manual in-line stabilization of the C-spine should simultaneously accompany airway assessment and management, with uncontrolled head tilt being avoided if possible.

More commonly the patient is conscious and simple questions regarding the site of any pain and the nature of any motor or sensory deficit can assist in localizing the affected area of the spinal cord (McLatchie & Lloyd-Parry 1997). Any neurological symptoms and signs need to be carefully recorded to facilitate accurate comparison when the player is re-evaluated.

If a cervical spine injury is immediately suspected, it is essential to calmly convey the situation to the player and gently prevent any active cervical movement. After completing an assessment of the airway, breathing and circulation, the player should be fitted with a sized semi-rigid collar and safely placed on a long spinal board (Newcombe et al 1995). However, if the patient has no peripheral symptoms, palpation of the cervical spine should be undertaken with the patient lying still. The location of tenderness should be carefully noted. Mild paraspinal tenderness is common, but direct midline tenderness especially if accompanied by midline swelling should be treated with utmost suspicion. If there is no pain or any neurological symptoms, the athlete may be allowed to sit up slowly and a further assessment of concussion and the cervical spine should be performed. At this stage the athlete can be requested to demonstrate a slow, controlled, active range of cervical motion. If there is a full, pain-free range of cervical motion with minimal tenderness, no peripheral neurological symptoms or signs and no signs of concussion, then the athlete may continue if he feels able to do so. If the initial assessment provokes any doubts in the player or physician, then it is preferable to immobilize the cervical spine (Newcombe et al 1995). By contrast, pain and/or limitation of cervical movements necessitates immobilization and removal from the field of play. Triple immobilization of the cervical spine involves use of a semi-rigid collar, long spinal board and blocks or tape. It is essential that these are available at every sports ground where contact sport is played (Newcombe et al 1995). When using a stretcher or spinal board, one person should carry each corner and the leader control the patient's head (Warren & Bailes 1998b). There is no clinical justification for using a semi-rigid collar in isolation without the two other components of full cervical immobilization. Prior to a hospital transfer it is important to ensure that the airway and breathing are secured, the patient has appropriate and full spinal immobilization in place and a full neurological assessment has been carried out and documented (Newcombe et al 1995, Warren & Bailes 1998b). In the event of a significant injury the game should be ceased until the patient is in a stable condition to be moved. This may require an ambulance or helicopter entering the ground to enable precipitous and safe transfer to a definitive care facility

Cardiac conditions in sport and exercise

Sudden cardiovascular death

Sudden cardiovascular death (SCD) is defined by the International Olympic Committee (IOC) Medical Commission as 'death occurring within one hour of the onset of symptoms in a person without a previously recognized cardiovascular condition that would appear fatal: this excludes cerebrovascular, respiratory, traumatic and drug related causes' (Oswald et al 2004). Cardiac deaths account for approximately 85% of sudden nontraumatic deaths among athletes (Maron et al 1996a)

and whilst considered a relatively rare occurrence, the death of a young, apparently healthy sportsperson results in considerable societal concern (Jensen-Urstad 1995). The prevalence of SCD in young athletes is estimated to be in the range of 1:100 000 to 1:300 000, and in older athletes 1:15 000 to 1:50 000 (Maron et al 1998). The majority of deaths occur during or just after significant physical exertion, implying that exercise is a trigger for fatal arrhythmias in susceptible individuals (Sharma et al 1997).

It is now well recognized that the risk factors for SCD differ for athletes either younger or older than 30 years of age (Futterman & Myerburg 1998, Maron et al 1996b). In the older age groups, coronary artery disease is the predominant cause of death. At autopsy in younger athletes, the most common structural cause of SCD is consistently hypertrophic obstructive cardiomyopathy (HOCM), accounting for 30 to 50% of deaths (Maron et al 1996b, Paffenbarger et al 1986). Other leading causes include congenital coronary artery anomalies (where the arteries arise from the wrong aortic sinus), arrhythymogenic right ventricular cardiomyopathy, left ventricular hypertrophy of indeterminate causation, myocarditis, ruptured aortic aneurysm (Marfan's syndrome) and tunneled coronary arteries (Maron 2003). A minority of individuals have normal cardiac morphology at autopsy and such deaths are likely to be due to either conduction disorders including Wolff Parkinson White syndrome or ion channel disorders such as prolonged QT and Brugada's syndrome (Maron 2003). Commotio cordis refers to sudden death following blunt trauma to the chest, inducing venticular fibrillation. This condition accounts for a significant proportion of sudden deaths in sport in the USA (Maron 2003), but as it is induced by trauma, it does not strictly fall within the definition of SCD.

HOCM is an autosomal dominant inherited condition, caused by a mutation in any one of 10 genes (Maron 2002). It is the most common genetic cardiovascular disease with a prevalence of approximately 1:500 individuals (Maron & Mitchell 1994). Morphogically, HOCM is characterized by ventricular hypertrophy, most commonly in an asymmetrical septal pattern (Sharma et al 1997). Histology typically shows myofibrillar and myocyte disorganization which precipitates a variety of pathophysiological disturbances and potential dysrhythmias. Two-dimensional echocardiography is generally the most reliable diagnostic tool, showing a hypertrophied but non dilated left ventricle (Maron 2002). The 12 lead ECG is abnormal in 75% to 95% of HOCM patients, with a wide spectrum of patterns described (Maron 2002).

Given the low incidence of SCD in young asymptomatic athletes, the value of routine screening continues to be heavily debated (Fuller et al 1997, Jensen-Urstad 1995). The American Heart Association guidelines for pre-participation screening (Maron et al 1996b), much used in North America, recommend a thorough history and examination but not a 12-lead ECG. Two major sets of guidelines have recently been released in the form of the Lausanne recommendations from the IOC Medical Commission (2004) and the European Society of Cardiology consensus statement (Corrado et al 2005) which both include the 12-lead ECG in the screening recommendations. The Lausanne recommendations suggest that participants under 35 years of age beginning competitive activity should undergo pre-participation cardiovascular screening that includes:

- A detailed personal and family history to rule out any potentially detectable cardiovascular condition
- A physical examination
- A 12-lead resting ECG after the onset of puberty.

They recommend that this screening battery is repeated at least every other year and that individuals with suspicious symptoms, adverse examination findings, a positive cardiac family history, or significant ECG changes, should be referred to an age appropriate cardiologist for further investigation (Oswald et al 2004).

There has been discussion for many years on the cost effectiveness of the use of the 12-lead ECG and echocardiography as part of a pre-sport cardiac screening program (Maron 2005). Italian law insists that every individual involved in competitive sport must undergo clinical evaluation as a condition of their eligibility to compete. Thus, there is a wealth of experience and data emerging from this country, suggesting that the 12-lead ECG may be as sensitive in detecting HOCM in a young population as echocardiography (Corrado et al 2005). This view, however, is not supported by all sports cardiologists, with some advocating that inevitable false positive ECG findings will negatively impact on both the available financial resources and the psychological status of affected athletes and their support group.

The athlete's heart

The concept of 'the athlete's heart' refers to the structural and functional adaptations that the heart undergoes in response to exercise. First described in the late nineteenth century in relation to cross country skiers (Urhausen & Kindermann 1999), it has subsequently been recognized as a physiological adaptation to stresses placed upon the cardiovascular system (Holly et al 1998, Mills et al 1997).

Endurance training subjects an athlete's heart to a volume overload stress. The result of this is an increased intracavity dimension involving all four chambers of the heart, with a concomitant increase in cardiac mass, known as eccentric hypertrophy (Pelliccia et al 1991). In addition, vagal tone increases and beta-adrenergic receptiveness decreases, resulting in a bradycardia (Holly et al 1998, Huston et al 1985, Stolt et al 1997). As a result of these adaptations, endurance trained athletes have characteristic ECG findings (Holly et al 1998, Stolt et al 1997) (Box 31.3). By comparison, strength training results in increased ventricular wall thickness, with little change in chamber volume, known as concentric hypertrophy (Pelliccia et al 1991). This is thought to result from an increase in afterload, as a result of vascular compression caused by the static muscular contraction.

Box 31.3 ECG findings in an endurance trained athlete that may be considered normal

Secondary to vagotonia
- Sinus bradycardia
- Sinus arrythmia
- Junctional escape beats
- AV conduction blocks (first degree, second degree Mobitz type one)

Secondary to cardiac mass
- Increased QRS voltage (S-V1 + R-V5 >35 mm)
- Prominent u waves
- Intraventricular delays (right bundle branch block, left anterior fascicle block)
- Early repolarization (upward displaced ST segment)
- Long QT Interval (normalizes when corrected for rate)

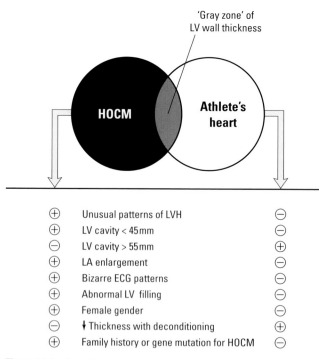

Figure 31.4 • Relationship between physiological hypertrophy and hypertrophic obstructive cardiomyopathy. (Reproduced from Maron B J, Pelliccia A, Spirito P 1995 Cardiac disease in young trained athletes. Insights into methods for distinguishing athlete's heart from structural heart disease, with particular emphasis on hypertrophic cardiomyopathy. Circulation 91:1596–1601.)

It is important to distinguish physiological ventricular hypertrophy from pathological cardiomyopathy. As has been noted above, HOCM is considered to be the leading cause of SCD among young athletes, and the distinction between the two entities often creates a diagnostic dilemma. Figure 31.4 illustrates the relationship between the two entities. With deconditioning, many of the ECG findings of the athlete's heart will resolve, and with exercise testing, any suspected abnormalities should disappear (Basilico 1999). Should exercise testing induce atypical cardiovascular changes, pathological conditions should be considered.

In summary, cardiac conditions are the leading cause of sudden death in otherwise fit individuals participating in exercise. Careful preparticipation screening (see Chapter 12), combined with an awareness of normal cardiac variations found in an athlete and an understanding of the demands of different sports, can assist in reducing the risk of sudden death.

Diabetes mellitus

Diabetes mellitis is a major cause of death and disability in the USA (Albright et al 2000, Steinbrook 2006) and has an estimated world wide prevalence of 5.1% or 194 million people (Gan 2003). It is a disease characterized by chronic hyperglycemia, due to defects in insulin secretion, insulin action or a combination of the two. Diabetes has two major subgroups. Type 1 diabetes results from a deficiency of endogenous insulin, and is common in childhood and adolescence. Management is predominantly pharmacological, with exogenous insulin replacement (Pierce 1999). Type 2 diabetes accounts for up to 90% of cases, with an incidence of approximately 3–5% in Europe but up to 40% in Oceanic countries (Gan 2003). Type 2 diabetes has a strong genetic basis and is primarily the result of reduced end organ sensitivity to insulin. This type of diabetes is managed with a combination of dietary manipulation, exercise and oral hypoglycemics (Colman et al 1999).

Diabetes may present with excessive urine losses, nocturnal urination, dehydration and increased thirst, as a result of elevated blood glucose levels. Weight loss, blurred vision, and recurrent infections are also common presentations (Gale 1990). Ketoacidotic or hyperosmolar coma may result from severely elevated blood glucose levels (Funk & Feingold 1995). There are several chronic complications of diabetes. Microvascular disease, resulting in both a retinopathy and nephropathy, as well as macrovascular diseases such as atherosclerosis, hypertension and hypertriglyceridemia are very common (Pierce 1999). Neuropathy involving either single or multiple peripheral nerves, as well as the autonomic nervous system, results in a high morbidity (Pierce 1999). Foot ulcers, secondary to both neuropathic and microvascular disease, are also common (Campbell et al 2000), as are infections resulting from both vascular disease and defective white cell function (Albright et al 2000). Cataracts are also frequently observed, as a result of sorbitol accumulation in the lens of the eye.

In 1999, the Australian Diabetes Society released new diagnostic criteria with a view to increasing the sensitivity of diabetes screening (Colman et al 1999). By detecting Type 2 diabetes earlier, it is anticipated that many of the chronic complications may be avoided.

It is well recognized that regular aerobic exercise results in improved lipoprotein profile, blood pressure and cardiovascular fitness (Diabetes Control and Complications Trial Research Group 1993, Pan et al 1997). As macrovascular disease is one of the major causes of morbidity and mortality in diabetes, exercise is believed to be of significant benefit (Zinman et al 1997). In addition, regular exercise has been shown to reduce an individual's insulin requirements, and the psychosocial benefits of exercise for the adolescent are invaluable (Zinman et al 1997). With particular regard to Type 2 diabetes, the potential benefits of exercise are substantial. An abundance of literature has summarized the potential metabolic benefits of aerobic exercise in Type 2 diabetes (Albright et al 2000, Di Loreto et al 2005, Eriksson 1999, Warburton et al 2006, Zinman et al 1997). These benefits include reduced blood glucose levels, improved insulin sensitivity, improved cardiovascular fitness, lowered blood pressure, improved lipid profile, improved body weight and improved stress management abilities and self-esteem. Additionally, there is increasing evidence that exercise may prevent or delay the onset of Type 2 diabetes (Zinman et al 1997).

Exercise and the diabetic

People with Type 1 diabetes, with no chronic complications and good blood glucose control, are able to perform in most forms and levels of sport and exercise (Zinman et al 1997). An exception to this, however, is scuba diving (Hazel 1994), which as a result of its unpredictable nature and dependence on a buddy system, make it an inappropriate activity for people with this condition (Gorman 1993). It is important that prior to the commencement of any exercise program, a full examination is performed. Particular attention must be paid to the cardiovascular, ocular, and neurological systems, as well as to the feet. It is recommended that individuals over the age of 35 years, or with a 15-year history of diabetes, undergo either a resting or exercise electrocardiogram (ECG) to exclude any underlying, silent, coronary artery disease (Zinman et al 1997). Baseline levels of renal function, glucose control and lipids should be performed (Eriksson 1999). Irregularities in the examination or investigative findings may alter the suitability of various exercise programs, and this requires individualized assessment (Zinman et al 1997).

Upon the initiation of an exercise program, it needs to be emphasized to the individual that the regular monitoring and subsequent adjustment of the therapeutic regimen is critical for ongoing safe participation (Zinman et al 1997). Education and understanding by the individual, family and training partners is fundamental to the success of an exercise program in this group of people (Draznin 2000).

Hypoglycemia is a common complication both during and up to 14 hours after exercise, and needs to be recognizable to both the individual and their training partners (Hernandez et al 2000). Common features of hypoglycemia include symptoms and signs secondary to both catecholamine release and central nervous system dysfunction. Sweating, shakiness, anxiety, palpitations, weakness, tremor, hunger, faintness and tachycardia can all occur secondary to catecholamine release. Confusion, irritability, headaches, abnormal behavior, weakness, diplopia, inappropriate affect, motor incoordination, convulsion and

Table 31.2 Guidelines for carbohydrate and insulin requirements before exercise (reproduced from Perlstein et al 1997 with the permission of the International Diabetes Institute, Australia)

Blood glucose levels before exercise	Exercise	Approximate amount of carbohydrate to eat prior to exercise[a]
<6 mmol/L	Short duration (30–45 min), low/moderate intensity (e.g. walking, aerobic dance)	25 g
	Short duration (30–45 min), high intensity (e.g. sprints, weight lifting)	25 g
	Moderate duration (60 min), moderate intensity, (e.g. cycling, basketball, tennis, swimming)	25–50 g
	Long duration (>75 min), low to moderate intensity/intermittent (e.g. marathon, triathlon, soccer, football)	50 g
6–10 mmol/L	Short duration (30–45 min), low/moderate intensity	0 g
	Short duration (30–45 min), high intensity	0 g
	Moderate duration (60 min), moderate intensity	0–25 g
	Long duration (>75 min), low to moderate intensity	25–50 g
10–15 mmol/L	Short duration (30–45 min), low/moderate intensity	0 g
	Short duration (30–45 min), high intensity	0 g
	Moderate duration (60 min), moderate intensity	0 g
	Long duration (>75 min), low to moderate intensity	0–25 g
>15 mmol/L, ketones absent	The effect of any exercise may be to raise blood glucose levels if there is not enough circulating insulin present. Knowing whether blood glucose levels were rising or falling in the few hours prior to exercise may help. If blood glucose levels are falling, exercise can be undertaken	
>15 mmol/L, ketones present	Rest and take some short acting insulin and delay exercise until blood glucose levels are under better control	

[a] Individuals have different responses to physical activity and food. The above recommendations are a guide and it is advisable for individuals to discuss these with a dietitian, diabetes nurse educator and/or doctor before undertaking any changes.

coma can occur secondary to central nervous system dysfunction. The risks of both hyperglycemia and hypoglycemia can be minimized with alterations in both the insulin regimen and carbohydrate intake, based on pre-exercise blood glucose levels. Guidelines for the manipulation of insulin dosage and carbohydrate intake are shown in Table 31.2. Exercise intensity and duration are the key variables to consider.

The keeping of an accurate exercise diary is critical in allowing an individual to assess responses to varying exercise intensities and insulin regimens (Fig. 31.5). It is recommended that blood glucose measurements be made immediately before, during, and after exercise in order to observe individual responses to differing regimens. It should be remembered that subcutaneous injections of insulin will be more rapidly absorbed from working muscles, and therefore injections into active limbs should be avoided (Koivisto & Felig 1978).

The maintenance of hydration with glucose-containing fluids and having carbohydrate rich foods available both during and following exercise will prevent intra-exercise, post exercise and nocturnal hypoglycaemia (Hernandez et al 2000, Zinman et al 1997). Low glycemic index (GI) foods prior to exercise, combined with high GI foods during exercise has been found to optimize a diabetic's blood glucose profile (Perlstein et al 1997). A 5–10 min low intensity warm-up and warm-down should be included in each exercise session in order to gradually prepare the cardiovascular, metabolic and musculoskeletal systems (Zinman et al 1997). To prevent podiatric complications, appropriate footwear and socks should be worn and regular inspection of feet should be mandatory (Campbell et al 2000). Any blisters or foot discomfort should be addressed rapidly, in order to prevent any progressive complications (e.g. foot ulcers) (Zinman et al 1997). The wearing of a diabetes identification bracelet, and not training alone are simple but important recommendations.

When exercising with Type 2 diabetes the risk of exercise induced hypoglycemia is reduced (Eriksson 1999). If the diabetes is being managed with diet control alone, then dietary manipulation prior to exercise may suffice. When requiring oral hypoglycemic medication, the dose may need to be reduced or withheld, and the timing of drug administration may need to be altered (Albright et al 2000). An individual's response to differing regimens should be closely monitored. In order to achieve health improvements, it is recommended that individuals with Type 2 diabetes exercise 3–5 times per week, at a low to moderate intensity (Constance & Clure 1996). Duration should begin at 10–15 min gradually increasing to approximately 60 min as tolerated (Albright et al 2000). Both aerobic and resistance training are recognized to offer significant benefits (Albright et al 2000).

COMPETITIVE ATHLETES

	Date	Exercise: Time	Exercise: Type	Exercise: Min	Exercise: Intensity	Exercise: Density (km)	Time / Blood glucose							Time / Insulin dose				Food/Fluid: Pre	Food/Fluid: During	Food/Fluid: Post	Weight: Pre	Weight: Post	Comments, e.g., cold weather, heart rate, injuries
Mon	3/3													7am / 10^{H}	12md / 8^{H}	6pm / 8^{H}	11pm / 12^{P}						
Tue	4/3	6pm	Cycle	90	H	45	7am / 6	12md / 5.5	6pm / 8.5	8pm / 9.9	11pm / 7.5			10	8	5	10	Jam sandwich 500 mL water	1 L dilute cordial, 1 banana	500 mL sports drink and dinner	76 kg	75 kg	
Wed	5/3													10	8	8	12						
Thur	6/3	6pm	Cycle	80	H	40	7am / 5	12md / 7.8	6pm / 13.0	8pm / 7.4	11pm / 6.0			10	8	6	10	1 glass juice, 500 mL water	1 L dilute cordial	1 can cola and dinner	–	–	Snack pre-bed: 1 cup milk and 2 raisin toast
Fri	7/3													10	8	8	12						
Sat	8/3	10am	Cycle	150	M	75	7am / 5	10am / 10.0	12:30 pm / 3.5	3pm / 7.0	11pm / 8.0			6	6	7	11	1/2 L water, 2 bananas	2 L dilute cordial, 10 dried apricots	See comments	75.5 kg	75.0 kg	Hypo 12:30pm after cycle. Ate jelly beans and lunch straight away. Felt fine
Sun	9/3													10	8	8	12						

Distance this week: 160 km

Cumulative distance: 1574 km for 2002

Codes : Intensity:
E – Easy
M – Moderate
H – Hard

Notes:

Figure 31.5 • Example of a training diary for a diabetic individual.

Table 31.3 Possible causes of recalcitrant fatigue in the athlete (reproduced from Brukner 1996 with the permission of Australian Family Physician)

Common causes	Less common causes	Causes not to be missed
Overtraining syndrome	Dehydration	Malignant disease
Viral illness	Exercise-induced asthma	Cardiac problems
URTI	Mg, Zn or B$_{12}$ deficiency	Bacterial endocarditis
Infectious mononucleosis	Postviral fatigue syndrome	Cardiac failure
Inadequate carbohydrate intake	Allergic disorders	Diabetes
Depletion of iron stores	Jet-lag	Hypothyroidism
Inadequate protein intake	Anemia	Renal failure
Insufficient sleep	Psychological stress	Neuromuscular disorders
	Anxiety	Infection
	Depression	Hepatitis A, B, C
	Medications	HIV
	Beta-blockers	Malaria
	Anxiolytics	Eating disorders
	Antihistamines	Anorexia
		Bulimia
		Pregnancy
		Postconcussive syndrome

The most frequent complication diabetics experience during exercise is a hypoglycemic episode. While this can be avoided with regular monitoring, the ability to recognize early signs and symptoms by both the individual and their training partners is vital. Should symptoms become apparent, the eating of high GI foods, and drinking glucose-containing fluid, is the most appropriate initial management. Should symptoms persist or progress, then medical advice should be sought.

In summary, it is well recognized that the benefits of exercise in diabetics outweigh the risks. With regular monitoring and by following the basic principles carefully, the risks associated with exercise may be minimized.

The tired athlete

While fatigue is a common reaction to hard and persistent training, ongoing fatigue that is not responsive to recovery warrants attention. There are a multitude of medical conditions that may result in prolonged tiredness. The most common causes in the highly trained athlete include overtraining syndrome (also termed the unexplained underperformance syndrome (Budgett et al 2000)), infections, sleep disturbance and dietary imbalances (Table 31.3) (Brukner 1996). Most significant, underlying medical conditions can be eliminated with a concise medical history and examination. However, in the absence of any overt medical condition a more comprehensive history will be required. Critical features to elucidate in the history from the athlete include nature of the fatigue (constant, sleepiness,

post-training, during training), associated recent illnesses, volume and intensity of training (including any modifications), amount of recovery time following sessions, dietary intake (carbohydrate, protein and fat, and relationship to training), fluid intake, quality and quantity of sleep and extracurricular psychosocial stresses.

Routine first line investigations for fatigued athletes may include full blood profile, electrolytes, blood glucose, renal and liver function tests, iron studies and urinalysis. Further investigations to consider include viral serology, vitamin and mineral status, thyroid function tests and creatine kinase assessment. If indicated, a chest radiograph or lung spirometry should be considered (Brukner 1996).

Overtraining syndrome

With adequate recovery from training, the body will adapt to increased demands (Wilmore & Costill 1994). A common principle in athletic training involves stressing the body as a stimulus for adaptation, known as progressive overload training (Wilmore & Costill 1994). However, if the recovery period is inadequate for the volume and intensity of training undertaken, then an athlete can experience an increase in fatigue and a reduction in performance. This temporary deterioration is known as over-reaching (Smith 2000) and by definition the affected athlete should recover with two weeks of relative rest (Budgett et al 2000). If the athlete fails to identify their over-reaching and modify their training appropriately, then an overtraining syndrome may develop (Fry et al 1991, Hedelin et al 2000).

The overtraining syndrome is characterized by a vast number of symptoms that can be categorized into psychological, physiological, immunological and biochemical (Fry et al 1991) (Box 31.4). The most common presenting symptoms of overtraining are fatigue, reduced performance, sleep disturbance, muscle soreness, recurrent injury and infection (Costill et al 1988, Fry et al 1991, Morgan et al 1988, Nieman et al 1995). Unlike the over-reached athlete, the overtrained athlete may take many months to recover (Hedelin et al 2000). There are several theories as to the etiology of the overtraining syndrome. These include autonomic nervous system dysfunction (Lehmann et al 1998), glutamine depletion (Kingsbury et al 1998, Smith & Norris 2000), tryptophan depletion (Smith 2000) and glycogen depletion (Snyder 1998). Smith (2000) attempted to integrate the existing theories into a single paradigm, proposing that the inflammatory cytokines released in response to normal training may be responsible for inducing each of the features observed in the overtraining syndrome. Hence excessive cytokine release following exercise induces a chronic systemic inflammatory state termed cytokine sickness. While the proposal is very attractive, it requires further consideration prior to being universally accepted.

If overtraining syndrome is suspected, the monitoring of testosterone, cortisol, creatine phosphokinase and immunological markers such as decreased neutrophil oxidative burst levels and salivary IgA (Mackinnon 2000) can assist in the monitoring of

Box 31.4 Symptoms of overtraining syndrome (reproduced from Fry et al 1991 with the permission of Adis International Ltd)

Physiological/performance
- Decreased performance
- Inability to meet previously attained performance standards/criteria
- Recovery prolonged
- Reduced toleration of loading
- Decreased muscular strength
- Decreased maximum work capacity
- Loss of coordination
- Decreased efficiency/decreased amplitude of movement
- Reappearance of mistakes already corrected
- Reduced capacity of differentiation and correcting technical faults
- Increased difference between lying and standing heart rate
- Abnormal T wave pattern in ECG
- Heart discomfort on slight exertion
- Changes in blood pressure
- Changes in heart rate at rest, exercise and recovery
- Increased frequency of respiration
- Perfuse respiration
- Decreased body fat
- Increased oxygen consumption at submaximal workloads
- Increased ventilation and heart rate at submaximal workloads
- Shift of the lactate curve towards the x-axis
- Decreased evening postworkout weight
- Elevated basal metabolic rate
- Chronic fatigue
- Insomnia with and without night sweats
- Feels thirsty
- Anorexia nervosa
- Loss of appetite
- Bulimia
- Amenorrhea/oligomenorrhea
- Headaches
- Nausea
- Increased aches and pains
- Gastrointestinal disturbances
- Muscle soreness/tenderness
- Tendinostic complaints
- Periosteal complaints
- Muscle damage
- Elevated C-reactive protein
- Rhabdomyolysis

Psychological/information processing
- Feeling of depression
- General apathy
- Decreased self-esteem/worsening feeling of self
- Emotional instability
- Difficulty in concentrating at work and training
- Sensitive to environmental and emotional stress
- Fear of competition
- Changes in personality
- Decreased ability to narrow concentration
- Increased internal and external distractability
- Decreased capacity to deal with large amounts of information
- Gives up when the going gets tough

Immunological
- Increased susceptibility to and severity of illness/colds/allergies
- Flu-like illnesses
- Unconfirmed glandular fever
- Minor scratches heal slowly
- Swelling of lymph glands
- One-day colds
- Decreased functional activity of neutrophils
- Decreased total lymphocyte counts
- Reduced response to mitogens
- Increased blood eosinophil count
- Decreased proportion of null (non-T, non-B lymphocytes)
- Bacterial infection
- Reactivation of herpes viral infection
- Significant variations in CD4:CD8 lymphocytes

Biochemical
- Negative nitrogen balance
- Hypothalamic dysfunction
- Flat glucose tolerance curves
- Depressed muscle glycogen concentration
- Decreased bone mineral content
- Delayed menarche
- Decreased hemoglobin
- Decreased serum iron
- Decreased serum ferritin
- Lowered TIBC
- Mineral depletion (Zn, Co, Al, Mn, Se, Cu, etc.)
- Increased urea concentrations
- Elevated cortisol levels
- Elevated ketosteroids in urine
- Low free testosterone
- Increased serum hormone binding globulin
- Decreased ratio of free testosterone to cortisol of more than 30%
- Increased uric acid production

the athlete's progress, but cannot be used to provide a firm diagnosis (Brukner 1996).

Initial management of the overtrained athlete involves exclusion of other possible causes of fatigue, and the recognition of the condition by both athlete and coach. Prolonged rest from training is the most important aspect of treatment, with return to training being gradual, progressive and guided by symptoms. Monitoring of morning heart rate may provide a simple guide to recovery from training, with an elevation of more than 6 beats per minute considered to be significant (Brukner & Khan 1993). Concurrently, issues such as injuries, nutrition, training program and psychosocial stresses should be addressed. Full recovery may take weeks to months (Hedelin et al 2000).

More recently, the concept of the overtraining syndrome has been redefined as unexplained underperformance syndrome (UPS) (Budgett et al 2000). The term UPS does not specify any set clinical criteria to facilitate diagnosis, but it has been adopted to stop the implication of 'training' or excessive training as necessarily the causative component of the condition, and encourages clinicians and researchers to investigate affected athletes with an open mind.

Prevention of overtraining syndrome or UPS requires that training programs be carefully constructed to incorporate the correct balance between load and recovery (Kuipers & Keizer 1988). Individuals respond differently to the same training load and have differing professional and personal pressures, which can all impact upon the response to training (Kuipers & Keizer 1988). It is important for training regimes to be personalized and take into account not only the training itself, but also any environmental, psychological and social factors that may affect training performance and recovery (Pyne et al 2000a). Educating coaches and athletes about the implications of overtraining syndrome is the most significant step in prevention. The athlete and coach should understand the importance of recognizing the overreached state before it progresses to overtraining and the implications this will have for rehabilitation time. Strategies such as periodization, cross-training, psychological skills training, dietary assistance, environmental manipulation, regular medical review and the use of regenerative techniques such as massage and hydrotherapy may all assist in the prevention of overtraining (Brukner 1996).

Travel medicine for the international athlete

The ease of modern air travel has enabled athletes to travel to competitions throughout the world with relative ease. In many situations, athletes may be accompanied by a team physician, but more often, the physical therapist or sports trainer will be the only traveling medical team member. There are three important phases in the provision of care for the traveling athlete: pre-travel, travel and on-location care (Young et al 1998). Prior to traveling it is important that the responsible medical officer be fully aware of any medical issues facing individual athletes and staff. A comprehensive history and examination should be performed prior to departure.

Vaccinations

It is important that a detailed travel itinerary is known in order to accurately plan for vaccinations (Young et al 1998). One of the major difficulties facing the medical practitioner is the short notice of impending travel often provided, making appropriate scheduling of vaccinations difficult. Athletes should, therefore, keep an accurate vaccination schedule in their training diary. Vaccinations which should be considered as mandatory include tetanus, diphtheria, measles, mumps, poliomyelitis and rubella. Those that should be considered on a more individualized basis

(dependent on the nature of the sport, ages and location being visited) include hepatitis A, hepatitis B, influenza, malaria, typhoid, Japanese encephalitis, cholera, rabies, meningococcus and yellow fever. It is important that all athletes have received their basic childhood vaccinations. It is also recommended that all traveling athletes be vaccinated against hepatitis A, and those involved in contact sports consider hepatitis B (Young et al 1998). The ever-changing distribution of diseases and disease vectors, as well as the increasing availability of international travel, ensures that the vaccination requirements of travel continue to change (World Health Organization 2001). It is important that an up-to-date vaccination schedule is consulted prior to travel.

Issues with air travel

Circadian rhythms are the body's daily rhythms that are synchronized to the day/night cycle. These rhythms control the body's physiological and psychological systems. Many components of sports performance such as flexibility, power output and muscle strength have been shown to vary with the time of day as a result of the circadian rhythm (Atkinson & Reilly 1996). Flights across time zones can result in de-synchronization of circadian rhythms, leading to circadian dysrhythmia or 'jet-lag'. Jet-lag is more pronounced when traveling over a greater number of time zones, and when traveling eastwards (Reilly et al 2001). Symptoms of jet-lag include disrupted sleep, gastrointestinal distress, headaches and general malaise. While anecdotally it would appear that jet-lag may impair performance, methodological difficulties have meant that the scientific substantiation of jet-lag impairing performance, is lacking (Youngstedt & O'Connor 1999). It is estimated that it takes one day to readjust to the new environment, for each time zone crossed (Loat & Rhodes 1989, Reilly et al 2001).

Jet-lag symptoms can be reduced with a number of simple strategies. In preparation for travel, adjusting one's sleeping pattern to the arrival time zone a few days prior to departure can reduce symptoms on arrival (Loat & Rhodes 1989). Sleeping well on the night prior to departure, minimizing time spent in transit with appropriate flight scheduling, and adjusting watches to the destination local time on boarding will also aid the traveler (Loat & Rhodes 1989, Young et al 1998). Either regular short sleep episodes or attempting to establish a new sleep-wake cycle in synchronization with the destination local time are both recommended, but need to be individualized (Young et al 1998). Use of relaxation techniques, ear plugs and eye shields may also assist in sleeping during and after the flight, by minimizing visual and auditory distractions (Young et al 1998). It has been suggested that following westward and eastward flights, competition be arranged in the morning and evenings, respectively, in order to optimize performance, by taking advantage of the circadian delay. Other means of minimizing jet-lag include avoiding alcohol, regularly mobilizing in the aircraft cabin and maintaining fluid and food intake. There is some suggestion that eating a high protein breakfast and a low protein/high carbohydrate dinner following a time zone change, may assist in resynchronization (Loat & Rhodes 1989).

The use of short-acting hypnotic medication or melatonin is considered useful in achieving sleep and assisting in establishing a new circadian rhythm. Melatonin is a peptide secreted by the pineal gland, which helps to induce sleep as the eyes register dusk (Waterhouse et al 1998). While it has been shown to reduce the subjective symptoms of jet-lag when taken before and after air travel (Herxheimer & Petrie 2001, Petrie et al 1993), it must be used carefully in order not to further upset the bodies circadian rhythm (Reilly et al 1998). Reilly et al (2001) showed no benefit of using low dose Temazepam on recovery from jet-lag, following a westerly flight over five time zones. As a result of the unpredictable individual effects, and the potential for prolonged drowsiness, the British Olympic Association Medical Committee advises against the use of hypnotics or melatonin in international travel (Reilly et al 1998). Under no circumstances should hypnotic medication or melatonin be used for the first time prior to a major competition.

On arrival, the risk of infection from oral–fecal contamination or insect vectors needs to be evaluated. If the water supply is suspected of being contaminated, then only sealed, bottled water should be used for drinking and teeth washing. Similarly, salads or other foods washed in tap water, as well as ice cubes should be avoided. If concerns regarding the water supply are expressed, the general rule of 'cook it, peel it, or leave it alone' should be applied. Drink bottles should be regularly cleaned, with bottled water, especially if sports drinks are being used. A brush should be taken for this purpose. Mosquitoes transmit parasites such as malaria, as well as arboviruses causing dengue fever, yellow fever and Japanese encephalitis (Bell et al 1995). While the Anopheline mosquitoes carrying malaria and the Aedes mosquitoes carrying dengue fever bite during the dusk and daylight hours respectively, similar preventative measures can be used. Use of light-colored, long-sleeved clothing, insect repellents and sleeping in nets is recommended in high-risk areas. Anti-malarial prophylactic medication requirements vary depending on the location and duration of stay, as well as an individuals' medical history, and should be discussed with a medical practitioner prior to departure.

Hot and humid climates place thermal demands on athletes, which require time to adapt. Acclimatization to heat may take up to two weeks, and until achieved may impair performance. If traveling to a particularly hot environment, it is recommended that at least two weeks be allowed for optimal acclimatization prior to competing. Training volume and intensity should be reduced on arrival, gradually increasing over two weeks, with training initially being performed at the coolest part of the day and progressively introducing the heat (Young et al 1998). Fluid intake should be increased during rest and activity, and both body weight and urine volume can be used to monitor fluid replacement. Light colored, loose fitting clothing and sunblock should be worn in order to minimize the risks of heat illness, and maximize the likelihood of successful performance. If traveling from sea level to compete at altitude, a similar period of acclimatization may be required. The alternative is to travel and compete within 24 hours of arrival.

Infections in athletes

Infectious conditions are common both in athletes and non-athletes. Upper respiratory tract, chest and generalized viral infections are the most common infection presentations to an elite sports medicine center (Fricker 1997). It has been shown that even a mild respiratory infection within six weeks of a major competition can have a significant impact on the competition outcome (Pyne et al 2000b). For this reason, it is important that athletes and support staff have an understanding of those infections to which athletes may be particularly susceptible.

Upper respiratory tract infections

While research suggests that well conditioned elite athletes may be at no greater risk of upper respiratory tract infections (URTI) than the general public (Fricker et al 2000), there is mounting evidence that transient alterations in the body's immune system as a result of intensive training, may predispose some athletes to infection (Gleeson 2000). Endurance athletes in particular may be at an increased risk of developing URTI during periods of heavy training and for 7–14 days after racing (Nieman 2000). While URTIs are commonly either viral or bacterial in origin, up to 80% are considered to be viral. Causative agents include the adenovirus, coxsackie virus, rhinovirus, coronavirus and others. Sore throat, conjunctivitis, headache, hoarseness, malaise and fever are the most common presenting symptoms. Management of the viral URTI is predominantly symptomatic including lozenges, paracetamol to control fevers, fluids to maintain hydration and relative rest. There is some evidence that zinc may reduce the duration of symptoms (Mossad et al 1996) and it is common practice to use a short course of high dose vitamin C (500 mg–1 g) for its antioxidant properties. The physician must however be aware of the interaction between vitamin C and the oral contraceptive, when used in this manner.

Epstein-Barr virus (EBV), the causative organism in glandular fever (infectious mononucleosis) in the young athlete, often presents with a thick exudative pharyngitis, lymphadenopathy, fever and malaise. Serology will allow confirmation of an acute infection and treatment is then supportive. EBV can result in a number of significant complications, including splenomegaly, which needs to be excluded before return to contact sport is permitted (Waninger & Harcke 2005). Should splenomegaly be detected clinically or on ultrasound investigation, contact sport is contraindicated for four weeks, or until the swelling is reduced, in order to prevent the theoretical risk of rupture (Young 1999).

Bacterial URTIs commonly present with an exudative tonsillitis and cervical lymphadenopathy, which require treatment with appropriate antibiotic medication. Many over-the-counter decongestants and mucolytic agents contain substances that are subject to restrictions or monitoring by the World Anti-Doping Agency (WADA). It is advisable for the treating physician to familiarize themselves with drugs listed in the current WADA code, as this list is reviewed annually (www.wada-ama.org).

Return to sport guidelines should be individualized. General principles are that if the illness is limited to the head, then it is acceptable to continue with moderate training, until symptoms have resolved. However, if there are generalized symptoms of fever, tachycardia, malaise, lymphadenopathy and fatigue, then all training should cease until symptoms have disappeared (Nieman 1993, Young 1998). The aim of this is to minimize the risk of complications such as myocarditis and post viral fatigue which may complicate an otherwise simple respiratory infection. Should fatigue persist following an URTI, it is recommended that exercise be very gradually resumed with light aerobic exercise at an intensity less than 65% of maximum heart rate. Subsequently, the frequency, duration and finally the intensity of exercise may be sequentially and gradually increased (Young 1999).

Blood-borne pathogens

The transmission of blood-borne viruses such as human immunodeficiency virus (HIV), hepatitis B (HBV) and hepatitis C (HCV) has been a major concern to sports people and support staff in recent years. Despite the high degree of public concern there has only been one reported case of HIV transmission as a result of a sporting injury (Torre et al 1990), and even this case is considered dubious (Mast et al 1995).

The concentration of HBV in blood is higher than that of HIV and it is more stable outside of the bloodstream, but there are still only limited examples of HBV transmission as a result of sports participation (AMSSM & AASM 1995, Kashiwagi et al 1982, Kordi & Wallace 2004). However, limited outbreaks have been recorded in a university American football team (Tobe et al 2000) and among Swedish cross country track finders (Ringertz & Zetterberg 1967) through open wounds sustained in both sports. Transmission in the sporting arena is most likely to occur when two open wounds are opposed, allowing direct contact between the blood of seropositive and seronegative individuals. Despite a relatively high incidence of bleeding wounds being documented in professional football of varying codes, the risk of HIV transmission has been estimated by various researchers to be 1 per 43 million games (range 1–85 million) (Kordi & Wallace 2004) whilst the corresponding figures for HBV range from 1 transmission every 10 000 games to 1 every 4.25 million games (Kordi & Wallace 2004). There are no known cases of HIV being transmitted via sweat or saliva (Feller & Flanigan 1997, 2000). Indeed, it is thought that off the field behavior of athletes may place them at greater risk of infection than bleeding episodes on the field (Feller & Flanigan 1997, Rich et al 1998). In 1995, the American Medical Society for Sports Medicine and the American Academy of Sports Medicine, in a joint position statement, outlined some specific preventative measures (AMSSM & AASM 1995) (Box 31.5). It is vital that medical practitioners and sports trainers are proactive in ensuring that sporting clubs with which they work employ these recommendations, in order to minimize risk of transmission of blood borne pathogens.

Box 31.5 Specific measures to prevent the transmission of blood borne pathogens (data from American Medical Society for Sports Medicine and American Academy of Sports Medicine (AMSSM & AASM 1995), with the permission of the American Journal of Sports Medicine)

- Pre-event dressing of all open wounds with occlusive dressings.
- Use of gloves, disinfectant, bleach, antiseptic, for washing/cleaning surfaces and clothing.
- Receptacles for contaminated clothing, bandages, dressing, needles, must be available on the side of the field of play and in the dressing rooms.
- Removal of players from play if active bleeding is present.
- Control of bleeding, covering of wound with occlusive dressing and change of blood stained clothing prior to return to play.
- Wearing of adequate, appropriate protective equipment by players.
- Athlete education and empowerment with responsibility to report wounds.
- Caregiver precautions including the using and changing of gloves between contacts.
- Covering of minor cuts and abrasions while on the field.
- Airway devices should be available for use in case of life threatening emergencies.
- Contaminated areas (e.g. mats) should be wiped down immediately and disinfected with bleach. The area should be dry before being re-used.
- Postevent, wounds should be reviewed and redressed.
- Soiled clothing and towels should be washed separately.
- All personnel involved in coaching and support of a team should be trained in basic first-aid

Cutaneous infections

Herpes simplex virus (HSV) is a commonly transmitted cutaneous infection in contact sports (Mast & Goodman 1997, Stacey & Atkins 2000). Transmission occurs via direct contact between infectious lesions or secretions, and broken skin. It is estimated that up to 15% of the population may be excreting HSV at any given time. HSV lesions manifest as painful vesicles that rapidly increase in number and ulcerate. Oral and topical antiviral agents are now available to treat HSV; however, once infected the virus may remain deactivated in the sensory nerve ganglion awaiting an opportunity to reappear. Players with active herpetic lesions should be prohibited from returning to play until the lesions are fully resolved (Stacey & Atkins 2000).

Streptococcal and staphylococcal bacterial outbreaks in sports teams have also been reported (Mast & Goodman 1997, Stacey & Atkins 2000). Direct contact with a discharging skin lesion or contact with an asymptomatic nasal carrier may result in vesicular, bullous or pustular skin lesions. Athletes in contact sports with bacterial skin lesions, which cannot be adequately covered, should be prohibited from play.

The warm, moist environment of the feet and groin, combined with constant friction in these areas predisposes athletes to fungal infections. These can be transmitted by direct contact or via infected skin scales in dressing rooms. Use of topical anti-fungal medication and using footwear in communal showers will help prevent the transmission of foot infections.

Summary

Unlike many common musculoskeletal problems encountered by physical therapists and physicians, medical problems in the sporting environment often create a great deal of anxiety. This chapter provided a detailed account of a select number of significant medical issues commonly encountered by a team medical or paramedical officer. A common theme throughout all the sections of this chapter has been 'if in doubt, refer on'. It is the authors' opinion that no one has ever had a sleepless night over, or had to defend, a decision to seek another opinion. Indeed the over-riding principle we should follow is 'first do no harm'.

Asthma attacks, epileptic seizures, concussive episodes and spinal cord injuries are all acute, serious conditions that physical therapists and athletic trainers can expect to encounter while working with a sporting team. The background and management of these conditions has been outlined in detail, but the initial management is very similar in each. The principles of safety, airways, breathing and circulation, followed by stabilization and transportation to an appropriate referral center are universal to these conditions. Thus, it is important that attendants are knowledgeable in cardiopulmonary resuscitation. Similarly, the nearest hospital to the sporting venue, and emergency phone numbers are mandatory knowledge.

Diabetes is a condition associated with a huge morbidity. Exercise has been shown to benefit the diabetic in a number of ways. With adequate preparation and support there is no reason why a diabetic athlete cannot compete at the top level in any number of sports. As medical professionals we should endeavor to expedite this through our association with sporting bodies.

Overtraining is a condition which is much easier to prevent than treat, and early recognition is critical in its management. The medical professional working with a team can play a pivotal role in preventing the development of this condition. The transmission of infection within the sporting environment is an area of increasing concern in the community. It is the responsibility of sporting organizations to provide a safe environment for athletes, and it is the role of the medical and paramedical professional to ensure that recommendations are instigated.

References

Albright A, Franz M, Hornsby G et al 2000 American College of Sports Medicine position stand. Exercise and type 2 diabetes. Medicine and Science in Sports and Exercise 32:1345–1360

AMSSM, AASM 1995 Human immunodeficiency virus (HIV) and other blood-borne pathogens in sports. Joint position statement. American Medical Society for Sports Medicine (AMSSM) and American Academy of Sports Medicine (AASM). American Journal of Sports Medicine 23:510–514

Anderson S, Daviskas E 2000 The mechanism of exercise-induced asthma is. . . Journal of Allergy and Clinical Immunology 106:453–459

Anderson S D, Holzer K 2000 Exercise-induced asthma: is it the right diagnosis in elite athletes? Journal of Allergy and Clinical Immunology 106:419–428

Asthma Management Handbook 2002 National Asthma Council of Australia

Atkinson G, Reilly T 1996 Circadian variation in sports performance. Sports Medicine 21:292–312

Aubry M R C, Cantu R, Dvorak J et al 2002 Summary and agreement statement of the First International Conference on Concussion in Sport, Vienna 2001. Recommendations for the improvement of safety and health of athletes who may suffer concussive injuries. British Journal of Sports Medicine 36:6–10

Basilico F C 1999 Cardiovascular disease in athletes. American Journal of Sports Medicine 27:108–121

Beck K C 1999 Control of airway function during and after exercise in asthmatics. Medicine and Science in Sports and Exercise 31:S4–S11

Bell D, Gilks C, Molyneux M et al 1995 Lecture notes on tropical medicine, 4th edn. Blackwell Sciences, Oxford

Brukner P 1996 Sports medicine. The tired athlete. Australian Family Physician 25:1283–1288

Brukner P, Khan K 1993 Clinical sports medicine 1. McGraw Hill, Roseville, Australia

Budgett R E, Newsholme E, Lehmann M et al 2000 Redefining the overtraining syndrome as the unexplained underperformance syndrome. British Journal of Sports Medicine 34:67–68

Campbell L V, Graham A R, Kidd R M et al 2000 The lower limb in people with diabetes. Position statement of the Australian Diabetes Society. Medical Journal of Australia 173:369–372

Cantu R C 1997 Stingers, transient quadriplegia, and cervical spinal stenosis: return to play criteria. Medicine and Science in Sports and Exercise 29:S233–S235

Cantu R C 1998a Epilepsy and athletics. Clinical Sports Medicine 17:61–69

Cantu R C 1998b Second-impact syndrome. Clinical Journal of Sports Medicine 17:37–44

Cantu R C 1998c Return to play guidelines after a head injury. Clinics in Sports Medicine 17:45–60

Colman P G, Thomas D W, Zimmet P Z et al 1999 New classification and criteria for diagnosis of diabetes mellitus. Position Statement from the Australian Diabetes Society, New Zealand Society for the Study of Diabetes, Royal College of Pathologists of Australasia and Australasian Association of Clinical Biochemists. Medical Journal of Australia 170:375–378

Constance A, Clure C 1996 Diabetes and exercise. A guide for health professionals, vol 2001, UP Diabetes Outreach Network. www.diabetesliving.com/manage/aguide.htm

Corrado D, Pelliccia A, Bjornstad H H et al 2005 Cardiovascular pre-participation screening of young competitive athletes for prevention of sudden death: proposal for a common European protocol. European Heart Journal 26:516–524

Costill D L, Flynn M G, Kirwan J P et al 1988 Effects of repeated days of intensified training on muscle glycogen and swimming performance. Medicine and Science in Sports and Exercise 20:249–254.

Crimi E, Milanese M, Oddera S et al 2001 Inflammatory and mechanical factors of allergen-induced bronchoconstriction in mild asthma and rhinitis. Journal of Applied Physiology 91:1029–1034

Deal E C Jr, McFadden E R Jr, Ingram R H Jr et al 1979 Esophageal temperature during exercise in asthmatic and nonasthmatic subjects. Journal of Applied Physiology 46:484–490

Diabetes Control and Complications Trial Research Group 1993 The effect of intensive treatment of diabetes on the development and progression of long-term complications in insulin-dependent diabetes mellitus. New England Journal of Medicine 329:977–986

Dickinson J W, Whyte G P, McConnell A K et al 2005a Impact of changes in the IOC-MC asthma criteria: a British perspective. Thorax 60:629–632

Dickinson J W, Whyte G P, McConnell A K et al 2005b Mid-expiratory flow versus FEV1 measurements in the diagnosis of exercise induced asthma in elite athletes. Thorax 61:111–114

Dickinson J W, Whyte G P, McConnell A K et al 2006 Screening elite winter athletes for exercise induced asthma: a comparison of three challenge methods. British Journal of Sports Medicine 40:179–183

Di Loreto C, Fanelli C, Lucidi P et al 2005 Make your diabetic patients walk: long-term impact of different amounts of physical activity on type 2 diabetes. Diabetes Care 28:1295–1302

Draznin M B 2000 Type 1 diabetes and sports participation. Physician and Sports Medicine 28: 49–56

Edelman J M, Turpin J A, Bronsky E A et al 2000 Oral montelukast compared with inhaled salmeterol to prevent exercise-induced bronchoconstriction. A randomized, double-blind trial. Exercise Study Group. Annals of Internal Medicine 132:97–104

Eriksson J G 1999 Exercise and the treatment of type 2 diabetes mellitus. An update. Sports Medicine 27:381–391

Fallon K 1997 Neurology. In: Fields K, Fricker P (eds) Medical problems in athletes. Blackwell Science, Boston, MA

Feller A, Flanigan T P 1997 HIV-infected competitive athletes. What are the risks? What precautions should be taken? Journal of General Internal Medicine 12:243–246

Feller A A, Flanigan T P 2000 HIV, infectious diseases, and competitive athletics. Medicine and Health, Rhode Island 83:56–59.

Fields K, Reimer C 1997 Pulmonary problems in athletes. In: K Fields, P Fricker (eds) Medical problems in athletes. Blackwell Science, Boston, MA

Finch C F, McIntosh A S, McCrory P 2001 What do under 15 year old schoolboy rugby union players think about protective headgear? British Journal of Sports Medicine 35:89–94

Fricker P 1997 Infectious problems in athletes: an overview. In: Fields K, Fricker P (eds) Medical problems in athletes. Blackwell Science, Boston, MA

Fricker P, Gleeson M, Flanagan A et al 2000 A clinical snapshot: do elite swimmers experience more upper respiratory illness than non-athletes? Clinical Exercise Physiology 2:155–158

Fry R W, Morton A R, Keast D 1991 Overtraining in athletes. An update. Sports Medicine 12:32–65

Fuller C M, McNulty C M, Spring D A et al 1997 Prospective screening of 5,615 high school athletes for risk of sudden cardiac death. Medicine and Science in Sports and Exercise 29:1131–1138

Funk J, Feingold K 1995 Disorders of the endocrine pancreas. In: McPhee S, Lingappa V, Ganong W et al (eds), Pathophysiology of disease. An introduction to clinical medicine. Appleton and Lange, Stamford, CT

Futterman L G, Myerburg R 1998 Sudden death in athletes: an update. Sports Medicine 26:335–350

Gale E 1990 Diabetes mellitus and other disorders of metabolism. In: Kumar P J, Clark M L (eds) Clinical medicine. Baillière Tindall, London

Gates J R, Spiegel R H 1993 Epilepsy, sports and exercise. Sports Medicine 15:1–5

Gan D 2003 Diabetes atlas, 2nd edn. International Diabetes Federation

Gavett S H, Koren H S 2001 The role of particulate matter in exacerbation of atopic asthma. International Archives of Allergy and Immunology 124:109–112

Gleeson M 2000 Mucosal immunity and respiratory illness in elite athletes. International Journal of Sports Medicine 21:S33–S43

Gorman D 1993 Fitness for diving. In: Gorman D (ed), Diving and hyperbaric medicine: course notes. Royal Adelaide Hospital Hyperbaric Medicine Unit, Adelaide

Grindel S H, Lovell M R, Collins M W 2001 The assessment of sport-related concussion: the evidence behind neuropsychological testing and management. Clinical Journal of Sports Medicine 11:134–143.

Hancock K 2001 Management issues in adult asthma. Australian Family Physician 30:114–119

Hazel J 1994 Australian Diabetes Society position statements: scuba diving. Australian Diabetes Society, Sydney

Hedelin R, Kentta G, Wiklund U et al 2000 Short-term overtraining: effects on performance, circulatory responses, and heart rate variability. Medicine and Science in Sports and Exercise 32:1480–1484

Helenius I J, Tikkanen H O, Sarna S et al 1998 Asthma and increased bronchial responsiveness in elite athletes: atopy and sport event as risk factors. Journal of Allergy and Clinical Immunology 101:646–652

Hernandez J M, Moccia T, Fluckey J D et al 2000 Fluid snacks to help persons with type 1 diabetes avoid late onset postexercise hypoglycemia. Medicine and Science in Sports and Exercise 32:904–910

Herxheimer A, Petrie K J 2001 Melatonin for preventing and treating jet lag (Cochrane Review). Cochrane Database of Systematic Reviews 1: CD001520

Hickey J C, Morris A L, Carlson L D et al 1967 The relation of mouth protectors to cranial pressure and deformation. Journal of the American Dental Association 74:735–740

Holly R G, Shaffrath J D, Amsterdam E A 1998 Electrocardiographic alterations associated with the hearts of athletes. Sports Medicine 25:139–148

Huston T P, Puffer J C, Rodney W M 1985 The athletic heart syndrome. New England Journal of Medicine 313:24–32

Jensen-Urstad M 1995 Sudden death and physical activity in athletes and nonathletes. Scandinavian Journal of Medicine and Science in Sports 5:279–284

International Olympic Committee Medical Commission 2004 Sudden cardiovascular death in sport. Lausanne recommendations. IOC Medical Committee, Lausanne

Johnston K, Barootes B, Barwitzki G et al 2000 Guidelines for assessment and management of sport-related concussion. Canadian Academy of Sport Medicine Concussion Committee. Clinical Journal of Sport Medicine 10:209–211

Johnston K M, McCrory P, Mohtadi N G et al 2001 Evidence-based review of sport-related concussion: clinical science. Clinical Journal of Sports Medicine 11:150–159

Kashiwagi S, Hayashi J, Ikematsu H et al 1982 An outbreak of hepatitis B in members of a high school sumo wrestling club. Journal of the American Medical Association 248:213–214

Kemp J P 2000 Leukotriene receptor antagonists for the treatment of asthma. Drugs 3:430–441

Kerr I L 1986 Mouth guards for the prevention of injuries in contact sports. Sports Medicine 3:415–427

Kingsbury K J, Kay L, Hjelm M 1998 Contrasting plasma free amino acid patterns in elite athletes: association with fatigue and infection. British Journal of Sports Medicine 32:25–32.

Knopfli B, Bar-Or O, Araujo C G et al 2005 Effect of ipratropium bromide on EIB in children depends on vagal activity. Medicine and Science in Sports and Exercise 37:354–359.

Koivisto V A, Felig P 1978 Effects of leg exercise on insulin absorption in diabetic patients. New England Journal of Medicine 298:79–83

Kordi R, Wallace W A 2004 Blood borne infections in sport: risks of transmission, methods of prevention, and recommendations for hepatitis B vaccination. British Journal of Sports Medicine 38:678–684

Kuipers H, Keizer H A 1988 Overtraining in elite athletes. Review and directions for the future. Sports Medicine 6:79–92

Lacroix V 1999 Exercise induced asthma. Physician and Sportsmedicine 27(12):75–92

Lehmann M, Foster C, Dickhuth H H et al 1998 Autonomic imbalance hypothesis and overtraining syndrome. Medicine and Science in Sports and Exercise 30:1140–1145

Loat C E, Rhodes E C 1989 Jet-lag and human performance. Sports Medicine 8:226–238

McCrea M, Kelly J, Kluge J et al 1997 Standardized assessment of concussion in football players. Neurology 48:586–588

McCrea M, Kelly J, Randolph C et al 1998 Standardized assessment of concussion (SAC): on-site mental status evaluation of the athlete. Journal of Head Trauma and Rehabilitation 13:27–35

McCrory P R 1997 Were you knocked out? A team physician's approach to initial concussion management. Medicine and Science in Sports and Exercise 29:S207–S212

McCrory P 1999 The eighth wonder of the world: the mythology of concussion management. British Journal of Sports Medicine 33:136–137

McCrory P 2001a Do mouthguards prevent concussion? British Journal of Sports Medicine 35:81–82

McCrory P 2001b Does second impact syndrome exist? Clinical Journal of Sports Medicine 11:144–149

McCrory P R, Berkovic S F 1998a Second impact syndrome. Neurology 50:677–683

McCrory P R, Berkovic S F 1998b Concussive convulsions. Incidence in sport and treatment recommendations. Sports Medicine 25:131–136

McCrory P, Johnson J, Meeuwisse W et al 2005 Summary and agreement statement of the 2nd International Conference on Concussion in Sport, Prague 2004. British Journal of Sports Medicine 39:196–204

McFadden E 1991 Asthma. In: Wilson J, Braunwald E, Isselbacher K et al (eds), Harrison's principles of internal medicine, vol 2. McGraw Hill, New York

McIntosh A S, McCrory P 2000 Impact energy attenuation performance of football headgear. British Journal of Sports Medicine 34:337–341

McIntosh A S, McCrory P, Comerford J 2000 The dynamics of concussive head impacts in rugby and Australian rules football. Medicine and Science in Sports and Exercise 32:1980–1984

Mackinnon L T 2000 Special feature for the Olympics: effects of exercise on the immune system: overtraining effects on immunity and performance in athletes. Immunology and Cell Biology 78:502–509

McLatchie G, Lloyd-Parry J 1997 Injuries to the neck and spine. Sports Exercise and Injury 3:183–190

McLaughlin D 1999 Epilepsy: key management issues. Australian Family Physician 28:889–896

Maddocks D L, Dicker G D, Saling M M 1995 The assessment of orientation following concussion in athletes. Clinical Journal of Sport Medicine 5:32–35

Marion D W, Domeier R, Dunham C M et al. 2000. Determination of cervical spine stability in trauma patients. Eastern Association for the Surgery of Trauma. www.east.org/tpg/chap3u.pdf

Maron B J 2002 Hypertrophic cardiomyopathy: a systematic review. Journal of the American Medical Association 287:1308–1320

Maron B J 2003 Sudden death in young athletes. New England Journal of Medicine 349:1064–1075

Maron B J 2005 How should we screen competitive athletes for cardiovascular disease? European Heart Journal 26:428–430

Maron B J, Mitchell J H 1994 Revised eligibility recommendations for competitive athletes with cardiovascular abnormalities. Journal of the American College of Cardiology 24:848–850

Maron B J, Shirani J, Poliac L C et al 1996a Sudden death in young competitive athletes. Clinical, demographic, and pathological profiles. Journal of the American Medical Association 276:199–204

Maron B J, Thompson P D, Puffer J C et al 1996b Cardiovascular preparticipation screening of competitive athletes. A statement for health professionals from the Sudden Death Committee (clinical cardiology) and Congenital Cardiac Defects Committee (cardiovascular disease in the young), American Heart Association. Circulation 94:850–856

Maron B J, Thompson P D, Puffer J C et al 1998 Cardiovascular preparticipation screening of competitive athletes: addendum: an addendum to a statement for health professionals from the Sudden Death Committee (Council on Clinical Cardiology) and the Congenital Cardiac Defects Committee (Council on Cardiovascular Disease in the Young), American Heart Association. Circulation 97:2294

Mast E E, Goodman R A 1997 Prevention of infectious disease transmission in sports. Sports Medicine 24:1–7

Mast E E, Goodman R A, Bond W W et al 1995 Transmission of bloodborne pathogens during sports: risk and prevention. Annals of Internal Medicine 122:283–285

Mickleborough T D, Lindley M R, Ray S et al 2005 Dietary salt, airway inflammation, and diffusion capacity in exercise-induced asthma. Medicine and Science in Sports and Exercise 37:904–914

Miller M G, Weiler J M, Baker R et al 2005 National athletic trainers' association position statement: management of asthma in athletes. Journal of Athletic Training 40:224–245

Mills J D, Moore G E, Thompson P D 1997 The athlete's heart. Clinical Journal of Sports Medicine 16:725–737

Moeller J 1996 Contraindications to athletic participation: cardiac, respiratory, and central nervous system conditions. Physician and Sportsmedicine 24:47–49, 53–54, 55–58

Morgan W P, Costill D L, Flynn M G et al 1988 Mood disturbance following increased training in swimmers. Medicine and Science in Sports and Exercise 20:408–414

Mossad S B, Macknin M L, Medendorp S V et al 1996 Zinc gluconate lozenges for treating the common cold. A randomized, double-blind, placebo-controlled study. Annals of Internal Medicine 125:81–88

Nakken K O 1999 Physical exercise in outpatients with epilepsy. Epilepsia 40:643–651

Newcombe R, Reid R, Smethills R et al Eds 1995 Head and neck injuries in football. Guidelines for prevention and management. Australian Government Publishing Service, Canberra

Nieman D 1993 Exercise and upper respiratory tract infection. Sports Medicine, Training and Rehabilitation 4:1–14

Nieman D C 2000 Is infection risk linked to exercise workload? Medicine and Science in Sports and Exercise 32 (7 suppl):S406–S411

Nieman D C, Henson D A, Sampson C S et al 1995 The acute immune response to exhaustive resistance exercise. International Journal of Sports Medicine 16:322–328

Oswald D, Dvorak J, Corrado et al 2004 Sudden cardiovascular death in sport. Lausanne recommendations. International Olympic Committee Medical Commission, Lausanne

Paffenbarger R S Jr, Hyde R T, Wing A L et al 1986 Physical activity, all-cause mortality, and longevity of college alumni. New England Journal of Medicine 314:605–613

Pan X R, Li G W, Hu Y H et al 1997 Effects of diet and exercise in preventing NIDDM in people with impaired glucose tolerance. The Da Qing IGT and Diabetes Study. Diabetes Care 20:537–544

Pelliccia A, Maron B J, Spataro A et al 1991 The upper limit of physiologic cardiac hypertrophy in highly trained elite athletes. New England Journal of Medicine 324:295–301

Perlstein R, McConell K, Hagger V 1997 Off to a flying start . . . insulin dependent diabetes and exercise. Everything you need to know. International Diabetes Institute, Caulfield, Victoria, Australia

Petrie K, Dawson A G, Thompson L et al 1993 A double-blind trial of melatonin as a treatment for jet lag in international cabin crew. Biological Psychiatry 33:526–530

Pierce NS 1999 Diabetes and exercise. British Journal of Sports Medicine 33:161–173

Provost-Craig M A, Arbour K S, Sestili D C et al 1996 The incidence of exercise-induced bronchospasm in competitive figure skaters. Journal of Asthma 33:67–71

Pyne D B, Gleeson M, McDonald W A et al 2000a Training strategies to maintain immunocompetence in athletes. International Journal of Sports Medicine 21:S51–S60

Pyne D B, McDonald W A, Gleeson M et al 2000b Mucosal immunity, respiratory illness, and competitive performance in elite swimmers. Medicine and Science in Sports and Exercise 33:348–353

Quinn D, Markus, R, Day R 2001 Antiepileptic therapy. Current Therapeutics 39:23–39

Reilly T, Maughan R, Budgett R 1998 Melatonin: a position statement of the British Olympic Association. British Journal of Sports Medicine 32:99–100

Reilly T, Atkinson G, Budgett R 2001 Effect of low-dose temazepam on physiological variables and performance tests following a westerly flight across five time zones. International Journal of Sports Medicine 22:166–174

Rich J D, Dickinson B P, Merriman N A et al 1998 Hepatitis C virus infection related to anabolic-androgenic steroid injection in a recreational weight lifter. American Journal of Gastroenterology 93:1598

Ringertz O, Zetterberg B 1967 Serum hepatitis among Swedish track finders. An epidemiologic study. New England Journal of Medicine 276:540–546

Rotem T, Lawson J S, Wilson S F et al 1998 Severe cervical spinal cord injuries related to rugby union and league football in New South Wales, 1984–1996. Medical Journal of Australia 168:379–381

Rundell K W, Wilber R L, Szmedra L et al 2000 Exercise-induced asthma screening of elite athletes: field versus laboratory exercise challenge. Medicine and Science in Sports and Exercise 32:309–316

Seward H G, Orchard J W, Hazard H et al 1993 Football injuries in Australia at the elite level. Medical Journal of Australia 159:298–301

Sharma S, Whyte G, McKenna W J et al 1997 Sudden death from cardiovascular disease in young athletes: fact or fiction? British Journal of Sports Medicine 31:269–276

Sirven J, Varrato J 1999 Physical activity and epilepsy. What are the rules? Physician and Sportsmedicine 27:63–64, 67–70

Smith D J, Norris S R 2000 Changes in glutamine and glutamate concentrations for tracking training tolerance. Medicine and Science in Sports and Exercise 32:684–689.

Smith L L 2000 Cytokine hypothesis of overtraining: a physiological adaptation to excessive stress? Medicine and Science in Sports and Exercise 32:317–331

Snyder A C 1998 Overtraining and glycogen depletion hypothesis. Medicine and Science in Sports and Exercise 30:1146–1150

Spiegel R, Gates J 1997 Epilepsy. In: Wikgren S (ed), ACSM's exercise management for persons with chronic diseases and disabilities. Human Kinetics, Champaign, IL

Spooner C, Rowe B H, Saunders L D 2000 Nedocromil sodium in the treatment of exercise-induced asthma: A meta-analysis. European Respiratory Journal 16:30–37

Stacey A, Atkins B 2000 Infectious diseases in rugby players: incidence, treatment and prevention. Sports Medicine 29:211–220

Steinbrook R 2006 Facing the diabetes epidemic – mandatory reporting of glycosylated hemoglobin values in New York City. New England Journal of Medicine 354:545–548

Stolt A, Kujala U M, Karjalainen J et al 1997 Electrocardiographic findings in female endurance athletes. Clinical Journal of Sports Medicine 7:85–89

Storms W 1999 Exercise-induced asthma: diagnosis and treatment for the recreational or elite athlete. Medicine and Science in Sports and Exercise 31:S33–S38

Tancredi G, Quattrucci S, Scalercio F et al 2004 3-min step test and treadmill exercise for evaluating exercise-induced asthma. European Respiratory Journal 23:569–574

Tang C, Rolland I M, Ward C et al 1996 Seasonal comparison of cytokine profiles in atopic asthmatics and atopic non-asthmatics. American Journal of Respiratory and Critical Care Medicine 154:1615–1622

Thien F C 1999 Leukotriene receptor antagonist drugs for asthma. Medical Journal of Australia 171:378–381

Thomas P 2001 Acute asthma. The management in the community. Australian Family Physician 30:100–105

Tobe K, Matsuura K, Ogura T et al 2000 Horizontal transmission of hepatitis B virus among players of a American football team. Archives of Internal Medicine 160:2541–2545

Torg J, Glasgow S 1991 Criteria for return to contact activities following cervical spine injury. Clinical Journal of Sports Medicine 1:12–26

Torg J, Ramsey-Emrhein J 1997 Suggested management guidelines for participation in collision activities with congenital, developmental, or postinjury lesions involving the cervical spine. Medicine and Science in Sports and Exercise 29:S256–S272

Torre D, Sampietro C, Ferraro G et al 1990 Transmission of HIV-1 infection via sports injury. Lancet 335:1105

Trost L F 3rd, Wender R C, Suter S S et al 2005 Management of epilepsy in adults. Diagnosis guidelines. Postgraduate Medicine 118:22–26

Urhausen A, Kindermann W 1999 Sports-specific adaptations and differentiation of the athlete's heart. Sports Medicine 28:237–244

van Linschoten R, Backx F J, Mulder O G et al 1990 Epilepsy and sports. Sports Medicine 10:9–19.

Waninger K N, Harcke H T 2005 Determination of safe return to play for athletes recovering from infectious mononucleosis. A review of the literature. Clinical Journal of Sports Medicine 15:410–416

Warburton D E, Nicol C W, Bredin S S 2006 Health benefits of physical activity: the evidence. Canadian Medical Association Journal 174:801–809

Warren W, Bailes J 1998a On field evaluation of athletic head injuries. Clinics in Sports Medicine 17:13–26

Warren W, Bailes J 1998b On field evaluation of athletic neck injury. Clinics in Sports Medicine 17:99–110

Waterhouse J, Reilly T, Atkinson G 1998 Melatonin and jet lag. British Journal of Sports Medicine 32:98–99

Weiler J M, Ryan E J 3rd 2000 Asthma in United States Olympic athletes who participated in the 1998 Olympic winter games. Journal of Allergy and Clinical Immunology 106:267–271

World Health Organization 2001 International Travel and Health. Vaccination requirements and health advice. World Health Organization, Geneva

Wilber R L, Rundell K W, Szmedra L et al 2000 Incidence of exercise-induced bronchospasm in Olympic winter sport athletes. Medicine and Science in Sports and Exercise 32:732–737

Williams C C, Bernhardt D T 1995 Syncope in athletes. Sports Medicine 19:223–234

Wilmore J, Costill D 1994 Physiology of sport and exercise. Human Kinetics, Champaign, IL

Young M 1998 What athletes often ask. Should I train when I have a cold and if not when can I return? British Journal of Sports Medicine 32:84

Young M 1999 How I treat: return to sport after post-viral fatigue. British Journal of Sports Medicine 33:173

Young M, Fricker P, Maughan R et al 1998 The traveling athlete: issues relating to the Commonwealth Games, Malaysia, 1998. Clinical Journal of Sports Medicine 8:130–135

Youngstedt S D, O'Connor P J 1999 The influence of air travel on athletic performance. Sports Medicine 28:197–207

Zeitoun M, Boguslaw W, Matsuzaka A et al 2004 Facial cooling enhances exercise-induced bronchoconstriction in asthmatic children. Medicine and Science in Sports and Exercise 36:767–771

Zinman B, Ruderman N, Campaigne B et al 1997 American College of Sports Medicine and American Diabetes Association joint position statement. Diabetes mellitus and exercise. Medicine and Science in Sports and Exercise 29:i–vi

Page numbers in **bold** refer to figures, tables or boxes.

A

A-band, 10
AAS *see* Anabolic androgenic steroids (AAS)
Abdominal examination, 197
Abdominal knee-ups, **156**
Abdominal organs, 43
Abductor pollicis longus (APL), 340
Abnormal foot pronation
  PFJ, 414
Abnormal impulse generating sites (AIGS), 94
Abuse injuries, 286
  diving injuries, 301–302
  shoulder, 297
  tennis injuries, 305
  throwing injuries, 300
  volleyball injuries, 304
AC *see* Alternating current (AC)
Accessory lateral collateral ligament (ALCL), 310
Accessory navicular
  children and adolescents, 472
Accessory ossicles
  children and adolescents, 472
Acclimatization, 193
ACE *see* Angiotensin converting enzyme (ACE) inhibitors
Acetabular labral tear
  children and adolescents, 466
Acetabulum
  fibrocartilaginous labrum, 373
Acetaminophen
  side effects with exercise, 491
Acetic acid
  iontophoresis, 223, **223**
Achilles peritendinous space, 32
Achilles tendinopathy
  classification, **453**
  clinical features, 452, **453**
  differential diagnosis, **453**
  eccentric exercise, 36
  rehabilitation, 452–453
  vascularity measurement, 34
Achilles tendonitis, 431
Achilles tendons, 32
  corticosteroids, 546
  insertion, 30
  Thompson's test, 199
ACI *see* Autologous chondrocyte implantation (ACI)
ACJ *see* Acromioclavicular joint (ACJ)
ACL *see* Anterior cruciate ligament (ACL)
Acromioclavicular joint (ACJ), 284
  mobilization, **293**
Acromioclavicular sprains
  children and adolescents, 474
Actin filaments, 10
Action potentials
  repeated, **13**
Active females, 499–524

Active range of motion (AROM)
  lower extremity musculotendinous injuries, 444
  shoulder injuries, 288
Activities of daily living
  lower extremity musculotendinous injuries, 444
Activities of Daily Living Scale of the Knee Outcome Survey, 212
Acute compartment syndrome, 432–433
Acute edema
  paratenon, 35
Acute fractures, 64–65
  rehabilitation, 65
Acute injuries
  children and adolescents, 466
    elbow, 476–477
    knee, 470
    shoulder and shoulder girdle, 474
    forearm, hand and wrist, 476
  team sports incidence, **238**
Acute lumbar pain evaluation, 264
Acute neck injury
  children and adolescents, 463
Acute pain, 136
Adolescents *see* Children and adolescents
Adrenaline (epinephrine), 95
Advisor
  fitness, 1–2
Aedes mosquitoes
  dengue fever, 593
Aerobic exercises, 390, **448**
  older adults guidelines, **493**
Aerobic fitness
  measurement, 163
Aerobic performance
  female athletes, 500–501
Age
  of athlete for clearance, 201
  balance, 487
  body function, 486–488
  bone, 485
  cardiovascular system, 486
  central nervous system, 485
  endurance, 486
  exercise skeletal effects, 73
  falls, 487–488
  flexibility, 487
  ligaments, 485
  maximal heart rate, 486
  mobility, 487
  muscle endurance, 487
  muscles, 485
  muscle strength, 486
  nervous system, 485
  peripheral nervous system, 485
  physiological effects, 484–485
  tendons, 485
Aggrecan, 28
Agility drills, 390–391

AIGS *see* Abnormal impulse generating sites (AIGS)
Air Carrier Access Act, 535
Air travel issues, 592–593
  disabled athletes, 535
Alar ligament test, **269**
ALCL *see* Accessory lateral collateral ligament (ALCL)
Alcohol, 554
  avoidance during NSAIDs use, 544
Alignment
  creep behavior, 47
  load-relaxation, 47
  stress fractures, 69
Allergies, 192
Alternating current (AC), 229
Amenorrhea, 195
  BMD, 510
  energy deficiency, 508
  female athletes, 503–504, 507
  stress fracture, **508**
American football
  preparticipation examination, 200
American Heart Association
  physical examination recommendations, 191, 198
American Physical Therapy Association, 2
  Clinical Research Agenda, 3–4
Amphiarthrodial symphysis pubis
  joint movement, 367
Amputee athletes, 531
Anabolic agents, 551
Anabolic androgenic steroids (AAS), 551
  side effects, **551**
Anabolic steroids, 550
Anaerobic power
  female athletes, 501
Analgesics, 542
  side effects with exercise
    non-opioid, **490**, 491
    opioid, **490**, 491
Anatomical malalignment
  children and adolescents, **460**, 461
Anconeus muscles, 311
Angina
  exercise, 494
Angiotensin converting enzyme (ACE) inhibitors
  side effects with exercise, **490**, 491
Ankle(s) *see also* Foot and ankle
  children and adolescents
    acute injuries, 470–472
    lateral sprains, 472
    ligaments, 470–471
    lateral sprains, 426–427, 472
    sprains, 427–428
      bracing, 426
Anopheline mosquitoes
  malaria, 593

Anorexia nervosa, 195
   female athletes, **504**, 504–507
   fluoxetine, 507
Anterior chest stretch on bolster, **292**
Anterior cruciate ligament (ACL)
   children and adolescents, 469
   closed-loop control mechanisms, 117–118
   drawer test, 289
   female athlete injury, **502**
      cost, 244
      etiology and mechanism, 244
      incidence, 243–244
      intervention effectiveness, 248
      neuromuscular training on high-risk
         mechanisms, 246–247, 248
      paradigm, 243–247
      potential modifiable mechanism and
         cutting techniques, 245
      potential modifiable mechanisms and
         landing techniques, 244–245
      preventive measures, 246, 248
      radiographic knee osteoarthritis, 244
      relationship of high-risk mechanism,
         245–246
      risk factors, 244
      underlying factors to high-risk
         mechanisms, 245
   grafts, 51
      comparison, **51**
   loading direction, 48
   mechanism of injury, 391
   nonoperative treatment, 391
   operative treatment, 391–392
   patella tendon autograft, 52
   postoperative training, 392–393
   reconstruction, 51
   tear, 43, 383
      children and adolescents, 469
      MRI, **565**
   testing, 385
Anterior drawer test, 289
Anterior glenohumeral subluxation, 472
Anterior hip structures
   figure-of-four position, **406**
Anterior muscle groups
   stretching, **446**
Anterior talofibular ligament (ATFL), 426
Anteroinferior test, 290
Anteromedial cortex
   tibia, calculated stresses, **64**
Anteroposterior laxity and stiffness
   knee joint, **54**
Anti-anxiety medications
   side effects with exercise, **490**
Antiarthritic medications, 542–543, 547
Anticoagulants
   for DVT, 437
Antidepressants
   side effects with exercise, **490**
Anti-estrogenic activity, 553
Antioxidant supplementation, 20
Antipsychotics
   side effects with exercise, **490**
Antiviral agents, 548
APL *see* Abductor pollicis longus (APL)
Apophyseal avulsion fracture hip/pelvis sites
   children and adolescents, **467**
Apophysitis
   children and adolescents, 470

Appendicular bone, 63
Aquatic rehabilitation
   osteoarthritis, 398
Arcuate complex
   test, 387
Arcuate ligament, 383
AROM *see* Active range of motion (AROM)
Arthometer testing, 387
Arthritis
   athlete, 396
   exercise for older adults, 494–495
Arthrodesis
   SIJ dysfunction, 372
Arthrography, 559–560
   wrist, **560**
Arthrolysis
   elbow, 335–336
Articular cartilage, 101
   aging, 485
   collagen, 102
   corticosteroids, 546
   defined, 102
   diarthrodial joints, 102
   lesion classification, **103**
   physiologic loading, 102
   polysaccharide, 101
   proteoglycans, 103
   rehabilitation principle, 107
   tensile properties, 102
Articular disk of triangular fibrocartilage tear
   ulnar wrist pain and impairment, 353–354
Aspirin, 547
Asthma, 578–579 *see also* Exercise-induced
   asthma (EIA)
ATFL *see* Anterior talofibular ligament (ATFL)
Athlete(s) *see also* Female athletes; Injured
   athletes
   age for clearance, 201
   amputees, 531
   arthritis, 396
   bacterial outbreaks, 594
   blood-borne pathogens, 594
   cerebral palsy, 529
   disabled, 525
   electrical stimulation for fracture repair,
      229
   endurance trained
      ECG, **586**
   ESWT, 230–232, **231**
      clinical evidence, 232
   groin injuries, 377–378
   HBV, 594
   HCV, 594
   heart, 586
   hip problems, 374–377
   HIV, 594
   hyperbaric oxygen, 230
   impaired muscled function treatment,
      226–228
   infections, 593–594
   international
      travel medicine, 592–593
      vaccinations, 592
   lasers, 229–230
   learning disabilities, 529–530
   motivation for returning to sport, 262
   pain tolerance, 138
   rehabilitation responsibility, 182
   return to play, 277–278

   staphylococcal bacterial outbreaks, 594
   streptococcal bacterial outbreaks, 594
   taping
      protection and rest, **349**
   tired, 590–591
   URTI, 593
   visual impairment, 530–531
   wheelchair, 532–534
Atlantoaxial motion test, **269**
Attendance at rehabilitation, 180
Attention control
   sports injury prevention, 173
Auditory system, 117
Augmented feedback, **128**
   simplification, segmentation and,
      130
Autografts, osteochondral defects, 105
Autologous chondrocyte implantation (ACI),
   105
   vs. mosaicplasty, 107
Autologous osteochondral grafting, 105
Avascular necrosis
   central wrist pain and impairment, 351
Avulsion fractures
   children and adolescents, 466–467
   thumb metacarpophalangeal joint, **478**
Axon
   arrangement, 83
   length, 82
   mechanosensitivity, 95
Axoplasm and blood flow, 88

B

Back
   inspection, **199**
Back pain
   exercise, 76, 514
   low
      children and adolescents, 462, **463**
      trunk muscle changes, **125**
   pregnancy, exercise, 514
Backstroke
   shoulder motion, 296
Balance, 426
   aging, 487
   exercises, 390
   training
      older adults, 492–493
Balance beam, **428**
Baseball players
   ITP, **325–327**
Basketball
   injuries incidence, **238**
   preparticipation examination, 200
Bench press, **157**
Bennet's fractures, 361
Benson's Relaxation Response, 183
Benzylic ester of hyaluronic acid, 106
Beta-2 agonists, 549, 552–553
   EIA, 580
Beta blockers, 554
   side effects with exercise, 490, **490**
Biceps brachii muscles, 310–311
Biceps tendon reflex, 315
Bicondylar sacroiliac joints
   joint movements, 366–367
Biglycan, 28, **29**

Biofeedback
    sports injury prevention, 173
Biopsychosocial model, 174–175
    of sport injury rehabilitation, **175**
Blocks *see also* Nerve(s), blocks
    epidural, **263**
        injection locations, **278**
    hardware, **263**
    injection locations, **278**
    selective nerve root, **263**
    SIJ, **263**
    sympathetic ganglion, **278**
Blood-borne pathogens, **594**
    athletes, 594
Blood pressure measurements
    children and adolescents, **197**
Blood supply
    axoplasm, 88
    hip joint, 374
    intrinsic
        nerve root, **85**
    tendons, 29
    wrist and hand, 338
BMD *see* Bone mineral density (BMD)
BMI *see* Body mass index (BMI)
Body composition
    athletic women, 499–500
Body function
    aging, 486
Body mass index (BMI), 195
Body-self neuromatrix, **135**
Bone(s), 59–77
    acute fractures, 64–65
    adaptation to mechanical loads, **61**
    aging, 485
    anatomy, 59
    appendicular, 63
    biomechanics, 62
    cells, 60
    clinical conditions, 64–75
    consolidation, 65
    constituents, 59
    cortical, **63**
    cortical and trabecular, 60
    exercise
        prescription, 73
        types, 74
    female athletes, 511–512
    Haversian, 60
    iliac, **366**
    imaging, 566–568
    innominate, 365
    inorganic component, 60
    lamellar, 60
    length *vs.* strength, 63
    loading, exercise prescription, 73
    macroscopic and microscopic appearance, 60
    mass, **507**
        DXA, 62
    material properties, 62
    mechanotransduction, 60–61
    mineral mass, 62
    modeling and remodeling, 61
    organic matrix, 59
    physical activity generating load, 63
    physiology, 60
    PT, 59–81
    response to local mechanical loading, 64
    scan, 560, **561**

stress fractures, 67, **67**
strain cycles, 64
strain distribution, 64
strain magnitude, 64
strain rate, 64
strength, exercise, 74
stress–strain curve, **63**
structural properties, 62
subchondral
    PFJ, 404–405
union, 65
union and consolidation times, **65**
whole body scan, **568**
Bone mineral density (BMD), 70, 71, 507
    amenorrhea, 510
    calcitonin, 512
    changes with age, **71**
    densitometry, 561
    measurement, 71
    medroxyprogesterone, 511
Bone–patellar tendon–bone allograft, 51
Bone–tendon junction, 29
Bony material
    shear stress distribution, **63**
Box jumps, 159
Brachialis muscles, 310–311
Brachioradialis muscles, 310–311
Bracing
    ankle sprain, 426
    stress fractures, 69
Breaststroke
    shoulder motion, 297
Bronchospasm
    exercise-induced, 194
Buckle-type force transducer, 13
Bulbous proteoglycan, 28
Bulimia nervosa, 195
    desipramine, 507
    female athletes, **504**, 504–506
    fluoxetine, 507
    imipramine, 507
Bump test, 432
Burners, 271–272
Bursitis, 375
Butterfly stroke
    shoulder motion, 296

C

Caffeine, 553
Calcaneal fat pad, 423
Calcaneonavicular coalition, **474**
Calcific tendinopathy, 35
Calcific tendonitis
    ESWT, 232
Calcified cartilage
    matrix composition and organization, 102
    zone, 102
Calcitonin
    BMD, 512
Calcitonin gene-related peptide (CGRP)
    nerves, 34
Calcium, 60
Calculated stresses
    tibia anteromedial cortex, **64**
Calpain, 19
Cannabinoids, 554
Capitellar osteochondritis dissecans, 475
Capsuloligamentous structures

elbow, 309–310
Carbohydrates
    requirements before exercise, **588**
Cardiac disease, 204, 585–587
    exercise
        older adults, 494
Cardiac history, 193
Cardiac muscles, 9
Cardiac output (CO), 163–164
Cardiovascular endurance training, 163–164
Cardiovascular system
    aging, 486
Carditis, 204
Carpal tunnel
    nerve and tendon gliding exercises, 95
Carpal tunnel syndrome (CTS), 338, 340–341,
        351–352
Carpometacarpal (CMC) joints, 340
    first grind for degenerative joint disease, **348**
Cartilage, 100–108 *see also* Articular cartilage
    anatomy, 100–101
    biomechanics, 102
    calcified
        matrix composition and organization, 102
        zone, 102
    chondroitin sulfate, 101
    conservative treatment, 106
    defects
        CPM, 104
        reconstructive techniques, 104–105
        regenerative techniques, 105
        reparative techniques, 104
    external load, 102
    functional properties, 100
    future development, 108
    glycosaminoglycans, 101
    growth, 461
    healing, 103
    imaging, 570
    keratan sulfate, 101
    lesions classification, 102–103
    maturation process biological phases, 107
    noncollagenous proteins, 101
    patellofemoral joint (PFJ), 404
    proteoglycans, 101
    rehabilitation, 107
    surgical procedure, 107–108
    treatment, 104–105
    type II collagen, 101
    water rehabilitation exercises, 107
Cartilaginous lesion
    morphological classifications, 103
    pathogenic cause classification, 103
Cathepsin
    lysomal, 19
Cathine, 553
CBSM *see* Cognitive behavioral stress
        management (CBSM)
Celecoxib, **543**, 545
Central nervous system
    aging, 485
    movement coordination, 115
    neurogenic pain, 95
    strategies, 116–120
Central pattern generators (CPG), 118
Central tendency, 217
Central wrist pain and impairment, 350–352
    algorithmic differential diagnosis and
        treatment, **343**

Central wrist pain and impairment (*contd.*)
avascular necrosis, 351
degenerative, 350
instability, 350–351
nerve compression, 351–352
synovitis, 351
tendonitis, 351–352
Cerebral palsy
athletes, 529
Cervical manipulation, 274
Cervical spine injury, 271–272, 584–585
Cervical spine tests, **269**
Cervicobrachial pain
neurodynamics, 95
C fibers
unmyelinated, 134
CGRP *see* Calcitonin gene-related peptide
(CGRP) nerves
Children and adolescents, 459–479 *see also*
Age
accessory navicular, 472
accessory ossicles, 472
acetabular labral tear, 466
ACL tears, 469
acromioclavicular sprains, 474
activity, **460**
acute injuries, 466
elbow, 475–476
acute neck injury, 463
anatomical malalignment, **460**, 461
ankles
acute injuries, 470–472
lateral sprains, 472
ligaments, 470–472
apophyseal avulsion fracture hip/pelvis
sites, **467**
apophysitis, 470
avulsion fractures, 466–467
blood pressure measurements, **197**
clavicle shaft fractures, 475
contusions, 466
coracoid fractures, **475**
diskoid lateral meniscus, 469
dislocations, 467
posterior hip, **467**
elbow, 475–476
overuse injuries, 475–476
endurance training, 165
FAI, 466
foot and ankle, 470–472
overuse injuries, 470–470
footwear, **460**
forearm, hand and wrist, 476–477
fractures, 467, 469–470
genetics, **460**, 461
growth, **460**
growth and maturation, 462
impingement, 472
joint laxity, 462
knee, 467–469
knee acute injuries, 469
knee ligament injuries, 469
low back pain, 462, **463**
meniscal injuries, 469
muscle strains, 466
musculotendinous imbalance, **460**, 461
os trigonum, 472
overuse injuries, 466, 467–468, 472–474
shoulder and shoulder girdle, 472–474

posterior hip dislocation, **467**
preparticipation examination, 196
prevention, 461
rehabilitation, 462
RICE, 462
risk factors, 460, **460**
sciatica, 465
shoulder and shoulder girdle, 472–474
shoulder dislocation and subluxation,
472–474
slipped capital femoral epiphysis, **465**,
465–466
snapping hip, 466
spine, 462–467
sternoclavicular separation, 474
stress fractures, 470
tarsal coalitions, 472
tendinitis, 470
traction apophysitis, 468
training errors, **460**
twisting injuries, 469
Cholesterol
high-density lipoprotein, 165
Chondrocytes
autologous transplantation, 105, 107
second-generation autologous
transplantation, 106, **106**
Chondroitin sulfate, 547
cartilage, 101
osteoarthritis, 397
Chronic exertional compartment syndrome
(CECS), 433
Chronic illness
exercise for older adults, 493–494
Chronic pain, 136–137
Cincinnati Knee Rating System, 209
Ciprofloxacin, 548
Circadian rhythms, 592
Circuit system of training, 162–163
Clavicle shaft fractures
children and adolescents, 475
Claw fist, **358**
Clenbuterol, 552
Climate
thermal demands, 593
Clinical outcomes
sport and exercise physical therapy, 206–218
assessment, **207**
collecting and analyzing, 215–217
data, 216–218
identification, 207–210
psychometrics, 211–212
Clinical prediction rule (CPR), 372
Clinic-based rehabilitation
adherence, 180
Closed chain exercises, 390, **447**
Closed-loop control system, **116**
basis, 121–122
changes, 121–122
mechanisms, 117
ACL, 117–118
problems, 117–118
movement, 116–117
problems, 121–122
sensory control, 116–117
CMC *see* Carpometacarpal (CMC) joints
CO *see* Cardiac output (CO)
Coach, fitness, 1–2
Cognitive appraisal models, **176**, 176–178

Cognitive-behavioral intervention
enhancing rehabilitation, 182
injured athlete, 183
pain management, 144
Cognitive behavioral stress management
(CBSM), 174
Cognitive reactions of injured athletes
characteristics, 178
Cognitive rehearsal, 183–184
Cognitive restructuring
rehabilitation, 184
Cognitive therapies
injury rehabilitation process, 144
pain management, 144
sports injury prevention, 173
Cohen's kappa statistic, 212
Cold
pain, injured athlete, 224
therapy, 275
Collagen, 27–28, 34, 59
articular cartilage, 102
bonding, **44**
content, 21–22
crosslinks helices, 28
degradation, 34
disruption, 35, 36
elastin and glycosaminoglycans, 43
electrical stimulation, 21–22
exercise, 32
fibers, 9
fibrils, **53**
ground substance, 34
ligaments, 43
in ligaments
hierarchical structure, **45**
structural arrangements, 44
synthesis, 32
tendon pain, 35, 36
transverse sections through, **53**
types, 43
Collateral ligaments
MCP joint, **339**
Common peroneal nerve, 435
Communication
injury management, 181
Compartment syndromes, 432–433,
435
Competition
classification, 527–526
Compression *see* RICE (rest, ice, compression,
elevation)
Compression test, **427**
Computed tomography (CT), 563
stress fractures, 67
navicular, 67
Concussion, **582**, 582–583
diagnosis, 582–583
history, 194
Maddock's questions, **583**
management, **583**
prevention, 584
returning to play after, 584
Congenital mimics of injuries
imaging, 573
Connectin, 17
Connective tissue
innervation, 93–94
neural, 86–87
peripheral nerve, **83**, 86

muscle immobilization, 21
sheaths, **83**
Connective tissue (perimysium), 9, 28–29
regeneration, 18–19
Consolidation
bone, 65
CONSORT guidelines, 3
Continuous passive motion (CPM)
cartilage defects, 104
Contraceptives
oral, athletic women, 503
Contractile elements
elastic properties, 16
regeneration, 17
Contractile process, 12–13
Controlled landing exercises, **429**
Contusions, 19
children and adolescents, 466
myositis ossificans, 450–451
quadriceps, 450–451
treatment protocols, **451**
Conus medullaris, **560**
Coracoid fractures
children and adolescents, **475**
Cord
normal deformation, **90**
Core muscles
training, 165–166
Core stability training programs, 165–166, **247**
Core strength and stability, 165–166
Corner injuries
posterolateral, 394–396
Coronary artery disease, 193
Cortical bone, 60
Stress–strain curve, **63**
Corticosteroids, 542, 546–547
Achilles tendon, 546
arachidonic acid metabolism, **543**
inhaled, 549
ITBFS, 454
pain management, 143–144
postinjection flare, 546
spinal injuries, 278
Corticotrophins, 552
COX-1 *see* Cyclooxygenase-1 (COX-1)
COX-2 *see* Cyclooxygenase-2 (COX-2)
CPG *see* Central pattern generators (CPG)
CPM *see* Continuous passive motion (CPM)
CPR *see* Clinical prediction rule (CPR)
Crank test, 290
Crash measures, 241
Creep, 31
Creep behavior
alignment, 47
Creep-elongation, **47**
Crepitus, 35
Crimp patterns
ligaments, 45
Cross-bridge detachment, 14
Crosslinks, 43
bond collagen helices, 28
Crunches, **156**
Cryotherapy
elbow injuries, 317
inflammation and edema, 229–230
pain management, 143
CT *see* Computed tomography (CT)
CTS *see* Carpal tunnel syndrome (CTS)
Cubital tunnel syndrome

neurodynamics, 95
Cutaneous infections, 594–595
Cyclic loading
tendon, 31
Cyclooxygenase-1 (COX-1)
inhibitors, 544
Cyclooxygenase-2 (COX-2)
inhibitors, 544
medications, 32

D

D band, 28
DC *see* Direct current (DC)
Debridement
SIJ dysfunction, 372
Decompressive surgery, 435
Decorin, 28, **29**
schematic diagrams, **29**
Deep vein thrombosis (DVT), 435–437
differential diagnosis, 436
prevention, 437
signs and symptoms, 436
treatment, 436–437
Deep (radial) zone, 101
Degeneration
tenocytes, 34
terminology, 32
Degenerative disorders
ulnar wrist pain and impairment, 353
Degenerative joint disease (DJD), 335,
346–347
first CMC grind for, **348**
Degradation
collagen, 34
Dehydroepiandrosterone (DHEA), 551–552
Delitto classification scheme, 264–267
DeLorme system of training, 162
Demonstration *vs.* instruction
teaching skills, 127–128
Dengue fever
Aedes mosquitoes, 593
Dentate ligaments, 86
Depression
pregnancy, exercise, 514
Depth jump, 158, **159**
DeQuervain's disease, 340, 347–349
factors affecting recovery, **350**
Finkelstein for, **348**
Desipramine
bulimia nervosa, 507
Desmin, 10
Dexamethasone
hips, 546
iontophoresis, **223**
DHEA *see* Dehydroepiandrosterone (DHEA)
DHLNL *see* Dihydroxylysinonorleucine
(DHLNL)
DHP *see* Dihydropyridine receptor (DHP)
Diabetes
gestational, 514–515
Diabetes mellitus, 587–589
exercise, 587–588
older adults, 494
hydration, **588**
training diary, **589**
Diagonal Pattern D2 Extension, **319**
Diagonal Pattern D2 Flexion, **319**
Diamorphine (heroin), 554

Diarrhea, 204
traveler's, 548
Diarthrodial joints
articular cartilage, 102
Dietary intake
stress fractures, 69
Digitalis
side effects with exercise, **490**
Digits
finger flexors, 340–341
Digit symbol substitution test (DSST), 584
Dihydropyridine receptor (DHP), 12
Dihydroxylysinonorleucine (DHLNL), 43
DIP *see* Distal interphalangeal (DIP) joints
Direct compression, 435
Direct current (DC), 229
Disability, 526
questionnaires, 258
Disability index
neck, **259**
Disabled athletes, 525
Disablement schemes
comparison, **208**
Discography
injection locations, **278**
Disk herniation
computed tomography, **563**
Diskogenic disease
imaging, 572
Diskoid lateral meniscus, **470**
children and adolescents, 469
Dislocations
children and adolescents, 467
posterior hip, **467**
shoulder, 472–473
elbow, 335
Lisfranc, 434
proximal interphalangeal joint, 355–356
Disordered eating
female athletes, 504–507
laboratory findings, **506**
Dispersion, 217
Dissociation
pain, 145
Distal interphalangeal (DIP) joints, 339
Distal radioulnar joint (DRUJ), 338
instability
ulnar wrist pain and impairment,
350–353
Distal radius
osteoporotic fractures, 343
Salter–Harris II fracture, **478**
Distal tibiofibular joint, 421
Diuretics, 553
side effects with exercise, **490**
Diving
biomechanics, 300–301
injuries
abuse injuries, 301–302
etiology, 301
misuse injuries, 302
overuse injuries, 301
training errors, 301–302
treatment, 301–302
DJD *see* Degenerative joint disease (DJD)
Doping, gene, 553
Doppler ultrasound, **34**
SIJ dysfunction, 371
Drawer test, 289

Drills
  agility, 390–391
  plyometric, **246**, 390, **449**
    elbow injuries, 322
Drugs
  antiarthritic, 542–543
  legal considerations, 550
  performance-enhancing, 550–555
    historical perspective, 550
  psychotropic
    side effects with exercise, **490**, 491
  testing, 554-555
DRUJ *see* Distal radioulnar joint (DRUJ)
DSST *see* Digit symbol substitution test
    (DSST)
Dual energy X-ray absorptiometry (DXA), 71
  bone mass, 62
  lumbar spine, **72**
Dura mater, 85, 86
  normal deformation, **90**
  ventral aspect, **88**
DVT *see* Deep vein thrombosis (DVT)
DXA *see* Dual energy X-ray absorptiometry
    (DXA)
Dynamic stability/neuromuscular control, 277
Dynamic training, 154–155

E

Ears
  examination, 196–197
Eating
  female athletes, 503–504
Eating disorders, 195
  female athletes, 504–507, **506**
  laboratory findings, **506**
EBP *see* Evidence-based practice (EBP)
EBV *see* Epstein-Barr virus (EBV)
ECBL *see* Extensor carpi brevis longus (ECBL)
Eccentric training, 156–158
ECG *see* Electrocardiography (ECG)
ECRL *see* Extensor carpi radialis longus
    (ECRL)
ECU *see* Extensor carpi ulnaris (ECU)
EDC *see* Extensor digitorum communis
    (EDC)
Edema
  acute, paratenon, 35
  cryotherapy, 229–230
  electrical stimulation, 229
  intravenous, nerve injuries, 92–93
  persistent endoneurial, 93
Education
  injury management, 181
  patient, older adults, 491
Effect size (ES), 217
  radar graph, **217**
Ege's test, 387
EIA *see* Exercise-induced asthma (EIA)
EIB *see* Exercise-induced bronchospasm
    (EIB)
Elasticity
  muscle, 16–17
Elastin
  ligaments, 44
Elbow, 308–337
  acute injuries, 476
  anatomy, 308–311

arthrolysis, 335–336
biomechanics in sport, 312–313
capsuloligamentous structures, 309–310
children and adolescents, 475–476, 477
  overuse injuries, 475–476
clinical examination, 314
dislocations, 335
displacement, **310**
flexion, **321–322**
  resisted, 289
fractures, 335
isometric tests results, **324**
manual resisted, **318**
musculotendinous structures, 310–311
neurological structures, 311–312
osseous structures, 308–309
rehabilitation, 315–323
sensory nerves, 315
sport-related injuries, 324–334
synovitis, 335
Elbow injuries
  cryotherapy, 317
  diagnostic images, 315
  history, 314
  lateral pivot shift test, 315
  laxity assessment, 315
  muscle testing, 314–315
  muscular endurance exercises, 318
  neurological testing, 315
  neuromuscular control exercises, 318, 322
  observation, 314
  palpation, 314
  plyometric drills, 322
  range of motion, 314
  rehabilitation, **316**
    advanced strengthening phase, 318–323
    immediate motion phase, 316–318
    intermediate motion phase, 318
    return-to-activity phase, 324
  special testing, 315
  strengthening exercises, 318, 322
  stretching exercises, 318
  valgus testing, 315
  varus testing, 315
Elderly *see* Older adults
Electrical stimulation, 275
  athletes, 229
  collagen content, 21–22
  fracture repair, 229
  inflammation and edema, 229
  injured athlete, 225–226
  lumbar, **277**
  motor and noxious, 225–226
  muscle belly, **446**
  neuromuscular, 390
  strength, 275
  tissue edema, 221
  transcutaneous nerve, 142, 225
Electroanalgesia
  pain, injured athlete, 224–225
Electrocardiography (ECG)
  endurance trained athlete, **586**
Electrophysical agents, 142–143, 220–232, 275
  impaired muscle function, 226–227
  inflammation and edema, 220–223
  ligament repair, 51
  pain, 224–225
  reduced tissue extensibility, 228
  tissue damage, 229–231

Elevation *see* RICE (rest, ice, compression,
    elevation)
Ely's test, 444
Empty can test, 289
Encouraged pain tolerance, 137
Endomysium, 14, 16
  muscle immobilization, 21
Endoneurial tubules
  integrity, 83
Endurance
  aging, 486
  physiological adaptations to, 163–164
Endurance trained athletes
  ECG, **586**
Endurance training
  adolescents, 165
  cardiovascular, 163–164
  children, 165
  exercise-based conditioning, 163–164
  injury prevention during, 165
  muscle adaptations, 164
  older adults, 165, 488, 492, **493**
  principles, 164–165
  rehabilitation, 163–164
Energy deficiency
  amenorrhea, 508
Enthesis, 30
  failure, 35
  fibrocartilaginous, 30
Enthesopathies, 35
Environmental pre-crash measures, 241
EPB *see* Extensor pollicis brevis (EPB)
Ephedrine, 553
Epicondylalgia
  lateral, neurodynamics, 95
Epicondylitis
  ESWT, 232
  medial, 475, 476
  medial and lateral, 324–327
  rehabilitation protocol, **329**
Epidural blocks, **263**
  injection locations, **278**
Epilepsy, 580–582
  exercise, 581–582
  management, 582
  seizure classification, **581**
Epimysium, 9, 14, 16
  muscle immobilization, 21
Epinephrine, 95
Epineurium
  sensory and motor roots, 85
EPL *see* Extensor pollicis longus (EPL)
EPO *see* Erythropoietin (EPO)
Epstein-Barr virus (EBV), 593
Equilibrium
  sensory modalities, 119
Equipment-related pre-crash measures, 241
ERT *see* Estrogen replacement therapy
    (ERT)
Erythropoietin (EPO), 552
ES *see* Effect size (ES)
Estimated change, 214
Estrogen replacement therapy (ERT), 510
ESWT *see* Extracorporeal shock wave therapy
    (ESWT)
Evidence-based practice (EBP), 3
  evaluation guidelines, **214**
  pelvis, 368
  SIJ, 371

Examination
eating disorder, **506**
female athletes, **506**
frequency, 191
genitourinary, 198
head, ears, eyes, nose and throat, 196–197
lung, 197
performing, 191–192
preparticipation, 190, 199–201
adolescent, 196
timing, 191
Excursion, 89–90
Exercise(s) *see also* Sports and exercise injuries
aerobic, 390, **448**
older adults guidelines, **493**
back pain, 76
balance, 390
benefits through aging process, 488
bone strength, 74
carpal tunnel, 95
cartilage, 107
closed chain, 390, **447**
collagen synthesis, 32
controlled landing, **429**
diabetes mellitus, 494, 587–588
effects on tendon, 32
elbow injuries, 318, 322
epilepsy, 581–582
gestational diabetes, pregnancy, 514–515
gliding, tendons, **352**
hip extension, **75**
hypertension, 494
injury, 3
insulin requirements, **588**
kinetic chain, 408–409, 431
ligaments, 52–53
PT, 52–58
strength, **54**
lumbar stabilization, **266**
muscular endurance, 318
nerve and tendon gliding, 95
neuromuscular control, 318, 322, 390
older adults
aerobic, **493**
angina, 494
arthritis, 494–495
cardiac disease, 494
chronic illness, 493–494
contraindications, 489, **489**
diabetes mellitus, 494
guidelines, 489
hypertension, 494
medication side effects, 489, **490**
osteoarthritis, 494
osteoporosis, 495
patient education, 491
peripheral vascular disease, 495
progression, **492**
risk assessment, 489
stretching, 491
warm-ups, 491
open chain, 390, **447**
osteoarthritis, 494
osteoporosis, 74–75, 495
pain management, 143
patient education, 491
peripheral vascular disease, 495
predicting success after, **266**
pregnancy, **512**, 512–514

back pain, 514
cardiac expenditure, 513
contraindications, 516, **516**
depression, 514
hemodynamics, 513
maternal effects, 514
musculoskeletal, 514
placental effects, 515
stress hormones, 514
prescription
bone loading, 73
clinical recommendations, 75
progression, **492**
progressive resistance, 468
proprioceptive, 390, 426
reactive neuromuscular control, 390
side effects with
ACE inhibitors, **490**, 491
acetaminophen, 491
anti-anxiety medications, **490**
beta blockers, 490
glucocorticoids, 491
hypoglycemic medications, 491
insulin, 491
non-opioid analgesics, 491
NSAIDs, 491
opioid analgesics, 491
psychotropic drugs, 491
skeletal effects
ages, 73
strengthening
elbow injuries, 318, 322
RTC, 294–296
stress hormones, 514
stretching, 491
elbow injuries, 318
stretch-shortening, 158
Supination, **322**
tendon gliding, 95
tendons response to, 32
therapies, 1–5
injury, 2
rehabilitation specialists and PT, 2
upper limb, **76**
warm-ups, 491
water rehabilitation, 107
weightbearing, **448**
scapular muscle stabilization, 294, **294**
Exercise-based conditioning and rehabilitation, 149–165
endurance training, 163–164
interval training, 163
sport and exercise injury management, 149–169
stabilization, 165–166
strength training, 149–161
Exercise-induced asthma (EIA), 549, 578–580, **579**
beta 2-agonists, 580
diagnosis, 579–580
management, 580
Exercise-induced bronchospasm (EIB), 194
Exercise injuries *see* Sports and exercise injuries
Exercise physical therapy
clinical outcomes, 206–218
assessment, **207**
collecting and analyzing, 215–217
identification, 207–210

psychometrics, 211–212
Extensor carpi brevis longus (ECBL), 340
Extensor carpi radialis longus (ECRL), 340, 349–350
Extensor carpi ulnaris (ECU), 340, 354
Extensor digitorum communis (EDC), 340
Extensor pollicis brevis (EPB), 340
Extensor pollicis longus (EPL), 340
Extensor supinator muscles, 311
Extensor tendons, 340
injuries, 360–361, **361**
External load
cartilage, 102
External Rotation at 0 Abduction, **319**
External rotation test, **427**
Extracellular matrix, 27–33, 34
sinusoidal pattern, 28
Extracorporeal shock wave therapy (ESWT)
athletes, 230–232, **231**
clinical evidence, 232
patient preparation and positioning, 231–232
calcific tendonitis, 232
epicondylitis, 232
plantar fasciitis, 232
tendonitis, 232
Extraneural fibrosis, 95
Extrinsic muscles
foot and ankle, 423
Eyes
examination, 196–197

F

Faber's (Patrick's) test, **375**
Facet joint
nerve blocks, **263**
injection locations, **278**
FAI *see* Femoral acetabular impingement (FAI)
Failed healing response, 32
Failure region, **46**
Fall on an outstretched hand (FOOSH), 343
Falls
aging, 487–488
reduction, 75
Family Education Rights and Privacy Act (FERPA), 201
Fascia latae muscles, 373
Fascicles, 9, 28, 83
bundles, 29
Fasciotomy
for CECS, 433
Fast-twitch fibers, 11
Fat pad
calcaneal, 423
metatarsal, 423
PFJ, 404
FCR *see* Flexor carpi radialis (FCR)
FCU *see* Flexor carpi ulnaris (FCU)
FDP *see* Flexor digitorum profundus (FDP)
FDS *see* Flexor digitorum superficialis (FDS)
Fear Avoidance Beliefs Questionnaire, 261, **261**
Feedback, **130**
augmented, **128**
simplification, segmentation, **130**
inaccurate
from movement, 122
motor learning, 128

Feedback (*contd.*)
  sensory
    reason for, 122
  types, 128
Feedforward control
  trunk stability, **120**
Female(s)
  ACL injuries paradigm, 243–247
  active, 499–524
  pain tolerance, 138
Female athletes, 195–196
  ACL injury, 502
  aerobic performance, 500–501
  amenorrhea, 503–504
  anaerobic power, 501
  anatomy and physiology, 499–502
  anorexia nervosa, **504**, 504–507
  body composition, 499–500
  bones, 511–512
  bulimia nervosa, **504**, 504–507
  disordered eating, 504–507
  eating, 503–504
    disorder, **506**
  heat tolerance, 501
  height, 499
  injury rates, 501–502
  laboratory findings
    disordered eating, **506**
  leanness, 506
  muscle tissue, 500
  neuromuscular control deficits, 244
  oral contraceptives, 503
  osteoporosis, 503–504
  skeleton, 501, **502**
  soccer players, **500**
  weight, 499
Female athlete triad, 195, 503–511
Femoral acetabular impingement (FAI)
  children and adolescents, 466
  imaging, 571
Femoral condyle
  MRI, **564**
Femoral tibial angle, **424**
FERPA *see* Family Education Rights and Privacy
    Act (FERPA)
Fetal effects
  pregnancy
    exercise, 515
FF *see* Forefoot (FF) to rearfoot (RF)
    alignment
Fiberoptics, 13
Fibrils, 28, 32
Fibroblasts, 43
  proliferation
    tendinopathy, **33**
    tendon, **32**
Fibrocartilage region
  unmineralized, 30
Fibrocartilaginous enthesis, 30
Fibrocartilaginous labrum
  acetabulum, 373
Fibromodulin, 28
Fibronectin, 44
Fibrosis
  intraneural, 93
  nerve injuries, 92–93
Figure-of-four position
  anterior hip structures, **406**
Filaments

types, 10
Finger flexors
  digits, 340–341
Finger injuries
  management, 355
Finger joints, 339
Finger tendons
  injury management, 359–362
Finkelstein for DeQuervain's, **348**
First carpometacarpal grind
  for DJD, **348**
Fitness
  aerobic measurement, 163
  coach or adviser, 1–2
  maintaining with stress fractures, 68
  principle, 154
    strength gains, 154
Flexibility
  aging, 487
Flexor carpi radialis (FCR), 346
  ultrasound, **562**
Flexor carpi ulnaris (FCU), 354
Flexor digitorum profundus (FDP), 340
Flexor digitorum superficialis (FDS), 340
Flexor pollicus longus (FLP), 341
Flexor pronator muscles, 311
Flexor tendons, 359–360, **360**
FLP *see* Flexor pollicus longus (FLP)
Fluoroscopy, 559
Fluoxetine
  anorexia nervosa, 507
  bulimia nervosa, 507
Follicle stimulating hormone (FSH), 507, **508**
Food
  female athletes, 503–504
FOOSH *see* Fall on an outstretched hand
    (FOOSH)
Foot
  abnormal pronation, PFJ, 414
  radiograph, **571**
Foot and ankle, 420–432
  arthrology, 420–422
  children and adolescents, 470–472
    overuse injuries, 470
  examination, 423–432
  extrinsic muscles, 423
  intrinsic muscles, 423
  non-weightbearing assessment, 425–426
  overuse injuries, 470
  sport-related injuries, 426–432
Football
  preparticipation examination, 200
Footwear
  children and adolescents, **460**
  stress fractures, 68
Force augmentation, 158
Force–deformation curve for ligament, **46**
Force–length relationship, 14, **14**
Force potential
  muscle, 15–16
Force–relaxation, **47**
Force–velocity relationship, 14–15, **15**
Forearm, hand and wrist
  acute injuries, 477
  children and adolescents, 476–477
  fractures, 477
Forefoot (FF) to rearfoot (RF) alignment, 425,
    425
Fractures

activity program, **70**
  acute, 64–65
    rehabilitation, 65
  athletes, 229
  avulsion, 466–467
    thumb metacarpophalangeal joint,
      478
  Bennet's, 361
  children and adolescents, 467, 469–470
    apophyseal avulsion, **467**
    avulsion, 466–467
    clavicle shaft, 475
    coracoid, **475**
  clavicle shaft
    children and adolescents, 475
  coracoid
    children and adolescents, **475**
  distal radius osteoporotic, 343
  elbow, 335
  electrical stimulation, 229
  forearm, 477
  greenstick, 461, **477**
  growth plate, **462**
  hand, 341–345, **359**, 477
  healing stages, **62**
  healing times, 65
  Jones, 431–432
  lower limb stress, **70**
  management principles, 65
  medial epicondyle avulsion, **477**
  metacarpal, 358
  osteoporotic compression, 575
  phalangeal, 358–359
  rehabilitation, **359**
  repair, 61–62
  Salter–Harris classification, **462**
  Salter–Harris II, 474
    distal radius, **478**
    proximal phalanx, **479**
  Salter–Harris III ulnar collateral ligament
    avulsion, **478**
  Salter I, **473**
  Salter IV, **471**
  scaphoid
    wrist and hand, 341–343
  shoulder and shoulder girdle
    children and adolescents, 474
  spinal stress, 255
  stress, 65–70
    amenorrhea, **508**
    hip, **559**
  tibial plateau, 396
  tibial stress, 432
  ulnar wrist pain and impairment, 350
  vertebral compression
    osteoporosis, 512
  wrist, 341–345, 350, 477
    treatment guidelines, **347**
Freestyle stroke
  shoulder motion, 296
Free weight
  advantages and disadvantages, **153**
  dumbbell exercise, **155**
Freiberg's infraction
  radiograph, **574**
Front (extension) or back (flexion)
  trunk, **122**
FSH *see* Follicle stimulating hormone (FSH)
Functional murmurs, 198

G

Gaenslen's test, 370
GAG see Glycosaminoglycans (GAG)
Gait
    angle, **424**
Galen, 42
Game interruption injuries, 242
Gastrocnemius muscle, 423
Gastrocnemius–soleus complex, 441
Gate control theory
    of pain, 134, **135**
Gene doping, 553
Genetics
    children and adolescents, **460**, 461
Genitourinary examination, 198
Gestational diabetes
    pregnancy exercises, 514–515
Glenohumoral joint (GHJ), 284–285
    anterior subluxation, 473
Glenoid
    radiograph, **569**
Glenoid labrum
    tests, 290
Gliding exercises
    carpal tunnel, 95
    nerves, 95
    tendons, 95, **352**
Global muscles, **121**
Globe Rating Scale, 391
Glucocorticosteroids, 546–547
    side effects with exercise, **490**, 491
Glucosamine, 547
    osteoarthritis, 397
Glutamate, 36
Gluteus maximus, 373
Gluteus medius
    weight bearing, **409**
Glycosaminoglycans (GAG)
    cartilage, 101
    collagen and elastin, 43
Goal setting
    implementation process, **182**
    injury management, 181
    rehabilitation, 184–185
Golf
    interval program, **328**
Golf swing
    elbow biomechanics, 313
Golgi tendon organs, 116
Gonadotrophin, 552
Gracilis test, 445
Grafts, 105
    types, 51
Greenstick fractures, 461, **477**
GRF see Ground reaction forces (GRF)
Grief response models, 175–176, **176**
Gripping rotatory impaction test (GRIT), 353
GRIT see Gripping rotatory impaction test (GRIT)
Groin, 365–381
    anatomy, 365–367
Groin injuries
    athlete, 377–378
        history, 378
        physical examination
        history, 378
Groin pain
    imaging, 571

Ground reaction forces (GRF), 64
Ground substance, 28
    collagen, 34
Growth
    children and adolescents, **460**
Growth cartilage, 461
Growth factors
    tendon repair, 37
Growth plate fractures
    Salter–Harris classification, **462**
Guyon's canal ulnar artery
    vascular thrombosis, 361

H

Haddon's matrix, 241, **241**
Hamstring muscles, 373, 441
    lateral test, 445
    medial test, 445
Hand, 338–364
    acute injuries, 477
    anatomy, 338–340
    blood supply, 338
    children and adolescents, 476–477
    degenerative disorders, 346–347
    examination, 341
    fractures, 341–345, 477
        rehabilitation, **359**
    nerve compression and traction, 349–350
    neurological and vascular structures, 341
    pain and impairment, 338–339
        instability, 345–346
        treatment, **345**
    provocative tests, **348**
    scaphoid fractures, 341–343
    sport-related injuries, 341–361
    stiffness treatment algorithm, **346**
    tendonitis, 347–349
Handball, team
    injuries incidence, **238**
Hardware blocks, **263**
Hashish, 554
Haversian bone, 60
HCV see Hepatitis C (HCV)
Head
    examination, 196–197
    injuries, 582
        imaging, 571–572
Healing
    failed response, 32
    monitoring, 17
    phases, **49**
    poor response in tendons, 36
Health Insurance Portability and Accountability Act (HIPPA), 201
Health professionals, 2
Health-related quality of life, 208–209
Heart
    athlete, 586
    examination, 198
Heart rate (HR), 163–164
    aging, 486
    responses to increased workload, **164**
Heat
    inflammatory process, 543
    pain, injured athlete, 224
    related illness, 193–194
    rubs, 546

tolerance, female athletes, 501
Heel pain
    neurodynamics, 95
Hegator, 42
Height
    athletic women, 499
Heparin
    for DVT, 436
Hepatitis C (HCV)
    athletes, 594
Heredity
    children and adolescents, **460**, 461
Heroin, 554
Herpes simplex virus (HSV), 594
hGH see Human growth hormone (hGH)
HHMD see Histidinohydroxymerodesmosine (HHMD)
High ankle sprains, 427–428
High-density lipoprotein cholesterol, 165
High intensity plyometrics, 159
High-intensity strength training
    older adults, **493**
High-load brief stressors (HLBS), 355
High-voltage pulsed galvanic electrical
    stimulation, **221**, 222
High-volt pulsed current (HVPC), 221
Hip(s), 365–381
    anatomy, 365–367
    anterior structures
        figure-of-four position, **406**
    apophyseal avulsion fracture, **467**
    children and adolescents, **467**
        snapping, 466
    dexamethasone, 546
    extension exercises, **75**
    external rotation test, **376**
    internal rotation test, **376**
    joint, 372–373
        blood supply, 374
        ligaments, 373
        movements, 372–373
        muscles, 373–374
        neurology, 374
    MRI, **566**
    pain, recurrent, 377
    patellofemoral joint, 409
    posterior dislocation, **467**
    problems
        in athletes, 374–377
        history, 374
        intervention, 376–377
        physical examination, 374–376
        prognosis, 376
    snapping, 466
    stress fracture, **559**
HIPPA see Health Insurance Portability and Accountability Act (HIPPA)
Hippocrates, 42
Histidinohydroxymerodesmosine (HHMD), 43
History
    preparticipation, 192
    respiratory, 194
    self-report, 192
HIV see Human immunodeficiency virus (HIV)
HLA see Human leukocyte antigen (HLA)
    tissue typing
HLBS see High-load brief stressors (HLBS)
HLNL see Hydroxylysinonorleucine (HLNL)

HOCM *see* Hypertrophic obstructive cardiomyopathy (HOCM)
Home-based rehabilitation
  adherence, 180–181
Hop tests, **388**, 388–389
Horizontal jump, **159**
Hormones, 552
  children and adolescents, **460**
  menstrual cycle, **509**
  stress and pregnancy, 514
Hot and humid climate
  thermal demands, 593
Hot packs, 275
  osteoporosis, 76
HP *see* Hydroxypyridinoline (HP)
HR *see* Heart rate (HR)
HSV *see* Herpes simplex virus (HSV)
Human growth hormone (hGH), 552
Human immunodeficiency virus (HIV)
  athletes, 594
Human leukocyte antigen (HLA) tissue
  typing, 35
Humeroradial joint, 309
Humeroulnar joint, 308–309
Humerus
  medial epicondyle, 309
Humidity
  thermal demands, 593
HVPC *see* High-volt pulsed current (HVPC)
HYAFF *see* Benzylic ester of hyaluronic acid
Hyalograft C, 106
Hyaluronic acid, 547
Hydration
  diabetes, **588**
Hydrotherapy
  osteoporosis, 76
Hydroxylysine, 43
Hydroxylysinonorleucine (HLNL), 43
Hydroxypyridinoline (HP), 43
Hyperbaric oxygen therapy, 542–543, 547
  athletes, 230
Hyperemia
  paratenon, 35
Hypertension exercise
  older adults, 494
Hypertrophic cardiomyopathy
  murmur of, 198
Hypertrophic obstructive cardiomyopathy
  (HOCM), 585
  vs. physiological hypertrophy, **586**
Hypoglycemia, 587–588
Hypoglycemic medications
  side effects with exercise, **490**, 491
Hypoxic tendinopathy, 35
Hysteresis
  schematic representation, **47**

IASP *see* International Association for the
  Study of Pain (IASP)
I-band, 10
Ice *see also* RICE (rest, ice, compression,
  elevation)
  osteoporosis, 76
Ice hockey
  injuries incidence, **238**
ICF *see* International Classification of
  Functioning and Disability (ICF)

ICIDH-2 *see* International Classification of
  Impairment, Disability and Health
  (ICIDH-2)
ICRS *see* International Cartilage Repair Society
  (ICRS)
Iliac bone, **366**
Iliofemoral ligaments, 373
Iliopsoas muscles, 373
Iliotibial band, 403, 441
Iliotibial band friction syndrome (ITBFS),
  444, 454
  corticosteroids, 454
  myofascial treatments, 454
  NSAID, 454
  stretching, 454
Imagery
  pain management, 145
  rehabilitation, 184
  sports injury prevention, 173
Imaging, 558–577
  anterior cruciate ligament tear, **565**
  bone, 566–568
  cartilage, 570
  choice of, **567**–568
  complications, 573–574
  congenital mimics of injuries, 573
  contraindications, **565**
  disk herniation, **564**
  diskogenic disease, 572
  femoroacetabular impingement, 571
  future developments, 575
  groin pain, 571
  head and neck injuries, 571–572
  injury types, 566–567
  internal impingement, 571
  ligaments, 569–570
  lumbar spine, 572, **573**
  modalities and techniques, 558–561
  myotendinous unit, 568
  needle guidance, 574–575
  nerve, 570
  pars defects, 572
  patellofemoral disease, 571
  pediatric injuries, 573
  stress fractures, 66–67, 570–571
    navicular, **67**
  therapeutics, 574–575
Imipramine
  bulimia nervosa, 507
Immobilization, 65
  exercise
    ligaments, 52–54
    strength, **54**
  muscle, 19–22
  remobilization, **54**
Immunization, 195
Impingement
  children and adolescents, 472
  femoral acetabular
    children and adolescents, 466
    imaging, 571
  internal
    imaging, 571
    shoulder injuries, 290
Inaccurate feedback
  from movement, 122
Infections
  athletes, 593–594
Inferior glide test, 290

Inflammation, 543
  cryotherapy, 229–230
  electrical stimulation, 229
  long-term peritendon, 35
  neural tissues, 93
  tendons, 35
Inhaled corticosteroids, 549
Injured athletes
  cognitive-behavioral intervention,
    183
  cognitive reactions of
    characteristics, 178
  motor and noxious electrical stimulation for
    pain, 225–226
  neurological screening for, **262**
  pain, 224–226
    electroanalgesia, 224–225
    sensory level stimulation, 225
    use of heat and cold, 224
  PT role, 182
  TENS for pain, 225
Injuries *see also* specific injury
  behavioral responses to, 179
  causation
    comprehensive model, **239**
  cognitive responses, 178
  congenital mimics of
    imaging, 573
  disuse, 17–22
  emotional responses to, 178
  history
    spinal injuries, 262
  and imaging, 566–567
  incidence
    specific sports, **238**
  management
    communication and rapport, 181
    education, 181
    goal setting and attainment, 181
    social support, 181
  mechanism, 17
  pain
    tendons, 36
  patterns
    sports, 461
  positive responses to, 179
  prevention, 236–248
    during endurance training, 165
    four-step sequence, **237**
    research methodology, 242
    sequence, 237–241
    stress management, 173
  psychological precursors, 171
  rates
    female athletes, 501–502
  rehabilitation
    adherence, 180–181
    cognitive therapies, 144
    psychology, 171–186
    psychosocial factors models, 174
    social support, 185
  repair
    ligaments, 48–51
  sport, exercise and physical activity, 3
  therapies, 2
  vulnerability
    interventions to produce, 173
Innervated connective tissue, 93–94
Innominate bone, 365

Insoles
    stress fractures, 68
Inspection
    lower extremity musculotendinous injuries,
        444
Instability
    central wrist pain and impairment,
        350–351
    tests
        prone, **268**
        shoulder, 289–290
    ulnar wrist pain and impairment, 354
Instruction, 127
    vs. demonstration
        teaching skills, 127–128
        verbal, 127–128
Insulin, 552
    requirements before exercise, **588**
    side effects with exercise, **490**, 491
Insulin-like growth factors, 552
Integrated Model of Psychological Response
        to the Sport Injury and Rehabilitation
        Process, 176, **177**
Interferential stimulation
    pain management, 142
Interferential therapy
    osteoporosis, 76
Intermolecular crosslinks, **44**
Internal impingement
    imaging, 571
    shoulder injuries, 290
Internal Rotation at 0 Abduction, **319**
Internal rotation resistance strength test
        (IRRS), 290
Internal System of Body Dynamics, 119
International Association for the Study of Pain
        (IASP), 133–134, 137
International athletes
    travel medicine, 592–593
    vaccinations, 592
International Cartilage Repair Society (ICRS),
        103
International Classification of Functioning
        and Disability (ICF), 208, 210,
        211, 215
International Classification of Impairment,
        Disability and Health (ICIDH-2),
        206, 208
International Federation of Sports
        Physiotherapy
    competencies, 2
Interphalangeal (IP) joints, 340
Intersection for intersection syndrome, **348**
Interval golf program, **328**
Interval tennis program, **328**
Interval throwing program (ITP)
    baseball players, **325–327**
Interval training
    exercise-based conditioning and
        rehabilitation, 163
Intraarticular facet joint injections, **263**
Intraneural fibrosis, 93
Intravenous edema
    nerve injuries, 92–93
Intrinsic blood supply
    nerve root, **85**
Intrinsic muscles
    foot and ankle, 423
Inverted subtalar joint

stretching, **430**
Iontophoresis, 222–223, **223**, **330**, 546
    acetic acid, 223
    efficacy, 222
    potassium iodide, 223
IP *see* Interphalangeal (IP) joints
IRRS *see* Internal rotation resistance strength
        test (IRRS)
Ischiofemoral ligaments, 373
Isokinetic dynamometer, 15
Isokinetic machines
    types, 152
Isokinetic strength training, 158, **448**
Isolated distal interphalangeal joint flexion and
        extension, **356**
Isolated proximal interphalangeal joint flexion
        and extension, **357**
Isometric tests
    elbow, **324**
Isometric torque, 15
Isometric training, 154
Isotopic bone scan (scintigraphy)
    stress fractures, 67
Isthmic spondylolysis, 255
ITBFS *see* Iliotibial band friction syndrome
        (ITBFS)
ITP *see* Interval throwing program (ITP)

J

Jet-lag, 592
    melatonin, 593
Joint(s) *see also* Patellofemoral joint (PFJ)
    acromioclavicular, 284
        mobilization, **293**
    anteroposterior laxity and stiffness, **54**
    articular cartilage, 102
    axes relationship to nerve structures, 89
    bicondylar sacroiliac, 366–367
    carpometacarpal, 340
    children and adolescents, 462
    degenerative disease, 335, 346–347
    diarthrodial, 102
    distal interphalangeal, 339
    distal radioulnar, 338
        instability, 350–353
    distal tibiofibular, 421
    facet, **263**
    finger, 339
    flexibility, 69
    glenohumoral, 284–284
        anterior subluxation, 473
    hip, 372–373
    humeroradial, 309
    humeroulnar, 308–309
    injections, intraarticular facet, **263**
    interphalangeal, 340
    inverted subtalar
        stretching, **430**
    isolated distal interphalangeal, **356**
    isolated proximal interphalangeal, **357**
    joint movements, 366–367
    knee, **54**
    laxity, 462
    manipulation and mobilizations, 274
    metacarpophalangeal, 339
        collateral ligaments, **339**
    metatarsalphalangeal, 422, **422**
        ultrasound, **563**

midcarpal, 338
midtarsal, 421–422
mobility testing, 271
movement
    amphiarthrodial symphysis pubis, 367
    SIJ, 366–367
    proximal interphalangeal, 339, **339**
        sprain and dislocation, 355–356
    proximal tibiofibular, 420
    radiocarpal, 338
    receptors, 116–117
        location and types, **116**
    sacroiliac
        articular surfaces, **366**
        bicondylar, 366–367
        blocks, **263**
        kinesiology, 365–366
    scapulothoracic, 284
    shoulder
        anatomy and biomechanics, 283
        mobility impairments, 292–293
    skeletal ligaments, 43
    spinal facet (zygapophyseal), 256
    stability
        control, 119–120, 124
        motor control, 118–119
        problems, 120
    sternoclavicular, 284
        mobilization, **293**
    stress fractures, 69
    subtalar, 421, **422**
        motion assessment, **425**
        neutral, **425**
    symphysis pubis
        kinesiology, 365–366
    talocrural, 421, **421**
    thumb
        injuries, 355
        metacarpophalangeal avulsion fractures,
            478
    tibiofemoral, 382
Joint-specific examination, 198
Jones fractures, 431–432
Jump training, 158

K

Keratan sulfate
    cartilage, 101
Kienbock's, 361
Kinematics
    patellofemoral joint, 403
Kinesiology
    sacroiliac joints, 365–366
    symphysis pubis joints, 365–366
Kinetic chain exercises, 408–409, 431
Kinetics
    patellofemoral joint, 403
Knee, 382–401
    acute injuries, 469–470
    anatomy and biomechanics, 382–383
    anterior view, **383**
    anteroposterior laxity and stiffness, **54**
    bony structure, 382–383
    children and adolescents, 467–469
    examination, 384–388
    flexion and extension
        small range, 409
    joint, **54**

Knee (*contd.*)
  ligaments, 383
    injuries, 469
    testing, 384–385
  menisci, 384
  MRI, **570**
  posterior view, **383**
  rehabilitation, 389–394
    phases, **389**, 389–390
    return-to-play phase, 390–391
Knee Outcome Survey-Activities of Daily
    Living Scale, 391

L

Laboratory findings
  eating disorder in female athletes, **506**
Lachman test, 385, **385**
Lactate, 36
Lamellar bone, 60
Laminin, 44
Lasers
  athletes, 229–230
  pain management, 142
Lateral ankle sprains, 426–427
  children and adolescents, 472
Lateral collateral ligament (LCL), 383
  testing, 385
Lateral epicondylalgia
  neurodynamics, 95
Lateral epicondylitis, 324–327
Lateral hamstrings test, 445
Lateral meniscus
  diskoid, **470**
    children and adolescents, 469
Lateral pivot shift test, 315
Lateral retinaculum, 403
Lateral ulnar collateral ligament (LUCL), 310
Laxity assessment
  elbow injuries, 315
Leanness
  female athletes, 506
Learning *see also* Motor learning
  sensory
    motor performance, 128
  skill
    training transfer, 128–129
Learning disabilities
  athletes, 529
Left lumbar shift, **265**
Leg(s) *see also* Lower legs; Lower limbs
  curls, **157**
  extension, **157**
  press, **157**
Legal considerations
  medications, 550
Leptin, 509–510
Leukotrienes, 550
Lever arms
  torque, **14**
LH *see* Luteinizing hormone (LH)
L'hermitte's sign, **268**
LHP *see* Long head of the biceps (LHP)
Lidocaine
  iontophoresis, **223**
Life Development Model, 179
Ligament(s), 42–54 *see also* Anterior cruciate
    ligament (ACL); Posterior cruciate
    ligament (PCL)

accessory lateral collateral, 310
aging, 485
alar test, **269**
ankles, 470–471
anterior talofibular, 426
arcuate, 383
biomechanics, 45–46
body tissue development, 42
children and adolescents, 469, 470–471
classification, 42
collagen, 43
  hierarchical structure, **45**
  structural arrangements, 44
collateral
  MCP joint, **339**
crimp patterns, 45
definition, 42
dentate, 86
derivation, 42
elastin, 44
exercises
  PT, 52–58
force–deformation curve for, **46**
grafts, 51–52
hip joint, 373
iliofemoral, 373
immobilization, remobilization and
    exercise, **54**
immobilization and exercise, 52–53
injuries
  classification, **49**
injury and repair, 48–51
ischiofemoral, 373
knee, 383
  injuries, 469
lateral collateral, 383
lateral ulnar collateral, 310
load–deformation characteristics, 45–46
LT, 338
medial collateral, 383
  age, 48
medial patellofemoral, 403
meniscofemoral, 383
morphology, 44
posterior oblique, 383
proteoglycans, 43–44
pubofemoral, 373
radial collateral, 310
remodeling phase, 50
repair, 54
  electrophysical modalities, 51
  with and without RICE management, **50**
repair phase, 50
sacrospinous, 367
sacrotuberous, 367
Salter–Harris III ulnar collateral
    avulsion fractures, **478**
SIJ, 367
skeletal, 43, **43**
SL, 338
spine, 256
sprains, 428
strain rate, 48
strength, 47, **54**
structural components, 48
structure and biochemistry, 42–43
subgroups, 43
suspensory abdominal organs, 43
testing, knee, 384–385

ulnar collateral, 309–310
  injuries, 331–332
  ultrastructural, 45
  viscoelastic behavior, 46–47
Ligamentum flavum
  load–deformation characteristics, **48**
Ligamentum teres, 373
Linear region, 46
Liniments, 546
Lipoid tendinopathy, 35
Lisfranc dislocation, 434
  NSAID, 434
  weight bearing, 434
Little League elbow, 475
Little League shoulder, 474
LLLD *see* Low load long duration (LLLD)
    stretch
Load
  physical activity generating
    bone, 63
    tendon, 31, 32, **32**
Load–deformation characteristics
  ligaments, 45–46
  ligamentum flavum, **48**
Loading direction
  ACL, 48
Load–relaxation
  alignment, 47
Local mechanical loading
  bone response to, 64
Local muscles, **121**
Long arm splint, **351**
Long head of the biceps (LHP), 285
Long-loop reflexes, 117
Long opponens splint, **347**
Long-term peritendon inflammation, 35
Loss of function
  inflammatory process, 543
Low back pain
  children and adolescents, 462, **463**
  trunk muscle changes, **125**
Lower extremity musculotendinous injuries
  activities of daily living, 444
  clinical examination, 444–445
  examination, 444–445
  general rehabilitation principles, 445–446
Lower legs, 420–432
  arthrology, 420–422
  compartments of, **433**
  examination, 423–432
  muscle contusion, 442–443 **443**, **451**
  muscle strain, 441, **442**
  muscle–tendon complexes, 440–441
  non-weightbearing assessment, 425–426
  sport-related injuries, 426–432
  tendinopathy, 443–444, **443**
Lower limbs
  muscle and tendon injury rehabilitation,
    440
    anatomy, 440
    musculotendinous injuries, 441–443
    rehabilitation, 444–453
  stress fractures
    activity program, **70**
Low load long duration (LLLD) stretch,
    316–317, **317**
LT *see* Lunotriquetral (LT) ligament
Lumbar
  classification scheme, 270

DXA scan, **72**
electrical stimulation, **277**
imaging, 572, **573**
injuries, 273–274
lower extremity pain
neurodynamics, 95
manipulation, 274–275
pain, acute
evaluation, 264
spine test, **268**
stabilization exercise program
predicting success after, **266**
Lumbopelvic manipulation, **275**
Lumican, 28
Lunge, **155**
Lung examination, 197
Lunotriquetral (LT) ligament, 338
Luteinizing hormone (LH), 507, **508**, **509**
Lysholm Knee Score, 209
Lysine, 43
Lysomal cathepsin, 19

M

Machines
advantages and disadvantages, **153**
weight exercises, **157**
Macrocycle, 153
Macrotraumatic repair
tendon repair, 37
Maddock's questions
concussion, **583**
Magnetic fields, 107
Magnetic resonance imaging (MRI), 562–564
anterior cruciate ligament tear, **565**
contraindications, **565**
femoral condyle, **564**
hip, **566**
knee, **570**
physis, **572**
stress fractures, 67
Malaria
Anopheline mosquitoes, 593
Males
maximal oxygen uptake, **163**
pain tolerance, 138
Mallet thumb, 361
Manually resisted scapular protraction, **294**
Manual resisted elbow and wrist flexion, **318**
Manual techniques
pain management, 143
Marfan's syndrome, 193
physical examination, 198
Marijuana, 554
Massage
plantar fasciitis, 430
soft tissue, osteoporosis, 76
Maternal effects
pregnancy, exercise, 514
Maximal heart rate
aging, 486
Maximal oxygen uptake
for males, **163**
Maximal voluntary isometric contraction
(MVIC), 390
McGill Pain Questionnaire (MPQ),
139, **140**
MCL *see* Medial collateral ligament (MCL)

McMurray's test, 387
MCP *see* Metacarpophalangeal (MCP) joint
Mechanical forces impact on physiology
neurodynamics, 92
Mechanoreceptors
for movement control, 116–117
Mechanosensitivity, 93–94
ulnar nerve, 89
Mechanotransduction
bone, 60–61
Medial and lateral epicondylitis,
324–327
Medial collateral ligament (MCL), 383
age, 48
mechanism of injury, 393
nonoperative treatment, 393
operative treatment, 393
postoperative treatment, 393
testing, 384–385
Medial epicondyle avulsion fractures, **477**
Medial epicondylitis, 475, 476
Medial hamstrings test, 445
Medial malleolus
tendons, 29
Medial patellofemoral ligament, 403
Medial retinaculum, 403
Median nerve, 311
compression, **352**
testing, **269**
Medical attention injuries, 242
Medical conditions and sports participation,
202–204
Medical history, 192–193
Medical imaging, 558–577
modalities and techniques, 558–561
Medical team examinations, 192
Medications, 541–557
antiarthritic, 542–543
COX-2, 32
legal considerations, 550
pain management, 143–144
side effects with exercise, **490**
Medroxyprogesterone
BMD, 511
Melatonin
circadian rhythm, 593
jet-lag, 593
Menarche, 195
Meninges
diagram, **86**
innervation, 86
Menisci
children and adolescents, 469
injuries, 469
knee, 384
mechanism of injury, 393
nonoperative treatment, 393
operative treatment, 393–394
postoperative treatment, 394
tests, 387
Meniscofemoral ligament, 383
Menstrual cycle, 503
hormone cycle, **509**
physiology, **508**
stress fractures, 69
Mental practice
motor performance, 128
sports injury prevention, 173
Mesocycles, 153

Metabolic demands
tendons, 29
Metacarpal fractures, 358
Metacarpophalangeal (MCP) joint, 339
collateral ligaments, **339**
Metatarsal fat pad, 423
Metatarsalphalangeal joint (MTP), 422, **422**
ultrasound, **563**
Methadone, 554
Microcycle, 153
Microtrauma
shoulder, 286
throwing injuries, 298–299
Midcarpal joints, 338
Middle zone, 101
Midtarsal joint, 421–422
Minimal detectable change, 214
Minitramp, 426, **427**, 431
Misuse injuries, 286
diving injuries, 302
shoulder, 298
tennis injuries, 305
throwing injuries, 300
volleyball injuries, 304
Mobility
aging, 487
Model of Meeuwisse, 241
Morphine, 554
Morphological classifications
cartilaginous lesion, 103
Mosaicplasty *vs.* ACI, 107
Mosquitoes
dengue fever, 593
malaria, 593
Motion assessment
subtalar joint, **425**
Motivation for return to sport, 262
Motoneuron excitability changes, 125–126
Motor and noxious electrical stimulation
pain, injured athlete, 225–226
Motor control, 115–130
application in PT low back pain, 129
changes in musculoskeletal injury and pain,
121–125
contemporary theories, 118
cycle, **126**
factors, 115–120
motor learning, 126–128
movement and stability, 118–119
musculoskeletal injury and pain, 121–124
organizational theories, 118
pain or changes, 126
postural and joint stability, 118–119
strategies, 116–120
training, 130
Motor learning
dosage, 128
feedback, 128
in management
sports-related injuries, 126–128
motor control, 126–128
practice
distribution, 128
of parts, 127
variability, 128
of whole, 127
stages, 126–127
strategies, 127
for musculoskeletal pain, 128

Motor performance
    mental practice, 128
    sensory learning, 128
Motor planning changes, 124–125
Motor roots
    epineurium, 85
Movement
    control
        and mechanoreceptors, 116–117
        vs. posture, 119
        coordination, 123–124
        sensory control of changes, 121–122
        stability and motor control, 118–119
MPQ *see* McGill Pain Questionnaire (MPQ)
M-region, 10
MRI *see* Magnetic resonance imaging (MRI)
MTP *see* Metatarsalphalangeal joint (MTP)
Mucoid tendinopathy, 35
Murmur of hypertrophic cardiomyopathy, 198
Muscle(s)
    adaptations following endurance training,
        164
    aging, 485
    anconeus, 311
    architecture, 15–16
    atrophy, 19
        reduction, 20
    belly, **446**
    biceps brachii, 310–311
    brachialis, 310–311
    brachioradialis, 310–311
    cardiac, 9
    children and adolescents
        acute injuries, 470–471
        lateral sprains, 472
        ligaments, 470–472
        strain, 466
    concentric and eccentric action
        lower extremity musculotendinous
            injuries, 444
    control system characteristics, 120–121
    contusion, thigh and lower leg, 442–443,
        443, 451
    core training, 165
    elasticity, 16–17
    electrical stimulation, **446**
    endurance, aging, 487
    extensor supinator, 311
    extrinsic, foot and ankle, 423
    fascia latae, 373
    fiber
        determination, 16
        trauma, 17
        type I *vs.* type II, 17
    flexibility, 444
    flexor pronator, 311
    foot and ankle, 423
    force measurements, 13–14
    force potential, 15–16
    fractures, 431–432
    gastrocnemius, 423
    global, **121**
    gluteus maximus, 373
    gross structure, 9–13
    hamstring, 373, 441
    hip joint, 373–374
    iliopsoas, 373
    immobilization, 19–22, **21**
        connective tissue, 21

endomysium, 21
epimysium, 21
perimysium, 21
type I and II fibers, 20
ultrastructural changes, 20
impaired function treatment in athletes,
    226–228
    electrophysical agents, 226–227
intrinsic, foot and ankle, 423
local, **121**
lower extremity musculotendinous injuries,
    444
lower limb, 440
    anatomy, 440
    musculotendinous injuries, 441–443
    rehabilitation, 444–453
patellofemoral joint, 403
pectineus, 373
pennate, 16
performance, 288–289
power, 15
pronator quadratus, 311
pronator teres, 311
PT, 9–25
receptors, location and types, **116**
rectus femoris, 373
sartorious, 373
sartorius, 441
scapular
    stabilization, 294
    strengthening, 293
shoulder injuries, 288–289
SIJ movement, 367–368
skeletal, 9
    organization, **10**
soleus, 423
spindles, 116
sprains
    bracing, 426
    shoes, 426
    taping, 426
stiffness, 119
strain
    children and adolescents, 466
    thigh and lower leg, 441–442, **442**
strengthening
    aging, 486
    NMES, 226–227
    stress fractures, 68
stress fractures, 69
tensor, 373
testing
    elbow injuries, 314–315
thigh
    strains, 441, 449–450
tightness, 444
tissue
    female athletes, 500
    lengthening effect, 22
triceps brachii, 311
trunk
    low back pain, **125**
    spine, 256
twitch, 13
types, 9
Muscle groups
    stretching
        anterior, **446**
        posterior, **446**

Muscle–tendon complexes
    thigh and lower leg, 440–441
Muscular endurance exercises
    elbow injuries, 318
Musculocutaneous nerve, 312
Musculoskeletal system
    examination, 198–199
    growth, **461**
    history, 195
    pain
        motor control, 121–125
        motor control changes, 121–124
        motor learning strategies, 128
    pregnancy and exercise, 514
Musculoskeletal tissue management principles
    physical therapies, 9–120
Musculotendinous imbalance
    children and adolescents, **461**, 462
    prevention, 449
Musculotendinous injuries
    lower limb muscle and tendon injury
        rehabilitation, 441–443
Musculotendinous junction, 29
Musculotendinous overuse, 35
Musculotendinous structures
    elbow, 310–311
MVIC *see* Maximal voluntary isometric
    contraction (MVIC)
Myelin nerve injuries, 92–93
Myelography, 559–560
Myofascial treatments
    ITBFS, 454
Myofibrils, 9
    regeneration, 18–19
Myosin, 10, **11**
Myositis ossificans rehabilitation, 451
Myotendinous unit imaging, 568
Myotubes, 18
Myxoid tendinopathy, 35

N

NADH-TR *see* Nicotinamide adenine
    dinucleotide-tetrazolium reductase
    (NADH-TR)
Nagi Disablement Model, 206, 207–208
Narcotics, 554
National High Blood Pressure Education
    Program, 196
Navicular accessory, 47
NCSP *see* Neutral calcaneal stance position
    (NCSP)
Nebulin, 10, 14
Neck
    acute injuries, 463
    children and adolescents, 463
    disability index, **259**
    injuries, 582
        imaging, 571–572
    range of motion, **199**
Nedocromil sodium, 549
Neovascularization, 36
Nerve(s), 82–96 *see also* Peripheral nerves
    blocks
        facet joint, **263, 278**
        transforaminal, **278**
        translaminar, **278**
    calcitonin gene-related peptide, 34

compression
  central wrist pain and impairment,
    351–352
  ulnar wrist pain and impairment, 354–355
compression and traction
  wrist and hand, 349–350
endings, tendons, 30
functional anatomy and physiology, 83–87
imaging, 570
injuries
  clinical features, **93**
  fibrosis, 92–93
  intravenous edema, 92–93
  myelin, 92–93
  nociceptive input, 95
  pain, 95
  venous congestion, 92–93
median, 311
  compression, **352**
  testing, **269**
mobilization technique, 96
musculocutaneous, 312
neurodynamics, 88–91
pathodynamics, 92–95
peripheral, aging, 485
radial, 311–312, 338
  testing, **269**
radial sensory, 349–350
regeneration, 44
root
  complexes, 84, **84**
  intrinsic blood supply, **85**
  normal deformation, **90**
  selective blocks, **263**
sensory, 312
  elbow, 315
sinu-vertebral, 93
structures relationship to joint axes, 89
supply to tendons, 29
ulnar, 311, 338
  mechanosensitivity, 89
  testing, **269**
  transposition, 331, **331**
Nerve and tendon gliding exercises
  carpal tunnel, 95
Nerve entrapment, 434–435
Nerve injuries
  treatment, 435
Nervi nervorum, 93
Nervous system
  aging, 485
  function, 82
Neural connective tissue
  innervation, 86–87
Neural container and mechanical interface,
    88–89
Neural inflammation
  spontaneous discharge, 95
Neural pathology
  recovery, 95
Neural tension, 270
Neural tissues
  inflammatory response, 93
  injury
    symptoms, **94**
Neurodynamics, 88–89
  cervicobrachial pain, 95
  clinical examination, 92
  cubital tunnel syndrome, 95

heel pain, 95
  lateral epicondylalgia, 95
  lumbar-lower extremity pain, 95
  mechanical continuum, 91–92
  mechanical forces impact on physiology,
    92
  nonuniform mechanics and order
    movement, 91
Neurogenic pain
  central nervous systems, 95
Neurokinin-1-receptor, 34
Neurological history, 194
Neuromatrix theory, 135–136
Neuromeningeal structures, 85–86
Neuromuscular control
  deficits, 244
  exercises, 390
    elbow injuries, 318, 322
    shoulder, 293
Neuromuscular electrical stimulation (NMES),
    390
  electrode placement, **227**, **228**
  muscle strengthening, 226–227
Neuromuscular training protocol, **246**, **247**
Neutral calcaneal stance position
    (NCSP), 424
Nicotinamide adenine dinucleotide-tetrazolium
    reductase (NADH-TR), 21
NMDAR *see* N-methyl-D-aspartate receptor
    (NMDAR)
NMES *see* Neuromuscular electrical
    stimulation (NMES)
N-methyl-D-aspartate receptor (NMDAR), 36
Noble compression test, 444
Nociceptive input
  nerve injury, 95
Nociceptive system, 134
Nociceptors, 134
  peripheral, **134**
Noncollagenous proteins, 59–60
  cartilage, 101
Nonlinear deformation, 45
Non-opioid analgesics
  side effects with exercise, **490**, 491
Nonreducible crosslinks, 43
Nonsteroidal anti-inflammatory drugs
    (NSAIDs), 543–547, **543**
  arachidonic acid metabolism, **543**
  choice of, 543–544
  clinical effects, 543
  ITBFS, 454
  Lisfranc dislocation, 434
  osteoarthritis, 397
  pain management, 143–144
  plantar fasciitis, 430
  side effects, 544
    with exercise, 491
  stress fractures, 68
  topical, 544
Nonuniform mechanics and order movement
  neurodynamics, 91
Noradrenaline (norepinephrine), 95, 514
Norandrostenedione, 552
Norepinephrine, 95, 514
Nose examination, 196–197
NRS *see* Numerical rating scale (NRS)
NSAID *see* Nonsteroidal anti-inflammatory
    drugs (NSAIDs)
Nuclear medicine, 560

Numerical rating scale (NRS), 139
  pain intensity, **139**
Nutraceuticals
  osteoarthritis, 397
Nutrition, 195

O

Ober's test, 444
O'Brien's active compression test, 290
Observed change, 214
OCD *see* Osteochondritis dissecans (OCD)
Older adults
  aerobic exercise guidelines, **493**
  angina, 494
  balance training, 492–493
  endurance training, 165, 488, 492, **493**
  exercise, 484–498, 494
    arthritis, 494–495
    cardiac disease, 494
    chronic illness, 493–494
    contraindications, 489, **489**
    diabetes mellitus, 494
    guidelines, 489
    hypertension, 494
    medication side effects, 489
    osteoarthritis, 494
    osteoporosis, 495
    patient education, 491
    peripheral vascular disease, 495
    progression, **492**
    risk assessment, 489
    warm-ups, 491
  high-intensity strength training, **493**
  men, 151
  physical activity
    epidemiology studies, 488
    psychological wellbeing, 488
  strength training, 150, 151, 488, 492
  stretching exercise, 491
  Tai Chi, 492–493, **493**
Olecranon osteophyte excision
  posterior, 331
Oligomenorrhea, 507
One-handed plyometric throws, **322**
Open chain exercises, 390, **447**
Open-loop control system, **116**
  centrally controlled, 118
  problems, 124–125
Open-loop feedforward manner, 120
Opioid analgesics
  side effects with exercise, **490**, 491
Optional External Rotation at 0 Abduction,
    319
Optional Internal Rotation at 0 Abduction, **319**
Oral contraceptives, 503
Oral supplements, osteoarthritis, 397
Organic matrix, bone, 59
Osgood–Schlatter disease, 468, **468**
Osseous structures, 308–309
Ossicles, 472
Osteitis pubis, 378
Osteoarthritis
  aquatic rehabilitation, 398
  chondroitin sulfate, 397
  exercise, 494
  glucosamine, 397
  nonoperative treatment, 396

Osteoarthritis (contd.)
  NSAID, 397
  nutraceuticals, 397
  older adults, 494
  operative treatment, 397
  oral supplements, 397
  postoperative treatment, 397–398
  weight bearing, 398
Osteochondral allografts, 105
Osteochondral autograft transfer, 105
Osteochondral defects
  autografts, 105
Osteochondral grafting
  autologous, 105
Osteochondritis dissecans (OCD), 334–335,
    468–469, **468**, **476**, 574
  capitellar, 475
  radiograph, **574**
Osteochondrosis, 361
Osteoclasts, 60
Osteopenia
  posture and flexibility, 75
Osteoporosis, 70–74, 195, 196, 485
  defined, 70
  diagnostic criteria, **73**
  education, 76
  exercise
    dosage, 74–75
    older adults, 495
  falls reduction, 75
  female athletes, 503–504
  hot packs, 76
  hydrotherapy, 76
  ice, 76
  interferential therapy, 76
  outcome measurements, **74**
  pain-relieving techniques, 76
  physical therapy assessment, 72
  physical therapy management, 73
  posture and flexibility, 75
  risk factors, **71**
  shortwave diathermy, 76
  signs and symptoms, 71
  soft tissue massage, 76
  subjective assessment, **73**
  TENS, 76
  vertebral compression fractures, 512
  WHO guidelines, **511**
Osteoporotic compression fractures, 575
Os trigonum, 472
Oswestry Low Back Pain Disability
    Questionnaire, 258, **260**
Outcomes data
  analyzing and interpreting, 216–217
  collection, 215–216
Outerbridge Morphological Classification,
    103
Out-of-competition testing, 554
Overhead sports
  preparticipation examination, 200
Overtraining syndrome, 590–591, **591**
Overuse injuries, 286
  ankle, 470
  children and adolescents, 466, 467–468
    elbow, 475–476
    foot and ankle, 470
  diving injuries, 301
  elbow, 475–476
  foot, 470

  patellofemoral pain, 467–468
  shoulder, 297
  tendon, 37
  tennis injuries, 305
  throwing injuries, 300
Oxford system of training, 162
Oxidative stress, 19
  decrease, 20
Oxycodone, 554
Oxygen uptake
  determined by, 164
  maximum for males, **163**

P

Pain, 133–146 *see also* Central wrist pain and
    impairment
  acute, 136
    lumbar, 264
  algorithmic differential diagnosis and
    treatment, **342**
  assessment, 138–141
  association, 145
  athlete, 224–226
  back
    exercise, 76
    pregnancy, 514
  cervicobrachial, 95
  chronic, 136–137
  classification, 137
  cycle, **126**
  descriptions, 136
  dissociation, 145
  electroanalgesia, 224–225
  electrophysical agents, 224–225
  encouraged tolerance, 137
  experience, 136–137
  gate control theory, 134, **135**
  groin imaging, 571
  heel, 95
  hip, recurrent prevention, 377
  and impairment
    radial wrist and hand, 338–339
    wrist and hand, 338–339
  inflammatory process, 542
  injured athlete, 224–226
  intensity
    numerical rating scale, **139**
    visual analog scale, **139**
  low back
    children and adolescents, 462, **463**
    trunk muscle changes, **125**
  lumbar-lower extremity, 95
  management, 142–145
    cognitive-behavioral approach, 144
    cognitive therapies, 144
    corticosteroids, 143–144
    cryotherapy, 143
    exercise, 143
    imagery, 145
    interferential stimulation, 142
    lasers, 142
    manual techniques, 143
    NSAID, 143–144
    osteoporosis, 76
    pharmacological agents, 143–144
    self-efficacy, 145
    sport and exercise injuries, 133–148

  stress fractures, 68
  superficial heat, 143
  ultrasound therapy, 142
  mechanisms, 133
    to affect motor control, **123**
  motor and noxious electrical stimulation,
    225–226
  motor control, 126
  musculoskeletal
    changes in, 121–125
    motor learning strategies, 128
  nerve injury, 95
  neurodynamics, 95
  neurogenic, CNS, 95
  parallel processing model, 136
  patellofemoral, **124**, 402, 405
    overuse injuries, 467–468
  perception and action systems, **135**
  perception threshold, 137
  PFJ, 404
  physical rehabilitation therapies, 142
  provocation test, 290
  radial wrist, **342**
  reconceptualizing, 144
  recurrent acute, 137
  referred, spinal injuries, 270–271
  sensory level stimulation, 225
  sport inventory, 142
  subacute, 137
  tendons, 35–36, 36
  TENS, 225
  theoretical perspectives, 134–135
  thresholds, 137–138
  tolerance, 137
    athletes, 138
    females, 138
    males, 138
  ulnar wrist, 352–355
  use of heat and cold, 224
  wrist and hand
    instability, 345–346
    treatment, **345**
Palmar arterial artery, 338
Palpation
  lower extremity musculotendinous injuries,
    444
  pulses, 198
Paracetamol, 547
Parallel processing model
  of pain distress, 136
Paratenon
  acute edema, 35
  hyperemia, 35
  with synovial cells, 29
Paratenonitis, 35
Pars defects
  imaging, 572
Participation
  screening for
    sport and exercise injuries, 190–205
Participation rates
  sport and recreational activities, 3
Passive range of motion
  shoulder injuries, 288
Patellar tendinopathy
  clinical features, 451–452
  rehabilitation, 452–453
Patellar tendon (PT)
  bone, 59–81

cartilage, 100–120
ligament exercises, 52–58
muscle, 9–25
nerves, 82–99
tendon gliding exercises, 26–41
transverse sections through collagen fibrils, **53**
ultrasound imaging, **34**
Patellofemoral joint (PFJ), 402–417
abnormal foot pronation, 414
applied anatomy, 402–404
cartilage, 404
dynamic examination, 405
examination, 405–406
in lying position, 405–406, **406**
in patellar position, 406, **407**
fat pad, 404
hip control, 409
investigations, 406–407
kinematics, 403
kinetics, 403
management, 407–413
multimodal physical therapy, 414–415
muscular structure, 403
observation, 405
pain sources, 404
physical therapy, 407–412
quadriceps retraining, 408–409
soft tissue structures, 403–404
strengthening programs, 407–408
stretching, 414
subchondral bone, 404–405
subjective examination, 405–406
synovium, 405
taping, 409–414
anterior tilt, **412**
evidence, 411
mediolateral tilt, 413
practice, 411–412
skin problems, **413**
thigh, **411**
weaning, **413**
tracking, 403–404
Patellofemoral pain (PFP)
overuse injuries, 467–468
Patellofemoral pain syndrome (PFPS), **124**,
402, 405
Pathogenic cause classification
cartilaginous lesion, 103
Patient education
exercise and older adults, 491
Patient satisfaction, 207
Patrick's test, **375**
PCL *see* Posterior cruciate ligament (PCL)
Pectineus muscles, 373
Pediatric injury imaging, 573
Pelvis, 365–381
anatomy, 365–367
apophyseal avulsion fracture, **467**
children and adolescents, **467**
clinical considerations, 368–371
control, stepping off step, **409**
evidence-based practice, 368
examination, 368–369
landmarks, **370**
obliquity, 369
problems
history, 368–369
pretest probability, 368–369, **369**
PEMF *see* Pulsed electromagnetic fields (PEMF)

Pennate muscles, 16
Percent agreement, 212
Performance-enhancing drugs, 550–555
historical perspective, 550
Perimysium, 9, 14, 16, 28–29
muscle immobilization, 21
regeneration, 18–19
Perineurial tissue, 85
Periodization, 153
Peripheral nerves
aging, 485
anatomy and physiology, 83
connective tissue innervation, 86
connective tissue sheaths, 83
injuries, **312**
trunk vascular networks, **89**
Peripheral nociceptors, **134**
Peripheral quantitative computed tomographic
(pQCT), **65**
Peripheral vascular disease
exercise, older adults, 495
Peritendinous structures, 29
Peroneal nerve, 435
Peroneal tendonitis, 429
Persistent endoneurial edema, 93
Perturbation training, 391, **392**
Pethidine, 554
PFJ *see* Patellofemoral joint (PFJ)
Phalanges
fractures, 358–359
proximal, Salter–Harris II fracture,
479
Pharmacological agents, 541–557
pain management, 143–144
Phasic pain, 136
Phenylpropanolamine, 553
Phonophoresis, 223–224
Physical activity
children and adolescents, **460**
epidemiology studies, 488
health benefits, 236
injury, 3
older adults, 488
epidemiology studies, 488
psychological wellbeing, 488
therapies, 1–5
injury, 2
rehabilitation specialists, 2
Physical examination
disordered eating
female athletes, **506**
Physical therapists, 2
role, 2
Physical therapy, 4
assessment, 72
clinical outcomes, 206–218
assessment, **207**
collecting and analyzing, 215–217
psychometrics, 211–212
clinical outcomes identification, 207–210
evidence base need, 3
musculoskeletal tissue management
principles, 9–120
osteoporosis, 72, 73
pain, 142
patellofemoral joint, 407–412
sports, 4–5
Physiological hypertrophy
vs. HOCM, **586**

Physiologic loading
articular cartilage, 102
Physiotherapy, 2
Physis MRI, **573**
Pia mater, 86
PIP *see* Proximal interphalangeal joint (PIP)
Pivot shift test, 386, **386**
Placental effects
pregnancy and exercise, 515
Plain film, 558–559
Plantar fasciitis, 429–431
ESWT, 232
massage, 430
NSAID, 430
stretching, 430
ultrasound, **562**
weight bearing, 430
Plyometrics, 158
drills, **246**, 390, **449**
elbow injuries, 322
high intensity, 159
throws one-handed, **322**
training considerations, 158–159
wrist flips, **322**
POL *see* Posterior oblique ligament (POL)
Polysaccharide
articular cartilage, 101
Poor healing response
in tendons, 36
Post-crash measures, 241–242
Posterior capsule mobilization, **292**
Posterior cruciate ligament (PCL), 383
injuries
mechanism of, 394
nonoperative treatment, 394–395
operative treatment, 395
postoperative treatment, 395–396
test, 386–387
Posterior drawer test, 289, 386, **386**
Posterior hip dislocation
children and adolescents, **467**
Posterior muscle groups
stretching, **446**
Posterior oblique ligament (POL), 383
testing, 385
Posterior olecranon osteophyte excision, 331
Posterior sag test, 386
Posterior superior iliac spine (PSIS), 368, 369
Posterior tibialis tendonitis, 428–429
Posterolateral corner injuries
mechanism of injury, 394
nonoperative treatment, 394–395
operative treatment, 395
postoperative treatment, 395–396
Postinjection flare
corticosteroids, 546
Postoperative rehabilitation
ulnar nerve transposition, **331**
Posture
control, 119, 124
equilibrium, 119
problems, 120
flexibility
osteopenia, 75
osteoporosis, 75
impairments, 292
improve, **76**
motor control, 118–119
movement control, 119

Posture (*contd.*)
  shoulder injuries, 287–288
  stability, 118–119
Potassium iodide
  iontophoresis, 223, **223**
Power
  defined, 151
  muscle, 15
  pQCT *see* Peripheral quantitative computed tomographic (pQCT)
PRE *see* Progressive resistance exercises (PRE)
Pre-crash measures, 241
Prednisone
  spinal injuries, 278
Pregnancy
  exercise, **512**, 512–514
    back pain, 514
    body temperature, 513
    cardiac expenditure, 513
    contraindications, 516, **516**
    depression, 514
    fetal effects, 515
    gestational diabetes, 514–515
    guidelines, 515
    hemodynamics, 513
    maternal effects, 514
    musculoskeletal, 514
    placental effects, 515
    stress hormones, 514
Preparticipation examination, 190, 199–201
  adolescent, 196
Preparticipation history, 192
Press-ups, **321**
Pressure receptors, 30
Prevention, 241
  assessing effectiveness, 242
  injury, 236–248
    research methodology, 242
    sequence, 237–241
  van Mechelen's sequence of, 242, 244
Procollagen, 28
Progression exercise, **492**
Progressive overload principle, 151
Progressive resistance exercises (PRE), 468
Proliferative tendon response, 32
Pronator quadratus muscles, 311
Pronator teres muscles, 311
Prone extension, **294**
Prone external rotation test, 387, **387**
Prone horizontal abduction, **320**
Prone instability test, **268**
Prone knee flexion test, **268**, 370
Prone rowing, **321**
Proprioceptive exercises, 390, 426
Prostaglandins
  inflammatory process, 542
Proteins
  noncollagenous, 59–60
    cartilage, 101
Proteoglycans, 28, **29**
  articular cartilage, 103
  bulbous, 28
  cartilage, 101
  ligaments, 43–44
Proximal interphalangeal joint (PIP), 339, **339**, 355–356
  injury and rehabilitation, 357
  sprain and dislocation, 355–356
Proximal phalanx

Salter–Harris II fracture, **479**
Proximal radial physis
  premature arrest, 475
Proximal tibiofibular joint, 420
Pseudoephedrine, 553
PSIS *see* Posterior superior iliac spine (PSIS)
Psychological models, 175–176
Psychotropic drugs
  side effects with exercise, **490**, 491
PT *see* Patellar tendon (PT)
PubMed, 371
Pubofemoral ligaments, 373
Pulmonary embolism
  and DVT, 437
Pulsed electromagnetic fields (PEMF), 229
Pulse palpation, 198
Push-ups, **321**
Pyramid system for strength training, 162

Q

Q angle, **424**
Q-T syndrome, 204
Quadriceps, **199**
  active test, 386, 444–445
  contusion, myositis ossificans, 450–451
  retraining, PFJ, 408–409
  strains, 449–450
  strength testing, 387–388
Quadriceps femoris, 440–441
Quadrupled semitendinosus autograft, 51
Quality of life
  assessment in ACL deficiency, 209
  health-related, 208–209
  SF-36 scales, **217**, 218
Quinolone, 548

R

Racket sports injuries, 304–305
  etiology, 305
  shoulder, 304
Radial collateral ligament (RCL), 310
Radial nerve, 311–312, 338
  testing, **269**
Radial sensory nerve (RSN), 349–350
  traction, **348**
Radial wrist
  pain and impairment, 338–339
    algorithmic differential diagnosis and treatment, **342**
Radial zone, 101
Radiocarpal joints, 338
Radiography
  feet, **571**
  Freiberg's infraction, **574**
  glenoid, **569**
  osteochondritis dissecans, **574**
  stress fractures, 67
Radius
  distal
    osteoporotic fractures, 343
    Salter–Harris II fracture, **478**
Range, 217
Range of motion (ROM), **199**
  active
    lower extremity musculotendinous injuries, 444
    shoulder injuries, 288

elbow injuries, 314
passive, 288
shoulder injuries, 288
Rapport
  injury management, 181
RCL *see* Radial collateral ligament (RCL)
Reactive neuromuscular control exercises, 390
Receptors, 116–117
Reconceptualizing pain, 144
Recovery, 152
Recreational activities
  participation rates, 3
Rectus femoris
  contracture test, 444
  muscles, 373
Recurrent acute pain, 137
Redness
  inflammatory process, 542
Reduced tissue extensibility, 228
Reducible crosslinks, 43
Reduction, 65
Referred pain
  spinal injuries, 270–271
Reflexes, 119
  changes, 122–123
  inhibition changes, 125–126
  response changes, 123
Regeneration
  connective tissue (perimysium), 18–19
  contractile elements, 17
  myofibrils, 18–19
Regenerative techniques
  cartilage defects, 105
Region of microfailure, **46**
Rehabilitation, 65 *see also* Exercise-based conditioning and rehabilitation
  Achilles tendinopathy, 452–453
  acute fractures, 65
  adherence
    injury, 180–181
    measurement, 180
  aquatic, osteoarthritis, 398
  athlete responsibility, 182
  attendance, 180
  cartilage, 107
  children and adolescents, 462
  clinic-based adherence, 180
  cognitive restructuring, 184
  elbow, 315–323
  elbow injuries, **316**
    advanced strengthening phase, 318–323
    immediate motion phase, 316–318
    intermediate motion phase, 318
    return-to-activity phase, 324
  epicondylitis, **329**
  goal setting and attainment, 184–185
  hand fractures, **359**
  home-based adherence, 180–181
  injuries
    cognitive therapies, 144
    psychology, 171–186
  knee
    phases, **389**, 389–390
    return-to-play phase, 390–391
  lower extremity musculotendinous injuries, 445–446
  lower limb injury, 440, 444–453
    musculotendinous injuries, 441–443
  muscle injury, 440, 444–453

musculotendinous injuries, 441–443
myositis ossificans, 451
osteoarthritis, 398
patellar tendinopathy, 452–453
physical pain, 142
PIP joint injury, **357**
postoperative ulnar nerve transposition, **331**
principles, 445–446
specialists, 2
sport injury, 2
  adherence, 181
  biopsychosocial model, **175**
systematic desensitization, 184
tendon injury, 440, 444–453
  musculotendinous injuries, 441–443
thigh muscle strains, 449–450
thumb MCM UCL, **356**
ulnar nerve transposition, **331**
water exercises cartilage, 107
Relaxation, 144–145
techniques, 183
Reliability clinical outcome, 212
Relocation test, 290
Remobilization ligament strength, **54**
Repair
fractures, 61–62
ligaments, 54
tendons, 36
Repeated action potentials, **13**
Resisted elbow flexion, 289
Resisted shoulder shrug deltoid strength, **199**
Resisted upper extremity elevation
reproducing diving movement, **302**
Respiratory history, 194
Responsiveness clinical outcomes, 213
Rest, ice, compression, elevation (RICE),
  50, 229
children and adolescents, 462
ligament repair, **50**
Resting calcaneal stance position (RCSP), 424
Rest intervals, 152
Retinaculum
lateral, 403
medial, 403
self-stretching, **414**
Retraining
quadriceps, PFJ, 408–409
VMO, 408–409
Return to sport
motivation for athletes, 262
Reverse empty can test, 289
Reverse Lasegue test, **268**
Reversibility principle
strength gains, 154
Rib mobility and dysfunction, 272
RICE (rest, ice, compression, elevation), 50a,
  229
children and adolescents, 462
ligament repair, **50**
Roentgen stereophonogrammetric analysis
  (RSA), 369
Rofecoxib, 544
ROM see Range of motion (ROM)
Rotator cuff (RTC), 284–289
muscular anatomy, 285
repairs, 291–292
strength assessment, 288–289
strengthening exercises, 294–296
tendinopathy, 36

Rowing
seated, 157
RSA see Roentgen stereophonogrammetric
  analysis (RSA)
RSN see Radial sensory nerve (RSN)
RTC see Rotator cuff (RTC)
Rubifacients, 546
Ryanodin receptor (RYR), 12

S

Sacroiliac joints (SIJ)
articular surfaces, 366
bicondylar joint movements, 366–367
blocks, 263
dysfunction
  arthrodesis, 372
  debridement, 372
  Doppler imaging, 371
  intervention, 371–372
  prognosis, 371
  recurrence prevention, 372
evidence-based practice, 371
kinesiology, 365–366
ligaments, 367
muscle movement, 367–368
Sacrospinous ligaments, 367
Sacrotuberous ligaments, 367
Sacrum, **366**
SAID (specific adaptation to imposed
  demands), 154, 390
Salter–Harris classification of growth plate
  fractures, **462**
Salter–Harris II fractures, 474
distal radius, **478**
proximal phalanx, **479**
Salter–Harris III ulnar collateral ligament
  avulsion fractures, **478**
Salter I fractures, **473**
Salter IV fractures, **471**
Sarcomere, 10, 14
Sartorius muscles, 373, 441
Satellite cells, **18**
self proliferating, 17
Satisfaction
patient, 207
Scanning electron micrograph
spinal cord, **86**
Scaphoid fractures
wrist and hand, 341–343
Scaphoid shift, **348**
Scapholunate advanced collapse (SLAC),
  344–345
Scapholunate (SL) ligament, 338
Scaption, **156**
external rotation, **320**
Scapular muscles
stabilization, 294
  prone on elbows, **295**
  push-up position, **295**
  quadruped, **295**
  upper extremities on wobble board, **295**
  upper extremities walkouts with stool, **296**
  upper extremities walkouts with Swiss
    ball, **295**
  weight-bearing exercises, 294, **294**
strengthening, 293
Scapular stabilizers, 285

Scapulothoracic (STJ) joint, 284
Scare tactics, 182
Scar tissue production, 18–19
SCD see Sudden cardiovascular death (SCD)
SCFE see Slipped capital femoral epiphysis
  (SCFE)
Scheuermann's disease, 463–464
School-based health centers, 192
Sciatica, 465
Sciatic nerve, 435
Scintigraphy
stress fractures, 67
SCJJ see Sternoclavicular joint (SCJJ)
Scoliosis check, **199**
Screening for participation
sport and exercise injuries, 190–205
Seated leg curls, **157**
Seated rows, **157**
Second-generation autologous chondrocyte
  transplantation, 106
operative technique, **106**
Second impact syndrome (SIS), 583
Sedative-hypnotics
side effects with exercise, **490**
Segmentation approach, 127
Seizure classification
epilepsy, **581**
Selective nerve root blocks, **263**
Self-efficacy pain management, 145
Self-report history, 192
Self-stretch to posterior capsule, **293**
SEM see Standard error of measurement
  (SEM)
Sensation threshold, 137
Sensory and motor roots
epineurium, 85
Sensory control of movement
changes, 121–122
Sensory deficits, 121–122
Sensory feedback
reason for, 122
Sensory learning
motor performance, 128
Sensory level stimulation
pain, injured athlete, 225
Sensory modalities
maintain equilibrium, 119
Sensory nerves, 312
elbow, 315
Sesmoiditis, 430–431
shoes, 431
SF-36
scales, **217**, 218
SFMPQ see Short-Form McGill Pain
  Questionnaire (SFMPQ)
Shear stress distribution
bony material, **63**
Shock wave therapy see Extracorporeal shock
  wave therapy (ESWT)
Shoes
ankle sprain, 426
children and adolescents, **460**
sesmoiditis, 431
stress fractures, 68
Short-Form McGill Pain Questionnaire
  (SFMPQ), **141**, 141–142
Short opponens splint, **349**
Shortwave diathermy
osteoporosis, 76

Shoulder, 283–307
  abduction
    to 90 degrees, **320**
    external rotation at 90 degrees, **322**
    sign, **269**
  abuse, 297
  acute injuries, 474–475
  anatomy and biomechanics, 283–284
  children and adolescents, 472–475
  clinical examination, 285–289
  dislocation and subluxation, 472–473
  flexion, 289
  fractures, 474
  impairments, 292–296
  injuries, 283–304
    abuse, 297
    acute, 474
    AROM, 288
    diving injuries, 300–301
    history and onset, 286–287
    internal impingement, 290
    muscle performance, 288–289
    objective examination, 287–288
    passive range of motion, 288
    posture, 287–288
    special tests, 289–290
    sports-related, 296–305
    strength assessment, 288–289
    subjective assessment, 286–287
    swimming, 296–297
    symptoms, 287
    throwing, 298–299
    upper quarter screening, 288
  instability tests, 289–290
  joint anatomy and biomechanics, 283
  joint mobility impairments, 292–293
  microtrauma, 286
  misuse injuries, 298
  motion
    backstroke, 296
    breaststroke, 297
    butterfly stroke, 296
  neuromuscular control, 293
  overuse injuries, 297, 472–474
  postural impairments, 292
  press, **156**
  racket sports injuries, 304–305
  scaption, **156**
  scapular stabilizers, 285
  soft tissue healing, **291**, 291–292
  swimmer's
    etiology, 297
    training errors, 297–298
    treatment, 297–298
  tennis injuries, 304–305
  treatment, 290–295
  volleyball injuries, 302–303
Sidelying External Rotation, **320**
Side support with knees extended, **277**
SIJ see Sacroiliac joints (SIJ)
Simplification, segmentation and augmented
    feedback, **130**
Simplification approach, 127, **127**
Sinding–Larsen–Johansson syndrome, 468, **468**
Single leg standing tests, 426
Sinusoidal pattern
  extracellular matrix, 28
Sinus tarsi syndrome, 433–434, **434**
Sinu-vertebral nerves, 93

SIP see Sport Inventory for Pain (SIP)
SIRAS see Sport Injury Rehabilitation
    Adherence Scale (SIRAS)
SIS see Second impact syndrome (SIS)
Sitting, 369
Skeletal injuries management, 355
Skeletal ligaments
  chemical composition, **43**
  functions, 43
  joints, 43
Skeletal muscles, 9
  organization, **10**
Skeleton
  female athletes, 501, **502**
Skill learning
  training transfer, 128–129
Skin, 198
  conditions, 194
  receptors, 117
SL see Scapholunate (SL) ligament
SLAC see Scapholunate advanced collapse
    (SLAC)
SLAP see Superior labral anterior posterior
    (SLAP)
Slipped capital femoral epiphysis (SCFE)
  children and adolescents, **465**, 465–466
Slow-twitch fibers, 11
Slump test, **268**, 445
Small range knee flexion and extension, 409
SMOC see Sports Medicine Observation Code
    (SMOC)
Snapping hip
  children and adolescents, 466
Soccer
  female players, **500**
  injuries incidence, **238**
  preparticipation examination, 200
Social support
  injury management, 181
  injury rehabilitation, 185
Sodium chloride
  iontophoresis, **223**
Sodium cromoglycate, 549
Soft tissue massage
  osteoporosis, 76
Soleus muscle, 423
Soreness
  exercise progression guidelines, **390**
Specialist certification process, 2
Specific adaptation to imposed demands
    (SAID), 390
  principle, 154
Specificity principle
  strength gains, 154
Spinal canal
  cross-section, **86**
  diagram, **86**
Spinal cord, 134, **134**
  cross-section, **86**
  diagram, **86**
  scanning electron micrograph, **86**
  strain behavior, **86**
Spinal facet (zygapophyseal) joint, 256
Spinal injuries
  acute lumbar pain evaluation, 264
  cervical spine tests, **269**
  emergency care, 256–258
  evaluation, 262–271
    instability, 265–267

problem complaint, 267
symptom behavior, 267
initial screening, 258–262
injury history, 262
joint mobility testing, 271
lumbar spine test, **268**
medical consultation, 278
movement response interpretation,
    264–265
neurological screening, 269–270
prednisone for, 278
referred pain, 270–271
stabilization exercises with criteria for
    progression, **267**
treatment-based classification schemes, 258
Spinal segments
  injection locations, **278**
Spine, 255–282
  anatomy and biomechanics, 255–257
  assessment, 256–258
  bony anatomy, 255–256
  children and adolescents, 462–467
  disc mechanics, 256
  injections, **263**
  ligaments, 256
  motions, **257**
  patient examination, 258–259
  questionnaires, 258, **259**, **260**
  stress fractures, 255
  treatment, 274–277
  trunk muscles, 256
Splint
  long arm, **351**
  long opponens, **347**
  short opponens, **349**
  wrist control, **349**
Spondylolisthesis, 273–274, 464, **464**
Spondylolysis, 273–274, **464**
  isthmic, 255
Sport Injury Rehabilitation Adherence Scale
    (SIRAS), 180, **180**
Sport Inventory for Pain (SIP), 142
Sports, 526
  acute injuries incidence, **238**
  classification, **201**
  lower extremity musculotendinous injuries,
    444
  physical therapy, 4–5
  rehabilitation specialists, 2
  team injury incidence, **238**
Sports and exercise and physical activity
  injury, 2, 3
  preparticipation screening exam, 191–200
  therapies, 1–5
    rehabilitation specialists, 2
Sports and exercise injuries
  cost, 171
  elbow, 324–334
  foot, ankle, lower leg, 426–432
  impact, 171
  managing, 115–236
    exercise-based conditioning and
      rehabilitation, 149–169
    motor control, 115–132
    pain, 133–148
    psychology, 171–190
  motor learning in management, 126–128
  rehabilitation
    psychology, 174–177

research design, 243
screening for participation, 190–205
determining clearance, 201–203
exam, 191–200
goals and objectives, 191
target audience, 190
study setting, 242–243
wrist and hand, 341–361
Sports and exercise physical therapy
clinical outcomes, 206–218
assessment, **207**
collecting and analyzing, 215–217
identification, 207–210
psychometrics, 211–212
Sports and physical therapy, 4
Sports and recreational activities
participation rates, 3
Sports injuries
categories, **240**
definition, 242
etiology, 239
extrinsic risk indicators, 239
incidence, 237–238
inciting events, 239
intrinsic risk indicators, 239
magnitude, 237
patterns, 461
prevention
attention control, 173
cognitive and biofeedback interventions, 173
imagery, 173
mental practice skills, 173
rehabilitation
adherence, 181
biopsychosocial model, **175**
severity, 238
Sports Medicine Observation Code (SMOC), 180
Sprains
acromioclavicular
children and adolescents, 474
ankle, 427–428
high ankle, 427–428
lateral ankle, 426–427
proximal interphalangeal joint, 355–356
spring ligament, 428
Spurling's test, **269**
Squat (Ege's test), **155**, 387
SRM *see* Standardized response mean (SRM)
Stability motor control, 118–119
Stabilization training, 275–276
Standard deviation, 217
Standard error of measurement (SEM), 212
Standardized response mean (SRM), 217
Standing flexion test, **370**
Staphylococcal bacterial outbreak in athletes, 594
Staphylococcus aureus infections, 194
Stepping off step
pelvic control, **409**
Sternoclavicular joint (SCJJ), 284
children and adolescents, 474
mobilization, **293**
separation, 474
Steroids, 545–546
anabolic, 550
androgenic, 551
side effects, **551**

with exercise, **490**, 491
Stimulants, 553–554
Stimulation
interferential pain management, 142
Stingers, 271–272
STJ *see* Scapulothoracic (STJ) joint
Straight leg raise, **268**
Straight leg raise test, 445
Strain(s), 62, 89–90
bone, 64
children and adolescents, 466
clinical features, 449–450
cycles, 64
distribution, 64
lower leg muscles, 441
magnitude, 64
muscles, 441, 449–450, 466
quadriceps, 449–450
rate, 64
rehabilitation, 449–450
thigh muscle, 441, 449–450
Strength, **247**
assessment
RTC, 288–289
shoulder injuries, 288–289
electrical stimulation, 275
exercises
elbow injuries, 318, 322
patellofemoral joint, 407–408
RTC, 294–296
scapular muscle, 293
gains
fitness principle, 154
reversibility principle, 154
specificity principle, 154
power gain, **160–161**
training, 275–276
common systems, 159–162
effects, **150**
exercise-based conditioning and rehabilitation, 149–161
high-intensity, **493**
isokinetic, **448**
men, 151
modes, 152
older adults, 150, 151, 488, 492, **493**
physiologic adaptations, 150–151
principles, 151–154
pyramid system for, 162
single-sets *vs.* multi-sets, 159–162
types, 154–158
Streptococcal bacterial outbreaks
athletes, 594
Stress, 62
calculated, tibia anteromedial cortex, **64**
hormones
pregnancy and exercise, 514
and injury model, **172**
management
cognitive behavioral, 174
injury prevention, 173
response
categories of variables, 172
shielding, 31
and strain curve, 31
cortical bone, **63**
tendons, 31
Stress fractures, 65–70
alignment features, 69

amenorrhea, **508**
biomechanical abnormalities, 68
biomechanical assessment, 69
bone scan, **67**
bracing, 69
children and adolescents, 470
computerized tomography, 67
defined, 65
diagnosis, 66
dietary intake, 69
footwear and insoles, 68
hip, **559**
imaging, 66–67, 570–571
isotopic bone scan (scintigraphy), 67
magnetic resonance imaging, 67
maintaining fitness, 68
menstrual status, 69
muscle and joint flexibility, 69
muscle strengthening, 68
navicular, CT, **67**
NSAID, 68
pain management, 68
phase II, 69–70
physical examination, 66
radiography, 67
requiring specific treatment, 70, **70**
risk factor
assessment, **66**
modification, 68
spinal, 255
surgery, 70
tibial, 432
training, 68
treatment, 67–68
Stretching, 275
anterior muscle groups, **446**
elbow injuries, 318
exercise for older adults, 491
inverted subtalar joint, **430**
ITBFS, 454
plantar fasciitis, 430
posterior muscle groups, **446**
reflexes, 119
and shortening exercises, 158
Striations, 10
Stroke volume (SV), 163–164
responses to increased workload, **164**
Subacromial space, 285, 289
Subacute pain, 137
Subchondral bone
PFJ, 404–405
Subluxation
shoulder, 472–473
Substance P, 36
Subtalar joint, 421, **422**
motion assessment, **425**
neutral, **425**
Sudden cardiovascular death (SCD), 585
Sulcus test, 290
Superficial heat pain management, 143
Superficial zone, 101
Superior labral anterior posterior (SLAP)
lesions, 290
prehension test, 290
Superset system, 162
Supination exercises, **322**
Supine thoracic manipulation, **271**
Supraspinatus tendons, 29
Surgical history, 192

Suspensory ligaments, abdominal organs, 43
SV *see* Stroke volume (SV)
Swelling inflammatory process, 542
Swimmer's shoulder
  etiology, 297
  training errors, 297–298
  treatment, 297–298
Swimming
  preparticipation examination, 200
  shoulder injuries, 296–297
Sympathetic ganglion blocks
  injection locations, **278**
Symphysis pubis joints
  amphiarthrodial movement, 367
  kinesiology, 365–366
Synemin, 10
Synovitis
  central wrist pain and impairment, 351
  elbow, 335
Synovium patellofemoral joint, 405
Systematic desensitization rehabilitation, 184

T

Tabletop intrinsic plus position, **358**
Tai Chi
  older adults, 492–493, **493**
Talocrural joint, 421, **421**
Taping
  ankle sprain, 426
  athlete, **349**
  patellofemoral joint, 409–414
    anterior tilt, **412**
    evidence, 411
    mediolateral tilt, 413
    skin problems, **413**
    weaning, **413**
  protection and rest, **349**
Tarsal coalitions
  children and adolescents, 472
Tarsal tunnel nerve entrapment, 435
Tarsal tunnel syndrome, 435
Teaching skills
  instruction *vs.* demonstration, 127–128
Team handball injuries incidence, **238**
Team sports acute injuries incidence, **238**
Teenagers *see* Children and adolescents
Tenascin, 44
Tendinitis, 470
Tendinopathic tendons, 34
Tendinopathy, 32, **32**, **33**
  fibroblast proliferation, **33**
  RTC, 36
  thigh and lower leg, 443–444, **443**
Tendinosis, **32**, 33
Tendon(s), 26–37
  Achilles, 32
    corticosteroids, 546
    insertion, 30
  aging, 485
  anatomy and histology, 26
  biceps, 315
  biomechanical properties, 30
  blood and nerve supply, 29
  calcification, 35
  cyclic loading, 31
  enthesis, **30**
  exercise effects, 32
  extensor, 340

injuries, 360–361, **361**
fibroblast proliferation, **32**
finger injuries, 359–362
flexor, 359–360, **360**
functions, 36
gliding exercises, **352**
  carpal tunnel, 95
  PT, 26–41
hierarchical and organization, **27**
inflammation, 35
injury rehabilitation, 36, 440
  anatomy, 440
  musculotendinous injuries, 441–443
  rehabilitation, 444–453
insertion, 30
length and size, 36
load, 31, 32, **32**
medial malleolus, 29
metabolic demands, 29
neovascularization, 34
nerve endings, 30
neurovascular structure, 34
nomenclature, **32**
overuse injuries, 37
pain, 35–36
  chemical and neurovascular sources, 36
  collagen disruption, 35, 36
  mechanisms, 36
  modulators, 36
  patellar
    transverse sections through collagen
      fibrils, **53**
    ultrasound imaging, **34**
pathology, 33–35
  new vessels, 34
  physiology, 36
  structural changes, 35
physiology, 31–32
poor healing response, 36
proliferative response, 32
repair, 36
  future direction, 37
  growth factors, 37
  macrotraumatic repair, 37
response to exercise, 32
stimuli adaptation, 31
stress–strain curve, 31
structures, 30
supraspinatus, 29
tendinopathic, 34
tensile loads, 31
tibialis posterior, 29
ultrastructural, 45
uncrimping, 31
viscoelastic time-dependent behaviors, 31
weakened, 31
Tendonitis
  Achilles, 431
  calcific, 232
  central wrist pain and impairment, 351–352
  ESWT, 232
  peroneal, 429
  posterior tibialis, 428–429
  ulnar wrist pain and impairment, 354
  wrist and hand, 347–349
Tendon organs
  type III Golgi, 30
Tennis
  biomechanics, 304

elbow biomechanics, 313
injuries
  abuse injuries, 305
  etiology, 304–305
  misuse injuries, 305
  overuse injuries, 305
  shoulder, 304–305
  training errors, 305
  treatment, 305
interval program, **328**
preparticipation examination, 200
Tenocytes, 27
  degeneration, 34
Tenosynovitis, 575
TENS *see* Transcutaneous electrical nerve
  stimulation (TENS)
Tensile injuries
  throwing injuries, 299
Tensile loads
  mechanical model, 91
  tendons, 31
Tensile properties
  articular cartilage, 102
Tensile strength, 32, 89–90
Tensile stress
  throwing injuries, 299
Tensor muscles, 373
Test(s)
  alar ligament, **269**
  anterior drawer, 289
  anteroinferior, 290
  arthometer, 387
  atlantoaxial motion, **269**
  Bump, 432
  cervical spine, **269**
  compression, **427**
  crank, 290
  digit symbol substitution, 584
  drawer, 289
  drug, 554
  Ege's, 387
  Ely's, 444
  empty can, 289
  external rotation, **427**
  Faber's (Patrick's), **375**
  Gaenslen's, 370
  gracilis, 445
  gripping rotatory impaction, 353
  hip external rotation, **376**
  hip internal rotation, **376**
  hop, **388**, 388–389
  inferior glide, 290
  instability shoulder, 289–290
  internal rotation resistance strength, 290
  isometric elbow, **324**
  joint mobility, 271
  Lachman, 385, **385**
  lateral hamstrings, 445
  lateral pivot shift, 315
  lumbar spine, **268**
  McMurray's, 387
  medial hamstrings, 445
  median nerve, **269**
  Noble compression, 444
  Ober's, 444
  O'Brien's active compression, 290
  out-of-competition, 554
  pain provocation, 290
  pivot shift, 386, **386**

posterior drawer, 289, 386, **386**
posterior sag, 386
prone external rotation, 387, **387**
prone instability, 268
prone knee flexion, 268, **370**
quadriceps active, 386, 444–445
quadriceps strength, 387–388
radial nerve, **269**
rectus femoris contracture, 444
relocation, 290
reverse empty can, 289
reverse Lasegue, 268
single leg standing, 426
SLAP prehension, 290
slump, 268, 445
Spurling's, **269**
standing flexion, **370**
straight leg raise, 445
sulcus, 290
Tinel's percussion, 349–350
Trendelenburg, **375**
ulnar nerve, **269**
valgus stress, 315, 384–385
varus, 315
varus stress, 385
vertebrobasilar artery, **269**
Wallace, 445
Tetanic stimulation, 13
TFCC see Triangular fibrocartilage complex (TFCC)
Theophylline, 550
Therapeutic agents, 541–550
Therapies
  evidence base need, 1
  sport, exercise and physical activity, 1–5
    injury, 2
    rehabilitation specialists, 2
Thermal demands
  hot and humid climate, 593
Thigh
  muscle contusion, 442–443, **443**, **451**
  muscle strains, 441, **442**
    clinical features and rehabilitation, 449–450
    muscle–tendon complexes, 440–441
    tendinopathy, 443–444, **443**
Thompson's test, Achilles tendon, 199
Thoracic extension, **76**
Thoracic injuries, 272–273
Thoracic outlet, 272–273
Thoracic spine mobilization, **300**
Threats, 182
Throat
  examination, 196–197
Thrombolytic agents, 541
Thrombospondin, 44
Thrower's Ten Program, **319–322**
Throwing
  biomechanics, 298
  injuries
    etiology, 298–299
    microtrauma, 298–299
    shoulder, 298–299
    tensile injuries, 299
    treatment, 299–300
  interval program
    baseball players, **325–327**
Thumb
  joint injury management, 355

mallet, 361
MCM UCL rehabilitation, **356**
metacarpophalangeal joint
  avulsion fractures, **478**
Tibia
  anteromedial cortex calculated stresses, **64**
  plateau fractures, 396
    mechanism of injury, 396
    nonoperative treatment, 396
    operative treatment, 396
    postoperative treatment, 396
  stress fractures, 432
Tibialis posterior tendons, 29
Tibialis tendonitis, 428–429
Tibial nerve, 435
Tibiofemoral joint, 382
Tibiofibular joint
  distal, 421
  proximal, 420
Time loss injuries, 242
Tinel's percussion testing, 349–350
Tired athletes, 590–591
Titin, 10, 14
Toe-phase, 45
Tomography, 559–560
Torque
  calculation, **14**
  lever arms, **14**
Trabecular bone, 60
Traction, 275
  apophysis, 462
  apophysitis, 468, **472**, 475
  children and adolescents, 468
  for radial sensory neuritis, 348
Training see also Endurance training; Strength, training
  cardiovascular endurance, 163–164
  circuit system of, 162–163
  core muscles, 165
  core stability, 165–166, **247**
  DeLorme system of, 162
  diabetes diary, **589**
  dynamic, 154–155
  eccentric, 158
  endurance, 152
  errors
    children and adolescents, **460**
    diving injuries, 301–302
  frequency, 152
  high-intensity strength
    older adults, **493**
  intensity, 151
  isokinetic strength, 158, **448**
  isometric, 154
  jump, 158
  motor control element, 130
  neuromuscular protocol, **246**, **247**
  Oxford system of, 162
  perturbation, 391, **392**
  plyometrics, 159
  stabilization, 275–276
  stress fractures, 68
  volume, 151–152
  weight, 75
Transcutaneous electrical nerve stimulation (TENS), 142
  injured athlete, 225
  osteoporosis, 76

pain, 225
Transducer
  buckle-type force, 13
Transforaminal nerve blocks
  injection locations, **278**
Transitional (middle) zone, 101
Translaminar nerve blocks
  injection locations, **278**
Transverse tubule-sarcoplasmic reticulum system, **12**
Trauma, muscle fibers, 17
Traveler's diarrhea, 548
Travel medicine for international athlete, 592–593
Treadmill-running program, 19
Treatment efficacy and tailoring rehabilitation goals, 182
Trendelenburg test, **375**
Triangular fibrocartilage complex (TFCC), 339, **339**
  tear, ulnar wrist pain and impairment, 353–354
Triceps brachii muscles, 311
Tricyclic antidepressants, 547
Triggered responses, 117
Trochlear groove, 309
Tropocollagen, 28
Tropomyosin, 10
Trunk
  feedforward control, **120**
  front (extension) or back (flexion), **122**
  muscles
    low back pain, **125**
    spine, 256
  peripheral nerve, 89
  stability, **120**
  vascular networks, 89
T-scores, 71
T-tubules, 12
Twisting injuries
  children and adolescents, 469
Type I collagen, 43
Type I fibers, 11
  muscle immobilization, 20
Type II collagen, 43
  cartilage, 101
Type II fibers, 11
  muscle immobilization, 20
Type III collagen, 37, 43
Type III Golgi tendon organs, 30
Type II Paccinian corpuscles, 30
Type I muscle fibers
  vs. type II muscle fibers, 17
Type I Ruffini corpuscles, 30
Type IV free nerve endings, 30

U

Ubiquitin-proteasome, 19
UCL see Ulnar collateral ligament (UCL)
Udry's recommendations, positive responses to injury, 179
Ulnar artery
  Guyon's canal, vascular thrombosis, 361
Ulnar collateral ligament (UCL), 309–310
  injuries, 331–332
    thumb metacarpophalangeal joint, 355
  instability tests, **332**
  lateral, 310

Ulnar collateral ligament (UCL) (*contd.*)
  reconstruction, 332–333
    postoperative rehabilitation, **334**
Ulnar nerve, 311, 338
  mechanosensitivity, 89
  testing, **269**
  transposition, 331
    postoperative rehabilitation, **331**
Ulnar neuropathy, 328–329
Ulnar wrist
  pain and impairment, 352–355
    algorithmic differential diagnosis and
      treatment, **344**
    articular disk of triangular fibrocartilage
      tear, 353–354
    degenerative disorders, 353
    distal radioulnar joint instability, 350–353
    fractures, 350
    instability, 354
    nerve compression, 354–355
    tendonitis, 354
Ultrasound (US), 223–224, **331**, 561–562, 575
  flexor carpi radialis, **562**
  in managing pain, 142
  metatarsalphalangeal joint, **563**
  patellar tendon, **34**
  plantar fascia, **562**
Union, bone, 65, **65**
Unmineralized fibrocartilage region, 30
Unmyelinated C fibers, 134
Upper limb exercises, **76**
Upper respiratory tract infections (URTI), 593
Upper thoracic manipulation, **270**
URTI *see* Upper respiratory tract infections
  (URTI)
US *see* Ultrasound (US)

V

Vaccinations for international athlete, 592
Valgus extension overload
  clinical test, **331**
Valgus stress, 328
  test, 315, 384–385, **385**
Validity
  clinical outcome, 211–212
Van Mechelen's sequence of prevention, 242,
  244
Variable resistance machines (VRM), 152
Variance, 217
Varus stress test, 385
Varus testing, 315
VAS *see* Visual analog scale (VAS)
Vascular endothelial growth factor (VEGF), 37
Vascular networks
  trunk peripheral nerve, **89**
Vascular thrombosis
  Guyon's canal ulnar artery, 361
Vastus longus (VL), 403
Vastus medialis longus (VML), 403
Vastus medialis oblique (VMO), 403
  retraining, 408–409
VEGF *see* Vascular endothelial growth factor
  (VEGF)

Venous congestion
  nerve injuries, 92–93
Verbal instruction, 127–128
Verbal rating scale (VRS), 139
Versican, 28
Vertebra
  anatomy, 255
  compression fractures
    osteoporosis, 512
Vertebrobasilar artery test, **269**
Vertical jump, **159**
Vestibular apparatus, 117
Vimentin, 10
Viscoelastic time-dependent behaviors
  tendons, 31
Vision history, 194
Visual analog scale (VAS), 139
  pain intensity, **139**
Visual impairment, 530–531
Visual system, 117
Vital signs, 196
Vitamin E, 20
VL *see* Vastus longus (VL)
VML *see* Vastus medialis longus (VML)
VMO *see* Vastus medialis oblique (VMO)
Volleyball
  biomechanics, 302–303
  injuries
    abuse injuries, 304
    etiology, 303–304
    incidence, **238**
    overuse injuries, 304
    shoulder, 302–303
    training errors, 304
    treatment, 304
  preparticipation examination, 200
VRM *see* Variable resistance machines (VRM)
VRS *see* Verbal rating scale (VRS)

W

Wallace test, 445
Warfarin
  for DVT, 437
Warm-ups
  exercise
    older adults, 491
Water rehabilitation exercises
  cartilage, 107
Waveforms, **229**
Weight
  athletic women, 499
Weight bearing
  exercises, **448**
    scapular muscle stabilization, 294, **294**
  gluteus medius, **409**
  Lisfranc dislocation, 434
  osteoarthritis, 398
  plantar fasciitis, 430
Weight-training program, 75
Western Ontario and McMaster Universities
  Osteoarthritis Index (WOMAC), 209
Wheelchair athletes, 532–534
Whole body bone scan, **568**

Whole-task practice, 127
Williams and Andersen model of stress and
  athletic injury, 172, 173
Wobble boards, 426, 431
WOMAC *see* Western Ontario and McMaster
  Universities Osteoarthritis Index
  (WOMAC)
World Anti-Doping Agency (WADA), 550–551
World anti-doping code, 550–551, **551**
World Health Organization (WHO)
  disablement models, 208, **211**
Wrestling preparticipation examination, 200
Wrist, 338–364 *see also* Central wrist pain and
  impairment; Ulnar wrist
  acute injuries, 477
  anatomy, 338–340
  arthrogram, **560**
  blood supply, 338
  children and adolescents, 476–477
  complex, 338
  control splint, **349**
  degenerative disorders, 346–347
  examination, 341
  extension, **322**
  flexion, **322**
    manual resisted, **318**
  fractures, 341–345, 477
    treatment guidelines, **347**
  nerve compression and traction, 349–350
  neurological and vascular structures, 341
  pain and impairment, 338–339
    instability, 345–346
    treatment, **345**
  plyometric flips, **322**
  provocative tests, **348**
  radial pain and impairment, **342**
  scaphoid fractures, 341–343
  sport-related injuries, 341–361
  stiffness treatment algorithm, **346**
  tendonitis, 347–349
Wry neck or facet syndrome, 272

X

X-rays, 558–559

Y

Young's modulus
  ligament biomechanics, 46
Youth *see* Children and adolescents

Z

Z-disks, 10, 11
Zeranol, 552
Zilpaterol, 552
Z-line, **12**, 17
Z-scores, 71
Zygapophyseal joint, 256